a LANGE medical book

Clinical
Anesthesiology

First Edition

G. Edward Morgan, MD
Department of Anesthesiology
University of Southern California
School of Medicine
Los Angeles

Maged S. Mikhail, MD
Department of Anesthesiology
University of Southern California
School of Medicine
Los Angeles

APPLETON & LANGE
Norwalk, Connecticut/San Mateo, California

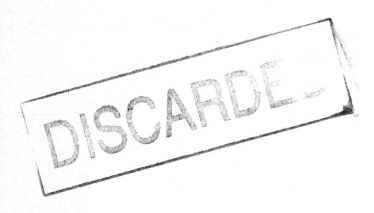

0-8385-1324-7

Notice: The authors and the publisher of this volume have taken care to make certain that the doses of drugs and schedules of treatment are correct and compatible with the standards generally accepted at the time of publication. Nevertheless, as new information becomes available, changes in treatment and in the use of drugs become necessary. The reader is advised to carefully consult the instruction and information material included in the package insert of each drug or therapeutic agent before administration. This advice is especially important when using new or infrequently used drugs. The publisher disclaims any liability, loss, injury, or damage incurred as a consequence, directly or indirectly, of the use and application of any of the contents of this volume.

Copyright © 1992 by Appleton & Lange
A Publishing Division of Prentice Hall

All rights reserved. This book, or any parts thereof, may not be used or
reproduced in any manner without written permission. For information,
address Appleton & Lange, 25 Van Zant Street, East Norwalk, Connecticut 06855.

92 93 94 95 96 / 10 9 8 7 6 5 4 3 2 1

Prentice Hall International (UK) Limited, *London*
Prentice Hall of Australia Pty. Limited, Sydney
Prentice Hall Canada, Inc., *Toronto*
Prentice Hall Hispanoamericana, S.A., *Mexico*
Prentice Hall of India Private Limited, *New Delhi*
Prentice Hall of Japan, Inc., *Tokyo*
Simon & Schuster Asia Pte. Ltd., *Singapore*
Editora Prentice Hall do Brasil Ltda., Rio de Janeiro
Prentice Hall, *Englewood Cliffs, New Jersey*

ISBN: 0-8385-1324-7
ISSN: 1058-4277

PRINTED IN THE UNITED STATES OF AMERICA

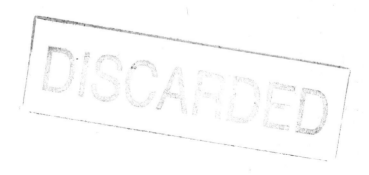

*The authors dedicate this book to their families,
especially to their wives,
Karen Morgan and May Mikhail,
who persevered and endured many sacrifices
in order to make this book possible.*

Table of Contents

III. REGIONAL ANESTHESIA & PAIN MANAGEMENT

IV. PHYSIOLOGY, PATHOPHYSIOLOGY, & ANESTHETIC MANAGEMENT

V. SPECIAL PROBLEMS

Foreword

Upon opening the cover of this book, your first reaction might be, "Oh no, not another textbook of anesthesia!" You may further ask, "What could this book offer me that is not readily available in the standard texts by Miller, Stoelting or Barash?" With the multitude of texts that have been written in recent years on the general subject of anesthesia, it seems almost inconceivable that a new textbook of anesthesia might have unique characteristics. However, such is the case with CLINICAL ANESTHESIOLOGY. What makes this book distinctive from its contemporaries? I will highlight its combination of features that makes it special, different, and a valuable resource in the library of every clinical anesthesiologist.

First, most comprehensive texts of anesthesia are multiauthored, which generally renders the text authoritative, but brings with it needless repetition and duplication that is almost impossible to eliminate. With the exception of three chapters, one on pain management and the other two on regional anesthesia, this book was authored entirely by two knowledgeable, experienced teachers and clinicians in our specialty. Professors G. Edward Morgan and M. Mikhail teach and practice anesthesia in one of the largest, busiest and most challenging environments in American medicine. The variety and complexity of anesthetic problems that these two encounter, either primarily or through their colleagues' experiences are enormous. As a result, they write principally from first-hand observations and experience, and there are no better teachers. The text is complete; nothing of consequence is omitted. The writing style is precise, concise and highly readable.

Second, this text is generously illustrated with tables and figures. When one is studying for retention, tables, figures and graphs collate and condense complex material into a visual image that is retained long after the descriptive words are forgotten. Professors Morgan and Mikhail have paid particular attention to making each illustration comprehensive in scope and content while remaining easily interpretable.

Finally, each chapter is enriched by a case summary which exemplifies the thrust of the chapter. As examples, the chapter on breathing systems contains a case summary of a patient who exhibits the manifestations of light anesthesia secondary to carbon dioxide retention from a malfunctioning expiratory valve in a circle system; the chapter on sympathetic nervous system pharmacology includes a case summary of the anesthetic management of a patient with a pheochromocytoma; and the chapter on anesthesia for thoracic surgery contains a case summary of the management of a patient with a mediastinal tumor and airway obstruction. The case summaries are well-chosen to highlight key problems of that topic, give vivid definition of critical considerations, and emphasize what might go awry and how to prevent or ameliorate it.

I commend the authors for having created a novel, valuable textbook of anesthesia that will enrich their readers' minds and skills beyond their expectations.

C. Philip Larson Jr., M.D.

Professor of Anesthesia and Surgery (Neurosurgery)
Stanford University School of Medicine
February 1991

Preface

Clinical Anesthesiology provides a concise, consistent presentation of the basic principles essential to the modern practice of anesthesia. It serves as a learning guide for the beginning clinician and a comprehensive review for the experienced practitioner.

All areas of clinical anesthesiology are discussed. The clinically relevant principles of pharmacology, physiology, and pathophysiology are emphasized. In areas of controversy, the viewpoints best supported by current literature are examined.

AUDIENCE

The text is written primarily for newcomers to the specialty. Medical students will find it ideal for an anesthesiology clerkship, yet detailed enough for reference after clerkship completion. Anesthesia residents will appreciate the book as an orientation text with a hands-on approach to clinical situations, affording a quick "night before" review of key points in the management of difficult cases. Board-eligible anesthesiologists will welcome the concise basic science summary and the board-type case presentations. Board-certified anesthesiologists will find the work a useful source of continuing education.

This book will also prove useful to practitioners in specialties outside anesthesiology. Internists will find it a useful reference to perioperative anesthetic risk factors and guidelines for preoperative optimization. Surgeons who are providing sedation for minor office procedures will benefit from the discussion of airway management, pharmacology and complications. It can also serve as an authoritative core text for dentists and nurse anesthetists.

ORGANIZATION AND SCOPE

The book is organized in five sections: Anesthesia Equipment and Monitors; Pharmacology; Regional Anesthesia and Pain Management; Physiology, Pathophysiology, and Anesthetic Management; and Special Problems. The topics of equipment, airway management, monitoring and pharmacology are introduced early since their understanding is requisite for patient safety. The regional anesthesia section emphasizes the techniques of performing nerve blocks and includes numerous illustrations.

Management of patients with specific medical problems is approached by organ system: basic physiology is reviewed (eg, intracranial pressure regulation), pathophysiology explained (space occupying cranial tumor), anesthetic management detailed (eg, hyperventilation), and relevant considerations of specialized surgical procedures examined (eg, air embolism in the sitting position).

The final section discusses topics of special interest to the anesthesiologist, and includes an introduction to critical care medicine.

FEATURES

The authors have attempted to develop a consistent presentation of their subject in all its major aspects, based on their experiences in clinical practice and teaching. In keeping with the Lange tradition, careful editing has resulted in a concise, highly readable text.

More than 300 illustrations amplify the text. Most of these superb drawings were created expressly for this book.

A case summary concludes each chapter, addressing the "why" aspects of clinical anesthesia. These summaries serve as a review and self-examination tool for the reader, and instill a logical approach to clinical situations.

References include relevant texts and key review articles, emphasizing material published since 1986.

ACKNOWLEDGEMENTS

The authors would like to thank and acknowledge the invaluable assistance of Dr Jim Ransom, Nancy Evans, Marge Bloom, Don Ramie, Merlin Hall, Becky Hainz-Baxter, and Alexander Kugushev. We would also like to thank our many colleagues both inside and outside the Department of Anesthesiology at the University of Southern California for their many helpful suggestions, especially Drs William Fulcher, Klane Hales, Georges Khoury, Kenneth Kuchta, Harry Lowe, Duraiyah Thangathurai, Dona Warner and, of course, the chairman John Viljoen.

Comments and suggestions for future editions can be sent to us in care of Appleton & Lange, 2755 Campus Drive, Suite 205, San Mateo, CA 94403.

G. Edward Morgan
Maged S. Mikhail

Los Angeles
November 1991

Section I
Anesthetic Equipment & Monitors

The Practice of Anesthesiology

1

The Greek philosopher Dioscorides is said to have first used the term anesthesia in the first century AD to describe the narcotic-like effects of the plant mandragora. The term subsequently appeared in Bailey's *An Universal Etymological English Dictionary* (1721) as "a defect of sensation" and again in the *Encyclopedia Britannica* (1771) as "privation of the senses." The present use of the term to denote the sleep-like state that makes possible painless surgery is credited to Oliver Wendell Holmes in 1846. In the United States, the term "anesthesiology" to denote the practice of anesthesia was first proposed in the second decade of this century to emphasize the growing scientific basis of the specialty. Although the specialty now rests on a scientific foundation that rivals any other, anesthesia remains very much a mixture of both science and art. Moreover, the practice of anesthesiology has expanded beyond rendering patients insensible to pain during surgery or obstetric delivery, causing the American Board of Anesthesiology to revise its definition in 1989 (Table 1–1). The specialty is unique in that it requires a working familiarity with most other specialties, including surgery and its subspecialties, internal medicine, pediatrics, and obstetrics as well as clinical pharmacology, applied physiology, and biomedical technology. The application of recent advances in biomedical technology in clinical anesthesia continues to make anesthesia an exciting and rapidly evolving specialty. The current popularity of the specialty is evidenced by the increasing number of physicians applying for training positions in anesthesiology, many of whom already have training and certification in other specialties.

This chapter reviews the history of anesthesia, its British and American roots, and the current scope of the specialty. The general approach to the preoperative evaluation of patients and documentation of the patient's anesthetic experience are also presented. The Case Discussion at the end of the chapter considers medicolegal aspects of the specialty.

THE HISTORY OF ANESTHESIA

Anesthetic practices date from ancient times, yet the evolution of the specialty began only in the mid 19th century and was not firmly established until just 50 years ago. Ancient civilizations had employed opium poppy, coca leaves, mandrake root, alcohol, and even phlebotomy (to the point of unconsciousness) to allow surgeons to operate. Interestingly, the ancient Egyptians used the combination of opium poppy (morphine) and hyoscyamus (hyoscyamine and scopolamine); a similar combination, morphine and scopolamine, is still used parenterally for premedication. "Regional anesthesia" in ancient times consisted of compression of nerve trunks (nerve ischemia) or application of cold (cryoanalgesia). The Incas may have practiced local anesthesia as their surgeons chewed coca leaves and spat saliva (presumably containing cocaine) into the operative wound. Surgical procedures were for the most part limited to caring for fractures, traumatic wounds, amputations, and the removal of bladder calculi. Amazingly, some civilizations were also able to perform trephination of the skull. A major qualification for a successful surgeon was speed.

The evolution of modern surgery was hampered not only by a poor understanding of disease processes, anatomy, and surgical asepsis but also by the lack of reliable and safe anesthetic techniques. These techniques evolved first with inhalation anesthesia, followed by local and regional anesthesia, and finally intravenous anesthesia.

INHALATIONAL ANESTHESIA

The first general anesthetics were inhalational agents: ether, nitrous oxide, and chloroform. Ether (really diethyl ether) was originally prepared by Valerius Cordus in 1540 but was not used as an anesthetic agent in humans until 1842, when Crawford W. Long and William E. Clark used it independently on patients. Four years later, in Boston, on October 16, 1846, William T.G. Morton conducted the first publicized demonstration of general anesthesia using ether. Nitrous oxide was discovered by Joseph Priestly in 1772, but its analgesic properties were first noted by Humphry Davy in 1800. Gardner Colton and Horace Wells are credited for having first used nitrous oxide as an anesthetic in humans in 1844. Chloroform was independently prepared by von Leibig, Guthrie, and Soubeiran in 1831. Although it was first used clinically as a general anesthetic by Holmes Coote in 1847,

Table 1–1. Definition of the practice of anesthesiology.[1]

1. Assessment, consultation, and preparation of patients for anesthesia
2. Rendering patients insensible to pain during surgical, obstetric, therapeutic, and diagnostic procedures
3. Monitoring and restoring homeostasis in perioperative and critically ill patients.
4. Diagnosing and treating painful syndromes
5. Management and teaching of cardiac and pulmonary resuscitation
6. Evaluating respiratory function and applying respiratory therapy
7. Teaching, supervising, and evaluating the performance of medical and paramedical personnel involved in anesthesia, respiratory care, and critical care
8. Conducting research at the basic and clinical science levels to explain and improve the care of patients in terms of physiologic function and drug response
9. Involvement in the administration of hospitals, medical schools, and outpatient facilities necessary to implement these responsibilities

[1]Adapted from the revised definition of the American Board of Anesthesiology, 1989.

chloroform was introduced into clinical practice by the obstetrician James Simpson, who administered it to his patients to relieve the pain of labor.

Nitrous oxide was the least popular of the three early inhalation anesthetics because of its relatively low potency and its tendency to cause asphyxia when used alone (Chapter 7). Interest in nitrous oxide did not revive until Edmund Andrews administered it in 20% oxygen in 1868. Nevertheless, it was overshadowed by the popularity of ether and chloroform. (It is ironic that nitrous oxide is the only one of these agents still in common use today.) Chloroform initially superseded ether in popularity in many areas, but reports of chloroform-related cardiac arrhythmias and hepatotoxicity eventually caused more and more practitioners to abandon it in favor of ether. Even with introduction of other inhalation anesthetics (ethyl chloride, ethylene, divinyl ether, cyclopropane, trichloroethylene, and fluroxene), ether remained the standard general anesthetic until the early 1960s. The only inhalational agent that rivaled ether's safety and popularity was cyclopropane. Unfortunately, both are highly combustible and have since been replaced by the nonflammable potent fluorinated hydrocarbons: halothane (discovered 1951, released 1956), methoxyflurane (discovered 1958, released 1960), enflurane (discovered 1963, released 1973), and isoflurane (discovered 1965, released 1981). New agents continue to be developed. One such agent, desflurane, has many of the desirable properties of isoflurane as well as the rapid uptake and elimination characteristics of nitrous oxide.

LOCAL & REGIONAL ANESTHESIA

The origin of modern local anesthesia is credited to Carl Koller, an ophthalmologist, who demonstrated the use of topical cocaine for surgical anesthesia of the eye in 1884. Cocaine had been isolated from the coca plant in 1855 by Gaedicke and later purified in 1860 by Albert Neimann. The surgeon William Halsted demonstrated in 1884 the use of cocaine for intradermal infiltration and nerve blocks (including the facial nerves, the brachial plexus, and the pudendal and posterior tibial nerves). August Bier is credited with the first spinal anesthetic in 1898; he used 3 mL of 0.5% cocaine intrathecally. He was also the first to describe intravenous regional anesthesia (Bier block) in 1908. Procaine was synthesized in 1904 by Alfred Einhorn and within a year found clinical use as a local anesthetic by Heinrich Braun. Braun was also the first the add epinephrine to prolong the action of local anesthetics. Caudal epidural anesthesia was introduced in 1901 by Ferdinand Cathelin and Jean Sicard. Lumbar epidural anesthesia was described first in 1921 by Fidel Pages and again in 1931 by Achille Dogliotti. Additional local anesthetics subsequently introduced clinically include dibucaine (1930), tetracaine (1932), lidocaine (1947), chloroprocaine (1955), mepivacaine (1957), prilocaine (1960), bupivacaine (1963), and etidocaine (1972). Ropivacaine, a new agent with the same duration of action as bupivacaine but perhaps less toxicity, may soon be available for clinical use.

INTRAVENOUS ANESTHESIA

Induction Agents

Intravenous anesthesia followed the invention of the hypodermic syringe and needle by Alexander Wood in 1855. Early attempts at intravenous anesthesia included the use of chloral hydrate (Oré in 1872), chloroform and ether (Burkhardt in 1909), and the combination of morphine and scopolamine (Bredenfeld in 1916). Barbiturates were synthesized in 1903 by Fischer and von Mering. The first barbiturate used for induction of anesthesia was diethylbarbituric acid (barbital), but it was not till the introduction of hexobarbital in 1927 that barbiturate induction became a popular technique. Thiopental was synthesized in 1932 by Volwiler and Tabern and first used clinically by John Lundy and Ralph Waters in 1934. Thiopental remains the most common induction agent for anesthesia. Methohexital was first used clinically in 1957 by V.K. Stoelting and is the only other barbiturate currently used for induction. Since the synthesis of chlordiazepoxide in 1957, the benzodiazepines—diazepam (1959), lorazepam (1971), and midazolam (1976)—have been extensively used for premedication, induction, supplementation of anesthesia, and intravenous sedation. Ketamine was synthesized in 1962 by Stevens and first used clinically in 1965 by Corssen and Domino; it was released in 1970. Ketamine was the first intravenous agent associated with minimal cardiac and respiratory depression. Etomidate was synthesized in 1964 and released in 1972; enthusiasm over its relative lack of circulatory and respiratory effects has been tempered by reports of adrenal suppression after even a single dose. The most recently released induction agent, propofol (diisopropylphenol, released in 1989), appears to be a major advance in outpatient anesthesia because of its short duration of action (Chapters 8 and 44).

Muscle Relaxants

The use of curare by Harold Griffith and Enid Johnson in 1942 was a milestone in anesthesia. Curare greatly facilitated endotracheal intubation and provided excellent abdominal relaxation for surgery. For the first time, surgery could be performed on patients without having to administer relatively large doses of anesthetic to produce muscle relaxation. These large doses often resulted in excessive circulatory and respiratory depression as well as prolonged emergence; moreover, they were often not tolerated by frail patients.

Other muscle relaxants soon introduced clinically included gallamine, decamethonium, metocurine, alcuronium, and pancuronium. Because these agents were often associated with significant side effects (Chapter 9), the search for the ideal muscle relaxant continued. Recently introduced agents that come close to this goal include vecuronium, atracurium, pipecuronium, and doxacurium. Succinylcholine was synthesized by Bovet in 1949 and released in 1951; it has become a standard agent for facilitating endotracheal intubation. Succinylcholine remains unparalleled in its rapid onset of profound muscle relaxation, but its occasional side effects have continued the search for a comparable substitute (Chapter 9). Mivacurium, a new short-acting nondepolarizing muscle relaxant that will be clinically available soon, has minimal side effects but still has a slow onset and longer duration of action than succinylcholine.

Opioids

Morphine was isolated from opium in 1805 by Sertürner and subsequently tried as an intravenous anesthetic (see above). The morbidity and mortality initially associated with high doses of opioids in early reports caused many anesthetists to avoid opioids and favor pure inhalational anesthesia. Interest in opioids in anesthesia returned following the synthesis of meperidine in 1939. The concept of "balanced" anesthesia was introduced by Lundy and others and evolved to consist of thiopental for induction, nitrous oxide for amnesia, meperidine (or any narcotic) for analgesia, and curare for muscle relaxation. In 1969, Lowenstein rekindled interest in opioid anesthesia by reintroducing the concept of high doses of narcotics as complete anesthetics. Morphine was initially employed, but fentanyl, sufentanil, and alfentanil were all subsequently used as sole agents. As experience grew with this technique, its limitations in reliably preventing patient awareness and suppressing autonomic responses during surgery were realized. Narcotics are now most commonly used in "balanced" tech-

niques (usually with nitrous oxide or a potent fluorinated hydrocarbon, or with both).

EVOLUTION OF THE SPECIALTY

British Origins

Following its first public demonstration in the United States, the use of ether quickly spread to England. John Snow became the first physician to take a full-time interest in this new anesthetic, for which he invented an inhaler. He was the first to scientifically investigate ether and the physiology of general anesthesia. (Snow was also a pioneer in epidemiology who helped stop a cholera epidemic in London by proving that the causative agent was transmitted by ingestion rather than inhalation.) In 1847, Snow published the first book on general anesthesia, *On the Inhalation of Ether.* When the anesthetic properties of chloroform were made known (see above), he also quickly investigated and developed an inhaler for that agent as well. He felt that an inhaler should be used in administering these agents in order to control the dose of the anesthetic. His second book, *On Chloroform and Other Anaesthetics,* was published posthumously in 1858. John Snow is generally considered the father of anesthesia.

After Snow's death, Joseph T. Clover took his place as England's leading physician anesthetist. Clover emphasized continuously monitoring the patient's pulse during anesthesia, a practice that was not widely accepted at the time. He was the first to use the jaw thrust maneuver for airway obstruction, first to have resuscitation equipment always available during anesthesia, and first to use a cricothyroid cannula (to save a patient with an oral tumor who developed complete airway obstruction). Sir Frederick Hewitt became England's foremost anesthetist at the turn of the century. He was responsible for many inventions, including the oral airway. Hewitt also wrote what many consider to be the first true textbook of anesthesia, which went through five editions. Snow, Clover, and Hewitt established a tradition of physician anesthetists that still exists in England. In 1893, the first organization of physician specialists in anesthesia, the Society of Anaesthetists, was formed by J.F. Silk in England.

American Origins

In the United States, few physicians had specialized in anesthesia by the turn of the century. The task of giving anesthesia was usually delegated to junior surgical house officers or medical students, who tended to be more interested in the surgical procedure than in monitoring the patient. Because of the shortage of physicians interested in the specialty in the United States, surgeons at both the Mayo Clinic and Cleveland Clinic trained and employed nurses as anesthetists. The first organization of physician anesthetists in the United States was the Long Island Society of Anesthetists in 1911. That society was eventually renamed the New York Society of Anesthetists and became national in

1936. It was subsequently renamed the American Society of Anesthetists and later, in 1945, the American Society of Anesthesiologists (ASA).

Three physicians stand out in the early development of anesthesia in the United States after the turn of the century: Arthur E. Guedel, Ralph M. Waters, and John S. Lundy. Guedel was the first to elaborate on the signs of general anesthesia after Snow's original description. He advocated cuffed endotracheal tubes and introduced artificial ventilation during ether anesthesia (later called "controlled respiration" by Waters). (The first elective endotracheal intubations during anesthesia were performed in the late 19th century by surgeons: Sir William MacEwen in Scotland, Joseph O'Dwyer in the United States, and Franz Kuhn in Germany.) Endotracheal intubation during anesthesia had been popularized in England by Sir Ivan Magill and Stanley Rowbotham in the 1920s. Ralph Waters added a long list of contributions to the specialty in the United States; the most important was insistence on proper training of specialists in anesthesia. Together with John Lundy, he introduced thiopental for induction of anesthesia.

Official Recognition

Widespread specialization in anesthesia did not take place until just before World War II. Ralph M. Waters was appointed the first professor of anesthesia in United States in 1933 at the University of Wisconsin, and in 1937 the American Board of Anesthesiology was established. In England, the first examination for the Diploma in Anaesthetics took place in 1935, and the first Chair in Anaesthetics was awarded to Sir Robert Macintosh in 1937 at Oxford University. Anesthesia became an officially recognized specialty in England only in 1947, when the Faculty of Anaesthetists of the Royal College of Surgeons was established.

THE SCOPE OF ANESTHESIA

The practice of anesthesia has changed dramatically since John Snow adopted the specialty. The modern anesthesiologist is now both a consultant and a primary care provider. The consultant role is appropriate because the primary goal of the anesthetist—to see the patient safely and comfortably through surgery—generally takes only a short time (minutes to hours). However, because anesthesiologists manage all "noncutting" aspects of the patient's care in the immediate perioperative period, they are also primary care providers. The "captain of the ship" doctrine, which held the surgeon responsible for every aspect of the patient's care perioperatively (including anesthesia), is no longer valid. The surgeon and anesthesiologist must function together effectively, but both are ulti-

mately answerable to the patient rather than to each other. Patients can select their own anesthesiologists, but their choices are usually limited by who is on the medical staff at a particular hospital, the surgeon's preference (if any), or the "on call" schedule for anesthesiologists on a given day.

The practice of anesthesia is no longer limited to the operating room nor even confined to rendering patients insensible to pain (Table 1–1). Anesthesiologists are now routinely asked to monitor, sedate, and provide general or regional anesthesia outside the operating room: in lithotripsy, magnetic resonance imaging, computerized tomography, fluoroscopy, electroconvulsive therapy, and cardiac catheterization units. Anesthesiologists have traditionally been pioneers in cardiopulmonary resuscitation and continue to be integral members of resuscitation teams. An increasing number of practitioners have subspecialized in cardiac anesthesia (Chapter 21), critical care (Chapter 48), neuroanesthesia (Chapter 26), obstetric anesthesia (Chapter 41), pediatric anesthesia (Chapter 42), and pain management (Chapter 18). Certification for special competence in critical care already exists and is being developed for pain management in the United States. Anesthesiologists are actively involved in administering and medically directing many operating rooms, intensive care units, and respiratory therapy departments. Moreover, they have assumed administrative and leadership positions on the medical staffs of hospitals and ambulatory care facilities.

PREOPERATIVE EVALUATION OF PATIENTS

As will become clear in later chapters, there is no one "standard anesthetic." Rather, an anesthetic plan (Table 1–2) should be formulated to optimally accommodate the patient's baseline physiologic state, including any medical and surgical illnesses, the planned procedure, drug sensitivities, previous anesthetic experiences, and psychologic makeup. To help formulate the anesthetic plan, a general outline for assessing patients preoperatively is an important starting point (Table 1–3). This assessment includes a pertinent history (including a review of previous medical records), a physical examination, and any indicated laboratory tests. Detailed discussions about evaluating patients with specific disorders and those undergoing unusual procedures are found throughout this book. The assessment is completed by classifying the patient according to the ASA physical status scale. Assessment of complicated patients may require consultations with other specialists to help determine if the patient is optimally ready for the procedure and to have their assistance if necessary in perioperative care. Following

Table 1–2. The anesthetic plan.

Premedication
Type of anesthesia
  General
    Airway management
    Induction
    Maintenance
    Muscle relaxation
  Local or regional anesthesia
    Technique
    Agents
  Monitored anesthesia care
    Supplemental oxygen
    Sedation
Intraoperative management
  Monitoring
  Positioning
  Fluid management
  Special techniques
Postoperative management
  Pain control
  Intensive care
    Postoperative ventilation
    Hemodynamic monitoring

Table 1–3. Routine preoperative anesthetic evaluation.

I. History
  1. Current problem
  2. Other known problems
  3. Medication history
    Allergies
    Drug intolerances
    Present therapy
      Prescription
      Nonprescription
    Nontherapeutic
      Alcohol
      Tobacco
      Illicit
  4. Previous anesthetics, surgery, and obstetric deliveries
  5. Family history
  6. Review of organ systems
    General (including activity level)
    Respiratory
    Cardiovascular
    Renal
    Gastrointestinal
    Hematologic
    Neurologic
    Endocrine
    Psychiatric
    Orthopedic
    Dermatologic
  7. Last oral intake
II. Physical examination
  1. Vital signs
  2. Airway
  3. Heart
  4. Lungs
  5. Extremities
  6. Neurologic examination
III. Laboratory evaluation: See Table 1–4.
IV. ASA classification: See Table 1–5.

---

the assessment, the anesthesiologist must discuss with the patient realistic options available for anesthetic management. Based on that discussion and the patient's wishes (reflected in the informed consent; see below), the final anesthetic plan is formulated.

The Preoperative History

The preoperative history should clearly establish the patient's present problem as well as the planned surgical, therapeutic, or diagnostic procedure. The presence and severity as well as the past and present treatments for known underlying medical problems must also be investigated. Because of the potential for drug interactions with anesthesia, a complete medication history should be elicited from every patient. This should include the use of tobacco and alcohol as well as illicit drugs such as marihuana, cocaine, and heroin. An attempt must also be made to distinguish between true drug allergies (often manifested as dyspnea or skin rashes) and drug intolerances (usually gastrointestinal upset). Detailed questioning about previous operations and anesthetics may uncover prior anesthetic complications. A family history of anesthetic problems may suggest a familial problem such as malignant hyperthermia (see Case Discussion in Chapter 42). A general review of organ systems is important in identifying undiagnosed medical problems. Questions should emphasize cardiovascular, pulmonary, endocrine, hepatic, renal, and neurologic function. A positive response to any of these questions should prompt more detailed inquiries to determine the extent of any organ impairment.

Physical Examination

The history and examination complement one another: The examination helps detect abnormalities not apparent from the history, while the history helps focus the examination on the organ systems that should be examined closely. Examination of healthy asymptomatic patients should minimally consist of measurement of vital signs (blood pressure, heart rate, respiratory rate, and temperature) and examination of the airway, heart, lungs, and extremities; standard techniques of inspection, auscultation, palpation, and percussion are used. An abbreviated neurologic examination is important when regional anesthesia is being considered and serves to document any subtle preexisting neurologic deficits. The patient's anatomy should be specifically evaluated for any planned procedures such as a nerve block, regional anesthesia, or invasive monitoring procedure; evidence of infection over or close to the site or significant anatomic abnormalities may contraindicate such procedures (Chapters 6 and 16).

The importance of examination of the airway cannot be overemphasized (Chapter 5). The patient's dentition should be inspected for loose or chipped teeth and the presence of caps, bridges, or dentures. A poor anesthesia mask fit should be expected in some edentulous patients and those with significant facial abnormalities. Micrognathia (a short distance between the chin and the hyoid bone), prominent upper incisors, a large tongue, limited range of motion of the temporal mandibular joint or cervical spine, or a short neck suggests that difficulty may be encountered in endotracheal intubation (Chapter 5).

Laboratory Evaluation

The utility of routine laboratory testing for healthy asymptomatic patients is doubtful when the history and physical examination fail to detect any abnormalities. Such routine testing is expensive and rarely alters perioperative management; moreover, abnormalities often are either ignored or result in unnecessary delays. Nonetheless, because of the current litigious environment in the United States, many physicians continue to order a hematocrit (or hemoglobin concentration), urinalysis, serum electrolyte measurements, coagulation studies, an electrocardiogram, and a chest x-ray on all patients.

A valuable preoperative test is one that implies an increased perioperative risk when it is abnormal and a reduced risk when the abnormality is corrected. The utility of a test in screening for disease depends on its sensitivity and specificity as well as the prevalence of the disease. Sensitive tests have a low rate of false-negative results, while specific tests have a low rate of false-positive results. The prevalence of a disease depends on the population tested and often depends on sex, age, genetic background, and lifestyle practices. Testing is therefore most effective when sensitive and specific tests are used in patients in whom the abnormality might be expected to occur. Accordingly, laboratory testing should be based on the presence or absence of underlying diseases and drug therapy as suggested by the history and physical examination. The nature of the procedure should also be taken into consideration. Thus, a baseline hematocrit is desirable in any patient about to undergo a procedure that may result in extensive blood loss requiring transfusion. General guidelines for preoperative testing of asymptomatic and seemingly healthy patients are given in Table 1–4.

Testing fertile women for an undiagnosed early pregnancy may be justified by the potentially teratogenic effects of anesthetic agents on the fetus (Chapter 41); pregnancy testing involves detection of human chorionic gonadotropin in urine or serum. Test-

ing for AIDS (detection of antibody against HIV) is highly controversial. Routine coagulation studies and urinalysis are not cost-effective in asymptomatic healthy patients.

Preventive Health Maintenance

Preoperative testing provides an excellent opportunity for preventive health maintenance. Preventive testing is generally indicated every 1–2 years and includes, in addition to a history and physical examination, testing stool for occult blood (patients over 40 years), breast examination and mammography (women over 40 years), a Papanicolaou smear (all women), and measurement of total serum cholesterol concentration (perhaps all patients).

ASA Physical Status Classification

In 1961 the ASA adopted a five-category physical status classification system (Table 1–5) for use in assessing a patient's preoperative status. Although this system was not intended as such, ASA physical status has since been shown to generally correlate with the perioperative mortality rate (Table 1–6). Because underlying disease is only one of many factors contributing to perioperative complications (see Chapter 45), it is not surprising that this correlation is not perfect. Nonetheless, the ASA physical status classification remains useful in planning anesthetic management, especially monitoring techniques (Chapter 6).

Informed Consent

The preoperative assessment culminates in giving the patient a reasonable explanation of the options available for anesthetic management: general, regional, local, or topical anesthesia or intravenous sedation. The term "monitored anesthesia care" (previously referred to as "local standby") is now commonly used and refers to monitoring the patient during a procedure performed with intravenous sedation or local anesthesia administered by the surgeon. Regardless of the technique chosen, consent must always be obtained for

Table 1–4. Routine preoperative laboratory evaluation of asymptomatic, apparently healthy patients.

1. Hematocrit or hemoglobin concentration:
   All menstruating women
   All patients over 60 years of age
   All patients who are likely to experience significant blood loss and may require transfusion
2. Serum glucose and creatinine (or blood urea nitrogen) concentration: all patients over 60 years of age
3. Electrocardiogram: all patients over 40 years of age
4. Chest radiograph: all patients over 60 years of age

Table 1–5. Preoperative classification of patients according to the American Society of Anesthesiologists.

Class	Definition
I	A normal healthy patient other than surgical pathology—without systemic disease.
II	A patient with mild systemic disease—no functional limitations.
III	A patient with moderate to severe systemic disturbance due to medical or surgical disease—some functional limitation but not incapacitating.
IV	A patient with severe systemic disturbance which poses a constant threat to life and is incapacitating.
V	A moribund patient not expected to survive 24 hours with or without surgery.
E	If the case is an emergency, the physical status is followed by the letter "E"—eg, "IIE."

Table 1–6. American Society of Anesthesiologists classification and perioperative mortality rates.

Class	Mortality Rate
I	0.06–0.08%
II	0.27–0.4%
III	1.8–4.3%
IV	7.8–23%
V	9.4–51%

general anesthesia in case other techniques prove inadequate.

If any procedure is performed without the patient's consent, the physician may be liable for assault and battery. When the patient is a minor or otherwise not competent to consent, the consent must be obtained from someone legally authorized to give it, such as a parent, guardian, or close relative. Although oral consent may be sufficient, written consent is usually advisable for medicolegal purposes. Moreover, consent must be *informed* to ensure that the patient (or guardian) has sufficient information about the procedures and their risks to make a reasonable and prudent decision whether to consent. It is generally accepted that not all risks need be detailed but only those that are realistic risks in similar patients with similar problems. It is generally advisable to inform the patient that some complications may be life-threatening.

The purpose of the preoperative visit is not only to gather important information and obtain informed consent—it also helps establish a healthy doctor-patient relationship. Moreover, an empathically conducted interview that answers important questions and lets the patient know what to expect has been shown to be at least as effective in relieving anxiety as some premedication drug regimens (Chapter 8).

DOCUMENTATION

Documentation is important both for quality assurance and for medicolegal purposes. Adequate documentation is essential for the defense of a malpractice action (see Case Discussion).

The Preoperative Note

The preoperative note should be written in the patient's chart and should describe all aspects of the preoperative assessment, including the medical history, past anesthetic history, medication history, the physical examination, laboratory results, ASA classification, and the recommendations of any consultants. Finally, the anesthetic plan together with the informed consent are described. The plan should be as detailed as possible and should include the use of specific procedures such as endotracheal intubation, invasive monitors (Chapter 6), and regional or hypotensive techniques. Documentation of informed conset usually takes the form of a narrative in the chart indicating that the plan, alternative plans, their advantages and disadvantages (including the risk of complications) were presented and understood and agreed to by the patient. Alternatively, the patient signs a special anesthesia consent form that contains the same information. A sample preanesthetic report form is illustrated in Figure 1–1. Although a completely handwritten note in the chart is acceptable, the use of a printed form lessens the likelihood of omitting important information.

The Intraoperative Anesthesia Record

The intraoperative anesthesia record (Figure 1–2) serves many purposes. It functions as a useful intraoperative monitor, a reference for future anesthetics for that patient, and a tool for quality assurance. This record should be as pertinent and accurate as possible. It should document all aspects of anesthetic care in the operating room, including the following:

(1) A preoperative check of the anesthesia machine and other equipment.
(2) A review or reevaluation of the patient immediately prior to induction of anesthesia.
(3) A review of the chart for new laboratory results or consultations.
(4) A review of the anesthesia and surgical consents.
(5) The time of administration, dosage, and route of intraoperative drugs.
(6) All intraoperative monitoring (including laboratory measurements, blood loss, and urine output).
(7) Intravenous fluid administration and transfusion.
(8) All procedures (such as intubation, placement of a nasogastric tube, or placement of invasive monitors).
(9) Routine and special techniques such as mechanical ventilation, hypotensive anesthesia, one-lung ventilation, high-frequency jet ventilation, or cardiopulmonary bypass.
(10) The timing and course of important events such as induction, positioning, surgical incision, and extubation.
(11) Unusual events or complications.
(12) The condition of the patient at the end of the procedure.

Vital signs are recorded graphically at least every 5 minutes. Other monitoring data are also usually entered graphically, while descriptions of techniques or complications are handwritten. Automated record-keeping systems are available, but their use is still not widespread. Unfortunately, the intraoperative anesthetic record is often inadequate to document critical incidents such as a cardiac arrest. In such cases, a

ANESTHESIOLOGY PHYSICIAN'S PREOPERATIVE REPORT

DATE:	TIME:	HT.	PREOP DIAGNOSIS:
AGE:	SEX: M F	WT.	PROPOSED OPERATION:

MEDICAL HISTORY   MEDICATIONS:
ALLERGIES:
INTOLERANCES:
DRUG USE: TOBACCO: ETOH:

PRESENT PROBLEM:

CARDIOVASCULAR

RESPIRATORY

DIABETES

NEUROLOGIC   RENAL

ARTHRITIS/MUSCULO-SKELETAL   HEPATIC

                                                  OTHER

PREVIOUS ANESTHETICS:

FAMILY HISTORY

LAST ORAL INTAKE

PHYSICAL EXAMINATION   BP   P   R   T

   HEART   EXTREMITIES

   LUNGS   NEUROLOGIC

   AIRWAY   OTHER

   TEETH

LABORATORY

   Hct/Hgb   ECG   CHEST X–RAY
   URINE
   LYTES: Na   Cl
           K   GLUCOSE   OTHER
           CO_2 BUN: CREATININE

PLAN   ☐ GEN.   INVASIVE MONITORS
             ☐
             ☐   SPECIAL TECHNIQUES

ASA CLASS   SIGNATURE _____ | _____ M.D.
                                              (RESIDENT)   (STAFF)

PATIENT CONSENT
ANESTHETIC ALTERNATIVES AND RISKS RANGING FROM TOOTH DAMAGE
TO LIFE THREATENING EVENTS HAVE BEEN EXPLAINED AND ACCEPTED.

                                                  NAME

PATIENT SIGNATURE
                                                  #

Figure 1–1. The preoperative note.

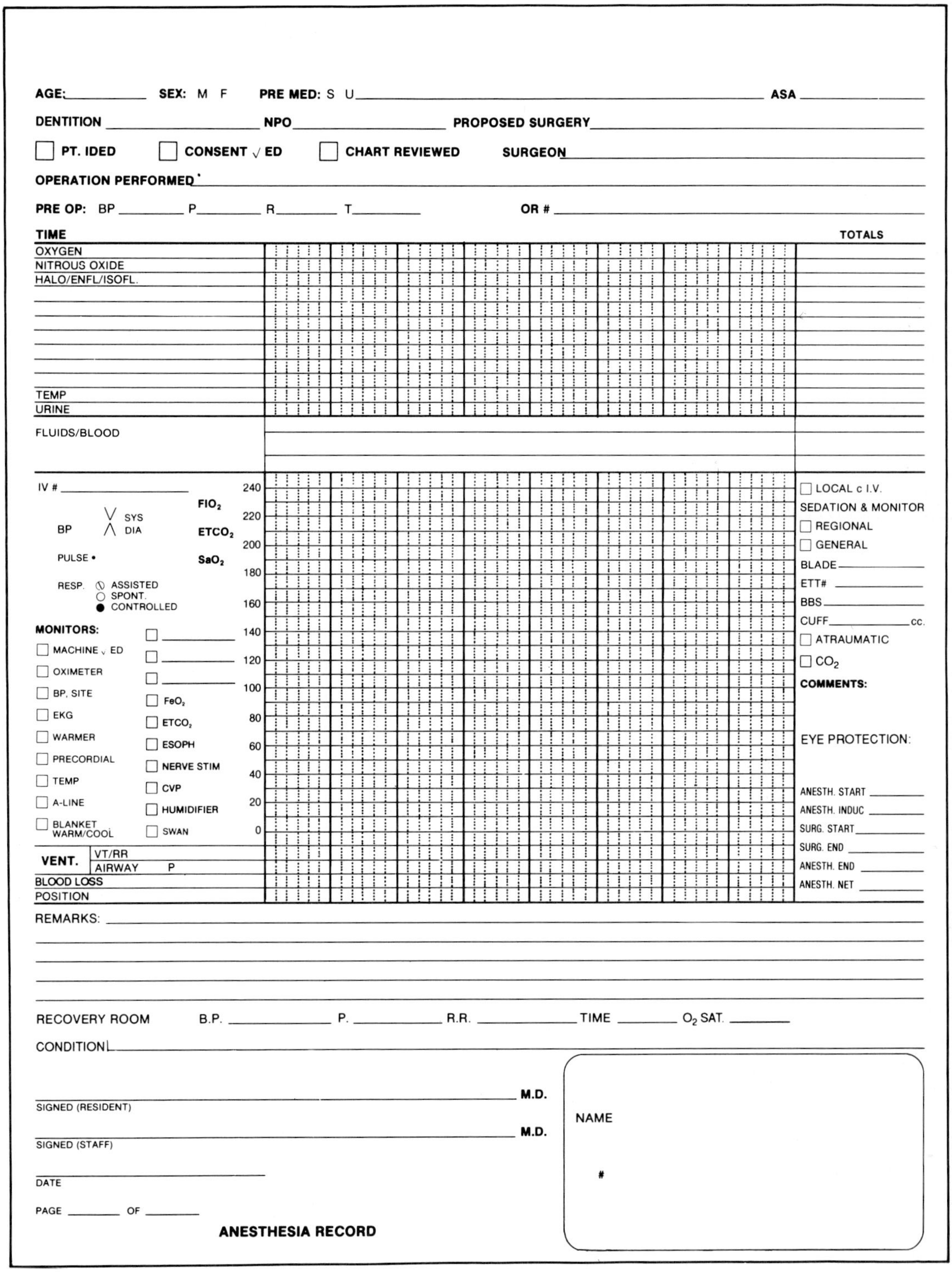

AGE:_____ SEX: M F   PRE MED: S U_____ ASA _____

DENTITION _____ NPO _____ PROPOSED SURGERY_____

☐ PT. IDED   ☐ CONSENT √ ED   ☐ CHART REVIEWED   SURGEON_____

OPERATION PERFORMED ._____

PRE OP: BP _____ P_____ R_____ T_____   OR # _____

TIME		TOTALS
OXYGEN		
NITROUS OXIDE		
HALO/ENFL/ISOFL.		
TEMP		
URINE		

FLUIDS/BLOOD

IV # _____   240
                FIO₂   220
    V SYS   200
BP ∧ DIA   ETCO₂
PULSE •   SaO₂   180
RESP. ⊘ ASSISTED   160
       ○ SPONT.
       ● CONTROLLED

MONITORS: ☐ _____ 140
☐ MACHINE √ ED ☐ _____ 120
☐ OXIMETER   ☐ _____ 100
☐ BP. SITE   ☐ FeO₂
☐ EKG   ☐ ETCO₂   80
☐ WARMER   ☐ ESOPH   60
☐ PRECORDIAL   ☐ NERVE STIM
☐ TEMP   ☐ CVP   40
☐ A-LINE   ☐ HUMIDIFIER 20
☐ BLANKET   ☐ SWAN   0
  WARM/COOL

VENT. VT/RR
       AIRWAY   P
BLOOD LOSS
POSITION

☐ LOCAL c I.V.
SEDATION & MONITOR
☐ REGIONAL
☐ GENERAL
BLADE_____
ETT#_____
BBS_____
CUFF_____cc.
☐ ATRAUMATIC
☐ CO₂
COMMENTS:

EYE PROTECTION:

ANESTH. START _____
ANESTH. INDUC _____
SURG. START _____
SURG. END _____
ANESTH. END _____
ANESTH. NET _____

REMARKS: _____
_____
_____
_____

RECOVERY ROOM   B.P. _____   P. _____   R.R. _____   TIME _____ O₂ SAT. _____

CONDITION∟_____

_____ M.D.
SIGNED (RESIDENT)

_____ M.D.
SIGNED (STAFF)

NAME

#

DATE _____

PAGE _____ OF _____

ANESTHESIA RECORD

Figure 1–2. The intraoperative anesthesia record.

9

ANESTHESIA POSTOP NOTES

IMMEDIATE POSTOP NOTE (BEFORE DISCHARGE FROM RECOVERY ROOM):

_____ NO COMPLICATIONS OF ANESTHESIA IMMEDIATELY APPARENT;
PATIENT HAS RECOVERED FROM IMMEDIATE EFFECTS OF
ANESTHESIA AND MAY BE TRANSFERRED TO WARD OR
OUTPATIENT DEPARTMENT.

_____ OTHER:

_____ M.D. _____
SIGNED   DATE   TIME

FOLLOW UP POSTOP NOTE: (AFTER DISCHARGE FROM RECOVERY ROOM, BEFORE DISCHARGE
FROM HOSPITAL):

_____ NO APPARENT POSTANESTHETIC COMPLICATIONS

_____ PATIENT DISCHARGED FROM HOSPITAL BY SURGEON PRIOR TO
POSTANESTHETIC VISIT.

_____ OTHER:

_____ M.D. _____
SIGNED   DATE   TIME

NAME

\#

CHART COPY

Figure 1–3. The postoperative note.

separate note in the patient's chart may be necessary to adequately document what happens. Careful recording of the course of events, actions taken, and their timing is necessary to avoid discrepancies between multiple simultaneous records (anesthesia record, nurses' notes, cardiopulmonary resuscitation record, and other physicians' entries in the medical record). Such discrepancies are frequently targeted as evidence of incompetence or dissembling by malpractice attorneys. Incomplete, inaccurate, or illegible records may subject physicians to unjustified legal liability.

Postoperative Notes

The anesthesiologist's immediate responsibility to the patient does not end until the patient has completely recovered from the effects of the anesthetic. After accompanying the patient to the postanesthesia care unit (PACU), the anesthesiologist should remain with the patient until normal vital signs have been established and the patient's condition is deemed stable (Chapter 47). Prior to discharge from the PACU, a discharge note should be written by the anesthesiologist to document (1) the patient's recovery from anesthesia, (2) any apparent anesthesia-related complications, and (3) the condition of the patient and (4) the disposition (discharge to an outpatient area, an inpatient ward, an intensive care unit, or even home). Inpatients should be seen again at least once within 48 hours after discharge from the PACU. Postoperative notes should document those visits, the condition of the patient, the presence or absence of any anesthesia-related complications, and any measures undertaken to treat complications.

CASE DISCUSSION: MEDICAL MALPRACTICE

A healthy 45-year-old man suffers a cardiac arrest during an elective inguinal hernia repair. Although cardiopulmonary resuscitation is successful, the patient is left with permanent mental status changes that preclude his return to work. Two years later, the patient files a complaint against the anesthesiologist, surgeon, and hospital.

What four elements must be proved by the plaintiff (patient) to establish negligence on the part of the defendant (physician or hospital)?

(1) Duty: Once a physician establishes a professional relationship with a patient, the physician owes that patient certain obligations such as adhering to the "standard of care."

(2) Breach of duty: If these obligations are not fulfilled, the physician has breached his duties to the patient.

(3) Causation: The plaintiff must demonstrate that the breach of duty was causally related to the injury. This "proximate cause" does not have to be the most important or immediate cause of the injury.

(4) Damages: An injury must result. The injury may cause general damages (eg, pain and suffering) or special damages (eg, loss of income).

How is the "standard of care" defined and established?

Individual physicians are expected to perform as any prudent and reasonable physician would in light of the surrounding circumstances. Being a specialist, the anesthesiologist is held to a higher standard of knowledge and skill with respect to the subject matter of that specialty than a general practitioner or a physician in another specialty. The standard of care is usually established by an expert witness. While most jurisdictions have extended the "locality rule" to encompass a national standard of care, the specific circumstances pertaining to each individual case are taken into account. The law recognizes that there are differences of opinion and varying schools of thought within the medical profession.

How is causation determined?

It is usually the plaintiff who bears the burden of proving (1) that the injury would not have occurred "but for" the negligence of the physician, or (2) that the physician's action was a "substantial factor" in causing the injury. An exception is the doctrine of *res ipsa loquitur* ("the thing speaks for itself"), which permits a finding of negligence based solely on circumstantial evidence. For "res ipsa" to apply in the present case summary, the plaintiff would have to establish that cardiac arrest does not ordinarily occur in the absence of negligence and that it could not have been due to something outside the control of the anesthesiologist. An important concept is that causation in civil cases need only be established by **a preponderance of the evidence** ("more likely than not")—as opposed to criminal cases, where all elements of a charged offense must be proved "beyond a reasonable doubt."

What factors influence the likelihood of a malpractice suit?

(1) **The physician-patient relationship:** This is particularly important for the anesthesiologist, who usually does not meet the patient until the night before or on the morning of surgery. Another problem is that the patient is unconscious while under the anesthesiologist's care. Thus, the preoperative and postoperative visits with the patient assume vital importance. While anesthesiologists have less long-term contact

with patients than other medical specialists, it is possible and desirable to make this contact meaningful. Family members should also be considered during these meetings, particularly if there has been an intraoperative complication.

(2) Adequacy of informed consent: Rendering care to a competent patient who does not consent constitutes assault and battery. However, consent is not enough. The patient should be informed of the contemplated procedure, including its reasonably anticipated risks, its possible benefits, and the therapeutic alternatives. The physician may be liable for a complication—even if it is not due to the negligent performance of a procedure—if a jury is convinced that a reasonable person would have refused treatment if properly informed of the possibility of the complication. This does not mean, of course, that a documented consent relieves physicians who violate the standard of care from liability.

(3) Quality of documentation: Careful documentation of the perioperative visits, informed consent, consultation with other specialists, intraoperative events, and postoperative care is absolutely essential. The viewpoint of many courts and juries is that "if it isn't written, it wasn't done." It goes without saying that medical records should never be intentionally destroyed or altered.

SUGGESTED READING

Cheng EY, Kay J (editors): *Manual of Anesthesia and the Medically Compromised Patient.* Lippincott, 1990. Blends the perspectives of internal medicine, critical care, and intraoperative anesthesia into perioperative evaluation and management.

Frost AM (editor): *Preanesthetic Assessment.* Anesthesiol Clin North Am 1990;8:No. 4. Anesthetic implications and preoperative management.

Little DM Jr: *Classical Anesthesia Files.* Wood Library–Museum of Anesthesiology (WLM), 1985.

Lyons AS, Petrucelli RJ: *Medicine: An Illustrated History.* Abrams, 1978. Muravchick S: *The Anesthetic Plan: From Physiologic Principles To Clinical Strategies.* Mosby Year Book, 1991. A good introduction to formulating anesthetic strategies that takes into account organ system dysfunction and emphasizes the role of the anesthesiologist as a consultant.

Smith WDA: *Under the Influence: A History of Nitrous Oxide and Oxygen Anesthesia.* Macmillan/WLM, 1982.

Sykes WS, Ellis RH: *Essays on the First Hundred Years of Anaesthesia,* 3 vols. Churchill Livingstone, 1982. This collection and other works of historical interest are available through the Wood Library–Museum of Anesthesiology, 515 Busse Highway, Park Ridge, IL 60068–3189.

Symposium on complications and medico-legal aspects of anaesthesia. Br J Anaesth 1987;59:813. British perspective on anesthetic complications and medical malpractice.

The Operating Room: Medical Gas Systems, Environmental Factors, & Electrical Safety

2

Anesthesiologists spend more time in operating rooms than any other group of physicians. Furthermore, anesthesiologists are responsible for protecting unconscious patients against a multitude of possible dangers during surgery. Some of these threats are unique to the operating room. As a result, no medical specialist has a greater responsibility than the anesthesiologist for the proper functioning of the operating room's medical gases, environmental factors (eg temperature, humidity, and ventilation), and electrical safety. This chapter describes the major features of operating rooms of special interest to anesthesiologists and the potential hazards associated with these systems. A case summary organizes some of this information into a protocol for testing a new operating room's medical gas pipeline system.

MEDICAL GAS SYSTEMS

The medical gases commonly used in operating rooms are oxygen, nitrous oxide, air, and nitrogen. While technically not a gas, vacuum exhaust for anesthetic waste gas disposal (scavenging) and surgical suction must also be provided and is considered an integral part of the medical gas system. Patients are endangered if medical gas systems, particularly oxygen, malfunction. The main features of medical gas systems are the source of the gases and the means of their delivery to the operating room. The anesthesiologist must understand both of these elements to prevent and detect medical gas depletion or supply line misconnection. Estimates of peak demand determine the

type of medical gas supply system that a particular hospital requires.

SOURCES OF MEDICAL GASES

Oxygen

A reliable supply of oxygen is a critical requirement in any surgical area. Medical grade oxygen (99% or 99.5% pure) is manufactured by fractional distillation of liquefied air. Oxygen is stored as a compressed gas at room temperature or refrigerated as a liquid. Most small hospitals store oxygen in banks of H-cylinders connected by a manifold (Figure 2–1). The number of cylinders in each bank depends on anticipated daily demand. The manifold contains valves that reduce the cylinder pressure (approximately 2000 pounds per square inch on the gauge [psig]) to line pressure (50 ± 5 psig) and automatically switch banks when one group of cylinders is exhausted.

A liquid oxygen storage system (Figure 2–2) is more economical for large hospitals. Liquid oxygen must be stored well below its critical temperature of −119°C since *gases may be liquefied by pressure only if stored below their critical temperature*. As a reserve, a large hospital may have a smaller liquid oxygen supply or a bank of compressed gas cylinders. The reserve should be capable of providing one day's oxygen requirement. In case of unanticipated hospital gas system failure, the anesthesiologist must always have available an emergency supply of oxygen in the operating room.

Most anesthesia machines accommodate one or two E-cylinders of oxygen (Table 2–1). As oxygen is expended, the cylinder's pressure falls in proportion to its content. A pressure of 1000 psig indicates an approximately half-full E-cylinder and represents 330 L of

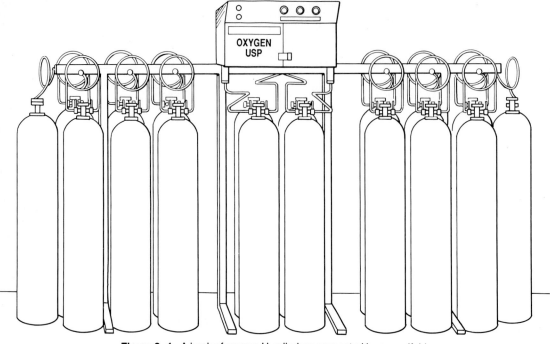

Figure 2–1. A bank of oxygen H-cylinders connected by a manifold.

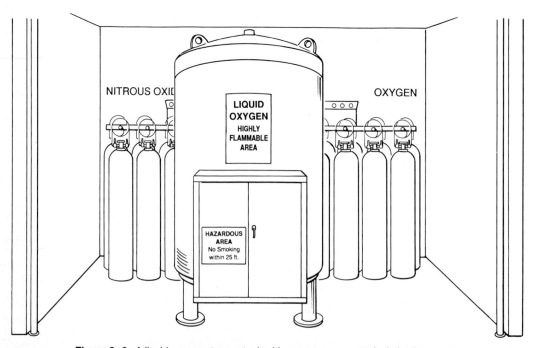

Figure 2–2. A liquid oxygen storage tank with reserve oxygen tanks in background.

Table 2–1. Characteristics of medical gas cylinders.

	E-Cylinder Capacity[1] (L)	H-Cylinder Capacity[1] (L)	Pressure[1] (psig)	Color (USA)	Color (Int'l)	Form
O_2	625–700	6000–8000	1800–2200	Green	White	Gas
Air	625–700	6000–8000	1800–2200	Yellow	White and black	Gas
N_2O	1590	15,900	745	Blue	Blue	Liquid
N_2	625–700	6000–8000	1800–2200	Black	Black	Gas

[1]Depending on the manufacturer.

oxygen at atmospheric pressure. If the oxygen is exhausted at a rate of 3 L/min, a half-full cylinder will be empty in 110 minutes. Oxygen cylinder pressure should be monitored before and periodically during use.

Nitrous Oxide

Nitrous oxide, the most commonly used anesthetic gas, is manufactured by heating ammonium nitrate (thermal decomposition). It is almost always stored by hospitals in large high-pressure cylinders (H-cylinders) connected by a manifold with an automatic crossover feature.

Since the critical temperature of nitrous oxide (36.5 °C) is above room temperature, it can be kept liquefied without an elaborate refrigeration system. If the temperature of liquefied nitrous oxide rises above its critical temperature, it will revert to its gaseous phase. Because nitrous oxide is not an ideal gas and is easily compressible, this transformation into a gaseous phase is not accompanied by a great rise in tank pressure. Nonetheless, all gas cylinders are equipped with an emergency pressure relief valve ("rupture disk") to prevent explosion under conditions of unexpectedly high gas pressure (eg, unintentional overfilling).

Bulk liquid storage of nitrous oxide is economical only in very large institutions. Although a disruption in supply is usually not catastrophic, most anesthesia machines have reserve nitrous oxide E-cylinders. Since these smaller cylinders also contain nitrous oxide in its liquid state, *the volume remaining in a cylinder is not proportionate to cylinder pressure.* By the time the liquid nitrous oxide is expended and the tank pressure begins to fall, only about 400 L of nitrous oxide remains. If liquid nitrous oxide is kept at a constant temperature (20 °C), it will vaporize at the same rate at which it is consumed and will maintain a constant pressure (745 psig) until the liquid is exhausted. *The only reliable way to determine residual volume of nitrous oxide is to weigh the cylinder.* For this reason, the tare weight (TW), or empty weight, of cylinders containing a liquefied compressed gas (eg, nitrous oxide) is often stamped on the shoulder of the cylinder.

Since energy is consumed in the conversion of a liquid to a gas (the latent heat of vaporization), the liquid nitrous oxide cools. The drop in temperature

results in a lower vapor pressure and lower cylinder pressure. The cooling is so pronounced at high flow rates that pressure regulators may freeze.

Air

The use of air is becoming more frequent in anesthesiology as the potential hazards of nitrous oxide and high concentrations of oxygen receive increasing attention. Cylinder air is medical grade and is obtained by blending oxygen and nitrogen. Dehumidified but unsterile air is provided to the hospital pipeline system by compression pumps. The inlets of these pumps must be distant from vacuum exhaust vents to minimize contamination. Because the critical temperature of air is −140.6 °C, it exists as a gas in pressurized cylinders.

Nitrogen

Although compressed nitrogen is not administered to patients, it provides power to many pieces of operating room equipment. It is most commonly stored in H-cylinders connected by a manifold.

Vacuum

A central hospital vacuum system usually consists of two independent suction pumps each capable of handling peak requirements. Traps at every user location prevent contamination of the system with foreign matter.

DELIVERY OF MEDICAL GASES

Medical gases are delivered from their central supply source to the operating room through a piping network. Gas pipes are usually constructed of seamless copper tubing. Internal contamination of the pipelines with dust, grease, or water must be avoided. The hospital's gas delivery system presents in the operating room as hose drops, gas columns, or elaborate articulating arms (Figure 2–3). Operating room equipment, including the anesthesia machine, interfaces with these pipeline system outlets by color-coded hoses. Quick coupler mechanisms, which vary in design with different manufacturers, connect one end of

A   B   C

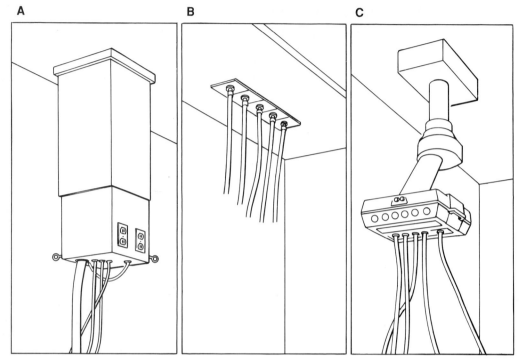

Figure 2–3. Typical examples of (A) gas columns, (B) ceiling hose drops, and (C) articulating arms. One end of a color-coded hose connects to the hospital medical gas supply system by way of a quick-coupler mechanism. The other end connects to the anesthesia machine through the diameter index safety system (DISS).

hose to a specific gas outlet. The other end connects to the anesthesia machine through a noninterchangeable **diameter index safety system (DISS)** fitting that prevents incorrect hose attachment.

E-cylinders of oxygen, nitrous oxide, and air attach directly to the anesthesia machine. To discourage incorrect cylinder attachments, a **pin index safety system (PISS)** has been adopted by cylinder manufacturers. Each gas cylinder (sizes A–E) has two holes in its cylinder valve that mate with corresponding pins in the yoke of the anesthesia machine (Figure 2–4). The relative positioning of the pins and holes is unique for each gas. This system can be defeated by placing multiple washers between the cylinder and yoke that prevent proper engagement of the pins and holes. Likewise, the pin index safety system is ineffective if yoke pins are damaged or the cylinder is filled with the wrong gas.

The functioning of medical gas supply sources and pipeline systems is constantly monitored by central alarm systems. Indicator lights and audible signals warn of changeover to secondary gas sources and abnormally high (eg, pressure regulator malfunction) or low (eg, supply depletion) pipeline pressures (Figure 2–5).

Despite a multitude of safety devices, alarms, and detailed regulations (established by the National Fire Protection Association, the Compressed Gas Association, and the Department of Transportation), anesthetic catastrophes continue to result from malfunctioning medical gas systems. Institution of periodic mandatory inspections of hospital gas delivery systems by independent agencies and increased involvement by anesthesiologists in gas system design could ameliorate this problem.

ENVIRONMENTAL FACTORS IN THE OPERATING ROOM

TEMPERATURE

The temperature in most operating rooms seems uncomfortably cold to many conscious patients and, at times, to conscious anesthesiologists. However, standing in surgical garb for hours under operating room lights can be an endurance course for scrub nurses and surgeons. As a general principle, the comfort of operating room personnel must be reconciled with patient needs. For example, small children and patients with large exposed surfaces (eg, thermal burns) constitute specific indications for an operating room temperature of 24°C or higher, since these patients lose heat rapidly and have a limited ability to compensate.

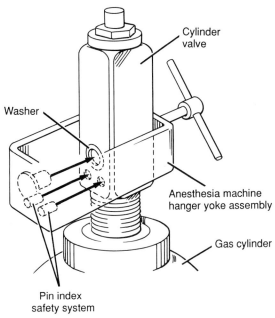

Figure 2–4. Pin index safety system (PISS) interlink between the anesthesia machine and gas cylinder.

HUMIDITY

In past decades, static discharges were a feared source of ignition in an operating room filled with flammable anesthetic vapors. Because increased humidity decreases the likelihood of static discharges, a relative humidity of at least 50% was recommended. Continued compliance with this requirement is anachronistic in this era of nonflammable anesthetic agents.

VENTILATION

A high rate of operating room air flow decreases contamination of the surgical site. These flow rates are usually achieved by blending recirculated air with fresh air. Although recirculation conserves energy costs associated with heating and air conditioning, it is unsuitable for anesthetic waste gas disposal. Therefore, a separate anesthetic gas scavenging system must always supplement operating room ventilation. Extreme rates of flow, such as produced by a laminar air system, have been proposed for procedures with particularly high risks of infection (eg, total hip replacement).

ELECTRICAL SAFETY

THE HAZARD OF ELECTROCUTION

The use of electronic medical equipment subjects patients and hospital personnel to the risk of electrocu-

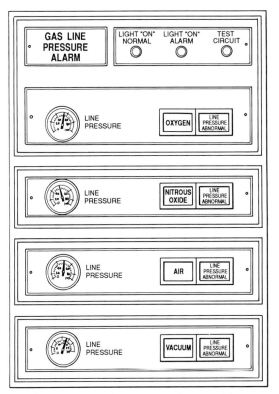

Figure 2–5. An example of a master alarm panel that monitors medical gas line pressure. (Courtesy of Ohio Medical Products.)

tion. Anesthesiologists must have at least a basic understanding of electrical hazards and their prevention.

Body contact with two conductive materials at different voltage potentials may complete a circuit and result in an electrical shock. Usually, one point of exposure is a "live" 110 V or 240 V conductor, and the circuit is completed through a second "ground" contact. For example, a grounded person need only contact one live conductor to complete a circuit and receive a shock. The additional conductor could be the frame of a patient monitor that has developed a fault to the "hot" side of the power line. A circuit is now complete between the power line (which is earth-grounded at the utility's pole-top transformer) through the victim and back to the ground (Figure 2–6). The physiologic effect of electrical current depends on the location, duration, frequency, and magnitude (more accurately, current density) of the shock.

Leakage current is present in all electrical equipment as a result of capacitive coupling, induction between internal electrical components, or defective insulation. Current can flow as a result of capacitive coupling between two conductive bodies (eg, a circuit board and its casing) even though they are not physically connected. Some monitors are doubly insulated to decrease the effect of capacitive coupling. Other monitors are designed to be connected to a low-impedance ground that will preferentially carry leakage current away from a person touching the instrument's case. The magnitude of such leakage is normally imperceptible to touch (less than 1 mA and well below the fibrillation threshold of 100 mA). However, if the current bypasses the high resistance offered by skin and is applied directly to the heart (micro-shock), current as low as 100 μA (*micro*amperes) may be fatal.

Cardiac pacing wires and invasive monitoring catheters provide a conductive pathway to the myocardial endothelium. In fact, blood and normal saline can serve as electrical conductors. The exact amount of current required to produce fibrillation depends upon the timing of the shock relative to the vulnerable period of heart repolarization (the T wave on the electrocardiogram). Even small differences in potential between the earth connections of two different electrical outlets in the same operating room might place a patient at risk for microelectrocution.

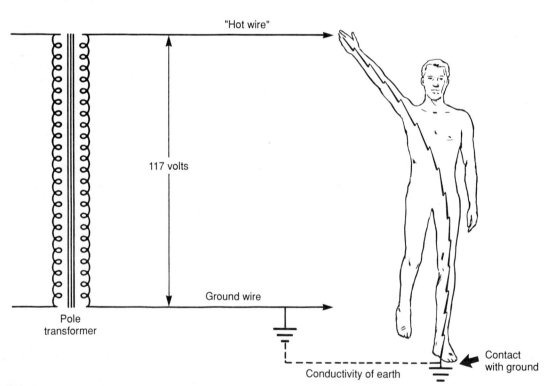

Figure 2–6. The setting for the great majority of electric shocks. An incidentally grounded person simultaneously contacts the "hot" wire of the electric service, usually via defective equipment that provides a pathway linking the hot wire to an exposed conductive surface. The complete electrical loop originates with the secondary of the pole transformer (the voltage source) and extends through the hot wire, the victim and the victim's contact with ground, the earth itself, the neutral ground rod at the service entrance, and, via the neutral (or ground) wire, back to the transformer. (Modified and reproduced, with permission, from Bruner J, Leonard PF: *Electricity, Safety, and the Patient.* Mosby Year Book, 1989.)

PROTECTION FROM ELECTRICAL SHOCK

Most patient electrocutions depend upon current flow from the live conductor of a grounded circuit through the body and back to a ground (Figure 2–6). This would be prevented if everything in the operating room were grounded except the patient. While direct patient grounds should be avoided, complete patient isolation is not feasible during surgery. Instead, the operating room power supply is isolated from grounds by an **isolation transformer** (Figure 2–7).

Unlike the utility company's pole-top transformer, the secondary wiring of an isolation transformer is *not* grounded and provides two live ungrounded voltage lines for operating room equipment. Equipment casing—but not the electrical circuits—is grounded through the longest blade of a three-pronged plug. If a live wire is now unintentionally contacted by a grounded patient, current will not flow since no circuit has been completed back to the secondary coil (Figure 2–8).

Of course, if both power lines are contacted, a circuit is completed and a shock is possible. To reduce the chance of two coexisting faults, a **line isolation monitor** (LIM) measures the potential for current flow from the isolated power supply to ground (Figure 2–9). Basically, the line isolation monitor determines the degree of isolation between the two power wires and the ground and predicts the amount of current that *could* flow if a short circuit were to develop. An alarm is activated if an unacceptably high current flow to ground becomes possible (usually 2 mA or 5 mA), but power is not interrupted unless a **ground leakage circuit breaker** (also called a ground-fault circuit-interrupter) is also activated. The latter is not installed in locations such as operating rooms, where discontinuation of life support systems is more hazardous than the risk of electrical shock. The alarm of the line isolation monitor merely indicates that the power supply has partially reverted to a grounded system. If an alarm is activated, the last piece of equipment that was plugged in is suspect and should be removed from service until it is repaired.

Even isolated power circuits do not provide complete protection from the small currents capable of causing microshock fibrillation. Modern equipment designs that decrease the possibility of microelectrocution include (1) double insulation of the chassis and casing, (2) ungrounded battery power supplies, and (3) patient isolation from equipment-connected grounds by using optical coupling or transformers.

SURGICAL DIATHERMY

Electrosurgical units generate an ultra-high-frequency electrical current that passes from a small active electrode (the cautery tip) through the patient and exits by way of a large plate electrode (the grounding pad or return electrode). The high current density at the cautery tip is capable of tissue coagulation or cutting, depending upon the electrical waveform. Ventricular fibrillation is prevented by the use of high electrical frequencies (0.1–3 million Hz) compared with line power (50–60 Hz). The large surface area of the

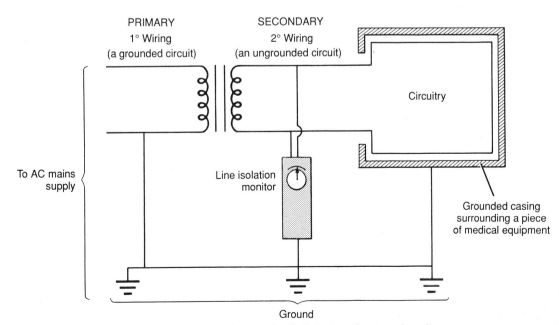

Figure 2–7. A circuit diagram of an isolation transformer and monitor.

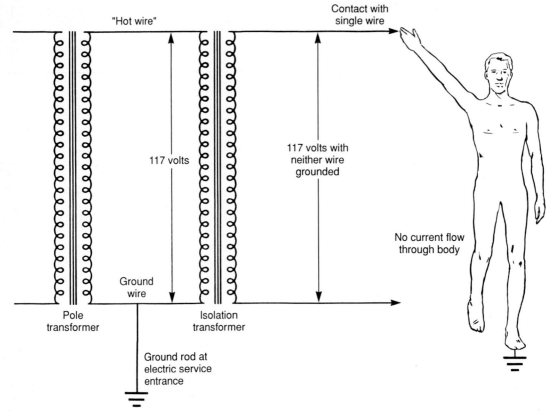

Figure 2–8. Even though a person is grounded, no shock results from contact with one wire of an isolated circuit. The individual is in simultaneous contact with two separate voltage sources but does not close a loop including either source. (Modified and reproduced, with permission, from Bruner J, Leonard PF: *Electricity, Safety, and the Patient.* Mosby Year Book, 1989.)

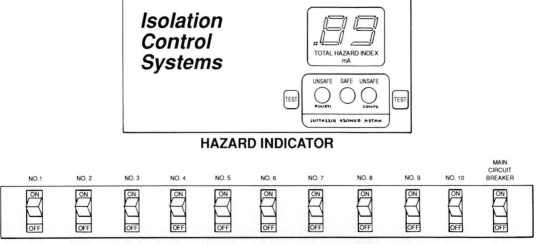

Figure 2–9. The panel of a line isolation monitor. (Courtesy of Ohio Medical Products.)

low-impedance return electrode avoids burns at the current's point of exit by providing a low current density (the concept of "exit" is technically incorrect, since the current is alternating).

Dysfunction of the return electrode may result from (1) disconnection from the electrosurgical unit, (2) inadequate patient contact, or (3) insufficient conductive gel. In these situations, the current will find another place to exit (eg, electrocardiogram pads or metal parts of the operating table), which may result in a burn (Figure 2–10). Precautions to prevent diathermy burns include proper return electrode placement that avoids bony protuberances and elimination of patient-to-ground contacts. Current flow through the heart may lead to pacemaker dysfunction. This can be minimized by placing the return electrode as close to the surgical field and as far away from the heart as practical.

Newer electrosurgical units are isolated from ground using the same principles as the isolated power supply ("isolated output" versus "ground-referenced" units). Although some electrosurgical units are capable of detecting return electrode malfunction, most alarm only if the return electrode is disconnected from the machine, regardless of the adequacy of its contact with the patient. Bipolar electrodes confine current propagation to a few millimeters, eliminating the need for a return electrode. Since pacemaker and electrocardiogram interference is possible, pulse and heart sounds should be closely monitored when any electrosurgical unit is used.

FIRES & EXPLOSIONS

There are three requisites for a fire or explosion: (1) a flammable agent (fuel), (2) a gas that supports combustion, and (3) a source of ignition. Flammable anesthetic agents (diethyl ether, divinyl ether, ethyl chloride, ethylene, and cyclopropane) are no longer used in the United States. However, the risk of fires or explosions has not been eliminated. Bowel gas, consisting of methane, hydrogen, and hydrogen sulfide, is highly flammable. Operating room supplies that have been reported to be combustible include endotracheal tubes, oxygen catheters, surgical drapes, benzoin aerosol, alcohol cleansing solutions, and even petroleum-based ointments (LacriLube). *If these substances ignite, they should be immediately removed from the patient* and extinguished. Burning surgical drapes are particularly difficult to extinguish, since they are designed to be water-resistant.

Both oxygen and nitrous oxide are capable of vig-

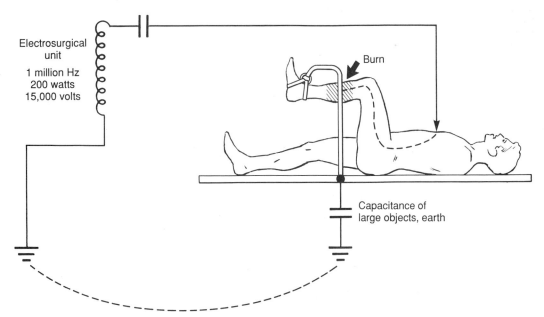

Figure 2–10. Electrosurgery—burn at unwanted site. If the intended "return path" is compromised, the circuit may be completed through other routes. Since the current is of high frequency, recognized conductors are not essential; capacitances can serve to complete gaps in the circuit. Current passing through the patient to a contact of small area may produce burn. (A leg drape would not be expected to offer protection in the example depicted.) Compared to the ground-referenced ESU, the "isolated output" electrosurgical unit (ESU) is much less likely to provoke burns at ectopic sites. "Ground-referenced" in this context applies to the ESU output and has nothing to do with isolated versus grounded power systems. (Modified and reproduced, with permission, from Bruner J, Leonard PF: *Electricity, Safety, and the Patient.* Mosby Year Book, 1989.)

orously supporting combustion; flammable agents that merely burn in air may explode in a mixture of nitrous oxide and oxygen. The accumulation of these agents under surgical drapes during head and neck surgery is particularly hazardous. Since the introduction of routine pulse oximetry, there is no reason to indiscriminately insufflate oxygen under surgical drapes.

Historically, static electricity has been the most feared source of ignition. Numerous hospital regulations have attempted to minimize this cause of anesthetic explosions by prohibiting the use in operating rooms of materials apt to cause static discharge (eg, nylon and wool), by installing conductive breathing circuits and flooring, and by maintaining relative humidity above 50%. Most of these antiquated guidelines are now disregarded. In fact, conductive flooring increases the risk of electrical hazards. More contemporary sources of ignition include electrical equipment such as the electrosurgical unit or laser. The use of diathermy near distended bowel or the laser near endotracheal tubes continues to provide proof that the danger of intraoperative explosion persists. The results of operating room fires are uniformly tragic.

CASE DISCUSSION: CHECKING OUT THE MEDICAL GAS SYSTEM IN A NEW OPERATING ROOM

A hospital has just dedicated its new obstetric wing, which includes two operating rooms. You are scheduled to deliver the first anesthetic.

Who is responsible for testing and certifying the medical gas delivery system?

No governmental or accreditation agency in the United States inspects hospital gas systems to enforce conformity with the National Fire Protection Associa-

tion 99 standard for health care facilities (the Canadian Standards Association certifies independent inspection firms in Canada). Ideally, third-party testing should certify that all aspects of the medical gas supply, piping, and outlet system comply with NFPA standards before use. Hospitals should have well-defined written policies for management, testing, control, and training of their medical gas systems. Although anesthesiologists are not responsible for hospital construction, they are responsible for intraoperative patient safety. In particular, the anesthesiologist is accountable for the portion of the medical gas system that extends from the wall outlet to the patient.

What elements of the medical gas system need to be tested?

A twenty-four-hour standing pressure test checks for system leaks and faulty pressure relief valves. Cross-connection of pipelines is prevented by pressurizing each gas system separately and confirming that pressure is present only at corresponding gas outlets. The content purity of each pipeline is verified by analysis of samples collected from each outlet. Excessive contamination by volatile gases or water moisture can usually be removed by high-flow nitrogen purging of the system. The anesthesiologist should double-check each ceiling outlet to make certain that the correct color-coded hose and quick-connect device are present. Gas line contents should be confirmed with an oxygen analyzer, gas chromatograph, or mass spectrometer. The vacuum system can be checked with a suction gauge capable of measuring negative pressure. Common problems include residual copper oxide particles inside the piping, improper joints, inadequate sizing, and component failure.

Can the new wing affect the preexisting operating room suites?

Whenever any new construction, remodeling, or expansion occurs near medical gas storage sites or pipelines, a high index of suspicion is justified regarding the use of medical gases throughout the hospital.

SUGGESTED READINGS

Blackburn JP: Explosions. In: *Scientific Foundations of Anaesthesia,* 4th ed. Scurr C, Feldman S (editors). Heinemann, 1990.

Bruner JMR, Leonard PF: *Electricity, Safety, and the Patient.* Mosby Year Book, 1989.

Dorsh JA, Dorsh SE: *Understanding Anesthesia Equipment.* Williams & Wilkins, 1984. A detailed discussion of compressed gases and medical gas delivery systems.

Heavner JE, et al: *Technical Manual Of Anesthesiology: An Introduction.* Raven Press, 1989. Overview of several aspects of anesthesia equipment, including medical gases.

Lisbon A: *Anesthetic Considerations in Setting Up a New Medical Facility.* International Anesthesiology Clinics, 1981. Installation and checkout of medical gas and operating room electrical systems.

The National Fire Protection Association: Provides publications on fire hazards (NFPA 53M-1979) and electrical systems (NFPA 76A-1977, 76B-1980, and 76C-1980). Can be obtained by writing to Post Office Box 9146, Quincy, MA 02269, or calling 1-800-735-0100.

Ward CS: *Anaesthetic Equipment: Physical Principles and Maintenance,* 2nd ed. Bailliere Tindall, 1985. Good reviews of medical gas systems and electrical hazards.

Breathing Systems

Breathing systems provide the final conduit for the delivery of anesthetic gases to the patient. In the modern practice of anesthesiology, breathing circuits link a patient to an anesthesia machine (Figure 3–1). Many modifications in circuit design have been developed, each with varying degrees of efficiency, convenience, and complexity. This chapter reviews the most important breathing systems: (1) insufflation, (2) open drop, (3) Mapleson circuits, (4) the circle system, and (5) resuscitation systems.

Most traditional attempts to classify breathing systems artificially consolidate functional aspects (eg, the extent of rebreathing) with physical characteristics (eg, the presence of unidirectional valves). Because these often contradictory classifications (eg, open, closed, semiopen, semiclosed) tend to result in confusion rather than understanding, they are avoided in this discussion.

INSUFFLATION

The term "insufflation" usually denotes the blowing of anesthetic gases across a patient's face. Although insufflation is categorized as a breathing system, it is better considered a technique that avoids direct connection between a breathing circuit and a patient's airway. Because children resist the placement of a face mask or intravenous line, insufflation is particularly valuable during pediatric inductions with inhalational anesthetics (Figure 3–2). Carbon dioxide accumulation under head and neck draping is a hazard of ophthalmic surgery performed with local anesthesia. Insufflation of oxygen and air across the patient's face at a high flow rate (> 10 L/min) avoids this problem (Figure 3–3). Since insufflation avoids any direct patient contact, there is no rebreathing of exhaled gases. However, ventilation cannot be controlled with this technique, and the inspired gas contains unpredictable amounts of entrained atmospheric air.

Insufflation can also be used as a means of maintaining arterial oxygenation during brief periods of apnea (eg, during bronchoscopy). Instead of blowing gases across the face, oxygen is directed into the lungs through a catheter placed in the trachea.

OPEN DROP ANESTHESIA

Although open drop anesthesia is not used in modern medicine, its historic significance and continued use in developing countries warrant a brief description here. A highly volatile anesthetic—most commonly ether or halothane—is dripped onto a gauze-covered mask applied to the patient's face. As the patient inhales, air passes through the gauze, vaporizes the liquid agent, and carries high concentrations of anesthetic to the patient. The vaporization lowers mask temperature, resulting in moisture condensation and a drop in anesthetic vapor pressure (vapor pressure is proportionate to temperature).

Deep levels of anesthesia will decrease minute ventilation and initiate a dangerous cycle of mask warming, increased vapor pressure, and higher concentrations of anesthetic. If sufficient CO_2 is trapped under the mask, rebreathing of anesthetic gases (apparatus dead space) becomes significant. The anesthetic vapors further dilute inspired oxygen content, creating a potentially hypoxic mixture. To minimize dead space and increase inspired oxygen concentration, supplemental oxygen can be administered under the mask.

Another characteristic of the open drop technique is the uncontrollable pollution of the operating room environment with anesthetic—a serious disadvantage if a flammable agent such as ether is being administered.

MAPLESON CIRCUITS

The insufflation and open drop systems have several disadvantages: (1) poor control of inspired gas concentration and depth of anesthesia, (2) inability to assist or control ventilation, (3) no conservation of exhaled heat or humidity, (4) difficult airway management during head and neck surgery, and (5) pollution of the operating room with large volumes of waste gas. The Mapleson systems solve some of these problems by incorporating additional components (ie, breathing tubes, fresh gas inlets, pressure relief valves, and breathing bags) into the breathing circuit. The relative location of these components determines circuit performance and is the basis of the Mapleson classification (Table 3–1).

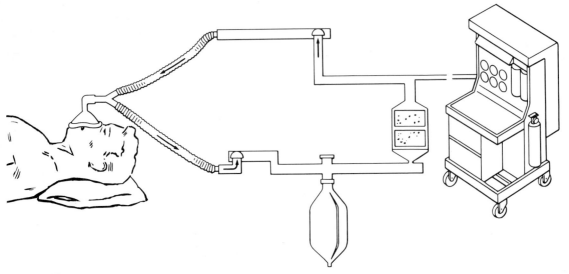

Figure 3–1 The relationship between the patient, the breathing system, and the anesthesia machine.

Components of Mapleson Circuits

A. Breathing Tubes: Corrugated breathing tubes composed of rubber (reusable) or plastic (disposable) connect the components of the Mapleson circuit to the patient (Figure 3–4). The large diameter of the tubes creates a low-resistance pathway and a potential reservoir for anesthetic gases. In order to minimize fresh gas flow requirements, the volume of the breathing tube in most Mapleson circuits should be at least as great as the patient's tidal volume.

The compliance of the breathing tubes partially determines the compliance of the circuit. (Compliance is defined as the change of volume produced by a specific change in pressure.) *Long breathing tubes with high compliance increase the difference between the volume of gas delivered to a circuit by a breathing bag or ventilator and the volume actually delivered to the patient.* For example, if a breathing circuit with a compliance of 8 mL gas/cm H_2O is pressurized during delivery of a tidal volume to 20 cm H_2O, 160 mL of the tidal volume will be lost to the circuit. Specifically, the 160 mL represents a combination of gas compression and breathing tube expansion. This is an important consideration in any circuit delivering positive-pressure ventilation through breathing tubes (eg, circle systems).

B. Fresh Gas Inlet: Gases from the anesthesia machine enter the circuit through the fresh gas inlet. As discussed below, the relative position of this component is a key differentiating factor in Mapleson circuit performance.

C. Pressure Relief Valve (Pop-Off Valve, Adjustable Pressure Limiting Valve): As anesthetic gases enter the breathing circuit, pressure will rise if gas inflow is greater than the combined uptake of the patient and the circuit. This pressure buildup is controlled by allowing gases to exit the circuit through a pressure relief valve. Exiting gases enter the operating room atmosphere or, preferably, a waste gas scavenging system. There are several designs of pressure relief valves, but all allow setting a variable pressure threshold for venting.

The pressure relief valve should be fully opened during spontaneous ventilation so that circuit pressure remains negligible throughout inspiration and expiration. Assisted and controlled ventilation require positive pressure during inspiration to expand the lungs. Partial closure of the pressure relief valve limits gas

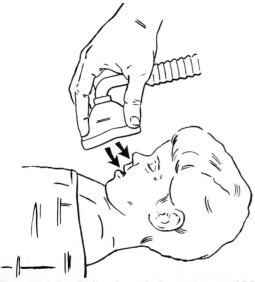

Figure 3–2 Insufflation of anesthetic agent across child's face during induction.

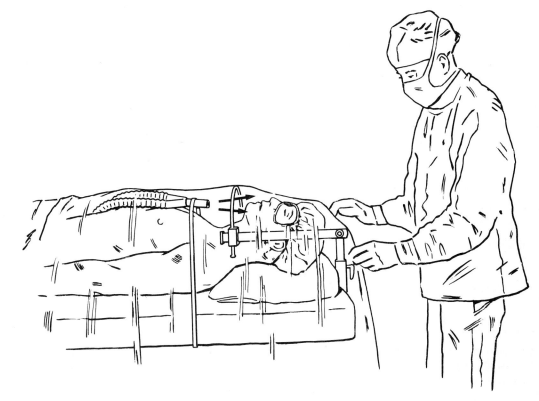

Figure 3–3 Insufflation of oxygen and air under head drape.

exit, permitting positive circuit pressures during breathing bag compressions.

D. Breathing Bag (Reservoir Bag): Breathing bags function as a reservoir of anesthetic gas and a method of generating positive-pressure ventilation. They are designed to increase in compliance as their volume increases. Three distinct phases of breathing bag filling are recognizable (Figure 3–5). After the nominal 3-L capacity of an adult breathing bag is achieved (phase I), pressure rises rapidly to a peak (phase II). Further increases in volume result in a plateau or even a slight decrease in pressure (phase III). This ceiling effect helps to protect the patient's lungs against high airway pressures if the pressure relief valve is unintentionally left in the closed position while fresh gas continues to flow into the circuit.

Performance Characteristics of Mapleson Circuits

Mapleson circuits are lightweight, inexpensive, simple, and do not require unidirectional valves. Breathing circuit efficiency is measured by the fresh gas flow required to eliminate CO_2 rebreathing. Because there are no unidirectional valves or CO_2 absorption in Mapleson circuits, rebreathing is prevented by venting exhaled gas through the pressure relief valve before inspiration. This usually requires high fresh gas flows.

Reexamine the drawing of a Mapleson A circuit in Figure 3–4. During spontaneous ventilation, alveolar gas containing CO_2 will be exhaled into the breathing tube or directly vented through an open pop-off valve. Before inhalation occurs, if the fresh gas flow exceeds alveolar minute ventilation, the alveolar gas remaining in the breathing tube will be forced to exit from the pressure release valve by the inflow of fresh gas. If the breathing tube volume is equal to or greater than the patient's tidal volume, the next inspiration will contain only fresh gas. Because a fresh gas flow equal to minute ventilation is sufficient to prevent rebreathing, the Mapleson A design is the most efficient Mapleson circuit for *spontaneous* ventilation.

However, positive pressure during *controlled* ventilation requires a partially closed pressure release valve. Although some alveolar and fresh gas exits through the valve during inspiration, no gas is vented during expiration. As a result, unpredictably high fresh gas flows are required to prevent rebreathing with a Mapleson A circuit during controlled ventilation.

Interchanging the position of the pressure relief valve and the fresh gas inlet transfers a Mapleson A into a Mapleson D circuit (Table 3–1). The latter system is efficient during controlled ventilation, since fresh gas flow now forces alveolar air *away* from the patient and *toward* the pressure relief valve. Therefore, simply moving components completely alters the fresh gas requirements of the Mapleson circuits.

Table 3–1. Classification and characteristics of Mapleson circuits.

Mapleson Class	Other Names	Diagram[1]	Required Fresh Gas Flows		Comments
			Spontaneous	Controlled	
A	Magill	Breathing tube — Pressure relief valve — Mask — Breathing bag — FGI	Equal to minute ventilation ($\approx$80 mL/kg/min)	Very high and difficult to predict	Poor choice during controlled ventilation.
B	Magill	FGI	2 × minute ventilation	2–2½ × minute ventilation	
C	Magill	FGI	2 × minute ventilation	2–2½ × minute ventilation	
D	Bain	FGI	2–3 × minute ventilation	1–2 × minute ventilation	Bain modification: Fresh gas tube inside breathing tube (see Fig 3–6).
E	Ayres T-piece	FGI	2–3 × minute ventilation	3 × minute ventilation (I:E = 1:2)	Exhalation tubing should provide a larger volume than tidal volume to prevent rebreathing. Scavenging is difficult.
F	Jackson-Reese	FGI — Pressure relief valve	2–3 × minute ventilation	2 × minute ventilation	A Mapleson E with a breathing bag connected to the end of the breathing tube to allow controlled ventilation and scavenging.

[1] FGI = Fresh gas inlet.

26

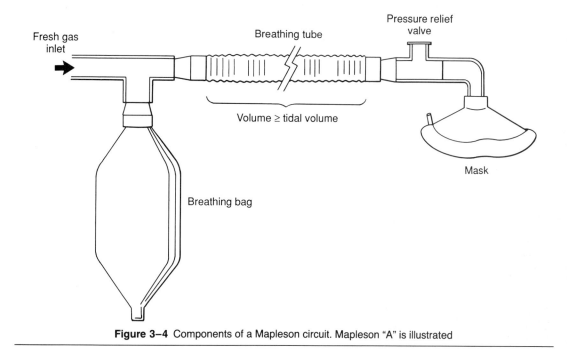

Figure 3–4 Components of a Mapleson circuit. Mapleson "A" is illustrated

The Bain system is a popular modification of the Mapleson D circuit that incorporates the fresh gas inlet tubing inside the breathing tube (Figure 3–6). This modification decreases the circuit's bulk and retains heat and humidity better than the Mapleson D as a result of partial warming of the inspiratory gas by countercurrent exchange with the warmer expired gases. A disadvantage of this coaxial circuit is the possibility of kinking or disconnection of the fresh gas inlet tubing. If unrecognized, either of these mishaps could result in significant rebreathing of exhaled gas.

THE CIRCLE SYSTEM

Although Mapleson circuits overcome some of the disadvantages of the insufflation and open drop systems, the high fresh gas flows required to prevent rebreathing result in (1) waste of anesthetic agent, (2) pollution of the operating room environment, and (3) loss of patient heat and humidity (Table 3–2). In an attempt to avoid these problems, the circle system adds more components to the breathing system.

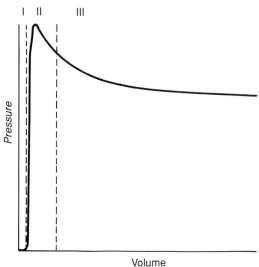

Figure 3–5 The increasing compliance and elasticity of breathing bags as demonstrated by their three phases of filling. (Reproduced, with permission, from Johnstone RE, Smith TC: Rebreathing bags as pressure limiting devices. Anesthesiology 1973;38:192.)

Table 3–2. Characteristics of breathing circuits.

	Insufflation and Open Drop	Mapleson	Circle
Complexity	Very simple	Simple	Complex
Control of anesthetic depth	Very poor	Poor	Good
Ability to scavenge	Very poor	Poor	Good
Conservation of heat and humidity	No	No	Yes[1]
Rebreathing of exhaled gases	No	No[1]	Yes[1]

[1]These properties depend upon the rate of fresh gas flow.

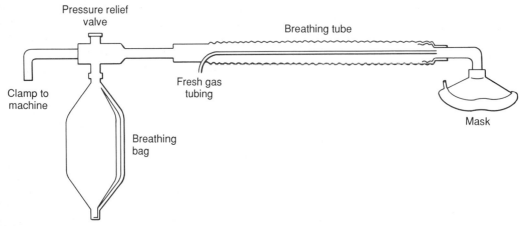

Figure 3–6 A Bain circuit is a Mapleson "D" design with the fresh gas tubing inside the corrugated breathing tube. (Redrawn and reproduced, with permission, from Bain JA, Spoerel WE: Flow requirements for a modified Mapleson "D" system during controlled ventilation. Can Anaesth Soc J 1973;20:629.)

Components of the Circle System

A. Carbon Dioxide Absorbent: Rebreathing alveolar gas conserves heat and humidity. However, the CO_2 in exhaled gas must be eliminated to prevent hypercapnia. Carbon dioxide chemically combines with water to form carbonic acid. Carbon dioxide absorbents (eg, soda lime or barium hydroxide lime) contain hydroxide salts that are capable of neutralizing carbonic acid (Table 3–3). Reaction end products include heat (the heat of neutralization), water, and calcium carbonate. Soda lime is the more common absorbent and is capable of absorbing 23 L of CO_2 per 100 g of absorbent. Its reactions are shown below:

$$CO_2 + H_2O \rightarrow H_2CO_3$$

$$H_2CO_3 + 2NaOH \rightarrow Na_2CO_3 + 2H_2O + Heat$$
$$\text{(a fast reaction)}$$

$$Na_2CO_3 + Ca(OH)_2 \rightarrow CaCO_3 + 2NaOH$$
$$\text{(a slow reaction)}$$

Note that the water and sodium hydroxide initially required are regenerated.

Color conversion of a pH indicator dye by increasing hydrogen ion concentration signals absorbent exhaustion (Table 3–4). Absorbent should be replaced when 50–70% has changed color. Although exhausted granules may revert to their original color if rested, no significant recovery of absorptive capacity occurs. Granule size is a compromise between the higher absorptive surface area of small granules and the lower resistance to gas flow of larger granules. The hydroxide salts are irritating to skin and mucous membranes. Increasing the hardness of soda lime by adding silica minimizes the risk of dust inhalation. Since barium hydroxide lime incorporates water into its structure (the water of crystallization), it is sufficiently hard without silica. Additional water is added to both types of absorbent during packaging to provide optimal conditions for carbonic acid formation.

Dry granules can absorb and later release significant amounts of volatile anesthetic. This property can be responsible for delayed induction or emergence. Trichloroethylene, an anesthetic no longer available in the United States, decomposes into neurotoxins (in-

Table 3–3. Comparison of soda lime and barium hydroxide lime.

	Soda Lime	Baralyme
Mesh size[1]	4–8	4–8
Method of hardness	Silica added	Water of crystallization
Content	Calcium hydroxide Sodium hydroxide Potassium hydroxide	Barium hydroxide Calcium hydroxide
Usual indicator dye	Ethyl violet	Ethyl violet
Absorptive capacity (liters of CO_2/100 g granules)	14–23	9–18

[1]Mesh size is the number of openings per linear inch in a wire screen that is used to grade particle size.

Table 3–4. Indicator dye changes signaling absorbent exhaustion.

Indicator	Color When Fresh	Color When Exhausted
Phenolphthalein	White	Pink
Ethyl violet	White	Purple
Clayton yellow	Red	Yellow
Ethyl orange	Orange	Yellow
Mimosa 2	Red	White

cluding phosgene gas) when exposed to soda lime and heat. Postoperative encephalitis and cranial nerve palsies have been traced to this toxic reaction.

B. Carbon Dioxide Absorbers: The granules of absorbent are contained within one or two canisters that fit snugly between a head and base plate. Together, this unit is called an absorber (Figure 3–7). Although bulky, double canisters permit more complete CO_2 absorption, less frequent absorbent changes, and lower gas flow resistance. To ensure complete absorption, a patient's tidal volume should not exceed the air space between absorbent granules, which is roughly equal to one-half the absorber's capacity. Indicator dye color is monitored through the absorber's transparent walls. Absorbent exhaustion preferentially occurs where exhaled gas enters the absorber and along the canister's smooth inner walls. Channeling through areas of loosely packed granules is minimized by an absorber baffle system. A trap at the base of the absorber collects dust and moisture. Some older absorbers have a bypass valve to allow absorbent change during ventilation. This bypass valve is easily overlooked and, if unintentionally left in the bypass position, may result in hypercapnia.

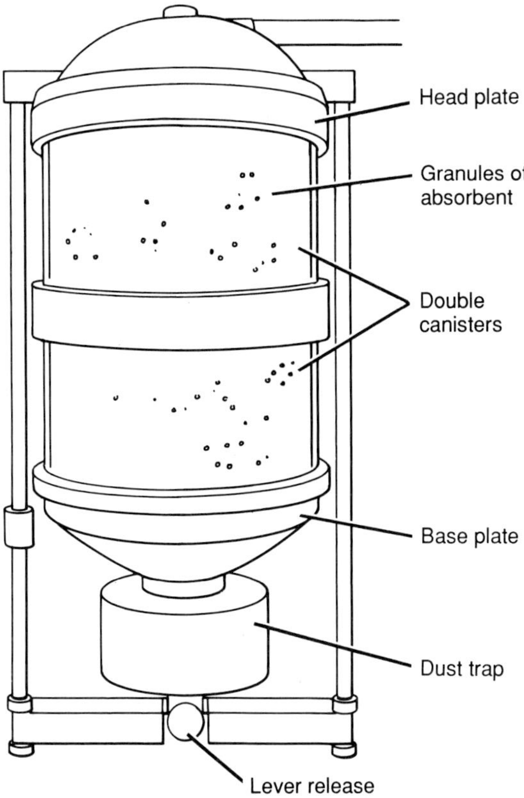

C. Unidirectional Valves: Unidirectional valves contain a rubber, plastic, or mica disk resting horizontally on an annular valve seat (Figure 3–8). Forward flow displaces the disk upward, permitting the gas to proceed through the circuit. Reverse flow pushes the disk against its seat, preventing reflux. Valve incompetence is usually due to warped disks or seat irregularities. The expiratory valve is especially vulnerable to damage since it is exposed to the humidity of alveolar gas.

Inhalation opens the inspiratory valve, allowing the patient to breath a mixture of fresh and exhaled gas that has passed through the CO_2 absorber. Simultaneously, the expiratory valve closes to prevent rebreathing of exhaled alveolar gas that still contains CO_2. The subsequent flow of gas away from the patient during exhalation opens the expiratory valve. This gas is vented through the pressure relief valve or rebreathed by the patient after passing through the absorber. Closure of the inspiratory valve during exhalation prevents expiratory gas from mixing with fresh gas in the inspiratory limb. Malfunction of either valve may allow rebreathing of CO_2, resulting in hypercapnia.

Optimization of Circle System Design

Although the major components of the circle system (unidirectional valves, fresh gas inlet, pressure relief

Figure 3–7 A carbon dioxide absorber.

Head plate

Granules of absorbent

Double canisters

Base plate

Dust trap

Lever release

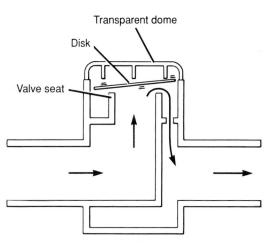

Transparent dome

Disk

Valve seat

Figure 3–8 A unidirectional valve.

valve, CO_2 absorber, and a breathing bag) can be placed in several configurations, one arrangement is preferred (Figure 3–9):

(1) Unidirectional valves should be close to the patient to prevent backflow into the inspiratory limb if a circuit leak develops. However, unidirectional valves should not be placed in the breathing tube Y-piece, since that makes it difficult to confirm proper orientation and intraoperative function.
(2) The fresh gas inlet is placed between the absorber and the inspiratory valve. Positioning downstream from the inspiratory valve would allow fresh gas to bypass the patient during exhalation and be wasted. Fresh gas introduced between the expiration valve and the absorber would be diluted by recirculating gas. Furthermore, inhaled anesthetics may be absorbed or released by soda lime granules, thus slowing induction and emergence.
(3) The pressure relief valve should be placed immediately before the absorber to conserve absorption capacity and to minimize venting of fresh gas.
(4) Resistance to exhalation is decreased by locating the breathing bag in the expiratory limb. Bag compression during controlled ventilation will vent alveolar gas through the pressure relief valve, conserving absorbent.

Performance Characteristics of the Circle System

A. Fresh Gas Requirement: With an absorber, the circle system prevents rebreathing of CO_2 even at fresh gas flows equal to the uptake of anesthetic gases and oxygen by the patient and the circuit itself (closed-system anesthesia). At fresh gas flows greater than 5 L/min, rebreathing is so minimal that a CO_2 absorber is usually unnecessary.

With low fresh gas flows, concentrations of oxygen and inhaled anesthetics can vary markedly between fresh gas (ie, gas in the fresh gas inlet) and inspired gas (ie, gas in the inspiratory limb of the breathing tubes), which is a mixture of fresh gas and exhaled gas that has passed through the absorber. Higher flows speed induction and recovery, compensate for leaks in the circuit, and decrease the risks of unanticipated gas mixtures.

B. Dead Space: Because of the unidirectional valves, apparatus dead space in a circle system is limited to the area distal to the point of inspiratory and expiratory gas mixing at the Y-piece. Unlike Mapleson circuits, the breathing tube length of a circle system does not directly affect dead space. Like Mapleson circuits, length does affect circuit compliance and thus the amount of tidal volume lost to the circuit during positive-pressure ventilation. Pediatric circle systems have a septum dividing the inspiratory and expiratory

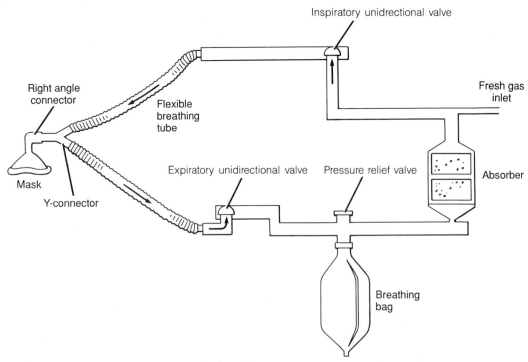

Figure 3–9 A circle system.

gas in the Y-piece and low-compliance breathing tubes to further reduce dead space.

C. Resistance: The unidirectional valves and absorber increase circle system resistance, especially at high respiratory rates and large tidal volumes. Nonetheless, even premature neonates can be successfully ventilated with circle systems.

D. Humidity and Heat Conservation: Medical gas delivery systems supply dehumidified gases to the anesthesia circuit at room temperature. In contrast, exhaled gas is saturated with water at body temperature. Therefore, the heat and humidity of inspired gas depends upon the relative proportion of rebreathed gas to fresh gas. High flows (5 L/min) are accompanied by low relative humidity, whereas low flows (< 0.5 L/min) allow greater water saturation. Absorbent granules provide a significant source of heat and moisture in the circle system.

Disadvantages of the Circle System

Most of the problems of Mapleson circuits are solved by the circle system. However, the improvements have led to other disadvantages: (1) greater size and less portability; (2) increased complexity, resulting in a higher risk of disconnection or malfunction; (3) increased resistance, dissuading some pediatric anesthesiologists from using the system; and (4) the difficulty of predicting inspired gas concentrations during low fresh gas flows.

RESUSCITATION BREATHING SYSTEMS

Resuscitation bags (Ambu bags or bag-mask units) are commonly used for emergency ventilation because of their simplicity, portability, and ability to deliver almost 100% oxygen (Figure 3–10). These resuscitators are unlike a Mapleson circuit or a circle system because they contain nonrebreathing valves. (Remember that a Mapleson system is considered valveless despite containing a nonrebreathing valve, while a circle system contains unidirectional valves that direct flow through an absorber but allow rebreathing of exhaled gases.)

High concentrations of oxygen can be delivered to a mask or endotracheal tube during spontaneous or controlled ventilation if a source of high fresh gas flow is connected to the inlet nipple. The **patient valve** opens during controlled or spontaneous inspiration to allow gas flow from the ventilation bag to the patient. Rebreathing is prevented by venting exhaled gas to the atmosphere through exhalation ports in this valve. The compressible, self-refilling ventilation bag also contains an **intake valve.** This valve closes during bag compression, permitting positive-pressure ventilation. The bag is refilled by flow through the fresh gas inlet and across the intake valve. Connecting a reservoir to the intake valve helps prevent the entrainment of room air. The **reservoir valve assembly** is really two unidirectional valves. The **inlet valve** allows ambient air to enter the ventilation bag if fresh gas flow is inadequate to maintain reservoir filling. Positive pressure in the reservoir bag opens the **outlet valve,** which vents oxygen if fresh gas flow is excessive.

There are several disadvantages to resuscitator breathing systems. First, they require fairly high fresh gas flows to achieve a high inspired oxygen concentration. FiO_2 is directly proportionate to the oxygen concentration and flow rate of the gas mixture supplied to the resuscitator (usually 100% oxygen) and inversely proportionate to the minute ventilation delivered to the patient. For example, a Laerdal resuscitator equipped with a reservoir requires a flow of 10 L/min to achieve an inspired oxygen concentration approaching 100% if a patient with a tidal volume of 750 mL is ventilated at a respiratory rate of 12 breaths/min. The maximum achievable tidal volumes are less than with a system that uses a 3-L breathing bag. In fact, most adult resuscitators have a maximum tidal volume of 1000 mL.

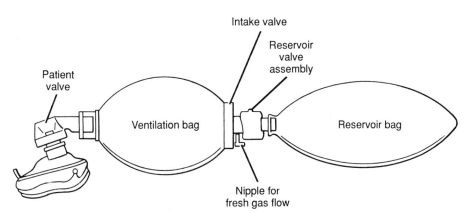

Figure 3–10 The Laerdal resuscitator. (Courtesy of Laerdal Medical Corp.)

Finally, although a normally functioning patient valve has low resistance to inspiration and expiration, exhaled moisture can cause valve sticking.

CASE DISCUSSION: UNEXPLAINED "LIGHT ANESTHESIA"

A massively obese but otherwise healthy 5-year-old girl presents for inguinal hernia repair. After uneventful induction of general anesthesia and endotracheal intubation, the patient is placed on a ventilator set to deliver a tidal volume of 7 mL/kg at a rate of 16 breaths/min. Despite delivery of 2% halothane in 50% nitrous oxide, tachycardia (145 beats/min) and mild hypertension (140/90 mm Hg) are noted. In order to increase anesthetic depth, fentanyl (3 µg/kg) is administered. Heart rate and blood pressure continue to rise and are accompanied by frequent premature ventricular contractions.

What should be considered in the differential diagnosis of this patient's cardiovascular changes?

The combination of tachycardia and hypertension during general anesthesia should always alert the anesthesiologist to the possibility of hypercapnia or hypoxia, which produce signs of increased sympathetic activity. These life-threatening conditions should be quickly and immediately ruled out by end-tidal CO_2 monitoring, pulse oximetry, or arterial blood gas analysis.

A common cause of intraoperative tachycardia and hypertension is an inadequate level of anesthesia. Normally, this is confirmed by movement. However, if the patient is paralyzed, there are few reliable indicators of light anesthesia. The lack of a response to a dose of narcotic should alert the anesthesiologist to the possibility of other, perhaps more serious causes.

Malignant hyperthermia is rare but must be considered in cases of unexplained tachycardia, especially if accompanied by premature contractions (see Case Discussion in Chapter 42). Certain **drugs** used in anesthesia (eg, pancuronium, ketamine, ephedrine) stimulate the sympathetic nervous system and can produce or exacerbate tachycardia and hypertension. Diabetic

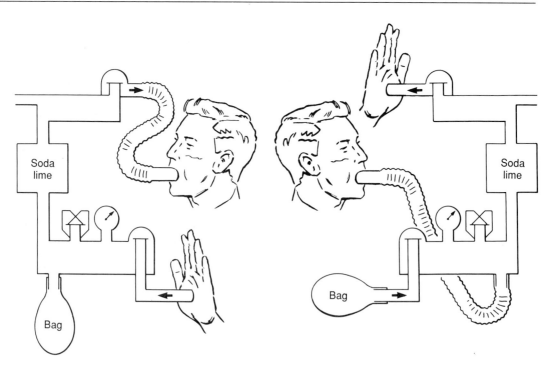

A. TEST FOR INHALATION VALVE   **B.** TEST FOR EXHALATION VALVE

Figure 3–11 How to connect the reservoir bag and corrugated tube for the competency test of inhalation **(A)** and exhalation **(B)** unidirectional dome valves. Heavy arrows indicate direction of flow through valves. (From Kim J, Kovac AL, Mathewson HS: A method for detection of incompetent unidirectional dome valves: A prevalent malfunction. Anesth Analg 1985;64:745. Reprinted with permission of the International Anesthesia Research Society.)

patients who become **hypoglycemic** from administration of insulin or long-acting oral hypoglycemic agents can have similar cardiovascular changes. Other **endocrine abnormalities** could also be considered: pheochromocytoma, toxic goiter, and carcinoid.

Could any of these problems be related to an equipment malfunction?

On some older models of anesthesia machines, it is necessary to turn on a master control switch in addition to the vaporizer control knob to activate the vaporizers. This is often true of copper kettle vaporizers. Briefly sniffing the anesthetic gas being delivered to the patient is an easy if not aesthetic method of confirming the presence of volatile agent. Nitrous oxide is more difficult to detect without sophisticated equipment, but an oxygen analyzer should provide a clue.

A misconnection of the ventilator could result in hypoxia or hypercapnia. Additionally, a malfunctioning unidirectional valve will increase circuit dead space and allow rebreathing of expired CO_2. Soda lime exhaustion or activation of an absorber bypass valve could also lead to rebreathing in the presence of a low fresh gas flow. Rebreathing of CO_2 can be detected during the inspiratory phase on a capnograph or mass spectrometer (see Chapter 6). If rebreathing appears to be due to an equipment malfunction, the patient should be disconnected from the anesthesia machine and ventilated with a resuscitation bag until repairs are possible.

How are unidirectional valves checked before the anesthesia machine is used?

The incidence of incompetent unidirectional valves has been found to approach 15%. There is a quick procedure for testing the function of these valves:

(1) First, disconnect the breathing tubes from the anesthesia machine, close the pressure release valve, and turn off all gas flow.
(2) To check inspiratory valve function, connect one end of a section of breathing tube to the inhalation outlet and occlude the exhalation outlet. If a breathing bag that is connected to its usual site fills when air is blown into the breathing tube, the inspiratory valve is incompetent (Figure 3–11A).
(3) To check expiratory valve function, connect one end of a section of breathing tube to the usual breathing bag site and cover the inhalation outlet. If a breathing bag connected to the exhalation outlet fills when air is blown into the breathing tube, the expiratory valve is incompetent (Figure 3–11B).

What are some other consequences of hypercapnia?

Hypercapnia has a multitude of effects, most of them masked by general anesthesia. Cerebral blood flow increases proportionately with arterial CO_2. This effect is dangerous in patients with increased intracranial pressure (eg, due to brain tumor). Extremely high levels of CO_2 (> 80 mm Hg) can produce unconsciousness.

Elevated serum CO_2 concentrations can overwhelm the blood's buffering capacity, leading to respiratory acidosis. This causes other anions such as Ca^{2+} and K^+ to shift extracellularly. Acidosis also shifts the oxyhemoglobin dissociation curve to the right.

Carbon dioxide is a powerful respiratory stimulant. In fact, for each mm Hg rise of $PaCO_2$ above baseline, normal subjects increase their minute ventilation by about 2–3 L/min. General anesthesia markedly decreases this response. Finally, severe hypercapnia can produce hypoxia by displacement of oxygen from alveoli as the body attempts to rid itself of CO_2.

SUGGESTED READINGS

Conway CM: Anaesthetic breathing systems. In: *Scientific Foundations of Anaesthesia*, 4th ed. Scurr C, Feldman S (editors). Heinemann, 1990. The British breathing system classification scheme.

Dorsch JA, Dorsch SE: *Understanding Anesthesia Equipment*. Williams & Wilkins, 1984. Detailed discussion of breathing systems in Chapters 5–8.

Petty C: *The Anesthesia Machine*. Churchill Livingstone, 1987. Contains a brief description of anesthesia circuits.

The Anesthesia Machine

No piece of equipment is more intimately associated with the practice of anesthesiology than the anesthesia machine. In essence, the anesthesiologist uses the anesthesia machine to control the patient's inspired gas mixture and gas exchange. Proper functioning of the machine is crucial for patient safety. In fact, the misuse and malfunction of anesthesia machines is a prominent cause of operative morbidity and death. In an attempt to increase the safety of anesthesia, a set of anesthesia machine requirements has been published by the American National Standards Institute. Nonetheless, preventable anesthetic mishaps are frequently traced to lack of familiarity with anesthetic equipment and failure to check machine function. This chapter is intended as an introduction to anesthesia machine design, function, and inspection.

OVERVIEW

Anesthesia machines have multiple functions that are performed by specific components (Figures 4–1 and 4–2), including the following:

(1) Receiving medical gases from attached cylinders or the hospital's gas delivery system (**gas inlets**)
(2) Reducing gas pressure (**pressure regulators**)
(3) Signaling low oxygen pressure (**oxygen pressure failure devices**)
(4) Controlling flow rate (**flow control valves and flowmeters**)
(5) Blending gases with volatile anesthetic agents (**vaporizers**)
(6) Delivering the final gas composition to the breathing circuit (**fresh gas outlet**)

Modern machines are equipped with **spirometers** that measure respiratory volumes within the breathing circuit, **ventilators with disconnect alarms, waste gas scavengers,** and **oxygen analyzers. Humidifiers** and **nebulizers** are available that connect between the anesthesia machine and the breathing circuit. Some newer models integrate a multitude of other monitors (eg, electrocardiographs, pulse oximeters, capnographs) that are traditionally considered separately (Chapter 5).

GAS INLETS & PRESSURE REGULATORS

Cylinders attached to the anesthesia machine's **hanger yolk assembly** are a high-pressure source of medical gases (Figure 4–1). The yolk assembly includes index pins (see the discussion of the pin index safety system in Chapter 2), a washer, a gas filter, and a check valve that prevents retrograde gas flow. Cylinder pressure is measured by a **Bourdon pressure gauge** (Figure 4–2). A flexible tube within this gauge straightens when exposed to gas pressure, causing a gear mechanism to move a needle pointer.

The high and variable gas pressure in a cylinder makes flow control difficult and potentially dangerous. To enhance safety and ensure preferential usage of pipeline gases, a **pressure regulator** reduces the cylinder gas pressure to below 50 psi. Two-stage pressure regulators (two one-stage regulators in series) further reduce any outlet pressure variations due to fluctuations in cylinder pressure.

The hospital's medical gas delivery system connects to the anesthesia machine through the diameter index safety system (see Chapter 2). Because the pipeline gases are supplied at pressures between 45 psi and 55 psi, they do not need to be further reduced. After passing through Bourdon pressure gauges and check valves, the pipeline gases share a common pathway with the cylinder gases.

OXYGEN PRESSURE FAILURE DEVICES & OXYGEN FLUSH VALVES

While the nitrous oxide and air lines directly connect with the flowmeters, the oxygen line passes by pressure failure devices, the oxygen flush valve, and the ventilator power outlet. If oxygen pressure falls below 25 psi (roughly 50% of normal), a **fail-safe valve** automatically closes the nitrous oxide and other gas lines to prevent accidental delivery of a hypoxic mixture to the patient (Figure 4–3). Additionally, a gas whistle or electric alarm sounds. It must be stressed that *only an oxygen pressure failure triggers these safety devices,* ie, they do not protect against other possible causes of hypoxic accidents.

The **oxygen flush valve** provides a high flow (35–75 L/min) of oxygen directly to the common gas out-

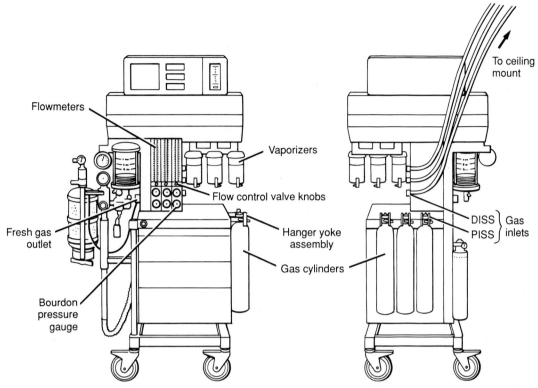

Figure 4–1. The anesthesia machine.

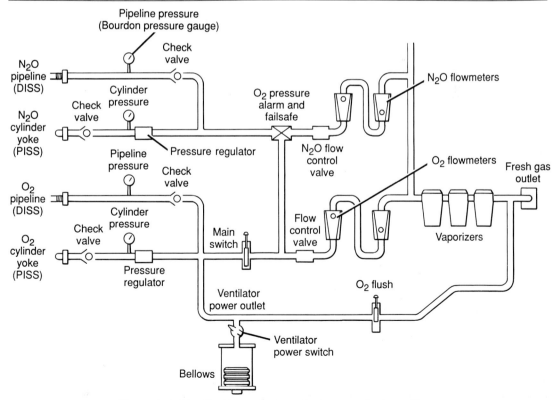

Figure 4–2. Simplified internal schematic of an anesthesia machine.

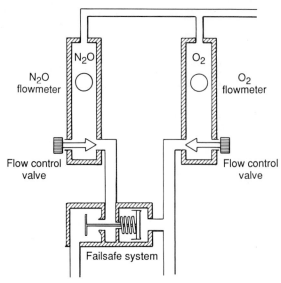

Figure 4–3. The "fail-safe system" controls the gas in its associated gas line in response to the pressure in the oxygen line. Its safety potential is limited. For example, it will permit the administration of hypoxic gas mixtures when the gas flow is erroneously composed so as not to contain a sufficient oxygen concentration, the oxygen flow control valve is accidentally adjusted downward, or the oxygen piping system contains a gas other than oxygen.

let, bypassing the flowmeters and vaporizers. Because oxygen is supplied at a line pressure of 45–55 psi, there is a real potential of lung barotrauma. For this reason, the flush valve must be used cautiously whenever a patient is connected to the breathing circuit. A protective rim limits the possibility of unintentional activation.

FLOW CONTROL VALVES, FLOWMETERS, & SPIROMETERS

Gas flows continuously from the anesthesia machine to the breathing circuit. The gas flow rate is determined by **flow control valves** and is measured by **flowmeters.** The tidal volume intermittently delivered to the patient from the breathing circuit is measured by a **spirometer** (respirometer).

When the knob of the flow control valve is turned counterclockwise, a pin is disengaged from its seat, allowing gas to flow through the valve (Figure 4–4). Stops in the full off and full on positions prevent valve damage. Touch- and color-coded control knobs make it harder to turn off or on the wrong gas (Figure 4–5).

The flowmeters on anesthesia machines are classified as **constant-pressure, variable orifice flowmeters.** An indicator ball, bobbin, or float is supported by the flow of gas through a tube (Thorpe tube) whose bore (orifice) is tapered. Near the bottom of the tube, where the diameter is small, a low flow of gas will result in sufficient pressure under the bobbin to raise it in the tube. As the bobbin rises, the orifice of the tube widens, allowing more gas to pass around the

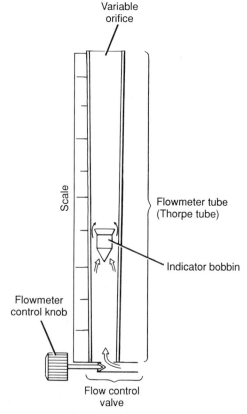

Figure 4–4. A constant-pressure variable orifice flowmeter (Thorpe type).

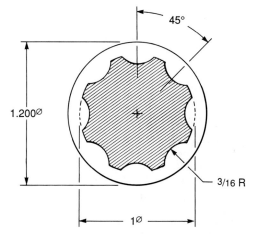

Figure 4–5. The touch-coded knob for the oxygen flow control valve reduces the possibility of operator error.

bobbin. The bobbin will quit rising when its weight is just supported by the difference in pressure between the top and the bottom of the bobbin. If flow is increased, the pressure under the bobbin increases, raising the bobbin higher in the tube until the pressure drop again just supports the bobbin's weight. This pressure drop is constant regardless of the flow rate or the position in the tube and depends upon the weight of the bobbin and its cross-sectional area. Stated another way, the higher the bobbin rises in the tube, the larger the tube's orifice and the greater the gas flow required to maintain a constant pressure drop.

Flowmeters are calibrated for specific gases, since the flow rate across a constriction depends upon the gas's viscosity at low laminar flows and its density at high turbulent flows. To minimize the effect of friction between the tube's wall and the bobbin, floats are designed to rotate constantly, which keeps them centered

in the tube. The effect of static electricity is reduced by coating the tube's interior with a conductive substance that grounds the system. Causes of flowmeter malfunction include dirt in the flow tube, less than perfectly vertical tube alignment, and sticking or concealment of a float at the top of a tube. Should a leak develop within or downstream from an oxygen flowmeter, a hypoxic gas mixture may be delivered to the patient. To lessen this risk, oxygen flowmeters should be positioned downstream (nearest the outlet) from the other medical gas flowmeters.

Not all flowmeters are constant-pressure ones. An adaptation of the Bourdon pressure gauge is commonly used to measure flow rates from free-standing gas cylinders. This device measures the pressure drop across a fixed orifice, which is proportionate to the square of the flow rate. This **fixed-orifice flowmeter** is inaccurate at low flow rates at low fixed rates or if flow is occluded.

The **pneumotachygraph** is another type of fixed orifice flowmeter. However, it measures varying or intermittent flows such as occur within a patient's breathing circuit instead of the constant flows within an anesthesia machine. A baffle chamber provides a slight resistance to air flow. The pressure drop across this resistance is sensed by a differential pressure transducer and is proportionate to the flow rate. Tidal volumes are derived by integrating the flow rates. Inaccuracies due to water condensation and temperature changes limit the clinical usefulness of this device.

The **Wright respirometer** also measures gas volumes within the breathing circuit (Figure 4–6). The flow of gas across vanes or rotators contained within the respirometer causes their rotation, which is measured electronically, photoelectrically, or mechanically. Most spirometers on modern anesthesia machines use this principle to measure minute ventilation and tidal volume. The Wright respirometer is prone to errors due to inertia, friction, and water condensation.

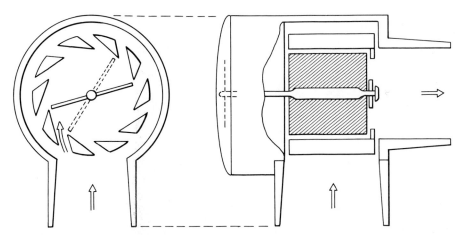

Figure 4–6. The Wright respirometer. (Reproduced, with permission, from Moshin WW et al: *Automatic Ventilation of the Lungs,* 2nd ed. Blackwell, 1969.)

VAPORIZERS

Volatile anesthetics (eg, halothane, isoflurane, and enflurane) are vaporized before being delivered to the patient. At a given temperature, the molecules of a volatile agent in a closed container are distributed between the liquid and gas phases. The gas molecules bombard the walls of the container, creating the vapor pressure of that agent. The higher the temperature, the greater the tendency for the liquid molecules to escape into the gaseous phase and the higher the vapor pressure. Vaporization requires energy (the heat of vaporization), which is supplied as a loss of heat from the liquid. As vaporization proceeds, liquid temperature drops and vapor pressure decreases unless heat is readily available to enter the system.

Vaporizers contain a chamber in which a carrier gas becomes saturated with volatile agent. Although many vaporizer models are available, only two representative models are examined in this chapter. In **copper kettle vaporizers,** the amount of carrier gas (oxygen) bubbled through the anesthetic is determined by a dedicated Thorpe tube flowmeter (Figure 4–7). A vapor-

izer circuit flow control valve separates the vaporizer circuit from the standard oxygen and nitrous oxide flowmeters. This valve should be off when the vaporizer circuit is not in use to prevent leakage and back-flushing of gas.

Copper is used as the construction metal because its relatively high specific heat (the quantity of heat required to raise the temperature of 1 g of substance by 1 °C) and thermal conductivity (the speed of heat conductance through a substance) enhance the vaporizer's ability to maintain a constant temperature.

All of the gas entering the vaporizer passes through anesthetic liquid and becomes saturated with vapor. One milliliter of liquid anesthetic is the equivalent of approximately 200 mL of anesthetic vapor. Because the vapor pressure of volatile anesthetics is greater than the partial pressure required for anesthesia, the saturated gas leaving a copper kettle must be diluted before it reaches the patient.

For example, the vapor pressure of halothane is 243 mm Hg at 20 °C, so the concentration of halothane exiting a copper kettle at 1 atm is 243/760, or 32%. If 100 mL of oxygen enters the kettle, roughly 150 mL of

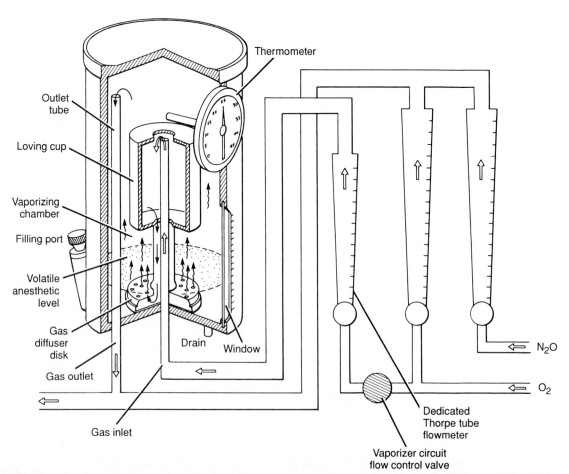

Figure 4–7. The copper kettle vaporizer. (Redrawn and reproduced, with permission, from Hill DW: *Physics Applied to Anaesthesia,* 4th ed. Butterworths, 1980.)

gas will exit, one-third of which is halothane vapor. In contrast, a partial pressure of only 7 mm Hg—or less than 1% concentration (7/760) at 1 atm—may be required for anesthesia. To deliver a 1% concentration of halothane, the 50 mL of halothane vapor and 100 mL of carrier gas that are leaving the copper kettle would have to be diluted with another 4850 mL of gas (5000 − 150 = 4850). As can be seen from this example, every 100 mL of oxygen passing through a halothane vaporizer translates into a 1% increase in concentration if total gas flow into the breathing circuit is 5 L/min. Since flow through this vaporizer determines the ultimate concentration of anesthetic, the copper kettle is classified as a **measured-flow vaporizer.** Isoflurane has an almost identical vapor pressure, so the same relationship between copper kettle flow, total gas flow, and anesthetic concentration exists.

On the other hand, enflurane has a vapor pressure of 175 mm Hg at 20 °C. Saturated gas leaving a copper kettle filled with enflurane at sea level has a concentration of 175/760, or 23%. Stated another way, 100 mL of oxygen will pick up 30 mL of enflurane vapor (30/130 = 23%). Thus, every 100 mL of oxygen passing through a copper kettle vaporizer filled with enflurane translates into a 1% increase in concentration if total gas flow into the breathing circuit is 3 L/min (30/3000 = 1%).

In general, the amount of vapor leaving a copper kettle depends on the vapor pressure of the anesthetic agent (VP), the flow rate of the carrier gas to the vaporizer (CG), and the barometric pressure (BP):

$$\text{Vapor output} = \frac{CG \times VP}{BP - VP}$$

For the enflurane example:

$$\frac{\text{Vapor}}{\text{output}} = \frac{(100 \text{ mL/min}) (175 \text{ mm Hg})}{(760 \text{ MM HG} - 175 \text{ mm Hg})} = 30 \text{ mL/min}$$

Percentage anesthetic concentration is found by dividing vapor output by total gas flow into the circuit:

$$\frac{\text{Anesthetic}}{\text{concentration}} = \frac{30 \text{ mL/vapor output}}{3000 \text{ mL/min total gas flow}} = 1\%$$

If total gas flow falls unexpectedly (eg, exhaustion of a nitrous oxide cylinder), volatile anesthetic concentration will rise to potentially dangerous levels.

The ability to accurately titrate the delivered concentration of anesthetic is crucial because of the severe consequences of overdosage. Modern **agent-specific vaporizers** are capable of delivering a constant concentration of agent regardless of temperature changes or flow through the vaporizer. Merely turning a single calibrated control knob counterclockwise (clockwise

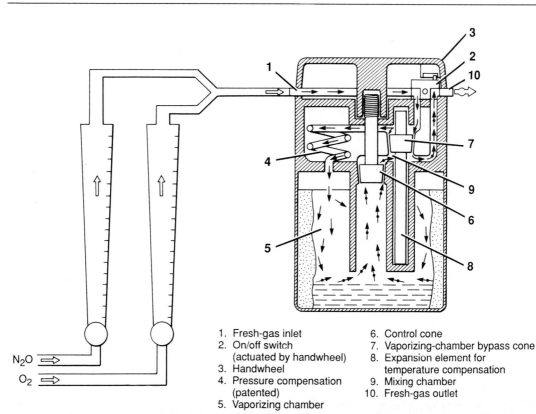

1. Fresh-gas inlet
2. On/off switch (actuated by handwheel)
3. Handwheel
4. Pressure compensation (patented)
5. Vaporizing chamber
6. Control cone
7. Vaporizing-chamber bypass cone
8. Expansion element for temperature compensation
9. Mixing chamber
10. Fresh-gas outlet

Figure 4–8. Agent-specific, variable bypass vaporizer.

in some older units) to the desired percentage divides the total gas flow into carrier gas, which flows over liquid anesthetic in a vaporizing chamber, and the balance, which exits the vaporizer unchanged (Figure 4–8). Because some of the entering gas is never exposed to anesthetic liquid, the agent-specific vaporizer is also known as a **variable bypass vaporizer.**

Temperature compensation is achieved by a strip composed of two different metals welded together. As the temperature increases, the strip bends as a result of unequal expansion (the metals have different coefficients of linear expansion), and less gas is shunted through the vaporizing chamber. Altering flow rates within a wide range does not affect anesthetic concentration because the same proportion of gas is exposed to the liquid. However, changing the gas composition from 100% oxygen to 70% nitrous oxide may result in a transient decrease in volatile anesthetic concentration owing to the greater solubility of nitrous oxide in volatile agents.

Because these vaporizers are agent-specific, filling with the wrong anesthetic must be avoided. For example, unintentionally filling a vaporizer with an anesthetic that has a higher vapor pressure or greater potency than the agent for which the vaporizer was designed could lead to anesthetic overdose. Excessive tilting of the vaporizer may flood the bypass area and lead to dangerously high anesthetic concentrations. Fluctuations in pressure due to positive-pressure ventilation may cause a reversed flow through the vaporizer, unpredictably changing agent delivery. This "pumping effect" is more pronounced with low gas flows. Design modifications in newer units limit the possibility of some of these problems.

Variable bypass vaporizers should be located outside of the circle system, between the flowmeters and the common gas outlet, to lessen the likelihood of concentration surges during use of the oxygen flush valve. An interlock or exclusion device prevents the concurrent use of more than one vaporizer. Older machines without this safety feature should have the vaporizers arranged in a specific order to lessen the risk of cross-contamination of agent if two vaporizers are on simultaneously. Based upon vapor pressures and potency, the following order from upstream to downstream is recommended: methoxyflurane-enflurane-isoflurane-halothane.

VENTILATORS & DISCONNECT ALARMS

Ventilators function by creating a pressure gradient between the proximal airway and the alveoli. Older units relied on the generation of negative pressure in the thorax (eg, iron lungs), while modern ventilators develop positive pressure in the upper airway. The ventilatory cycle is divided into four phases: inspiration, the transition from inspiration to expiration, expiration, and the transition from expiration to inspiration. Ventilators are classified on the basis of their functioning during these phases.

During inspiration, mechanical ventilators generate tidal volumes by producing gas flow along a pressure gradient. Either pressure (**constant pressure generators**) or flow rate (**constant flow generators**) may remain constant throughout the cycle regardless of changes in lung mechanics (Figures 4–9A and 4–9B). **Nonconstant generators** produce pressures or flow rates that vary during the cycle but remain consistent from breath to breath. For instance, a ventilator that generates a flow pattern resembling a half cycle of a sine wave would be classified as a nonconstant flow generator (Figure 4–9C). An increase in airway resistance or a decrease in lung compliance would increase peak inspiratory pressure but would not alter the flow rate generated by this type of ventilator.

Termination of the inspiratory phase can be triggered by the attainment of a preset limit of time duration, inspiratory pressure, or tidal volume. **Time-cycled ventilators** allow tidal volume and peak inspiratory pressure to vary depending on lung compliance. Tidal volume is adjusted by setting inspiratory duration and inspiratory flow rate (eg, the Airshields ventilator). **Pressure-cycled ventilators** will not cycle from the inspiratory phase to the expiratory phase until a preset pressure is reached. If a large circuit leak decreases peak pressures significantly, a pressure-cycled ventilator may remain in the inspiratory phase indefinitely. On the other hand, a small leak may not result in a markedly decreased tidal volume because cycling will be delayed until the pressure limit is met. Because of their use of a Venturi jet, pressure-cycled ventilators increase flow at the expense of decreasing inspired oxygen content (eg, the small Bird ventilator models used to deliver IPPB therapy). **Volume-cycled ventilators** vary inspiratory duration and pressure in order to deliver a preset volume (usually there is a safety pressure limit). Many anesthesia ventilators are volume-limited but time cycled (eg, Drager AV-E ventilator).

The expiratory phase of most ventilators reduces airway pressure to atmospheric. Therefore, flow out of the lungs is passive and determined chiefly by airway resistance and lung compliance. Positive end-expired pressure can be created by retarding expiratory gas flow. A few older ventilator models were able to generate negative expiratory pressures. This feature is rarely used today because of the potential for premature airway closure.

The next inspiratory phase usually begins after a preset time interval (**controlled ventilation**), but in some machines it can be triggered by a negative pressure generated by the patient (**assisted ventilation**). **Intermittent mandatory ventilation (IMV)** allows patients to breath spontaneously between controlled breaths. In contrast to assisted-controlled ventilation, the patient receiving intermittent mandatory ventilation does not necessarily receive the preset tidal volume during the spontaneous breaths. **Synchronized**

A. CONSTANT PRESSURE   **B**. CONSTANT FLOW   **C**. NONCONSTANT FLOW

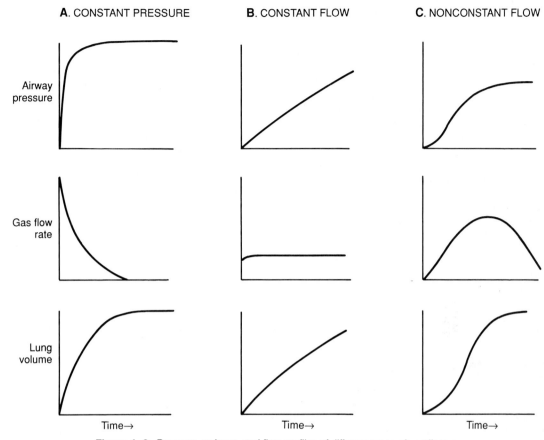

Figure 4–9. Pressure, volume, and flow profiles of different types of ventilators.

intermittent mandatory ventilation (SIMV) helps prevent "fighting the ventilator" by providing mandatory breaths when the patient initiates spontaneous ventilation.

There are structural similarities between many different types of ventilators used in anesthesiology. Tidal volume is delivered from a bellows assembly that consists of a rubber bellows and its clear plastic enclosure. A **standing (ascending) bellows** is preferred since it draws attention to a circuit disconnection by collapsing (Figure 4–10A). In contrast, a **hanging (descending) bellows** continues to fill by gravity even though it is no longer connected to the breathing circuit (Figure 4–10B).

The bellows takes the place of the breathing bag in the anesthesia circuit. Pressurized oxygen from the ventilator power outlet (Figure 4–2) is routed to the space between the inside wall of the enclosure and the outside wall of the bellows. The increased pressure causes the pleated bellows to compress, forcing the anesthetic gas it contains into the breathing circuit. Therefore, there are two distinct circuits within the ventilator that are separated by the bellows wall: the external high-pressure oxygen circuit that powers the ventilator and an internal extension of the anesthesia breathing circuit.

Oxygen is consumed to power the ventilator at a rate at least equal to minute ventilation. Thus, if oxygen fresh gas flow is 2 L/min and a ventilator is delivering 6 L/min to the circuit, a total of at least 8 L/min of oxygen is being consumed. This should be kept in mind if the hospital's medical gas system fails and cylinder oxygen is required.

By using an electronic control box, modern anesthesia ventilators are capable of delivering a wide range of tidal volumes, peak inspiratory pressures, respiratory rates, inspiratory plateaus, inspiratory-to-expiratory ratios, intermittent sighs, and positive end-expiratory pressures. These ventilators require compressed oxygen to power the bellows and electricity (often with battery backup) to power the control box.

Alarms should be an integral part of all anesthesia ventilators. *Whenever a ventilator is used, a disconnect alarm must be activated.* Breathing circuit disconnection, a leading cause of anesthetic accidents, is detected by a drop in peak circuit pressure. Other useful ventilator alarms signal excessive airway pressure, low oxygen supply pressure, and inability of the ventilator to deliver the desired minute ventilation.

Whenever a ventilator is used, the circle system's pressure relief valve should be closed or functionally removed from the circuit. Ventilators commonly used

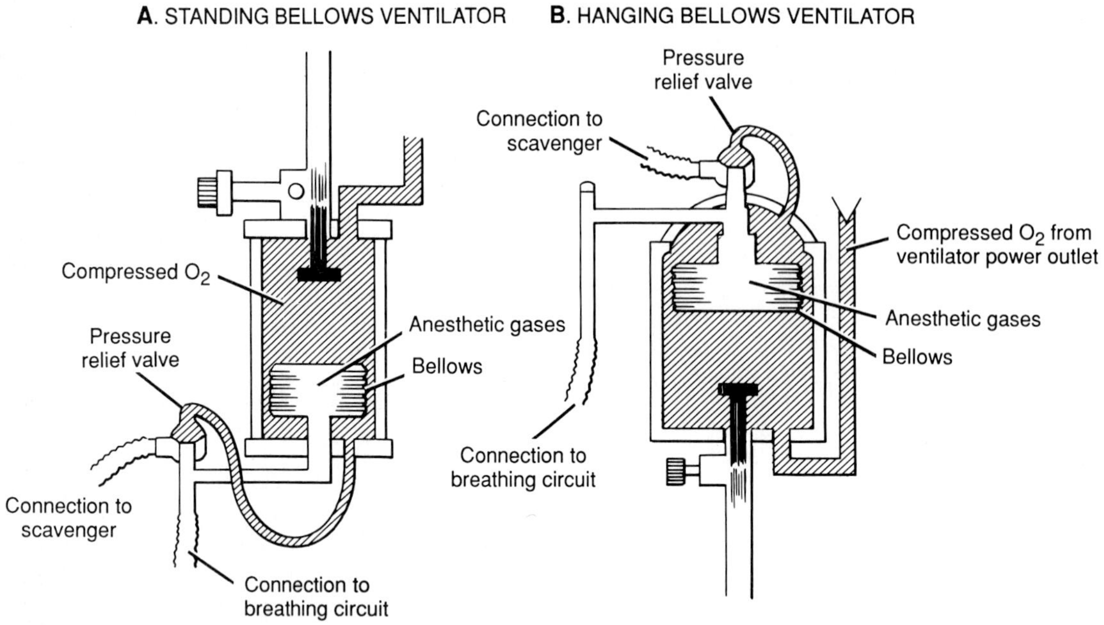

A. STANDING BELLOWS VENTILATOR   **B**. HANGING BELLOWS VENTILATOR

Figure 4–10. Two types of bellows are available on anesthesia ventilators. Standing bellows **(A)** collapse if there is a leak greater than the fresh gas flow, while hanging bellows **(B)** refill and continue to cycle. Shading indicates the external high-pressure oxygen circuit that powers the ventilator and closes the pressure relief valve during inspiration. The unshaded gases in the bellows are part of the anesthetic breathing circuit.

in anesthesia contain their own pressure relief valve that remains closed during inspiration so that positive pressure can be generated. When the ventilator bellows are refilled during expiration, circuit pressure rises and the ventilator's pressure relief valve opens. Sticking of this valve results in abnormally elevated airway pressure. In contrast, if the breathing circuit's pressure relief valve is not fully closed or is not functionally removed from the system, airway pressures may be inadequate to ventilate the patient.

Because the ventilator's pressure relief valve is closed during inspiration, the circuit's fresh gas flows contribute to the tidal volume delivered to the patient. For example, if the fresh gas flow is 6 L/min, the inspiratory-to-expiratory ratio is 1:2, and the respiratory rate is 10 breaths/min, each tidal volume will include 200 mL in addition to the ventilator's output:

$$\frac{(6000 \text{ mL/min}) (33\%)}{10 \text{ breaths/min}} = 200 \text{ mL/breath}$$

Therefore, increasing fresh gas flow increases minute ventilation. Likewise, the use of the oxygen flush valve during the inspiratory cycle of a ventilator must be avoided because the pressure relief valve is closed and the surge of circuit pressure will be transferred to the patient's lungs.

A leak in the bellows can transmit high oxygen pressure to the patient's airway, perhaps resulting in barotrauma. This may be detected by noticing a higher than expected inspired oxygen concentration. Miscon-

necting ventilator hoses on the anesthesia machine and the breathing circuit has resulted in hypoxic brain injury. Other potential problems include electrical failure, flow obstruction, electromagnetic interference, and valve malfunction.

WASTE GAS SCAVENGERS

Waste gas scavengers dispose of gases that have been vented from the breathing circuit by a pressure release valve. Pollution of the operating room environment with anesthetic gases may pose a health hazard to surgical personnel (Chapter 45). Although it is difficult to define "safe" levels of exposure, the National Institute for Occupational Safety and Health (NIOSH) recommends limiting the room concentration of nitrous oxide to 25 ppm and halogenated agents to 2 ppm (0.5 ppm if nitrous oxide is also being used). Reduction to these trace levels is only possible with properly functioning waste gas scavenging systems.

To avoid the buildup of pressure, excess gas volume is vented through the pressure relief valve in the breathing circuit or the ventilator. Both of these valves should be connected to hoses (transfer tubing) leading to the scavenging interface (Figure 4–11). The outlet of the scavenging system can be a direct line to the outside (passive scavenging), a line to the air conditioning system beyond any point of recirculation, or a connection to the hospital's vacuum system (active scavenging). The latter method is the most reliable

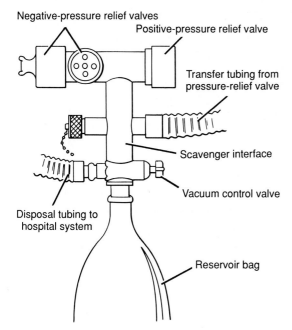

Negative-pressure relief valves

Positive-pressure relief valve

Transfer tubing from pressure-relief valve

Scavenger interface

Vacuum control valve

Disposal tubing to hospital system

Reservoir bag

Figure 4–11. Waste gas scavenging system.

but also the most complex. Negative- and positive-pressure relief valves protect the patient from the negative pressure of the vacuum system or positive pressure from an obstruction in the disposal tubing. A reservoir bag accepts waste gas overflow when the vacuum's capacity is exceeded.

The vacuum control valve should be adjusted to allow the evacuation of 10–15 L of waste gas per minute. This rate is adequate for periods of high fresh gas flow (ie, induction and emergence) yet minimizes the risk of transmitting negative pressure to the breathing circuit during lower flow conditions (maintenance).

HUMIDIFIERS & NEBULIZERS

Relative humidity is the ratio of the mass of water present in a volume of gas (**absolute humidity**) to the maximum amount of water possible at a particular temperature. Inhaled gases are normally warmed to body temperature and saturated with water by the upper respiratory tract (100% relative humidity = 44 mg H_2O/L at 37 °C). Endotracheal intubation and high fresh gas flows bypass this normal humidification system and expose the lower airways to dry (< 10 mg H_2O/L), room temperature gases. Humidification of gases by the lower respiratory tract leads to dehydration of mucosa, altered ciliary function, inspissation of secretions, and even ventilation/perfusion mismatching due to atelectasis. Body heat is lost during ventilation in order to warm and, more importantly, to humid-

ify dry gases. (The heat of vaporization of water = 560 kcal/g of water vaporized.)

Humidifiers added to the breathing circuit minimize water and heat loss. The simplest designs are the **condenser humidifier** and the **heat and moisture exchanger** (Figure 4–12). These devices do not add heat and vapor but rather conserve some of the heat and water vapor that is exhaled. Depending on design, they may increase apparatus dead space and breathing circuit resistance, which could be significant in pediatric patients.

Pass-over or **bubble-through humidifiers** expose gas to a cold or hot water bath. Because increasing temperature increases the capacity of a gas to hold water vapor, water baths heated by a thermostatically controlled element are more effective humidifiers. The hazards of these units include thermal lung injury (inhaled gas temperature should be monitored), nosocomial infection, increased airway resistance, and an increased likelihood of circuit disconnection. Nonetheless, in cases where the risk of intraoperative hypothermia is unacceptable, these humidifiers effectively provide heat and moisture. These humidifiers are particularly valuable in children since they help prevent hypothermia and plugging of small endotracheal tubes by dried secretions. Of course, any design that increases airway dead space should be avoided in pediatric patients.

Nebulizers suspend (aerosolize) water particles into a spray. The size of the droplets depends on the method of nebulization: **high-pressure jet nebulizers** produce droplets 5–30 μm in diameter, while **ultrasonic nebulizers** create droplets of 1–10 μm. The former entrains a water stream by the Bernoulli effect (similar to the Venturi effect) and breaks it up with a high-velocity gas jet. Jet nebulizers are often used in recovery rooms to provide an aerosol at room temperature with high water content. Ultrasonic nebulizers are so efficient that they possess the potential for overhydration. Their primary usefulness is for the delivery of bronchodilator drugs to peripheral airways and the mobilization of secretions during respiratory therapy.

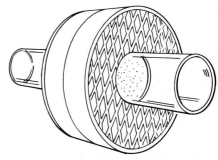

Figure 4–12. The condenser humidifier is an "artificial nose" that attaches between the endotracheal tube and the right-angle connector of the breathing circuit. (Courtesy of Terumo Corp.)

OXYGEN ANALYZERS

General anesthesia should never be performed without an oxygen analyzer in the breathing circuit. Oxygen concentration can be measured electrochemically, by paramagnetic analysis, or by mass spectrometry (Chapter 6). Two electrochemical sensors are available: the **galvanic cell** (a fuel cell) and the **polarographic cell** (a Clark electrode). Both contain cathode and anode electrodes embedded in an electrolyte gel separated from the sample gas by an oxygen-permeable membrane. As oxygen reacts with the electrodes, a current is generated that is proportionate to the oxygen partial pressure in the sample gas. The galvanic and polarographic sensors differ in the composition of their electrodes and electrolyte gel. The components of the galvanic cell are capable of providing enough chemical energy so that the reaction does not require an external power source. The differences between galvanic and polarographic sensors are summarized in Table 4–1.

A third type of oxygen sensor, the **paramagnetic sensor,** has a higher initial cost than the electrochemical sensors. However, paramagnetic devices have no consumable parts and are able to self-calibrate. Additionally, their response time is fast enough to differentiate between inspired and expired oxygen concentrations.

All oxygen analyzers should have a low-level alarm that is automatically activated by turning on the analyzer. The sensor can be placed into the inspiratory or expiratory limb of the circle system's breathing circuit but not the fresh gas line. Owing to the patient's oxygen consumption, the expiratory limb has a slightly lower oxygen partial pressure compared with the inspiratory limb, especially at low fresh gas flows. The increased humidity of expired gas does not significantly affect most modern sensors.

ANESTHESIA MACHINE CHECKOUT LIST

Machine malfunction is a significant cause of anesthesia accidents. A routine inspection of anesthesia

equipment before each use increases operator familiarity and confirms proper functioning. The United States Food and Drug Administration has made available a generic checkout procedure for anesthesia gas machines and breathing systems (Table 4–2). This procedure should be modified as necessary depending on the specific equipment being used. Note that the entire checkout does not need to be repeated between cases on the same day. Nonetheless, the conscientious use of a checkout list is mandatory before each anesthetic procedure.

CASE DISCUSSION: DETECTION OF A LEAK

After induction of general anesthesia and intubation of a 70-kg man for elective surgery, a standing bellows ventilator is set to deliver a tidal volume of 700 mL at a rate of 10 breaths/min. Within a few minutes, the anesthesiologist notices that the bellows fails to rise to the top of its clear plastic enclosure during expiration. Shortly thereafter, the disconnect alarm is triggered.

Why has the ventilator bellows fallen and the disconnect alarm sounded?

Fresh gas flow into the breathing circuit is inadequate to maintain the circuit volume required for positive-pressure ventilation. In a situation of *no* fresh gas flow, the volume in the breathing circuit will slowly fall owing to the constant uptake of oxygen by the patient (metabolic oxygen consumption) and absorption of expired CO_2. An absence of fresh gas flow could be due to exhaustion of the hospital's oxygen supply (remember the function of the fail-safe valve) or failure to turn on the anesthesia machine's flow control valves. These possibilities can be ruled out by examining the oxygen Bourdon pressure gauge and the flowmeters. A more likely explanation is a gas leak that exceeds the rate of fresh gas flow. Leaks are particularly important in closed circuit anesthesia (Chapter 8 Case Discussion).

How can the size of the leak be estimated?

When the rate of fresh gas inflow equals the rate of gas outflow, the circuit's volume will be maintained. Therefore, the size of the leak can be estimated by increasing fresh gas flows until there is no change in the height of the bellows from one expiration to the next. If the bellows collapses despite a high rate of fresh gas inflow, a complete circuit disconnection should be considered. The site of the disconnection must be determined immediately and repaired to prevent hypoxemia and hypercapnia. A resuscitation bag can be used to ventilate the patient if there is a delay in correcting the situation.

Table 4–1. Comparison of galvanic and polarographic sensors.

Property	Galvanic	Polarographic
Anodes	Lead	Silver
Cathodes	Silver or gold	Platinum or gold
Electrolyte solution	KOH	KCl
Cost	Expensive electrodes	Expensive initial cost
Response time	Slow	Fast
Warm-up time	None	A few minutes
Servicing requirements	Sensors	Electrolyte and membranes
Power source	Chemical reaction	Batteries

Table 4-2. Anesthesia apparatus checkout recommendations.

(This checkout, or a reasonable equivalent, should be conducted before administering anesthesia. This is a guideline which users are encouraged to modify to accommodate differences in equipment design and variations in local clinical practice. Such local modifications should have appropriate peer review. Users should refer to the operator's manual for special procedures or precautions.)

*1. Inspect anesthesia machine for:
   Machine identification number
   Valid inspection sticker
   Undamaged flowmeters, vaporizers, gauges, supply hoses
   Complete, undamaged breathing system with adequate CO_2 absorbent
   Correct mounting of cylinders in yokes
   Presence of cylinder wrench

*2. Inspect and turn on:
   Electrical equipment requiring warm-up (ECG/pressure monitor, oxygen monitor, etc)

*3. Connect waste gas scavenging system:
   Adjust vacuum as required

*4. Check that:
   Flow-control valves are off
   Vaporizers are off
   Vaporizers are filled (not overfilled)
   Filler caps are sealed tightly
   CO_2 absorber bypass (if any) is off

*5. Check oxygen (O_2) cylinder supplies:
   a. Disconnect pipeline supply (if connected) and return cylinder and pipeline pressure gauges to zero with O_2 flush valve.
   b. Open O_2 cylinder; check pressure; close cylinder and observe gauge for evidence of high pressure leak.
   c. With the O_2 flush valve, flush to empty piping.
   d. Repeat as in b and c above for second O_2 cylinder, if present.
   e. Replace any cylinder less than about 600 psig. At least one should be nearly full.
   f. Open less full cylinder.

*6. Turn on master switch (if present)

*7. Check nitrous oxide (N_2O) and other gas cylinder supplies:
   Use same procedure as described in 5a and 5b above, but open and CLOSE flow-control valve to empty piping.
   Note: N_2O pressure below 745 psig indicates that the cylinder is less that one-quarter full.

*8. Test flowmeters:
   a. Check that float is at bottom of tube with flow-control valves closed (or at minimum O_2 flow if so equipped).
   b. Adjust flow of all gases through their full range and check for erratic movements of floats.

*9. Test ratio protection/warning system (if present):
   Attempt to create hypoxic O_2/N_2O mixture, and verify correct change in gas flows and/or alarm.

*10. Test O_2 pressure failure system:
   a. Set O_2 and other gas flows to mid range.
   b. Close O_2 cylinder and flush to release O_2 pressure.
   Verify that all flows fall to zero. Open O_2 cylinder.
   c. Close all other cylinders and bleed piping pressures.
   d. Close O_2 cylinder and bleed piping pressure.
   CLOSE FLOW CONTROL VALVES.

Table 4-2. (Continued)

*11. Test central pipeline gas supplies:
   a. Inspect supply hoses (should not be cracked or worn). Connect supply hoses, verifying correct color coding.
   b. Adjust all flows to at least mid range.
   Verify that supply pressures hold (45–55 psig).
   c. Shut off flow control valves.

*12. Add any accessory equipment to the breathing system:
   Add PEEP valve, humidifier, etc, if they might be used (if necessary remove after step 18 until needed).

13. Calibrate O_2 monitor:
   *a. Calibrate O_2 monitor to read 21% in room air.
   *b. Test low alarm.
   c. Occlude breathing system at patient end; fill and empty system several times with 100% O_2.
   d. Check that monitor reading is nearly 100%.

14. Sniff inspiratory gas: There should be no odor.

*15. Check unidirectional valves:
   a. Inhale and exhale through a surgical mask into the breathing system (each limb individually, if possible).
   b. Verify unidirectional flow in each limb.
   c. Reconnect tubing firmly.

**16. Test for leaks in machine and breathing system:
   a. Close APL (pop-off) valve and occlude system at patient end.
   b. Fill system via O_2 flush until bag just full, but negligible pressure in system. Set O_2 flow to 5 L/min.
   c. Slowly decrease O_2 flow until pressure *no longer rises* above about 20 cm N_2O. This approximates total leak rate, which should be no greater than a few hundred mL/min (less for closed circuit techniques).
   CAUTION: Check valves in some machines make it imperative to measure flow in step c above when pressure *just stops rising.*
   d. Squeeze bag to pressure of about 50 cm H_2O and verify that system is tight.

17. Exhaust valve and scavenger system:
   a. Open APL valve and observe release of pressure. Occlude breathing system at patient end and verify that negligible positive or negative pressure appears with either zero or 5 L/min flow and exhaust relief valve (if present) opens with flush flow.

18. Test ventilator:
   a. If switching valve is present, test function in both bag and ventilator mode.
   b. Close APL valve if necessary and occlude system at patient end.
   c. Test for leaks and pressure relief by appropriate cycling (exact procedure will vary with type of ventilator).
   d. Attach reservoir bag at mask fitting, fill system and cycle ventilator. Assure filling/emptying of bag.

19. Check for appropriate level of patient suction.

20. Check, connect, and calibrate other electronic monitors.
   Check final position of all controls.

21. Turn on and set other appropriate alarms for equipment to be used. (Perform next two steps as soon as is practical.)

22. Set O_2 monitor alarm limits.

23. Set O_2 monitor alarm limits.

24. Set airway pressure and/or volume monitor alarm limits (if adjustable).

*If an anesthetist uses the same machine in successive cases, the steps marked with an asterisk (*) need not be repeated or may be abbreviated after the initial checkout.
**A vaporizer leak can only be detected if the vaporizer is turned on during this test. Even then, a relatively small but clinically significant leak may still be obscured.

Where are the most likely locations of a breathing circuit disconnection or leak?

Frank disconnections occur most frequently between the right-angle connector and the endotracheal tube, while leaks are most commonly traced to the base plate of the CO_2 absorber. In the intubated patient, leaks often occur in the trachea around an uncuffed endotracheal tube or an inadequately filled cuff. However, there are numerous potential sites of disconnection or leak within the anesthesia machine and the breathing circuit. Every addition to the breathing circuit, such as a humidifier, increases the likelihood of a leak.

How can these leaks be detected?

Leaks can be conceptualized as occurring proximal to the fresh gas outlet (ie, within the anesthesia machine) or distal to the fresh gas inlet (ie, within the breathing circuit). Leaks within the anesthesia machine are less common and can be ruled out by a simple test. Pinching the tubing that connects the machine's fresh gas outlet to the circuit's fresh gas inlet creates a back pressure that will obstruct the forward flow of fresh gas from the anesthesia machine. This is indicated by a drop in the height of the flowmeter bobbins. Upon release of the fresh gas tubing, the bobbins should briskly rebound and settle at their original height. If there is a substantial leak within the machine, obstructing the fresh gas tubing will not result in any back pressure, and the bobbins will not drop. Correcting a leak within the machine usually requires removing it from service.

How are leaks in the breathing circuit detected?

Any connection within the breathing circuit is a potential site of a gas leak. A quick survey of the circuit may reveal a loosely attached breathing tube or a cracked oxygen analyzer adaptor. Less obvious causes include detachment of the tubing used by the disconnect alarm to monitor circuit pressures, an open pressure relief valve, or an improperly adjusted scavenging unit. Leaks can usually be identified audibly or by applying a soap solution to suspect connections and looking for bubble formation.

Are gas leaks preventable?

Leaks within the anesthesia machine and breathing circuit are usually detectable if the machine and circuit have undergone an established checkout procedure. For example, step 16 of the FDA recommendations (Table 4–2) will reveal most significant leaks.

SUGGESTED READINGS

Dorsch JA, Dorsch SE: *Understanding Anesthesia Equipment: Construction, Care and Complications.* Williams & Wilkins, 1984. The anesthesia machine is covered in many chapters of this classic reference.

Heavner JE et al: *Technical Manual Of Anesthesiology: An Introduction.* Raven Press, 1989. Chapter 3 presents an overview of anesthesia machine design.

Mushin WW, Jones PL: *Physics for the Anesthetist.* Blackwell, 1987. Discusses many of the principles underlying the design of anesthesia machines.

Parbrook GD, Davis PD, Parbrook EO: *Physics and Measurement in Anesthesia.* Appleton-Century-Crofts, 1986. Physical principles related to the anesthesia machine.

Petty C: *The Anesthesia Machine.* Churchill Livingstone, 1987.

Ward CS: *Anaesthetic Equipment: Physical Principles and Maintenance,* 2nd ed. Bailliere Tindall, 1985. A thorough review of many types of anesthesia equipment, some of which are no longer used.

Airway Management

Adept airway management is an essential skill for an anesthesiologist. This chapter reviews the anatomy of the upper respiratory passages, describes necessary equipment, and presents techniques and complications of laryngoscopy, intubation, and extubation. Patient safety depends upon a thorough understanding of each of these topics.

ANATOMY

Successful mask ventilation, intubation, cricothyrotomy, and regional anesthesia of the larynx require detailed knowledge of airway anatomy. There are two openings to the human airway: the nose, which leads to the **nasopharynx;** and the mouth, which leads to the **oropharynx.** These passages are separated anteriorly by the palate, but they join posteriorly (Figure 5–1). At the base of the tongue, the **epiglottis** functionally separates the **larynx,** which leads to the trachea, from the **hypopharynx,** which leads to the esophagus. The epiglottis prevents aspiration by covering the **glottis** (the opening of the larynx) during swallowing. The larynx is a cartilaginous skeleton held together by ligaments and muscle. The larynx is composed of nine cartilages (Figure 5–2): **thyroid, cricoid, epiglottic,** and (in pairs) **arytenoid, corniculate,** and **cuneiform.**

The sensory supply to the upper airway is derived from the cranial nerves (Figure 5–3). The mucous membranes of the nose are innervated by the ophthalmic division of the trigeminal nerve anteriorly **(anterior ethmoidal nerve)** and by the maxillary division posteriorly **(sphenopalatine nerves).** The **palatine nerves** provide sensory fibers from the trigeminal nerve and the facial nerve to the hard and soft palate. The tongue is supplied by the **facial nerve** (anterior two-thirds) and **glossopharyngeal nerve** (posterior third). The glossopharyngeal nerve also innervates the roof of the pharynx, the tonsils, and the undersurface of the soft palate. The **vagus nerve** provides sensation to the airway below the epiglottis. The **superior laryngeal branch** of the vagus divides into an **external** (motor) and **internal** (sensory) **laryngeal nerve.** The latter provides sensory supply to the larynx between the epiglottis and the vocal cords. Another branch of the vagus, the **recurrent laryngeal nerve,** innervates the larynx below the vocal cords and the trachea.

All of the muscles confined to the larynx are innervated by the **recurrent laryngeal nerve** except the cricothyroid muscle, which is innervated by the **external** (motor) **laryngeal nerve.** The posterior cricoarytenoid muscles abduct the vocal cords, while the lateral cricoarytenoid muscles are the principal adductors.

Phonation involves complex simultaneous actions by several laryngeal muscles. Damage to the motor nerves innervating the larynx leads to a spectrum of speech disorders (Table 5–1). Because the superior laryngeal nerve provides only motor innervation to the cricothyroid muscle (by way of the external laryngeal nerve), unilateral denervation causes very subtle clinical findings. Bilateral palsy of the superior laryngeal nerve may result in hoarseness or easy tiring of the voice, but airway control is not jeopardized.

Unilateral paralysis of a recurrent laryngeal nerve results in paralysis of the ipsilateral vocal cord, causing a deterioration in voice quality. *Acute* bilateral recurrent laryngeal nerve palsy can result in stridor and respiratory distress due to the remaining unopposed tension of the cricothyroid muscle (assuming an intact superior laryngeal nerve). Airway problems are less frequent in *chronic* bilateral recurrent laryngeal nerve loss because of the development of various compensatory mechanisms (eg, atrophy of the laryngeal musculature).

Bilateral vagal nerve injury affects both the superior and the recurrent laryngeal nerves. Thus, bilateral vagal denervation produces flaccid, midpositioned vocal cords similar to those seen after succinylcholine administration. Although phonation is severely impaired in these patients, airway control is rarely a problem.

EQUIPMENT

Oral & Nasal Airways

Loss of pharyngeal muscle tone in anesthetized patients allows the tongue and epiglottis to fall back against the posterior wall of the pharynx (Figure 5–4). Artificial airways inserted through the mouth or nose create an air passage between the tongue and the posterior pharyngeal wall (Figure 5–5). Awake or lightly anesthetized patients may cough or even develop laryngospasm during airway insertion if laryngeal reflexes are intact. Placement of an oral airway is sometimes fa-

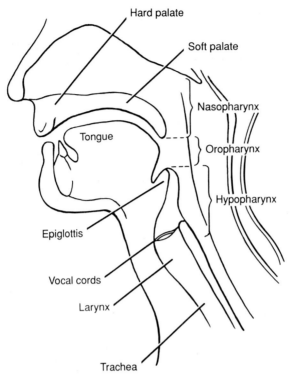

Figure 5–1. Anatomy of the airway.

cilitated by depressing the tongue with a tongue blade. The distance between the tip of the nose and the ear lobe approximates the correct length of an oral airway.

Nasal airways should be approximately 2–4 cm longer than oral airways. Because of the risk of epistaxis, nasal airways should not be used in anticoagulated patients or in children with prominent adenoids. Any tube inserted through the nose (eg, nasal airways, nasogastric catheters, and nasotracheal tubes) should be lubricated and advanced at an angle perpendicular to the face to avoid traumatizing the turbinates or the roof of the nose. Nasal airways are usually better tolerated than oral airways in lightly anesthetized patients.

Mask Design & Technique

A face mask delivers anesthetic gas from a breathing circuit to a patient by creating an airtight seal with the patient's face (Figure 5–6). The rim of the mask is contoured and conforms to a variety of facial features. The mask's 22-mm orifice attaches to the breathing circuit through a right-angle connector. Several mask designs are available. Transparent bodies allow observation of exhaled, humidified gas and immediate recognition of vomiting. Black rubber masks are often pliable enough to adapt to uncommon facial bone structures. Retaining hooks surrounding the orifice attach to a head strap so that the mask does not have to be continually held in place by the anesthesiologist. Some pediatric masks are specially designed to minimize apparatus dead space (Figure 5–7).

Effective ventilation requires both a gas-tight mask fit and a patent airway. Continued deflation of the breathing bag when the pressure relief valve is closed usually indicates a substantial leak around the mask. In contrast, the generation of high breathing circuit pressures with minimal chest movement and breath sounds implies an obstructed airway. Both of these problems are usually resolved by proper mask technique.

By holding the mask with the left hand, one can use the right hand to generate positive-pressure ventilation by squeezing the breathing bag. The mask is held against the face by downward pressure on the mask body exerted by the left thumb and index finger (Figure 5–8). The middle and ring finger grasp the mandible to extend the atlanto-occipital joint. Finger pressure should be placed on the bony mandible and not on the soft tissues supporting the base of the tongue, which may obstruct the airway. The little finger slides under the angle of the jaw and thrusts it anteriorly.

In difficult situations, two hands may be needed to provide adequate jaw thrust and create a mask seal. Therefore, an assistant may be needed to squeeze the breathing bag. In such cases, the thumbs hold the mask down while the fingertips or knuckles displace the jaw forward (Figure 5–9). It is often difficult to form an adequate mask fit with the cheeks of edentulous patients. Leaving dentures in place or packing the buccal cavities with gauze may help. Positive-pressure ventilation should normally be limited to 20 cm H_2O to avoid stomach inflation.

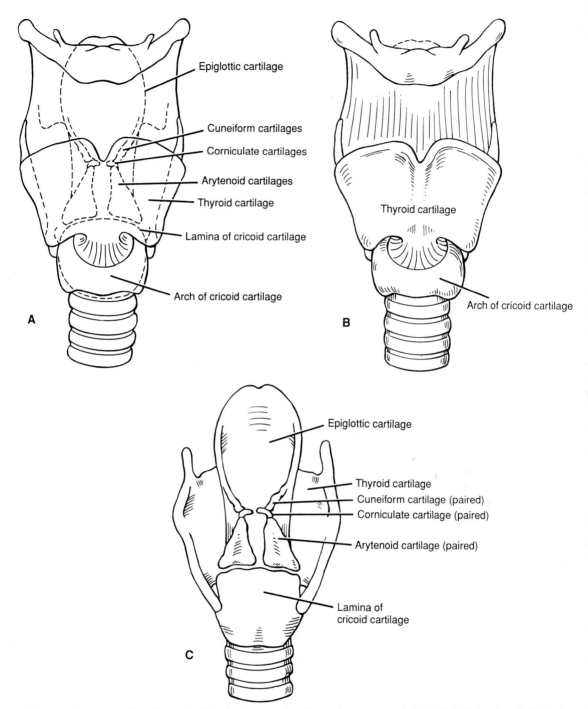

Figure 5–2. Laryngeal cartilages. **A:** The nine laryngeal cartilages (superimposed view). **B:** Anterior view. **C:** Posterior view. (Modified and reproduced, with permission, from Hollinshead WH: *Textbook of Anatomy,* 4th ed. Harper & Row, 1985.)

Most patients' airways can be maintained with a face mask, an oral or nasal airway, and a face strap. Mask ventilation for long periods may result in pressure injury to branches of the trigeminal or facial nerves. Face mask and face strap position should be regularly changed to prevent ischemic injury. Corneal abrasions and excessive pressure on the eye should be avoided.

Endotracheal Tubes

Endotracheal tubes deliver anesthetic gases directly into the trachea. Standards govern endotracheal tube

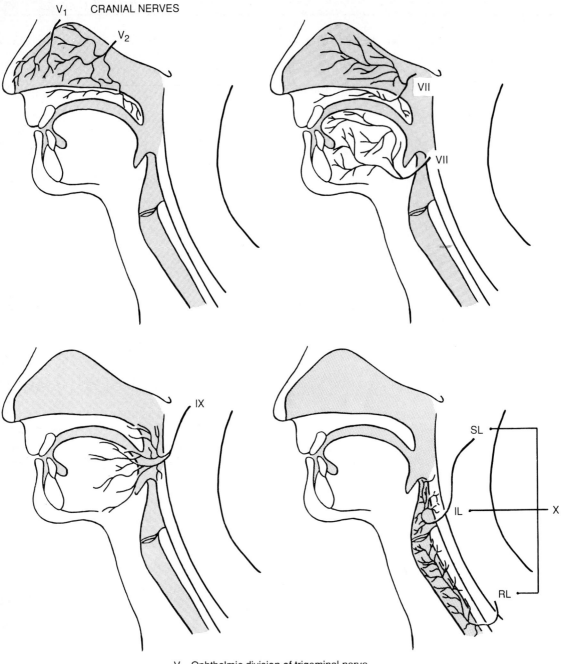

CRANIAL NERVES

V_1 Ophthalmic division of trigeminal nerve
(anterior ethmoidal nerve)

V_2 Maxillary division of trigeminal nerve
(sphenopalatine nerves)

VII Facial nerve

IX Glossopharyngeal nerve

X Vagus nerve
— SL Superior laryngeal branch of
the vagus nerve
— IL Internal laryngeal nerve
— RL Recurrent laryngeal nerve

Figure 5–3. Sensory nerve supply of the airway.

Table 5–1. The effects of laryngeal nerve injury on the voice.

Nerve	Effect of Nerve Injury
Superior laryngeal nerve	
Unilateral	Minimal effects
Bilateral	Hoarseness, tiring of voice
Recurrent laryngeal nerve	
Unilateral	Hoarseness
Bilateral	
Acute	Stridor, respiratory distress
Chronic	Aphonia
Vagal nerve	
Unilateral	Hoarseness
Bilateral	Aphonia

manufacture (American National Standard for Anesthetic Equipment; ANSI Z–79). Polyvinyl chloride is the material most commonly used in making endotracheal tubes. Tracheal tubes marked "I.T." or "Z–79" are implant-tested to ensure nontoxicity. The shape and rigidity of endotracheal tubes can be altered by inserting a stylet. The patient end of the tube is beveled to aid visualization and insertion through the vocal cords. Murphy tubes have a hole (the "Murphy eye") to lessen the risk of complete tube occlusion (Figure 5–10).

Resistance to air flow depends primarily on tube diameter but is also affected by tube length and curvature. Endotracheal tube size is usually designated in millimeters of *internal* diameter or, less commonly, in the French scale (external diameter in millimeters multiplied by 3). The choice of tube diameter is always a compromise between maximizing flow with a large size and minimizing airway trauma with a small size (Table 5–2).

Most adult endotracheal tubes have a cuff inflation system consisting of a valve, pilot balloon, inflating tube, and cuff (Figure 5–10). The valve prevents air loss after cuff inflation. The pilot balloon provides a gross indication of cuff inflation. The inflating tube connects the valve to the cuff and is incorporated into the tube's wall. By creating a seal, endotracheal tube cuffs permit positive-pressure ventilation and reduce the likelihood of aspiration. Uncuffed tubes are usually used in children to minimize the risk of pressure injury and postintubation croup (Chapter 42).

There are two major types of cuffs: high-pressure (low volume) and low-pressure (high volume). High-pressure cuffs are associated with more ischemic damage to the tracheal mucosa and are less suitable for intubations of long duration. Low-pressure cuffs may increase the likelihood of sore throat (larger mucosal contact area), aspiration, spontaneous extubation, and difficult insertion (due to the floppy cuff). Nonetheless, because of a decreased incidence of severe mucosal damage, low-pressure cuffs are more commonly recommended.

Cuff pressure depends on many factors: (1) inflation volume, (2) the diameter of the cuff in relation to the trachea, (3) tracheal and cuff compliance, and (4) intrathoracic pressure (eg, cuff pressures increase with coughing). Cuff pressure may rise during general anesthesia as a result of the diffusion of nitrous oxide from the tracheal mucosa into the endotracheal tube cuff.

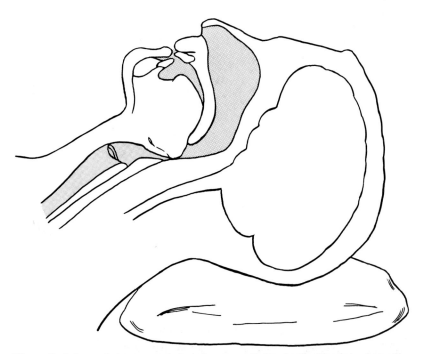

Figure 5–4. Loss of airway muscle tone in an anesthetized patient leads to obstruction.

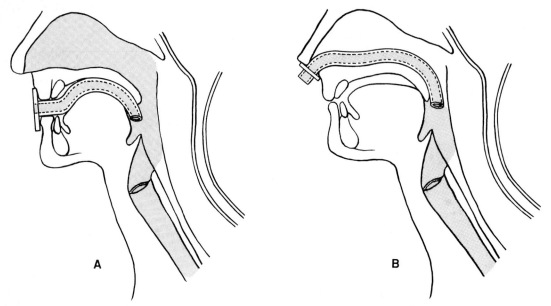

Figure 5–5. Proper positioning of an oral **(A)** and nasal **(B)** airway. (Modified and reproduced, with permission, from Dorsch JA, Dorsch SE: *Understanding Anesthesia Equipment: Construction, Care, and Complications.* Williams & Wilkins 1984.)

Rigid Laryngoscopes

A laryngoscope is an instrument used to examine the larynx and intubate the trachea. The handle usually contains batteries to light a bulb on the blade (Figure 5–11). The Macintosh and Miller blades are the most popular curved and straight designs in the United States. The choice of blade depends on personal preference and patient anatomy. Because no blade is perfect for all situations, the clinician should become familiar and proficient with a variety of blade designs (Figure 5–12).

Flexible Fiberoptic Laryngoscopes

In some situations—eg, patients with poor range of motion of the temporomandibular joint or those with certain congenital upper airway anomalies—direct laryngoscopy with a rigid laryngoscope is undesirable or impossible. A flexible fiberoptic laryngoscope allows indirect visualization of the larynx in such cases (Figure 5–13). This instrument is constructed of coated glass fibers that transmit light and images by internal reflection—ie, a light beam becomes trapped within a fiber and exits unchanged at the opposite end. The insertion tube contains two bundles of fibers, each consisting of 10,000–15,000 fibers. One bundle transmits light from the light source (light source bundle) while the other provides a high-resolution image (image bundle). Directional manipulation of the insertion tube is accomplished with an angulation wire. Aspiration channels are convenient for suctioning secretions, insufflating oxygen, or instilling local anesthetic. However, aspiration channels can be difficult to clean,

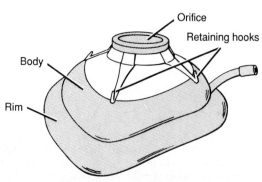

Figure 5–6. An adult face mask.

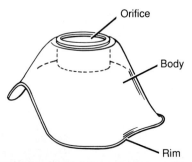

Figure 5–7. The Rendell-Baker-Soucek pediatric face mask has a shallow body and minimal dead space.

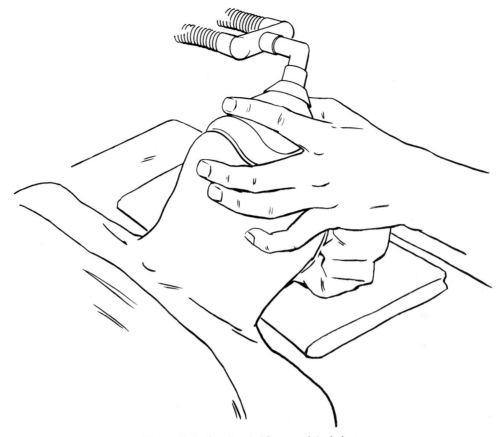

Figure 5–8. One-handed face mask technique.

provide a nidus for infection, and require a larger-diameter insertion tube.

TECHNIQUES OF DIRECT LARYNGOSCOPY & INTUBATION

Indications for Intubation

Inserting a tube into the trachea has become a routine part of general anesthesia. However, intubation is not a risk-free procedure, and not all patients receiving general anesthesia require it. In general, intubation is indicated for patients who are at risk for aspiration and in those undergoing surgical procedures involving body cavities or the head and neck. Mask ventilation is usually satisfactory for short minor procedures (eg, cystoscopy, eye examination under anesthesia).

Preparation for Rigid Laryngoscopy

Preparation for intubation includes checking equipment and properly positioning the patient. The endotracheal tube should be examined. The tube's cuff inflation system can be tested by inflating the cuff with a 10-mL syringe. Maintenance of cuff pressure *after detaching the syringe* ensures proper cuff and valve func-

tion. Some anesthesiologists cut the endotracheal tube to a preset length to lessen the risk of endobronchial intubation or occlusion due to tube kinking (Table 5–2). The connector should be pushed into the tube as far as possible to lessen the likelihood of disconnection. If a stylet is used, it should be inserted into the endotracheal tube, which is then bent to resemble a hockey stick (Figure 5–14). This shape facilitates intubation of an anteriorly positioned larynx. The desired blade is locked onto the laryngoscope handle, and bulb function is tested. The light intensity should remain constant even if the bulb is slightly jiggled. A blinking light signals a poor electrical contact, while fading indicates low batteries. An extra handle, blade, endotracheal tube (one size smaller), and stylet should be immediately available. The proper functioning of a suction unit should be ensured in case of unexpected secretions, bleeding, or vomiting.

Successful intubation often depends on correct patient positioning. The patient's head should be level with the anesthesiologist's xiphoid process to prevent unnecessary back strain during laryngoscopy. Rigid laryngoscopy displaces pharyngeal soft tissues to create a direct line of vision from the mouth to the glottic opening. Moderate head elevation and exten-

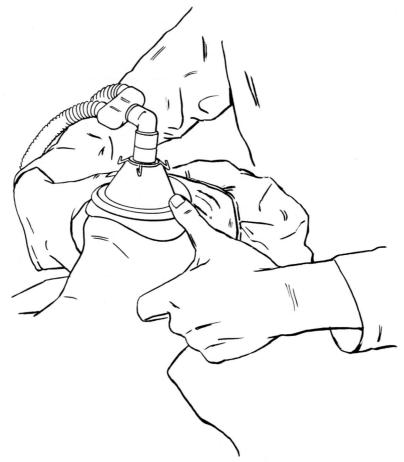

Figure 5–9. A difficult airway can often be managed with a two-handed technique.

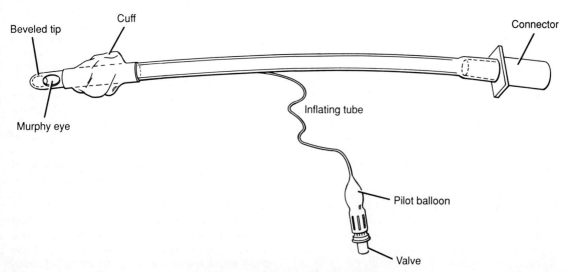

Figure 5–10. Murphy endotracheal tube.

Table 5-2. Oral endotracheal tube size guidelines.

Age	Internal Diameter (mm)	Cut Length (cm)
Full-term infant	3.5	12
Children	$4 + \dfrac{\text{Age}}{4}$	$14 + \dfrac{\text{Age}}{2}$
Adult Female Male	 7–7.5 7.5–8	 24 24

sion of the atlanto-occipital joint places the patient in the desired "sniffing position" (Figure 5–15). The lower portion of the cervical spine is actually flexed by resting the head on a pillow.

Preparation for induction and intubation also involves the question of routine preoxygenation. Preoxygenation with several deep breaths of 100% oxygen provides an extra margin of safety in case the patient is not easily ventilated after induction. Preoxygenation can be omitted in patients who object to the face mask and are free of pulmonary disease.

Orotracheal Intubation

The laryngoscope is held in the left hand. With the patient's mouth opened widely, the blade is introduced into the right side of the oropharynx with care to avoid the teeth. The tongue is swept to the left and up into the floor of the pharynx by the blade's flange. The tip of a curved blade is usually inserted into the vallecula, while the straight blade tip covers the epiglottis. With either blade, the handle is raised up and away from the patient in a plane perpendicular to the patient's mandible to expose the vocal cords (Figure 5–16). Leverage

on the teeth is avoided. The endotracheal tube is taken with the right hand, and its tip is passed through the abducted vocal cords. The endotracheal tube cuff should lie in the upper trachea but beyond the larynx. The laryngoscope is withdrawn, again with care to avoid tooth damage. The cuff is inflated with the least amount of air necessary to create a seal during positive-pressure ventilation.

After intubation, the chest and epigastrium are immediately auscultated and a capnographic tracing is monitored to ensure intratracheal location (Figure 5–17). If there is doubt about whether the tube is in the esophagus or trachea, it is prudent to remove the tube and ventilate the patient with a mask. Otherwise, the tube is taped to secure its position (Figure 5–18). Although the persistent detection of CO_2 by a capnograph is the best confirmation of tracheal placement of an endotracheal tube, it cannot exclude endobronchial intubation due to overinsertion. The earliest manifestation of endobronchial intubation is an increase in peak inspiratory pressure. Proper tube location can be reconfirmed by palpating the cuff in the sternal notch while compressing the pilot balloon with the other hand. The cuff should not be felt above the level of the cricoid cartilage, since a prolonged intralaryngeal location may result in postoperative hoarseness. Tube position can be documented by chest radiography, but this is not usually required.

The description presented here assumes an unconscious patient. Oral intubation is usually poorly tolerated by awake patients. However, intravenous sedation, application of local anesthetic spray in the oropharynx, and constant reassurance will improve patient acceptance.

A failed intubation should not be followed by repeated attempts that are merely "more of the same." Something must be changed to increase the likelihood of success, such as repositioning the patient, decreasing tube size, adding a stylet, selecting a different blade, attempting a nasal route, or requesting the assistance of another anesthesiologist. If the patient is also difficult to ventilate with a mask, preparations must be made for possible emergency tracheostomy or cricothyrotomy (Figure 5–19).

Nasotracheal Intubation

Nasal intubation is similar to oral intubation except that the endotracheal tube is advanced through the nose into the oropharynx before laryngoscopy. The nostril through which the patient breathes most easily is selected for preparation. Phenylephrine nose drops (0.5% or 0.25%) vasoconstrict vessels and shrink mucous membranes. If the patient is awake, local anesthetic drops and nerve blocks can also be utilized (see Case Discussion).

An endotracheal tube lubricated with water-soluble jelly is introduced along the floor of the nose, below the inferior turbinate, *at an angle perpendicular to the face*. The tube's bevel should be directed laterally away from the turbinates. In order to make certain that

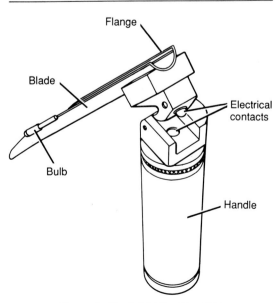

Figure 5–11. A rigid laryngoscope.

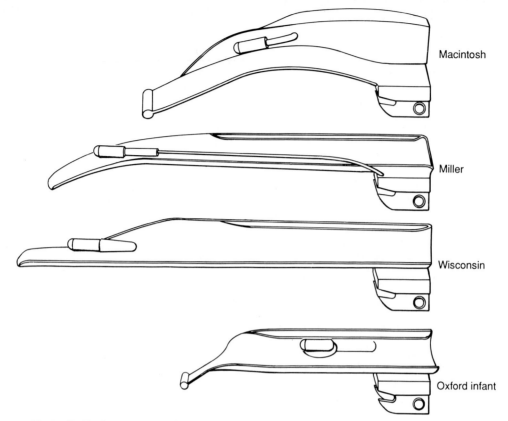

Macintosh

Miller

Wisconsin

Oxford infant

Figure 5–12. An assortment of laryngoscope blades: Macintosh, Miller, Wisconsin, Oxford infant.

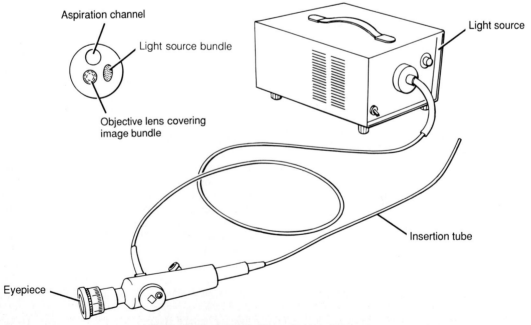

Aspiration channel

Light source bundle

Objective lens covering image bundle

Light source

Insertion tube

Eyepiece

Figure 5–13. A flexible fiberoptic bronchoscope.

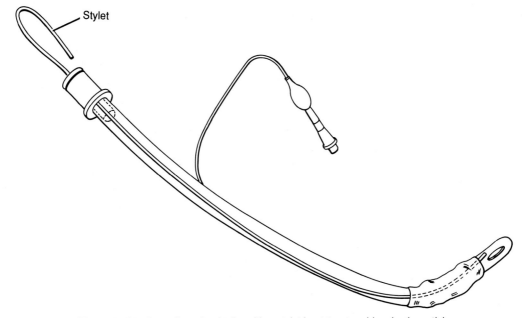

Figure 5–14. An endotracheal tube with a stylet bent to resemble a hockey stick.

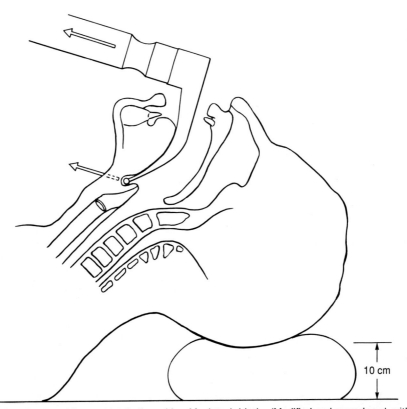

Figure 5–15. The "sniffing" position and intubation with a Macintosh blade. (Modified and reproduced, with permission, from Dorsch JA, Dorsch SE: *Understanding Anesthesia Equipment: Construction, Care, and Complications.* Williams & Wilkins 1984.)

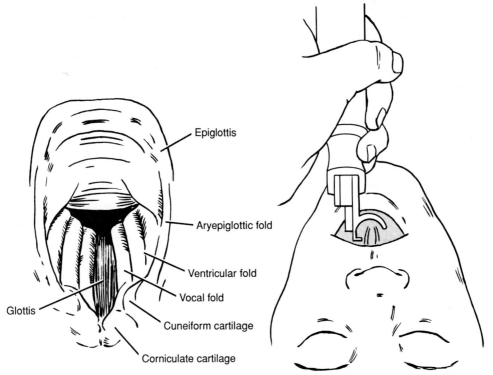

Figure 5–16. Typical view of the glottis during laryngoscopy with a curved blade. (Modified and reproduced, with permission, from Barash PG: *Clinical Anesthesia*. Lippincott, 1989.)

the tube passes along the floor of the nasal cavity, it should be pulled cephalad (Figure 5–20). The tube is gradually advanced until its tip can be visualized in the oropharynx. Laryngoscopy, as we have seen, reveals the abducted vocal cords. Passage of the tip of the tube through the vocal cords may be facilitated by manipulation with Magill forceps. Nasal passage of endotracheal tubes, airways, or nasogastric catheters is dangerous in patients with severe midfacial trauma because there is a risk of intracranial placement.

Flexible Fiberoptic Nasal Intubation

Both nostrils are prepared with vasoconstrictive drops. The nostril through which the patient breathes more easily is identified. A large red rubber nasal airway (eg, 36F) is inserted into the other nostril. The breathing circuit can be directly connected to the end of this nasal airway in order to administer 100% oxygen during laryngoscopy. If the patient is unconscious and not breathing spontaneously, the mouth can be taped and respiration controlled through the single nasal airway. *When this technique is used, adequacy of ventilation and oxygenation should be confirmed by capnography and pulse oximetry.*

The endotracheal tube is lubricated and inserted into the other nostril the length of a nasal airway. The lubricated shaft of the fiberoptic scope is introduced into the endotracheal tube lumen. *The single most important*

rule during endoscopy is to always advance the scope into a lumen—do not advance it if only the wall of the endotracheal tube or mucous membrane is visualized. As the tip of the fiberoptic instrument passes through the distal end of the endotracheal tube, the epiglottis or glottis should be visible. The tip of the laryngoscope is manipulated as needed to pass the abducted cords.

There is no need to hurry, since the patient's ventilation and oxygenation are being monitored. If either becomes inadequate, the fiberoptic scope is withdrawn in order to ventilate the patient with a mask. Having an assistant thrust the jaw forward or apply cricoid pressure may improve visualization in difficult cases. If the patient is breathing spontaneously, pulling the tongue forward with a clamp may also facilitate intubation.

Once in the trachea, the scope is advanced to within sight of the carina. The presence of tracheal rings and the carina is proof of proper positioning. The endotracheal tube is slipped over the fiberoptic shaft. Proper endotracheal tube position is confirmed by viewing the tip of the tube above the carina before the fiberoptic scope is withdrawn.

TECHNIQUES OF EXTUBATION

Judging when to remove an endotracheal tube is part of the art of anesthesiology that develops with experi-

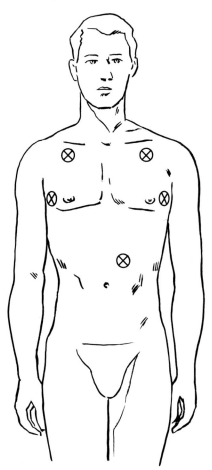

Figure 5–17. Sites for auscultation of breath sounds at the apices and over the stomach.

lessened by pretreatment with 1.5 mg/kg of intravenous lidocaine 1–2 minutes before suctioning and extubation, deep extubation may be preferable in patients who cannot tolerate these effects. On the other hand, deep extubation would be contraindicated in a patient at risk for aspiration or one whose airway may be difficult to control after removal of the endotracheal tube.

Regardless of whether the tube is removed when the patient is deeply anesthetized or awake, the patient's pharynx should be thoroughly suctioned before extubation in order to lessen the risk of aspiration or laryngospasm. In addition, patients should be ventilated with 100% oxygen in case it becomes difficult to establish an airway after the endotracheal tube is removed. Just prior to extubation, the endotracheal tube is untaped and its cuff deflated. Whether the tube is removed when the patient is at end-expiration or end-inspiration is controversial and probably not very important. The tube is withdrawn in a single, smooth motion, and a face mask is usually applied to deliver 100% oxygen until the patient is stable enough for transportation to the recovery room. In some institutions, oxygen delivery by face mask is maintained during the period of transportation.

COMPLICATIONS OF LARYNGOSCOPY & INTUBATION

The complications of laryngoscopy and intubation are usually due to (1) errors of tube positioning, (2) airway trauma, (3) physiologic responses to airway instrumentation, or (4) tube malfunction. These complications can occur during laryngoscopy and intubation, while the tube is in place, or following extubation (Table 5–3).

Errors of Endotracheal Tube Positioning

Unintentional esophageal intubation can produce catastrophic results. Detection of this complication depends on (1) direct visualization of the tip of the endotracheal tube passing through the vocal cords, (2) careful auscultation for the presence of bilateral breath sounds and the absence of gastric gurgling, (3) analysis of exhaled gas for the presence of CO_2 (the most reliable method), (4) chest radiography, or (5) fiberoptic bronchoscopy.

Even though the tube is confirmed to be in the trachea, it may not be correctly positioned. Overinsertion usually results in intubation of the right main stem bronchus due to its less acute angle with the trachea. Clues to the diagnosis of endobronchial intubation include (1) unilateral breath sounds, (2) detection of unexpected hypoxia with pulse oximetry (unreliable with high inspired oxygen concentrations), (3) inability to palpate the endotracheal tube cuff in the sternal notch

ence. In general, extubation is best performed when a patient is either "deeply anesthetized" or "awake." In either case, spontaneous ventilation and adequate recovery from muscle relaxants should be established prior to extubation. Extubation during a "light" plane of anesthesia (ie, a state between deep and awake) is avoided because of the increased risk of laryngospasm. The distinction between deep and light anesthesia is usually apparent during pharyngeal suctioning: Any reaction to suctioning (eg, breath-holding, coughing) signals a light plane of anesthesia, while no reaction is characteristic of a deep plane. Similarly, eye opening or purposeful movements imply that the patient is "awake."

Extubating an awake patient is usually associated with coughing ("bucking") on the endotracheal tube. This reaction increases the heart rate, central venous pressure, arterial blood pressure, intracranial pressure, and intraocular pressure. It may also cause wound dehiscence and bleeding. The presence of an endotracheal tube in an awake asthmatic patient often triggers bronchospasm. While these consequences may be

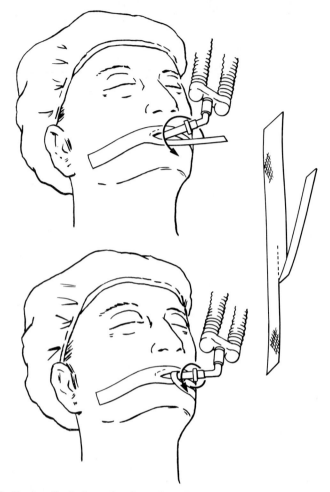

Figure 5–18. A method of securing the endotracheal tube with waterproof adhesive tape.

during cuff inflation, and (4) poor breathing bag compliance.

In contrast, inadequate insertion depth will position the cuff in the larynx, predisposing the patient to laryngeal trauma. This can be detected by palpating the cuff over the thyroid cartilage or by radiography of the neck.

Since no single technique protects against all of these possibilities for misplacing an endotracheal tube, it is suggested that minimal testing should include chest auscultation, cuff palpation, and routine capnography.

If the patient is repositioned, tube placement must be reconfirmed. Neck extension or lateral rotation moves an endotracheal tube away from the carina, while neck flexion moves the tube toward the carina.

Airway Trauma

Instrumentation with a metal laryngoscope blade and insertion of a stiff endotracheal tube often traumatizes delicate airway tissues. Although tooth damage is the most common cause of malpractice claims against anesthesiologists, laryngoscopy and intubation can lead to a range of complications from sore throat to tracheal stenosis. Most of these are due to prolonged external pressure on delicate airway structures. When these pressures exceed the capillary-arteriolar blood pressure (approximately 30 mm Hg), tissue ischemia may lead to a sequence of inflammation, ulceration, granulation, and stenosis.

Postintubation croup due to glottic or tracheal edema is particularly serious in children. Vocal cord paralysis due to cuff compression or other traumatization of the recurrent laryngeal nerve results in hoarseness and increases the risk of aspiration. Some of these complications may be lessened by using an endotracheal tube shaped to conform to the anatomy of the airway (eg, Lindholm Anatomical Tracheal Tube). Applying water-soluble lubricant to the tip or cuff of the orotracheal tube does not decrease the incidence of postoperative sore throat or hoarseness. Smaller tubes (size 6.5 in women and size 7.0 in men) are associated with fewer complaints of postoperative sore throat.

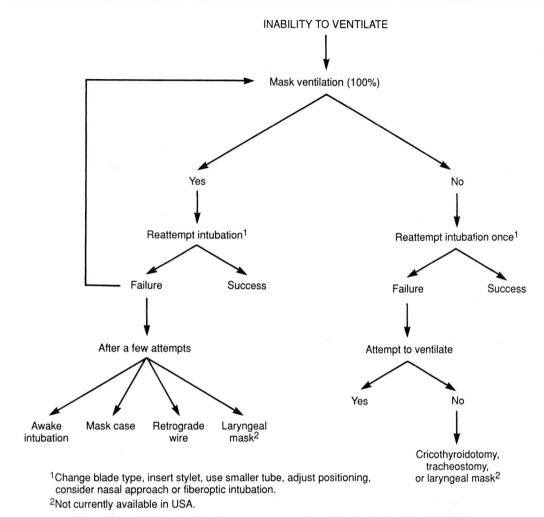

INABILITY TO VENTILATE

Mask ventilation (100%)

Yes — No

Reattempt intubation[1]

Failure — Success

After a few attempts

Awake intubation — Mask case — Retrograde wire — Laryngeal mask[2]

Reattempt intubation once[1]

Failure — Success

Attempt to ventilate

Yes — No

Cricothyroidotomy, tracheostomy, or laryngeal mask[2]

[1]Change blade type, insert stylet, use smaller tube, adjust positioning, consider nasal approach or fiberoptic intubation.
[2]Not currently available in USA.

Figure 5–19. Algorithm for management of unanticipated difficult intubation.

Physiologic Responses to Airway Instrumentation

Laryngoscopy and intubation violate the patient's protective airway reflexes and predictably lead to hypertension and tachycardia. These hemodynamic changes can be attenuated by intravenous administration of lidocaine (1.5 mg/kg 1–2 minutes before laryngoscopy), alfentanil (10–20 μg/kg 2–3 minutes before laryngoscopy), or fentanyl (3–8 μg/kg 4–5 minutes before laryngoscopy). Hypotensive agents, including sodium nitroprusside, nitroglycerin, hydralazine, and propranolol, have also been shown to effectively prevent the transient hypertensive response. Cardiac dysrhythmias—particularly ventricular bigeminy—are not uncommon during intubation and usually indicate light anesthesia.

Laryngospasm is a forceful involuntary spasm of the laryngeal musculature caused by sensory stimulation of the superior laryngeal nerve. Triggering stimuli include pharyngeal secretions or passing an endotracheal

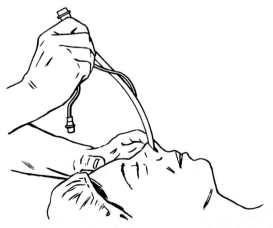

Figure 5–20. Cephalad traction on the tube will help direct its tip inferiorly along the floor of the nasal cavity.

Table 5–3. Complications of intubation.

During laryngoscopy and intubation
  Malpositioning
    Esophageal intubation
    Endobronchial intubation
    Laryngeal cuff position
  Airway trauma
    Tooth damage
    Lip, tongue or mucosal laceration
    Sore throat
    Dislocated mandible
    Retropharyngeal dissection
  Physiologic reflexes
    Hypertension, tachycardia
    Intracranial hypertension
    Intraocular hypertension
    Laryngospasm
  Tube malfunction
    Cuff perforation
While the tube is in place
  Malpositioning
    Unintentional extubation
    Endobronchial intubation
    Laryngeal cuff position
  Airway trauma
    Mucosal inflammation and ulceration
    Excoriation of nose
  Tube malfunction
    Ignition
    Obstruction
Following extubation
  Airway trauma
    Edema and stenosis (glottic, subglottic, or tracheal)
    Hoarseness (vocal cord granuloma or paralysis)
    Laryngeal malfunction and aspiration
  Physiologic reflexes
    Laryngospasm

tube through the larynx during extubation. Although possible in the awake patient, laryngospasm is usually prevented by extubating patients either deeply asleep or fully awake. Treatment of laryngospasm includes providing gentle positive-pressure ventilation with 100% oxygen or administering intravenous lidocaine (1–1.5 mg/kg). If laryngospasm persists and hypoxia develops, succinylcholine (0.25–1 mg/kg) should be given in order to paralyze the laryngeal muscles and allow controlled ventilation. The large negative intrathoracic pressures generated by the struggling patient in laryngospasm can result in development of pulmonary edema even in healthy young adults.

While laryngospasm represents an abnormally sensitive reflex, aspiration can result from depression of laryngeal reflexes following prolonged intubation and general anesthesia. Bronchospasm is another reflex response to intubation and is most common in asthmatic patients. Bronchospasm can sometimes be a clue to endobronchial intubation. Other pathophysiologic effects of intubation include increased intracranial and intraocular pressures.

Endotracheal Tube Malfunction

Endotracheal tubes do not always function as intended. The risk of polyvinyl chloride tube ignition in an O_2/N_2O-enriched environment was mentioned in Chapter 2. Valve or cuff damage is not unusual and should be excluded prior to insertion. Endotracheal tube obstruction can result from kinking, foreign body aspiration, or thick pulmonary secretions.

CASE DISCUSSION: EVALUATION & MANAGEMENT OF A DIFFICULT AIRWAY

A 17-year-old girl presents for emergency drainage of a submandibular abscess.

What are some important anesthetic considerations during the preoperative evaluation of a patient with an abnormal airway?

Induction of general anesthesia followed by direct laryngoscopy and oral intubation is dangerous, if not impossible, in several situations (Table 5–4). To determine the optimal intubation technique, the anesthesiologist must carefully examine the patient's airway.

If a facial deformity is severe enough to preclude a good mask seal, positive-pressure ventilation may be impossible. Furthermore, patients with hypopharyn-

Table 5–4. Conditions associated with difficult intubations.

Tumors
  Cystic hygroma
  Hemangioma
  Hematoma
Infections
  Submandibular abscess
  Peritonsillar abscess
  Epiglottitis
Congenital anomalies
  Pierre Robin syndrome
  Treacher Collins' syndrome
  Laryngeal atresia
  Goldenhar's syndrome
  Craniofacial dysostosis
Foreign body
Trauma
  Laryngeal fracture
  Mandibular or maxillary fracture
  Inhalation burn
  Cervical spine injury
Obesity
Inadequate neck extension
  Rheumatoid arthritis
  Ankylosing spondylitis
  Halo traction
Anatomic variations
  Micrognathia
  Prognathism
  Large tongue
  Arched palate
  Short neck
  Prominent upper incisors

geal disease are more dependent on awake muscle tone to maintain airway patency. These two groups of patients should not be allowed to become apneic for any reason—including induction of anesthesia, sedation, or muscle paralysis—until their airway is secured.

If there is abnormal limitation of the temporomandibular joint that may not improve with muscle relaxation, a nasal approach should be considered. Infection confined to the floor of the mouth usually does not preclude nasal intubation. But if the hypopharynx is involved to the level of the hyoid bone, any translaryngeal attempt will be difficult. Other clues to a potentially difficult laryngoscopy include a distance between the tip of the patient's mandible and hyoid bone of less than 7 cm and a poorly visualized uvula during voluntary tongue protrusion (Figure 5–21).

The anesthesiologist should also evaluate the patient for signs of airway obstruction (eg, chest retraction, stridor) and hypoxia (agitation, restlessness, anxiety, lethargy). Aspiration pneumonitis is more likely if the patient has recently eaten or if pus is draining from an abscess into the mouth. In either case, techniques that ablate laryngeal reflexes (eg, topical anesthesia) should be avoided.

In this case, physical examination reveals extensive facial edema that limits the mandible's range of motion. Mask fit does not appear to be impaired. Lateral radiographs of the head and neck suggest that the in-

fection has spread over the larynx. Frank pus is observed in the mouth.

Which intubation technique is indicated?

Routine oral and nasal intubations have been described for anesthetized patients. Both of these can also be performed in awake patients. Whether the patient is awake or asleep or whether intubatation is to be oral or nasal, it can be performed with rigid laryngoscopy, fiberoptic visualization, or a "blind" technique. Thus, there are at least 12 methods of translaryngeal intubation (eg awake/nasal/fiberoptic). Furthermore, tracheostomy or cricothyrotomy can be lifesaving methods of airway preservation.

Because in this patient intubation may be difficult, there is pus draining into the mouth, and positive-pressure ventilation may be impossible, induction of anesthesia should be delayed until after the airway has been secured. The submandibular location of the abscess suports the choice of a nasal approach and probably excludes rigid laryngoscopy. Therefore, the alternatives are (1) awake/nasal/fiberoptic intubation or (2) awake/nasal/blind intubation. This final decision depends upon the availability of a fiberoptic bronchoscope and personnel experienced in its use.

Regardless of which alternative is chosen, preparation for tracheostomy should be readied. This includes

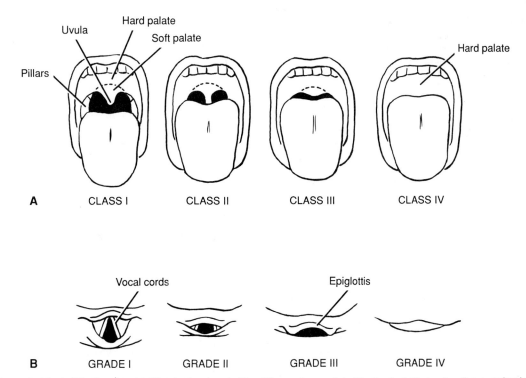

Figure 5–21. A difficult orotracheal intubation (grade III or IV) may be predicted by the inability to visualize certain pharyngeal structures (class III or IV) during the preoperative examination. (Reproduced, with permission, from Mallamdati SR: Clinical signs to predict difficult tracheal intubation (hypothesis). Can Anaesth Soc J 1983;30:316.)

(1) a team of experienced surgeons in the operating room, (2) all necessary equipment available and unwrapped, and (3) sterile preparation and draping of the neck.

What premedication would be appropriate for this patient?

Any loss of consciousness or interference with airway reflexes could result in airway obstruction or aspiration. Glycopyrrolate would be a good choice of premedication since it minimizes upper airway secretions without crossing the blood-brain barrier (Chapter 11). Parenteral sedatives could be very carefully titrated or omitted entirely. Management of patients at risk for aspiration is the subject of the case discussion presented in Chapter 15.

Describe a "blind" nasotracheal intubation.

An endotracheal tube is lubricated with lidocaine jelly and deformed for a few minutes to exaggerate its curvature (Figure 5–22). The patient's head should be placed in the sniffing position. The tip of the tube is gently introduced into the nares at a plane perpendicular to the face. Air movement through the tube should be continually felt, heard, or monitored by capnography. The tube is incrementally advanced during inspiration. If the patient's respirations continue but no air flow is detected through the tube, the tip has passed the glottis and is in the esophagus. In that case, the tube must be withdrawn and advanced again. Breath-holding and coughing signal close proximity to the larynx, and tube advancement should continue with each inspiration.

If the tube does not easily enter the trachea, several maneuvers may enhance success. After advancement

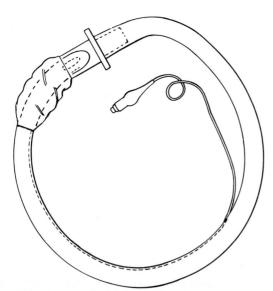

Figure 5–22. An endotracheal tube is bent to exaggerate its curvature so that it will pass anteriorly into the larynx during a blind nasal intubation.

to an area near the glottis, a stylet that has been bent to resemble a hockey stick can be inserted through the tube to direct its tip more anteriorly. Extension of the head will also tend to guide the tube more anteriorly, while head rotation will move the tip laterally. Laryngeal or cricoid pressure may beneficially change the relationship between the tip and the glottis. Inflation of the endotracheal tube cuff in the hypopharynx may also force the tip anteriorly. If the tube persistently slips into the esophagus, voluntary tongue protrusion will inhibit swallowing and may move the tongue and the tube anteriorly.

After intubation is confirmed, intravenous induction may proceed. At the end of the procedure, the patient should be totally awake, with protective airway reflexes intact, before extubation is attempted. Necessary equipment and personnel should be available for unexpected reintubation.

What nerve blocks could be helpful during an awake intubation?

Bilateral superior laryngeal nerve blocks and a transtracheal block would anesthetize the airway below the epiglottis (Figure 5–23). The hyoid bone is located, and 3 mL of 2% lidocaine is infiltrated 1 cm below each greater cornu where the superior laryngeal nerves penetrate the thyrohyoid membrane.

A transtracheal block is performed by identifying and penetrating the cricothyroid membrane while the neck is extended. After confirmation of an intratracheal position by aspiration of air, 4 mL of 4% lidocaine is injected into the trachea at end-expiration. A deep inhalation and cough immediately following injection distributes the anesthetic throughout the trachea. While these blocks may allow the awake patient to better tolerate intubation, they also obtund protective reflexes and may lead to aspiration.

Because of this patient's increased risk for aspiration, local anesthesia should be limited to the nasal passages. Four percent cocaine has no advantages compared with a mixture of 4% lidocaine and 0.25% phenylephrine and can cause cardiovascular side effects. The maximum safe dose of local anesthetic should be calculated and not exceeded (Chapter 14). Local anesthetic is applied to the nasal mucosa with cotton-tipped applicators until a red rubber nasal airway that has been lubricated with lidocaine jelly can be placed into the nares with minimal discomfort.

Why be prepared for emergency tracheostomy?

Laryngospasm is always a possible complication of intubation in the nonparalyzed patient even if the patient remains awake. Laryngospasm may make positive-pressure ventilation with a mask impossible. If succinylcholine is administered to break the spasm, the consequent relaxation of pharyngeal muscles may lead to upper airway obstruction and continued inability to ventilate. In this situation, emergency tracheostomy may be lifesaving.

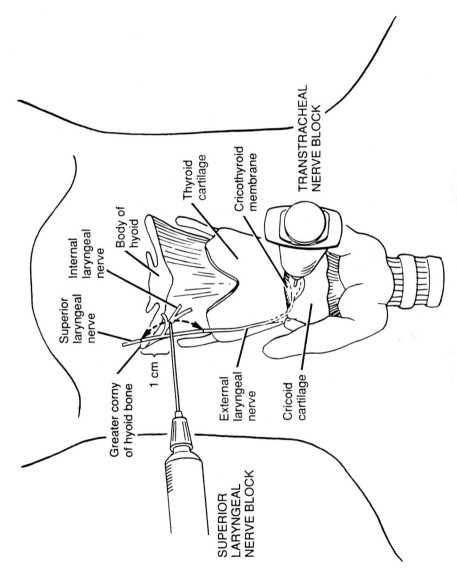

Figure 5–23. Superior laryngeal nerve block and transtracheal block.

What are some alternative techniques that might be successful?

Other possible strategies include the retrograde passage of a wire or epidural catheter through the cricothyroid membrane. The catheter is guided cephalad into the pharynx and out through the nose or mouth.

An endotracheal tube is passed over the catheter, which is withdrawn after the tube has entered the larynx. Another possibility is cricothyrotomy, which is described in Chapter 46. Either of these techniques would have been difficult in the patient described in this case owing to the swelling and anatomic distortion of the neck that can accompany a submandibular abscess.

SUGGESTED READINGS

Berry FA: *Anesthetic Management of Difficult and Routine Pediatric Patients*. Churchill Livingstone, 1986.

Crosby ET, Lui AL: The adult cervical spine: Implications for airway management. Can J Anaesth 1990;37:77. A review of the preoperative assessment of the abnormal airway, with emphasis on intubation of patients with unstable cervical spines.

Dorsch SA, Dorsch SE: *Understanding Anesthesia Equipment: Construction, Care and Complications*. Williams & Wilkins, 1984. Endotracheal tubes, laryngoscopes, face masks, and airways.

Ellis H, Feldman S: *Anatomy for Anaesthetists*. Blackwell, 1983. Includes a chapter on airway anatomy.

Gorback MS (editor): *Emergency Airway Management*. BC Decker, 1990.

Latto IP, Rosen M: *Difficulties in Tracheal Intubation*. Bailliere Tindall, 1985.

McIntyre JWR: Laryngoscope design and the difficult adult tracheal intubation. Can J Anaesth 1989;36:94. Relates choice of anesthetic blade (eg, Miller versus Macintosh) to the anatomic peculiarities of the individual patient.

Ovassapian A: *Fiberoptic Airway Endoscopy in Anesthesia and Critical Care*. Raven Press, 1990. Extensively illustrated.

Patil VU, Stehling LC, Zauder HL: *Fiberoptic Endoscopy in Anesthesia*. Year Book, 1983.

Patient Monitors

6

One of the primary responsibilities of an anesthesiologist is to act as a guardian for the anesthetized patient during surgery. In fact, "Vigilance" is the motto of the American Society of Anesthesiologists. Because vigilance implies monitoring, minimal standards of intraoperative monitoring have been adopted by the American Society of Anesthesiologists (see accompanying box). An understanding of the technology of sophisticated monitoring equipment—including cost-benefit considerations—is required for optimal vigilance. This chapter reviews the indications, contraindications, techniques and complications, and clinical considerations relevant to the most important anesthetic monitors.

CARDIAC MONITORS

ARTERIAL BLOOD PRESSURE

The rhythmic contractions of the left ventricle result in pulsatile arterial pressures. The peak pressure generated during systolic contraction is the **systolic arterial blood pressure** (SBP); the trough pressure during diastolic relaxation is the **diastolic arterial blood pressure** (DBP). **Pulse pressure** is the difference between the systolic and diastolic pressures. The time-weighted average of arterial pressures during a pulse cycle is the **mean arterial pressure** (MAP). Mean arterial pressure can be estimated by application of the following formula:

$$MAP = \frac{(SBP) + 2(DBP)}{3}$$

Measurements of arterial blood pressure are greatly affected by sampling site. As a pulse moves peripherally through the arterial tree, wave reflection distorts the pressure waveform, leading to an exaggeration of systolic and pulse pressures (Figure 6–1). For example, radial artery systolic pressure is usually higher than aortic systolic pressure because of the former's more distal location. In contrast, radial artery pressures are often lower than aortic pressures following car-

diopulmonary bypass because of a decrease in the hand's vascular resistance. The level of the sampling site relative to the heart will alter measurement of blood pressure because of the effect of gravity (Figure 6–2). Because noninvasive (palpation, Doppler, auscultation, oscillometry, plethysmography) and invasive (arterial cannulation) methods of blood pressure determination differ greatly, they are discussed separately.

1. NONINVASIVE ARTERIAL BLOOD PRESSURE MONITORING

Indications

General or regional anesthesia is an absolute indication for arterial blood pressure measurement. The techniques and frequency of pressure determination depend largely on the patient's condition and the type of surgical procedure. An auscultatory measurement every 3–5 minutes is adequate in most cases. However, auscultation may be unreliable because of problems such as morbid obesity, in which case a Doppler or oscillometric technique may be preferable.

Contraindications

Although some method of blood pressure measurement is mandatory, techniques that rely on a blood pressure cuff are best avoided in extremities with vascular abnormalities (eg, dialysis shunts) or intravenous lines.

Techniques & Complications

A. Palpation: Systolic blood pressure can be determined by (1) locating a palpable peripheral pulse; (2) inflating a blood pressure cuff proximal to the pulse until flow is occluded; (3) releasing cuff pressure by 2 or 3 mm Hg per heartbeat; and (4) measuring the cuff pressure at which pulsations are again palpable, the systolic pressure. This method tends to underestimate systolic pressure because of the insensitivity of touch and the delay between flow under the cuff and distal pulsations. Palpation does not provide a diastolic or mean arterial pressure. The equipment required is simple and inexpensive (Figure 6–3).

B. Doppler Probe: By substituting a Doppler probe for the anesthesiologist's finger, arterial blood pressure measurement becomes sensitive enough to be useful in obese patients, those who are in shock, and in

Standards for Basic Intraoperative Monitoring
(January 1, 1991)

These standards apply to all anesthesia care although, in emergency circumstances, appropriate life support measures take precedence. These standards may be exceeded at any time based on the judgment of the responsible anesthesiologist. They are intended to encourage high-quality patient care, but observing them cannot guarantee any specific patient outcome. They are subject to revision from time to time, as warranted by the evolution of technology and practice. This set of standards addresses only the issue of basic intraoperative monitoring, which is one component of anesthesia care. In certain rare or unusual circumstances, (1) some of these methods of monitoring may be clinically impractical, and (2) appropriate use of the described monitoring methods may fail to detect untoward clinical developments. Brief interruptions of continual§ monitoring may be unavoidable. *Under extenuating circumstances, the responsible anesthesiologist may waive the requirements marked with an asterisk (*); it is recommended that when this is done, it should be so stated (including the reasons) in a note in the patient's medical record.* These standards are not intended for application to the care of the obstetric patient in labor or in the conduct of pain management.

Standard I

Qualified anesthesia personnel shall be present in the room throughout the conduct of all general anesthetics, regional anesthetics, and monitored anesthesia care.

Objective: Because of the rapid changes in patient status during anesthesia, qualified anesthesia personnel shall be continuously present to monitor the patient and provide anesthesia care. In the event there is a direct known hazard (eg, radiation) to the anesthesia personnel that might require intermittent remote observation of the patient, some provision for monitoring the patient must be made. In the event that an emergency requires the temporary absence of the person primarily responsible for the anesthetic, the best judgment of the anesthesiologist will be exercised in comparing the emergency with the anesthetized patient's condition and in the selection of the person left responsible for the anesthetic during the temporary absence.

Standard II

During all anesthetics, the patient's oxygenation, ventilation, circulation, and temperature shall be continually evaluated.

OXYGENATION

Objective: To ensure adequate oxygen concentration in the inspired gas and the blood during all anesthetics.

Methods:

(1) Inspired gas: During every administration of general anesthesia using an anesthesia machine, the concentration of oxygen in the patient breathing system shall be measured by an oxygen analyzer with a low concentration limit alarm in use.*

pediatric patients (Figure 6–4). The Doppler effect is the apparent shift in the frequency of sound waves when a wave source moves relative to the observer. For example, the pitch of a train's whistle increases as the train approaches and decreases as it departs. The reflection of sound waves off a moving object similarly causes an apparent frequency shift. A Doppler probe transmits an ultrasonic signal that is reflected by underlying tissue. Because red blood cells move through an artery, a Doppler frequency shift will be detected by the probe. The difference between transmitted and received frequency is represented by the Doppler's characteristic swishing sound, which indicates blood flow. Because air reflects ultrasound, a coupling gel (but not corrosive electrode jelly) must be applied between the Doppler probe and the skin. Correct positioning of the probe directly above an artery is crucial, since the beam must pass through the vessel wall. In-

(2) Blood oxygenation: During all anesthetics, a quantitative method of assessing oxygenation such as pulse oximetry shall be employed.* Adequate illumination and exposure of the patient is necessary to assess color.

VENTILATION
Objective: To ensure adequate ventilation of the patient during all anesthetics.
Methods:
(1) Every patient receiving general anesthesia shall have the adequacy of ventilation continually evaluated. While qualitative clinical signs such as chest excursion, observation of the reservoir breathing bag, and auscultation of breath sounds may be adequate, quantitative monitoring of the CO_2 content and/or volume of expired gas is encouraged.
(2) When an endotracheal tube is inserted, its correct positioning in the trachea must be verified by clinical assessment and by identification of CO_2 in the expired gas.* End-tidal CO_2 analysis, in use from the time of endotracheal tube placement, is encouraged.
(3) When ventilation is controlled by a mechanical ventilator, there shall be in continuous use a device that is capable of detecting disconnection of components of the breathing system. The device must give an audible signal when its alarm threshold is exceeded.
(4) During regional anesthesia and monitored anesthesia care, the adequacy of ventilation shall be evaluated, at least, by continual observation of qualitative clinical signs.

CIRCULATION
Objective: To ensure the adequacy of the patient's circulatory function during all anesthetics.
Methods:
(1) Every patient receiving anesthesia shall have the electrocardiogram continuously displayed from the beginning of anesthesia until preparing to leave the anesthetizing location.*
(2) Every patient receiving anesthesia shall have arterial blood pressure and heart rate determined and evaluated at least every 5 minutes.*
(3) Every patient receiving general anesthesia shall have, in addition to the above, circulatory function continually evaluated by at least one of the following: palpation of a pulse, auscultation of heart sounds, monitoring of a tracing of intra-arterial pressure, ultrasound peripheral pulse monitoring, or pulse plethysmography or oximetry.

BODY TEMPERATURE
Objective: To aid in the maintenance of appropriate body temperature during all anesthetics.
Methods: There shall be readily available a means to continuously measure the patient's temperature. When changes in body temperature are intended, anticipated, or suspected, the temperature shall be measured.

§Note that "continual" is defined as "repeated regularly and frequently in steady rapid succession," whereas "continuous" means "prolonged without any interruption at any time."

terference due to probe movement or electrocautery is an annoying distraction. Only systolic pressures can be reliably determined with the Doppler technique.

A variation of Doppler technology uses a piezoelectric crystal to detect lateral arterial wall movement due to the intermittent opening and closing of vessels between systolic and diastolic pressure. Thus, this instrument (Arteriosonde) detects both systolic and diastolic pressures.

C. Auscultation: Inflation of a blood pressure cuff to a pressure between systolic and diastolic pressures will partially collapse an underlying artery, producing turbulent flow and the characteristic **Korotkoff sounds.** These sounds are audible through a stethoscope placed under—or just beyond—the distal third of an inflated blood pressure cuff. The Diasyst is a specially molded rubber stethoscope that is secured under the cuff with Velcro fasteners (Figure 6–5). Sys-

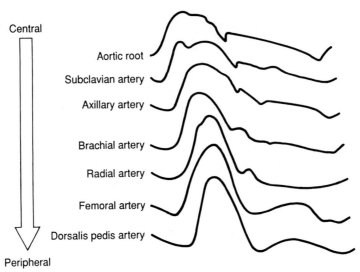

Figure 6–1. Changes in configuration as a waveform moves peripherally. (Reproduced, with permission, from Blitt CD: *Monitoring in Anesthesia and Critical Care Medicine,* 2nd ed. Churchill Livingstone, 1990.)

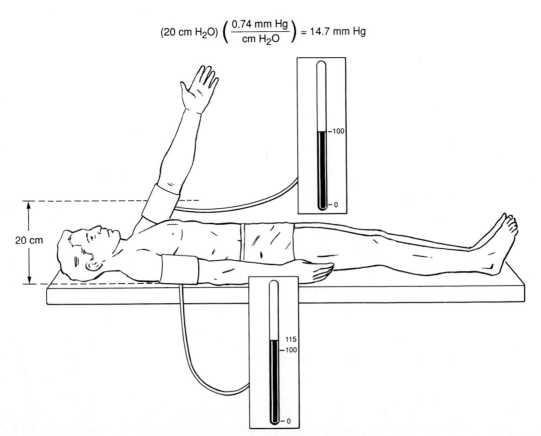

Figure 6–2. The difference in blood pressure (mm Hg) at two different sites of measurement equals the height of an interposed column of water (cm H_2O) multiplied by a conversion factor (1 cm H_2O = 0.74 mm Hg).

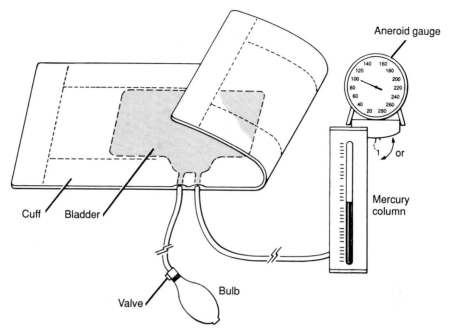

Figure 6–3. Equipment required for arterial blood pressure measurement by palpation.

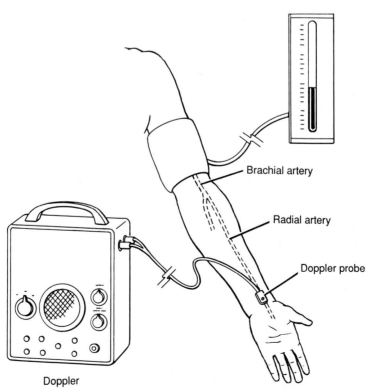

Figure 6–4. A Doppler probe secured over the radial artery will sense red blood cell movement as long as the blood pressure cuff is below systolic pressure. (Courtesy of Parks Medical Electronics.)

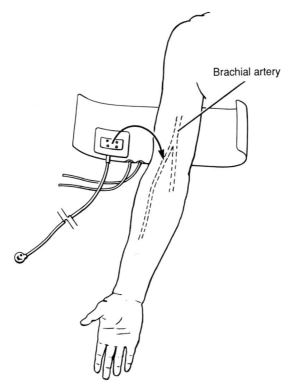

Brachial artery

Figure 6–5. The Diasyst—a type of stethoscope. (Modified and reproduced, with permission, from Cohen DD, Robbins LS: Blood pressure monitoring in the anesthetized patient: A new stethoscope device. Anesth Analg 1966;45:93.)

tolic blood pressure coincides with the onset of Korotkoff sounds, while diastolic pressure is variably determined as their muffling or disappearance. Occasionally, Korotkoff sounds cannot be heard through part of the range from systolic to diastolic pressure. This **auscultatory gap** is most common in hypertensive patients and can lead to a falsely low measurement.

Korotkoff sounds are often difficult to auscultate during episodes of hypotension or marked peripheral vasoconstriction. In these situations, the subsonic frequencies associated with them can be detected by a microphone and amplified to indicate systolic and diastolic pressures. Motion artifact and electrocautery interference limit the usefulness of this method (Infrasonde).

D. Oscillometry: Arterial pulsations cause oscillations in cuff pressure. These oscillations are small if the cuff is inflated above systolic pressure. However, when the cuff pressure decreases to systolic pressure, the pulsations are transmitted to the entire cuff and the oscillations markedly increase. Maximal oscillation occurs at the mean arterial pressure, after which oscillations decrease. Because some oscillations are present above and below arterial blood pressure, observation of a mercury or aneroid manometer is a gross and unreliable measurement. Automated blood pressure monitors electronically measure the pressures at which the oscillation amplitudes change (Figure 6–6). A microprocessor derives systolic, mean, and diastolic pressures by using an algorithm. Machines that demand identical, consecutive pulse waves for measurement confirmation may be unreliable during arrhythmias (eg, atrial fibrillation). Oscillometric monitors should not be used on patients being perfused with a heart-lung machine. Nonetheless, the speed, accuracy, and versatility of oscillometric devices have greatly improved.

E. Plethysmography: Arterial pulsations transiently increase the blood volume in an extremity. A finger photoplethysmograph, consisting of a light-emitting diode and a photoelectric cell, detects changes in finger volume. If the pressure in a proximally placed cuff exceeds systolic pressure, the pulsations and changes in volume cease. The Finapres (*finger-arterial-pressure*) plethysmograph continuously measures the minimum pressures required in a small finger cuff to maintain a constant finger volume. A solenoid-controlled air pump rapidly modulates cuff pressures, which are displayed as a beat-to-beat tracing. Although this monitor's measurements usually correspond to intra-arterial determinations, plethysmography does not work well in patients with poor peripheral perfusion (eg, those with peripheral vascular disease or hypothermia).

F. Arterial Tonometry: Arterial tonometry non-

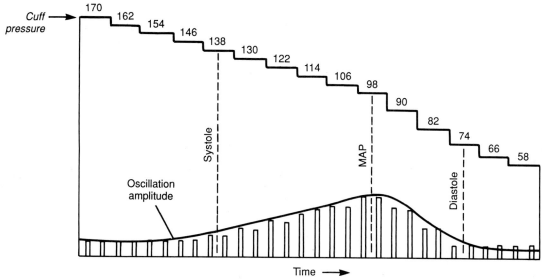

Figure 6–6. Oscillometric determination of blood pressure.

invasively measures beat-to-beat arterial blood pressure by sensing the pressure required to partially flatten a superficial artery that is supported by a bony structure (eg, radial artery). A tonometer consisting of several independent pressure transducers is applied to the skin overlying the artery (Figure 6–7). The contact stress between the pressure transducer directly over the artery and the skin reflects intraluminal pressure. Continuous pulse recordings result in a tracing very similar to an invasive arterial blood pressure waveform. Current limitations on this technology include sensitivity to movement artifact and the need for frequent calibration.

Clinical Considerations

Adequate oxygen delivery to vital organs must be maintained during anesthesia. Unfortunately, instruments to monitor specific organ perfusion and oxygenation are complex and expensive, and for that reason arterial blood pressure is assumed to reflect organ blood flow. But flow also depends on vascular resistance:

$$\text{Flow} = \frac{\text{Pressure gradient}}{\text{Vascular resistance}}$$

Thus, arterial blood pressure should be viewed as an indicator—but not a measure—of end organ perfusion.

The accuracy of any method of blood pressure measurement that involves a blood pressure cuff depends upon proper cuff size (Figure 6–8). The cuff's rubber bladder should extend at least halfway around the extremity. Additionally, the width of the cuff should be

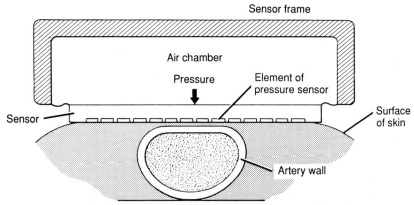

Figure 6–7. Tonometry is a new method of continuous (beat-to-beat) arterial blood pressure determination. The sensors must be positioned directly over the artery.

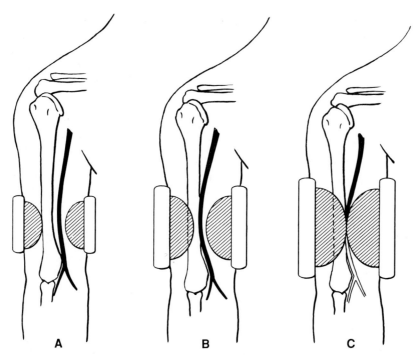

Figure 6–8. Blood pressure cuff width influences the pressure readings. Three cuffs, all inflated to the same pressure, are shown. The narrowest cuff *(A)* will require more pressure and the widest cuff *(C)* less pressure to occlude the brachial artery for determination of systolic pressure. Therefore, a large overestimation of systolic pressure can be the consequence of using a cuff that is too narrow. The wider cuff may give an underestimation of the systolic pressure, but the error with a cuff 20% too wide is not as great as with a cuff 20% too narrow. (Reproduced, with permission, from Gravenstein JS, Paulus DA: *Monitoring Practice in Clinical Anesthesia.* Lippincott, 1982.)

20–50% greater than the extremity's diameter (Figure 6–9).

Automated blood pressure monitors, utilizing one or a combination of methods described above, are becoming more frequently used in anesthesiology. A self-contained air pump inflates the cuff at predetermined intervals. Overzealous use of these automated devices has resulted in nerve palsies and extensive extravasation of intravenously administered fluids. In case of equipment failure, an alternative method of blood pressure determination must be immediately available.

2. INVASIVE ARTERIAL BLOOD PRESSURE MONITORING

Indications

Indications for invasive arterial pressure monitoring by catheterization include (1) elective hypotension, (2) anticipation of wide intraoperative blood pressure swings, (3) end organ disease necessitating precise beat-to-beat blood pressure regulation, and (4) multiple analyses of arterial blood gases.

Contraindications

Catheterization should be avoided if possible in arteries without documented collateral blood flow or in extremities where there is a suspicion of preexisting vascular insufficiency (eg, Raynaud's phenomenon).

Techniques & Complications

A. Selection of Artery for Cannulation: Several arteries are available for percutaneous catheterization.

1. The **radial artery** is commonly cannulated because of its superficial location and collateral flow. However, 5% of patients have incomplete palmar arches and lack adequate collateral blood flow. **Allen's test** is a simple—but not completely reliable—method for determining the adequacy of ulnar collateral circulation in case of radial artery thrombosis. First, the patient exsanguinates the hand by making a fist. While the operator occludes the radial and ulnar arteries with fingertip pressure, the patient relaxes the blanched hand. Collateral flow through the hand's arterial arches is confirmed by flushing of the thumb within 5 seconds after pressure on the ulnar artery is released. Delayed return of normal coloration indicates an equivocal test (5–10 seconds) or insufficient collateral circulation (> 10 seconds). Alternatively, blood flow distal to the radial artery occlusion can be detected by palpation, Doppler, plethysmography, or pulse oximetry. Unlike Allen's test, these methods of determining the adequacy of collateral circulation do not require patient cooperation.

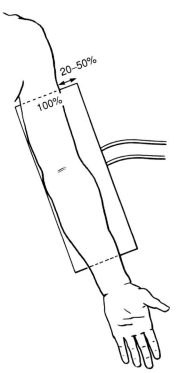

20–50%

100%

Figure 6–9. The width of the blood pressure cuff should be 20–50% greater than the diameter of the patient's extremity.

2. Ulnar artery catheterization is more difficult because of the artery's deeper and more tortuous course. Because of the risk of compromising blood flow to the hand, it should not be considered if the ipsilateral radial artery has been punctured but unsuccessfully cannulated.

3. The **brachial artery** is large and easily identifiable in the antecubital fossa. Its proximity to the aorta provides less waveform distortion. Being near the elbow predisposes brachial artery catheters to kinking.

4. The **femoral artery** is prone to pseudoaneurysm and atheroma formation but often provides an access of last resort in burn or trauma victims. Aseptic necrosis of the head of the femur is a rare but tragic complication of femoral artery cannulation in children.

5. The **dorsalis pedis** and **posterior tibial arteries** are at some distance from the aorta and therefore have distorted waveforms. Modified Allen tests should be performed to document adequate collateral flow around these arteries.

6. The **axillary artery** is surrounded by the axillary plexus, so that nerve damage can result from a hematoma or traumatic cannulation. Air or thrombi will quickly gain access to the cerebral circulation during retrograde flushing of the left axillary artery.

B. Technique of Radial Artery Cannulation: One technique of radial artery cannulation is illustrated in Figure 6–10. Supination and extension of the wrist provide optimal exposure of the radial artery. The pressure tubing-transducer system should be nearby and already flushed with heparinized saline (0.5–1 unit of heparin per milliliter of saline) to ensure easy connection after cannulation. The radial pulse is palpated and the artery's course is determined by lightly pressing the *tips* of the index and middle fingers of the anesthesiologist's nondominant hand over the area of maximal impulse. After preparing the skin with iodophor and alcohol solution, 0.5 mL of lidocaine is infiltrated directly above the artery with a 25- or 27-gauge needle. A 20- or 22-gauge Teflon catheter-over-needle assembly penetrates the skin at a 45-degree angle and is directed toward the point of palpation. Upon blood flashback, the needle is lowered to a 30-degree angle and advanced another 2 mm to make certain that the tip of the catheter is well into the vessel lumen. The catheter is advanced over the needle, which is then withdrawn. Applying pressure with the two palpating fingertips prevents blood from spurting until the tubing is firmly connected. Waterproof tape or suture keeps the catheter in place.

C. Complications: Complications of intra-arterial monitoring include hematoma, vasospasm, arterial thrombosis, embolization of air bubbles or thrombi, skin necrosis overlying the catheter, nerve damage, infection, and unintentional intra-arterial drug injection. Complications are more apt to occur after repeated attempts at cannulation. The risks are minimized when the ratio of catheter to artery size is small, heparinized saline is continuously infused at a rate of 2–3 mL/h, flushing of the catheter is limited, and meticulous attention is paid to aseptic technique. By placing a pulse oximeter on the ipsilateral index finger, adequacy of perfusion can be continually monitored during radial artery cannulation.

Clinical Considerations

Because intra-arterial cannulation provides continuous, beat-to-beat blood pressure measurement, it is considered the "gold standard" of blood pressure monitoring techniques. However, the quality of the transduced waveform depends on the dynamic characteristics of the catheter-tubing-transducer system (Figure 6–11). False readings can lead to inappropriate therapeutic interventions. An intra-arterial catheter also provides access for sampling arterial blood gases.

A complex waveform, such as an arterial pulse, can be expressed as a summation of simple sine and cosine waves **(Fourier analysis).** The catheter-tubing-transducer system must be capable of responding adequately to the highest frequency of the arterial waveform for faithful reproduction (Figure 6–12). Stated another way, the natural frequency of the measuring system must exceed the natural frequency of the arterial pulse (approximately 16–24 Hz).

Catheter-tubing-transducer systems must also prevent hyperresonance artifact caused by reverberation of pressure waves within the system. A **dampening coefficient β** of 0.6–0.7 is optimal. The natural frequency and dampening coefficient can be determined

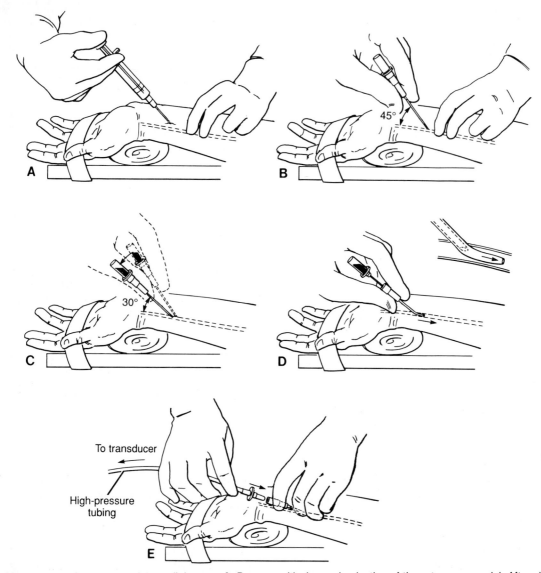

Figure 6–10. Cannulation of the radial artery. **A:** Proper positioning and palpation of the artery are crucial. After skin preparation, local anesthetic is infiltrated with a 25-gauge needle. **B:** A 20- or 22-gauge catheter is advanced through the skin at a 45-degree angle. **C:** Flashback of blood signals entry into the artery, and the catheter-needle assembly is lowered to a 30-degree angle and advanced 2 mm to ensure an intraluminal catheter position. **D:** The catheter is advanced over the needle, which is withdrawn. **E:** Proximal pressure with middle and ring fingers prevents blood loss, while the arterial tubing Luer-lock connector is secured to the intra-arterial catheter.

by examining tracing oscillations after a high-pressure flush (Figure 6–13).

System dynamics are improved by minimizing tubing length, eliminating unnecessary stopcocks, removing air bubbles, and using low-compliance tubing. Although smaller diameter catheters lower natural frequency, they tend to improve underdampened systems and are less apt to result in vascular complications. If a large catheter totally occludes an artery, reflected waves can distort pressure measurements.

Pressure transducers have evolved from bulky, reusable instruments to miniaturized, disposable chips.

Transducers convert the mechanical energy of a pressure wave into an electrical signal. Most are based upon the **strain gauge** principle: stretching a wire or silicone crystal changes its electrical resistance. The sensing elements are arranged as a Wheatstone bridge circuit so that the voltage output is proportionate to the pressure applied to the diaphragm.

Transducer accuracy depends upon correct calibration and zeroing procedures. A stopcock at the level of the desired point of measurement—usually the midaxillary line—is opened, and the zero switch on the monitor is activated. If the patient's position is altered by

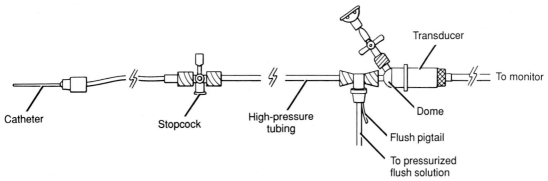

Figure 6–11. The catheter-tubing-transducer system.

raising or lowering the operating room table, the transducer must either be moved in tandem or zeroed to the new level of the midaxillary line. The arterial pressure in the brain of a patient in a sitting position differs significantly from left ventricular pressure. In this circumstance, cerebral pressure is determined by zeroing the transducer at the level of the ear, which approximates the circle of Willis. The transducer's zero should be regularly checked to eliminate "drift" from temperature changes.

External calibration of a transducer compares the transducer's reading with a mercury column (Figure 6–14). If necessary, the monitor's preamplifier may be adjusted to give a reading within 5% of the mercury column. The calibration switch present on some monitors only checks internal electrical circuits and does not calibrate the transducer.

Digital readouts of systolic and diastolic pressures are a running average of the highest and lowest measurements within a certain time interval. Since motion or cautery artifacts can result in some very misleading numbers, the arterial waveform should always be monitored. The shape of the arterial wave gives clues

to several hemodynamic variables. Rate of upstroke indicates contractility; rate of downstroke indicates peripheral vascular resistance; and exaggerated variations in size during respirations suggest hypovolemia. Mean arterial pressure is calculated by integrating the area under the pressure curve.

ELECTROCARDIOGRAPHY

Indications

All patients should have intraoperative electrocardiographic monitoring.

Contraindications

None.

Techniques & Complications

Lead selection determines the diagnostic sensitivity of the ECG. The electrical axis of lead II parallels the atria, resulting in the greatest P wave voltages of any surface lead. This orientation enhances dysrhythmia diagnosis and inferior wall ischemia detection. Lead

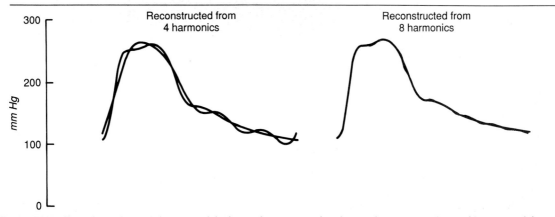

Figure 6–12. This illustration overlays an original waveform onto a four-harmonic reconstruction **(left)** and an eight-harmonic reconstruction **(right).** Note that the higher harmonic plot more closely resembles the original waveform. (Reproduced, with permission, from Saidman LS, Smith WT: *Monitoring in Anesthesia.* Butterworths, 1984.)

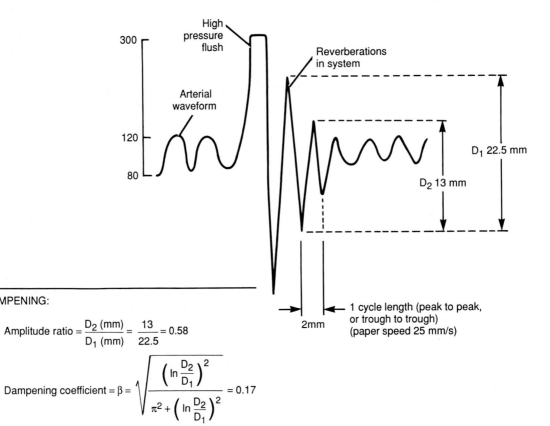

DAMPENING:

Amplitude ratio $= \dfrac{D_2 \text{ (mm)}}{D_1 \text{ (mm)}} = \dfrac{13}{22.5} = 0.58$

Dampening coefficient $= \beta = \sqrt{\dfrac{\left(\ln \dfrac{D_2}{D_1}\right)^2}{\pi^2 + \left(\ln \dfrac{D_2}{D_1}\right)^2}} = 0.17$

Amplitude ratio (D_2/D_1)	Dampening coefficient
.9	.034
.8	.071
.7	.113
.6	.160
.5	.215
.4	.280
.3	.358
.2	.456
.1	.591

NATURAL FREQUENCY:

Natural frequency $= fn = \dfrac{1}{2\pi} \sqrt{\dfrac{\pi D^2 \, \Delta P}{4\rho \, L\Delta V}} = \dfrac{\text{Paper speed (mm/sec)}}{\text{Length of 1 cycle (mm)}}$

$= \dfrac{25 \text{ mm/sec}}{2 \text{ mm}} = 12.5 \text{ HZ}$

D = Internal diameter of tubing

ρ = Density of blood

L = Length of tubing

$\dfrac{\Delta P}{\Delta V}$ = Compliance ("stiffness") of system

Figure 6–13. Dampening and natural frequency of a transducer system can be determined by a high-pressure flush test. (Modified and reproduced, with permission, from Blitt CD: *Monitoring in Anesthesia and Critical Care Medicine,* 2nd ed. Churchill Livingstone, 1990.)

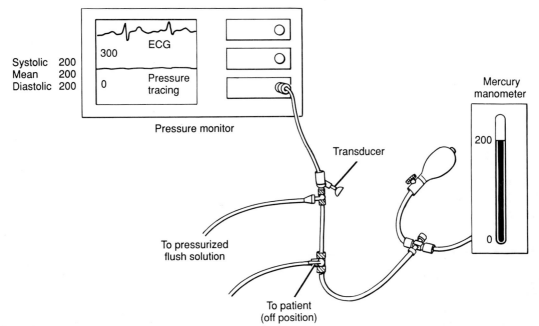

Figure 6–14. External calibration of a transducer with a mercury manometer. The system is pressurized to 200 mm Hg and deflated in increments of 50 mm Hg. Sterility must be maintained, and introduction of air into the pressure tubing must be avoided. The transducer should read within 5% of the mercury column.

V_5 lies over the fifth intercostal space at the anterior axillary line, and this position is a good compromise for detecting anterior and lateral wall ischemia. A true V_5 lead is possible only on operating room electrocardiographs with at least five lead wires, but a modified V_5 can be monitored by rearranging the standard three limb lead placement (Figure 6–15). Ideally, since each lead provides unique information, leads II and V_5 should be monitored simultaneously by an electrocardiograph with two channels. If only a single-channel machine is available, the preferred lead for monitoring depends upon the location of any prior infarction or ischemia. Esophageal leads are even better than lead II for dysrhythmia diagnosis but have not yet gained general acceptance in the operating room.

The electrocardiograph contacts the patient's body through silver chloride electrodes (Figure 6–16). Conductive gel lowers the skin's electrical resistance, which can be further decreased by cleansing the site of application with alcohol or a degreasing agent. Needle electrodes are used only if the silver chloride disks are unsuitable (eg, an extensively burned patient).

Clinical Considerations

The ECG is a recording of the electrical potentials generated by myocardial cells. Its routine intraoperative use allows detection of dysrhythmias, myocardial ischemia, conduction abnormalities, pacemaker malfunction, and electrolyte disturbances. Because of the small voltage potentials being measured, artifact rejection remains a major problem of electrocardiography. Patient or lead wire movement, electrosurgical units,

60-cycle interference, and faulty electrodes can simulate dysrhythmias. Monitoring filters incorporated into the amplifier may lessen artifacts but can lead to distortion of the ST segment and confuse the diagnosis of ischemia. Digital readout of heart rate may be misleading because of the monitor's misinterpretation of artifacts or large T waves—often seen in pediatric patients—as QRS complexes.

Depending on equipment availability, a preinduction rhythm strip should be printed or frozen on the monitor's screen to compare with intraoperative tracings. To properly interpret ST segment changes, the electrocardiograph must be standardized so that a 1-mV signal results in a 10-mm deflection. Newer units continuously analyze ST segments for early detection of myocardial ischemia. The audible beep associated with each QRS complex should be set loud enough for detection of rate and rhythm changes when the anesthesiologist's visual attention is diverted to other responsibilities. Some electrocardiographs are capable of intrepreting dysrhythmias and storing aberrant QRS complexes for further analysis. However, the interference caused by electrosurgical units has limited the usefulness of automated arrhythmia analysis in the operating room.

CENTRAL VENOUS CATHETERIZATION

Indications

Central venous catheterization is indicated for (1) monitoring central venous pressure for the fluid

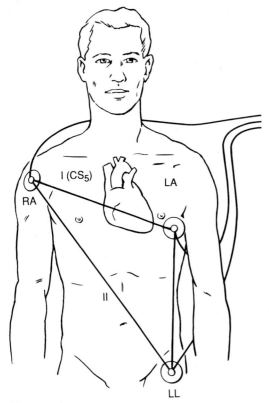

Figure 6–15. Anterior and lateral ischemia can be detected placing the left arm lead (LA) at the V_5 position. When lead I is selected on the monitor, a modified V_5 lead (CS_5) is displayed. Lead II allows detection of dysrhythmias and inferior wall ischemia.

management of hypovolemia and shock, (2) infusion of caustic drugs and hyperalimentation, (3) aspiration of air embolism, (4) insertion of transcutaneous pacing leads, and (5) gaining venous access in patients with poor peripheral veins.

Contraindications

Contraindications include renal cell tumor extension into the right atrium or fungating tricuspid valve vegetations. Other contraindications relate to the cannulation site. For example, internal jugular vein can-

nulation is relatively contraindicated in patients who are anticoagulated or who have had an ipsilateral carotid endarterectomy because of the possibility of unintentional carotid artery puncture.

Techniques & Complications

Measurement of central venous pressure involves introducing a catheter into a vein so that the catheter's tip lies just above the junction of the superior vena cava and the right atrium. Because this location exposes the catheter tip to intrathoracic pressure, inspiration will increase or decrease central venous pressure depending on whether ventilation is controlled or spontaneous. Measurement of central venous pressure is made with a water column (cm H_2O) or, preferably, an electronic transducer (mm Hg). Most clinicians measure venous pressures during end-expiration.

Cannulation is possible at various sites. Long-term catheterization of the subclavian vein is associated with a low incidence of bacteremia. This is offset by a significant risk of pneumothorax during insertion. The right internal jugular vein provides a combination of accessibility and safety (Table 6–1). There are at least three different cannulation techniques: (1) catheter over a needle (similar to peripheral catheterization), (2) catheter through a needle (requiring a large bone needle stick), and (3) catheter over a guide wire (Seldinger's technique). The latter is illustrated in Figures 6–17A to 6–17D and described below.

The patient is placed in the Trendelenburg position to decrease the risk of air embolism and to distend the internal jugular vein. The two heads of the sternocleidomastoid muscle and the clavicle form three sides of a triangle (Figure 6–17A). Venous catheterization requires full aseptic technique. After preparing the skin with iodophor solution, a 25-gauge needle is used to infiltrate the apex of the triangle with local anesthetic. The internal jugular vein is found by advancing the 25-gauge needle—or a 23-gauge needle in heavier patients—toward the ipsilateral nipple at an angle of 30 degrees to the skin (Figure 6–17B). Aspiration of blood confirms the vein's location. The possibility of carotid puncture is ruled out by transducing the waveform or comparing the blood's color or PaO_2 with an arterial sample. An 18-gauge thin-wall needle is advanced along the same path as the locator needle. When free blood flow is achieved, a J-wire with a 3-mm radius of curvature is introduced (Figure 6–

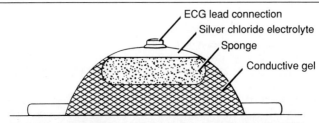

Figure 6–16. A cross-sectional view of a silver chloride electrode.

Table 6–1. Relative rating of central venous access technique.
(In each category, 1 = best, 5 = worst.)

	Basilic	External Jugular	Internal Jugular	Subclavian	Femoral
Ease of cannulation	1	2	4	5	3
Long-term use	4	3	2	1	5
Success rate (pulmonary artery catheter placement)	4	5	1	2	3
Complications (technique-related)	1	2	4	5	3

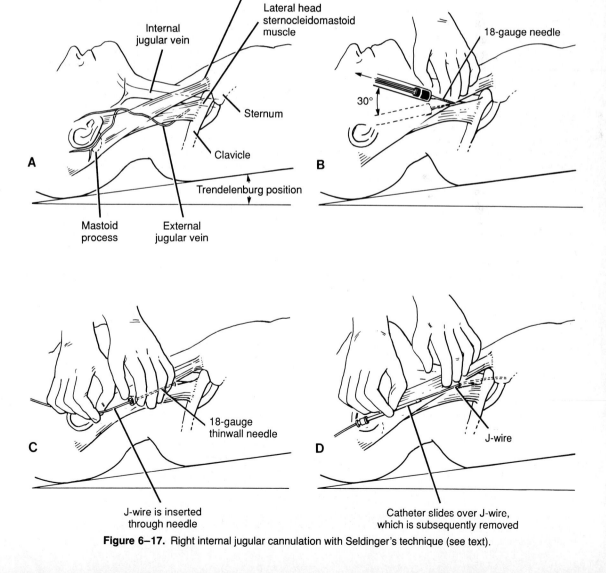

Figure 6–17. Right internal jugular cannulation with Seldinger's technique (see text).

17C). The needle is removed, and a catheter—preferably Silastic—is advanced over the wire (Figure 6–17D). The catheter is then secured, and sterile dressings are applied. Correct location is confirmed with a chest radiograph. The catheter's tip should not be allowed to migrate into the heart chambers.

The risks of central venous cannulation include infection, air embolism, dysrhythmias (indicating that the catheter tip is in the right atrium or ventricle), hematoma, pneumothorax, hemothorax, hydrothorax, chylothorax, cardiac perforation, cardiac tamponade, trauma to nearby nerves and arteries, embolization, and thrombosis. Some of these complications can be attributed to poor technique.

Clinical Considerations

Normal cardiac function requires adequate ventricular filling by venous blood. Central venous pressure approximates right atrial pressure, which is a major determinant of right ventricular end-diastolic volume. In healthy hearts, right and left ventricular performance is parallel, so that left ventricular filling can also be judged by central venous pressure.

The shape of the central venous waveform corresponds to the events of cardiac contraction (Figure 6–18): *a* waves due to atrial contraction are absent in atrial fibrillation and exaggerated in junctional rhythms (cannon waves); *c* waves are due to tricuspid valve elevation during early ventricular contraction; *v* waves reflect venous return against a closed tricuspid valve; and the *x* and *y* descents are probably caused by the downward displacement of the ventricle during systole and tricuspid valve opening during diastole.

PULMONARY ARTERY CATHETERIZATION

Indications

As familiarization with pulmonary artery catheters increases, so do the indications for their insertion (Table 6–2). Basically, pulmonary artery catheterization is indicated whenever it is necessary to know cardiac indices, preload, volume status, or the degree of mixed venous blood oxygenation.

Contraindications

Relative contraindications to pulmonary artery catheterization include complete left bundle branch block (because of the risk of complete heart block), Wolff-Parkinson-White syndrome, and Ebstein's malformation (because of possible tachyarrhythmias). A catheter with pacing capability is better suited to these situations. A balloon-flotation catheter may serve as a nidus of infection in septic patients or thrombus formation in those prone to hypercoagulation.

Techniques & Complications

Although various pulmonary artery catheters are available, the most popular design integrates four lumens into a 7F catheter, 110 cm long, with a polyvinylchloride body (Figure 6–19). The lumens house the following features: (1) wiring to connect the thermistor near the catheter tip to a thermodilution cardiac output computer; (2) an air channel for inflation of the balloon; (3) a proximal passage for infusions, cardiac output injections, and measurements of right atrial pressures; and (4) a distal passage for aspiration of

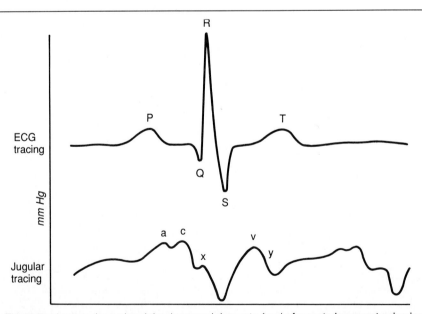

Figure 6–18. The upward waves *(a, c, v)* and the downward descents *(x, y)* of a central venous tracing in relation to the electrocardiogram. (Reproduced, with permission, from Gravenstein JS, Paulus DA: *Monitoring Practice in Clinical Anesthesia.* Lippincott, 1982.)

Table 6–2. Indications for pulmonary artery catheterization.

Cardiac disease
    Coronary artery disease with left ventricular dysfunction or recent infarction
    Valvular heart disease
    Heart failure (eg cardiomyopathy, pericardial tamponade, cor pulmonale)
Pulmonary disease
    Acute respiratory failure (eg adult respiratory distress syndrome)
    Severe chronic obstructive pulmonary disease
Complex fluid management
    Shock
    Sepsis
    Acute renal failure
    Acute burn patients
    Hemorrhagic pancreatitis
Specific surgical procedures
    Coronary artery bypass grafting
    Valve replacement
    Pericardiectomy
    Aortic cross clamping (eg aortic aneurysm repair)
    Sitting craniotomies
    Portal systemic shunts
High-risk obstetrics
    Severe toxemia
    Placental abruption

mixed venous blood samples and measurements of pulmonary artery pressure.

Insertion of a pulmonary artery catheter requires central venous access, which can be accomplished by the Seldinger technique, described above. Instead of a central venous catheter, a dilator and sheath are threaded over the guide wire. The sheath's lumen accommodates the pulmonary artery catheter after removal of the dilator and guide wire (Figure 6–20).

Prior to insertion, the flotation catheter is checked by inflating and deflating its balloon and irrigating the proximal and distal lumens with heparinized saline. The distal port is connected to a transducer which is zeroed to the patient's midaxillary line.

The catheter is advanced through the sheath and into the left internal jugular vein. At approximately 15 cm, the distal tip should enter the right atrium, and a central venous tracing that varies with respiration confirms an intrathoracic position. The balloon is inflated with air according to the manufacturer's recommendations (usually 1.5 mL). Once the catheter is in the right atrium, the balloon must always be inflated during catheter advancement to protect the endocardium from the catheter tip and to allow the right ventricle's cardiac output to direct the catheter's forward migration. Conversely, the balloon is always deflated during withdrawal. During advancement, the electrocardiograph is monitored for dysrhythmias. Transient ectopy due to irritation of the right ventricular endocardium by the balloon and catheter tip is common but rarely requires treatment with intravenous lidocaine. A sudden increase in the *systolic* pressure on the distal tracing indicates a right ventricular location of the catheter tip (Figure 6–21). Entry into the pulmonary artery normally occurs by 35–45 cm and is heralded by a sudden increase in *diastolic* pressure.

To prevent catheter knotting, the balloon should be deflated and the catheter withdrawn if pressure changes do not occur at expected distances. In particularly difficult cases (low cardiac output, pulmonary hypertension, or congenital heart anomalies), flotation of the catheter may be enhanced by having the patient inhale deeply; by positioning the patient in a head-up, right lateral tilt position; by injecting iced saline through the proximal lumen to stiffen the catheter (increasing the risk of perforation); or by administering a small dose of inotropic agent to increase cardiac output.

After attaining a pulmonary artery position, minimal catheter advancement results in a pulmonary capillary wedge waveform. The pulmonary artery tracing should reappear when the balloon is deflated. Wedging before maximal balloon inflation signals an overwedged position, and the catheter should be

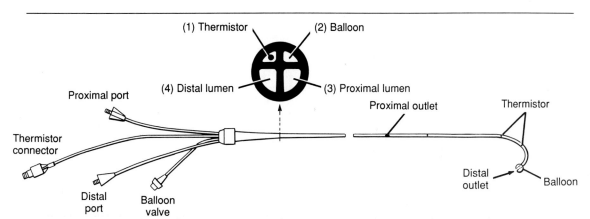

Figure 6–19. Balloon-tipped pulmonary artery flotation catheter (Swan-Ganz catheter). (Reproduced, with permission, from Blitt CD: Monitoring in Anesthesia and Critical Care Medicine, 1nd ed. Churchill Livingstone, 1990.)

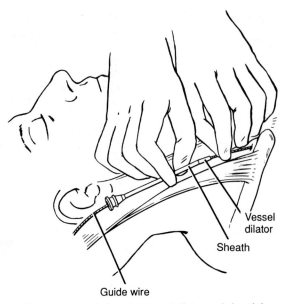

Figure 6–20. A percutaneous introducer consisting of a vessel dilator and sheath is passed over the guide wire.

slightly withdrawn (with the balloon down, of course). Because pulmonary artery rupture carries a 50–70% mortality rate and usually occurs because of balloon overinflation, the frequency of wedge readings should be minimized. Pulmonary artery pressure—not wedge pressure—should be continuously monitored to detect catheter migration.

Correct catheter position can be confirmed by a lateral chest radiograph. Although most catheters migrate caudally and to the right side, occasionally a catheter will wedge anterior to the vena cava. In this position, true pulmonary capillary pressures may be less than alveolar pressures, resulting in spuriously elevated measurements.

The numerous complications of pulmonary artery catheterization include those associated with central venous cannulation plus bacteremia, endocarditis, thrombogenesis, pulmonary infarction, pulmonary artery rupture (especially in patients who are anticoagulated, elderly, female, or have pulmonary hypertension), catheter knotting, dysrhythmias, conduction abnormalities, and pulmonary valvular damage. Even

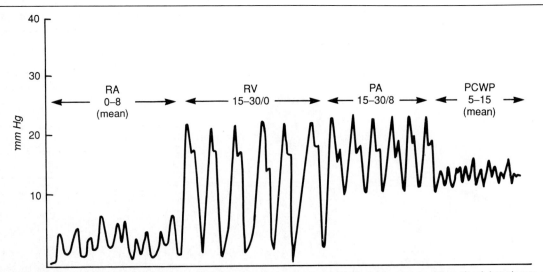

Figure 6–21. Normal pressure values and waveforms as a pulmonary artery catheter is advanced from the right atrium to a wedged position in a pulmonary artery.

nominal hemoptysis should not be ignored, since it may herald pulmonary artery rupture. Prompt placement of a double-lumen endotracheal tube may maintain adequate oxygenation by the unaffected lung.

Clinical Considerations

The introduction of Swan-Ganz pulmonary artery catheters into the operating room revolutionized the intraoperative management of critically ill patients. Catheterization of the pulmonary artery allows more precise estimations of left ventricular preload than central venous catheterization or physical examination. Additionally, it allows sampling of mixed venous blood and detection of air embolism and myocardial ischemia. Catheters with self-contained thermistors measure cardiac output, from which a multitude of hemodynamic values can be derived (Table 6–3). New catheter designs incorporate electrodes that allow intracavitary electrocardiography and pacing. Optional fiberoptic bundles can continuously determine the oxygen saturation of mixed venous blood.

Starling demonstrated the relationship between left ventricular function and left ventricular end-diastolic muscle fiber length, which is usually proportionate to end-diastolic volume. If compliance is not abnormally decreased (eg, by myocardial ischemia, overload, or pericardial tamponade), left ventricular end-diastolic *pressure* should also reflect fiber length. In the presence of a normal mitral valve, left atrial pressure approaches left ventricular pressure during diastolic filling. The left atrium connects with the right side of the heart through the pulmonary vasculature. The distal lumen of a correctly wedged pulmonary artery catheter is isolated from right-sided pressures by balloon inflation. Its distal opening is exposed only to capillary pressure, which—in the absence of high airway pressures or pulmonary vascular disease—equals left atrial pressure. In fact, aspiration through the distal port during balloon inflation samples arterialized blood. This string of assumptions and relationships forms the rationale for monitoring pulmonary capillary wedge pressure—ie, it is an indirect method of measuring left ventricular fiber length and, therefore, ventricular function.

While central venous catheterization accurately reflects right ventricular function, a pulmonary artery catheter is indicated if either ventricle is markedly depressed, causing disassociation of right- and left-sided hemodynamics. Central venous pressures are not predictive of pulmonary capillary pressures in patients with ejection fractions less than 0.50. However, even pulmonary artery wedge pressures do not always predict left ventricular end-diastolic pressures (Table 6–4).

CARDIAC OUTPUT

Indications

Patients who benefit from measurements of pulmonary artery pressure also benefit from cardiac output determination. In fact, to completely use the information available from flotation catheters, cardiac outputs must be obtained (Table 6–3). For these reasons, any patient being exposed to the risks of pulmonary artery catheterization should receive the benefits of cardiac output measurements. Perfection of noninvasive techniques may eventually lead to routine intraoperative cardiac output monitoring.

Contraindications

Cardiac output measurement by thermodilution adds no contraindications beyond those for pulmonary artery catheterization.

Techniques & Complications

A. Thermodilution: The injection of a quantity (2.5, 5, or 10 mL) of fluid that is below body temperature (usually room temperature or iced) into the right atrium changes the temperature of blood in contact with a thermistor in the pulmonary artery. The degree

Table 6–3. Hemodynamic variables derived from pulmonary artery catheterization data.

Variable	Formula	Normal	Units
Cardiac index	$\dfrac{\text{Cardiac output (L/min)}}{\text{Body surface area (m}^2\text{)}}$	2.8–4.2	L/min/m²
Total peripheral resistance	$\dfrac{\text{MAP (mm Hg)} - \text{CVP (mm Hg)} \times 80}{\text{Cardiac output (L/min)}}$	1200–1500	Dynes-s-cm^{-5}
Pulmonary vascular resistance	$\dfrac{\text{PA} - \text{PCWP} \times 80}{\text{Cardiac output (L/min)}}$	100–300	Dynes-s-cm^{-5}
Stroke volume	$\dfrac{\text{Cardiac output (L/min)} \times 1000}{\text{Heart rate (beats/min)}}$	60–90	mL/beat
Stroke index (SI)	$\dfrac{\text{Stroke volume (mL/beat)}}{\text{Body surface area}}$	30–65	mL/beat/m²
Right ventricular stroke-work index	0.0136 (PA − CVP) × SI	5–10	g-m/beat/m²
Left ventricular stroke-work index	0.0136 (MAP − PCWP) × SI	45–60	g-m/beat/m²

Table 6–4. Pulmonary capillary wedge pressure wrongly estimates left ventricular end-diastolic pressure in certain conditions.

PCWP > LVEDP
 1. Mitral stenosis
 2. Left atrial myxoma
 3. Pulmonary venous obstruction
 4. Elevated alveolar pressure
PCWP < LVEDP
 1. Decreased left ventricular compliance (stiff ventricle or LVEDP > 25 mm Hg)
 2. Aortic insufficiency

---

of change is inversely proportionate to cardiac output: Temperature change is minimal if there is a high blood flow but pronounced if flow is low. Plotting the temperature change as a function of time produces a **thermodilution curve.** Cardiac output is determined by a computer that integrates the area under the curve. Accurate measurements depend upon (1) rapid and smooth injection at end-expiration, (2) precisely known injectate temperature and volume, (3) correct entry of the calibration factors for the specific type of pulmonary artery catheter and injectate used into the cardiac output computer, and (4) avoidance of measurements during electrocautery. Tricuspid regurgitation and cardiac shunts invalidate results because only right ventricular output is actually being measured. Rapid infusion of iced injectate has rarely resulted in cardiac dysrhythmias. Other possible complications involve those of central venous cannulation and pulmonary artery catheterization.

B. Dye Dilution: If indocyanine green dye is injected through a central venous catheter, its appearance in the arterial circulation can be measured by analyzing arterial samples with a densitometer. The area under the resulting **dye indicator curve** is related to cardiac output. The dye-dilution technique introduces the problems of indicator recirculation, arterial blood sampling, and background tracer buildup.

C. Ultrasonography: A two-dimensional image of the heart can be obtained by passing a probe containing piezoelectric crystals into the esophagus. **Transesophageal echocardiography** assesses left ventricular filling (end-diastolic volume and end-systolic volume), ejection fraction, wall motion abnormalities, and contractility. It is a sensitive indicator of myocardial ischemia and air embolism (including paradoxic air embolism).

Pulsed Doppler is a related technology that measures the velocity of aortic blood flow. Combined with transesophageal echocardiography, which determines aortic cross-sectional area, this instrument can measure stroke volume and cardiac output. Further applications of ultrasonography include **transesophageal Doppler color flow mapping,** which evaluates valvular function and intracardiac shunting. Blood flow information is represented by color (indicating direction of flow) and intensity (indicating velocity of flow).

The major limitation of all of these systems is their expense.

Continuous-wave suprasternal Doppler also measures aortic blood velocity. Instead of requiring transesophageal echocardiography, it uses a nomogram based on the patient's age, sex, and weight to estimate aortic cross-sectional area for cardiac output calculations. While considerably less expensive, the use of a nomogram introduces the possibility of error, particularly in patients with aortic disease.

D. Thoracic Bioimpedance: Changes in thoracic volume cause changes in thoracic resistance (bioimpedance). If thoracic bioimpedance changes are measured following ventricular depolarization, stroke volume can be continuously determined. This noninvasive technique requires four pairs of electrocardiographic electrodes in order to inject sample microcurrents and to sense bioimpedance on both sides of the chest. Disadvantages of thoracic bioimpedance include susceptibility to electrical interference and reliance upon correct electrode positioning. As with suprasternal Doppler, the accuracy of this technique is questionable in several groups of patients, including those with aortic valve disease or previous heart surgery.

E. Fick Principle: The amount of oxygen consumed by an individual equals the difference between arterial and venous oxygen content multiplied by cardiac output:

$$\text{Oxygen consumption} = \text{Arterial/venous } O_2 \text{ difference} \times \text{Cardiac output}$$

Therefore,

$$\text{Cardiac output} = \frac{\text{Oxygen consumption}}{\text{Arterial/venous } O_2 \text{ content difference}} = \frac{\dot{V}O_2}{C_aO_2 - C_vO_2}$$

Mixed venous and arterial oxygen content are easily determined if a pulmonary artery catheter and arterial line are in place. Oxygen consumption can be calculated from the difference between oxygen content in inspired and expired gas. Variations of the Fick principle are the basis of all indicator-dilution methods of cardiac output determination.

Clinical Considerations

Cardiac output measurements allow calculation of many indices that reflect the function of the entire circulatory system. Pulmonary artery pressures are difficult to interpret without knowing cardiac output. For instance, a patient with normal blood pressure and pulmonary capillary wedge pressure may have poor vital organ perfusion due to a low cardiac output and high systemic vascular resistance. Effective pharmacologic manipulation of preload, afterload, and contractility depends upon accurate determination of cardiac output.

RESPIRATORY SYSTEM MONITORS

PRECORDIAL & ESOPHAGEAL STETHOSCOPES

Indications

Many anesthesiologists believe that all anesthetized patients should be monitored with a precordial or esophageal stethoscope.

Contraindications

Instrumentation of the esophagus should be avoided in patients with esophageal varices or strictures.

Techniques & Complications

A precordial stethoscope (Wenger chestpiece) is a heavy, bell-shaped piece of metal placed over the chest or suprasternal notch. Although its weight tends to maintain its position, double-sided adhesive disks provide an acoustic seal to the patient's skin (Figure 6–22). Various chestpieces are available, but the child size works well for most patients. The stethoscope is connected to the anesthesiologist by extension tubing. A molded monaural earpiece allows simultaneous monitoring of the stethoscope and the operating room environment. Complications of precordial monitoring are extremely unlikely, though local allergic reactions, skin abrasion, and pain during removal of the adhesive disk rarely occur.

The esophageal stethoscope is a soft plastic catheter (8–24F) with balloon-covered distal openings (Figure 6–23). Although the quality of breath and heart sounds is much better with an esophageal stethoscope, its use is limited to intubated patients. Temperature probes and even electrocardiographic leads have been incorporated into stethoscope design. Placement through the mouth or nose can occasionally cause mucosal irritation and bleeding. Rarely, the stethoscope slides into the trachea instead of the esophagus, resulting in a gas leak around the endotracheal tube cuff.

Clinical Considerations

The information provided by a precordial or esophageal stethoscope includes confirmation of ventilation, quality of breath sounds (eg, wheezing), regularity of heart rate, and quality of heart tones (muffled tones are associated with decreased cardiac output). However, the confirmation of bilateral breath sounds after endotracheal intubation should be made with a more sensitive binaural stethoscope.

BREATHING CIRCUIT PRESSURE & EXHALED TIDAL VOLUME

Indications

Both of these respiratory parameters are routinely measured during general anesthesia.

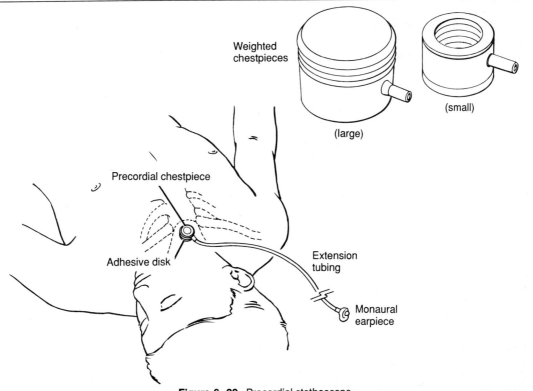

Figure 6–22. Precordial stethoscope.

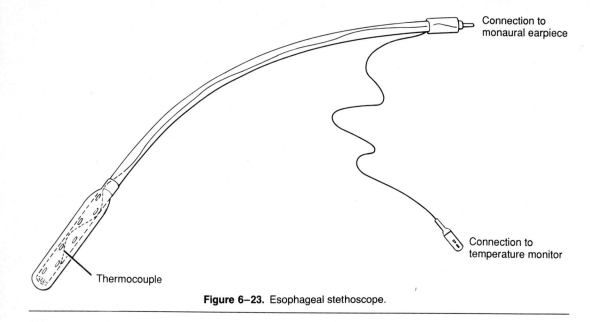

Connection to
monaural earpiece

Connection to
temperature monitor

Thermocouple

Figure 6–23. Esophageal stethoscope.

Contraindications

None.

Techniques & Complications

A pressure gauge usually measures breathing circuit pressure somewhere between the expiratory and inspiratory unidirectional valves, the location depending upon the model of anesthetic machine. A Wright respirometer measures exhaled tidal volume at the expiratory limb of the breathing tubes, just before the expiratory valve (Figure 4–6). Since both devices require connection to the breathing circuit, they increase the potential for a circuit leak or disconnection.

Clinical Considerations

Breathing circuit pressure usually reflects airway pressure. A rise in pressure may signal worsening pulmonary compliance, an increase in tidal volume, or an obstruction in the breathing circuit. A drop in pressure may indicate an improvement in compliance, a decrease in tidal volume, or a leak in the circuit. However, if the circuit pressure is being measured at the CO_2 absorber, it will not always mirror the pressure in the patient's airway. For example, clamping the expiratory limb of the breathing tubes during exhalation will prevent the patient's breath from exiting the lungs. Despite this persistence in airway pressure, a pressure gauge at the absorber will read zero due to the intervening one-way valve.

Changes in exhaled tidal volume usually represent changes in ventilator settings but can also be due to circuit leaks, disconnections, or ventilator malfunction. The Wright respirometer is prone to errors due to inertia, friction, and water condensation (see Chapter 4). Furthermore, the measurement of tidal volumes

includes gas that has been lost to the circuit in the form of gas compression and breathing tube expansion. This difference between the volume of gas delivered to the circuit and the volume of gas actually reaching the patient becomes significant with long compliant breathing tubes, high airway pressures, and rapid respiratory rates.

PULSE OXIMETRY

Indications

Pulse oximeters are mandatory intraoperative monitors. They are particularly useful when frequent measurements of patient oxygenation are required because of preexisting lung disease (eg, bleomycin toxicity), the nature of the surgical procedure (eg, hiatal hernia repair), or the requirements of special anesthetic technique (eg, one-lung anesthesia). Pulse oximeters are also helpful in monitoring neonates at risk for retinopathy of prematurity.

Contraindications

None.

Techniques & Complications

Pulse oximeters combine the principles of oximetry and plethysmography to noninvasively measure oxygen saturation in arterial blood. A sensor containing light sources (two light-emitting diodes) and a light detector (a photodiode) is placed across a finger, toe, ear lobe, or any other perfused tissue that can be transilluminated.

Oximetry depends upon the observation that oxygenated and reduced hemoglobin differ in their absorption of red and infrared light (**Lambert-Beer law**). Specifically, oxyhemoglobin (HbO_2) absorbs more infrared light (eg, 990 nm), while deoxyhemoglobin absorbs more red light (eg, 660 nm). Since deoxy-hemoglobin absorbs more red light, it appears blue or cyanotic to the naked eye. Thus, the change in light absorption during arterial pulsations is the basis of oximetry determinations (Figure 6–24). The ratio of the absorptions at a red and infrared wavelength is analyzed by a microprocessor to give the oxygen saturation reading. Arterial pulsations are identified by plethysmography, allowing correction for light absorption by nonpulsating venous blood and tissue. Heat from the light source or sensor pressure may rarely result in tissue damage if the monitor is not periodically moved. No user calibration is required.

Clinical Considerations

In addition to oxygen saturation, pulse oximeters provide an indication of tissue perfusion (pulse amplitude) and measure heart rate. Because oxygen saturation is normally close to 100%, only gross abnormalities are detectable in most anesthetized patients. For example, endobronchial intubation will usually go undetected in the absence of lung disease or low inspired oxygen concentrations. Depending upon a particular patient's oxygen-hemoglobin dissociation curve, a 90% saturation may indicate a PaO_2 of less than 65 mm Hg.

Because carboxyhemoglobin (COHb) and oxy-hemoglobin absorb light at 660 nm identically, pulse oximeters that only compare two wavelengths of light will register a falsely high reading in patients suffering from carbon monoxide poisoning. Methemoglobin has the same absorption coefficient at both red and infrared wavelengths. The resulting 1:1 absorption ratio corresponds to a saturation reading of 85%. Thus, met-hemogobinemia causes a falsely low saturation reading when SaO_2 is actually greater than 85% and a falsely high reading if SaO_2 is actually less than 85%. In contrast, fetal hemoglobin and bilirubin do not affect pulse oximeter function.

Most pulse oximeters are inaccurate at low oxygen saturations. Ear probes detect changes in saturation sooner than finger probes. Causes of pulse oximetry artifact include the following: (1) excessive ambient light; (2) motion; (3) methylene blue dye; (4) venous pulsations in a dependent limb; (5) low perfusion (eg, low cardiac output, very low hemoglobin, hypothermia, increased systemic vascular resistance); and (6) leakage of light from the light-emitting diode to the photodiode, bypassing the arterial bed (optical shunting). Nevertheless, pulse oximetry can be an invaluable aid to the rapid diagnosis of catastrophic hypoxemia, as may occur in unrecognized esophageal intubation. It furthers the goal of monitoring oxygen delivery to vital organs.

END-TIDAL CARBON DIOXIDE ANALYSIS

Indications

Determination of end-tidal CO_2 concentration to confirm adequate ventilation is useful during all anesthetic techniques. Ventilator control of intracranial hypertension by lowering $PaCO_2$ is easily monitored by expired CO_2 analysis. A rapid fall of end-tidal CO_2 is a sensitive indicator of air embolism, a major complication of sitting craniotomies.

Contraindications

None.

Techniques & Complications

There are two types of capnographs in common use. Both rely on the absorption of infrared light by CO_2 (Figure 6–25).

A. Flow-Through (Mainstream): Flow-through capnographs measure CO_2 passing through an adaptor placed in the breathing circuit (Figure 6–26). Infrared light transmission through the gas is measured and CO_2 concentration determined by the monitor. Because of problems with drift, older flow-through models self-zeroed during inspiration. Thus, they were incapable of detecting inspired CO_2, as would occur with a breathing circuit malfunction (eg, sticking unidirectional valves or absorber exhaustion). The weight of the sensor causes traction on the endotracheal tube, and its radiant heat generation has caused skin burns. Newer designs have addressed these problems.

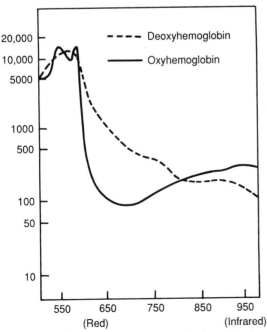

Figure 6–24. Oxyhemoglobin and deoxyhemoglobin differ in their absorption of red and infrared light.

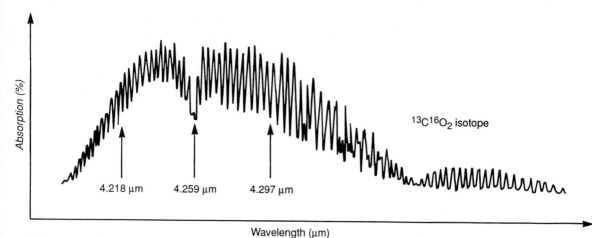

Figure 6–25. Absorption spectrum for CO_2. (Reproduced, with permission, from Scurr C, Feldman S: *Scientific Foundations of Anesthesia.* Year Book, 1982.)

B. Aspiration (Sidestream): Aspiration capnographs continuously suction gas from the breathing circuit into a sample cell within the monitor (Figure 6–27). Carbon dioxide concentration is determined by comparing infrared light absorption in the sample cell with a chamber free of CO_2. Continuous aspiration of anesthetic gas essentially represents a leak in the breathing circuit that will contaminate the operating room unless it is scavenged or returned to the breathing system. High sampling rates usually increase sensitivity. However, if tidal volumes are small (eg, pediatric patients), a high rate of aspiration may entrain fresh gas from the circuit and dilute end-tidal CO_2 measurement. These units are zeroed to room air, but calibration requires a source of known CO_2 concentra-

tion (usually 5%). Expiratory valve malfunction is detected by the presence of CO_2 in inspired gas. Although inspiratory valve failure also results in rebreathing CO_2, this is not as readily apparent since part of the inspiratory volume will still be free of CO_2, causing the monitor to read zero during part of the inspiratory phase. Aspiration units are prone to water precipitation in the aspiration tube or sampling cell that can cause obstruction of the sampling line and erroneous readings.

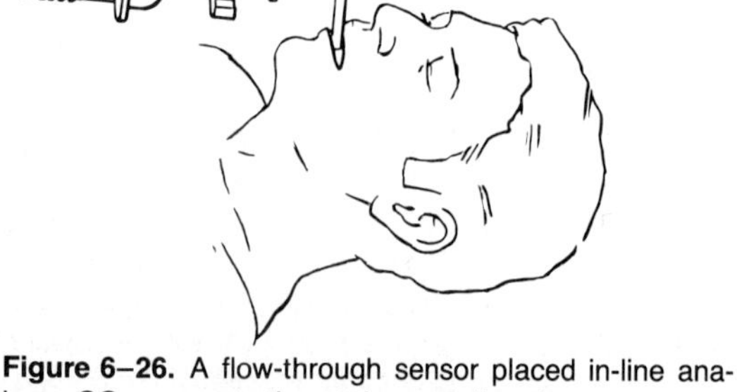

Clinical Considerations

Other gases (eg, nitrous oxide) also absorb infrared light, leading to a "pressure broadening" effect. To minimize the error introduced by nitrous oxide, various modifications and filters have been incorporated into monitor design. Capnographs rapidly and reliably indicate esophageal intubation—a common cause of anesthetic catastrophe. While there may be some CO_2 in the stomach from swallowing expired air, this should be washed out within a few breaths. Sudden cessation of CO_2 during the expiratory phase may indicate a circuit disconnection. The increased metabolic rate caused by malignant hyperthermia causes a marked rise in end-tidal CO_2.

The gradient between end-tidal CO_2 and arterial CO_2 (normally 2–5 mm Hg) reflects alveolar dead space (alveoli that are ventilated but not perfused). Any significant reduction in lung perfusion (air embolism, upright positions, decreased cardiac output, or decreased blood pressure) increases alveolar dead space, dilutes expired CO_2, and lessens end-tidal CO_2. True capnographs (as opposed to capnometers) display a waveform of CO_2 concentration that allows recognition of a variety of conditions (Figure 6–28).

In summary, the capnograph is a valuable monitor of the respiratory, cardiac, and anesthetic breathing systems.

Figure 6–26. A flow-through sensor placed in-line analyzes CO_2 concentration at the sampling site.

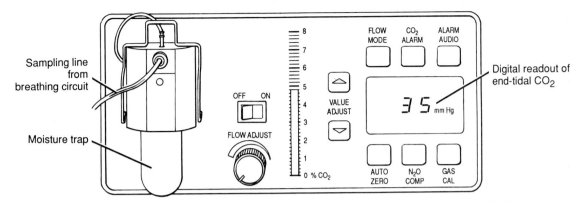

Figure 6–27. An aspiration capnometer draws gas from the breathing circuit into a sample chamber within the monitor. A capnograph would also display a waveform.

TRANSCUTANEOUS OXYGEN & CARBON DIOXIDE MONITORS

Indications

Although useful in the management of many critically ill patients, transcutaneous gas monitors have gained widest acceptance in pediatric intensive care units.

Contraindications

None.

Techniques & Complications

A sensor containing a CO_2 or oxygen (Clark) electrode—or both—and a heating element is attached to the skin (Figure 6–29). The oxygen electrode senses alterations in gas composition by changes in electrical conductivity of an electrolyte solution (polarography). Most CO_2 electrodes measure changes in pH:

$$pH = 0.97(\log PCO_2)$$

The heating element vasodilates ("arteriolizes") capillary vessels and increases gas diffusion by liquefying the stratum corneum. Dry standard gases and room air can be used for calibration and zeroing. Depending on blood flow, skin thickness, and heat settings, most sensors require 15–30 minutes to reach a stable plateau. Sensor location should be changed every 2

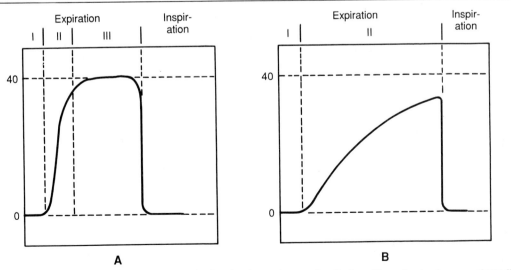

Figure 6–28. **A:** A normal capnograph demonstrating the three phases of expiration: Phase I—dead space; phase II—mixture of dead space and alveolar gas; phase III—alveolar gas plateau. **B:** Capnograph of a patient with severe chronic obstructive pulmonary disease. No plateau is reached before the next inspiration. The gradient between end-tidal CO_2 and arterial CO_2 is increased.

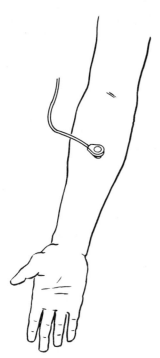

Figure 6–29. A transcutaneous oxygen sensor attached to a patient's forearm.

hours to prevent skin burns, especially if perfusion is low.

Clinical Considerations

Transcutaneous sensors actually measure cutaneous partial pressures, which approach arterial values if cardiac output and perfusion are adequate. $P_{tc}O_2$ (P_sO_2) is approximately 75% of PaO_2, and $P_{tc}CO_2$ (P_sCO_2) is 130% of $PaCO_2$. A gradual drop in $P_{tc}O_2$ may be due to a lower PaO_2 or a decrease in skin perfusion. *The lack of consistent correlation between $P_{tc}O_2$ and Pa_{O2} should not be viewed as a fault of this technology but rather as an early warning of inadequate tissue perfusion.* The $P_{tc}O_2$ index is the ratio of $P_{tc}O_2$ to PaO_2 and varies proportionately with cardiac output and peripheral blood flow. A rapid drop in $P_{tc}O_2$ to 21 mm Hg indicates a displaced sensor that is exposed to room air.

Transcutaneous monitoring has not gained the popularity of pulse oximetry because of its warm-up time, difficulties of sensor maintenance, and complex interpretation. This is unfortunate, because it is a true indicator of tissue—albeit skin—oxygen delivery. Pulse oximetry and transcutaneous oxygen should be viewed as complimentary, not competing technologies. For example, a fall in $P_{tc}O_2$ in the face of unchanging SaO_2 is a strong indication of poor tissue perfusion. Conjunctival oxygen sensors may increase interest in this technology, since they appear to be capable of noninvasively estimating arterial pH.

ANESTHETIC GAS ANALYSIS

Indications

Analysis of anesthetic gases could be useful during any procedure requiring general anesthesia.

Contraindications

There are no contraindications, though high costs have prevented widespread deployment of these units.

Techniques & Complications

The most common techniques for analyzing multiple anesthetic gases involve mass spectrometry, Raman spectroscopy, or infrared absorption. A vacuum pump inside a mass spectrometer draws a gas sample from a side port in a breathing circuit elbow, through long tubing 1 mm in diameter, into the analyzer. Because of cost considerations, one mass spectrometer is usually shared by several operating rooms (a multiplexed system), and an inlet selector valve automatically switches sampling from one room to the next. The gas sample is ionized by an electron beam and passed through a magnetic field. The ions with the highest mass-to-charge ratio are least deflected and follow a curved path of greatest radius (Figure 6–30). The spectrum of ion deflection forms the basis of analysis. Gases with identical molecular weights (CO_2 and N_2O) are differentiated by the deflection of the fragments generated during electron beam bombardment.

Raman spectroscopy identifies and measures gas concentrations by analyzing the intensity of light emitted when a gas sample returns to its unexcited state

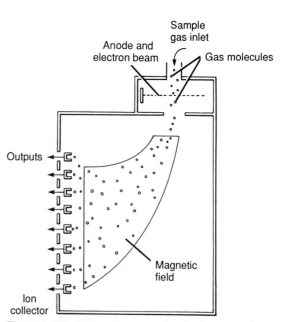

Figure 6–30. The mass spectrometer ionizes a gas sample and exposes it to a magnetic field. The degree of ion deflection determines its identity.

after being energized by a laser beam. Infrared units utilize a technique similar to that described for capnography.

Clinical Considerations

Although dedicated units are available, most mass spectrometers service more than one operating room. Therefore, gas samples are usually analyzed sequentially and results updated every 1–2 minutes. Newer units continuously measure CO_2 by infrared analysis and share the advantages of a separate capnograph. Other gases identified and quantified include nitrogen, oxygen, nitrous oxide, halothane, enflurane, and isoflurane. Rising end-tidal nitrogen quantitatively detects air embolism or leakage of air into the breathing system. Measurement of volatile agents guards against unintentional overdosage due to vaporizer malfunction or unintentional vaporizer misfilling. For example, an enflurane vaporizer partially filled with halothane will deliver a higher than expected anesthetic dose due to the differences in potency and vapor pressure of these agents.

One of mass spectrometry's disadvantages is that the constant suctioning of sample gas complicates the measurement of oxygen consumption during closed system techniques. In the presence of small tidal volumes or valveless Mapleson circuits, a high sampling rate may entrain fresh gas and dilute expired concentrations. The future of mass spectrometry may include the capability of noninvasive measurement of lung volume and cardiac output.

Mass spectrometers and Raman spectroscopy are equally accurate despite their basic technologic differences. Raman spectroscopy has the possible added advantages of a faster response time, self-calibration, and increased durability. Furthermore, the currently available Raman unit (the Rascal) is a stand-alone monitor that is not shared by multiple operating rooms.

Stand-alone units are also available that measure the concentration of volatile anesthetic by quartz oscillation or infrared absorption instead of mass spectrometry or Raman spectroscopy. Although less expensive, most of these are unable to detect improperly filled vaporizers since they cannot distinguish between agents. Newer units that utilize multiple wavelengths of infrared light and other variations of infrared technology are able to discriminate between volatile agents.

NEUROLOGIC SYSTEM MONITORS

ELECTROENCEPHALOGRAPHY

Indications

The electroencephalogram (EEG) is occasionally used during cerebrovascular surgery, cardiopulmonary bypass, and controlled hypotension to confirm the adequacy of cerebral oxygenation. Monitoring the depth of anesthesia with a full 16-lead, 8-channel EEG is rarely warranted considering the availability of simpler techniques (eg, lower esophageal contractility).

Contraindications

None.

Techniques & Complications

The EEG is a recording of electrical potentials generated by cells in the cerebral cortex. Although standard electrocardiographic electrodes can be used, silver disks containing a conductive gel are preferred. Platinum or stainless steel needle electrodes traumatize the scalp and have high impedance (resistance) but can be sterilized and placed in a surgical field. Electrode position (montage) is governed by the international 10–20 system (Figure 6–31). Electric potential differences between combinations of electrodes are filtered, amplified, and displayed by an oscilloscope or pen recorder.

Clinical Considerations

Acceptance of intraoperative electroencephalographic monitoring has been limited by its space requirements, difficult interpretation, and equivocal efficacy. The changes that accompany ischemia, such as decreased high-frequency activity, can be mimicked by hypothermia, anesthetic agents, electrolyte disturbances, and marked hypocapnia. Nonetheless, detection of electroencephalographic changes should lead to

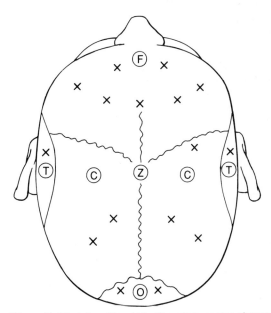

Figure 6–31. International 10–20 system montage letters refer to cranium location. F = frontal; C = coronal; T = temporal; O = occipital; Z = middle.

an immediate review of possible causes of cerebral ischemia before irreversible brain damage has a chance to occur.

The voluminous data generated by electroencephalography can be processed by several mathematical techniques (eg, periodic, aperiodic, and power spectrum analysis) to simplify interpretation. Unfortunately, this computer-assisted analysis usually sacrifices some degree of sensitivity. Monitors that only process information from one pair of electrodes inadequately detect focal ischemia. As automated processing and displays become more sophisticated, intraoperative electroencephalography will become more practical.

EVOKED POTENTIALS

Indications

Indications for intraoperative monitoring of evoked potentials include surgical procedures associated with possible neurologic injury: cardiopulmonary bypass, carotid endarterectomy, spinal fusion with Harrington rods, abdominal aortic aneurysm, and craniotomy. Global ischemia due to anesthetic overdose or hypoxia is detectable. Evoked potential monitoring facilitates probe localization during stereotactic neurosurgery.

Contraindications

Although there are no specific contraindications, this modality is severely limited by the availability of monitoring sites, equipment, and trained personnel.

Techniques & Complications

Evoked potential monitoring noninvasively assesses neural function by measuring electrophysiologic responses to sensory stimulation. Commonly monitored evoked potentials are visual, auditory, and somatosensory (Table 6–5). Only the latter is considered in this discussion.

A brief electrical current is delivered to a sensory or mixed peripheral nerve by a pair of electrodes. If the intervening pathway is intact, an evoked potential will be transmitted to the contralateral sensory cortex. This potential is measured by the international 10–20 scalp electrode montage. To differentiate the cortical response to a specific stimulus, multiple responses are averaged and background noise is eliminated. Evoked potentials are represented by a plot of voltage versus time. The resulting waveforms are analyzed for their **poststimulus latency** (the time between stimulation and potential detection) and **peak amplitude.** These are compared with baseline tracings. The significance of any change must be determined. Complications of evoked potential monitors are infrequent but include electrical shock, skin irritation, and pressure ischemia at the sites of electrode application.

Clinical Considerations

Evoked potentials are altered by many variables other than neural damage. The effect of anesthetics is complex and not easily summarized. In general, balanced anesthetic techniques (nitrous oxide, relaxants, and narcotics) cause minimal changes, while volatile agents (halothane, enflurane, and isoflurane) are best avoided. **Early-occurring (specific)** evoked potentials are less affected by anesthetics than **late-occurring (nonspecific)** responses. Physiologic (eg, blood pressure, temperature, and oxygen saturation) and pharmacologic factors should be kept as constant as possible.

Persistent obliteration of evoked potentials is predictive of postoperative neurologic deficiency. Unfortunately, because of their different anatomic pathways, *sensory* (dorsal spinal cord) evoked potential preservation does not guarantee normal *motor* (ventral spinal cord) function.

MISCELLANEOUS MONITORS

TEMPERATURE

Indications

The temperature of patients undergoing general anesthesia should be monitored. Very brief procedures (eg, under 15 minutes) may be an exception to this guideline.

Contraindications

There are no contraindications, though a particular monitoring site may be unsuitable in certain patients.

Table 6–5. Characteristics and uses of evoked potentials.

Type	Stimulus	Method of Delivering Stimulus	Surgical Procedure
Visual	Flashing lights	Light-emitting goggles	Pituitary tumor resection
Auditory	Clicks, tones	Ear transducer	Cerebellopontine angle tumor resection
Somatosensory	Electrical current	Electrodes	Spinal cord surgery

Techniques & Complications

Intraoperatively, temperature is usually measured by a thermistor or thermocouple. **Thermistors** are semiconductors whose resistance predictably decreases with warming. A **thermocouple** is a circuit of two dissimilar metals joined so that a potential difference is generated when the metals are at different temperatures. Disposable thermocouple and thermistor probes are available for monitoring the temperature of the tympanic membrane, rectum, nasopharynx, esophagus, bladder, and skin.

Complications of temperature monitoring are usually related to trauma caused by the probe (eg, rectal or tympanic membrane perforation).

Clinical Considerations

Each monitoring site has advantages and disadvantages. The **tympanic membrane** reflects brain temperature because the auditory canal's blood supply is the external carotid artery. Trauma during insertion and cerumen insulation detract from the routine use of tympanic probes. **Rectal** temperatures have a slow response to changes in *core temperature* (central blood temperature). **Nasopharyngeal** probes are prone to cause epistaxis but accurately measure core temperature if placed adjacent to the nasopharyngeal mucosa. Likewise, the thermistor on a **pulmonary artery catheter** measures core temperature. There is a variable correlation between **axillary** temperature and core temperature depending on skin perfusion. Liquid crystal adhesive strips placed on the **skin** are inadequate indicators of core body temperature during surgery. **Esophageal** temperature sensors, often incorporated into esophageal stethoscopes, provide the best combination of economy, performance, and safety. To avoid measuring the temperature of tracheal gases, the temperature sensor should be positioned behind the heart in the lower third of the esophagus. Conveniently, heart sounds are most prominent at this location.

URINE OUTPUT

Indications

Urinary bladder catheterization is the only reliable method of monitoring urine output. Insertion of a urinary catheter is indicated in patients with congestive heart failure, renal failure, advanced hepatic disease, or shock. Catheterization is routine in some surgical procedures such as cardiac surgery, aortic or renal vascular surgery, craniotomy, or procedures in which large fluid shifts are expected. Lengthy surgeries and intraoperative diuretic administration are other possible indications. Occasionally, postoperative bladder catheterization is indicated in patients having difficulty voiding in the recovery room after general or regional anesthesia.

Contraindications

Bladder catheterization should be avoided in patients at high risk for infection (eg, total hip replacement).

Techniques & Complications

Bladder catheterization is usually performed by surgical or nursing personnel. To avoid unnecessary trauma, a urologist should catheterize patients suspected of having abnormal urethral anatomy. A soft rubber Foley catheter is inserted into the bladder transurethrally and connected to a disposable calibrated collection chamber. To avoid urine reflux, the chamber should remain at a level below the bladder. Complications of catheterization include urethral trauma and urinary tract infections. Rapid decompression of a distended bladder can cause hypotension. Suprapubic catheterization with plastic tubing inserted through a large bone needle is an uncommon alternative.

Clinical Considerations

Urine output is a reflection of kidney perfusion and function. It is an indicator of renal, cardiovascular, and fluid volume status. Inadequate urine output (**oliguria**) is often arbitrarily defined as urine output of less than 0.5 mL/kg/h but actually is a function of the patient's concentrating ability and osmotic load. Urine electrolyte composition, osmolality, and specific gravity aid in the differential diagnosis of oliguria (Chapter 48).

PERIPHERAL NERVE STIMULATION

Indications

Because of the variation in patient sensitivity to neuromuscular blockade, the neuromuscular function of all patients receiving nondepolarizing muscle relaxants should be monitored. Additionally, peripheral nerve stimulation is helpful in assessing paralysis during rapid sequence inductions or during continuous infusions of succinylcholine. Finally, peripheral nerve stimulators can locate nerves to be blocked by regional anesthesia and can determine the extent of sensory blockade.

Contraindications

There are no contraindications to neuromuscular monitoring, though certain sites may be precluded by the surgical procedure.

Techniques & Complications

A peripheral nerve stimulator delivers a current of variable frequency to a pair of electrodes—either electrocardiographic silver chloride disks or subcutaneous needles—placed over a peripheral motor nerve. The evoked mechanical or electrical response of the innervated muscle is observed. Although electromyography provides a fast, accurate, and quantitative measure of neuromuscular transmission, visual or tactile observation of muscle contraction is adequate for clinical practice. The ulnar nerve's stimulation of the adductor pollicis muscle is most commonly monitored (Figure 6–32). Since it is the blockade of the neuromuscular junction that needs to be monitored, direct stimulation of muscle should be avoided by placing electrodes over the course of the nerve and not the muscle itself. To deliver a supramaximal stimulation to the underlying nerve, peripheral nerve stimulators must be capable of generating a 50-mA current across a 1000-ohm load. This current is quite uncomfortable for a conscious patient. Complications of nerve stimulation are limited to skin irritation and abrasion at the site of electrode attachment.

Clinical Considerations

The degree of neuromuscular blockade is monitored by applying various patterns of electrical stimulation (Figure 6–33). All stimuli are 200 μs in duration, of square-wave pattern, and of equal current intensity. A **twitch** is a single pulse that is delivered every second to every 10 seconds (1–0.1 Hz). Increasing blockade results in decreased evoked response to twitch stimulation.

Train-of-four stimulation denotes four successive twitch stimuli in 2 seconds (2 Hz). The twitches in a train-of-four pattern progressively fade as relaxation increases. The ratio of the responses to the first and fourth twitch is a sensitive indicator of nondepolarizing muscle relaxation. Because it is difficult to estimate the train-of-four ratio, it is more convenient to visually observe the sequential disappearance of the twitches, since this also correlates with the extent of blockade. Disappearance of the fourth twitch represents a 75% block, the third twitch an 80% block, and the second twitch a 90% block. Clinical relaxation usually requires 75–95% neuromuscular blockade.

Tetany at 50 or 100 Hz is a sensitive test of neuromuscular function. Sustained contraction for 5 seconds indicates adequate but not necessarily complete reversal from neuromuscular blockade. **Double-burst stimulation** (DBS) represents two variations of tetany that are less painful to the patient. The DBS$_{3,3}$ pattern of nerve stimulation consists of three short-lasting (200 μs), high-frequency bursts separated by 20-ms intervals (50 Hz) and followed 750 ms later by another three bursts. DBS$_{3,2}$ consists of three 200-μs impulses at 50 Hz followed 750 ms later by two such impulses. Double-burst stimulation is more sensitive than train-of-four stimulation in the clinical evaluation of fade.

Since muscle groups differ in their sensitivity to muscle relaxants, the peripheral nerve stimulator cannot replace direct observation of the muscles that need to be relaxed for a specific surgical procedure (eg, the diaphragm). Furthermore, recovery of adductor pollicis function does not exactly parallel recovery of muscles required to maintain an airway. Other indicators of adequate recovery include sustained head life, an inspiratory effort of 25 cm H_2O, and a forceful hand grip. Peripheral nerve stimulation is further considered in Chapter 9.

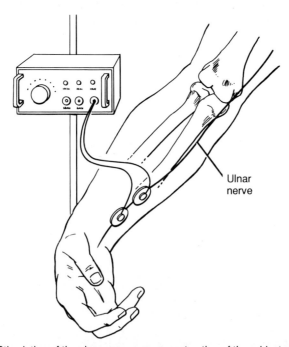

Figure 6–32. Stimulation of the ulnar nerve causes contraction of the adductor pollicis muscle.

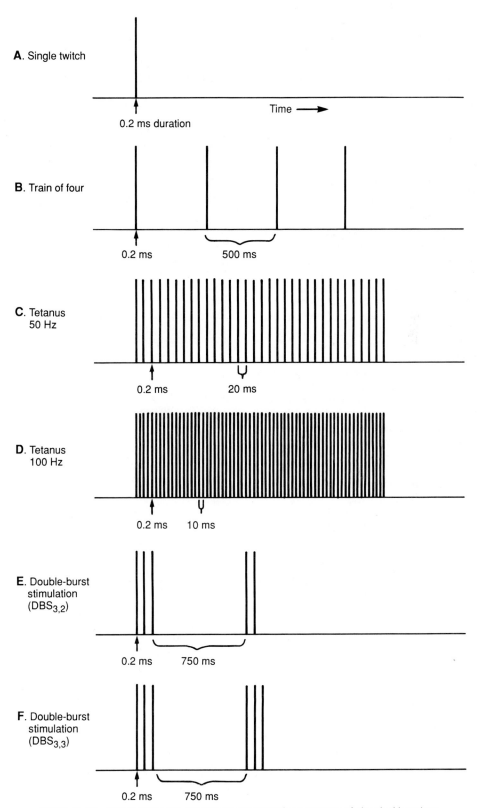

Figure 6–33. Peripheral nerve stimulators create various patterns of electrical impulses.

CASE DISCUSSION: MONITORING THE SEDATED PATIENT

A healthy 18-year-old man is scheduled for cosmetic rhinoplasty in a plastic surgeon's office. The surgeon plans to infiltrate with local anesthetic and requests your presence to provide intravenous sedation and monitoring.

Is the continuous presence of anesthesia personnel required during "standby" cases?

Absolutely yes. The term "standby anesthesia" is a misnomer that has been replaced with "monitored anesthesia care." Sedated patients need to be continuously monitored to prevent a multitude of unforeseen complications such as apnea or emesis.

Which monitors should be considered mandatory in this case?

Adequacy of oxygenation can be grossly assessed by observing skin and nail color. Continuous auscultation of breath sounds with a precordial stethoscope will identify airway obstruction due to excessive sedation. Electrocardiography, intermittent arterial blood pressure measurements, and palpation of a peripheral pulse will help to ensure adequate circulation. Conversation with the patient assesses level of consciousness.

Which other monitors may provide valuable information?

Pulse oximetry will warn of hypoxia but not hypoventilation. Aspiration end-tidal CO_2 analyzers can be adapted to local cases by connecting the collection tubing to a site near the patient's mouth. Although entrainment of room air precludes exact measurements, this technique provides a qualitative indicator of ventilation. In addition to providing information regarding the circulation, keeping a finger on the radial pulse will help to reassure an anxious patient.

Further monitoring as needed.

Soon after the beginning of surgery, it becomes clear that the patient will not lie still despite administration of sedative drugs. Which additional monitors would be required if this patient were converted to general anesthesia?

The oxygen concentration of the patient's inspired or expired gas should be measured. Some method for continuous monitoring of temperature must be available. If a ventilator is used, it must be equipped with a disconnect alarm. Pulse oximetry is mandatory and end-tidal CO_2 monitoring is strongly recommended.

In summary, the patient should receive the same level of care in the plastic surgeon's office as he would receive in a hospital operating room.

What factors affect the degree of monitoring?

The two fundamental determinants are the patient's physical status and the surgical procedure. For example, an elderly patient with many medical problems requires more intensive monitoring for the same procedure than a healthy young adult, and the young adult would require more monitoring for a brain tumor resection in the sitting position than for a rhinoplasty.

SUGGESTED READINGS

Ali HA: Monitoring of neuromuscular function. Chapter 4 in: *Muscle Relaxants: Basic and Clinical Aspects,* 2nd ed. Katz RL (editor). Grune & Stratton, 1985. Discussion of peripheral nerve stimulation.

Atlee JL: *Perioperative Cardiac Dysrhythmias: Mechanisms, Recognition, Management.* Year Book, 1985.

Blitt CD: *Monitoring in Anesthesia and Critical Care Medicine,* 2nd ed. Churchill Livingstone, 1990. All aspects of patient monitoring during anesthesia.

Dorsch JA, Dorsch SE: *Understanding Anesthesia Equipment: Construction, Care and Complications.* Williams & Wilkins, 1984. Includes an excellent discussion on capnographs and mass spectrometers.

Gravenstein JS, Paulus DA: *Monitoring Practice in Clinical Anesthesia.* Lippincott, 1982.

Lake CL (editor): *Clinical Monitoring.* Saunders, 1990. Reviews the physiology and physics needed for understanding current monitoring technology.

May WS et al: *Capnography in the Operating Room.* Raven Press, 1985. Illustrates and explains 30 sample capnographs.

Mushin WW, Jones PL: *Physics for the Anaesthetist.* Blackwell, 1987. See annotation, next item.

Scurr C, Feldman S: *Scientific Foundations of Anaesthesia,* 4th ed. Heinemann, 1990. This book and the previous explain the physics underlying the development of many anesthetic monitors, including the transducer, Doppler, and thermistor.

Tremper KK, Barker SJ: Pulse oximetry. Anesthesiology 1989;70:98. Uses and limitations.

Section II
Clinical Pharmacology

Inhalational Anesthetics

7

Nitrous oxide, chloroform, and ether were the first universally accepted general anesthetics. Although chloroform and ether have long been abandoned in the United States (chiefly because of problems with toxicity and flammability), five inhalational agents continue to be used in clinical anesthesiology: (1) nitrous oxide, (2) halothane, (3) methoxyflurane, (4) enflurane, and (5) isoflurane. Desflurane is a new volatile anesthetic that will be available for clinical use in the near future.

The course of general anesthesia can be divided into three phases: (1) induction, (2) maintenance, and (3) emergence. Inhalational anesthetics are particularly useful in the induction of pediatric patients unwilling to accept an intravenous line. In contrast, adults usually prefer rapid induction with intravenous agents. Regardless of the patient's age, anesthesia is often maintained with inhalational agents. Emergence depends chiefly upon the pulmonary elimination of these agents.

Because of their unique route of administration, inhalational anesthetics have useful pharmacologic properties not shared by other anesthetic agents. For instance, exposure to the pulmonary circulation allows a more rapid appearance of drug in arterial blood than intravenous administration. The study of the relationship between a drug's dose, tissue concentration, and elapsed time is called **pharmacokinetics.** The study of drug action, including toxic responses, is called **pharmacodynamics.**

After a general description of the pharmacokinetics (how a body affects a drug) and pharmacodynamics (how a drug affects a body) of inhalational anesthetics, this chapter presents the clinical pharmacology of individual agents.

PHARMACOKINETICS OF INHALATIONAL ANESTHETICS

Although the mechanism of action of inhalational anesthetics remains obscure, it is assumed that their ultimate effect depends upon attainment of a therapeutic tissue concentration in the brain. However, there are many steps between the administration of an anesthetic from a vaporizer and its deposition in the brain (Figure 7–1).

FACTORS AFFECTING INSPIRATORY CONCENTRATION (F_I)

The fresh gas leaving the anesthesia machine mixes with gases in the breathing circuit before being inspired by the patient. Thus, the patient is not necessarily receiving the concentration set on the vaporizer. The actual composition of the inspired gas mixture depends mainly on the fresh gas flow rate, the volume of the breathing system, and any absorption by the machine or breathing circuit. The higher the fresh gas flow rate, the smaller the breathing system volume, and the lower the circuit absorption, the closer the inspired gas concentration will be to the fresh gas concentration. Clinically, these attributes translate into quicker induction and recovery times.

FACTORS AFFECTING ALVEOLAR CONCENTRATION (F_A)

Uptake

If there were no uptake of anesthetic agent by the body, the alveolar gas concentration (F_A) would rapidly approach the inspired gas concentration (F_I). However, since anesthetic agent is taken up by the pulmonary circulation during induction, alveolar concentrations lag behind inspired concentrations (F_A/F_I < 1.0). The greater the uptake, the slower the rate of rise of the alveolar concentration and the lower the F_A/F_I ratio.

Because the concentration of a gas is directly proportionate to its partial pressure, the alveolar partial pressure will also be slow to rise. The alveolar partial pressure is important because it determines the par-

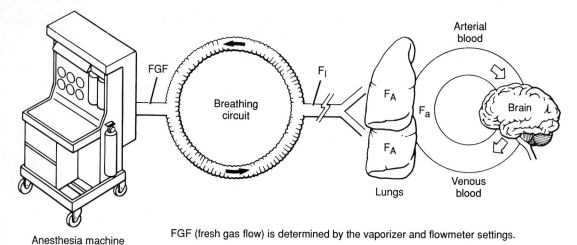

FGF (fresh gas flow) is determined by the vaporizer and flowmeter settings.

F_I (inspired gas concentration) is determined by (1) FGF rate; (2) breathing circuit volume; and (3) circuit absorption.

F_A (alveolar gas concentration) is determined by (1) uptake (uptake = $\lambda_{b/g} \times C(A-V) \times \dot{Q}$); (2) ventilation; and (3) the concentration effect and second gas effect:
      a) concentrating effect
      b) augmentation inflow effect

F_a (arterial gas concentration) is affected by ventilation/perfusion mismatching.

Figure 7–1. Inhalational anesthetic agents must pass through many barriers between the anesthesia machine and the brain.

tial pressure of anesthetic in the blood and, ultimately, in the brain. Similarly, the partial pressure of the anesthetic in the brain is directly proportionate to its brain tissue concentration, which we have already accepted as determining clinical effect. *Therefore, the greater the uptake of anesthetic agent, the greater the discrepancy between inspired and alveolar concentrations, and the slower the rate of induction.*

Three factors affect anesthetic uptake: (1) solubility in the blood, (2) alveolar blood flow, and (3) the partial pressure difference between alveolar gas and venous blood. Insoluble agents such as nitrous oxide are taken up by the blood less avidly than soluble agents such as halothane. As a consequence, the alveolar concentration of nitrous oxide rises faster than that of halothane, and induction is faster. The relative solubilities of an anesthetic in air, blood, and tissues are expressed as **partition coefficients** (Table 7–1). Each coefficient is the ratio of the concentrations of the anesthetic in two phases at equilibrium. Equilibrium is defined as equal partial pressures in the two phases. For instance, the blood/gas partition coefficient ($\lambda_{b/g}$) of nitrous oxide at 37 °C is 0.47. In other words, at equilibrium, 1 mL of blood contains 0.47 as much nitrous oxide as 1 mL of alveolar gas even though the partial pressures are the same. Stated another way, blood has 47% of the

capacity for nitrous oxide compared with the gas phase. Nitrous oxide is much less soluble in blood than halothane, which has a blood/gas partition coefficient at 37 °C of 2.4. Thus, almost five times more halothane than nitrous oxide must be dissolved to raise the partial pressure of blood. The higher the blood/gas coefficient, the greater the anesthetic's solubility and the greater its uptake by the pulmonary circulation. As a consequence of this high solubility, alveolar partial pressure rises more slowly, and induction is prolonged. Since fat/blood partition coefficients are greater than 1, it is not surprising that blood/gas solubility is increased by postprandial lipidemia and decreased by anemia.

The second factor affecting uptake is alveolar blood flow, which in the absence of pulmonary shunting is essentially equal to cardiac output. If the cardiac output drops to zero, so will anesthetic uptake. As cardiac output increases, anesthetic uptake increases, the rise in alveolar partial pressure slows, and induction is delayed. *The effect of changing cardiac output is less pronounced for insoluble anesthetics, since so little is taken up regardless of alveolar blood flow.* Low-output states predispose patients to overdosage with soluble agents, since the rate of rise in alveolar concentrations will be markedly increased. Higher than anticipated

Table 7–1. Partition coefficients of volatile anesthetics at 37 °C.

Agent	Blood/Gas	Brain/Blood	Muscle/Blood	Fat/Blood
Nitrous oxide	0.47	1.1	1.2	2.3
Halothane	2.4	2.9	3.5	60
Methoxyflurane	12	2.0	1.3	49
Enflurane	1.9	1.5	1.7	36
Isoflurane	1.4	2.6	4.0	45
Desflurane	0.42	1.3	2.0	27

levels of a volatile anesthetic which is also a myocardial depressant (eg, halothane) may create a positive feedback loop by lowering cardiac output even further.

The final factor affecting uptake of anesthetic by the pulmonary circulation is the partial pressure difference between alveolar gas and venous blood. This gradient depends upon tissue uptake. If anesthetic did not pass into organs, such as the brain, venous and alveolar partial pressures would become identical and there would be no pulmonary uptake. The transfer of anesthetic from blood to tissues is determined by three factors analogous to systemic uptake: tissue solubility of the agent (tissue/blood partition coefficient), tissue blood flow, and the partial pressure difference between arterial blood and the tissue.

Tissues can be assigned into four groups based upon their solubility and blood flow (Table 7–2). The highly perfused **vessel-rich group** (brain, heart, liver, kidney, and endocrine organs) is the first to take up appreciable amounts of anesthetic. However, moderate solubility and small volume limit the capacity of this group, so it is also the first to fill (ie, arterial and tissue partial pressures are equal). The **muscle group** (skin and muscle) is not as well perfused, so uptake is slower. In addition, it has a greater capacity owing to a larger volume, and uptake will be sustained for hours. Perfusion of the **fat group** nearly equals that of the muscle group, but the tremendous solubility of anesthetic in fat leads to a total capacity (tissue/blood solubility × tissue volume) that would take days to fill. The minimal perfusion of the **vessel-poor group** (bone, ligaments, teeth, hair, and cartilage) results in insignificant uptake.

Anesthetic uptake produces a characteristic curve that relates the rise in alveolar concentration to time (Figure 7–2). The shape of this graph is determined by the uptakes of individual tissue groups (Figure 7–3). The initial steep rate of uptake is due to unopposed filling of the alveoli by ventilation. The rate of rise slows as the vessel-rich group—and eventually the muscle group—reach their capacity.

Ventilation

The lowering of alveolar partial pressure by uptake can be countered by increasing alveolar ventilation. In other words, by constantly replacing anesthetic taken up by the pulmonary bloodstream, alveolar concentration will be better maintained. *The effect of increasing ventilation will be most obvious in raising the F_A/F_I for soluble anesthetics,* since they are more subject to uptake. Since the F_A/F_I is already high for insoluble agents, increasing ventilation has minimal effect. In contrast to the effect of anesthetics on cardiac output, anesthetics that depress ventilation (eg, halothane) will decrease the rate of rise in alveolar concentration and create a negative feedback loop.

Concentration

The effects of uptake can also be lessened by increasing the inspired concentration. Interestingly, increasing the inspired concentration not only increases the alveolar concentration but also increases its rate of rise (increases F_A/F_I). This has been termed the **concentration effect,** which is really the result of two phenomena. The first (confusingly) is called the **concentrating effect.** If 50% of an anesthetic is taken up

Table 7–2. Tissue groups based on perfusion and solubilities.

Characteristic	Vessel-Rich	Muscle	Fat	Vessel-Poor
% Body weight	10	50	20	20
% Cardiac output	75	19	6	0
Perfusion (mL/min/100 g)	75	3	3	0
Relative solubility	1	1	20	0

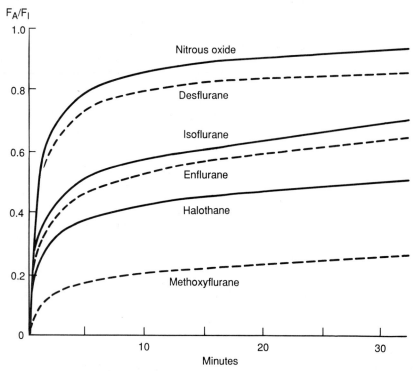

Figure 7–2. F_A rises toward F_I faster with nitrous oxide (an insoluble agent) than with methoxyflurane (a soluble agent). (See Figure 7–2 for explanation of abbreviations.) (Modified and reproduced, with permission, from Eger EL II: *Isoflurane [Forane]: A Reference and Compendium.* Ohio Medical Products, 1981.)

by the pulmonary circulation, an inspired concentration of 20% (20 parts of anesthetic per 100 parts of gas) will result in an alveolar concentration of 11% (10 parts of anesthetic remaining in a total volume of 90 parts of gas). On the other hand, if the inspired con-

centration is raised to 80% (80 parts per 100), the alveolar concentration will be 67% (40 parts of anesthetic remaining in a total volume of 60 parts). Thus, even though 50% of the anesthetic is taken up in both examples, *a higher inspired concentration results in a*

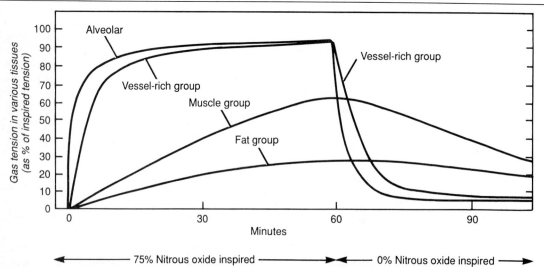

Figure 7–3. The rise and fall in alveolar partial pressure precedes that of other tissues. (Modified and reproduced, with permission, from Cowles AL et al: Uptake and distribution of inhalation anesthetic agents in clinical practice. Anesth Analg 1968;4:404.)

disproportionately higher alveolar concentration. In this example, increasing the inspired concentration fourfold results in a sixfold increase in alveolar concentration. The extreme case is an inspired concentration of 100% (100 parts of 100), which, despite a 50% uptake, will result in an alveolar concentration of 100% (50 parts remaining in a total volume of 50 parts).

The second phenomenon responsible for the concentration effect is the **augmented inflow effect.** Using the example above, the 10 parts of absorbed gas must be replaced by an equal volume of the 20% mixture to prevent alveolar collapse. Thus, the alveolar concentration becomes 12% (10 plus 2 parts of anesthetic in a total of 100 parts of gas). In contrast, after absorption of half of the anesthetic in the 80% gas mixture, 40 parts of 80% gas must be inspired. This further increases the alveolar concentration from 67% to 72% (40 plus 32 in a volume of 100).

The concentration effect is more significant with nitrous oxide than with the volatile anesthetics, since the former can be used in much higher concentrations. Nonetheless, a high concentration of nitrous oxide will augment not only its own uptake but also that of a concurrently administered volatile anesthetic by the same mechanism. The concentration effect one gas has upon another is called the **second gas effect.**

FACTORS AFFECTING ARTERIAL CONCENTRATION (Fa)

Ventilation/Perfusion Mismatch

Normally, alveolar and arterial anesthetic partial pressures are assumed to be equal. The existence of ventilation/perfusion mismatching will increase the alveolar-arterial difference. Mismatch acts like a restriction to flow: It raises the pressure in front of the restriction, lowers the pressure beyond the restriction, and reduces the flow through the restriction. The overall effect is an increase in the alveolar partial pressure (especially for highly soluble agents) and a decrease in the arterial partial pressure (especially for poorly soluble agents). Thus, an endobronchial intubation or a right-to-left intracardiac shunt will slow the rate of induction with nitrous oxide more than with halothane.

FACTORS AFFECTING ELIMINATION

Recovery from anesthesia depends upon a lowering of the brain tissue concentration. Anesthetic can be eliminated by biotransformation, transcutaneous loss, or exhalation. Biotransformation usually accounts for a minimal increase in the rate of decline of alveolar partial pressure. Its greatest impact is on the elimination of soluble anesthetics that undergo extensive metabolism (eg, methoxyflurane). The greater biotransformation of halothane compared with enflurane accounts for halothane's faster elimination despite its

being more soluble. Diffusion of anesthetic through the skin is insignificant.

The most important route for elimination of inhalational anesthetics is the alveolus. Many of the factors that speed induction also speed recovery: elimination of rebreathing, high fresh gas flows, low anesthetic circuit volume, low absorption by the anesthetic circuit, decreased solubility, and increased ventilation. Nitrous oxide elimination is so rapid that it dilutes alveolar oxygen and CO_2. The resulting **diffusion hypoxia** is prevented by administering 100% oxygen for 5–10 minutes after discontinuing nitrous oxide. Rate of recovery is usually faster than induction because tissues that have not reached equilibrium will continue to take up anesthetic until the alveolar partial pressure falls below tissue partial pressure. For instance, fat will continue to take up anesthetic and hasten recovery until its partial pressure exceeds alveolar partial pressure. This redistribution is not as available after a long anesthetic—thus, the speed of recovery depends also upon the length of time the anesthetic has been administered.

PHARMACODYNAMICS OF INHALATIONAL ANESTHETICS

THEORIES OF ANESTHETIC ACTION

General anesthesia is an altered physiologic state characterized by loss of consciousness, analgesia of the entire body, amnesia, and some degree of muscle relaxation. The multitude of substances capable of producing general anesthesia is remarkable: inert elements (xenon), simple inorganic compounds (nitrous oxide), halogenated hydrocarbons (halothane), and complex organic structures (barbiturates). A unifying theory explaining anesthetic action would have to accommodate this diversity of structure. In fact, different agents probably produce anesthesia by quite different methods. For instance, opioids are known to interact with stereospecific receptors, while inhalational agents do not have a predominant "structure-activity" relationship (opiate receptors may mediate some minor inhalational anesthetic effects).

There does not appear to be a single macroscopic site of action that is shared by all inhalational agents. Specific brain areas affected by various anesthetics include the reticular activating system, the cerebral cortex, the cuneate nucleus, the olfactory cortex, and the hippocampus. Additionally, spinal cord impulses are inhibited.

At a microscopic level, synaptic transmission is much more sensitive to general anesthetic agents than axonal conduction, though small-diameter nerve axons may be vulnerable. Both presynaptic and postsynaptic mechanisms are plausible.

The **unitary hypothesis** proposes that all inhalational agents share a common mechanism of action at the molecular level. This is supported by the observation that the anesthetic potency of inhalational agents correlates directly with their lipid solubility (**Meyer-Overton rule**). The implication is that anesthesia results from molecules dissolving at specific hydrophobic sites. Of course, not all lipid-soluble molecules are anesthetics (some are actually convulsants), and the correlation between anesthetic potency and lipid solubility is only approximate (Figure 7–4).

Neuronal membranes contain a multitude of hydrophobic sites in their phospholipid bilayer. Anesthetic binding to these sites could expand the bilayer beyond a critical amount, altering membrane function (**critical volume hypothesis**). While this theory is probably an oversimplification, it explains an interesting phenomenon: the reversal of anesthesia by increased pressure. Laboratory animals exposed to elevated hydrostatic pressure develop a resistance to anesthetic effects. Perhaps the pressure is displacing a number of molecules from the membrane, increasing anesthetic requirements.

Anesthetic binding might significantly modify membrane structure. Two theories suggest disturbances in membrane form (the **fluidization theory of anesthesia** and the **lateral phase separation theory**), while another proposes decreases in membrane conductance. Altering membrane structure could produce anesthesia in a number of ways. For instance, electrolyte permeability could be changed by disrupting ion channels. Alternatively, hydrophobic membrane proteins might undergo conformational changes. In either event, synaptic function could be inhibited.

MINIMUM ALVEOLAR CONCENTRATION

The alveolar concentration of an inhaled anesthetic that prevents movement in 50% of patients in response

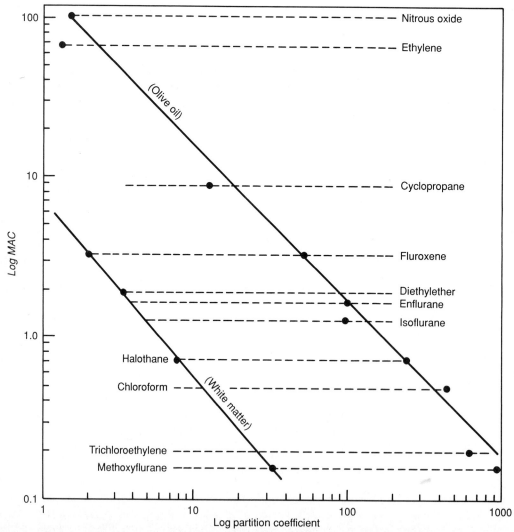

Figure 7–4. There is good but not perfect correlation between anesthetic potency and lipid solubility. (Modified and reproduced, with permission, from Lowe HJ, Hagler K: *Gas Chromatography in Biology and Medicine.* Churchill, 1969.)

to a standardized stimulus (eg, surgical incision) is the **minimum alveolar concentration** (MAC). MAC is a useful measure because it mirrors brain partial pressure, allows comparisons of potency between agents, and provides a standard for experimental evaluations (Table 7–3). Nonetheless, it should be considered a statistical average that has limited value in managing individual patients, especially during times of rapidly changing alveolar concentrations (eg, induction).

The MAC values for different anesthetics are roughly additive. For example, a mixture of 0.5 MAC of nitrous (53%) and 0.5 MAC of halothane (0.37%) approximates the degree of central nervous depression of 1.0 MAC of enflurane (1.68%). In contrast to central nervous system depression, the degree of myocardial depression may not be equivalent at the same MAC: 0.5 MAC of halothane causes more myocardial depression than 0.5 MAC of nitrous oxide.

MAC represents only one point on the dose-response curve—it is the equivalent of an ED50. MAC multiples are clinically useful if the dose-response curves of the anesthetics being compared are parallel, straight, and continuous for the effect being predicted. For instance, roughly 1.3 MAC of any of the volatile anesthetics (eg, for halothane: $1.3 \times 0.74\% = 0.96\%$) has been found to prevent movement in about 95% of patients (an approximation of the ED95).

MAC can be altered by several physiologic and pharmacologic variables (see Table 7–4). MAC is not affected by species, sex, or duration of anesthesia.

CLINICAL PHARMACOLOGY OF INHALATIONAL ANESTHETICS (Table 7–5)

NITROUS OXIDE

Physical Properties

Nitrous oxide (N_2O; laughing gas) is the only inorganic anesthetic gas in clinical use (Table 7–3). It is

Table 7–3. Properties of modern inhalational anesthetics.

Agent	Structure	MAC%[1]	Vapor Pressure (mm Hg @ 20 °C)	Blood/Gas Partition Partition Coefficient
Nitrous oxide	N=N \ / O	105[2]	—	0.47
Halothane (Fluothane)	F Cl | | F−C−C−H | | F Br	0.74	243	2.4
Methoxyflurane (Penthrane)	H F Cl | | | H−C−O−C−C−H | | | H F Cl	0.16	22.5	12.0
Enflurane (Ethrane)	F F Cl | | | H−C−O−C−C−H | | | F F F	1.68	175	1.9
Isoflurane (Forane)	F H F | | | H−C−O−C−C−F | | | F Cl F	1.15	240	1.4
Desflurane	F H F | | | H−C−O−C−C−F | | | F F F	6.0	681	0.42

[1]These MAC values are for 30- to 55-year-old human subjects and are expressed as a percentage of 1 atm. High altitude requires a higher inspired concentration of anesthetic to achieve to same partial pressure.
[2]A concentration greater than 100% means that hyperbaric conditions are required to achieve 1.0 MAC.

Table 7–4. Factors affecting MAC.

Variable	Effect on MAC	Comments
Temperature		
Hypothermia	↓	
Hyperthermia	↓	↑ if > 42 °C
Age		
Young	↑	
Elderly	↓	
Alcohol		
Acute intoxication	↓	
Chronic abuse	↑	
Anemia		
Hematocrit < 10%	↓	
PaO₂		
<40 mm Hg	↓	
PaCO₂		
>95 mm Hg	↓	Due to < pH in CSF
Thyroid		
Hyperthyroid	N/C	
Hypothyroid	N/C	
Blood pressure		
MAP < 40 mm Hg	↓	
Electrolytes		
Hypercalcemia	↓	
Hypernatremia	↑	Due to altered CSF
Hyponatremia	↓	Due to altered CSF
Pregnancy	↓	
Drugs		
Local anesthetics	↓	Except cocaine
Opioids	↓	
Ketamine	↓	
Barbiturates	↓	
Benzodiazepines	↓	
Verapamil	↓	
Lithium	↓	
Sympatholytics		
Methyldopa	↓	
Reserpine	↓	
Clonidine	↓	
Sympathomimetics		
Amphetamine		
Chronic	↓	
Acute	↑	
Cocaine	↑	
Ephedrine	↑	

colorless and essentially odorless. Although nonexplosive and nonflammable, nitrous oxide is as capable as oxygen of supporting combustion. Unlike the potent volatile agents, nitrous oxide is a gas at room temperature and ambient pressure. However, nitrous oxide can be kept as a liquid under pressure because its critical temperature lies above room temperature (see Chapter 2).

Effects on Organ Systems

A. Cardiovascular: The circulatory effects of nitrous oxide are explained by its tendency to stimulate the sympathetic nervous system. Even though nitrous oxide directly depresses myocardial contractility in vitro, arterial blood pressure, cardiac output, and heart rate are essentially unchanged or slightly elevated in vivo. Myocardial depression may be unmasked in patients with coronary artery disease or severe hypovolemia. Constriction of pulmonary vascular smooth muscle increases pulmonary vascular resistance, which results in an elevation of right atrial pressure. Despite vasoconstriction of cutaneous vessels, peripheral vascular resistance is not significantly altered. Because nitrous oxide increases endogenous catecholamine levels, it may be associated with a higher incidence of epinephrine-induced dysrhythmias.

B. Respiratory: Nitrous oxide increases respiratory rate (tachypnea) and decreases tidal volume as a result of central nervous system stimulation and perhaps activation of pulmonary stretch receptors. The net effect is a minimal change in minute ventilation and resting arterial CO₂ levels. **Hypoxic drive,** the ventilatory response to arterial hypoxemia that is mediated by peripheral chemoreceptors in the carotid bodies, is markedly depressed by even small amounts of nitrous oxide. This has serious implications in the recovery room, where patients with low arterial oxygen tensions may go unrecognized.

C. Cerebral: By increasing cerebral blood flow, nitrous oxide produces a mild elevation of intracranial pressure. Nitrous oxide also increases cerebral oxygen consumption (CMRO₂). Levels of nitrous oxide below the MAC provide analgesia in dental surgery and other minor procedures.

D. Neuromuscular: In contrast to other inhalational agents, nitrous oxide does not provide significant muscle relaxation. In fact, at high concentrations in hyperbaric chambers, nitrous oxide causes skeletal muscle rigidity. Nitrous oxide is probably not a triggering agent of malignant hyperthermia.

E. Renal: Nitrous oxide appears to decrease renal blood flow by increasing renal vascular resistance. This leads to a drop in glomerular filtration rate and urinary output.

F. Hepatic: Hepatic blood flow probably falls during nitrous oxide anesthesia, but to a lesser extent than with the volatile agents.

Biotransformation & Toxicity

During emergence, almost all nitrous oxide is eliminated by exhalation. A small amount diffuses out through the skin. Biotransformation is limited to less than 0.01% that undergoes reductive metabolism in the gastrointestinal tract by anaerobic bacteria.

By irreversibly oxidizing the cobalt atom in vitamin B₁₂, nitrous oxide inhibits enzymes that are vitamin B₁₂-dependent. These enzymes include methionine synthetase, which is necessary for myelin formation; and thymidylate synthetase, which is necessary for DNA synthesis. Prolonged exposure to anesthetic concentrations of nitrous oxide can result in bone marrow depression (megaloblastic anemia) and even neurologic deficiencies (peripheral neuropathies and pernicious anemia). Because of possible teratogenic effects, nitrous oxide is probably best avoided in pregnant patients. Nitrous oxide may also alter the immu-

Table 7–5. Clinical pharmacology of inhalational anesthetics.

	Nitrous Oxide	Halothane	Methoxyflurane	Enflurane	Isoflurane	Desflurane
Cardiovascular						
Blood pressure	N/C	↓↓	↓↓	↓↓	↓↓	↓↓
Heart rate	N/C	↓	↑	↑	↑	N/C or ↑
Systemic vascular resistance	N/C	N/C	N/C	↓	↓↓	↓↓
Cardiac output[1]	N/C	↓	↓	↓↓	N/C	N/C or ↓
Respiratory						
Tidal volume	↓	↓	↓	↓	↓	↓
Respiratory rate	↑	↑↑	↑↑	↑↑	↑	↑
PaCO$_2$						
Resting	N/C	↑	↑	↑↑	↑	↑
Challenge	↑	↑	↑	↑↑	↑	↑
Cerebral						
Blood flow	↑	↑↑	↑	↑	↑	↑
Intracranial pressure	↑	↑↑	↑	↑↑	↑	↑
Seizures	↓	↓	↓	↑	↓	↓
Neuromuscular						
Nondepolarizing blockade[2]	↑	↑↑	↑↑	↑↑↑	↑↑↑	↑↑↑
Renal						
Renal blood flow	↓↓	↓↓	↓↓	↓↓	↓↓	?
Glomerular filtration rate	↓↓	↓↓	↓↓	↓↓	↓↓	?
Urinary output	↓↓	↓↓	↓↓	↓↓	↓↓	?
Hepatic						
Blood flow	↓	↓↓	↓↓	↓↓	↓	?
Metabolism[3]	0.004%	15–20%	50%	2–5%	0.2%	<0.1%

[1] Controlled ventilation.
[2] Depolarizing blockade is probably also prolonged by these agents, but this is usually not clinically significant.
[3] Metabolism = percentage of absorbed anesthetic undergoing metabolism.

nologic response to infection by affecting chemotaxis and motility of polymorphonuclear leukocytes.

Contraindications

Although nitrous oxide is insoluble compared to other inhalational agents, it is 35 times more soluble in blood than nitrogen. Thus, it tends to diffuse into air-containing cavities more rapidly than nitrogen is absorbed by the bloodstream. For instance, if a patient with a 100-mL pneumothorax inhales 50% nitrous oxide, the gas content of the pneumothorax will tend to approach that of the bloodstream. Since nitrous oxide will diffuse into the cavity more rapidly than the air (principally nitrogen) diffuses out, the pneumothorax expands until it contains 100 mL of air and 100 mL of nitrous oxide. If the walls surrounding the cavity are rigid, pressure rises instead of volume. Examples of conditions where nitrous oxide might be hazardous include air embolism, pneumothorax, acute intestinal obstruction, intracranial air (tension pneumocephalus following dural closure or pneumoencephalography), pulmonary air cysts, intraocular air bubbles, and tympanic membrane grafting. Nitrous oxide will even diffuse into endotracheal tube cuffs, increasing the pressure against the tracheal mucosa.

Because of the effect of nitrous oxide on the pulmonary vasculature, it should be avoided in patients with pulmonary hypertension. Obviously, nitrous oxide is of limited value in patients requiring high inspired oxygen concentrations.

Drug Interactions

Because the relatively high MAC of nitrous oxide prevents its use as a complete general anesthetic, it is frequently used in combination with the more potent volatile agents. The addition of nitrous oxide decreases the requirements of these other agents. While nitrous oxide should not be considered a benign carrier gas, it does attenuate the circulatory and respiratory effects of volatile anesthetics in adults. Nitrous oxide potentiates neuromuscular blockade, but less so than the volatile agents (Chapter 9). The concentration of nitrous oxide flowing through a vaporizer can influence the concentration of volatile anesthetic delivered. For example, decreasing nitrous oxide concentration (ie, increasing oxygen concentration) increases the concentration of volatile agent despite a constant vaporizer setting. This discrepancy is due to the relative solubilities of nitrous oxide and oxygen in liquid volatile anesthetics. The second gas effect has been discussed.

HALOTHANE

Physical Properties

Halothane is a halogenated alkane (Figure 7–3). The carbon-fluoride bonds are responsible for its nonflammable and nonexplosive nature. Thymol preservative and amber-colored bottles retard spontaneous oxidative decomposition.

Effects on Organ Systems

A. Cardiovascular: A dose-dependent reduction of arterial blood pressure is due to direct myocardial depression. Two MAC of halothane results in a 50% decrease of blood pressure and cardiac output. Cardiac depression—due to interference with intracellular calcium utilization—causes an increase in right atrial pressure. Although halothane is a coronary artery vasodilator, coronary blood flow decreases owing to the drop in systemic arterial pressure. Adequate myocardial perfusion is usually maintained, since oxygen demand also drops. Normally, hypotension inhibits baroreceptors in the aortic arch and carotid bifurcation, causing a decrease in vagal stimulation and a compensatory rise in heart rate. Halothane blunts this reflex. Slowing of sinoatrial node conduction may result in a junctional rhythm or bradycardia. Halothane sensitizes the heart to the dysrhythmogenic effects of epinephrine, so that doses of epinephrine above 1.5 μg/kg should be avoided. Although organ blood flow is redistributed, systemic vascular resistance is unchanged.

B. Respiratory: Halothane typically causes rapid, shallow breathing. The increased respiratory rate is not enough to counter the decreased tidal volume, so alveolar ventilation drops and resting $PaCO_2$ is elevated. **Apneic threshold,** the highest $PaCO_2$ at which a patient remains apneic, also rises because the difference between it and resting $PaCO_2$ is not altered by general anesthesia. Similarly, halothane limits the increase in minute ventilation that normally accompanies a rise in $PaCO_2$. Halothane's ventilatory effects are probably due to central (medullary depression) and peripheral (intercostal muscle dysfunction) mechanisms. These changes are exaggerated by preexisting lung disease and attenuated by surgical stimulation. The increase in $PaCO_2$ and the decrease in intrathoracic pressure that accompanies spontaneous ventilation with halothane partially reverse the cardiac output, arterial blood pressure, and heart rate depression described above. Hypoxic drive is severely depressed by even low concentrations of halothane (0.1 MAC).

Halothane is considered a bronchodilator, since it often reverses asthma-induced bronchospasm. This action is not inhibited by propranolol, a β-adrenergic blocking agent. Halothane also depresses clearance of mucus from the respiratory tract **(mucociliary function),** promoting postoperative hypoxemia and atelectasis.

C. Cerebral: By dilating cerebral vessels, halothane lowers cerebral vascular resistance and increases cerebral blood flow. **Autoregulation,** the maintenance of constant cerebral blood flow during changes in arterial blood pressure, is blunted. Concomitant rises in intracranial pressure can be prevented by establishing hyperventilation *prior to* halothane administration. Cerebral activity is decreased, leading to electroencephalographic slowing and reduced metabolic oxygen requirements.

D. Neuromuscular: Halothane relaxes skeletal muscle and potentiates nondepolarizing neuromuscular blocking drugs. Halothane, like the other potent volatile anesthetics, is a triggering agent of malignant hyperthermia.

E. Renal: By decreasing arterial blood pressure, halothane reduces renal blood flow, glomerular filtration rate, and urine output. Because the reduction in renal blood flow is greater than the reduction in glomerular filtration rate, the filtration fraction is increased. Preoperative hydration limits these changes.

F. Hepatic: Halothane causes hepatic blood flow to decrease in proportion to the depression of cardiac output. Hepatic artery vasospasm has been reported during halothane anesthesia. The metabolism and clearance of some drugs (eg, fentanyl, phenytoin, verapamil) appear to be impaired by halothane. Other evidence of hepatic cellular dysfunction includes sulfobromophthalein (BSP) dye retention and minor liver transaminase elevations.

Biotransformation & Toxicity

Halothane is oxidized in the liver to its principal metabolite, trifluoroacetic acid. Bromide, another oxidative metabolite, has been incriminated but is an improbable cause of postanesthetic changes in mental status. In the absence of oxygen, reductive metabolism may result in hepatotoxic end products that covalently bind to tissue macromolecules. This is especially apt to occur following enzyme induction by phenobarbital. Elevated fluoride levels signal significant anaerobic metabolism.

Postoperative hepatic dysfunction has several causes: (1) viral hepatitis, (2) impaired hepatic perfusion, (3) preexisting liver disease, (4) hepatocyte hypoxia, (5) sepsis, (6) hemolysis, (7) benign postoperative intrahepatic cholestasis, and (8) drug-induced hepatitis. **Halothane hepatitis** is extremely rare (1:35,000 cases) and is a diagnosis of exclusion. Patients exposed to multiple halothane anesthetics at short intervals, middle-aged obese women, and persons with a familial predisposition to halothane toxicity or a prior personal history of toxicity are considered to be at increased risk.

The hepatic lesion seen in humans—centrilobular necrosis—also occurs in rats pretreated with an enzyme inducer (phenobarbital) and exposed to halothane under hypoxic conditions ($FiO_2 < 14\%$). This "halothane hypoxic model" implies hepatic damage due to reductive metabolites or hypoxia. However, more recent models have produced necrosis without hypoxia (the isoniazid and triiodothyronine models).

Other evidence points to an immune mechanism. For instance, some signs of the disease indicate an allergic reaction (eg, eosinophilia, rash, and fever) and do not appear until a few days after exposure. Furthermore, an antibody that binds to hepatocytes previously exposed to halothane has been isolated from patients with halothane-induced hepatic dysfunction.

Immunologic and metabolic mechanisms are not

necessarily mutually exclusive. For instance, reductive metabolites could bind to hepatocytes, initiating a cell-damaging hypersensitivity response. Alternatively, the existence of different mechanisms might explain the range of halothane-associated hepatic dysfunction from subclinical liver damage to fatal hepatic necrosis.

Contraindications

It would seem prudent to withhold halothane from patients with unexplained liver dysfunction following previous exposure. Because halothane hepatitis appears to affect only adults and children past puberty, some anesthesiologists choose other volatile anesthetics in these patients. There is no compelling evidence associating halothane with worsening of preexisting liver disease.

Halothane should be used with great caution in patients with intracranial mass lesions because of the possibility of intracranial hypertension.

Hypovolemic patients and some patients with severe cardiac disease (aortic stenosis) may not tolerate halothane's negative inotropic effects. Sensitization of the heart to catecholamines limits the usefulness of halothane when exogenous epinephrine is administered or in patients with pheochromocytoma.

Drug interactions

The myocardial depression seen with halothane is exacerbated by β-adrenergic blocking agents (eg, propranolol) and calcium channel-blocking agents (eg, verapamil). Tricyclic antidepressants and monoamine oxidase inhibitors have been associated with blood pressure fluctuations and dysrhythmias, though neither represents an absolute contraindication. The combination of halothane and aminophylline has resulted in serious ventricular dysrhythmias.

METHOXYFLURANE

Physical Properties

Methoxyflurane, a halogenated methylethyl ether, is a colorless anesthetic with a sweet, fruity odor. It is light-sensitive and stabilized with butylated hydroxytoluene. As with other modern volatile anesthetics, methoxyflurane is nonexplosive and nonflammable at clinical concentrations. It is the most potent of the inhalational agents, but its high solubility (leading to breathing circuit absorption) and low vapor pressure at room temperature (maximum inspired concentration of 3%) limit its rate of induction.

Effects on Organ Systems

A. Cardiovascular: Methoxyflurane depresses cardiac contractility, lowering cardiac output and arterial blood pressure. Unlike halothane, methoxyflurane does not alter the carotid baroreflex, and the heart rate usually rises.

B. Respiratory: Despite an increased respiratory rate, methoxyflurane reduces minute ventilation by lowering tidal volume. Resting $PaCO_2$ is elevated. Methoxyflurane has mild bronchodilating properties. Mucociliary function is depressed.

C. Cerebral: Methoxyflurane vasodilates the cerebral vasculature, increasing cerebral blood flow and intracranial pressure. Cerebral metabolic requirements are reduced.

D. Neuromuscular: Methoxyflurane relaxes skeletal muscle.

E. Renal: Methoxyflurane resembles other volatile anesthetics by causing a fall in renal blood flow and glomerular filtration rate. It is unclear whether these changes are entirely due to lower perfusion pressure or partially result from impaired autoregulation of renal blood flow. Postoperative high-output renal failure is a distinguishing feature of methoxyflurane anesthesia (see Biotransformation and Toxicity, below).

F. Hepatic: Methoxyflurane depresses hepatic blood flow.

Biotransformation & Toxicity

Methoxyflurane is metabolized to a greater extent than any other inhalational agent. Oxidative metabolites include free fluoride (F^-) and oxalic acid. While both of these end products are nephrotoxic, fluoride is responsible for the **vasopressin-resistant high-output renal failure** that characterizes methoxyflurane toxicity. A fluoride level of 50 μmol/L, the threshold for renal dysfunction, is achievable after 2.5–3 MAC-hours of exposure (1 MAC-hour is 1 MAC sustained for 1 hour). Methoxyflurane metabolism is greater in obese and elderly patients and can be induced by a variety of drugs.

Fluoride directly inhibits tubular function (eg, chloride transport in the ascending loop of Henle), leading to a concentrating defect. Clinical signs of methoxyflurane nephrotoxicity include (1) polyuria resistant to vasopressin; (2) increased serum osmolality, sodium, creatinine, and BUN; (3) decreased urinary clearance of creatinine and urea nitrogen; and (4) urine hypo-osmolality.

Methoxyflurane has been rarely associated with postoperative hepatic dysfunction.

Contraindications

Nephrotoxicity has severely limited the usefulness of methoxyflurane. In fact, it is presented here more as a model of nephrotoxicity than as a modern anesthetic agent. Patients with any degree of preexisting renal dysfunction represent a clear contraindication. Even in healthy patients, exposure should be limited to 2 MAC-hours.

Drug Interactions

Methoxyflurane should be avoided in patients receiving other nephrotoxic drugs (eg, aminoglycoside antibiotics). Several drugs, including phenobarbital, isoniazid, and ethanol, induce methoxyflurane metabolism, resulting in higher than expected fluoride levels. Methoxyflurane potentiates nondepolarizing muscle relaxants.

ENFLURANE

Physical Properties

Enflurane is a halogenated ether. It has a mild, sweet, ethereal odor and is nonflammable at clinical concentrations.

Effects on Organ Systems

A. Cardiovascular: Enflurane, like halothane, depresses myocardial contractility. Arterial blood pressure, cardiac output, and myocardial oxygen consumption are lowered. Unlike halothane, systemic vascular resistance is decreased, while the heart rate usually rises. Enflurane sensitizes the heart to the dysrhythmic effects of epinephrine, but doses up to 4.5 μg/kg are usually well tolerated.

B. Respiratory: Enflurane shares most of halothane's respiratory properties: (1) decreased minute ventilation despite an increase in respiratory rate, (2) increased resting $PaCO_2$, (3) decreased response to hypercapnia, (4) abolishment of hypoxic drive, (5) depressed mucociliary function, and (6) bronchodilatation.

Enflurane causes marked respiratory depression—at 1 MAC, resting $PaCO_2$ is 60 mm Hg. Even assisted ventilation (supplementing respiratory rate or tidal volume during spontaneous ventilation) will not lower the $PaCO_2$ much below 55 mm Hg because of the unchanged relationship between resting $PaCO_2$ and apneic threshold.

C. Cerebral: Enflurane increases cerebral blood flow and intracranial pressure. Interestingly, enflurane has been shown to increase the secretion of cerebrospinal fluid and the resistance to cerebrospinal fluid outflow. During deep enflurane anesthesia, high-voltage, fast-frequency electroencephalographic changes can progress to a spike-and-wave pattern culminating in frank tonic-clonic seizures. This epileptiform activity is exacerbated by high anesthetic concentrations and hypocapnia. Therefore, hyperventilation is not recommended to attenuate enflurane-induced intracranial hypertension. Cerebral metabolic requirements are decreased by enflurane unless seizure activity is initiated.

D. Neuromuscular: Enflurane relaxes skeletal muscle.

E. Renal: Renal blood flow, glomerular filtration rate, and urinary output fall during enflurane anesthesia. A metabolite of enflurane is nephrotoxic (see Biotransformation and Toxicity, below).

F. Hepatic: The decrease in hepatic blood flow with enflurane is similar to that caused by equipotent doses of other volatile anesthetics.

Biotransformation & Toxicity

Fluoride is an end product of enflurane metabolism. However, defluorination is much less than with meth-oxyflurane, and detectable renal dysfunction is unlikely. After almost 10 MAC-hours, fluoride concentrations in healthy patients average less than 40 μmol/L, causing a mild reduction in renal concentrating ability.

The evidence of postoperative hepatic damage following enflurane anesthesia is circumstantial at best.

Contraindications

Enflurane should probably be avoided in patients with preexisting kidney disease even though deterioration in renal function is unlikely. Similarly, another inhalational agent should probably be chosen for patients with seizure disorders. Precautions concerning intracranial hypertension, hemodynamic instability, and malignant hyperthermia are shared with halothane.

Drug Interactions

Isoniazid (but not phenobarbital, ethanol, or phenytoin) induces enflurane defluorination. This may be clinically significant in so-called **"rapid acetylators,"** ie, patients with an autosomal dominant trait that increases the rate of hepatic acetylation.

Nondepolarizing blocking agents are potentiated.

ISOFLURANE

Physical Properties

Isoflurane is a nonflammable volatile anesthetic with a pungent ethereal odor. Although it is a chemical isomer of enflurane, it has different physicochemical properties (Table 7–3).

Effects on Organ Systems

A. Cardiovascular: Isoflurane causes minimal cardiac depression in vivo. Cardiac output is maintained by a rise in heart rate due to partial preservation of carotid baroreflexes. Mild β-adrenergic stimulation increases skeletal muscle blood flow, decreases systemic vascular resistance, and lowers arterial blood pressure. Coronary blood flow is also affected. Dilatation of normal coronary arteries may divert blood away from fixed, stenotic lesions. There is conflicting evidence about whether this **"coronary steal syndrome"** causes regional myocardial ischemia during episodes of tachycardia or drops in perfusion pressure. Some anesthesiologists are avoiding the use of high concentrations of isoflurane in patients with coronary artery disease.

B. Respiratory: Respiratory depression during isoflurane anesthesia resembles that of other volatile anesthetics, except that tachypnea is less pronounced. Despite a tendency to irritate upper airway reflexes, isoflurane is considered a good bronchodilator.

C. Cerebral: At concentrations greater than 1 MAC, isoflurane increases cerebral blood flow and intracranial pressure. These effects are less pronounced than with other volatile agents and are reversed by hyperventilation. In contrast to halothane, the hyperventilation does not have to be instituted prior to isoflurane in order to prevent intracranial hypertension. Isoflurane reduces cerebral metabolic oxygen requirements, and at 2 MAC it produces an electrically silent electroencephalogram.

D. Neuromuscular: Isoflurane relaxes skeletal muscle.

E. Renal: Isoflurane decreases renal blood flow, glomerular filtration rate, and urine output in somewhat the same way as other volatile anesthetics.

F. Hepatic: Total hepatic blood flow (hepatic artery and portal vein flow) is reduced during isoflurane anesthesia. However, hepatic oxygen supply may be better maintained with isoflurane than halothane due to preservation of hepatic artery perfusion. Liver function tests are minimally affected.

Biotransformation & Toxicity

Isoflurane is metabolized to one-tenth the extent of enflurane. Trifluoroacetic acid is the principal end product. Although serum fluoride fluid levels may rise (peak < 5 μmol/L), nephrotoxicity is extremely unlikely even in the presence of enzyme inducers. This limited metabolism also minimizes any possible risk of significant hepatic dysfunction.

Contraindications

Isoflurane presents no unique contraindications other than the controversy concerning the possibility of coronary steal. Patients with severe hypovolemia may not tolerate its vasodilating effects.

Drug Interactions

Epinephrine can be safely administered in doses up to 4.5 μg/kg. Nondepolarizing muscle relaxants are potentiated by isoflurane.

DESFLURANE
(I-653)

Physical Properties

Desflurane's structure is very similar to that of isoflurane. In fact, the only difference is the substitution of a fluorine atom for isoflurane's chlorine atom. However, that "minor" change has profound effects on the physical properties of the drug. For instance, the vapor pressure of desflurane at 20 °C is 681 mm Hg. Thus, it boils at room temperature at high altitudes (eg, Denver, Colorado). This problem has been dealt with by development of a special desflurane vaporizer. Furthermore, the low solubility of desflurane in blood and body tissues causes a very rapid wash-in and wash-out of anesthetic. Wake-up times are reported to be approximately half as long as those observed following isoflurane. This is principally attributable to a blood/gas partition coefficient (0.42) that is even lower than that of nitrous oxide (0.47). While desflurane is roughly one-fourth as potent as the other volatile agents, it is 17 times more potent than nitrous oxide. A high vapor pressure, an ultrashort duration of

action, and moderate potency are desflurane's most characteristic features.

Effects on Organ Systems

A. Cardiovascular: The cardiovascular effects of desflurane appear to be similar to those of isoflurane. Increasing the dose is associated with a decline in systemic vascular resistance that leads to a fall in arterial blood pressure. Cardiac output remains relatively unchanged or slightly depressed at 1–2 MAC. There is a moderate rise in heart rate, central venous pressure, and pulmonary artery pressure that often does not become apparent at low doses. In contrast to isoflurane, desflurane does not increase coronary artery blood flow and does not appear to contribute to a coronary steal phenomenon. Desflurane does not sensitize the myocardium to epinephrine-induced dysrhythmias.

B. Respiratory: Desflurane causes a decrease in tidal volume and an increase in respiratory rate. There is an overall decrease in alveolar ventilation that causes a rise in resting $PaCO_2$. Like other modern volatile anesthetic agents, desflurane depresses the ventilatory response to increasing $PaCO_2$. Desflurane is mildly irritating to the airway.

C. Cerebral: Like the other volatile anesthetics, desflurane decreases cerebral vascular resistance, increases cerebral blood flow, and is associated with an increase in intracranial pressure at normotension and normocapnia. However, the cerebral vasculature remains responsive to changes in $PaCO_2$, so that intracranial pressure can be lowered by hyperventilation. Cerebral oxygen consumption is decreased during desflurane anesthesia. Thus, during periods of desflurane-induced hypotension (mean arterial pressure = 60 mm Hg), cerebral blood flow is adequate to maintain aerobic metabolism despite a low cerebral perfusion pressure. The effect on the electroencephalogram is similar to that of isoflurane.

D. Neuromuscular: Desflurane is associated with a dose-dependent decrease in the response to train-of-four and tetanic peripheral nerve stimulation.

E. Renal: There is no evidence of any nephrotoxic effects due to exposure to desflurane.

F. Hepatic: Hepatic function tests are unaffected, and there is no evidence of hepatic injury following desflurane anesthesia.

Biotransformation & Toxicity

Desflurane undergoes minimal metabolism in humans. Serum and urine inorganic fluoride levels following desflurane anesthesia are essentially unchanged from preanesthetic levels. There is insignificant percutaneous loss.

Contraindications

Desflurane shares many of the contraindications of other modern volatile anesthetics: severe hypovolemia, malignant hyperthermia, and intracranial hypertension.

Drug Interactions

Desflurane potentiates nondepolarizing muscle relaxants to the same extent as isoflurane.

CASE DISCUSSION: CLOSED-CIRCUIT ANESTHESIA*

A 22-year-old man weighing 70 kg is scheduled for arthroscopy under general anesthesia. You and your attending staff are considering a closed-circuit anesthetic technique.

Describe closed-circuit anesthesia and tell how it differs from other techniques.

Anesthesia systems may be classified as non-rebreathing, partial rebreathing, or total rebreathing techniques. In nonrebreathing systems (open systems), the fresh gas flow into the breathing circuit exceeds the patient's minute ventilation. All gases not absorbed by the patient are exhausted through the pressure relief valve; there is no flow through the CO_2 absorber; and no gas is rebreathed by the patient.

In partial rebreathing systems (semi-open or semi-closed), the fresh gas flow into the breathing circuit is less than the minute ventilation provided to the patient but greater than the rate of uptake of all gases by the patient. The difference between the fresh gas flow and patient uptake is equal to the exhaust volume from the pressure relief valve. Therefore, exhaled gas can take one of three courses: It can be (1) evacuated by the pressure relief valve, (2) absorbed by the CO_2 absorber, or (3) rebreathed by the patient.

A total rebreathing system (closed system) does not evacuate any gas through the pressure relief valve. This has many implications: (1) all exhaled gases except CO_2 are rebreathed; (2) expired CO_2 must be eliminated by the CO_2 absorber to prevent hypercapnia; and (3) the total amount of fresh gas delivered to the system must nearly equal the amount of gas taken up by the patient's lungs. The fresh gas flow required to maintain the desired alveolar partial pressure of anesthetic agent and oxygen depends upon anesthetic uptake and metabolic rate. This flow rate is achieved by maintaining (1) a constant circuit volume, as reflected in an unchanging end-expiratory breathing bag volume or ventilator bellows height; and (2) a constant expired oxygen concentration.

What are the advantages and disadvantages of closed-circuit anesthesia?

Rebreathing anesthetic gases conserves heat and humidity, decreases anesthetic waste (pollution and cost), demonstrates the principles of anesthetic uptake,

and allows early detection of circuit leaks and metabolic changes. However, some anesthesiologists consider closed-circuit techniques to impose a greater risk of hypoxia, hypercapnia, and anesthetic overdose. Without question, closed-circuit anesthesia requires a high level of vigilance and a comprehensive understanding of pharmacokinetics. Some of the newer anesthetic machines cannot deliver low flows because they have mandatory oxygen flow rates greater than metabolic oxygen consumption or do not allow the administration of potentially hypoxic gas mixtures.

Is any special equipment necessary for closed-circuit anesthesia?

General anesthesia should never be performed without an oxygen analyzer in the breathing circuit. During low-flow anesthesia, the oxygen concentrations in the expiratory limb may be significantly lower than in the inspiratory limb owing to the patient's oxygen consumption. Therefore, expiratory oxygen concentration should be measured whenever the anesthesia system is closed. Gas leaks in the anesthetic system will interfere with estimations of nitrous oxide and oxygen consumption. These leaks are proportionate to mean airway pressure and inspiratory time. Modern circle systems have over 20 potential sites of leaks, including the absorber, tubing connections, unidirectional valves, rubber hoses, and breathing bag (see Chapter 4 Case Discussion). Vaporizers and flowmeters must be accurate at low flows and varying circuit pressures. An alternative to a vaporizer is direct injection of volatile agent into the *expiratory* limb of the breathing circuit.

How are oxygen requirements predicted during closed-circuit anesthesia?

Anesthesia establishes a basal metabolic rate that is dependent upon the patient's weight and body temperature. Basal metabolic oxygen consumption ($\dot{V}O_2$) equals 10 times a patient's weight in kilograms to the three-quarters power:

$$\dot{V}O_2 = 10kg^{3/4}$$

For a 70-kg patient, oxygen consumption is–

$$\dot{V}O_2 = 10 \times (24.2) = 242 \text{ mL } O_2/\text{min}$$

Oxygen requirements decrease by 10% for each degree below 37.6 °C:

$$\dot{V}O_2 \text{ at } 36.6 \text{ °C} = 242 - 24 = 218 \text{ mL } O_2/\text{min}$$
$$\dot{V}O_2 \text{ at } 35.6 \text{ °C} = 218 - 22 = 196 \text{ mL } O_2/\text{min}$$

This is only a model for prediction. *Actual oxygen requirements vary, and must be determined for each patient.* For instance, hypovolemic shock, hypothyroidism, and aortic cross-clamping are associated

---

*The authors would like to thank Harry S. Lowe, MD, for his contribution to this Case Discussion.

with decreased metabolic oxygen consumption. In contrast, malignant hyperthermia, hyperthyroidism, thermal burns, and sepsis lead to greater than predicted oxygen requirements. Increasing depth of anesthesia does not significantly alter basal metabolic rate until tissue perfusion is compromised.

What is the relationship between oxygen consumption and CO_2 production?

Carbon dioxide production is approximately 80% of oxygen consumption (ie, respiratory ratio = 0.8):

$$\dot{V}CO_2 = 8kg^{3/4} = 194 \text{ mL } CO_2/min$$

How much ventilation is required to maintain normocapnia?

Minute ventilation is the sum of alveolar ventilation and ventilation of anatomic dead space and equipment dead space. Normocapnia is approximately a 5.6% alveolar concentration of CO_2:

$$\frac{40 \text{ mm Hg}}{760 \text{ mm Hg} - 47 \text{ mm Hg}} = 5.6\%$$

Thus, alveolar ventilation must be sufficient to dilute the 194 mL of expired CO_2 to a concentration of 5.6%:

$$\dot{V}_A = \frac{\dot{V}CO_2}{5.6\%} = \frac{194 \text{ mL/min}}{5.6\%} = 3393 \text{ mL/min}$$

Anatomic dead space is estimated as 1 mL/kg/breath:

$$\text{Anatomic dead space} = \text{Weight} \times 1 \text{ mL/kg}$$
$$= 70 \text{ mL/breath}$$

Equipment dead space consists primarily of the ventilation lost to expansion of the breathing circuit during positive-pressure ventilation. This can be estimated if the circuit compliance and peak airway pressure are known:

$$\text{Equipment dead space}$$
$$= \text{Compliance} \times \text{Pressure}$$
$$= (10 \text{ mL/cm } H_2O) \times (20 \text{ cm } H_2O)$$
$$= 200 \text{ mL/breath}$$

Therefore, at a respiratory rate of 10 breaths/min, total ventilation as measured by a spirometer should be $\dot{V}_T = 3393 + 700 + 2000 = 6093$ mL/min, and tidal volume would equal 609 mL.

How is the uptake of a volatile anesthetic predicted?

Anesthetic uptake by the pulmonary circulation depends upon the agent's blood/gas partition coefficient ($\lambda_{b/g}$), the alveolar/venous difference (CA–v), and the cardiac output ($\dot{Q}$):

$$\text{Uptake} = \lambda_{b/g} \times C(A - v) \times (\dot{Q})$$

The blood/gas partition coefficients of anesthetic agents have been experimentally determined (Table 7–1). At the beginning of an anesthetic procedure, the venous concentration of anesthetic is zero, so the alveolar-venous difference is equal to the alveolar concentration. The alveolar concentration required for surgical anesthesia is typically 1.3 MAC (Table 7–3). Cardiac output (dL/min) is related to metabolic rate and oxygen consumption:

$$\dot{Q} = 2kg^{3/4}$$

Thus, the rate of halothane uptake ($\dot{Q}_{an}$) by the pulmonary circulation at the end of the first minute of anesthesia can be predicted:

$$\dot{Q}_{an} \text{ at 1 min} = (2.4) \times (1.3)(.75) \times (2)(24.2)$$
$$= 113 \text{ mL of vapor}$$

As organs fill with anesthetic, the rate of uptake declines. An empirical mathematical model that closely fits observed uptake demonstrates the fall in uptake as being inversely proportionate to the square root of time (the **square root of time model**). In other words, the uptake at 4 minutes is one-half that at 1 minute and twice that at 16 minutes. Thus, the rate of uptake in our example would be 112 mL/min (112 ÷ 1) at the end of the first minute, 56 mL/min (112 ÷ 2) at the end of the fourth minute, and 28 mL/min (112 ÷ 4) at the end of the 16th minute. In general, the rate of uptake at any time *(t)* is—

$$\dot{Q}_{an} \text{ at } t \text{ min} = (\dot{Q}_{an} \text{ at 1 min}) \times t^{-1/2}$$

How can the amount of anesthetic taken up be predicted from the rate of uptake?

The cumulative anesthetic dose at any time *t* can be determined by integrating the rate function (finding the area under the FA/FI curve):

$$\text{Cumulative uptake} = 2 - (\dot{Q}_{an} \text{ at 1 min}) \times t^{1/2}$$

Therefore, at 1 minute the total amount of anesthetic that has been taken up is 224 mL; a total of 448 mL is taken up by 4 minutes; and 672 mL is taken up by 9 minutes. Stated another way, 226 mL is required to maintain a constant alveolar concentration during each square root of time interval. This quantity is called the **unit dose.**

What is a "priming dose"?

The breathing circuit, the patient's functional residual capacity, and the arterial circulation must be "primed" with anesthetic before tissue uptake can begin. The amount of anesthetic required to prime the breathing circuit and the functional residual capacity is equal to their combined volume (approximately 100 dL) multiplied by the desired alveolar concentration (1.3 MAC). Likewise, the amount of anesthetic required to prime the arterial circulation is equal to the blood volume—roughly equal to cardiac output—multiplied by the desired concentration and the blood/gas partition coefficient. For simplicity, these two priming doses are considered to be equal to 1 unit dose. Thus, during the first minute of anesthesia, 2 unit doses are administered: one as a priming dose and the other for tissue uptake.

By what methods can a unit dose of anesthetic be administered during a square root of time interval?

The 224 mL of halothane vapor can be administered by a copper kettle vaporizer or an agent-specific variable bypass vaporizer, or it can be directly injected in liquid form into the expiratory limb of the anesthesia circuit. Because the vapor pressure of halothane is 243 mm Hg at 20 °C, the concentration of halothane exiting a copper kettle is $243 \div 760$, or 32%. Therefore, 477 mL of oxygen must enter a copper kettle during one interval for 224 mL of halothane vapor to exit (see the vapor output equation in Chapter 4):

$$224 \text{ mL} \times \frac{760 - 243}{243} = 477 \text{ mL}$$

Modern agent-specific vaporizers deliver a constant concentration of agent regardless of flow. Therefore, if the total flow (nitrous oxide, oxygen, and anesthetic vapor) is 5 L during one time interval, a 4.5% concentration is required:

$$\frac{224 \text{ mL}}{5000 \text{ mL}} = 4.5\%$$

Direct injection into the circuit from a glass syringe with a metal stopcock is an easy way to administer volatile agents. Each milliliter of liquid halothane, methoxyflurane, isoflurane, or enflurane represents approximately 200 mL of vapor. Thus, a little over 1 mL needs to be injected during one time interval:

$$\frac{224 \text{ mL vapor}}{200 \text{ mL vapor/mL liquid}} = 1.12 \text{ mL liquid}$$

Can nitrous oxide uptake be predicted in a similar manner?

Similar predictions can be made for nitrous oxide with two qualifications. First, 1.3 MAC (approximately 137% N_2O) cannot be delivered at atmospheric pressure due to hypoxia. Second, because 30% of the blood supply to highly perfused organs is shunted, only 70% of the predicted nitrous oxide is actually taken up by blood recirculating through the lungs. Therefore, a shunt factor of 0.7 is introduced into the uptake equation:

$$\text{Uptake } N_2O = 0.7 \times 0.47 \times \%N_2O \times \dot{Q}$$

For a 70-kg patient at 65% nitrous oxide—

$$\dot{Q}_{an} \text{ at 1 min} = 0.7 \times 0.47 = 65 = (2)(24.2)$$
$$= 1035 \text{ mL/min}$$

The unit dose for nitrous oxide would be—

$$\text{Unit dose} = 2 \times \dot{Q}_{an} \text{ at 1 min} = 2070 \text{ mL}$$

A large priming dose is required:

$$\text{Circuit prime} = (\text{FRC} + \text{Circuit volume}) \times 65\%$$
$$= (100\text{dL})(0.65) = 65 \text{ dL}$$

$$\text{Arterial prime} = \text{Blood volume} \times \lambda_{b/g} = 65\%$$
$$= (50\text{dL})(0.45)(0.65) = 15 \text{ dL}$$

$$\text{Total prime} = 80 \text{ dL} = 8\text{L}$$

Therefore, in the first minute of a nitrous oxide anesthetic procedure, several liters of nitrous oxide would be administered. In clinical practice, nitrous oxide is empirically administered in amounts sufficient to maintain circuit volume as judged by constant breathing bag size or the height of a ventilator's standing bellows. If expired oxygen concentration falls below acceptable levels, the metabolic oxygen flow (242 mL/min) is increased. Sixty-five percent nitrous oxide anesthesia would be supplemented with intravenous or volatile agents. Since MAC is additive, 0.65 MAC of volatile anesthetic is required to attain a total of 1.3 MAC.

Briefly describe the first few minutes of a closed-circuit anesthetic procedure with nitrous oxide and halothane.

After preoxygenation, intravenous induction, and intubation, oxygen flow is set to the predicted metabolic oxygen requirement (242 mL/min). At the same time, nitrous oxide is administered at 6–8 L/min to prime the circuit and the patient's functional residual capacity. When expired oxygen drops to 40%, the nitrous oxide is reduced to match the calculated rate of uptake (2070 mL per square root of time interval), and the pressure relief valve is closed. If the ventilator bellows or breathing bag indicates an increasing or decreasing circuit volume, the nitrous oxide flowmeter is adjusted accordingly. If the expired oxygen concentration falls too low, the oxygen flow rate is increased. The priming and unit dose of volatile anesthetic can be administered by either of the methods described. Dosing intervals and amounts are only predictions. The correct dose for each patient is determined by the clinical signs of anesthetic depth: blood pressure, heart rate, respiratory rate, tearing, pupillary changes, diaphoresis, movement, etc.

SUGGESTED READINGS

Attia RR, Grogono AW, Domer FR (editors): *Practical Anesthetic Pharmacology.* Appleton-Century-Crofts, 1987. Includes many tables comparing the physical, chemical, and pharmacologic properties of inhalational anesthetics.

Brown BR: Development of concepts of hepatotoxicity of halogenated anesthetics. Semin Anesth 1988;7:47. Historical review of the hepatotoxicity of anesthetic agents from chloroform to modern volatile agents.

Covino BG et al (editors): *Effects of Anesthesia.* American Physiological Society, 1985. A collection of fairly technical articles on the molecular basis of anesthetic agents and their pulmonary and cardiac effects.

Eger EI: *Anesthetic Uptake and Action.* Williams & Wilkins, 1974. The most complete single source of information regarding uptake and distribution of inhalational anesthetics.

Hans-Joachim P: Isoflurane and coronary hemodynamics. Anesthesiology 1989;71:960. An overview of the controversy of coronary steal.

Lowe HJ, Ernst EA: *The Quantitative Practice of Anesthesia: Use of The Closed Circuit.* Williams & Wilkins, 1981. Authoritative work on closed-circuit anesthesia which eloquently presents the square root of time model.

Marshall BE, Longnecker DE: General anesthetics. Chapter 14 in: *Goodman and Gilman's The Pharmacologic Basis of Therapeutics,* 8th ed. Gilman AG, Goodman LS (editors). Pergamon, 1990.

Saidman LJ: The role of desflurane in the practice of anesthesia. (Editorial.) Anesthesiology 1991;74:399. This issue of *Anesthesiology* contains the results of many early investigations of the human pharmacology of desflurane.

Stoelting RK: *Pharmacology and Physiology in Anesthetic Practice.* Lippincott, 1987. One of the best discussions of the clinical pharmacology of volatile anesthetic agents. Does not include desflurane.

Nonvolatile Anesthetic Agents

General anesthesia is not limited to the use of inhaled agents. Numerous drugs that are administered orally, intramuscularly, and intravenously augment or produce an anesthetic state within their therapeutic dosage range. Preoperative sedation is often accomplished by way of oral or intramuscular routes, while induction and maintenance of anesthesia usually involve intravenous administration. This chapter begins with a review of the pharmacologic principles of pharmacokinetics and pharmacodynamics and how they apply to this class of drugs. The clinical pharmacology of several anesthetic agents is presented: barbiturates, benzodiazepines, opioids, ketamine, etomidate, propofol, and droperidol.

PHARMACOLOGIC PRINCIPLES

PHARMACOKINETICS

As explained in Chapter 7, pharmacokinetics is the study of the relationship between a drug's dose, tissue concentration, and time since administration. Simply stated, it describes how the body affects a drug. Pharmacokinetics is defined by four parameters: **absorption, distribution, biotransformation,** and **excretion. Elimination** implies drug removal by both biotransformation and excretion. **Clearance** is a measurement of the rate of elimination.

Absorption

There are many possible routes of systemic drug absorption: oral, sublingual, rectal, inhalational, transdermal, subcutaneous, intramuscular, and intravenous. Absorption, the process by which a drug leaves its site of administration to enter the bloodstream, is affected by the physical characteristics of the drug (solubility, pK_a, and concentration) and the site of absorption (circulation, pH, and surface area). Absorption differs from **bioavailability,** which is the fraction of unchanged drug that reaches the systemic circulation. For instance, nitroglycerin is well absorbed by the gastrointestinal tract. However, it has low bioavailability when administered orally since it is extensively metabolized by the liver before it can reach the systemic circulation and the myocardium (**first-pass hepatic metabolism).**

Oral administration is convenient, economical, and relatively tolerant of dosage error. However, it is unreliable since it (1) depends upon patient cooperation, (2) exposes the drug to first-pass hepatic metabolism, and (3) allows interference by gastric pH, enzymes, motility, food, and other drugs.

The nonionized forms of drugs are preferentially absorbed. Therefore, an acidic environment favors the absorption of acidic drugs ($A^- + H^+ \rightarrow AH$), while an alkaline environment favors basic drugs ($BH^+ \rightarrow H^+ + B$). Regardless of ionization considerations, the large surface area of the small intestine provides a preferential site of absorption for most drugs compared with the stomach.

Because the veins of the mouth drain into the superior vena cava, **sublingual** or **buccal** drug absorption bypasses the liver and first-pass metabolism. **Rectal** administration is an alternative to oral medication in patients who are uncooperative (eg, pediatric patients) or unable to tolerate oral ingestion. Because the venous drainage of the rectum bypasses the liver, first-pass metabolism is less significant than with small intestinal absorption. However, rectal absorption can be erratic, and many drugs cause irritation of the rectal mucosa. Absorption of **inhalational** agents is discussed in Chapter 7.

Transdermal drug administration has the advantage of prolonged and continuous absorption with a minimal total drug dose. However, the stratum corneum serves as an effective barrier to all but small, lipid-soluble drugs (eg, clonidine, nitroglycerin, and scopolamine).

Parenteral injection includes **subcutaneous, intramuscular,** and **intravenous** routes of administration. Subcutaneous and intramuscular absorption depends upon diffusion from the site of injection to the circulation. The rate of diffusion depends upon the blood flow to the area and the carrier vehicle (eg, solutions are absorbed faster than suspensions). Irritating preparations can cause pain and tissue necrosis. Intravenous injection completely bypasses the process of absorption, since the drug is placed directly into the bloodstream.

Distribution

Distribution plays a key role in clinical pharmacology since it is a major determinant of end-organ drug concentration. A drug's distribution depends primarily upon (1) organ perfusion, (2) protein binding, and (3) lipid solubility.

After absorption, a drug is distributed by the bloodstream throughout the body. Highly perfused organs (the **vessel-rich group**) have the initial opportunity to take up a proportionately large amount of drug compared with less perfused organs (the **muscle, fat,** and **vessel-poor groups**). Thus, even though the total mass of the vessel-rich group is small, it can account for substantial initial drug uptake (Table 8–1).

As long as a drug is bound to a plasma protein, it is unavailable for uptake by an organ regardless of the extent of perfusion to that organ. Albumin often binds acidic drugs (eg, barbiturates), while α_1-acid glycoprotein binds basic drugs (local anesthetics). If these proteins are diminished (eg, albumin in severe liver disease) or if the protein binding sites are occupied (eg, other drugs), the amount of free drug available for tissue uptake is increased.

Availability of a drug to a specific organ does not ensure uptake by that organ. For instance, the permeation by ionized drugs into the central nervous system is limited by pericapillary glial cells and endothelial cell tight junctions, which constitute the **blood-brain barrier.** Lipid-soluble, un-ionized molecules pass freely through lipid membranes. Other factors, such as molecular size and tissue binding—especially by the lung—can also influence drug distribution.

After the highly perfused organs are saturated during initial distribution, the greater mass of the less perfused organs will continue to take up drug from the bloodstream. As plasma concentration falls, some drug will leave the highly perfused organs to maintain equilibrium. This **redistribution** from the vessel-rich group is responsible for termination of effect of many anesthetic drugs. For example, *awakening from the effects of thiopental is not due to metabolism or excretion but rather to redistribution of the drug from brain to muscle.* As a corollary, if the less perfused organs are saturated from repeated doses of drug, redistribution cannot occur and awakening will depend to a greater extent upon drug elimination. Thus, rapid-acting drugs such as thiopental and fentanyl may become long-acting after repeated administration or when a large single dose is given.

Table 8–1. Tissue group composition, relative body mass, and percentage of cardiac output.

Tissue Group	Composition	% Body Mass	% Cardiac Output
Vessel-rich	Brain, heart, liver, kidney, endocrine glands	10	75
Muscle	Muscle, skin	50	19
Fat	Fat	20	6
Vessel-poor	Bone, ligament, cartilage	20	0

The *apparent* volume into which a drug has been distributed is called its **volume of distribution (V_d)** and is determined by dividing the dose of drug administered by the resulting plasma concentration:

$$V_d = \frac{Dose}{Concentration}$$

This calculation is complicated by the need to adjust for the effects of drug elimination and continual redistribution. A small volume of distribution implies relative confinement of the drug to the intravascular space, which leads to a high plasma concentration (eg, the V_d of pancuronium = 10 L in a 70-kg person). Causes for a small volume of distribution include high protein binding or ionization. On the other hand, the apparent volume of distribution may exceed total body water (approximately 40 L). Explanations for this include high solubility or binding of the drug in tissues other than plasma (eg, the V_d of fentanyl = 350 L). *Therefore, the volume of distribution does not represent a real volume but rather reflects the volume of plasma that would be necessary to account for the observed plasma concentration.*

Biotransformation

Biotransformation is the alteration of a substance by metabolic processes. The end products of biotransformation are usually—but not necessarily—inactive and water-soluble. The latter property allows excretion by the kidney. The liver is the primary organ of biotransformation.

Metabolic biotransformation can be divided into phase I and phase II reactions. **Phase I reactions** convert a parent drug into more polar metabolites through oxidation, reduction, or hydrolysis. **Phase II reactions** couple (conjugate) a parent drug or a phase I metabolite with an endogenous substrate (eg, glucuronic acid) to form a highly polar end product that can be eliminated in the urine. Although this is usually a sequential process, phase I metabolites may be excreted without undergoing phase II biotransformation, and a phase II reaction can precede a phase I reaction.

Hepatic clearance is the rate of elimination of a drug due to liver biotransformation. More specifically, clearance is the volume of plasma cleared of drug per unit time and is expressed in milliliters per minute. The hepatic clearance depends upon the hepatic blood flow and the fraction of drug removed from the blood by the liver (**hepatic extraction ratio**). Drugs that are efficiently cleared by the liver have a high hepatic extraction ratio, and their clearance is proportionate to hepatic blood flow. On the other hand, drugs with a low hepatic extraction ratio are poorly cleared by the liver, and their clearance is limited by the capacity of the hepatic enzyme systems. Therefore, the effect of liver disease on drug pharmacokinetics depends upon the drug's hepatic extraction ratio and the disease's propensity to alter hepatic blood flow or hepatocellular function.

Excretion

The kidney is the principal organ of excretion. Non-protein bound drugs freely cross from plasma into the glomerular filtrate. The nonionized fraction of drug will be reabsorbed in the renal tubules, while the ionized portion will be excreted. Thus, alterations in urine pH can alter renal excretion. The kidney also actively secretes some drugs. **Renal clearance** is the rate of elimination of a drug due to kidney excretion. Renal failure changes the pharmacokinetics of many drugs by altering protein binding, volumes of distribution, and clearance rates.

Relatively few drugs depend on biliary excretion, since they are usually reabsorbed in the intestine and are consequently excreted in the urine. Delayed toxic effects from some drugs may be due to this **enterohepatic recirculation** (eg, fentanyl).

The lung is responsible for excretion of volatile agents such as inhalational anesthetics (Chapter 7).

Compartment Models

Compartment models offer a simple way to characterize the distribution and elimination of drugs in the body. A compartment can be conceptualized as a group of tissues that possess similar pharmacokinetics. For example, plasma and the vessel-rich group could represent the **central compartment,** while muscle, fat, and skin could represent the **peripheral compartment.** Having said this, it must be stressed that compartments are conceptual and do not represent actual tissues.

A **two-compartment model** correlates well with the distribution and elimination phases of many drugs (Figure 8–1). After an intravenous bolus, the plasma concentration of a drug will instantaneously rise. The initial rapid decline in plasma concentration, called the **distribution phase,** or **alpha phase,** corresponds to the redistribution of drug from the plasma and the vessel-rich group of the central compartment to the less perfused tissues of the peripheral compartment. As distribution slows, elimination of drug from the central compartment is responsible for a continued—but less steep—decline in plasma concentration called the **elimination phase** or **beta phase.** Elimination half-life is proportionate to the volume of distribution and inversely proportionate to the rate of clearance. The plasma concentration curves of many drugs are better characterized by a **three-compartment model** consisting of a central compartment and two peripheral compartments. Plasma concentration following a bolus administration of a drug can be expressed by a triexponential equation:

$$Cp(t) = Ae^{-\alpha t} + Be^{-\beta t} + Ce^{-\gamma t}$$

where $Cp(t)$ = plasma concentration at time t and A, B, and C are fractional coefficients that denote the relative contributions of each of three hybrid rate constants (α corresponding to the rapid distribution half-life, β to the slow-distribution half-life, and γ to the

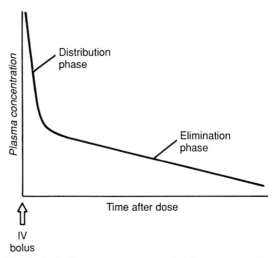

Figure 8–1. Two-compartment model demonstrates the distribution phase (α phase) and the elimination phase (β phase). During the distribution phase, drug moves from the central compartment to the peripheral compartment. The elimination phase consists of metabolism and excretion.

elimination half-life). Therefore, drug plasma concentration is determined by six pharmacokinetic parameters and not just half-lives, as is often assumed.

Rates of distribution and biotransformation can usually be described in terms of **first-order kinetics.** In other words, a constant fraction or percentage of drug is distributed or metabolized per unit of time regardless of plasma concentration. For instance, 10% of a drug may be biotransformed hourly whether the plasma concentration is 10 μg/mL or 100 μg/mL. However, if the concentration of drug exceeds the biotransformation capacity, then a constant amount of drug may be metabolized per unit time **(zero-order kinetics).** Using a similar example, 500 μg of drug might be metabolized each hour regardless of whether the plasma concentration were 10 μg/mL or 100 μg/mL. Alcohol metabolism can be predicted by zero-order kinetics.

Compartment models allow the prediction of pharmacokinetic variables (eg, elimination half-life) and explain clinically important differences between similar drugs. They are less accurate predictors of individual responses to drugs.

PHARMACODYNAMICS

Pharmacodynamics is the study of the therapeutic and toxic organ system effects of drugs (how a drug affects a body). The extent of these effects determines a drug's efficacy, potency, and therapeutic ratio. However, pharmacodynamics also inquires into mechanisms of action, drug interactions, and structure-activity relationships. Understanding dose-response curves and drug receptors provides a framework to help explain these diverse parameters of pharmacodynamics.

Dose-Response Curves

Dose-response curves express the relationship between drug dose and pharmacologic effect. Drug dose or steady-state plasma concentration is plotted on the abscissa (*x* axis) and is represented in linear (Figure 8–2A) or logarithmic scale (Figure 8–2B). Pharmacologic effect is plotted on the ordinate (*y* axis) in terms of absolute units (Figure 8–2A) or as a fraction of maximal effect (Figure 8–2B). The position of the dose-response curve along the abscissa is an indication of drug **potency.** The maximal effect of the drug relates to its **efficacy.** The slope of the dose-response curve reflects receptor-binding characteristics. The influence of pharmacokinetics in dose-response curves can be minimized by studying the relationship of blood concentration to pharmacologic response.

The **median effective dose** (ED50) is the dose of drug required to produce a given effect in 50% of the population. Note that the ED50 is *not* the dose required to produce one-half the maximal effect. The ED50 of inhalational anesthetics is the same as the minimum alveolar concentration (see Chapter 7). The **median lethal dose** (LD50) is the dose that results in death in 50% of the population exposed to that dose. The **therapeutic index** is the ratio of the median lethal dose to the median effective dose (LD50:ED50).

Drug Receptors

Drug receptors are macromolecules—usually proteins embedded into cell membranes—that interact with a drug to mediate characteristic intracellular changes. The mechanism of action of several (not all) drugs depends upon interaction with a receptor. Endogenous substances (eg, hormones) or exogenous substances (eg, drugs) that directly change cell function by binding to receptors are called **agonists. Antagonists** also bind to the receptors but without causing a direct effect on the cell. The pharmacologic effect of antagonist drugs depends upon the subsequent inability of agonist substances to activate the receptors. **Competitive antagonists** reversibly bind to receptors and can be displaced by higher concentrations of agonists. **Noncompetitive (irreversible) antagonists** bind to the receptor with such affinity that even high concentrations of agonists cannot reverse the receptor blockade. Competition of two drugs for the same receptor is one source of drug interactions.

Receptors affect cell function either directly (eg, by changing transmembrane ion flux) or by controlling the production of another regulatory molecule (eg, the second-messenger cAMP). Individual variability in response to receptor binding is a significant cause of inconsistency in drug responsiveness. Continued activation of a receptor often leads to **hyporeactivity,** while lack of stimulation results in **hyperreactivity.** Chemical structure determines the degree of affinity between a drug and a receptor (**structure-activity relationship).** Minor changes in molecular configuration can have dramatic effects on clinical pharmacology.

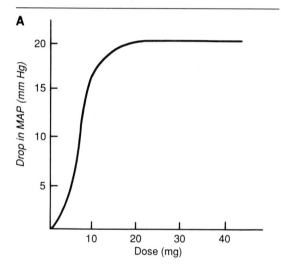

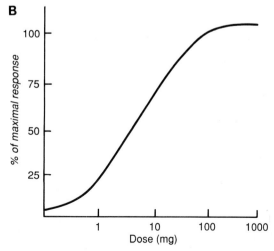

Figure 8–2. The shapes of dose-response curves depend on whether the dose or steady-state plasma concentration (C_CPSS) is plotted on a linear **(A)** or logarithmic **(B)** scale.

SPECIFIC NONVOLATILE ANESTHETIC AGENTS

BARBITURATES

Mechanisms of Action

Barbiturates depress the reticular activating system, a complex polysynaptic network of neurons and regulatory centers located in the brainstem that controls several vital functions, including consciousness. In clinical concentrations, barbiturates preferentially affect the function of nerve synapses as opposed to nerve axons. They suppress transmission of excitatory neurotransmitters (eg, acetylcholine) and enhance transmission of inhibitory neurotransmitters (eg, γ-aminobutyric acid). Specific mechanisms include interfering with transmitter release (presynaptic) and stereoselectively interacting with receptors (postsynaptic).

Structure-Activity Relationships

Barbiturates are barbituric acid derivatives (Figure 8–3). Substitution at the number 5 carbon (C_5) deter-

mines hypnotic potency and anticonvulsant activity. For example, a long branched chain conveys more potency than a short straight chain. Likewise, the **phenyl** group in *phenobarbital* is anticonvulsive compared with the **methyl** group in *methohexital*. Replacing the **oxygen** at C_2 (*oxybarbiturates*) with a **sulfur** atom (*thiobarbiturates*) increases lipid solubility. As a result, thiopental and thiamylal have greater potency, more rapid onset of action, and shorter durations of action than pentobarbital and secobarbital. The short duration of action of methohexital is related to the methyl substitution at N_1. The sodium salts of the barbiturates are water-soluble but markedly alkaline (pH of 2.5% thiopental > 10) and relatively unstable (2-week shelf-life for 2.5% thiopental solution). Con-

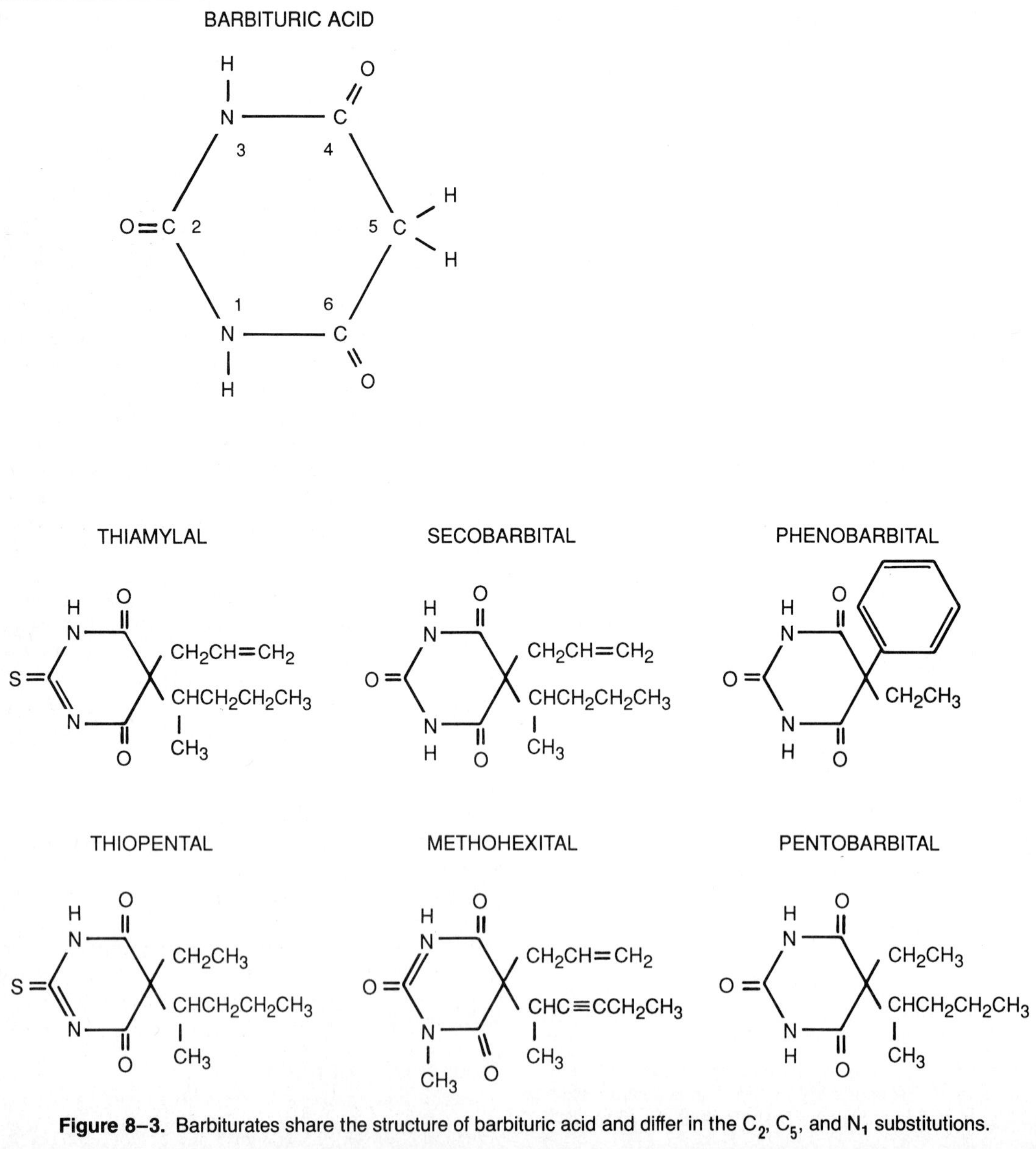

Figure 8–3. Barbiturates share the structure of barbituric acid and differ in the C_2, C_5, and N_1 substitutions.

centrations higher than recommended cause an unacceptable incidence of pain on injection and venous thrombosis.

Pharmacokinetics

A. Absorption: In clinical anesthesiology, barbiturates are most frequently administered intravenously for induction of general anesthesia in adults. Exceptions include rectal thiopental or methohexital for induction in children and intramuscular pentobarbital or secobarbital for premedication of all age groups.

B. Distribution: The duration of action of highly lipid-soluble barbiturates (thiopental, thiamylal, and methohexital) is determined by redistribution, not metabolism or elimination. For example, although thiopental is highly protein-bound (80%), its great lipid solubility and high nonionized fraction (60%) account for maximal brain uptake within 30 seconds. If the central compartment is contracted (eg, hypovolemic shock), if the serum albumin is low (eg, severe liver disease), or if the nonionized fraction is increased (eg, acidosis), higher brain and heart concentrations will be achieved for a given dose. Subsequent redistribution to the peripheral compartment—specifically, the muscle group—lowers plasma and brain concentration to 10% of peak levels within 20–30 minutes (Figure 8–4). This pharmacokinetic profile correlates with clinical experience—patients typically lose consciousness within 30 seconds and awaken within 20 minutes. In contrast to the rapid initial distribution half-life of a few minutes, the elimination half-life of thiopental ranges from 3 hours to 12 hours. Thiamylal and methohexital have similar distribution patterns, while less lipid-soluble barbiturates have much longer distribution half-lives and durations of action. Repetitive administration of barbiturates will saturate the peripheral compartments, so that redistribution cannot occur and

duration of action will become more dependent on elimination.

C. Biotransformation: Biotransformation of barbiturates principally involves hepatic oxidation to inactive, water-soluble metabolites. Because of greater hepatic extraction, methohexital is cleared by the liver three to four times more rapidly than thiopental or thiamylal. While redistribution is responsible for the awakening from a single dose of any of these lipid-soluble barbiturates, full recovery of psychomotor function is more rapid following methohexital owing to its enhanced metabolism.

D. Excretion: High protein binding decreases barbiturate glomerular filtration, while high lipid solubility tends to increase renal tubular reabsorption. Except for the less bound and less lipid-soluble agents such as phenobarbital, renal excretion is limited to water-soluble end products of hepatic biotransformation. Methohexital is excreted in the feces.

Effects on Organ Systems

A. Cardiovascular: Induction doses of intravenously administered barbiturates cause a fall in blood pressure and an elevation in heart rate. Depression of the medullary vasomotor center vasodilates peripheral capacitance vessels, which increases peripheral pooling of blood and decreases venous return to the right atrium. The tachycardia is probably due to a central vagolytic effect. Cardiac output is often maintained by a rise in heart rate and increased myocardial contractility due to compensatory baroreceptor reflexes. Sympathetically induced vasoconstriction of resistance vessels may actually increase peripheral vascular resistance. However, in the absence of an adequate baroreceptor response (eg, hypovolemia, congestive heart failure, or β-adrenergic blockade), cardiac output and arterial blood pressure may fall dramatically owing to uncompensated peripheral pooling and unmasked direct myocardial depression. Patients with poorly controlled hypertension are particularly prone to wide swings in blood pressure during induction. Thus, the cardiovascular effects of barbiturates vary markedly depending on volume status, baseline autonomic tone, and preexisting cardiovascular disease. A slow rate of injection and adequate preoperative hydration attenuate these changes in many patients.

B. Respiratory: Barbiturate depression of the medullary ventilatory center decreases the ventilatory response to hypercapnia and hypoxia. Apnea usually follows an induction dose of barbiturate. During awakening, tidal volume and respiratory rate are decreased. Barbiturates do not completely depress noxious airway reflexes, and bronchospasm in asthmatic patients or laryngospasm in lightly anesthetized patients is not uncommon following airway instrumentation. Laryngospasm and hiccuping is more common after methohexital than after thiopental.

C. Cerebral: Barbiturates constrict the cerebral vasculature, causing a decrease in cerebral blood flow

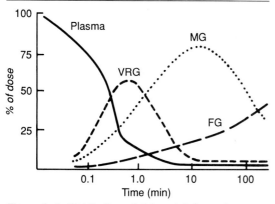

Figure 8–4. Distribution of thiopental from plasma, to vessel-rich group (VRG), to muscle group (MG), and finally to fat group (FG). (Modified and reproduced, with permission, from Price HL et al: The uptake of thiopental by body tissues and its relation to the duration of narcosis. Clin Pharmacol Ther 1960;1:16.)

and intracranial pressure. The drop in intracranial pressure exceeds the decline in arterial blood pressure, so that **cerebral perfusion pressure** (CPP) is usually increased (CPP = cerebral artery pressure minus the greater of cerebral venous pressure or intracranial pressure). The decrease in cerebral flow is not detrimental, since barbiturates induce an even greater decline in **cerebral oxygen consumption** (up to 50% of normal). Alterations in cerebral activity and oxygen requirements are reflected by changes in the EEG, which progresses from low-voltage fast activity with small doses to high-voltage slow activity and electrical silence (isoelectric) with very large doses of barbiturate (30–40 mg/kg of thiopental). This effect of barbiturates may protect the brain from transient episodes of focal ischemia (eg, cerebral embolism) but probably not from global ischemia (eg, cardiac arrest).

The degree of central nervous system depression induced by barbiturates ranges from mild sedation to unconsciousness, depending on the dose administered (Table 8–2). Unlike narcotics, barbiturates do not selectively impair the perception of pain. In fact, they sometimes appear to have an **antianalgesic effect** by lowering the pain threshold. Small doses occasionally cause a state of excitement and disorientation that can be disconcerting when sedation is the objective. Barbiturates do not produce muscle relaxation, and some induce involuntary skeletal muscle contractions (eg, methohexital). Relatively small doses of thiopental (50–100 mg intravenously) rapidly control most grand mal seizures. Acute tolerance and physiologic dependence on the sedative effect of barbiturates develop quickly.

D. Renal: Barbiturates reduce renal blood flow and glomerular filtration rate in proportion to the fall in blood pressure.

E. Hepatic: Hepatic blood flow is decreased. Chronic exposure to barbiturates has opposing effects on drug biotransformation. Induction of hepatic enzymes increases the rate of metabolism of some drugs (eg, digitoxin), while combination with the cytochrome P-450 enzyme system interferes with the biotransformation of others (eg, tricyclic antidepressants). The induction of aminolevulinic acid synthetase stimulates the formation of porphyrin (an intermediary in heme synthesis), which may precipitate **acute intermittent porphyria** or **variegate porphyria** in susceptible individuals.

F. Immunologic: Anaphylactic and anaphylactoid allergic reactions are rare. Sulfur-containing thiobarbiturates evoke mast cell histamine release in vitro, while oxybarbiturates do not. For this reason, some anesthesiologists prefer methohexital over thiopental or thiamylal in asthmatic or atopic patients.

Drug Interactions

Contrast media, sulfonamides, and other drugs that occupy the same protein-binding sites as thiopental will increase the amount of free drug available and potentiate the organ system effects of a given dose.

Ethanol, narcotics, antihistamines, and other central nervous system depressants potentiate the sedative effects of barbiturates.

BENZODIAZEPINES

Mechanisms of Action

Benzodiazepines interact with specific receptors in the central nervous system, particularly in the cerebral cortex. Benzodiazepine receptor binding enhances the inhibitory effects of various neurotransmitters. For example, benzodiazepine receptor binding facilitates γ-aminobutyric acid receptor binding, which increases the membrane conductance of chloride ions. This causes a change in membrane polarization that inhibits normal neuronal function.

Structure-Activity Relationships

The chemical structure of benzodiazepines includes a benzene ring and a seven-member diazepine ring (Figure 8–5). Substitutions at various positions on these rings affect potency and biotransformation. The imidazole ring of midazolam contributes to its water solubility at low pH. The insolubility of diazepam and lorazepam in water requires parenteral preparations to contain propylene glycol, which has been associated with venous irritation.

Pharmacokinetics

A. Absorption: Benzodiazepines are commonly administered orally, intramuscularly, and intra-

Table 8–2. Uses and dosages of commonly used barbiturates.

Agent	Use	Route	Concentration	Dose
Thiopental, thiamylal	Induction Sedation	IV IV	2.5% 2.5%	3–6 mg/kg 0.5–1.5 mg/kg
Methohexital	Induction Sedation Induction	IV IV Rectal (children)	1% 1% 10%	1–2 mg/kg 0.2–0.4 mg/kg 25 mg/kg
Secobarbital, pentobarbital	Premedication	Oral IM Rectal suppository	5%	2–4 mg/kg[1] 2–4 mg/kg[1] 3 mg/kg

[1]Maximum dose 150 mg.

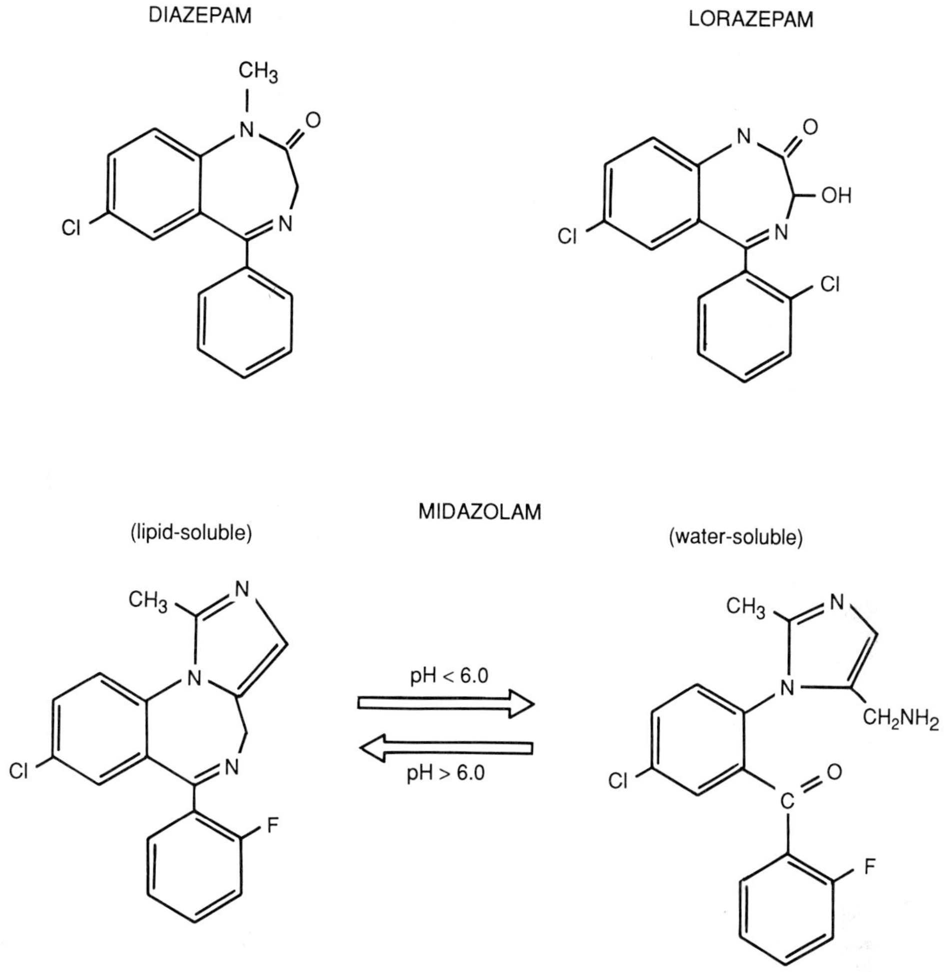

DIAZEPAM

LORAZEPAM

MIDAZOLAM

(lipid-soluble)

(water-soluble)

pH < 6.0

pH > 6.0

Figure 8–5. The structures of commonly used benzodiazepines share a seven-member diazepine ring. (Modified and reproduced, with permission, from White PF: Pharmacologic and clinical aspects of preoperative medication: Anesth Analg 1986;65:963. With permission from the International Anesthesia Research Society.)

venously to provide sedation or induction of general anesthesia (Table 8–3). Diazepam and lorazepam are well absorbed from the gastrointestinal tract, with peak plasma levels usually achieved in 1 and 2 hours, respectively. Midazolam is not approved for oral administration.

Intramuscular injection of diazepam is painful and unreliable. In contrast, midazolam and lorazepam are well absorbed after intramuscular injection, with peak levels achieved in 30 and 90 minutes, respectively.

Induction of general anesthesia obviously relies upon intravenous administration.

B. Distribution: Diazepam is quite lipid-soluble and rapidly penetrates the blood-brain barrier. Although midazolam is water-soluble at low pH, its imidazole ring closes at physiologic pH, causing an increase in its lipid solubility (Figure 8–5). The moderate lipid solubility of lorazepam accounts for its slower brain uptake and onset of action. Redistribution

is fairly rapid for the benzodiazepines (initial distribution half-life = 3–10 minutes) and, similar to the barbiturates, is responsible for awakening. Although midazolam is frequently used as an induction agent, none of the benzodiazepines can match the rapid onset and short duration of action of thiopental. All three benzodiazepines are highly protein-bound (90–98%).

C. Biotransformation: The benzodiazepines rely upon the liver for biotransformation into water-soluble glucuronide end products. The phase I metabolites of diazepam are pharmacologically active.

Slow hepatic extraction and a large volume of distribution result in a long elimination half-life for diazepam (30 hours). Although lorazepam also has a low hepatic extraction ratio, its lower lipid solubility limits its volume of distribution, resulting in a shorter elimination half-life (15 hours). Nonetheless, the clinical duration of lorazepam is often quite prolonged owing to a very high receptor affinity. In contrast, midazolam

Table 8–3. Uses and dosages
of commonly used benzodiazepines.

Agent	Use	Route	Dose
Diazepam	Premedication	Oral	0.2–0.5 mg/kg[1]
	Sedation	IV	0.04–0.2 mg/kg
	Induction	IV	0.3–0.6 mg/kg
Midazolam	Premedication	IM	0.07–0.15 mg/kg
	Sedation	IV	0.01–0.1 mg/kg
	Induction	IV	0.1–0.4 mg/kg
Lorazepam	Premedication	Oral	0.05 mg/kg[2]
		IM	0.03–0.05 mg/kg[2]
	Sedation	IV	0.03–0.04 mg/kg[2]

[1]Maximum dose 15 mg.
[2]Not recommended for children.

shares diazepam's volume of distribution, but its elimination half-life (2 hours) is the shortest of the group because of its high hepatic extraction ratio.

D. Excretion: The metabolites of benzodiazepine biotransformation are excreted chiefly in the urine. Enterohepatic circulation produces a secondary peak in diazepam plasma concentration 6–12 hours following administration.

Organ System Effects

A. Cardiovascular: The benzodiazepines display minimal cardiovascular depressant effects even at induction doses. Arterial blood pressure, cardiac output, and peripheral vascular resistance usually decline slightly, while the heart rate sometimes rises. Midazolam tends to reduce blood pressure and peripheral vascular resistance more than diazepam.

B. Respiratory: Benzodiazepines depress the ventilatory response to CO_2. This depression is usually insignificant unless the drugs are administered intravenously or in association with other respiratory depressants. Although apnea may be less common than following barbiturate induction, even small intravenous doses of diazepam and midazolam have resulted in respiratory arrest. The steep dose-response curve and high potency of midazolam necessitate careful titration. Ventilation must be monitored in all patients receiving intravenous benzodiazepines, and resuscitation equipment must be immediately available.

C. Cerebral: Benzodiazepines reduce cerebral oxygen consumption, cerebral blood flow, and intracranial pressure but not to the extent the barbiturates do. They are very effective in preventing and controlling grand mal seizures. Oral sedative doses often produce antegrade amnesia, a useful premedication property. The mild muscle-relaxant properties of these drugs is mediated at the spinal cord level, not at the neuromuscular junction. The antianxiety, amnesic, and sedative effects seen at low doses progress to stupor and unconsciousness at induction doses. Compared to thiopental, induction with benzodiazepines is associated with a slower loss of consciousness and a

prolonged recovery. Benzodiazepines do not have direct analgesic properties.

Drug Interactions

Flumazenil (an imidazobenzodiazepine) is a specific benzodiazepine receptor antagonist that effectively reverses most of the central nervous system effects of benzodiazepines. It is extensively and rapidly metabolized by the liver, leading to a relatively short half-life ($t_{1/2} = 1$ hour). The intravenous dosage is 0.1–1 mg. Side effects of reversal include anxiety, headache, nausea, vomiting, and potential resedation.

Cimetidine binds to cytochrome P-450 and reduces the metabolism of diazepam.

Heparin displaces diazepam from protein binding sites and increases the free drug concentration (200% increase after 1000 units of heparin).

The combination of opioids and diazepam markedly reduces arterial blood pressure and peripheral vascular resistance. This synergistic interaction is especially pronounced in patients with ischemic or valvular heart disease.

Benzodiazepines reduce the minimum alveolar concentration of volatile anesthetics up to a ceiling of 30%.

Ethanol, barbiturates, and other central nervous system depressants potentiate the sedative effects of the benzodiazepines.

OPIOIDS

Mechanisms of Action

Opioids bind to specific receptors located throughout the central nervous system and other tissues. Four major types of opioid receptor have been identified: **mu** (μ) (with subtypes μ-1 and μ-2), **kappa** (κ), **delta** (δ), and **sigma** (σ) (Table 8–4). While opioids provide some degree of sedation, they are most effective at producing analgesia. The pharmacodynamic properties of specific opioids depend upon which receptor is bound, the binding affinity, and whether the receptor is activated. Although both opioid agonists and antagonists bind to opioid receptors, only agonists are capable of receptor activation. Agonist-antagonists (eg, nalbuphine, nalorphine, butorphanol, and pentazocine) are drugs that have opposite actions at different receptor types. The pure opioid antagonist naloxone is discussed in Chapter 15.

Endorphins, enkephalins, and **dynorphins** are endogenous peptides that bind to opioid receptors. These three families of opioid peptides differ in their protein precursors, anatomic distributions, and receptor affinities.

Opioid receptor activation inhibits the presynaptic release and postsynaptic response to excitatory neurotransmitters (eg, acetylcholine and substance P) from nociceptive neurons. The cellular mechanism for these effects may involve alterations in potassium and

Table 8–4. Classification of opioid receptors.[1]

Receptor	Clinical Effect	Agonists
Mu	Supraspinal analgesia (μ-1) Respiratory depression (μ-2) Physical dependence Muscle rigidity	Morphine Met-enkephalin[2] Beta-endorphin[2]
Kappa	Sedation Spinal analgesia	Morphine Nalbuphine Butorphanol Dynorphin[2]
Delta	Analgesia Behavioral Epileptogenic	Leu-enkephalin[2] Beta-endorphin[2]
Sigma	Dysphoria Hallucinations Respiratory stimulation	Pentazocine Nalorphine Ketamine?

[1]Note: The relationships between receptor, clinical effect, and agonist are more complex than indicated in this table. For example, pentazocine is an antagonist at mu receptors, a partial agonist at kappa receptors, and an agonist of sigma receptors.
[2]Endogenous opioid.

calcium ion conductance. Peripheral nerve conduction is not affected, though transmission of pain impulses is interrupted at the level of the dorsal horn of the spinal cord. Modulation of a descending inhibitory pathway from the periaqueductal gray through the nucleus raphe magnus to the dorsal horn of the spinal cord may also play a role in opioid analgesia.

Structure-Activity Relationships

Opioid receptor interaction is shared by a chemically diverse group of compounds. Nonetheless, there are common structural characteristics which are highlighted in Figure 8–6. Small molecular changes can convert an agonist into an antagonist. The levorotatory isomers are generally more potent than the dextrorotatory isomers.

Pharmacokinetics

A. Absorption: Rapid and complete absorption follows the intramuscular injection of morphine and meperidine, with peak plasma levels usually obtained after 20–60 minutes. Oral transmucosal fentanyl citrate absorption ("fentanyl lollipop") is an effective method of producing analgesia and sedation.

B. Distribution: Table 8–5 summarizes the physical characteristics that determine distribution and uptake of opioid anesthetics. The distribution half-lives of all of the narcotics are fairly rapid (5–20 minutes). However, the low fat solubility of morphine slows passage across the blood-brain barrier, with the result that its onset of action is slow and its duration of action is prolonged. This contrasts with the high lipid solubility of fentanyl and sufentanil, which allows a rapid onset and short duration of action. Interestingly,

alfentanil has the most rapid onset of action and the shortest duration of action, even though it is less lipid-soluble than fentanyl. The high fraction of alfentanil that is nonionized at physiologic pH and its small volume of distribution increase the amount of drug available for binding in the brain. Redistribution terminates the action of small doses of all of these drugs, while larger doses must depend on biotransformation to adequately lower plasma levels. Alfentanil has the shortest distribution half-life.

C. Biotransformation: All of the opioids depend primarily upon the liver for biotransformation. Their high hepatic extraction ratio causes their clearance to be dependent upon liver blood flow. The small volume of distribution of alfentanil is responsible for a 50% shorter elimination half-life ($1^{1}/_{2}$ hours) compared with the other opioids. Morphine undergoes conjugation with glucuronic acid to form morphine 3-glucuronide and morphine 6-glucuronide. Meperidine is N-demethylated to normeperidine, an active metabolite associated with seizure activity. The end products of fentanyl, sufentanil, and alfentanil are inactive.

D. Excretion: The end products of morphine and meperidine biotransformation are eliminated by the kidneys, with less than 10% undergoing biliary excretion. Because 5–10% of morphine is excreted unchanged in the urine, renal failure prolongs its duration of action. The accumulation of morphine metabolites (morphine 3-glucuronide and morphine 6-glucuronide) in patients with renal failure has been associated with prolonged narcosis. Similarly, renal dysfunction increases the chance of toxic effects from normeperidine accumulation. A late secondary peak in fentanyl plasma levels occurs up to 4 hours after the last intravenous dose and may be explained by enterohepatic recirculation or mobilization of sequestered drug. Metabolites of sufentanil are excreted in urine and bile.

Organ System Effects

A. Cardiovascular: In general, opioids do not seriously impair cardiovascular function. Meperidine tends to increase heart rate (it is structurally similar to atropine), while high doses of morphine, fentanyl, sufentanil, and alfentanil are associated with a vagus-mediated bradycardia. With the exception of meperidine, the opioids do not depress cardiac contractility. Nonetheless, arterial blood pressure often falls as a result of bradycardia, venodilatation, and decreased sympathetic reflexes. Additionally, meperidine and morphine evoke histamine release in some individuals that can lead to profound drops in arterial blood pressure and systemic vascular resistance. The effects of histamine release can be minimized in susceptible patients by slow opioid infusion, adequate intravascular volume, or pretreatment with H_1 and H_2 histamine antagonists (see Chapter 15).

Intraoperative hypertension during opioid anesthe-

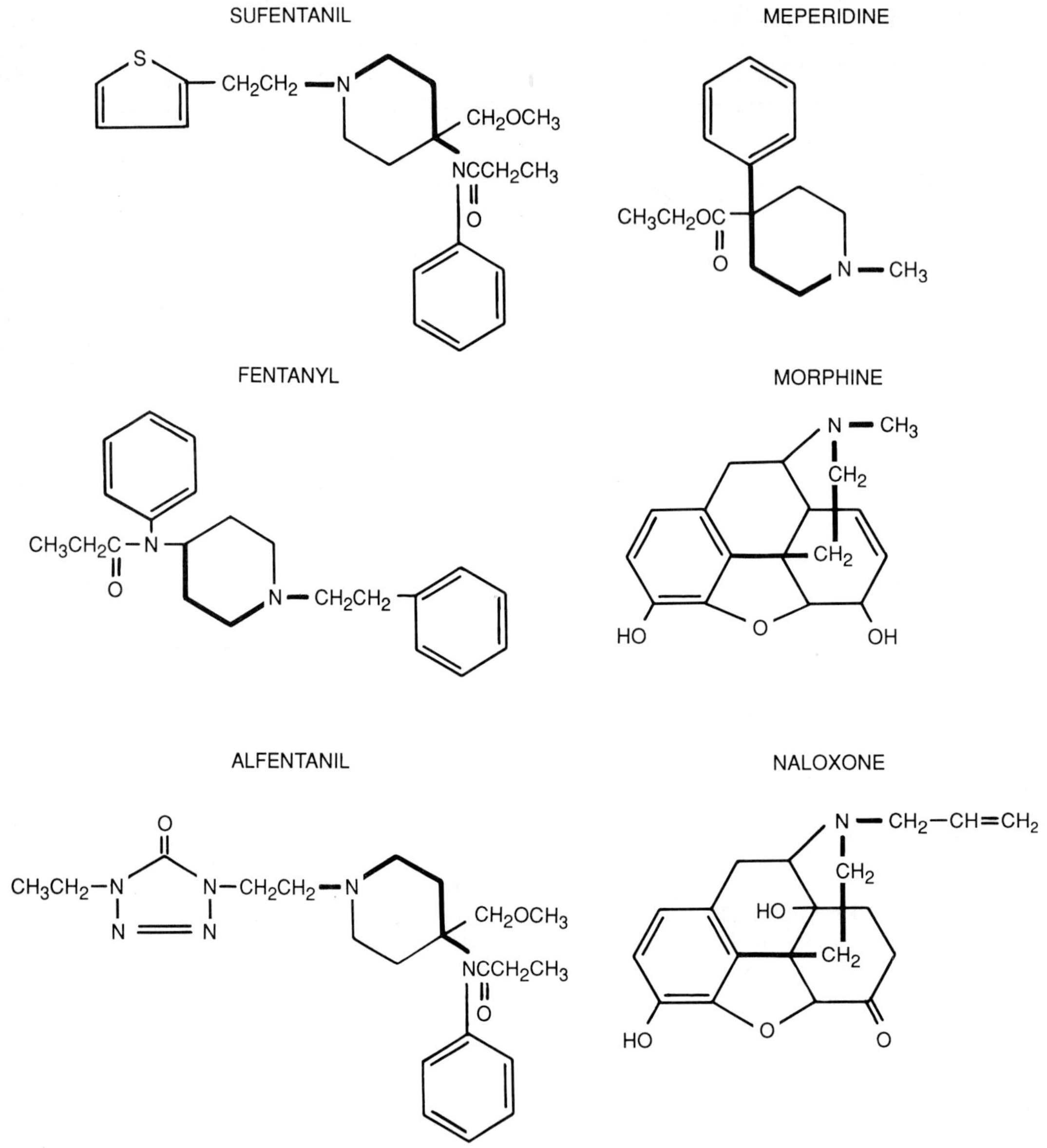

SUFENTANIL

MEPERIDINE

FENTANYL

MORPHINE

ALFENTANIL

NALOXONE

Figure 8–6. Opioid agonists and antagonists share part of their chemical structure, which is outlined in bold.

sia, particularly morphine and meperidine, is not un-common. It is often attributable to inadequate anesthetic depth and can be controlled with the addition of vasodilators or volatile anesthetic agents. The combination of opioids with other anesthetic drugs (eg, nitrous oxide, diazepam, barbiturates, and volatile agents) can result in significant myocardial depression.

B. Respiratory: Opioids depress ventilation, particularly respiratory rate. Resting $PaCO_2$ increases and the response to a CO_2 challenge is blunted, resulting in a shift of the CO_2 response curve downward and to the right (Figure 8–7). These effects are mediated through the respiratory centers in the brainstem. The

apneic threshold—the highest $PaCO_2$ at which a patient remains apneic—is elevated, and **hypoxic drive** is decreased. Morphine and meperidine can cause histamine-induced bronchospasm in susceptible patients. Opioids (particularly fentanyl, sufentanil, and alfentanil) can induce chest wall rigidity severe enough to prevent adequate ventilation. This centrally mediated muscle contraction is most frequent after large drug boluses and is effectively treated with muscle relaxants.

C. Cerebral: Opioids reduce cerebral oxygen consumption, cerebral blood flow, and intracranial pressure, but to a lesser extent than barbiturates or benzodiazepines. These effects presume a mainte-

Table 8–5. Physical characteristics of opioids that determine distribution.

Agent	Nonionized Fraction	Protein Binding	Lipid Solubility
Morphine	++	++	+
Meperidine	+	+++	++
Fentanyl	+	+++	++++
Sufentanil	++	++++	++++
Alfentanil	++++	++++	+++

Key: + = very low; ++ = low; +++ = high; ++++ = very high.

nance of normocapnia by artificial ventilation. The effect of opioids on the EEG is minimal, though high doses are associated with slow delta wave activity. High doses of fentanyl may rarely be associated with seizure activity, though this is not well documented. One study suggests that sufentanil may transiently increase cerebral blood flow, while others have challenged this finding. Stimulation of the medullary chemoreceptor trigger zone is responsible for a high incidence of nausea and vomiting. Physical dependence is a significant problem associated with repeated opioid administration. Unlike the barbiturates or benzodiazepines, relatively large doses of opioids are required to render patients unconscious (Table 8–6). Regardless of the dose, opioids do not reliably produce amnesia. Intravenous opioids have been the mainstay of pain control for over a century. The relatively recent use of opioids in epidural and subdural spaces has revolutionized pain management (see Chapter 18).

D. Gastrointestinal: Opioids slow gastric emptying time by reducing peristalsis. Biliary colic may result from opioid-induced contraction of the sphincter of Oddi. Biliary spasm may mimic a common bile duct stone on cholangiography and is effectively reversed with the pure opioid antagonist naloxone.

E. Endocrine: The stress response to surgical stimulation is measured in terms of the secretion of specific hormones, including catecholamines, antidiuretic hormone, and cortisol. Opioids block the release of these hormones more completely than do volatile anesthetics. This is particularly true of the more potent opioids such as fentanyl, sufentanil, and alfentanil. Patients with ischemic heart disease especially may benefit from attenuation of the stress response.

Drug Interactions

The combination of opioids—particularly meperidine—and monoamine oxidase inhibitors may result in respiratory arrest, hypertension or hypotension, coma, and hyperpyrexia. The cause of this dramatic interaction is not understood.

Barbiturates, benzodiazepines, and other central nervous system depressants can have synergist cardiovascular, respiratory, and sedative effects with opioids.

KETAMINE

Mechanisms of Action

Ketamine has multiple effects throughout the central nervous system, including blocking polysynaptic reflexes in the spinal cord and inhibiting excitatory neurotransmitter effects in selected areas of the brain. In contrast to the depression of the reticular activating

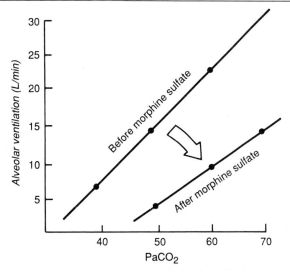

Figure 8–7. Opioids depress ventilation. This is graphically displayed by a shift of the CO_2 curve downward and to the right.

Table 8–6. Uses and dosages of commonly used opioids.

Agent	Use	Route	Dose[1]
Morphine	Premedication	IM	0.05–0.2 mg/kg
	Intraoperative anesthesia	IV	0.1–1 mg/kg
	Postoperative analgesia	IM	0.05–0.2 mg/kg
		IV	0.03–0.15 mg/kg
Meperidine	Premedication	IM	0.5–1 mg/kg
	Intraoperative anesthesia	IV	2.5–5 mg/kg
	Postoperative analgesia	IM	0.5–1 mg/kg
		IV	0.2–0.5 mg/kg
Fentanyl	Intraoperative anesthesia	IV	2–150 μg/kg
	Postoperative analgesia	IV	0.5–1.5 μg/kg
Sufentanil	Intraoperative anesthesia	IV	0.25–30 μg/kg
Alfentanil	Intraoperative anesthesia		
	Loading dose	IV	8–100 μg/kg
	Maintenance infusion	IV	0.5–3 μg/kg/min

[1]**Note:** The wide range of opioid dosages reflects a large therapeutic index and depends upon which other anesthetics are simultaneously administered. The relative potencies of fentanyl, sufentanil, and alfentanil are estimated to be 1:9:1/7.

system induced by the barbiturates, ketamine functionally "dissociates" the thalamus (which relays sensory impulses from the reticular activating system to the cerebral cortex) from the limbic cortex (which is involved with the awareness of sensation). While some brain neurons are inhibited, others are tonically excited. Clinically, this state of **dissociative anesthesia** causes the patient to appear conscious (eg, eye opening, swallowing, muscle contracture) but unable to process or respond to sensory input. The existence of specific ketamine receptors and interactions with opioid receptors has been postulated.

Structure-Activity Relationships

Ketamine (Figure 8–8) is a structural analogue of phencyclidine (PCP). It is one-tenth as potent yet retains many of phencyclidine's "psychotomimetic" effects. The increased anesthetic potency of one isomer implies the existence of stereospecific receptors.

Pharmacokinetics

A. Absorption: Ketamine is administered intravenously or intramuscularly (Table 8–7). Peak plasma levels are usually achieved within 10–15 minutes after intramuscular injection.

B. Distribution: Compared with thiopental, ketamine is more lipid-soluble, less protein-bound, and equally ionized at physiologic pH. These characteristics, along with a ketamine-induced increase in cerebral blood flow and cardiac output, lead to rapid brain uptake and subsequent redistribution (distribution half-life = 10–15 minutes). Once again, awakening is due to redistribution to peripheral compartments.

C. Biotransformation: Ketamine is biotransformed in the liver to several metabolites, some of which retain anesthetic activity (eg, norketamine). Induction of hepatic enzymes may partially explain the development of tolerance in patients who receive mul-

tiple doses of ketamine. Extensive hepatic uptake (hepatic extraction ratio of 0.9) explains ketamine's relatively short elimination half-life (2 hours).

D. Excretion: End products of biotransformation are renally excreted.

Organ System Effects

A. Cardiovascular: In sharp contrast to other anesthetic agents, ketamine increases arterial blood pressure, heart rate, and cardiac output (Table 8–8). These indirect cardiovascular effects are due to central stimulation of the sympathetic nervous system. Accompanying these changes are increases in pulmonary artery pressure and myocardial work. For these reasons, ketamine should be avoided in patients with coronary artery disease, uncontrolled hypertension, congestive heart failure, and arterial aneurysms. The direct myocardial depressant effects of large doses of ketamine are unmasked by sympathetic blockade (eg, spinal cord transection) or exhaustion of catecholamine stores (eg, severe end-stage shock). Nonetheless, ketamine's indirect stimulatory effects are often beneficial to patients with acute hypovolemic shock.

B. Respiratory: Ventilatory drive is minimally affected by the customary induction doses of ketamine, though rapid intravenous bolus administration or pretreatment with opioids occasionally produces apnea. Ketamine is a potent bronchodilator, making it a good induction agent for asthmatic patients. Although upper airway reflexes remain largely intact, patients at increased risk for aspiration pneumonitis should be intubated (see Case Discussion, Chapter 15). The increased salivation associated with ketamine can be attenuated by premedication with an anticholinergic agent.

C. Cerebral: Consistent with its cardiovascular effects, ketamine increases cerebral oxygen consumption, cerebral blood flow, and intracranial pressure.

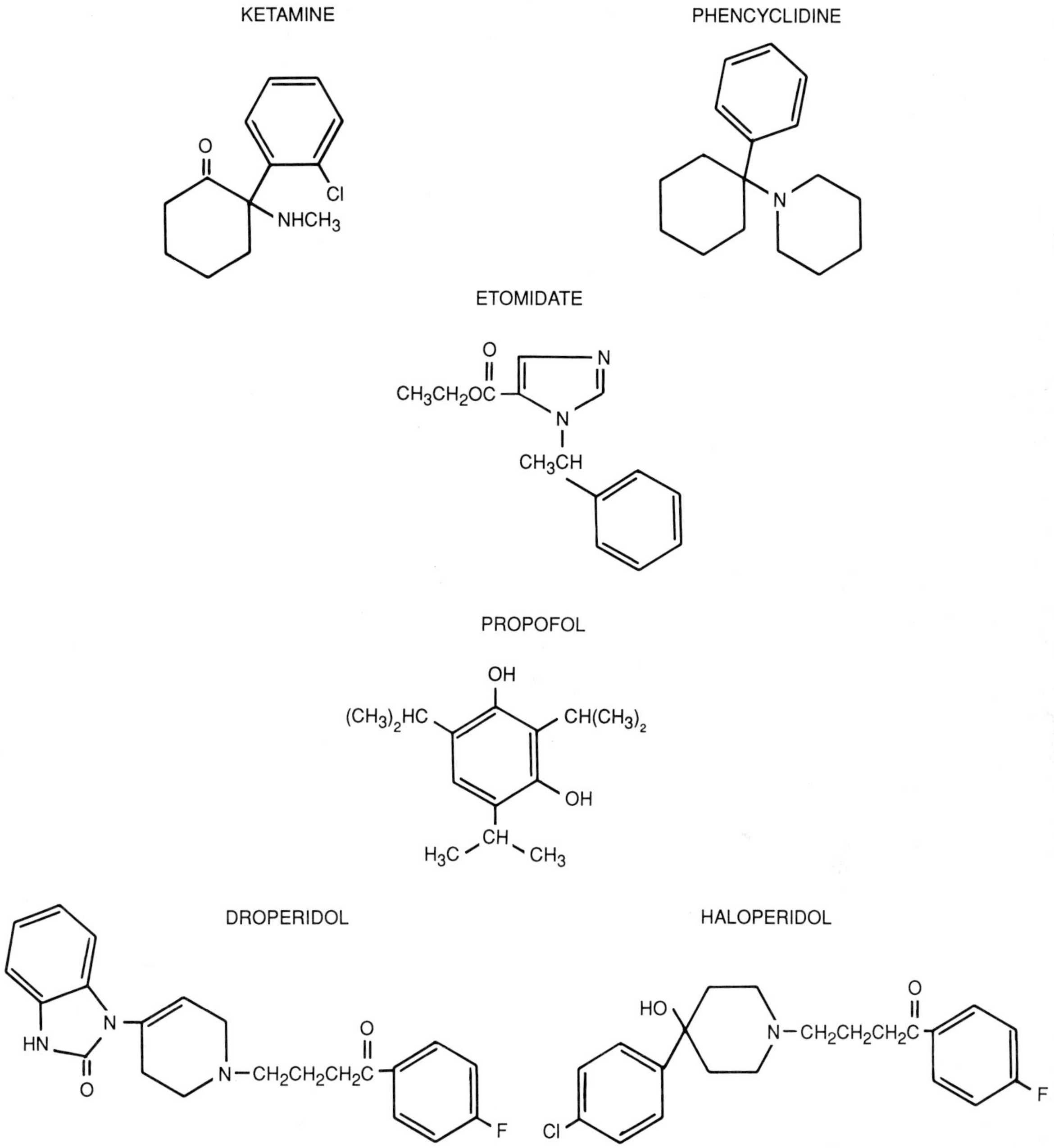

KETAMINE

PHENCYCLIDINE

ETOMIDATE

PROPOFOL

DROPERIDOL

HALOPERIDOL

Figure 8–8. The structures of ketamine, etomidate, propofol, and droperidol. Note the similarities between ketamine and phencyclidine and between droperidol and haloperidol.

These effects preclude its use in patients with space-occupying intracranial lesions. Myoclonic activity is associated with increased subcortical electrical activity, which is not apparent on surface electroencephalography. Undesirable psychotomimetic side effects (eg, illusions, disturbing dreams, and delirium) during emergence and recovery are less common in children and in patients premedicated with benzodiazepines. Of the nonvolatile agents, ketamine is the closest to being a "complete anesthetic" since it induces a state of analgesia, amnesia, and unconsciousness.

Drug Interactions

Nondepolarizing muscle relaxants are potentiated by ketamine (see Chapter 9).

The combination of theophylline and ketamine may predispose patients to seizures.

Table 8–7. Uses and dosages of ketamine, etomidate, propofol, and droperidol.

Agent	Use	Route	Dose
Ketamine	Induction	IV IM	1–2 mg/kg 3–5 mg/kg
Etomidate	Induction	IV	0.2–0.5 mg/kg
Propofol	Induction Maintenance infusion	IV IV	1–2.5 mg/kg 3–12 mg/kg/h
Droperidol	Premedication Sedation Antiemetic	IM IV IV	0.04–0.07 mg/kg 0.02–0.07 mg/kg 0.05 mg/kg[1]

[1]Maximum adult dose without prolonging emergence is 1.25–2.5 mg.

Diazepam attenuates ketamine's cardiostimulatory effects and prolongs its elimination half-life.

Propranolol, phenoxybenzamine, and other sympathetic antagonists unmask the direct myocardial depressant effects of ketamine.

Ketamine produces myocardial depression when given to patients anesthetized with halothane or, to a lesser extent, other volatile anesthetics.

Lithium may prolong the duration of action of ketamine.

ETOMIDATE

Mechanisms of Action

Etomidate depresses the reticular activating system and mimics the inhibitory effects of γ-aminobutyric acid. Unlike barbiturates, it may have disinhibitory effects on parts of the nervous system that control extrapyramidal motor activity. This disinhibition is responsible for a 30–60% incidence of myoclonus.

Structure-Activity Relationships

Etomidate, which contains a carboxylated imidazole, is structurally unrelated to other anesthetic agents (Figure 8–8). The imidazole ring provides water solubility in acidic solutions and lipid solubility at physiologic pH. Etomidate is dissolved in propylene glycol. This solution often causes pain on injection that can be attenuated by prior injection of lidocaine.

Pharmacokinetics

A. Absorption: Etomidate is available only for

Table 8–8. Summary of nonvolatile anesthetic organ system effects.

Agent	Cardiovascular		Respiratory		Cerebral		
	HR	MAP	Vent	B'dil	CBF	CMRO$_2$	ICP
Barbiturates							
Thiopental	↑↑	↓↓	↓↓↓	↓	↓↓↓	↓↓↓	↓↓↓
Thiamylal	↑↑	↓↓	↓↓↓	↓	↓↓↓	↓↓↓	↓↓↓
Methohexital	↑↑	↓↓	↓↓↓	0	↓↓↓	↓↓↓	↓↓↓
Benzodiazepines							
Diazepam	0/↑	↓	↓↓	0	↓↓	↓↓	↓↓
Lorazepam	0/↑	↓	↓↓	0	↓↓	↓↓	↓↓
Midazolam	↑	↓↓	↓↓	0	↓↓	↓↓	↓↓
Opioids							
Meperidine*	↑	*	↓↓↓	*	↓	↓	↓
Morphine*	↓	*	↓↓↓	*	↓	↓	↓
Fentanyl	↓↓	↓	↓↓↓	0	↓	↓	↓
Sufentanil	↓↓	↓	↓↓↓	0	↓	↓	↓
Alfentanil	↓↓	↓↓	↓↓↓	0	↓	↓	↓
Ketamine	↑↑	↑↑	↓	↑↑↑	↑↑↑	↑	↑↑↑
Etomidate	0	↓	↓	0	↓↓↓	↓↓↓	↓↓↓
Propofol	0	↓↓↓	↓↓↓	0	↓↓↓	↓↓↓	↓↓↓
Droperidol	↑	↓↓	0	0	↓	0	↓

*The effects of meperidine and morphine on MAP and bronchodilatation depend upon the extent of histamine release.

Abbreviations:
HR = heart rate
MAP = Mean arterial pressure
Vent = Ventilatory drive
B'dil = Bronchodilatation
CBF = Cerebral blood flow
CMRO$_2$ = Cerebral oxygen consumption
ICP = Intracranial pressure

Key:
0 = no effect
↓ = decrease (mild, moderate, marked)
↑ = increase (mild, moderate, marked).

intravenous administration and is used chiefly for induction of general anesthesia (Table 8–7).

B. Distribution: Despite being highly protein-bound, etomidate is characterized by a very rapid onset of action owing to its high lipid solubility and large nonionized fraction at physiologic pH. Redistribution is responsible for decreasing plasma concentration to awakening levels.

C. Biotransformation: Hepatic microsomal enzymes and plasma esterases rapidly hydrolyze etomidate to an inactive metabolite. The rate of biotransformation is five times greater for etomidate than for thiopental.

D. Excretion: The end product of hydrolysis is primarily excreted in the urine.

Organ System Effects

A. Cardiovascular: Etomidate has minimal effects on the cardiovascular system. A mild reduction in peripheral vascular resistance is responsible for a slight decline in arterial blood pressure. Myocardial contractility and cardiac output are usually unchanged. Etomidate does not release histamine.

B. Respiratory: Ventilation is affected less with etomidate than with barbiturates or benzodiazepines. Even induction doses usually do not result in apnea unless opioids have also been administered.

C. Cerebral: Etomidate decreases the cerebral metabolic rate, cerebral blood flow, and intracranial pressure to the same extent as thiopental. Because of minimal cardiovascular effects, cerebral perfusion pressure is well maintained. Electroencephalographic changes resemble those associated with barbiturates. Postoperative nausea and vomiting are more common than following barbiturate induction, but can be minimized by antiemetic medications. Etomidate is a sedative-hypnotic but lacks analgesic properties.

D. Endocrine: Induction doses of etomidate transiently inhibit enzymes involved in cortisol and aldosterone synthesis. Long-term infusions lead to adrenocortical suppression that may be associated with an increased mortality rate in critically ill patients.

Drug Interactions

Fentanyl increases the plasma level and prolongs the elimination half-life of etomidate.

Opioids decrease the myotonic contractions characteristic of an etomidate induction.

PROPOFOL

Mechanisms of Action

The mechanism by which propofol induces a state of general anesthesia has not been described.

Structure-Activity Relationships

Propofol (2,6-diisopropylphenol) consists of a phenol ring with two isopropyl groups attached (Figure 8–

8). Altering side chain length of this alkylphenol influences potency, induction, and recovery characteristics. Propofol is not water-soluble, but a 1% aqueous solution (10 mg/mL) is available for intravenous administration as an oil-in-water emulsion containing soybean oil, glycerol, and egg lecithin. Egg allergy is not a contraindication, since the reaction is usually to a yolk component whereas lecithin is contained in egg white. This formulation can cause pain during injection, which can be attenuated by prior injection of lidocaine. More importantly, since the propofol formulation is preservative-free, good sterile technique must be observed in preparation and handling. Sepsis and death have been linked to contaminated propofol preparations.

Pharmacokinetics

A. Absorption: Propofol is available only for intravenous administration for the induction of general anesthesia (Table 8–7).

B. Distribution: The high lipid solubility of propofol results in an onset of action which is almost as rapid as that of thiopental (one arm-to-brain circulation time). Awakening from a single bolus dose is also rapid owing to a very short initial distribution half-life (2–8 minutes). Some investigators feel that recovery from propofol is more rapid and accompanied by less "hangover" than recovery from methohexital, thiopental, or etomidate. This would make it a good agent for outpatient anesthesia. A lower induction dose is recommended in elderly patients owing to a smaller volume of distribution.

C. Biotransformation: The clearance of propofol exceeds hepatic blood flow, implicating the existence of extrahepatic metabolism. This exceptionally high clearance rate probably contributes to relatively rapid recovery after a continuous infusion. Conjugation in the liver results in inactive metabolites. The pharmocokinetics of propofol do not appear to be affected by moderate cirrhosis.

D. Excretion: Although metabolites of propofol are primarily excreted in the urine, chronic renal failure does not affect clearance of the parent drug.

Organ System Effects

A. Cardiovascular: The major cardiovascular effect of propofol is a decrease in arterial blood pressure owing to a drop in systemic vascular resistance, cardiac contractility, and preload. Hypotension is more pronounced than with thiopental but is usually reversed by the stimulation accompanying laryngoscopy and intubation. Factors exacerbating the hypotension include large doses, rapid injection, and old age. Changes in heart rate and cardiac output are usually transient and insignificant in healthy patients. Patients with impaired ventricular function may experience a significant drop in cardiac output owing to decreases in ventricular filling pressures and contractility. Although myocardial oxygen consumption and coronary blood flow decrease to a similar extent, coronary sinus lactate production increases in some patients. This indicates a regional mismatch between myocardial oxygen supply and demand.

B. Respiratory: Like the barbiturates, propofol is a profound respiratory depressant that usually causes apnea following an induction dose.

C. Cerebral: Propofol decreases cerebral blood flow and intracranial pressure. In patients with elevated intracranial pressure, propofol can cause a critical reduction in cerebral perfusion pressure ($<$ 50 mm Hg) because the drop in cerebral artery pressure can exceed the drop in intracranial pressure. Propofol does not have anticonvulsant properties. Induction is occasionally accompanied by excitatory phenomena such as muscle twitching, spontaneous movement, or hiccuping. Propofol decreases intraocular pressure.

Drug Interactions

Nondepolarizing muscle relaxants may be potentiated by previous formulations of propofol containing Cremophor. Newer formulations do not share this interaction.

Alfentanil concentrations may be increased by concomitant administration of propofol.

DROPERIDOL

Mechanisms of Action

Droperidol antagonizes the activation of dopamine receptors. For example, in the central nervous system, the caudate nucleus and the medullary chemoreceptor trigger zone are affected. Droperidol also interferes with transmission mediated by serotonin, norepinephrine, and γ-aminobutyric acid. These central actions account for droperidol's tranquilizer and antiemetic properties. Peripheral actions include α-adrenergic blockade (see Chapter 12).

Structure-Activity Relationships

Droperidol, a butyrophenone, is structurally related to haloperidol (Figure 8–8). Differences between the two drugs explain the neuroleptic characteristics of the former and the antipsychotic activity of the latter.

Pharmacokinetics

A. Absorption: Although droperidol is occasionally administered intramuscularly as part of a premedication regimen, it is usually given intravenously (Table 8–7).

B. Distribution: Despite a rapid distribution phase ($t_{1/2}$ = 10 minutes), the sedative effects of droperidol are delayed by a relatively high molecular weight and extensive protein binding, which hinder penetration of the blood-brain barrier. A prolonged duration of action (3–24 hours) may be explained by tenacious receptor binding.

C. Biotransformation: Droperidol is extensively metabolized in the liver, as evidenced by a hepatic clearance as rapid as that of ketamine and etomidate.

D. Excretion: The end products of biotransformation are excreted primarily in the urine.

Organ System Effects

A. Cardiovascular: Droperidol's mild α-adrenergic blocking effects decrease arterial blood pressure by peripheral vasodilatation. Hypovolemic patients can experience exaggerated blood pressure declines. The alpha-blocking actions may be responsible for an antidysrhythmic effect. Patients with pheochromocytoma should not receive droperidol because it can induce catecholamine release from the adrenal medulla, resulting in severe hypertension.

B. Respiratory: Droperidol, administered in usual dosages and alone, does not significantly depress respiration and may actually stimulate hypoxic ventilatory drive.

C. Cerebral: Droperidol decreases cerebral blood flow and intracranial pressure by inducing cerebral vasoconstriction. However, droperidol does not reduce cerebral oxygen consumption—unlike the barbiturates, benzodiazepines, and etomidate. The EEG is not markedly changed. Droperidol is a potent antiemetic, though delayed awakening limits its intraoperative use to low doses (0.05 mg/kg to a maximum of 2.5 mg). The antidopaminergic activity of droperidol rarely precipitates extrapyramidal reactions (eg, oculogyric crises, torticollis, and agitation), which can be treated with diphenhydramine. Nonetheless, droperidol should be avoided in patients with Parkinson's disease.

Although patients premedicated with droperidol appear placid and sedated, they are often extremely apprehensive and fearful. For this reason, droperidol has fallen into disfavor as a premedication. The addition of an opioid decreases the incidence of dysphoria. Droperidol is a tranquilizer, and it does not produce analgesia, amnesia, or unconsciousness at usual doses. The combination of fentanyl with droperidol (Innovar) produces a state characterized by analgesia, immobility, and variable amnesia (**neuroleptanalgesia**). The addition of nitrous oxide leads to unconsciousness and general anesthesia (**neuroleptanesthesia**) similar to the dissociative state induced by ketamine.

Drug Interactions

Droperidol antagonizes the effects of levodopa and may precipitate parkinsonian symptoms.

The renal effects of dopamine are countered by droperidol.

Theoretically, droperidol could antagonize the central α-adrenergic action of clonidine and precipitate rebound hypertension.

Droperidol attenuates the cardiovascular effects of ketamine.

CASE DISCUSSION: PREMEDICATION OF THE SURGICAL PATIENT

An extremely anxious 17-year-old woman presents for uterine dilatation and curettage. She demands to be asleep before going to the operating room and does not want to remember anything.

What are the goals of administering preoperative medication?

Anxiety is a normal emotional response to impending surgery. Minimizing anxiety is usually the major goal of preoperative medication. For many patients, the preoperative interview with the anesthesiologist allays fears more effectively than sedative drugs. Other psychologic objectives of preoperative medication include preoperative pain relief and perioperative amnesia.

There may also be specific medical indications for preoperative medication: prophylaxis against aspiration pneumonitis (eg, antacids), prevention of allergic reactions (eg, antihistamines), or decreasing upper airway secretions (eg, anticholinergics). Thus, the goals of preoperative medication are dependent upon many factors, including the health and emotional status of the patient, the proposed surgical procedure, and the anesthetic plan. For this reason, the choice of anesthetic premedication is not routine and must follow a thorough preoperative evaluation.

What is the difference between sedation and anxiety relief?

This distinction is well illustrated by the paradoxic effects of droperidol. Patients may appear to an observer to be adequately sedated but upon questioning may be quite anxious. Anxiety relief can only be measured by the patient.

Do all patients require preoperative medication?

No—customary levels of preoperative anxiety do not harm most patients. Some patients dread intramuscular injections, and others find altered states of consciousness more unpleasant than "nervousness." If the surgical procedure is brief, the effects of some sedatives may extend into the postoperative period and prolong recovery time. This is especially troublesome for patients undergoing ambulatory surgery. Specific contraindications for sedative premedication include severe lung disease, hypovolemia, impending airway obstruction, increased intracranial pressure, and depressed baseline mental status. Premedication with sedative drugs should never be given before informed consent has been obtained.

Which patients are most likely to benefit from preoperative medication?

Some patients are quite anxious despite the preoperative interview. Separation of young children from their parents is often a traumatic ordeal, especially if they have endured multiple prior surgeries. Chronic drug abusers may benefit from a premedication to lessen the risk of withdrawal reactions. Medical conditions such as coronary artery disease or hypertension may be aggravated by psychologic stress.

How does preoperative medication influence the induction of general anesthesia?

Some preoperative medications (eg, opioids) lessen anesthetic requirements and can "smooth" induction. However, intravenous administration of these medications just prior to induction is a more reliable method of achieving the same benefits.

What governs the choice between the preoperative medications commonly administered?

After the goals of premedication have been determined, the clinical effects of the agents dictate choice. For instance, in a patient experiencing preoperative pain due to a femoral fracture, the analgesic effects of an opioid (eg, morphine or meperidine) will lessen the discomfort associated with transportation to the operating room and positioning on the operating room table. Respiratory depression, orthostatic hypotension, and nausea detract from the desirability of opioid premedication.

Barbiturates are effective sedatives but lack analgesic properties and can produce respiratory depression. Benzodiazepines relieve anxiety, often provide amnesia, and are relatively free of side effects. However, like barbiturates, they are not analgesics. Diazepam and lorazepam are available orally. Intramuscular midazolam has a rapid onset (30 minutes) and short duration (90 minutes). Dysphoria, prolonged sedation, and α-adrenergic blockade limit the clinical usefulness of droperidol.

Other preoperative medications are discussed in subsequent chapters: anticholinergics in Chapter 11; antihistamines, metoclopramide, and antacids in Chapter 15.

Which factors must be considered in selecting the anesthetic premedication for this patient?

First, it must be made clear to the patient that, for safety reasons, anesthesia is not induced outside the operating room. Long-acting agents such as morphine or droperidol would not be a good choice for an outpatient procedure. Lorazepam and diazepam can also affect mental function for several hours. One alternative is to establish an intravenous line in the preoperative holding area and titrate small doses of midazolam, with or without fentanyl, using slurred speech as an end point. At that time, the patient can be taken to the operating room. Vital signs—particularly respiratory rate—must be continuously monitored.

SUGGESTED READINGS

Corssen G, Reves JG, Stanley TH: *Intravenous Anesthesia and Analgesia*. Lea & Febiger, 1987. History and clinical pharmacology of nonvolatile anesthetic agents.

Feldman SA, Scurr CF, Paton W: *Drugs in Anaesthesia: Mechanisms of Action*. Arnold, 1987. The cellular and subcellular mechanisms of hypnotics, general anesthetics, and opioids.

Fragen RJ (editor): *Drug Infusions in Anesthesiology*. Raven Press, 1991. The pharmacokinetic and hardware information necessary to fully utilize intravenous drug delivery systems.

Reich DL, Silvay G: Ketamine: An update on the first twenty-five years of clinical experience. Can J Anaesth 1989;36:186. Evolution of the multiple uses of ketamine.

Sebel PS, Lowdon JD: Propofol: A new intravenous anesthetic. Anesthesiology 1989;71:260. Pharmacology and clinical uses.

Stanski DR, Watkins WD: *Drug Disposition in Anesthesia*. Grune & Stratton, 1982.

Stoelting RK: *Pharmacology and Physiology in Anesthetic Practice*. Lippincott, 1987.

Verderame M: *Handbook of CNS Agents and Local Anesthetics*. CRC Press, 1986. Includes many drugs still undergoing investigation. Monographs highlight commonly used drugs.

White PF: What's new in intravenous anesthetics? Anesth Clin North Am 1988;6:297.

Muscle Relaxants

9

Skeletal muscle relaxation can be produced by deep inhalational anesthesia, regional nerve block, or neuromuscular junction blocking agents (commonly called muscle relaxants). In 1942, Harold Griffith published the results of a study using a refined extract of curare (a South American arrow poison) during anesthesia. Muscle relaxants rapidly became a routine part of the anesthesiologist's drug arsenal. As Griffith noted, it is important to realize that neuromuscular junction blocking agents produce paralysis, not anesthesia. In other words, muscle relaxation does not ensure unconsciousness, amnesia, or analgesia. This chapter reviews the principles of neuromuscular transmission and presents the mechanisms of action, physical structure, routes of elimination, recommended dosages, and side effects of several muscle relaxants.

NEUROMUSCULAR TRANSMISSION

The region of approximation between a motor neuron and a muscle cell is the **neuromuscular junction** (Figure 9–1). The cell membranes of the neuron and muscle fiber are separated by a narrow gap, the **synaptic cleft.** As a nerve's action potential depolarizes its terminal, an influx of calcium ions into the nerve cytoplasm allows **storage vesicles** to fuse with the **terminal membrane** and release their contents of acetylcholine (ACh). The ACh molecules diffuse across the synaptic cleft to bind with **nicotinic cholinergic receptors** on a specialized portion of the muscle membrane, the **motor endplate.**

Each ACh receptor consists of six protein subunits, two of which are identical and capable of binding ACh molecules. If both binding sites are occupied by ACh, a conformational change in the subunits opens an ion channel in the core of the receptor (Figure 9–2).

Cations flow through the open channel (sodium and calcium in, potassium out), generating an **endplate potential.** The contents of a single vesicle, a quantum of ACh, produce a **miniature endplate potential.** If enough receptors are occupied by ACh, the endplate potential will be sufficiently strong to depolarize the perijunctional membrane. Sodium channels within

this portion of the muscle membrane open when a voltage is developed across them, as opposed to endplate receptors that open when acetylcholine is applied. The resulting action potential propagates along the muscle membrane and T tubule system, opening sodium channels and releasing calcium from the sarcoplasmic reticulum. This intracellular calcium allows the contractile proteins actin and myosin to interact, bringing about muscle contraction.

ACh is rapidly hydrolyzed into acetate and choline by the substrate-specific enzyme **acetylcholinesterase.** This enzyme (also called specific cholinesterase and true cholinesterase) is embedded into the motor endplate membrane immediately adjacent to the ACh receptors. Eventually, the receptors' ion channels close, causing the endplate to repolarize. When action potential generation ceases, the sodium channels in the muscle membrane also close. Calcium is resequestered in the sarcoplasmic reticulum, and the muscle cell relaxes.

DISTINCTIONS BETWEEN DEPOLARIZING & NONDEPOLARIZING BLOCKADE

Neuromuscular blocking agents are divided into two classes: depolarizing and nondepolarizing (Table 9–1). This division reflects distinct differences in (1) mechanism of action, (2) response to peripheral nerve stimulation, and (3) reversal of block.

MECHANISM OF ACTION

Depolarizing muscle relaxants physically resemble ACh and therefore bind to ACh receptors, generating a muscle action potential. *However, unlike ACh, these drugs are not metabolized by acetylcholinesterase.* Thus, their concentration in the synaptic cleft does not fall as rapidly, resulting in a prolonged depolarization of the muscle endplate.

Continuous endplate depolarization causes muscle relaxation in the following way. As has been ex-

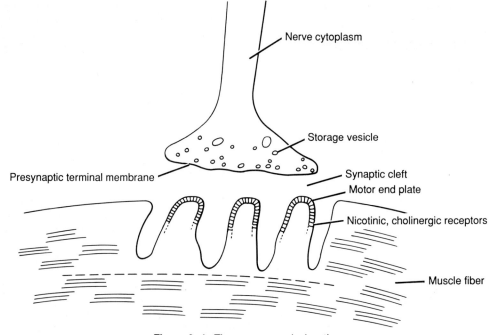

Figure 9–1. The neuromuscular junction.

plained, an endplate potential of sufficient strength will result in generation of an action potential in the neighboring perijunctional muscle membrane. However, the subsequent opening of perijunctional sodium channels is time-limited. After initial excitation and opening, these ion channels close. Furthermore, these sodium channels cannot reopen until the endplate repolarizes, which is not possible as long as a depolarizer continues to bind to ACh receptors. Once the perijunctional channels close, the action potential disappears and the membrane downstream returns to its resting state, resulting in muscle relaxation. This is a **phase I block.**

Nondepolarizing muscle relaxants also bind to ACh receptors but are incapable of inducing the conformational change necessary for ion channel opening.

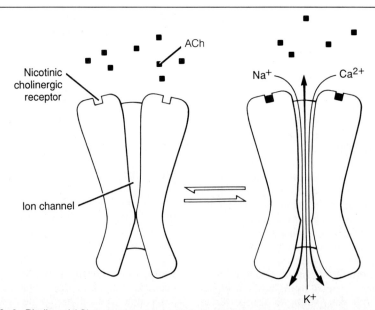

Figure 9–2. Binding of ACh to receptors on muscle endplate causes channel opening and ion flux.

Table 9–1. Depolarizing and nondepolarizing muscle relaxants.

Depolarizing	Nondepolarizing
Short-acting	Long-acting
Succinylcholine	Tubocurarine
Decamethonium	Metocurine
	Doxacurium
	Pancuronium
	Pipecuronium
	Gallamine
	Intermediate-acting
	Atracurium
	Vecuronium
	Short-acting
	Mivacurium

Since ACh is precluded from binding to its receptors, no endplate potential develops.

RESPONSE TO PERIPHERAL NERVE STIMULATION

The use of peripheral nerve stimulators to monitor neuromuscular function was discussed in Chapter 6. Four patterns of electrical stimulation with supramaximal square-wave pulses were considered:

(1) Tetanus: A sustained stimulus of 50–100 Hz (pulses per second), usually lasting 5 seconds.
(2) Twitch: A single pulse 0.2 ms in duration.
(3) Train of four: A series of four twitches in 2 seconds (2-Hz frequency), each 0.2 ms in duration.

(4) Double-burst stimulation: Three short-lasting (0.2 ms), high-frequency stimulations separated by a 20-ms interval (50 Hz) and followed 750 ms later by either two (DBS$_{3,2}$) or three (DBS$_{3,3}$) additional impulses (Figure 6–33).

The occurrence of **fade,** a gradual diminution of evoked response during prolonged or repeated nerve stimulation, is indicative of a nondepolarizing block (Table 9–2). Fade may be due to a prejunctional effect of nondepolarizing relaxants that reduces the amount of ACh in the nerve terminal which is available for release during stimulation (blockade of ACh mobilization).

The ability of tetanus stimulation during a partial nondepolarizing block to increase the evoked response to a subsequent twitch is termed **posttetanic potentiation.** This phenomenon may relate to a compensatory increase in ACh mobilization subsequent to tetanus stimulation.

In contrast, a phase I depolarization block does not exhibit fade during tetanus or train of four, nor does it demonstrate posttetanic potentiation. However, if enough depolarizer is administered, the quality of the block changes to resemble a nondepolarizing block. This so-called **phase II block** appears to be caused by ionic and conformational changes that accompany prolonged muscle membrane depolarization.

REVERSAL OF BLOCK

Because depolarizing muscle relaxants are not metabolized by acetylcholinesterase, they diffuse away

Table 9–2. Evoked responses during depolarizing (phase I and phase II) and nondepolarizing block.

Evoked Stimulus	Depolarizing Block		Nondepolarizing Block
	Phase I	Phase II	
Train-of-four	Constant but diminished	Fade	Fade
Tetanus	Constant but diminished	Fade	Fade
Posttetanic potentiation	Absent	Present	Present

from the neuromuscular junction and are hydrolyzed in the plasma and liver by another enzyme: **pseudo-cholinesterase** (nonspecific cholinesterase, plasma cholinesterase). Fortunately, this is a fairly rapid process, since no specific agent to reverse a depolarizing blockade is available.

With the exception of mivacurium, nondepolarizing agents are not significantly metabolized by either acetylcholinesterase or pseudocholinesterase. Reversal of their blockade depends upon redistribution, gradual metabolism and excretion of the relaxant by the body, or administration of specific reversal agents. These reversal drugs inhibit acetylcholinesterase enzyme activity. This inhibition increases the amount of ACh available at the neuromuscular junction to compete with the nondepolarizing agents. Clearly, the reversal agents would not be of benefit in reversing a depolarizing block. In fact, by increasing neuromuscular junction ACh concentration and inhibiting pseudocholinesterase, *cholinesterase inhibitors prolong depolarization blockade.*

DEPOLARIZING MUSCLE RELAXANTS

SUCCINYLCHOLINE

The only depolarizing muscle relaxant in general use today is succinylcholine.

Physical Structure

Muscle relaxants owe their paralytic properties to mimicry of acetylcholine. For example, all are quaternary ammonium compounds. In fact, succinylcholine—also called suxamethonium and diacetylcholine—consists of two joined acetylcholine molecules (Figure 9–3). This copycat structure is responsible for succinylcholine's mechanism of action, side effects, and metabolism.

Metabolism & Excretion

The continued popularity of succinylcholine is due to its rapid onset of action (30–60 seconds) and short duration of action (typically less than 10 minutes). Its rapid onset of action is largely due to its low lipid solubility (all muscle relaxants are highly charged and water-soluble) and the relative overdose that is usually administered.

As soon as succinylcholine enters the circulation, most of it is rapidly metabolized by pseudocholinesterase into succinylmonocholine. This process is so efficient that only a fraction of the injected dose ever reaches the neuromuscular junction. As drug serum levels fall, succinylcholine molecules diffuse away from the neuromuscular junction, limiting the duration of action.

The duration of action can be prolonged by increasing the dose or by decreasing metabolism. The latter may result from hypothermia, low enzyme levels, or genetically abnormal enzyme action. Hypothermia decreases the rate of hydrolysis. Low enzyme levels (measured as units per liter) are capable of doubling or tripling the duration of blockade. Causes of low enzyme levels include pregnancy, liver disease, and certain drugs (Table 9–3). In contrast, the presence of genetically abnormal enzyme can have profound consequences.

One in 500 patients has one normal and one abnormal gene, resulting in a slightly prolonged block. Even fewer (1:3000) have two abnormal genes (homozygous atypical) that produce an enzyme with 1/100 the normal affinity for succinylcholine. These patients will have very prolonged blockade (6–8 hours) following administration of succinylcholine. Of the recognized abnormal genes, the dibucaine variant is the most common.

Dibucaine, a local anesthetic, inhibits normal pseudocholinesterase activity by 80% but only inhibits the homozygous atypical enzyme by 20%. The heterozygous enzyme is characterized by an intermediate 40% inhibition. The percentage inhibition of pseudocholinesterase activity is termed the **dibucaine number.** The dibucaine number is proportionate to pseudocholinesterase function and has no relationship to the amount of enzyme. Therefore, adequacy of pseudocholinesterase can be determined in the laboratory quantitatively in units per liter (a minor factor) and qualitatively by dibucaine number (the major factor). Prolonged paralysis from succinylcholine due to abnormal pseudocholinesterase (atypical cholinesterase) should be treated with continued mechanical ventilation until muscle function returns to normal.

Drug Interactions

The effects of muscle relaxants can be modified by concurrent drug therapy (Table 9–4). Succinylcholine is involved in two interactions deserving special comment.

A. Cholinesterase Inhibitors: Although cholinesterase inhibitors reverse nondepolarizing paralysis, they markedly prolong a depolarizing phase I block by two mechanisms. First, by inhibiting acetylcholinesterase, they lead to a higher acetylcholine concentration at the nerve terminal which intensifies depolarization. Secondly, they reduce the hydrolysis of succinylcholine by inhibiting pseudocholinesterase. Organophosphate pesticides cause an irreversible inhibition of acetylcholinesterase and can prolong the action of succinylcholine by 20–30 minutes.

B. Nondepolarizing Relaxants: In general, small doses of nondepolarizing relaxants antagonize a depolarizing phase I block. Because the drugs occupy some ACh receptors, depolarization by succinylcholine is partially precluded. An exception to this interaction is pancuronium, which augments succinylcholine blockade by inhibiting pseudocholinesterase.

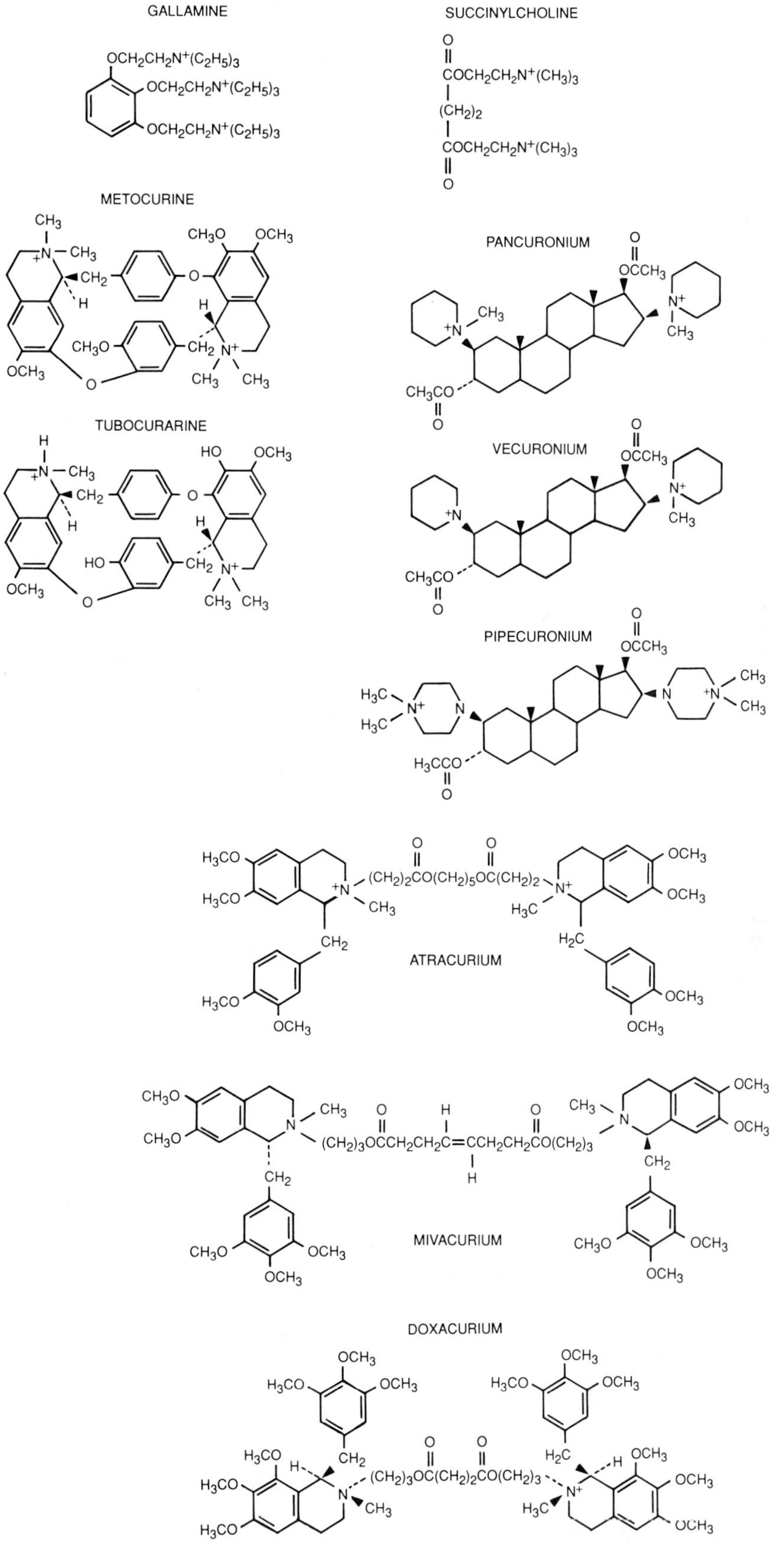

Figure 9–3. Chemical structures of neuromuscular blocking agents.

Table 9–3. Drugs causing quantitative decreases in pseudocholinesterases.

Drug	Uses
Echothiophate	Irreversible cholinesterase inhibitor used for treatment of glaucoma
Neostigmine, pyridostigmine	Reversible cholinesterase inhibitors
Hexafluorenium	A seldom used nondepolarizer
Phenelzine	A monoamine oxidase inhibitor
Cyclophosphamide, mechlorethamine	Antineoplastic agents
Trimethaphan	An antihypertensive

If enough depolarizing agent is administered to develop a phase II block, a nondepolarizer will potentiate paralysis. Similarly, an intubating dose of succinylcholine reduces nondepolarizer dosage requirements for at least 30 minutes.

Dosages

Because of its rapid onset and short duration, many clinicians feel that succinylcholine is still the drug of choice for routine intubations. Certainly, succinylcholine remains unequaled during rapid-sequence inductions or emergency intubations. The adult dosage for intubation is usually 1–1.5 mg/kg intravenously. Re-

peated small boluses (10 mg) or a succinylcholine drip (1 g in 500 or 1000 mL, titrated to effect) are employed during some surgical procedures that require brief but intense paralysis (eg, otolaryngologic endoscopies). Methylene blue indicator dye is often added to succinylcholine drips to prevent confusion with other intravenous fluids. In addition, neuromuscular function should be constantly monitored with a nerve stimulator to prevent overdosage and the development of phase II block. The introduction of intermediate-duration nondepolarizing relaxants (eg, vecuronium, atracurium) has detracted from this technique.

Since succinylcholine is not lipid-soluble, its distribution is limited to the extracellular space. Infants and neonates have an increased extracellular space on a per kilogram basis when compared with adults. Therefore, pediatric dosage requirements are often greater than for adults. If succinylcholine is administered *intramuscularly* to children, a dose as high as 4–5 mg/kg does not always produce complete paralysis.

Side Effects & Clinical Considerations

Succinylcholine is a relatively safe drug, assuming its many potential complications are understood and avoided.

A. Cardiovascular: Because of the resemblance of muscle relaxants to acetylcholine, it is not surprising that they affect cholinergic receptors besides those at the neuromuscular junction. The entire parasym-

Table 9–4. Potentiation (+) and inhibition (−) of neuromuscular blocking agents by other drugs.

Drug	Effect on Depolarizing Blockade	Effect on Nondepolarizing Blockade	Comments
Antibiotics	+	+	Streptomycins, colistin, polymyxin, tetracycline, lincomycin, clindamycin
Anticonvulsants	?	+	Phenytoin, carbamazepine
Antidysrhythmics	+	+	Quinidine, lidocaine, calcium channel blockers
Antihypertensives	+	+	Trimethaphan, nitroglycerin (only affects pancuronium)
Cholinesterase inhibitors	+	−	Neostigmine, pyridostigmine, edrophonium
Dantrolene	?	+	Used in treatment of malignant hyperthermia (has quaternary ammonium group)
Furosemide <10 μg/kg 1–4 mg/kg	 + −	 + −	Biphasic effect depending on dose
Inhalational anesthetics	+	+	Isoflurane and enflurane > halothane > N_2O
Ketamine	?	+	
Local anesthetics	+	+	
Lithium carbonate	+	?	Causes prolonged onset and duration of succinylcholine; one case report of prolonged block with nondepolarizer
Magnesium sulfate	+	+	Used for preeclampsia and eclampsia of pregnancy

pathetic nervous system and parts of the sympathetic nervous system (sympathetic ganglions, adrenal medulla, and sweat glands) depend upon acetylcholine as neurotransmitter.

Succinylcholine not only stimulates nicotinic cholinergic receptors at the neuromuscular junction—it stimulates all acetylcholine receptors. Stimulation of nicotinic receptors in parasympathetic and sympathetic ganglia and muscarinic receptors in the sinoatrial node of the heart can increase or decrease blood pressure and heart rate.

A succinylcholine metabolite, succinylmonocholine, excites cholinergic receptors in the sinoatrial node, resulting in bradycardia. Although children are particularly susceptible, bradycardia is commonly seen in adults if a second dose of succinylcholine is administered. Intravenous atropine (0.02 mg/kg in children, 0.4 mg in adults) is often given prophylactically in children and *always* before a second dose of succinylcholine. Other arrhythmias such as nodal bradycardia and ventricular ectopy have been reported.

B. Fasciculations: The onset of paralysis by succinylcholine is usually signaled by visible motor unit contractions called **fasciculations.** Fasciculations can be prevented by pretreatment with a small dose of nondepolarizing relaxant. Since this pretreatment antagonizes a depolarizing block, a higher dose of succinylcholine is subsequently required (1.5 mg/kg).

C. Hyperkalemia: Normal muscle releases enough potassium during succinylcholine-induced depolarization to raise serum potassium by 0.5 meq/L. While this is usually insignificant in patients with normal baseline potassium levels, *a life-threatening potassium elevation is possible in patients with burn injury, massive trauma, severe intra-abdominal infection, neurologic disorders (spinal cord injury, encephalitis, stroke, Guillain-Barré syndrome, severe Parkinson's disease), and tetanus.* In denervation injuries, acetylcholine receptors develop outside the neuromuscular junction. These extrajunctional receptors allow succinylcholine to effect widespread depolarization and extensive potassium release. Life-threatening potassium release is *not* reliably prevented by pretreatment with a nondepolarizer.

D. Muscle Pains: Patients who have received succinylcholine have an increased incidence of postoperative myalgia. This complaint is most common in healthy female outpatients. Pregnancy and extremes of age seem to be protective. The efficacy of nondepolarizing pretreatment is controversial.

E. Intragastric Pressure Elevation: Abdominal wall muscle fasciculations increase intragastric pressure, which is offset by an increase in lower esophageal sphincter tone. Therefore, the risk of gastric reflux or pulmonary aspiration is probably not increased by succinylcholine. Pretreatment with nondepolarizers abolishes the rise in gastric pressure but also prevents the increase in lower esophageal sphincter tone.

F. Intraocular Pressure Elevation: Extraocular muscle differs from other striated muscle by having multiple motor endplates on each cell. Prolonged membrane depolarization and contraction of extraocular muscles following succinylcholine administration raises intraocular pressure and could compromise an injured eye. The intraocular pressure elevation is not always prevented by nondepolarizer pretreatment.

G. Malignant Hyperthermia: Succinylcholine is a potent triggering agent in patients susceptible to malignant hyperthermia, a hypermetabolic disorder of skeletal muscle. Paradoxic contraction of jaw musculature (trismus) following succinylcholine administration is often a premonitory sign (see Chapter 42 Case Discussion).

H. Generalized Contractions: Patients afflicted with myotonia may develop myoclonus after succinylcholine administration.

I. Prolonged Paralysis: As discussed above, patients with low levels of normal pseudocholinesterase may have a longer than normal duration of action, while patients with atypical pseudocholinesterase will experience markedly prolonged paralysis. This is a dangerous complication if ventilation is not adequately maintained.

J. Intracranial Pressure: Succinylcholine may lead to an activation of the EEG and increases in cerebral blood flow and intracranial pressure in some patients. The increase in intracranial pressure can be attenuated by maintaining good airway control, instituting hyperventilation, and pretreating with a nondepolarizing muscle relaxant.

NONDEPOLARIZING MUSCLE RELAXANTS
(Table 9-5)

Unique Pharmacologic Characteristics

In contrast to depolarizing muscle relaxants, there is a wide selection of nondepolarizers. Choice of a particular drug depends upon its unique characteristics.

A. Autonomic Side Effects: In clinical doses, the nondepolarizers significantly differ in their effects on nicotinic and muscarinic cholinergic receptors. Tubocurarine and, to a lesser extent, metocurine block autonomic ganglia. This compromises the sympathetic nervous system's ability to increase heart contractility and rate in response to hypotension and other intraoperative stresses. In contrast, pancuronium and gallamine block vagal muscarinic receptors in the sinoatrial node, resulting in tachycardia. Gallamine's potent vagolytic effect has severely limited its clinical usefulness. Atracurium, mivacurium, doxacurium, vecuronium, and pipecuronium are devoid of significant autonomic effects in their recommended dosage ranges.

Table 9–5. A summary of the pharmacology of nondepolarizing muscle relaxants.

Relaxant	Metabolism	Primary Excretion	Onset	Duration	Histamine Release	Vagal Blockade	Relative Potency[1]
Tubocurarine	Insignificant	Renal	+ +	+ + +	+ + +	0	1
Metocurine	Insignificant	Renal	+ +	+ + +	+ +	0	2
Atracurium	+ + +	Insignificant	+ +	+ +	+	0	1
Mivacurium	+ + +	Insignificant	+ +	+	+	0	2.5
Doxacurium	Insignificant	Renal	+	+ + +	0	0	10
Pancuronium	+	Renal	+ +	+ + +	0	+	5
Pipecuronium	+	Renal	+ +	+ + +	0	0	6
Vecuronium	+	Biliary	+ +	+ +	0	0	5

[1]For example, pancuronium and vecuronium are five times *more* potent than tubocurarine or atracurium.
Key: Onset: + = slow, + + = moderately rapid (succinylcholine would be + + +)
Duration: + = short, + + + = long
Histamine release: 0 = no effect, + + + = marked effect
Vagal blockade: 0 = no effect, + = some effect

B. Histamine Release: Histamine release from mast cells can result in hypotension from peripheral vasodilatation, skin flushing, and bronchospasm. Nondepolarizers capable of triggering histamine release are tubocurarine 14 > metocurine > atracurium and mivacurium. Slow injection rates and H_1 and H_2 antihistamine pretreatment ameliorate these side effects.

C. Dependence on Hepatic Metabolism: Only pancuronium and vecuronium are metabolized to any significant degree by the liver. Liver failure prolongs pancuronium blockade. Atracurium and mivacurium, while extensively metabolized, depend on extrahepatic mechanisms.

D. Dependence on Renal Clearance: Metocurine and gallamine are almost entirely dependent on renal excretion, and their use in renal failure is therefore ill-advised. However, since these agents are ionized, they may be removed by dialysis. Tubocurarine, doxacurium, pancuronium, vecuronium, and pipecuronium are partially excreted by the kidneys, and their action is prolonged in patients with renal failure. Atracurium and mivacurium are eliminated independently of kidney function.

E. Suitability for Intubation: None of the currently available nondepolarizing agents have an onset of action as rapid as that of succinylcholine. For this reason, they are less suitable for rapid-sequence inductions in patients at risk for aspiration. However, if succinylcholine is contraindicated, onset may be quickened by employing a larger dose or a "priming dose." Although a larger intubating dose speeds onset, it is accompanied by an exaggeration of side effects and a prolongation of blockade. For example, a dose of 0.15 mg/kg of pancuronium may produce intubating conditions in 90 seconds—but at the cost of more pronounced hypertension and tachycardia—and a block that may be irreversible for more than 45 minutes.

Since the introduction of shorter-acting agents, the efficacy of a **priming dose** has been popularized. Ten to 15 percent of the usual intubating dose given 5 minutes before induction will theoretically occupy enough receptors so that paralysis will quickly follow when the balance of relaxant is administered. A priming dose does not usually lead to clinically significant paralysis because that requires 75–80% of the receptors be blocked (a neuromuscular **margin of safety**). However, in some patients the priming dose occupies enough receptors to produce dyspnea. In this situation, induction of anesthesia should proceed without delay. Use of a priming dose has allowed conditions suitable for intubation 90 seconds after induction. If succinylcholine is contraindicated, vecuronium and mivacurium appear to be good choices for rapid-sequence inductions because of (1) minimal side effects at high doses, (2) intermediate duration of action, and (3) possible priming dose efficacy.

F. Suitability for Preventing Fasciculations: To prevent fasciculation, 10–15% of a nondepolarizer intubating dose can be administered 5 minutes before succinylcholine. While most nondepolarizers have been successfully used for this purpose, tubocurarine appears to be the most efficacious (**precurarization**). Because of the antagonism between depolarizers and a phase I block, the subsequent dose of succinylcholine should be raised to 1.5 mg/kg.

G. Potentiation by Inhalational Anesthetics: Volatile agents decrease nondepolarizer dosage requirements by at least 15%. The actual degree of this postsynaptic augmentation depends upon both the inhalational anesthetic (isoflurane and enflurane > halothane > N_2O/O_2/narcotic) and the muscle relaxant employed (tubocurarine and pancuronium > vecuronium and atracurium).

H. Potentiation by Other Nondepolarizers: Some combinations of nondepolarizers (eg, tubocurarine with pancuronium) produce a greater than additive neuromuscular blockade. Some of these combinations have the added advantage of offsetting side effects, eg, the attenuation of tubocurarine's hypotensive effect by pancuronium. The lack of augmentation by closely related compounds (eg, vecuronium and pancuronium) lends credence to the theory that potentiation results from slightly differing mechanisms of action.

General Pharmacologic Characteristics

Some variables affect all nondepolarizing muscle relaxants.

A. Temperature: Hypothermia prolongs blockade by decreasing metabolism (eg, pancuronium, vecuronium, atracurium) and delaying excretion (eg, tubocurarine, metocurine, pancuronium).

B. Acid-Base Balance: Respiratory acidosis generally potentates a nondepolarizing blockade and antagonizes its reversal. This could prevent complete neuromuscular recovery in a hypoventilating postoperative patient. Conflicting findings regarding the neuromuscular effects of other acid-base changes may be due to coexisting alterations in extracellular pH, intracellular pH, or electrolyte concentrations.

C. Electrolyte Abnormalities: Hypokalemia and hypocalcemia augment a nondepolarizing block. The response of a patient with hypercalcemia is unpredictable. Hypermagnesemia, as may be seen in preeclamptic patients being managed with magnesium sulfate, potentiates blockade.

D. Age: Neonates have an increased sensitivity to nondepolarizing relaxants because of their immature neuromuscular junctions. This sensitivity does not necessarily decrease dosage requirements, since the neonate's extracellular space is increased, providing a larger volume of distribution.

E. Drug Interactions: Many drugs augment nondepolarizing blockade (Table 9–4). They have multiple sites of interaction: prejunctional structures, postjunctional cholinergic receptors, and muscle membranes.

F. Concurrent Disease: The presence of neurologic or muscular disease can have profound effects on an individual's response to muscle relaxants (Table 9–6).

G. Muscle Groups: The diaphragm is the muscle most resistant to relaxants. While a fortuitous safety feature, persistent diaphragmatic contractions can be disconcerting in the face of complete adductor pollicis paralysis, which is the muscle most commonly monitored. Glottic musculature is also quite resistant to blockade, as is often confirmed during laryngoscopy.

Considering the multitude of factors influencing the duration and magnitude of muscle relaxation, it becomes clear that an individual's response to neuromuscular blocking agents should be monitored. Dosage recommendations, including those that follow, should be considered guidelines that require modification for individual patients.

TUBOCURARINE

Physical Structure

Tubocurarine (*d*-tubocurarine) is a monoquaternary compound with a tertiary amine group (Figure 9–3). The quaternary ammonium group mimics ACh and is

Table 9–6. Diseases with altered responses to muscle relaxants.

Disease	Response to Depolarizers	Response to Nondepolarizers
Amyotrophic lateral sclerosis	Contracture	Hypersensitivity
Autoimmune disorders (systemic lupus erythematosus, polymyositis, dermatomyositis)	Hypersensitivity	Hypersensitivity
Burn injury	Hyperkalemia	Resistance
Familial period paralysis (hyperkalemic)	Myotonia and hyperkalemia	Hypersensitivity?
Hemiplegia	Hyperkalemia	Resistance on affected side
Muscular denervation (peripheral nerve injury)	Hyperkalemia and contracture	Normal response or resistance
Muscular dystrophy (Duchenne type)	Hyperkalemia and malignant hyperthermia	Hypersensitivity
Myasthenia gravis	Resistance and proneness to phase II block	Hypersensitivity
Myasthenic syndrome	Hypersensitivity	Hypersensitivity
Myotonia (dystrophica, congenita, paramyotonia)	Generalized muscular contractions	Normal or hypersensitivity

responsible for receptor binding, while the cumbersome ring structure prevents receptor activation.

Metabolism & Excretion

Tubocurarine is not metabolized to a significant extent. Elimination is primarily renal (50% of injected dose in the first 24 hours) and secondarily biliary (10%).

Dosages

For intubation, 0.5–0.6 mg/kg of tubocurarine is administered slowly over 3 minutes. Intraoperative relaxation is achieved with a dose of 0.15 mg/kg initially, followed by incremental doses of 0.05 mg/kg. The average 70-kg patient usually receives a 9-mg loading dose followed by 3-mg increments every 20–30 minutes.

Initial dosage requirements are not usually less in children, though subsequent doses may be less frequently required. Neonates can display a marked variation in response.

Tubocurarine is packaged as 3 mg/mL and does not require refrigeration.

Side Effects & Clinical Considerations

A. Hypotension and Tachycardia: These cardiovascular effects are primarily related to histamine release. Of secondary importance is tubocurarine's ability to block autonomic ganglia.

B. Bronchospasm: This also is related to increased histamine levels, and tubocurarine is best avoided in asthmatics.

METOCURINE

Physical Structure

Metocurine is a derivative of tubocurarine and is also known as dimethyl tubocurarine. Tubocurarine and metocurine share many pharmacologic properties and side effects because their structures are so closely related.

Metabolism & Excretion

Like tubocurarine, metocurine is not metabolized and is primarily excreted by the kidneys (50% in the first 24 hours). Biliary excretion plays a minor role (< 5%).

Dosages

Conditions suitable for intubation are achieved by administering 0.3 mg/kg over 1–2 minutes to minimize side effects. Intraoperative relaxation is provided by 0.08 mg/kg initially, followed by incremental doses of 0.03 mg/kg.

Dosage considerations are similar to those described for tubocurarine in pediatric patients. Regardless of age, metocurine is twice as potent as tubocurarine.

Metocurine is packaged in 20-mL vials containing 2 mg/mL and does not require refrigeration.

Side Effects & Clinical Considerations

In equipotent doses, metocurine releases half as much histamine as tubocurarine. Nonetheless, if large doses are administered, side effects include hypotension and tachycardia, bronchospasm, and allergic reactions. Patients allergic to iodine (eg, those with fish allergies) may be hypersensitive to metocurine preparations since they too contain iodide (eg, Metubine Iodide).

ATRACURIUM

Physical Structure

Like all muscle relaxants, atracurium has a quaternary group. However, a benzyl isoquinoline structure is responsible for its unique method of degradation.

Metabolism & Excretion

Atracurium is so extensively metabolized that less than 10% is excreted unchanged by renal and biliary routes. Because of extensive metabolism, atracurium's pharmacokinetics are independent of renal and hepatic function. Two separate processes are responsible for metabolism.

A. Ester Hydrolysis: This action is catalyzed by nonspecific esterases, not acetylcholinesterase or pseudocholinesterase.

B. Hoffmann Elimination: Spontaneous nonenzymatic chemical breakdown occurs at physiologic pH and temperature.

Dosages

A dose of 0.5 mg/kg is administered intravenously over 30–60 seconds for intubation. Intraoperative relaxation is achieved with 0.25 mg/kg initially, then in incremental doses of 0.1 mg/kg every 10–20 minutes. An infusion of 5–10 μg/kg/min can effectively replace intermittent boluses.

Although dosage requirements do not significantly vary with age, atracurium may be shorter-acting in children and infants than in adults.

Atracurium is available as a solution of 10 mg/mL. It must be stored at 2–8 °C, since it loses 5–10% of its potency for each month it is exposed to room temperature.

Side Effects & Clinical Considerations

Atracurium triggers the release of histamine to a lesser extent than either tubocurarine or metocurine.

A. Hypotension and Tachycardia: Cardiovascular side effects are unusual unless doses in excess of 0.5 mg/kg are administered. A slow rate of injection minimizes histamine release.

B. Bronchospasm: Atracurium should be avoided in asthmatic patients. Nonetheless, severe bronchospasm is possible even in patients without a history of asthma.

C. Laudanosine Toxicity: Laudanosine is a breakdown product of atracurium's Hoffmann elimination that has been associated with central nervous system excitation, resulting in elevation of the minimum alveolar concentration and even precipitation of seizures. These are probably irrelevant considerations unless a patient has received an extremely high total dose or has hepatic failure (laudanosine is metabolized by the liver).

D. pH and Temperature Sensitivity: Because of its unique metabolism, atracurium's duration of action can be markedly prolonged in hypothermic or acidotic patients.

E. Chemical Incompatibility: Atracurium will precipitate as a free acid if it is introduced into an intravenous line containing an alkaline solution such as thiopental.

MIVACURIUM

Physical Structure

Mivacurium is a benzyl isoquinoline derivative.

Metabolism & Excretion

Mivacurium, like succinylcholine, is metabolized by pseudocholinesterase. It is only minimally metabolized by true cholinesterase. This introduces the possibility of prolonged action in patients with atypical cholinesterase. Mivacurium does not appear to be dependent on normal renal or hepatic function. Despite being hydrolyzed by pseudocholinesterase, mivacurium can be effectively antagonized by cholinesterase inhibitors.

Dosages

The usual intubating dose of mivacurium is 0.2 mg/kg. Steady-state infusion rates for intraoperative relaxation vary with pseudocholinesterase levels but can be initiated at 2 μg/kg/min. Children require higher dosages than adults when dosage is calculated in terms of body weight rather than surface area.

Side Effects & Clinical Considerations

Mivacurium releases histamine to about the same degree as atracurium. The consequent cardiovascular side effects can be minimized by slow injection over 1 minute. Nonetheless, patients with cardiac disease may rarely experience a significant drop in arterial blood pressure after doses larger than 0.15 mg/kg despite a slow injection rate. Mivacurium's onset time is similar to that of the intermediate-acting nondepolarizing relaxants (2–3 minutes). Its principal advantage is its brief duration of action (20–30 minutes), which is

still 2–3 times longer than a phase I block from succinylcholine.

DOXACURIUM

Physical Structure

Doxacurium is a benzyl isoquinoline compound closely related to mivacurium and atracurium.

Metabolism & Excretion

This long-acting relaxant undergoes slow hydrolysis by plasma cholinesterase. Because its primary route of excretion is renal (70%), the duration of action of doxacurium is prolonged in patients with renal disease. Hepatobiliary excretion appears to play a minor role in doxacurium clearance.

Dosages

Adequate conditions for tracheal intubation within 5 minutes require 0.05 mg/kg. Intraoperative relaxation is achieved with an initial dose of 0.02 mg/kg followed by doses of 0.005 mg/kg. Doxacurium may be given in similar weight-adjusted dosages to young and elderly patients.

Side Effects & Clinical Considerations

Doxacurium is essentially devoid of cardiovascular side effects. It has an onset of action slightly slower than that of other long-acting nondepolarizing relaxants (4–6 minutes), while its duration of action is similar to that of pancuronium (60–90 minutes).

PANCURONIUM

Physical Structure

Pancuronium consists of a steroid ring on which two modified acetylcholine molecules are positioned (Figure 9–3). To an ACh receptor, pancuronium resembles acetylcholine enough to bind but not enough to open the lock.

Metabolism & Excretion

Unlike tubocurarine or metocurine, pancuronium is metabolized (deacetylated) by the liver, but to a limited degree. Its metabolic products have some neuromuscular blocking activity. Excretion is primarily renal (40%), though some is cleared by the bile (10%). Not surprisingly, pancuronium elimination is slowed and neuromuscular blockade is prolonged by renal failure. Patients with cirrhosis may require a higher initial dose due to an increased volume of distribution but have lower maintenance requirements due to a decreased rate of plasma clearance.

Dosages

Pancuronium is half as potent as doxacurium. A dose of 0.08–0.12 mg/kg of pancuronium provides adequate relaxation for intubation in 2–3 minutes. Intraoperative relaxation is achieved by administering 0.04 mg/kg initially followed every 20–40 minutes by 0.01 mg/kg.

Children may require moderately higher doses of pancuronium.

Pancuronium is available as a solution of 1 or 2 mg/mL and is stored at 2–8 °C.

Side Effects & Clinical Considerations

A. Hypertension and Tachycardia: These cardiovascular effects are caused by the combination of vagal blockade and catecholamine release from adrenergic nerve endings. Pancuronium should be given with caution to patients in whom an increased heart rate would be particularly detrimental (eg, coronary artery disease or idiopathic hypertrophic subaortic stenosis).

B. Dysrhythmias: Increased atrioventricular conduction and catecholamine release increase the likelihood of ventricular dysrhythmias in predisposed individuals. The combination of pancuronium, tricyclic antidepressants, and halothane has been reported to be particularly dysrhythmogenic.

C. Allergic Reactions: Patients who are hypersensitive to bromides may demonstrate allergic reactions to pancuronium (pancuronium bromide).

VECURONIUM

Physical Structure

Vecuronium is pancuronium minus a quaternary methyl group (a monoquaternary relaxant). This minor structural change beneficially alters side effects without affecting potency.

Metabolism & Excretion

Vecuronium is metabolized to a small extent by the liver. Unique among relaxants, vecuronium depends primarily upon biliary excretion and secondarily (25%) upon renal excretion. While it is a good drug for renal failure patients, its duration of action is somewhat prolonged. Vecuronium's brief duration of action is explained by its shorter elimination half-life and more rapid clearance when compared with pancuronium.

Dosages

Vecuronium is equipotent with pancuronium, and the intubating dose is 0.08–0.12 mg/kg. A dose of 0.04 mg/kg initially followed by increments of 0.01 mg/kg every 15–20 minutes provides intraoperative relaxation. Alternatively, an infusion of 1–2 μg/kg/min produces good maintenance of relaxation.

Age does not affect initial dose requirements, though subsequent doses are required less frequently in neonates and infants. The duration of action of vecuronium may be prolonged in postpartum patients owing to alterations in hepatic blood flow or liver uptake.

Vecuronium is packaged as 10 mg of powder which is reconstituted with 5 or 10 mL of preservative-free water immediately before use. Unused portions are discarded after 24 hours.

Side Effects & Clinical Considerations

A. Cardiovascular: Even at doses of 0.28 mg/kg, vecuronium is devoid of significant cardiovascular effects.

B. Liver Failure: Although it is dependent upon biliary excretion, vecuronium's duration of action is not prolonged in patients with cirrhosis unless doses greater than 0.15 mg/kg are given.

PIPECURONIUM

Physical Structure

Pipecuronium has a steroidal structure very similar to that of pancuronium.

Metabolism & Excretion

Like other long-acting nondepolarizers, metabolism of pipecuronium plays a minor role. Elimination depends upon excretion, which is primarily renal (70%) and secondarily biliary (20%). The duration of action is increased in patients with renal failure.

Dosages

Pipecuronium is slightly more potent than pancuronium, and the usual intubating dose ranges from 0.06 to 0.1 mg/kg. Likewise, maintenance relaxation doses can be reduced by approximately 20% compared with pancuronium. Infants require less pipecuronium on a per kilogram basis than children or adults.

Side Effects & Clinical Considerations

The principal advantage of pipecuronium over pancuronium is its lack of cardiovascular side effects. Pipecuronium is not associated with histamine release. Onset of action and duration of action are similar for both drugs.

CASE DISCUSSION: DELAYED RECOVERY FROM GENERAL ANESTHESIA

A 72-year-old man has undergone general anesthesia for transurethral resection of the prostate. Twenty minutes after conclusion of the procedure, he is still intubated and shows no evidence of spontaneous respiration or consciousness.

What is your general approach to this diagnostic dilemma?

Clues to the solution of complex clinical problems are usually found in a pertinent review of the past medical history, past surgical history, history of drug ingestions, physical examination, and laboratory results. In this case, the perioperative anesthetic management should also be considered.

What medical illnesses predispose a patient to delayed awakening or prolonged paralysis?

Chronic hypertension alters cerebral blood flow autoregulation and decreases the brain's tolerance to episodes of hypotension. Liver disease reduces hepatic drug metabolism and biliary excretion, resulting in prolonged drug action. Reduced serum albumin levels increase free drug (active drug) availability. Hepatic encephalopathy can alter consciousness. Kidney disease lessens the renal excretion of many drugs. Uremia can also affect consciousness. Diabetics are prone to hypoglycemia and hyperosmotic, hyperglycemic, nonketotic coma. A prior stroke or *symptomatic* carotid bruit increases the risk of intraoperative cerebral vascular accident. Right-to-left heart shunts, especially in children with congenital heart disease, allow air emboli to pass directly from the venous circulation to the systemic (possibly cerebral) arterial circulation. A paradoxic air embolism can result in permanent brain damage. Severe hypothyroidism is associated with impaired drug metabolism and, rarely, myxedema coma.

Does an uneventful history of general anesthesia narrow the differential?

Hereditary atypical pseudocholinesterase is ruled out by uneventful prior general anesthesia, assuming succinylcholine was administered. Decreased levels of normal enzyme would not result in postoperative apnea unless the surgery was of very short duration. Malignant hyperthermia does not typically present as delayed awakening, though prolonged somnolence is not unusual. Uneventful prior anesthetics *do not* rule out malignant hyperthermia. Individuals unusually sensitive to anesthetic agents (eg, geriatric patients) may have a history of delayed emergence.

How do drugs that a patient takes at home affect awakening from general anesthesia?

Drugs that decrease minimum alveolar concentration, such as reserpine or methyldopa, predispose to anesthetic overdose. Acute ethanol intoxication decreases barbiturate metabolism and acts independently as a sedative. Drugs that decrease liver blood flow, such as cimetidine, will limit hepatic drug metabolism. Antiparkinsonism drugs and tricyclic antidepressants have anticholinergic side effects that augment the sedation produced by scopolamine. Long-acting

sedatives, such as the benzodiazepines, can delay awakening.

Does anesthetic technique alter wake-up?

Preoperative medications can affect awakening. In particular, anticholinergics (with the exception of glycopyrrolate, which does not cross the blood-brain barrier), narcotics, and sedatives can interfere with postoperative recovery. Patients with low cardiac output may have delayed absorption of intramuscular injections.

Anesthetic maintenance techniques influence the recovery rate. Specifically, nitrous-narcotic (eg, N_2O/fentanyl) techniques tend to be associated with rapid return of the *early* signs of awakening such as eye opening or response to verbal commands. However, nitrous-narcotic and volatile anesthetics do not significantly differ in the time required for complete recovery.

Intraoperative hyperventilation is a common cause of postoperative apnea. Since volatile agents raise the apneic threshold, the $PaCO_2$ at which spontaneous ventilation ceases, moderate postoperative hypoventilation may be required to stimulate the respiratory centers. Severe intraoperative hypotension or hypertension may lead to cerebral hypoxia and edema.

Hypothermia decreases minimum alveolar concentration, antagonizes muscle relaxation reversal, and limits drug metabolism. Arterial hypoxia or severe hypercapnia ($PaCO_2 > 70$ mm Hg) can alter consciousness.

Certain surgical procedures such as carotid endarterectomy, cardiopulmonary bypass, and intracranial procedures are associated with an increased incidence of postoperative neurologic deficits. Transurethral resection of the prostate is associated with hyponatremia due to the dilutional effects of absorbed irrigating solution.

What clues does a physical examination provide?

Pupil size is not always a reliable indicator of central nervous system integrity. However, fixed and dilated pupils in the absence of anticholinergic medication or ganglionic blockade (eg, trimethaphan) may be an ominous sign. Response to physical stimulation such as a forceful jaw thrust may differentiate somnolence from paralysis. Peripheral nerve stimulation will also differentiate paralysis from coma.

What specific laboratory findings would you order?

Arterial blood gases and serum electrolytes, particularly sodium, may be helpful. CT scanning may be recommended by a neurologic consultant.

What therapeutic interventions should be considered?

Supportive mechanical ventilation should be continued in the unresponsive patient. Naloxone, physostigmine, doxapram, or aminophylline may be indicated depending upon the probable cause of the delayed emergence.

SUGGESTED READINGS

Katz RL (editor): *Muscle Relaxants: Basic and Clinical Aspects.* Grune & Stratton, 1985.

Norman J (editor): *Neuromuscular Blockade. Clinics in Anesthesiology.* Saunders, 1985. Many aspects of neuromuscular pharmacology, including theories of muscle relaxant action.

Smith NT, Corbascio AN: *Drug Interactions in Anesthesia.* Lea & Febiger, 1986. Interactions between muscle relaxants and other drugs.

Stanski DR, Watkins WD: *Drug Disposition in Anesthesia.* Grune & Stratton, 1982. Pharmacokinetic principles and their relevance to muscle relaxant administration.

Cholinesterase Inhibitors

10

The primary clinical use of cholinesterase inhibitors, also called anticholinesterases, is to reverse non-depolarizing muscle blockade. However, this drug group has effects on cholinergic receptors beyond the neuromuscular end plate. This chapter reviews cholinergic pharmacology, explores the mechanisms of acetylcholinesterase inhibition, and presents the clinical pharmacology of commonly used cholinesterase inhibitors (neostigmine, edrophonium, pyridostigmine, and physostigmine).

CHOLINERGIC PHARMACOLOGY

The term "cholinergic" refers to the effects of the neurotransmitter acetyl*choline,* as opposed to the "adrenergic" effects of norepinephrine (nor*adrenaline*). Acetylcholine is synthesized in the nerve terminal by the enzyme choline acetyltransferase, which catalyzes the reaction between acetylcoenzyme A and choline (Figure 10–1). After its release, acetylcholine is rapidly hydrolyzed by acetylcholinesterase (true cholinesterase) into acetate and choline.

Acetylcholine is the neurotransmitter for (1) the entire parasympathetic nervous system (parasympathetic ganglions and effector cells), (2) parts of the sympathetic nervous system (sympathetic ganglions, adrenal medulla, and sweat glands), (3) some neurons in the central nervous system, and (4) somatic nerves innervating skeletal muscle (Figure 10–2).

Cholinergic receptors have been subdivided into two major groups depending upon their reaction to the alkaloids muscarine and nicotine (Figure 10–3). Nicotine stimulates the autonomic ganglia and skeletal muscle receptors **(nicotinic receptors),** while muscarine activates end-organ effector cells in bronchial smooth muscle, salivary glands, and the sinoatrial node **(muscarinic receptors).** Nicotinic receptors are blocked by nondepolarizing muscle relaxants (Chapter 9), while muscarinic receptors are blocked by anticholinergic drugs such as atropine (Chapter 11). Although nicotinic and muscarinic receptors differ in their response to some agonists (eg, nicotine and muscarine) and some antagonists (eg, pancuronium and

atropine), they both respond to acetylcholine (Table 10–1). *The primary goal of muscle relaxant reversal is to maximize nicotinic transmission while at the same time minimizing muscarinic side effects.*

MECHANISM OF ACTION

Neuromuscular transmission depends on acetylcholine binding to nicotinic cholinergic receptors on the motor end plate. Nondepolarizing muscle relaxants act by competing with acetylcholine for these binding sites, thereby blocking neuromuscular transmission. Reversal of blockade depends upon either gradual diffusion, metabolism, and excretion from the body of the nondepolarizing relaxant or upon specific reversal agents. The cholinesterase inhibitors *indirectly* increase the amount of acetylcholine available to compete with the nondepolarizing agent, thereby reestablishing neuromuscular transmission.

Cholinesterase inhibitors inactivate acetylcholinesterase by reversibly binding to the enzyme. The stability of the bond influences the duration of action: **edrophonium's** electrostatic attraction and hydrogen bonding are short-lived, while the covalent bonds of **neostigmine** and **pyridostigmine** are longer-lasting. This difference in duration of action can be overcome by adjustments in dosages. Reversible cholinesterase inhibitors are also used in the diagnosis and treatment of myasthenia gravis.

Another class of cholinesterase inhibitors, the **organophosphates,** form very stable "irreversible" bonds to the enzyme. The use of organophosphates such as echothiophate to treat glaucoma can result in a significant prolongation of blockade from succinylcholine, because these drugs also inhibit pseudocholinesterase (Chapter 38).

Mechanisms of action other than acetylcholinesterase inactivation may contribute to the restoration of neuromuscular function. For example, neostigmine has a direct (but weak) agonist effect on nicotinic receptors. Furthermore, acetylcholine mobilization and release by the nerve may be enhanced.

In excessive doses, acetylcholinesterase inhibitors can paradoxically potentiate a nondepolarizing neuromuscular blockade by plugging the ion channel in the core of the acetylcholine receptor. Additionally, these drugs prolong the depolarization blockade of

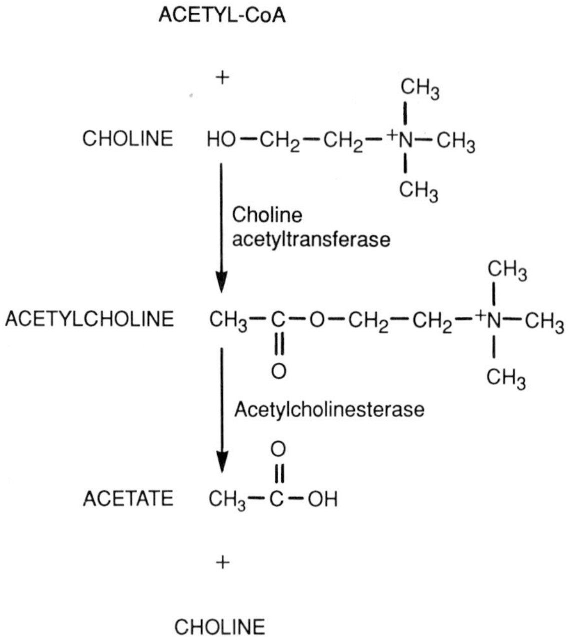

ACETYL-CoA

Figure 10-1. The synthesis and hydrolysis of acetylcholine.

succinylcholine. Two mechanisms may explain this latter effect: (1) an increase in acetylcholine, which increases motor end plate depolarization; and (2) inhibition of pseudocholinesterase (plasma cholinesterase) activity. Neostigmine itself can cause a weak depolarizing neuromuscular blockade.

CLINICAL PHARMACOLOGY

General Pharmacologic Characteristics

The increase in acetylcholine caused by cholinesterase inhibitors affects not only the nicotinic receptors of skeletal muscle (Table 10–2). Cholinesterase inhibitors can act at cholinergic receptors of several other organ systems, including the following: (1) Cardiovascular receptors: The predominant muscarinic effect on the heart is a vagal-like bradycardia that can progress to sinus arrest. (2) Pulmonary receptors: Muscarinic stimulation can result in bronchospasm (smooth muscle contraction) and increased respiratory tract secretions. (3) Cerebral receptors: Physostigmine is a cholinesterase inhibitor that crosses the blood-brain barrier and can cause diffuse activation of the EEG by stimulating muscarinic and nicotinic receptors within the central nervous system. (4) Gastrointestinal receptors: Muscarinic stimulation increases peristaltic activity (esophageal, gastric, and intestinal) and glandular secretions (eg, salivary and parietal).

Unwanted muscarinic side effects are minimized by prior or concomitant administration of anticholinergic medications such as atropine sulfate or glycopyrrolate (Chapter 11).

The pharmacokinetics of the cholinesterase inhibitors are similar. Differences in onset, potency, and duration in patients with normal renal and hepatic function are better explained by pharmacodynamics (eg, affinity and bonding to acetylcholinesterase) than by pharmacokinetics (eg, distribution half-lives or rates of elimination). Clearance is due both to hepatic metabolism (25–50%) and to renal excretion (50–75%). Thus, any prolongation of action of a nondepolarizing muscle relaxant due to renal or hepatic insufficiency will probably be accompanied by an increase in the duration of action of a cholinesterase inhibitor.

Dose requirements of cholinesterase inhibitors depend on the degree of neuromuscular block that is being reversed. This is usually estimated by the response to peripheral nerve stimulation. The time required to fully reverse a nondepolarizing block depends on several factors, including the dose of cholinesterase inhibitor administered and the extent of the blockade before reversal. As a rule, no amount of cholinesterase inhibitor can immediately reverse a block so intense that there is no response to tetanic peripheral nerve stimulation. Excessive dosages of cholinesterase inhibitors may actually prolong recovery. The time to recovery of neuromuscular function does not depend on when antagonism is attempted.

The use of a peripheral nerve stimulator to monitor recovery from neuromuscular blockade is discussed in Chapters 6 and 9. In general, the higher the frequency

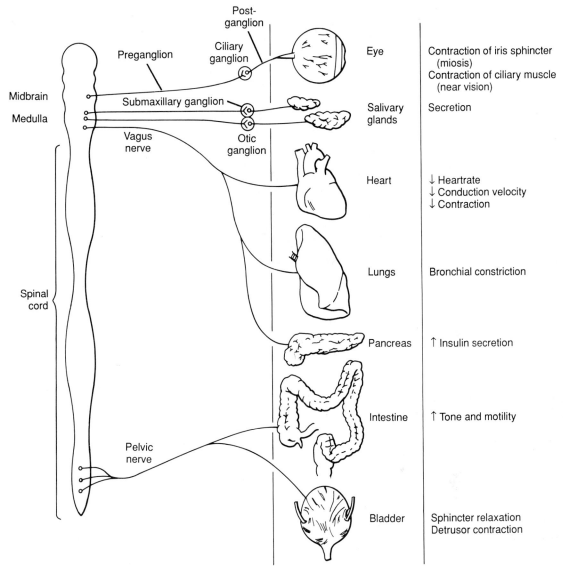

Figure 10–2. The parasympathetic nervous system uses acetylcholine as preganglionic and postganglionic neurotransmitter.

of stimulation, the greater the sensitivity of the test (100 Hz tetanus > 50 Hz or train of four > single-twitch height). Since peripheral nerve stimulation is uncomfortable, alternative tests of neuromuscular function must be used in awake patients. These also vary in sensitivity (sustained head lift > inspiratory force > vital capacity > tidal volume). Therefore, the suggested end points of recovery are sustained tetanus for 5 seconds in response to a 100-Hz stimulus in asleep patients or sustained head lift in awake patients. If neither of these end points is achieved, the patient should remain intubated and ventilation should continue to be supported.

SPECIFIC ANTICHOLINERGIC AGENTS

NEOSTIGMINE

Physical Structure

Neostigmine consists of a carbamate moiety and a quaternary ammonium group (Figure 10–4). The former provides covalent bonding to acetylcholines-

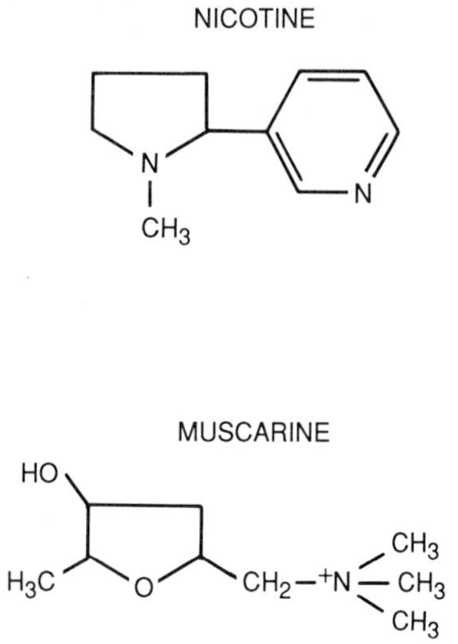

NICOTINE

MUSCARINE

Figure 10–3. The molecular structures of nicotine and muscarine. Compare these alkaloids with acetylcholine (Fig 10–1).

terase, which leads to prolonged inhibition. The latter renders the molecule lipid-insoluble, so that it cannot pass through the blood-brain barrier.

Dosages & Packaging

The maximum recommended dose of neostigmine is 0.08 mg/kg (up to 5 mg in adults), but smaller amounts often suffice (Table 10–3). Neostigmine is most commonly packaged as 10 mL of a 1 mg/mL solution,

Table 10–1. Characteristics of cholinergic receptors.

	Nicotinic	Muscarinic

Location	Autonomic ganglia
	  Sympathetic ganglia
	  Parasympathetic
	    ganglia
	Skeletal muscle
		Glands
		  Lacrimal
		  Salivary
		  Gastric
		Smooth muscle
		  Bronchial
		  Gastrointestinal
		  Bladder
		  Blood vessels
		Heart
		  SA mode
		  AV node

Agonists	Acetylcholine Nicotine	Acetylcholine Muscarine
Antagonists	Nondepolarizing relaxants Pancuronium Tubocurarine Vecuronium Atracurium Metocurine Mivacurium Pipecuronium Doxacurium	Antimuscarinics Atropine Scopolamine Glycopyrrolate

Table 10–2. Muscarinic side effects of cholinesterase inhibitors.

Organ System	Muscarinic Side Effects
Cardiovascular	Decreased heart rate, dysrhythmias
Pulmonary	Bronchospasm, bronchial secretions
Cerebral	Diffuse excitation[1]
Gastrointestinal	Intestinal spasm, increased salivation
Genitourinary	Increased bladder tone
Ophthalmologic	Pupillary constriction

[1] Only applies to physostigmine.

though 0.5 mg/mL and 0.25 mg/mL concentrations are available also.

Clinical Considerations

The effects of neostigmine (0.04 mg/kg) are usually apparent in 5–10 minutes and last over an hour. Pediatric and elderly patients appear to be more sensitive to its effects, experiencing a more rapid onset and having a decreased dosage requirement. The duration of action is prolonged in geriatric patients. Muscarinic side effects are minimized by prior or concomitant administration of an anticholinergic agent. The onset of action of glycopyrrolate (0.2 mg glycopyrrolate per 1 mg of neostigmine) is similar to that of neostigmine and is associated with less tachycardia than atropine (0.4 mg of atropine per 1 mg of neostigmine). Neostigmine is also used to treat myasthenia gravis, urinary bladder atony, and paralytic ileus.

PYRIDOSTIGMINE

Physical Structure

Pyridostigmine is structurally similar to neostigmine except that the quaternary ammonium is incorporated into the phenol ring. Pyridostigmine shares neostigmine's covalent binding to acetylcholinesterase and its lipid insolubility.

Dosages & Packaging

Pyridostigmine is one-fifth as potent as neostigmine and may be administered in dosages up to 0.4 mg/kg (20 mg in adults). It is available as a solution of 5 mg/mL.

Clinical Considerations

The onset of action of pyridostigmine is slower (10–15 minutes) and its duration longer (> 2 hours) than those of neostigmine. Equivalent doses of anticholinergic medications are required to prevent bradycardia. Again, glycopyrrolate (0.05 mg of glycopyrrolate per 1 mg of pyridostigmine) is preferred owing to its slower onset of action compared with atropine (0.1 mg of atropine per 1 mg of pyridostigmine).

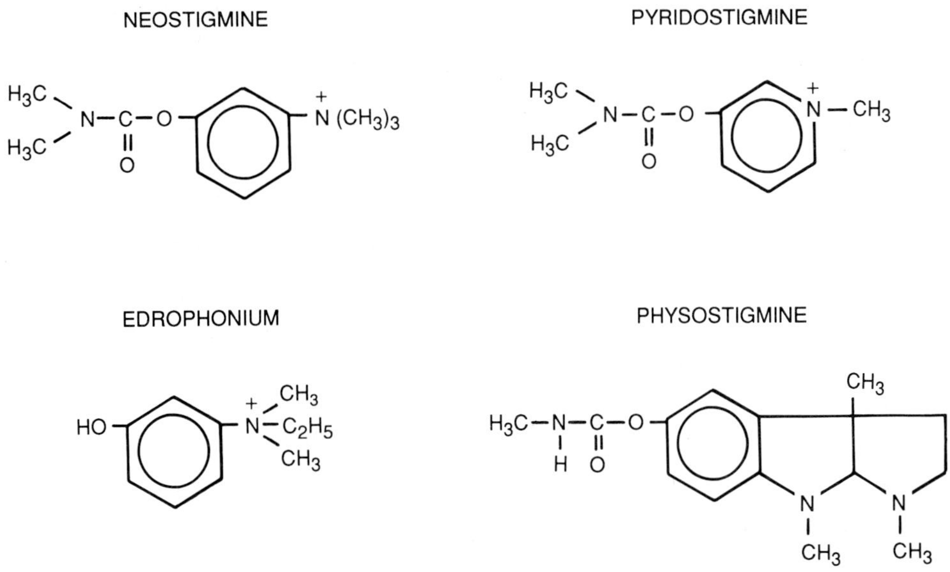

NEOSTIGMINE

PYRIDOSTIGMINE

EDROPHONIUM

PHYSOSTIGMINE

Figure 10–4. Molecular structures of neostigmine, pyridostigmine, edrophonium, and physostigmine.

EDROPHONIUM

Physical Structure

Because it lacks a carbamate group, edrophonium must rely on noncovalent bonding to the acetylcholinesterase enzyme. Lipid solubility is limited by the quaternary ammonium group.

Dosages & Packaging

Edrophonium is less than one-tenth as potent as neostigmine. The recommended dosage range is 0.5–1 mg/kg. Edrophonium is available as a solution containing 10 mg/mL.

Clinical Considerations

Edrophonium has the most rapid onset of action (1–2 minutes) and the shortest duration of effect of any of the cholinesterase inhibitors. Low doses should not be used, because longer-acting muscle relaxants may outlast edrophonium's effects. Higher doses prolong the duration of action to over 1 hour. Patients at the extremes of age are not more sensitive to edrophonium reversal (as is the case with neostigmine). Edrophonium may not be as effective at reversing intense neuromuscular blockade as neostigmine. In equipotent doses, edrophonium's muscarinic effects are less pronounced than those of neostigmine or pyridostigmine, requiring only half the amount of anticholinergic agent. Edrophonium's rapid onset is well matched to that of atropine (0.014 mg of atropine per 1 mg of edrophonium). Although glycopyrrolate (0.007 mg per 1 mg of edrophonium) can also be used, it should be given several minutes prior to edrophonium to avoid the possibility of bradycardia.

Table 10–3. The choice and dose of cholinesterase inhibitor determines the choice and dose of anticholinergic.

Cholinesterase Inhibitor	Usual Dose of Cholinesterase Inhibitor	Recommended Anticholinergic	Usual Dose of Anticholinergic per mg of Cholinesterase Inhibitor
Neostigmine	0.04–0.08 mg/kg	Glycopyrrolate	0.2 mg
Pyridostigmine	0.1–0.4 mg/kg	Glycopyrrolate	0.05 mg
Edrophonium	0.5–1 mgu/kg	Atropine	0.014 mg
Physostigmine	0.01–0.03 mg/kg	Usually not necessary	—

PHYSOSTIGMINE

Physical Structure

Physostigmine, a tertiary amine, has a carbamate group but no quaternary ammonium. Therefore, it is lipid-soluble and is the only cholinesterase inhibitor available for clinical use that freely passes the blood-brain barrier.

Dosages & Packaging

The dose of physostigmine is 0.01–0.03 mg/kg. It is packaged as a solution containing 1 mg/mL.

Clinical Considerations

Physostigmine's lipid solubility and central nervous system penetration limit its usefulness as a reversal agent for nondepolarizing blockade. For the same reasons, it is effective in the treatment of central anticholinergic toxicity due to overdoses of atropine or scopolamine (Chapter 11). In addition, physostigmine reverses some of the central nervous system depression and delirium from benzodiazepines and volatile anesthetics. These effects are transient, and repeat doses may be required. Bradycardia is infrequent in the recommended dosage range, but atropine or glycopyrrolate should be immediately available. Because glycopyrrolate does not cross the blood-brain barrier, it will not reverse the central nervous system effects of physostigmine (Chapter 11). Other possible muscarinic side effects include excessive salivation, vomiting, and convulsions. In contrast to other cholinesterase inhibitors, physostigmine is almost completely metabolized by plasma esterases, so that renal excretion is not important.

CASE DISCUSSION: RESPIRATORY FAILURE IN THE RECOVERY ROOM

A 66-year-old woman weighing 85 kg is brought to the recovery room following cholecystectomy. Her anesthetic included isoflurane and pancuronium for muscle relaxation. At the conclusion of the procedure, the anesthesiologist administered 6 mg of morphine sulfate for postoperative pain control and 3 mg of neostigmine with 0.6 mg of glycopyrrolate to reverse any residual neuromuscular blockade. The dose of cholinesterase inhibitor was empirically based on "clinical judgment." Although she was apparently breathing normally on arrival in the recovery room, the patient's tidal volume progressively diminished. Arterial blood gas measurements revealed a $PaCO_2$ of 62 mm Hg, a PaO_2 of 110 mm Hg, and a pH of 7.26 on an FIO_2 of 40%.

What drugs administered to this patient could explain her hypoventilation?

Isoflurane, morphine sulfate, and pancuronium all interfere with a patient's ability to maintain a normal ventilatory response to an elevated $PaCO_2$.

Why would the patient's breathing worsen in the recovery room?

Possibilities include the delayed onset of action of morphine sulfate, lack of sensory stimulation in the recovery area, fatigue of respiratory muscles, and splinting due to upper abdominal pain.

Could the patient still have residual neuromuscular blockade?

If the dose of neostigmine was not determined by the response to a peripheral nerve stimulator or if the recovery of muscle function was inadequately tested after the reversal drugs were given, persistent neuromuscular blockade is possible. For instance, assume that the patient had minimal or no response to initial tetanic stimulation at 100 Hz. Even the maximal dose of neostigmine (5 mg) may not adequately reverse the paralysis. Because of enormous patient variability, the response to peripheral nerve stimulation must always be monitored when nondepolarizing muscle relaxants are administered. Even if partial reversal was achieved, paralysis may worsen if the patient hypoventilates. Other factors besides respiratory acidosis that impair the reversal of nondepolarizing muscle relaxants include (1) intense neuromuscular paralysis, (2) electrolyte disturbances (hypermagnesemia, hypokalemia, and hypocalcemia), (3) hypothermia (< 32 °C), (4) drug interactions (Table 9–4), (5) metabolic alkalosis (due to accompanying hypokalemia and hypocalcemia), and (6) coexisting diseases (Table 9–6).

How could the extent of reversal be tested?

Tetanic stimulation is a sensitive but uncomfortable test of neuromuscular transmission in an awake patient. Because of its shorter duration of action, double-burst stimulation is better tolerated by conscious patients than tetanus. Many other tests of neuromuscular transmission, such as vital capacity and tidal volume, are insensitive since they may appear normal when 70–80% of receptors are still blocked. In fact, 70% of receptors may remain blocked despite an apparently normal response to train-of-four stimulation. However, the ability to sustain a head lift for 5 seconds indicates that less than 33% of receptors are occupied by muscle relaxant.

What treatment would you suggest?

Ventilation should be assisted to reduce the respiratory acidosis. Even if diaphragmatic function appears to be grossly adequate, residual blockade can lead to airway obstruction and poor airway protection. More neostigmine (with an anticholinergic) could be administered up to a maximum recommended dose of 5 mg.

If this does not adequately reverse paralysis, mechanical ventilation and airway protection should be instituted and continued until neuromuscular function is fully restored.

SUGGESTED READINGS

Connelly R: Muscle relaxant antagonists. Chapter 13 in: *Muscle Relaxants: Basic And Clinical Aspects.* Katz RL (editor). Grune & Stratton, 1985. Answers many questions regarding nondepolarizing muscle relaxant reversal.

Stoelting RK: *Pharmacology and Physiology in Anesthetic Practice.* Lippincott, 1987. An up-to-date presentation of cholinesterase inhibitors.

Taylor P: Anticholinesterase agents. Chapter 7 in: *The Pharmacological Basis of Therapeutics,* 8th ed. Gilman AG et al (editors). Pergamon, 1990. A good reference source for the structure-function relationships and multiple therapeutic uses of this class of drug.

Watanabe AM: Cholinoceptor-activating drugs. Chapter 7 in: *Basic & Clinical Pharmacology,* 4th ed. Katzung BG (editor). Appleton & Lange, 1987.

11

Anticholinergic Drugs

One group of cholinergic antagonists has already been discussed: the nondepolarizing neuromuscular blocking agents. These drugs act chiefly at the **nicotinic receptors** in skeletal muscle. This chapter presents the pharmacology of drugs that block **muscarinic receptors.** Although the classification "anticholinergic" usually refers to this latter group, a more precise term would be "antimuscarinic."

The mechanism of action and clinical pharmacology are introduced for three common anticholinergics: (1) atropine, (2) scopolamine, and (3) glycopyrrolate. The clinical uses of these drugs in anesthesia relate to their effect on the cardiovascular, respiratory, cerebral, gastrointestinal, and other organ systems (Table 11–1).

MECHANISMS OF ACTION

Anticholinergics are esters of an aromatic acid combined with an organic base (Figure 11–1). The ester linkage is essential for effective binding of the anticholinergics to the acetylcholine receptors. This competitively blocks binding by acetylcholine and precludes receptor activation. The cellular effects of acetylcholine, which are mediated through second messengers such as cyclic guanosine monophosphate (cGMP), are prevented. The tissue receptors vary in their sensitivity to blockade. In fact, muscarinic receptors are not homogeneous, and receptor subgroups have been identified (eg M_1 and M_2 receptors).

CLINICAL PHARMACOLOGY

General Pharmacologic Characteristics

In clinical doses, only muscarinic receptors are blocked by the anticholinergic drugs discussed in this chapter. The extent of the anticholinergic effect depends on the degree of baseline vagal tone. Several organ systems are affected:

A. Cardiovascular: Blockade of muscarinic receptors in the sinoatrial node results in tachycardia. This effect is especially useful in reversing bradycardia due to vagal reflexes (eg, baroreceptor reflex, peritoneal stimulation, or oculocardiac reflex). A tran-

sient slowing of heart rate in response to low doses of anticholinergics has been reported. The mechanism of this paradoxic response may be a weak peripheral *agonist* effect, suggesting that these drugs are not pure antagonists. Facilitation of conduction through the atrioventricular node shortens the PR interval on the ECG and often decreases heart block due to vagal activity. Atrial dysrhythmias and nodal rhythms occasionally occur. Anticholinergics have little effect on ventricular function or peripheral vasculature because of the paucity of direct cholinergic innervation of these areas despite the presence of cholinergic receptors. Large doses of anticholinergic agents can result in dilatation of cutaneous blood vessels ("atropine flush").

B. Respiratory: The anticholinergics inhibit the secretions of the respiratory tract mucosa from the nose to the bronchi. This drying effect was more important before the advent of less irritating inhalational agents. Relaxation of bronchial smooth musculature reduces airway resistance and increases anatomic dead space. These effects are particularly pronounced in patients with chronic obstructive pulmonary disease or asthma.

C. Cerebral: Anticholinergic medications can cause a spectrum of central nervous system effects ranging from stimulation to depression, depending on drug choice and dosage. Stimulation may present as excitation, restlessness, or hallucinations. Depression can cause sedation and amnesia. Physostigmine, a cholinesterase inhibitor that crosses the blood-brain barrier, promptly reverses these actions.

D. Gastrointestinal: Salivary secretions are markedly reduced by anticholinergic drugs. Gastric secretions are also decreased, but larger doses are necessary. Decreased intestinal motility and peristalsis prolong gastric emptying time. Lower esophageal sphincter pressure is reduced. Overall, the anticholinergic drugs are not especially advantageous in the prevention of aspiration pneumonitis (see Chapter 15 Case Discussion).

E. Ophthalmic: Anticholinergics cause mydriasis (pupillary dilatation) and cycloplegia (inability to accommodate to near vision). Nonetheless, acute angle-closure glaucoma is unlikely following systemic administration of most anticholinergic drugs.

Table 11–1. Pharmacologic characteristics of anticholinergic drugs.

	Atropine	Scopolamine	Glycopyrrolate
Tachycardia	+++	+	++
Bronchodilatation	++	+	++
Sedation	+	+++	0
Antisialagogue effect	++	+++	+++

Key:
0   = No effect
+   = Minimal effect
++   = Moderate effect
+++ = Marked effect

F. Genitourinary: Anticholinergics may decrease ureter and bladder tone due to smooth muscle relaxation and lead to urinary retention, particularly in elderly men with prostatic hypertrophy.

G. Thermoregulation: Inhibition of sweat glands may lead to a rise in body temperature ("atropine fever").

H. Immune-Mediated Hypersensitivity: Decreasing intracellular cGMP would theoretically be useful in the treatment of hypersensitivity reactions. Clinically, anticholinergics appear to have little efficacy in these situations.

SPECIFIC ANTICHOLINERGIC DRUGS

ATROPINE

Physical Structure

Atropine is a tertiary amine consisting of tropic acid (an aromatic acid) and tropine (an organic base). The naturally occurring levorotatory form is active, but the commercial mixture is racemic (Figure 11–1).

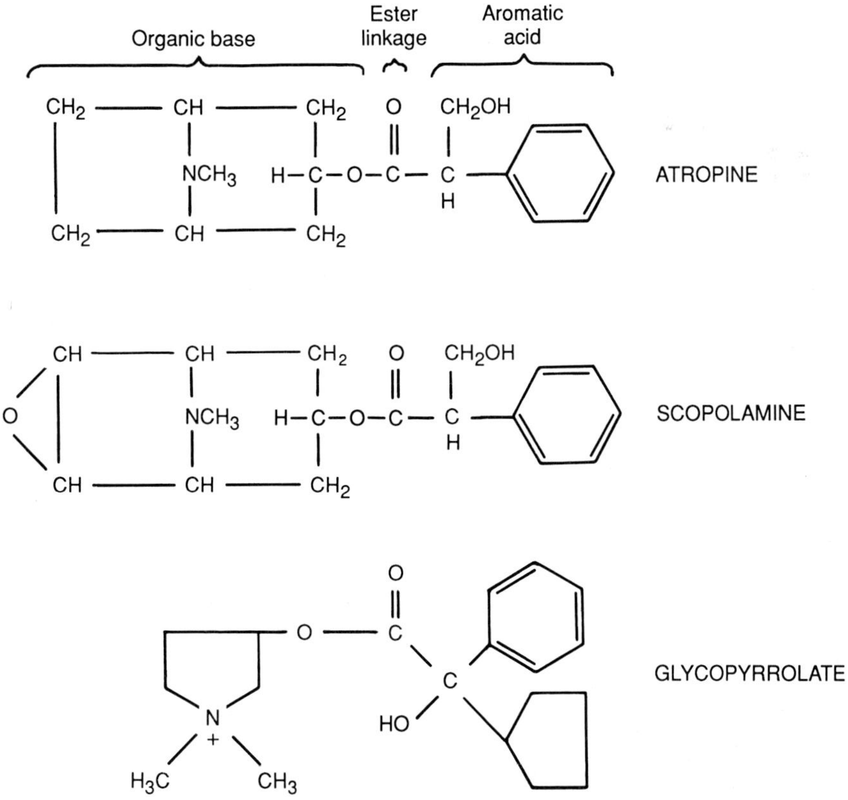

Figure 11–1. Physical structures of anticholinergic drugs.

Dosages & Packaging

As a premedication, atropine is administered intravenously or intramuscularly in a dosage range of 0.01–0.02 mg/kg up to the usual adult dose of 0.4–0.6 mg. Larger intravenous doses up to 2 mg may be required to completely block the cardiac vagal nerves in the treatment of severe bradycardia. The appropriate dose for minimizing the side effects of cholinesterase inhibitors during reversal of nondepolarizing blockade is presented in Chapter 10. Atropine sulfate is available as solutions for injection containing 0.05, 0.1, 0.3, 0.4, 0.5, 0.8, and 1 mg/mL.

Clinical Considerations

Atropine has particularly potent effects on the heart and bronchial smooth muscle and is the most efficacious anticholinergic for treating bradyarrhythmias. Patients with coronary artery disease may not tolerate the increased myocardial oxygen demand and decreased oxygen supply associated with tachycardia caused by atropine. A derivative of atropine (ipratropium bromide) is available in a metered-dose inhaler for the treatment of bronchospasm. The central nervous system effects of atropine are minimal after usual dosages, even though this tertiary amine can rapidly cross the blood-brain barrier. Toxic doses are associated with excitatory reactions.

SCOPOLAMINE

Physical Structure

Scopolamine differs from atropine by incorporating an oxygen bridge into the organic base to form scopine.

Dosages & Packaging

The premedication dose of scopolamine is the same as that of atropine. Scopolamine is usually given intramuscularly. Scopolamine hydrobromide is available as solutions containing 0.3, 0.4, and 1 mg/mL.

Clinical Considerations

Scopolamine is a more potent antisialagogue and causes greater central nervous system effects than atropine. Clinical dosages usually result in drowsiness and amnesia, though restlessness and delirium are possible. The sedative effects may be desirable for premedication but can interfere with awakening following short procedures. Scopolamine has the added virtue of preventing motion sickness. The lipid solubility allows transdermal absorption. Because of pronounced ocular effects, scopolamine is best avoided in patients with closed-angle glaucoma.

GLYCOPYRROLATE

Physical Structure

Glycopyrrolate is a synthetic quaternary ammonium containing mandelic acid in the place of tropic acid.

Dosages & Packaging

The usual dose of glycopyrrolate is one-half that of atropine. For instance, the premedication dose is 0.005–0.01 mg/kg up to 0.2–0.3 mg in adults. Glycopyrrolate for injection is packaged as a solution of 0.2 mg/mL.

Clinical Considerations

Because of a quaternary structure, glycopyrrolate cannot cross the blood-brain barrier and is almost always devoid of central nervous system and ophthalmic activity. Potent inhibition of salivary gland and respiratory tract secretions is the primary rationale for using glycopyrrolate as a premedication. Heart rate usually increases after intravenous but not intramuscular administration. Glycopyrrolate has a longer duration of action than atropine (2–4 hours versus 30 minutes after intravenous administration).

CASE DISCUSSION: CENTRAL ANTICHOLINERGIC SYNDROME

An elderly patient is scheduled for enucleation of a blind, painful eye. Scopolamine, 0.4 mg intramuscularly, is administered as premedication. In the preoperative holding area, the patient becomes agitated and disoriented. The only other medication the patient has received is 1% atropine eye drops.

How many milligrams of atropine are in 1 drop of a 1% solution?

A 1% solution contains 1 g dissolved in 100 mL, or 10 mg/mL. Eye droppers vary in the number of drops formed per milliliter of solution but average 20 drops/mL. Therefore, 1 drop usually contains 0.5 mg of atropine.

How are ophthalmic drops systemically absorbed?

Absorption by vessels in the conjunctival sac is similar to subcutaneous injection. More rapid absorption is possible by the nasolacrimal duct mucosa.

What are the signs and symptoms of anticholinergic poisoning?

Reactions from an overdose of anticholinergic medication involve several organ systems. The **"central anticholinergic syndrome"** refers to central nervous system changes that range from unconsciousness to hallucinations. Agitation and delirium are not unusual in elderly patients. Other systemic manifestations include dry mouth, tachycardia, "atropine flush," "atropine fever," and impaired vision.

What other drugs possess anticholinergic activity that could predispose patients to the central anticholinergic syndrome?

Tricyclic antidepressants, antihistamines, and antipsychotics have antimuscarinic properties that could potentiate the side effects of anticholinergic drugs.

What drug is an effective antidote to anticholinergic overdosage?

Cholinesterase inhibitors indirectly increase the amount of acetylcholine available to compete with anticholinergic drugs at the muscarinic receptor. Neostigmine, pyridostigmine, and edrophonium possess a quaternary ammonium group that prevents penetration of the blood-brain barrier. Physostigmine, a tertiary amine, is lipid-soluble and effectively reverses central

anticholinergic toxicity. An initial dose of 0.01–0.03 mg/kg may have to be repeated after 15–30 minutes.

Should this case be canceled or allowed to proceed?

Enucleation due to a painful eye is clearly an elective procedure. The most important question that must be addressed for elective cases is whether the patient is "optimally medically managed." In other words, would canceling surgery allow further "fine tuning" of any medical problems. For example, if this anticholinergic overdose is accompanied by tachycardia, it would probably be prudent to postpone surgery in this elderly patient. On the other hand, if the patient's mental status responds to physostigmine and there appear to be no other significant anticholinergic side effects, surgery could proceed.

SUGGESTED READINGS

Brown JH: Atropine, scopolamine, and related antimuscarinic drugs. Chapter 8 in: *Goodman and Gilman's The Pharmacological Basis of Therapeutics,* 8th ed. Gilman AG et al (editors): Pergamon, 1990. Mechanisms of action, structure-activity relationships, and therapeutic uses.

Katzung BG: Cholinoceptor-blocking drugs. Chapter 8 in: *Basic and Clinical Pharmacology,* 4th ed. Katzung BG (editor). Appleton & Lange, 1989.

Stoelting RK: *Pharmacology and Physiology in Anesthetic Practice.* Lippincott, 1987.

12

Adrenergic Agonists & Antagonists

The three previous chapters presented the pharmacology of drugs that affect cholinergic activity. This chapter introduces an analogous group of agents that interact at adrenergic receptors—**adrenoceptors.** The clinical effects of these drugs can be deduced from an understanding of adrenoceptor physiology and a knowledge of which receptors each drug activates or blocks.

ADRENOCEPTOR PHYSIOLOGY

The term "adrenergic" originally referred to the effects of epinephrine (*adren*aline), as opposed to the "cholinergic" effects of acetyl*choline*. It is now known that norepinephrine (noradrenaline) is the neurotransmitter responsible for most "adrenergic" activity of the sympathetic nervous system. With the exception of eccrine sweat glands and some blood vessels, norepinephrine is released by postganglionic sympathetic fibers at end-organ tissues (Figure 12–1). In contrast, as was explained in Chapter 10, acetylcholine is released by preganglionic sympathetic fibers and all parasympathetic fibers.

Norepinephrine is synthesized in the cytoplasm and packaged into vesicles of sympathetic postganglionic fibers (Figure 12–2). After release by a process of exocytosis, the action of norepinephrine is terminated by (1) reuptake into the postganglionic nerve ending (inhibited by tricyclic antidepressants), (2) diffusion from receptor sites, or (3) metabolism by monoamine oxidase (inhibited by monoamine oxidase inhibitors) and catechol-O-methyltransferase (Figure 12–3). Prolonged adrenergic activation leads to desensitization and hyporesponsiveness to further stimulation.

Adrenergic receptors are divided into two general categories: alpha and beta. Each of these has been further subdivided into at least two subtypes: α_1 and α_2, β_1 and β_2.

Alpha$_1$ Receptors

Alpha$_1$ receptors are postsynaptic adrenoceptors located in smooth muscle throughout the body, including the eye, lung, blood vessels, uterus, gut, and genitourinary system. Activation of these receptors increases intracellular calcium ion concentration, which leads to muscle contraction. Thus, α_1 agonists are associated with mydriasis (contraction of the radial eye muscles), bronchoconstriction, vasoconstriction, uterine contracture, and contraction of sphincters in the gastrointestinal and genitourinary tracts. Alpha$_1$ stimulation also inhibits insulin secretion and stimulates glycogenolysis and gluconeogenesis. The myocardium may possess α_1 receptors that have slightly positive inotropic and negative chronotropic effects. Nonetheless, the most important cardiovascular effect of α_1 stimulation is vasoconstriction, which increases peripheral vascular resistance and arterial blood pressure.

Alpha$_2$ Receptors

In contrast to α_1 receptors, α_2 receptors are located chiefly on the presynaptic nerve terminal. Activation of these adrenoceptors inhibits adenylyl cyclase activity. This decreases the entry of calcium ions into the neuronal terminal, which limits subsequent exocytosis of storage vesicles containing norepinephrine. Thus, α_2 receptors create a negative feedback loop that inhibits further norepinephrine release from the neuron. Additionally, vascular smooth muscle contains postsynaptic α_2 receptors that produce vasoconstriction. More importantly, stimulation of postsynaptic α_2 receptors in the central nervous system causes sedation and reduces sympathetic outflow, which leads to peripheral vasodilatation and lower blood pressure.

Beta$_1$ Receptors

The most important β_1 receptors are located on postsynaptic membranes in the heart. Stimulation of these receptors activates adenylyl cyclase, which converts ATP to cAMP and initiates a kinase phosphorylation cascade. The end result is cardiac stimulation, manifested by increased heart rate, conduction, and contractility.

Beta$_2$ Receptors

Beta$_2$ receptors are chiefly postsynaptic adrenoceptors located in smooth muscle and gland cells. They share a common mechanism of action with β_1 recep-

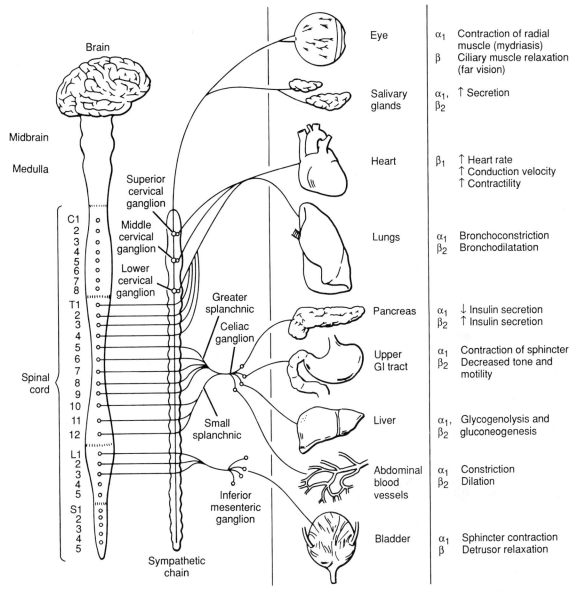

Figure 12–1. The sympathetic nervous system. Organ innervation, receptor type, and response to stimulation. The origin of the sympathetic chain is the thoracoabdominal (T1–L3) spinal cord, in contrast to the craniosacral distribution of the parasympathetic nervous system. Another anatomic difference is the greater distance from the sympathetic ganglion to the visceral structures.

tors: adenylyl cyclase activation. Despite this commonality, β_2 stimulation relaxes smooth muscle, resulting in bronchodilatation, vasodilatation, and relaxation of the uterus (tocolysis), bladder, and gut. Glycogenolysis, gluconeogenesis, and insulin release are stimulated. Beta$_2$ agonists activate the sodium-potassium pump, which drives potassium intracellularly and can induce hypokalemia and dysrhythmias.

ADRENERGIC AGONISTS

Adrenergic agonists interact with varying specificity (selectivity) at alpha and beta adrenoceptors (Table 12–1). Overlapping of activity complicates prediction of clinical effects. For example, epinephrine stimu-

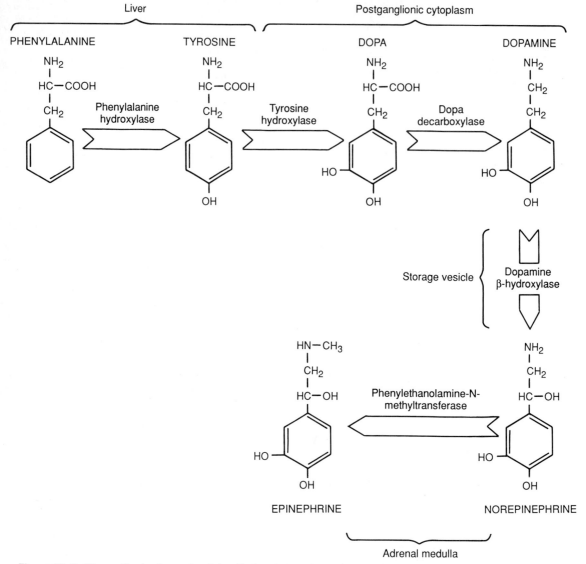

Figure 12–2. The synthesis of norepinephrine. Hydroxylation of tyrosine to DOPA is the rate-limiting step. Dopamine is actively transported into a storage vesicle. Norepinephrine can be converted to epinephrine in the adrenal medulla.

lates α_1, α_2, β_1, and β_2 adrenoceptors. Its net effect on arterial blood pressure depends on the balance between α_1 vasoconstriction, α_2 and β_2 vasodilatation, and β_1 inotropic influences. Moreover, this balance changes at different dosages.

Adrenergic agonists can also be categorized as direct or indirect. **Direct agonists** bind to the receptor, while **indirect agonists** increase endogenous neurotransmitter release. Mechanisms of indirect action include increased release or decreased reuptake of norepinephrine. The differentiation between direct and indirect mechanisms of action is particularly important in patients who have abnormal endogenous norepinephrine stores, as may occur with some antihyper-

tensive medications or with monoamine oxidase inhibitor therapy. Intraoperative hypotension in these patients should be treated with direct agonists, since their response to indirect agonists will be altered.

Another feature distinguishing adrenergic agonists from each other is their chemical structures. Adrenergic agonists that have a 3,4-dihydroxybenzene structure are known as **catecholamines.** These drugs are typically short-acting owing to metabolism by monoamine oxidase and catechol-O-methyltransferase. The naturally occurring catecholamines are epinephrine, norepinephrine, and dopamine.

Adrenergic agonists commonly used in anesthesiology are individually discussed below. Note that the

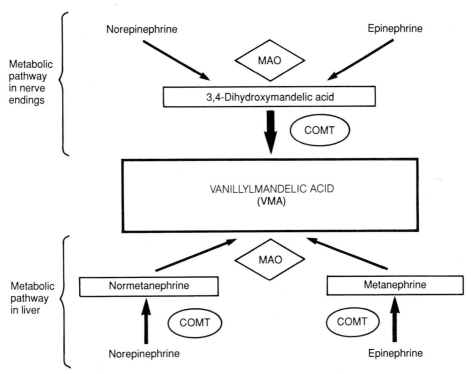

Figure 12–3. Sequential metabolism of norepinephrine and epinephrine. Monoamine oxidase (MAO) and catechol-O-methyltransferase (COMT) produce a common end product, vanillylmandelic acid (VMA).

recommended doses for continuous infusion are expressed as $\mu g/kg/min$ for some agents and $\mu g/min$ for others. In either case, these recommendations should be regarded only as guidelines, since individual responses are quite variable.

PHENYLEPHRINE

Clinical Considerations

Phenylephrine is a noncatecholamine with predominantly direct α_1 agonist activity (high doses may stimulate α_2 and β receptors). Peripheral vasoconstriction with a concomitant rise in systemic vascular resistance and arterial blood pressure is phenylephrine's primary effect. Reflex bradycardia can reduce cardiac output. Coronary blood flow is increased, but renal blood flow falls (Table 12–2).

Dosage & Packaging

Small intravenous boluses of 50–100 μg (0.5–1 $\mu g/kg$) of phenylephrine rapidly reverse blood pressure reductions due to peripheral vasodilatation (eg, spinal anesthesia). A continuous infusion (100 $\mu g/mL$ at a rate of 0.25–1 $\mu g/kg/min$) will maintain arterial blood pressure, but at the expense of renal blood flow. Phenylephrine must be diluted from a 1% solution (10 mg/1 mL ampule).

Table 12–1. Receptor selectivity of adrenergic agonists.

Drug	α_1	α_2	β_1	β_2
Methoxamine	+++	+	0	0
Phenylephrine	+++	+	+	0
Metaraminol[1]	+++	?	++	0
Methyldopa	+	+++	0	0
Clonidine	+	+++	0	0
Epinephrine[2]	++	++	+++	++
Ephedrine[1]	++	?	++	+
Norepinephrine[2]	++	++	++	0
Dopamine[2]	++	++	++	+
Mephentermine[1]	+	?	++	+
Isoproterenol	0	0	+++	+++
Dobutamine	0/+	0	+++	+
Terbutaline	0	0	+	+++

[1]The primary mode of action of metaraminol, ephedrine, and mephentermine is indirect stimulation.
[2]The α_1 effects of epinephrine, norepinephrine, and dopamine become more prominent at high doses.
Key:
 0 = No effect
 + = Agonist effect (mild, moderate, marked)
 ? = Unknown effect

Table 12–2. Organ system effects of adrenergic agonists.

Drug	Heart Rate	Mean Arterial Pressure	Cardiac Output	Peripheral Vascular Resistance	Broncho-dilatation	Renal Blood Flow
Phenylephrine	↓	↑↑↑	↓	↑↑↑	0	↓↓↓
Methyldopa	↓	↓↓	↓	↓↓	0	↑
Ephinephrine	↑↑	↑	↑↑	↑/↓	↑↑	↓↓
Ephedrine	↑↑	↑↑	↑↑	↑	↑↑	↓↓
Norepinephrine	↓	↑↑↑	↓/↑	↑↑↑	0	↓↓↓
Dopamine	↑/↑↑	↑	↑↑↑	↑	0	↑↑↑
Isoproterenol	↑↑↑	↓	↑↑↑	↓↓	↑↑↑	↓/↑
Dobutamine	↑	↑	↑↑↑	↓	0	↑

Key:
0 = No effect
↑ = Increase (mild, moderate, marked)
↓ = Decrease (mild, moderate, marked)

METHYLDOPA & CLONIDINE

Clinical Considerations

Methyldopa, an analogue of levodopa, enters the norepinephrine synthesis pathway and is converted to α-methylnorepinephrine and α-methylepinephrine. These false transmitters activate alpha adrenoceptors, particularly central α_2 receptors. As a result, norepinephrine release and sympathetic tone are diminished. A fall in peripheral vascular resistance is responsible for a drop in arterial blood pressure (peak effect within 4 hours). Renal blood flow is maintained or increased.

Because of similar mechanisms of action, methyldopa may be useful in treating the side effects of rebound hypertension due to clonidine withdrawal. Side effects of α_2 agonists that reflect a central mechanism of action include sedation and decreased anesthetic requirements. In fact, investigational studies with clonidine have shown it to be a very effective analgesic when administered intravenously or epidurally. An important side effect of methyldopa is that about 20% of patients will develop a positive Coombs test, causing difficulty in blood cross-matching. Although methyldopa and clonidine are adrenergic agonists, they are also considered to be **sympatholytic** because sympathetic outflow is reduced.

Dosage & Packaging

Methyldopa is available for intravenous administration (50 mg/mL). The dose is 250–1000 mg administered over a 30-minute period every 6 hours. Currently, clonidine is available only as an oral or transdermal preparation. Oral clonidine has been used as premedication (5 μg/kg).

EPINEPHRINE

Clinical Considerations

Direct stimulation of β_1 receptors by epinephrine raises cardiac output and myocardial oxygen demand by increasing contractility and heart rate (increased rate of spontaneous phase 4 depolarization). Alpha$_1$ stimulation decreases splanchnic and renal blood flow but increases coronary and cerebral perfusion pressure. Systolic blood pressure rises, though β_2-mediated vasodilatation in skeletal muscle may lower diastolic pressure. Beta$_2$ stimulation also relaxes bronchial smooth muscle.

Epinephrine administration is the principal pharmacologic treatment for anaphylaxis and ventricular fibrillation (Chapters 45 and 46). Complications of epinephrine administration include cerebral hemorrhage, coronary ischemia, and ventricular dysrhythmias. Volatile anesthetics, particularly halothane, potentiate the dysrhythmic effects of epinephrine.

Dosage & Packaging

In emergency situations (eg, shock or allergic reactions), epinephrine is administered as an intravenous bolus of 0.05–1 mg depending on the severity of cardiovascular compromise. To improve myocardial contractility or heart rate, a continuous infusion is prepared (1 mg in 250 mL D$_5$W; 4 μg/mL) and run at a rate of 2–20 μg/min. Some local anesthetic solutions containing epinephrine at a concentration of 1:200,000 (5 μg/mL) or 1:100,000 (10 μg/mL) are characterized by less systemic absorption and a longer duration of action. Epinephrine is available in vials at a concentration of 1:1000 (1 mg/mL) and prefilled syringes at a concentration of 1:10,000 (0.1 mg [100 μg]/mL). A 1:100,000 (10 μg/mL) concentration is available for pediatric use.

EPHEDRINE

Clinical Considerations

The cardiovascular effects of ephedrine are similar to those of epinephrine: blood pressure, heart rate, contractility, and cardiac output increase. Likewise, ephedrine is also a bronchodilator. However, there are important differences: Ephedrine has a longer duration of action because it is a noncatecholamine, is much less potent, has indirect and direct actions, and stimulates the central nervous system (raises minimum alveolar concentration).

Ephedrine is commonly used as a vasopressor during anesthesia. As such, its administration should be viewed as a temporizing measure while the cause of hypotension is determined and remedied. Unlike direct-acting α_1 agonists, ephedrine does not decrease uterine blood flow. This makes it the preferred pressor for most obstetric uses. Ephedrine has also been reported to possess antiemetic properties.

Dosage & Packaging

Ephedrine is administered as a bolus of 2.5–10 mg to adults (0.1 mg/kg in children). Subsequent doses are increased to offset the development of tachyphylaxis, which is probably due to depletion of norepinephrine stores. It is available in 1 mL ampules containing 25 or 50 mg.

NOREPINEPHRINE

Clinical Considerations

Direct α_1 stimulation in the absence of β_2 activity induces intense vasoconstriction of arterial and venous vessels. Increased myocardial contractility due to β_1 effects may contribute to a rise in arterial blood pressure, but elevated afterload and reflex bradycardia prevent any elevation in cardiac output. Decreased renal blood flow and increased myocardial oxygen requirements limit the usefulness of norepinephrine to the treatment of refractory shock requiring potent vasoconstriction to maintain tissue perfusion pressure. Norepinephrine has been employed with an alpha-blocker (eg, phentolamine) in an attempt to take advantage of its beta activity without the profound vasoconstriction caused by its alpha stimulation. Extravasation of norepinephrine at the site of intravenous administration can cause tissue necrosis.

Dosage & Packaging

Norepinephrine is administered as a continuous infusion (4 mg of base in 500 mL D_5W; 8 $\mu g/mL$) at a rate of 2–20 $\mu g/min$. Ampules contain 4 mg of norepinephrine base in 4 mL of solution.

DOPAMINE

Clinical Considerations

Dopamine is a nonselective, direct and indirect adrenergic agonist whose clinical effects vary markedly with dose. Small doses ($<$ 2 $\mu g/kg/min$) have minimal adrenergic effects but activate dopaminergic receptors. Stimulation of these non-

adrenergic receptors (specifically, DA_1 receptors) vasodilates the renal vasculature and promotes diuresis. At moderate doses (2–10 $\mu g/kg/min$), β_1 stimulation increases myocardial contractility, heart rate, and cardiac output. Myocardial oxygen demand typically increases more than supply. Alpha$_1$ effects become prominent at higher doses (10–20 $\mu g/kg/min$), causing an increase in peripheral vascular resistance and a fall in renal blood flow. Dopamine's indirect effects are due to release of norepinephrine, which it resembles at doses above 20 $\mu g/kg/min$.

Dopamine is commonly used in the treatment of shock to improve cardiac output, support blood pressure, and maintain renal function. It is often used in combination with a vasodilator (eg, nitroglycerin or nitroprusside), which reduces afterload and further improves cardiac output (Chapter 13). The chronotropic and dysrhythmogenic effects of dopamine limit its usefulness in some patients.

Dosage & Packaging

Dopamine is administered as a continuous infusion (400 mg in 1000 mL D_5W; 400 $\mu g/mL$) at a rate of 1–20 $\mu g/kg/min$. It is most commonly supplied in 5 mL ampules containing 200 or 400 mg.

ISOPROTERENOL

Clinical Considerations

Isoproterenol is a pure beta agonist. Beta$_1$ effects increase heart rate, contractility, and cardiac output. Beta$_2$ stimulation decreases peripheral vascular resistance and diastolic blood pressure. Myocardial oxygen demand increases, while oxygen supply falls, making isoproterenol a poor choice of inotrope in many situations. Isoproterenol may reverse atropine-resistant bradycardia, third-degree heart block, or excessive beta blockade until a pacemaker can be inserted. More β_2-selective agents (eg, terbutaline) have replaced its use as a bronchodilator. Isoproterenol may decrease pulmonary vascular resistance in some patients with pulmonary hypertension and can be quite useful in patients with mitral valve disease.

Dosage & Packaging

An infusion of isoproterenol (1 mg in 500 mL D_5W; 2 $\mu g/mL$) is administered at a rate of 1–20 $\mu g/min$. It is available in 1, 5, and 10 mL ampules containing 0.2 mg/mL.

DOBUTAMINE

Clinical Considerations

Dobutamine is a relatively selective β_1 agonist. Its primary cardiovascular effect is a rise in cardiac output due to increased myocardial contractility. A slight decline in peripheral vascular resistance due to β_2 activation usually prevents much rise in arterial blood pressure. Left ventricular filling pressure decreases, while coronary blood flow increases. Heart rate increases are less marked than with other beta agonists. These favorable effects on myocardial oxygen balance make dobutamine a good choice for patients with the combination of congestive heart failure and coronary artery disease, particularly if peripheral vascular resistance and heart rate are already elevated.

Dosage & Packaging

Dobutamine is administered as an infusion (1 g in 250 mL; 4 mg/mL) at a rate of 2–20 μg/kg/min. It is supplied in 20 mL vials containing 250 mg.

ADRENERGIC ANTAGONISTS

Adrenergic antagonists bind but do not activate adrenoceptors. They act by preventing adrenergic agonist activity. Like the agonists, the antagonists differ in their spectrum of receptor interaction (Table 12–3).

PHENTOLAMINE

Clinical Considerations

Phentolamine produces a competitive (reversible) blockade of alpha receptors. Alpha$_1$ antagonism and direct smooth muscle relaxation are responsible for peripheral vasodilatation and a decline in arterial blood pressure. The drop in blood pressure provokes reflex tachycardia. This tachycardia is augmented by antagonism of α_2 receptors in the heart because α_2 blockade promotes norepinephrine release by eliminating the negative feedback loop. These cardiovascular effects are usually apparent within 2 minutes and last up to 15 minutes. As with all of the adrenergic antagonists, the extent of the response to receptor blockade depends

Table 12–3. Receptor selectivity of adrenergic antagonists.

Drug	α_1	α_2	β_1	β_2
Prazosin	– –	0	0	0
Phenoxybenzamine	– –	–	0	0
Phentolamine	– –	– –	0	0
Labetalol[1]	–	0	– –	– –
Metoprolol	0	0	– – –	–
Esmolol	0	0	– – –	–
Propranolol	0	0	– – –	– – –

[1]Labetalol may also have some β_2 agonist activity.
Key:
 0 = No effect
 – = Antagonist effect (mild, moderate, marked)

upon the degree of existing sympathetic tone. Reflex tachycardia and postural hypotension limit the usefulness of phentolamine to the treatment of hypertension due to excessive alpha stimulation (eg, pheochromocytoma or clonidine withdrawal).

Dosage & Packaging

Phentolamine is administered intravenously as intermittent boluses (1–5 mg in adults) or as a continuous infusion (10 mg in 100 mL D$_5$W; 100 μg/mL). To prevent tissue necrosis following extravasation of intravenous fluids containing an alpha agonist (eg, norepinephrine), 5–10 mg of phentolamine in 10 mL of normal saline can be locally infiltrated. Phentolamine is packaged as a lyophilized powder (5 mg).

LABETALOL

Clinical Considerations

Labetalol blocks α_1, β_1, and β_2 receptors. The ratio of alpha to beta blockade has been estimated to be approximately 1:7 following intravenous administration. This mixed blockade reduces peripheral vascular resistance and arterial blood pressure. Heart rate and cardiac output are usually slightly depressed or unchanged. Thus, labetalol lowers blood pressure without reflex tachycardia because of its combination of alpha and beta effects. Peak effect usually occurs within 5 minutes after an intravenous dose. Left ventricular failure, paradoxic hypertension, and bronchospasm have been reported.

Dosage & Packaging

The initial recommended dose of labetalol is 0.1–0.25 mg/kg administered intravenously over 2 minutes. Twice this amount may be given at 10-minute intervals until the desired blood pressure response is obtained. Labetalol can also be administered as a slow continuous infusion (200 mg in 250 mL D$_5$W) at a rate of 2 mg/min. However, owing to its long elimination half-life (elimination half-life > 5 hours), prolonged infusions are not recommended. Labetalol is available in 20 and 40 mL containers (5 mg/mL).

ESMOLOL

Clinical Considerations

Esmolol is an ultra-short-acting selective β_1 antagonist that reduces heart rate and, to a lesser extent, blood pressure. It has been successfully employed to prevent tachycardia and hypertension in response to perioperative stimuli such as intubation, surgical stimulation, and emergence. Esmolol is as effective as propranolol in controlling the ventricular rate of patients with atrial fibrillation or flutter. Although esmolol is considered to be cardioselective, at higher doses it inhibits β_2 receptors in bronchial and vascular smooth muscle.

Its short duration of action is due to rapid redistribution (distribution half-life = 2 minutes) and hydrolysis by red blood cell esterase (elimination half-life = 9 minutes). Side effects can be reversed within minutes by discontinuing infusion. As with all β_1 antagonists, esmolol should be avoided in patients with sinus bradycardia, heart block greater than first-degree, cardiogenic shock, or overt heart failure.

Dosage & Packaging

Esmolol is administered as a bolus (0.2–0.5 mg/kg) for short-term therapy, such as attenuating the cardiovascular response to laryngoscopy and intubation. Long-term treatment is typically initiated with a loading dose of 0.5 mg/kg administered over 1 minute, followed by a continuous infusion of 50 μg/kg/min to maintain the therapeutic effect. If this fails to produce a sufficient response within 5 minutes, the loading dose may be repeated and the infusion increased by increments of 50 μg/kg/min every 5 minutes to a maximum of 200 μg/kg/min.

Esmolol is supplied as multidose vials for bolus administration containing 10 mL of drug (10 mg/mL). Ampules for continuous infusion (2.5 g in 10 mL) are also available but must be diluted prior to administration to a concentration of 10 mg/mL.

PROPRANOLOL

Clinical Considerations

Propranolol nonselectively blocks β_1 and β_2 receptors. Arterial blood pressure is lowered by several mechanisms, including decreased myocardial contractility, lowered heart rate, and diminished renin release. Cardiac output and myocardial oxygen demand are reduced. Propranolol is particularly useful during myocardial ischemia related to increased blood pressure and heart rate. Impedance of ventricular ejection is beneficial in patients with obstructive cardiomyopathy and aortic aneurysm. Propranolol slows atrioventricular conduction and stabilizes myocardial membranes, though the latter effect may not be significant at clinical doses. Propranolol is particularly effective in slowing the ventricular response to supraventricular tachycardia, and it occasionally controls recurrent ventricular tachycardia or fibrillation due to myocardial ischemia. Propranolol blocks the β-adrenergic effects of thyrotoxicosis and pheochromocytoma.

Side effects include bronchospasm (β_2 antagonism), congestive heart failure, bradycardia, and atrioventricular heart block (β_1 antagonism). Propranolol may worsen the myocardial depression of volatile anesthetics (eg, enflurane) or unmask the negative inotropic characteristics of indirect cardiac stimulants (eg, ketamine). Concomitant administration of propranolol and verapamil (a calcium channel blocker) synergistically depresses heart rate, contractility, and atrioventricular node conduction. Abrupt discontinuation of propranolol therapy for 24–48 hours may trig-

ger a withdrawal syndrome characterized by hypertension, tachycardia, and angina pectoris. This effect appears to be caused by an increase in the number of β-adrenergic receptors ("up-regulation"). Propranolol is extensively protein-bound, and cleared by hepatic metabolism. Its elimination half-life of 100 minutes is quite long compared to that of esmolol.

Dosage & Packaging

Individual dosage requirements of propranolol depend upon baseline sympathetic tone. Generally, propranolol is titrated to desired effect, beginning with 0.5 mg and progressing by 0.5 mg increments every 3–5 minutes. Total doses rarely exceed 0.15 mg/kg. Propranolol is supplied in 1 mL ampules containing 1 mg.

CASE DISCUSSION: PHEOCHROMOCYTOMA

A 45-year-old man with a history of paroxysmal attacks of headache, hypertension, sweating, and palpitations is scheduled for resection of an abdominal pheochromocytoma.

What is a pheochromocytoma?

A pheochromocytoma is a vascular tumor of chromaffin tissue (most commonly the adrenal medulla) that produces and secretes norepinephrine and epinephrine. The diagnosis and management of pheochromocytoma are based upon the effects of abnormally high circulating levels of these endogenous adrenergic agonists.

How is the diagnosis of pheochromocytoma made in the laboratory?

Urinary excretion of vanillylmandelic acid (an end product of catecholamine metabolism), norepinephrine, and epinephrine are often markedly increased. The total plasma concentration of catecholamines may also be elevated. The location of the tumor can be determined by MRI, CT scan, ultrasound, or scintigraphy.

What pathophysiology is associated with chronic elevations of norepinephrine and epinephrine?

Alpha$_1$ stimulation increases peripheral vascular resistance and arterial blood pressure. Hypertension can lead to intravascular volume depletion (increasing hematocrit), renal failure, and cerebral hemorrhage. Elevated peripheral vascular resistance also increases myocardial work, which predisposes patients to myocardial ischemia, ventricular hypertrophy, and congestive heart failure. Prolonged exposure to epinephrine and norepinephrine may lead to a catecholamine-induced cardiomyopathy. Hyperglycemia results from decreased insulin secretion in the face of increased glycogenolysis and gluconeogenesis. $Beta_1$ stimulation increases automaticity and ventricular ectopy.

Which adrenergic antagonists might be helpful in controlling the effects of norepinephrine and epinephrine hypersecretion?

Phenoxybenzamine, an α_1 antagonist, effectively reverses the vasoconstriction, resulting in a drop in arterial blood pressure and an increase in intravascular volume (hematocrit drops). Glucose intolerance is often corrected. Phenoxybenzamine can be administered orally and is longer-acting than phentolamine, another α_1 antagonist. For these reasons, phenoxybenzamine is often administered to control symptoms preoperatively.

Intravenous phentolamine is often used intraoperatively to control hypertensive episodes. However, compared with some other hypotensive agents (Chapter 13), phentolamine has a slow onset and long duration of action. Furthermore, tachyphylaxis often develops.

$Beta_1$ blockade with an agent such as propranolol is recommended for patients with tachycardia or ventricular dysrhythmias.

Why should α_1 receptors be blocked with phenoxybenzamine before administration of a beta antagonist?

If beta receptors are blocked first, norepinephrine and epinephrine will produce unopposed alpha stimulation. $Beta_2$-mediated vasodilation will not be able to offset α_1 vasoconstriction, and peripheral vascular resistance would increase. This may explain the paradoxic hypertension that has been reported in a few patients with pheochromocytoma treated with labetalol. Finally, the myocardium might not be able to handle its already elevated work load without the inotropic effects of β_1 stimulation.

Which anesthetic agents should be specifically avoided?

Succinylcholine-induced fasciculations of the abdominal musculature will increase intra-abdominal pressure, which might cause release of catecholamines from the tumor. Ketamine is a sympathomimetic and would exacerbate the effects of adrenergic agonists. Halothane sensitizes the myocardium to the dysrhythmogenic effects of epinephrine. Vagolytic drugs (eg, anticholinergics, pancuronium, or gallamine) will worsen the imbalance of autonomic tone. Since histamine provokes catecholamine secretion by the tumor, drugs associated with histamine release (eg, tubocurarine, atracurium, morphine sulfate, and meperidine) are best avoided. Vecuronium or pipecuronium are probably the muscle relaxants of choice. Although droperidol is an alpha antagonist, it has been associated with hypertensive crises in some patients with pheochromocytoma. Pheochromocytoma is further considered in Chapter 36.

SUGGESTED READINGS

Fahmy NR: Drugs that affect the autonomic nervous system. Chapter 9 in: *Practical Anesthetic Pharmacology.* Attia RR, Grogono AW, Domer FR (editors). Appleton & Lange, 1987. Overview of adrenergic and cholinergic pharmacology.

Maze M, Tranquilli W: Alpha-2 adrenoceptor agonists: Defining the role in clinical anesthesia. Anesthesiology 1991;74:581. Review of a class of drug that may find a multitude of uses in clinical anesthesia.

Merin RG: New drugs: Beta-adrenergic blockers. Semin Anesth 1988;7:75.

Merin RG: Pharmacology of the autonomic nervous system. Chapter 14, in: *Anesthesia,* 3rd ed. Miller RD (editor). Churchill Livingstone, 1990. Anatomy, physiology, and pharmacology.

Runciman WB: Adrenoceptor agonists. Chapter 9 in: *Drugs in Anaesthesia: Mechanisms of Action.* Feldman SA, Scurr CF, Paton W (editors). Arnold, 1987.

Runciman WB: Adrenoceptor antagonists. Chapter in: *Drugs in Anaesthesia: Mechanisms of Action.* Feldman SA, Scurr CF, Paton W (editors). Arnold, 1987. Two chapters provide a detailed explanation of the mechanisms and effects of adrenergic receptor stimulation and blockade.

Stoelting RK: *Pharmacology and Physiology in Anesthetic Practice.* Lippincott, 1987. Contains several chapters on topics related to adrenergic pharmacology: Chapter 12 (Sympathomimetics); Chapter 14 (Alpha- and Beta-Adrenergic Receptor Antagonists); Chapter 15 (Antihypertensive Drugs); and Chapter 42 (Physiology of the Autonomic Nervous System).

Hypotensive Agents

13

A multitude of drugs are capable of lowering blood pressure, including volatile anesthetics (Chapter 7) and sympathetic antagonists (Chapter 12). This chapter examines four additional agents that are particularly useful to the anesthesiologist for intraoperative control of arterial blood pressure: (1) hydralazine, (2) sodium nitroprusside, (3) nitroglycerin, and (4) trimethaphan (Figure 13–1; Table 13–1). All of these drugs lower blood pressure by dilating peripheral vessels. Nonetheless, they are not identical in their mechanisms of action, clinical uses, routes of metabolism, effects on organ systems, and drug interactions.

HYDRALAZINE

Mechanism of Action

Hydralazine relaxes arteriolar smooth muscle, causing dilatation of precapillary resistance vessels. The mechanism of this effect may be interference with calcium utilization or activation of guanylyl cyclase (see Sodium Nitroprusside).

Clinical Uses

Intraoperative hypertension is usually controlled with an intravenous dose of 5–20 mg. The onset of action is within 15 minutes, and the antihypertensive effect usually lasts 2–4 hours. Continuous infusions (0.25–1.5 $\mu g/kg/min$) are less frequently used owing to the rather slow onset and long duration of action. Hydralazine is frequently used to control the hypertension of eclampsia.

Metabolism

Hydralazine undergoes acetylation and hydroxylation in the liver.

Effects on Organ Systems

A. Cardiovascular: The lowering of peripheral vascular resistance causes a drop in arterial blood pressure. The body reacts to the fall in blood pressure by increasing heart rate, myocardial contractility, and cardiac output. These compensatory responses can be detrimental to patients with coronary artery disease and are minimized by the concurrent administration of a β-adrenergic antagonist. Conversely, the decline in afterload often proves beneficial to patients in congestive heart failure.

B. Cerebral: Hydralazine is a potent cerebral vasodilator and inhibitor of cerebral blood flow autoregulation. Unless blood pressure is markedly reduced, cerebral blood flow and intracranial pressure will rise.

C. Renal: Because renal blood flow is usually maintained or increased by hydralazine, it is often selected for patients with renal disease. Renin secretion by juxtaglomerular cells is stimulated.

Drug Interactions

Hydralazine may induce enflurane defluorination, increasing its potential for nephrotoxicity.

SODIUM NITROPRUSSIDE

Mechanism of Action

Sodium nitroprusside relaxes both arteriolar and venous smooth muscle. Its primary mechanism of action is shared with other organic nitrates (eg, hydralazine and nitroglycerin). These drugs form nitric oxide, which activates guanylyl cyclase. This enzyme is responsible for the synthesis of guanosine 3′,5′-monophosphate (cGMP), which controls the phosphorylation of several proteins, including some involved in smooth muscle contraction.

Clinical Uses

Sodium nitroprusside is a potent and consistent antihypertensive. It is usually diluted to a concentration of 100 $\mu g/mL$ and administered as a continuous intravenous infusion (0.5–10 $\mu g/kg/min$). Its extremely rapid onset of action (1–2 minutes) and its fleeting duration of action allow precise titration of arterial blood pressure. A bolus of 1–2 $\mu g/kg$ minimizes blood pressure elevation during laryngoscopy but can cause transient hypotension in some patients. The potency of this drug requires frequent blood pressure measurements—or, preferably intra-arterial monitoring—and the use of mechanical infusion pumps. Solutions of sodium nitroprusside must be protected from light because of photodegradation.

Metabolism

After parenteral injection, sodium nitroprusside enters red blood cells, where it receives an electron from the iron of oxyhemoglobin (Fe^{2+}). This nonenzymatic

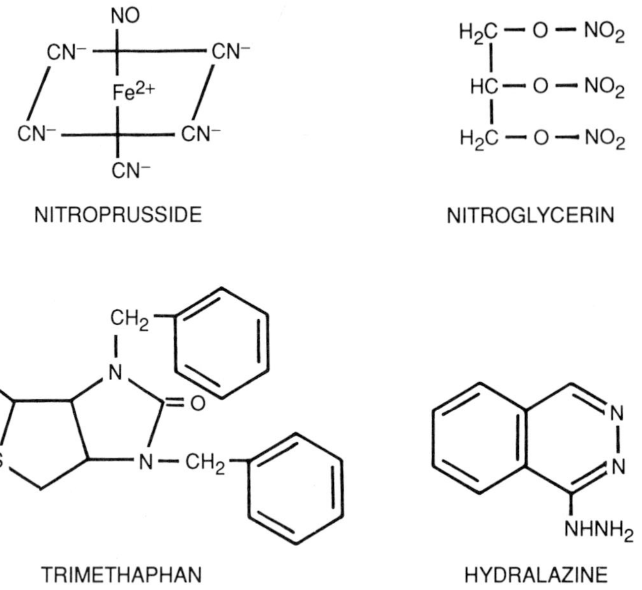

Figure 13–1. Structures of hypotensive agents.

electron transfer results in an unstable nitroprusside radical and methemoglobin (Fe^{3+}). The former moiety spontaneously decomposes into 5 cyanide ions and the active nitroso (N=O) group.

The cyanide ions can be involved in one of three possible reactions: (1) binding to methemoglobin to form cyanmethemoglobin; (2) undergoing a reaction in the liver and kidney catalyzed by the enzyme rhodanase (thiosulfate + cyanide → thiocyanate); or (3) binding to tissue cytochrome oxidase, which interferes with normal oxygen utilization (Figure 13–2).

The last of these reactions is responsible for the development of acute cyanide toxicity, which is characterized by metabolic acidosis, cardiac dysrhythmias, and increased venous oxygen content (due to the inability to metabolize oxygen). Another early sign of cyanide toxicity is the resistance to the hypotensive effects of increasing doses of sodium nitroprusside (tachyphylaxis). Cyanide toxicity can usually be avoided if the cumulative dose of sodium nitroprusside is less than 0.5 mg/kg/h. The treatment of cyanide toxicity depends upon increasing the kinetics of the two reactions by administering sodium thiosulfate (150 mg/kg over 15 minutes) or 3% sodium nitrate (5 mg/kg over 5 minutes), which oxidizes hemoglobin to methemoglobin.

Table 13–1. Comparative pharmacology of hypotensive agents.

	Hydralazine	Nitroprusside	Nitroglycerin	Trimethaphan
Organ effects				
Heart rate	↑↑↑	↑↑	↑	↑
Preload	0	↓↓↓	↓↓↓	↓↓
Afterload	↓↓↓	↓↓↓	↓↓	↓↓
Cerebral blood flow, intracranial pressure	↑↑	↑↑	↑↑	0
Kinetics				
Onset	5–10 min	1 min	1 min	3 min
Duration	2–4 hours	5 min	5 min	10 min
Metabolism	Liver	Blood, kidney	Blood, liver	?Blood
Dose				
Bolus	5–20 mg	50–100 μg	50–100 μg	NA
Infusion (μg/kg/min)	0.25–1.5	0.5–10	0.5–10	10–100

Key:
0 = No change
↑ = Increase (slight, moderate, marked)
↓ = Decrease (slight, moderate, marked)
NA = Not applicable

SNP + Oxyhemoglobin $\longrightarrow$ (SNP)$^-$ + Methemoglobin
(SNP)$^-$ $\longrightarrow$ 5CN$^-$

CN$^-$ + Methemoglobin $\longrightarrow$ Cyanmethemoglobin

or

$$CN^- + Thiosulfate \xrightarrow{\text{Rhodanase, vitamin B}_{12}} Thiocyanate$$

or

CN$^-$ + Cytochrome oxidase $\longrightarrow$ Cyanide toxicity

Figure 13–2. The metabolism of sodium nitroprusside.

Thiocyanate is slowly cleared by the kidney. Accumulation of large amounts of thiocyanate (eg, patients with renal failure) may result in a milder toxic reaction that includes thyroid dysfunction, muscle weakness, nausea, hypoxia, and an acute toxic psychosis. In contrast, the risk of cyanide toxicity is not increased by renal failure. Methemoglobinemia due to excessive doses of sodium nitroprusside or sodium nitrate can be treated with methylene blue (1–2 mg/kg of a 1% solution over 5 minutes), which reduces methemoglobin to hemoglobin.

Effects on Organ Systems

A. Cardiovascular: The combined dilatation of venous and arteriolar vascular beds by sodium nitroprusside results in reductions of preload and afterload. Arterial blood pressure falls owing to the decrease in peripheral vascular resistance. Although cardiac output is usually unchanged in normal patients, the reduction in afterload may increase cardiac output in patients with congestive heart failure, mitral regurgitation, or aortic regurgitation. In contrast to pure afterload reduction by hydralazine, sodium nitroprusside reduces preload, which decreases myocardial work and the likelihood of ischemia. In opposition to any favorable changes in myocardial oxygen requirements are reflex-mediated responses to the fall in arterial blood pressure. These include tachycardia (less than with hydralazine) and increased myocardial contractility. Additionally, dilatation of coronary arterioles by sodium nitroprusside may result in an intracoronary steal of blood flow away from ischemic areas that are already maximally dilated.

B. Cerebral: Sodium nitroprusside dilates cerebral vessels. Cerebral blood flow will increase unless arterial blood pressure is markedly reduced. The resulting increase in cerebral blood volume tends to increase intracranial pressure, especially in patients with reduced intracranial compliance (eg, brain tumors). This intracranial hypertension can be minimized by slow administration of sodium nitroprusside and institution of hypocapnia.

C. Respiratory: The pulmonary vasculature also dilates in response to sodium nitroprusside infusion. Reductions in pulmonary artery pressure may decrease the perfusion of some normally ventilated alveoli, in-creasing physiologic dead space. By dilating pulmonary vessels, sodium nitroprusside may prevent the normal vasoconstrictive response of the pulmonary vasculature to hypoxia (hypoxic pulmonary vasoconstriction). Both of these effects tend to mismatch pulmonary ventilation to perfusion and decrease arterial oxygenation.

D. Renal: In response to decreased arterial blood pressure, renin and catecholamines are released during nitroprusside administration. This hormonal response, which can lead to a pressure rebound after discontinuation of the drug, is blocked by propranolol. Renal function is fairly well maintained during sodium nitroprusside infusion despite moderate drops in arterial blood pressure and renal perfusion.

Drug Interactions

Sodium nitroprusside does not directly interact with muscle relaxants. Nonetheless, a decrease in muscle blood flow due to arterial hypotension could indirectly delay the onset and prolong the duration of neuromuscular blockade. By inhibiting phosphodiesterase, aminophylline increases cGMP and potentiates the hypotensive effects of these agents.

NITROGLYCERIN

Mechanism of Action

Nitroglycerin relaxes vascular smooth muscle, with venous dilatation predominating over arterial dilatation. Its mechanism of action is presumably similar to sodium nitroprusside.

Clinical Uses

Nitroglycerin relieves myocardial ischemia, hypertension, and ventricular failure. Like sodium nitroprusside, nitroglycerin is commonly diluted to a concentration of 100 µg/kg and administered as a continuous intravenous infusion (0.5–10 µg/kg/min). Glass containers and special intravenous tubing are recommended because of the adsorption of nitroglycerin to polyvinylchloride. Nitroglycerin can also be administered by a sublingual (peak effect in 4 minutes) or transdermal (sustained release for 24 hours) route.

Metabolism

Nitroglycerin undergoes rapid reductive hydrolysis in the liver and blood by glutathione-organic nitrate reductase. One metabolic product is nitrite, which can covert hemoglobin (Fe^{2+}) to methemoglobin (Fe^{3+}). Significant methemoglobinemia is rare and can be treated with intravenous methylene blue (1–2 mg/kg over 5 minutes).

Effects on Organ Systems

A. Cardiovascular: Nitroglycerin reduces myocardial oxygen demand and increases myocardial oxygen supply by several mechanisms:

(1) The pooling of blood in the large capacitance vessels reduces venous return and preload. The accompanying decrease in ventricular end-diastolic pressure reduces myocardial oxygen demand and increases endocardial perfusion.

(2) Any afterload reduction due to arteriolar dilatation will decrease end-systolic pressure, also decreasing oxygen demand. Of course, a fall in diastolic pressure may lower coronary perfusion pressure and actually decrease myocardial oxygen supply.

(3) Nitroglycerin redistributes coronary blood flow to ischemic areas of the subendocardium.

(4) Coronary artery spasm may be relieved.

The beneficial effect of nitroglycerin in patients with coronary artery disease contrasts with the coronary steal phenomenon seen with sodium nitroprusside.

A drop in preload decreases cardiac output in the absence of congestive heart failure. Preload reduction makes nitroglycerin an excellent drug for the relief of cardiogenic pulmonary edema. Heart rate is unchanged or minimally increased. Rebound hypertension is less likely than following discontinuation of sodium nitroprusside.

B. Cerebral: The effects of nitroglycerin on cerebral blood flow and intracranial pressure are similar to those of sodium nitroprusside. Headache from dilatation of cerebral vessels is a common side effect of nitroglycerin.

C. Respiratory: In addition to the dilating effects on the pulmonary vasculature previously described for sodium nitroprusside, nitroglycerin relaxes bronchial smooth muscle.

Drug Interactions

Nitroglycerin has been reported to potentiate the neuromuscular blockade produced by pancuronium.

TRIMETHAPHAN

Mechanism of Action

Trimethaphan produces peripheral vasodilatation by direct smooth muscle relaxation and by blockade of acetylcholine receptors in autonomic ganglia. Two other groups of cholinergic antagonists have been described in previous chapters: the antinicotinic nondepolarizing neuromuscular blocking agents (Chapter 9) and the antimuscarinic drugs (Chapter 11). Like the nondepolarizing agents, trimethaphan competitively blocks nicotinic receptors. However, these nicotinic receptors are located in autonomic ganglia instead of skeletal muscle. Because both sympathetic and parasympathetic ganglia are cholinergic, trimethaphan results in a mixed autonomic blockade.

Clinical Uses

Trimethaphan is used to control arterial blood pressure and to manage autonomic hyperreflexia (a syndrome of massive sympathetic discharge seen in patients with upper spinal cord injuries). A continuous intravenous infusion of 0.1% trimethaphan (1 mg/mL) is titrated to the desired blood pressure response (usually 10–100 μg/kg/min). Trimethaphan acts rapidly, but its duration of action is longer than that of sodium nitroprusside. Tachyphylaxis is common after prolonged administration.

Metabolism

Trimethaphan does not depend upon the kidney or liver for its termination of action. Because trimethaphan interferes with plasma cholinesterase activity, it has been postulated that this enzyme may play a role in its metabolism.

Effects on Organ Systems

A. Cardiovascular: Trimethaphan decreases arterial blood pressure by arteriolar and venous dilatation. The latter decreases venous return to the heart and lowers cardiac output. This characteristic is valuable when increases in cardiac output are best avoided (eg, dissecting aortic aneurysm repair). Heart rate often increases, not from sympathetic reflexes but because of parasympathetic ganglionic blockade. Patients are particularly susceptible to postural hypotension (eg, reverse Trendelenburg). In the event of sudden hypotension due to acute blood loss, trimethaphan's sympathetic ganglion blocking action will prevent restoration of cardiac output by abolishing the arterial baroreflex response. This may provide a lower margin of safety than nitroprusside or nitroglycerin in some clinical situations.

B. Cerebral: Trimethaphan is a highly ionized quaternary ammonium and does not easily pass the blood-brain barrier. Unlike the other peripheral vasodilators discussed in this chapter, trimethaphan is not associated with cerebral vasodilatation. Nonetheless, cerebral blood flow is usually adequately maintained at mean arterial pressures above 60 mm Hg. Pupillary dilatation accompanying ganglionic blockade can interfere with the interpretation of neurologic examinations.

C. Renal and Gastrointestinal: Trimethaphan's parasympathetic effects can result in urinary retention and paralytic ileus following prolonged infusions.

D. Endocrine: In contrast to sodium nitroprusside, trimethaphan-induced hypotension does not activate catecholamine and renin release. However, trimethaphan can cause histamine release.

Drug Interactions

Trimethaphan inhibits plasma cholinesterase and can double the duration of action of succinylcholine. Since both autonomic ganglia and skeletal neuromuscular junctions contain nicotinic cholinergic receptors, it is not surprising that trimethaphan also potentiates nondepolarizing muscle blockade.

CASE DISCUSSION: CONTROLLED HYPOTENSION

A 59-year-old man is scheduled for total hip arthro-plasty under general anesthesia. The surgeon requests a controlled hypotensive technique.

What is controlled hypotension, and what are its advantages?

Controlled hypotension is the elective lowering of arterial blood pressure. The primary advantages of this technique are minimization of surgical blood loss and better wound visualization.

How is controlled hypotension achieved?

The primary methods of electively lowering blood pressure are proper positioning, positive-pressure ventilation, and administration of hypotensive drugs. Positioning involves elevation of the surgical site so that the blood pressure at the wound is selectively reduced. The increase in intrathoracic pressure that accompanies positive-pressure ventilation lowers venous return, cardiac output, and mean arterial pressure. Numerous pharmacologic agents effectively lower blood pressure: volatile anesthetics, sympathetic antagonists, calcium channel blockers, and the peripheral vasodilators discussed in this chapter. Owing to their rapid onset and short duration of action, sodium nitroprusside, nitroglycerin, and trimethaphan have the advantage of precise control. An additional method of producing hypotension is creation of a high sympathetic block with an epidural or spinal anesthetic.

What surgical procedures might benefit most from a controlled hypotensive technique?

Controlled hypotension has been successfully used during cerebral aneurysm repair, brain tumor resection, total hip arthroplasty, radical neck dissection, radical cystectomy, and other operations associated with significant blood loss. Controlled hypotension may allow safer surgery of patients whose religious beliefs prohibit blood transfusions (eg, Jehovah's Witnesses). Decreasing extravasation of blood may improve the result of some plastic surgery procedures.

What are some relative contraindications to controlled hypotension?

Some patients have predisposing illnesses that lessen the margin of safety for adequate organ perfusion: severe anemia, hypovolemia, atherosclerotic vascular disease, renal or hepatic insufficiency, cerebrovascular disease, and uncontrolled glaucoma.

What are the possible complications of controlled hypotension?

As the above list of contraindications suggests, the risks of low arterial blood pressure include cerebral thrombosis, hemiplegia, acute tubular necrosis, massive hepatic necrosis, myocardial infarction, cardiac arrest, and blindness from retinal artery thrombosis.

What is a safe level of hypotension?

This depends on the patient. Healthy young individuals tolerate mean arterial pressures as low as 50–60 mm Hg without complications. On the other hand, chronically hypertensive patients have altered autoregulation of cerebral blood flow and may tolerate a mean arterial pressure no more than 25% lower than baseline. Patients with a history of transient ischemic attacks may not tolerate any decline in cerebral perfusion.

What special monitoring is indicated during controlled hypotension?

Intra-arterial blood pressure monitoring is strongly recommended. Central venous monitoring and measurement of urinary output by an indwelling catheter are indicated if extensive surgery is anticipated. Monitors of neurologic function (eg, electroencephalography) have not gained widespread acceptance.

SUGGESTED READINGS

Bennett DR (editor-in-chief): *AMA Drug Evaluations Annual*. American Medical Association, 1991. An excellent reference source with unbiased information on clinical pharmacology.

Gerber JG, Nies AS: Antihypertensive agents and the drug therapy of hypertension. Chapter 33 in: *Goodman and Gilman's The Pharmaceutical Basis of Therapeutics*. 8th ed. Gilman AG et al (editors). Pergamon, 1990.

Lake CL: *Cardiovascular Anesthesia*. Springer-Verlag, 1985. The chapter entitled "Pharmacology of Cardiac Drugs" describes the utility of hypotensive agents during cardiothoracic surgery.

Miller ED: Deliberate hypotension. Chapter 43, in: *Anesthesia*, 3rd ed. Miller RD (editor). Churchill Livingstone, 1990.

Stoelting RK: *Pharmacology and Physiology in Anesthetic Practice*. Lippincott, 1987. Relevant chapters include discussions of other, less frequently used hypotensive agents.

14

Local Anesthetics

Regional anesthetic techniques depend on a group of drugs—local anesthetics—that produce transient loss of sensory, motor, and autonomic function in a discrete portion of the body. This chapter presents the mechanism of action, structure-activity relationships, and clinical pharmacology of local anesthetic drugs. Commonly used nerve blocks are presented in Section III (Chapters 16 and 17).

THEORIES OF LOCAL ANESTHETIC ACTION

Nerve cells maintain a **resting membrane potential** by active transport and passive diffusion of ions. The sodium-potassium pump transports sodium out of the cell and potassium into the cell. This creates a concentration gradient that favors the extracellular diffusion of potassium and the intracellular diffusion of sodium. However, the cell membrane is much more permeable to potassium than to sodium, so a relative excess of negatively charged ions (anions) accumulates intracellularly. This accounts for the negative resting potential difference (-70 mV polarization).

After chemical, mechanical, or electrical excitation, an impulse is conducted along a nerve axon. The impulse propagation is usually accompanied by depolarization of the nerve membrane. If the depolarization exceeds the **threshold level** (a membrane potential of -55 mV), sodium channels in the membrane are activated, allowing a sudden and spontaneous influx of sodium ions. This increase in sodium permeability causes a relative excess of positively charged ions (cations) intracellularly, resulting in a membrane potential of $+35$ mV. A consequent drop in sodium permeability (due to inactivation of the sodium channels) and an increase in potassium conductance (allowing more potassium to exit the cell) return the membrane to its resting potential. Baseline concentration gradients are eventually reestablished by the sodium-potassium pump. These changes in axon membrane potential are collectively called the **action potential.**

Most local anesthetics bind to sodium channels in the inactivated state, preventing subsequent channel activation and the large transient sodium influx associated with membrane depolarization. This does not alter the resting membrane potential or the threshold

level, but it slows the rate of depolarization. The action potential is not propagated, because the threshold level is never attained. Specific receptors in the interior of the sodium channels are probably the specific site of local anesthetic action.

Some local anesthetics may penetrate the membrane, causing membrane expansion and channel distortion analogous to the critical volume hypothesis of general anesthetics (Chapter 7). Alternatively, the surface charge theory postulates that partial penetration by local anesthetics of the axonal membrane could increase the transmembrane potential and inhibit depolarization.

STRUCTURE-ACTIVITY RELATIONSHIPS

Local anesthetics consist of a **lipophilic group**—usually a benzene ring—separated from a **hydrophilic group**—usually a tertiary amine—by an intermediate chain which includes an **ester or amide linkage.** Local anesthetics are weak bases that usually carry a positive charge at the tertiary amine group at physiologic pH. The nature of the intermediate chain is the basis of the classification of local anesthetics as esters or amides (Table 14–1). Physicochemical properties of local anesthetics depend upon the substitutions in the aromatic ring, the type of linkage in the intermediate chain, and the alkyl groups attached to the amine nitrogen.

Potency correlates with lipid solubility. Stated another way, potency depends upon the ability of the local anesthetic to penetrate a hydrophobic environment. In general, potency and hydrophobicity increase with an increase in the total number of carbon atoms in the molecule. More specifically, potency is increased by adding a halide to the aromatic ring (2-chloroprocaine versus procaine), an ester linkage (procaine versus procainamide), and large alkyl groups on the tertiary amine nitrogen (etidocaine versus lidocaine). **Cm** is the minimum concentration of local anesthetic that will block nerve impulse conduction and is analogous to the minimum alveolar concentration (MAC) of inhalational anesthetics. This measure of relative potency is affected by several factors, including (1) fiber size, type, and myelination; (2) pH (acidic pH antagonizes block); (3) frequency of nerve stimulation (access of local anesthetic to the sodium receptor is enhanced by repeatedly opening the sodium channel); and (4) electrolyte concentrations (hypokalemia and hypercalcemia antagonize blockade).

Onset of action depends upon many factors, including the relative concentration of the nonionized lipid-soluble form (B) and the ionized water-soluble form (BH$^+$). The pH at which the amount of ionized and nonionized drug is equal is the **pK$_a$** of the drug. For instance, the pK$_a$ of lidocaine is 7.8. When lidocaine is exposed to a higher hydrogen ion concentration (eg, a pH of 7.4), more than half of it will exist as the charged cation form (BH$^+$).

Although both forms of local anesthetic are involved in blockade, only the lipid-soluble form diffuses across the neural sheath (epineurium) and nerve membrane. Local anesthetics with a pK$_a$ closer to physiologic pH will have a higher concentration of nonionized base that can pass through the nerve cell membrane, and onset will be more rapid. Once inside the cell, the nonionized base will reach an equilibrium with its ionized form. Only the charged cation actually binds to the receptor within the sodium channel. However, not all local anesthetics exist in a charged form (eg, benzocaine). These anesthetics probably act by one of the alternative mechanisms (eg, expanding the lipid membrane).

The importance of the ionized and nonionized forms has many clinical implications. Local anesthetic solutions are prepared commercially as the water-soluble hydrochloride salt (pH 6–7). Epinephrine is unstable in alkaline environments, so local anesthetic solutions containing it are made even more acidic (pH 4–5). Because of the lower concentration of free base, these commercial preparations have a slower onset than if epinephrine is added at the time of use. Similarly, the extracellular base:cation ratio is decreased and onset is delayed when local anesthetics are injected into acidic (eg, infected) tissues. Tachyphylaxis—the decreased efficacy of repeated doses—is explained by the eventual consumption of local extracellular buffering capacity by the acidic local anesthetic solution. Conversely, if carbonated solutions of local anesthetic are used rather than the hydrochloride salts, onset of action may be shortened. This appears to be due to improved intracellular distribution of the ionized form. Likewise, the addition of a small amount of sodium bicarbonate to a local anesthetic solution may speed onset and improve the quality of blockade.

Onset of action of local anesthetics in *isolated* nerve fiber preparations directly correlates with pK$_a$. However, *clinical* onset of action is not necessarily identical for local anesthetics with the same pK$_a$. Other factors, such as ease of diffusion through connective tissue, can affect the onset of action in vivo.

Duration of action is associated with plasma protein binding (α_1 acid glycoprotein), presumably because the local anesthetic receptor is also a protein. The pharmacokinetic factors that determine absorption also affect duration of action.

CLINICAL PHARMACOLOGY

Pharmacokinetics

A. Absorption: Absorption of local anesthetics depends upon blood flow, which is determined by the following factors.

1. Site of injection–The rate of systemic absorption is proportionate to the vascularity of the site of injection: intravenous > tracheal > intercostal > caudal > paracervical > epidural > brachial plexus > sciatic > subcutaneous.

2. Presence of vasoconstrictors–The addition of epinephrine—or, less commonly, phenylephrine or norepinephrine—causes vasoconstriction at the site of administration. The consequent decreased absorption enhances neuronal uptake, prolongs duration of action, and limits toxic side effects. The effects of vasoconstrictors are more pronounced with shorter-acting agents. For example, the addition of epinephrine to lidocaine usually extends the duration of anesthesia by at least 50%, but epinephrine has no significant effect when added to bupivacaine, whose long duration of action is due to a high degree of protein binding.

3. Local anesthetic agent–Local anesthetics that are highly tissue-bound are more slowly absorbed (eg, etidocaine). The agents also vary in their intrinsic vasodilator properties.

B. Distribution: Distribution depends upon organ uptake, which is determined by the following factors.

1. Tissue perfusion–The highly perfused organs (brain, lung, liver, kidney, and heart) are responsible for initial rapid uptake (alpha phase), which is followed by a slower redistribution (beta phase) to moderately perfused tissues (muscle and gut). In particular, the lung extracts significant amounts of local anesthetic.

2. Tissue:blood partition coefficient–Strong plasma protein binding tends to retain anesthetic in the blood, while high lipid solubility facilitates tissue uptake.

3. Tissue mass–Muscle provides the greatest reservoir for local anesthetic agents due to its large mass.

C. Metabolism and Excretion: The metabolism and excretion of local anesthetics differ depending upon their structure.

1. Esters–Ester local anesthetics are predominantly metabolized by pseudocholinesterase (plasma cholinesterase). Ester hydrolysis is very rapid. The water-soluble metabolites are excreted in the urine. One metabolite, *p*-aminobenzoic acid, has been associated with allergic reactions. Patients with genetically abnormal pseudocholinesterase are at increased risk for toxic side effects, since metabolism is slower. Cerebral spinal fluid lacks esterase enzymes, so the termination of action of intrathecally injected ester local anesthetics depends upon their absorption into the bloodstream. In contrast to other ester anesthetics, co-

Table 14–1. Physicochemical properties of local anesthetics.

Generic (Proprietary)	Structure Ring-Chain-Amine	Potency and Lipid Solubility	pK_a	Duration and Protein Binding	Uses	Maximum Dose (mg/kg)
Amides						
Bupivacaine (Marcaine)	(structure: 2,6-dimethylphenyl–NHCO–piperidine, C_4H_9)	++++	8.1	++++	Epidural, caudal Spinal Infiltration Peripheral nerve block	3
Dibucaine (Nupercaine)	(structure: quinoline OC_4H_9, –CONHCH$_2$–N(C_2H_5)(C_2H_5))	++++	8.8	++++	Spinal Topical	1
Etidocaine (Duranest)	(structure: 2,6-dimethylphenyl–NHCOCH(C_2H_5)–N(C_2H_5)(C_3H_7))	++++	7.7	++++	Epidural, caudal Infiltration Peripheral nerve block	4
Lidocaine (Xylocaine)	(structure: 2,6-dimethylphenyl–NHCOCH$_2$–N(C_2H_5)(C_2H_5))	++	7.8	++	Epidural, caudal Spinal Infiltration Peripheral nerve block Topical	4.5[1] 7[2]
Mepivacaine (Carbocaine)	(structure: 2,6-dimethylphenyl–NHCO–piperidine, CH_3)	++	7.6	++	Epiural, caudal Infiltration Peripheral nerve block	4.5[1] 7[2]

Drug	Structure					
Prilocaine (Citanest)		++	7.8	++	Epidural, caudal Infiltration Peripheral nerve block	8
Esters Chloroprocaine (Nesacaine)[3]		+	9.0	+	Epidural, caudal Infiltration Peripheral nerve block	12
Cocaine		++	8.7	++	Topical	3
Procaine (Novacaine)		+	8.9	+	Spinal Infiltration Peripheral nerve block	12
Tetracaine (Pontocaine)		++++	8.2	+++	Spinal Topical	3

[1]Maximum dose without epinephrine.
[2]Maximum dose with epinephrine.
[3]Chloroprocaine is metabolized too rapidly to measure lipid solubility or protein binding. It has a rapid onset of action despite a high pK_a.

caine is partially metabolized in the liver and partially excreted unchanged in the urine.

2. Amides—Amide local anesthetics are metabolized by microsomal enzymes in the liver. The rate of metabolism depends on the specific agent (prilocaine > lidocaine > bupivacaine) but is much slower than ester hydrolysis. Decreases in hepatic function (eg, cirrhosis of the liver) or liver blood flow (eg, congestive heart failure) will reduce the metabolic rate and predispose patients to systemic toxicity. Very little drug is excreted unchanged by the kidneys, though metabolites are dependent upon renal clearance.

Metabolites of prilocaine (o-toluidine derivatives), which accumulate after large doses of drug (> 10 mg/kg), convert hemoglobin to methemoglobin. Neonates of mothers who have received prilocaine epidural anesthesia during labor and patients with limited cardiopulmonary reserve are particularly susceptible to the alteration in oxygen transport. Benzocaine, a common ingredient in local anesthetic sprays, also can cause methemoglobinemia. Treatment of significant methemoglobinemia includes intravenous administration of methylene blue (1–2 mg/kg of 1% solution over 5 minutes). Methylene blue reduces methemoglobin (Fe^{3+}) to hemoglobin (Fe^{2+}).

Effects on Organ Systems

Since blockade of sodium channels affects action potential propagation throughout the body, it is not surprising that local anesthetics have the capability for systemic toxicity. While organ system effects are discussed for these drugs as a group, it must be recognized that individual drugs differ in their pharmacology.

Toxicity is often directly proportionate to potency. Maximal safe dosages are listed in Table 14–1. Mixtures of local anesthetics should be considered to have roughly additive toxic effects: A solution containing 50% of the toxic dose of lidocaine with 50% of the toxic dose of bupivacaine will have 100% of the toxic effects of either drug.

A. Cardiovascular: In general, local anesthetics depress myocardial automaticity (spontaneous phase 4 depolarization) and reduce the duration of the refractory period. Myocardial contractility and conduction velocity are depressed at higher concentrations. These effects result from direct cardiac muscle membrane changes (ie, cardiac sodium channel blockade) and inhibition of the autonomic nervous system. Smooth muscle relaxation causes some degree of arteriolar dilatation. The ensuing combination of bradycardia, heart block, and hypotension may culminate in cardiac arrest. *Cardiac dysrhythmia or circulatory collapse is often the presenting sign of local anesthetic overdose during general anesthesia.*

Lower concentrations of lidocaine provide effective treatment for some types of ventricular dysrhythmias. Myocardial contractility and arterial blood pressure are generally unaffected by usual intravenous doses (1.5 mg/kg). The hypertension associated with laryngoscopy and intubation is attenuated in some patients by intravenous administration of lidocaine (1.5 mg/kg) 1–3 minutes prior to instrumentation.

Unintentional intravascular injection of bupivacaine during regional anesthesia has produced severe cardiotoxic reactions, including hypotension, atrioventricular heart block, and dysrhythmias, including ventricular fibrillation. Pregnancy, hypoxemia, and respiratory acidosis are predisposing risk factors. Electrophysiologic studies have demonstrated that bupivacaine is associated with more pronounced depolarization changes than lidocaine. Furthermore, bupivacaine's high degree of protein binding makes resuscitation prolonged and difficult.

Cocaine's cardiovascular reactions are unlike any other local anesthetic. Adrenergic nerve terminals normally reabsorb norepinephrine after its release. Cocaine inhibits this reuptake, thereby potentiating the effects of adrenergic stimulation. Cardiovascular responses to cocaine include hypertension and ventricular ectopy. The latter contraindicates its use in patients anesthetized with halothane. Cocaine is the only clinically available local anesthetic to produce vasoconstriction when applied topically.

B. Respiratory: Lidocaine depresses hypoxic drive (the ventilatory response to low PaO_2). Apnea can result from phrenic and intercostal nerve paralysis or depression of the medullary respiratory center following direct exposure to local anesthetic agents (eg, postretrobulbar apnea syndrome). Local anesthetics relax bronchial smooth muscle. Intravenous lidocaine (1.5 mg/kg) may be effective in blocking the reflex bronchoconstriction sometimes associated with intubation.

C. Cerebral: The central nervous system is especially vulnerable to local anesthetic toxicity and is the site of premonitory signs of overdose in awake patients. Early symptoms are circumoral numbness, tongue paresthesia, and dizziness. Sensory complaints may include tinnitus and blurred vision. Excitatory signs (eg, restlessness, agitation, nervousness, paranoia) often precede central nervous system depression (eg, slurred speech, drowsiness, unconsciousness). Muscle twitching heralds the onset of tonic-clonic seizures. Respiratory arrest often follows. The excitatory reactions are a result of selective blockade of inhibitory pathways. By decreasing cerebral blood flow and drug exposure, benzodiazepines and hyperventilation raise the threshold of local anesthetic-induced seizures. Thiopental (1–2 mg/kg) quickly and reliably terminates seizure activity. Adequate ventilation and oxygenation must be maintained.

Intravenous lidocaine (1.5 mg/kg) decreases cerebral blood flow and attenuates the rise in intracranial pressure that accompanies intubation in patients with decreased intracranial compliance. Infusions of lidocaine and procaine have been used to supplement general anesthetic techniques, since they are capable of reducing the minimum alveolar concentration of volatile anesthetics by up to 40%.

Cocaine stimulates the central nervous system and

usually causes a sense of euphoria. Overdosage is heralded by restlessness, emesis, tremors, convulsions, and respiratory failure.

Local anesthetics only temporally block neuronal function. Nonetheless, large volumes of chloroprocaine unintentionally injected into the subarachnoid instead of the epidural space have caused prolonged neurologic deficit. The cause of this local tissue toxicity may be the low pH of the combination of chloroprocaine and its preservative, sodium bisulfite. Chloroprocaine administered epidurally has been associated with back pain.

D. Immunologic: True hypersensitivity reactions to local anesthetic agents—as distinct from systemic toxicity due to excessive plasma concentration—are quite uncommon. Esters are more likely to induce an allergic reaction because they are derivatives of *p*-aminobenzoic acid, a known allergen. Commercial multidose preparations of amides often contain methylparaben, which has a chemical structure similar to that of *p*-aminobenzoic acid. This preservative may be responsible for the rare allergic responses to amide agents. The signs and treatment of allergic drug reactions are discussed in Chapter 45.

Drug Interactions

Nondepolarizing muscle relaxant blockade is potentiated by local anesthetics.

Succinylcholine and ester-type local anesthetics depend on pseudocholinesterase for metabolism. Concurrent administration may potentiate the effects of both drugs.

Dibucaine, an amide local anesthetic, inhibits pseudocholinesterase and is used to detect genetically abnormal enzyme (Chapter 9).

Pseudocholinesterase inhibitors can lead to decreased metabolism of ester-type local anesthetics (Table 9–3).

Cimetidine and propranolol decrease hepatic blood flow and lidocaine clearance. Higher lidocaine blood levels increase the potential for systemic toxicity.

Opioids (eg, fentanyl, morphine) and α_2-adrenergic agonists (eg, epinephrine, clonidine) potentiate local anesthetic pain relief.

CASE DISCUSSION: LOCAL ANESTHETIC OVERDOSE

An 18-year-old woman in the active stage of labor requests an epidural anesthetic for delivery. Immediately following the epidural injection of 12 mL of 2% lidocaine, the patient complains of lip numbness and becomes very apprehensive.

What is your presumptive diagnosis?

The temporal relationship of the numbness and apprehension to the administration of local anesthetic suggests an unintentional intravascular injection. These prodromal signs do not always precede a seizure.

What prophylactic measures should be immediately taken?

Because hypocapnia increases the seizure threshold of local anesthetics, the patient should be instructed to hyperventilate. Simultaneously, a very small dose of thiopental sodium (50 mg) could be intravenously administered. Unconsciousness should be strictly avoided, because pregnant patients are considered to have a "full stomach." The patient should already be receiving supplemental oxygen.

If symptoms progress to a generalized convulsion, what treatment should be initiated?

The laboring patient is always considered to be at risk for aspiration (Chapter 41). Therefore, protecting the airway is of utmost importance. Immediate administration of succinylcholine should be followed by a rapid-sequence intubation (see Chapter 15 Case Discussion). While the succinylcholine will eliminate tonic-clonic activity, it will not address the underlying cerebral excitability. An anticonvulsant such as diazepam (2.5–10 mg) or thiopental sodium (another 50–75 mg) should be administered. *It is clear from this sequence of events that whenever large doses of local anesthetic are administered, the same drugs and equipment must be available as for a general anesthetic.*

What could have been expected if a large dose of bupivacaine had been given intravascularly instead of lidocaine?

Bupivacaine is more cardiotoxic than lidocaine, especially in the presence of acute respiratory acidosis. Ventricular dysrhythmias and conduction disturbances may lead to cardiac arrest and death. Bupivacaine is considered a more potent cardiac sodium channel blocker because the channels recover more slowly than after lidocaine blockade. Bretylium should be considered as the preferred alternative to lidocaine in the treatment of local anesthetic-induced ventricular tachyarrhythmias. Isoproterenol may effectively reverse some of the electrophysiologic abnormalities characteristic of bupivacaine toxicity. Although total dose rather than concentration determines toxicity, the Food and Drug Administration no longer recommends 0.75% bupivacaine for anesthesia during labor. The reason for the higher incidence of cardiotoxicity during pregnancy is unclear.

What could have prevented the toxic reaction described?

The risk of intravascular injection of toxic doses of local anesthetic during epidural anesthesia is mini-mized by using an adequate test dose (Chapter 16), fractionation of the therapeutic dose into safe aliquots, and administering the minimum total dose of local anesthetic possible.

SUGGESTED READINGS

Adams HJ, Ronfeld RA, Takman BH: Local anesthetic agents. In: *CRC Handbook of CNS Agents and Local Anesthetics.* Verderame M (editor). CRC Press, 1986. Stresses the basic chemical pharmacology of anesthetic agents.

Butterworth JF, Strichartz GR: Molecular mechanisms of local anesthetics: A review. Anesthesiology 1990;72:711. Recent advances in electrophysiologic techniques have contributed to understanding of local anesthetic action.

Covino BG, Scott DB: Pharmacological considerations. Chapter 3 in: *Handbook of Epidural Anaesthesia and Analgesia.* Grune & Stratton, 1985.

Covino BG: Local anesthetic agents. Chapter 4 in: *Practical Anesthetic Pharmacology,* 2nd ed. Attia RR, Grogono AW, Domer FR (editors). Appleton & Lange, 1987.

Ritchie JM, Greene NM: Local anesthetics. Chapter 15 in: *Goodman and Gilman's The Pharmacological Basis of Therapeutics,* 8th ed. Gilman AG et al (editors). Pergamon, 1990.

Scott DB, Cousins MJ: Clinical pharmacology of local anesthetic drugs. In: *Neural Blockade in Clinical Anesthesia and Management of Pain.* Cousins MJ, Bridenbaugh D (editors). Lippincott, 1980.

Adjuncts to Anesthesia

15

This final pharmacology chapter describes several drugs of particular interest to the anesthesiologist. Because the first three (diphenhydramine, cimetidine, and ranitidine) are histamine receptor antagonists, the physiology of histamine is briefly reviewed. Diphenhydramine represents the classic antihistaminic drug. Cimetidine and ranitidine are helpful in the preoperative preparation of patients at risk for aspiration pneumonitis. Two other drugs commonly utilized to prevent aspiration (metoclopramide and antacids) are introduced. The chapter concludes with a discussion of a respiratory stimulant (doxapram) and an opiate antagonist (naloxone).

HISTAMINE RECEPTOR ANTAGONISTS

Histamine Physiology

Histamine is synthesized throughout the body by decarboxylation of the amino acid histidine. The highest concentrations of histamine are found in the storage granules of mast cells and basophils. Histamine release (degranulation) can be triggered by chemical, mechanical, or immunologic stimulation. Histamine is metabolized primarily by histamine-N-methyltransferase to inactive metabolites which are excreted in the urine. This enzymatic reaction is inhibited by droperidol. The organ system effects of histamine are mediated through two types of receptors (H_1 and H_2):

A. Cardiovascular: Histamine reduces arterial blood pressure but increases heart rate and myocardial contractility. The drop in blood pressure is attributed to peripheral arteriolar dilatation (combined H_1 and H_2 receptor stimulation). The tachycardia and inotropic effects are due to direct H_2 receptor stimulation, catecholamine release from the adrenal medulla, and activation of the baroreceptor reflex.

B. Respiratory: Histamine constricts bronchiolar smooth muscle. This response to H_1 receptor stimulation is exaggerated in patients with bronchial asthma.

C. Gastrointestinal: Activation of H_2 receptors in parietal cells increases gastric acid secretion. Stimulation of H_1 receptors leads to contraction of intestinal smooth muscle.

D. Dermal: The classic wheal-and-flare response

of the skin to histamine results from increased capillary permeability and vasodilatation.

E. Immunologic: Histamine is a major mediator of type 1 hypersensitivity reactions (Chapter 45).

1. H_1 RECEPTOR ANTAGONISTS (Diphenhydramine)

Mechanism of Action

Diphenhydramine (an ethanolamine) is an example of a diverse group of drugs that competitively block H_1 receptors (Table 15-1). Many drugs with H_1 antagonist properties also have considerable antimuscarinic, or atropine-like, activity (eg, dry mouth).

Clinical Uses

Like other H_1 receptor antagonists, diphenhydramine has a multitude of therapeutic uses: suppression of allergic symptoms (eg, urticaria, rhinitis, conjunctivitis), prevention of motion sickness, treatment of vestibular disturbances (eg, Meniere's disease), and production of sedation. Some of these actions are predictable from the discussion of histamine physiology, while others are due to the drug's antimuscarinic effects. Although H_1 blockers prevent the bronchoconstrictive response to histamine, they are ineffective in the treatment of bronchial asthma, which is primarily due to other mediators. Likewise, H_1 blockers will not prevent the hypotensive effect of histamine unless an H_2 blocker is administered concomitantly. Thus, the usefulness of H_1 blockers during an acute anaphylactic reaction is quite limited. The antiemetic and mild hypnotic effects of antihistaminic drugs have led to their use for premedication (particularly diphenhydramine, promethazine, and hydroxyzine).

Dosages

The usual adult dose of diphenhydramine is 50 mg (0.5-1.5 mg/kg) orally, intramuscularly, or intravenously every 4-6 hours. The dosages of other H_1 antagonists are listed in Table 15-1.

Drug Interactions

The sedative effects of H_1 antagonists can potentiate other central nervous system depressants such as barbiturates and narcotics.

Table 15–1. Properties of commonly used H_1 antagonists.

Drug	Route	Dose	Duration	Sedation	Antiemetic
Diphenhydramine (Benadryl)	PO, IM, IV	50–100 mg	3–6 hours	+++	++
Dimenhydrinate (Dramamine)	PO, IM, IV	50–100 mg	3–6 hours	+++	++
Chlorpheniramine (Chlor-Trimeton)	PO, IM, IV	2–12 mg 5–20 mg	4–8 hours	++	0
Hydroxyzine (Atarax, Vistaril)	PO, IM	25–100 mg	4–12 hours	+++	++
Promethazine (Phenergan)	PO, IM, IV	12.5–50 mg	4–12 hours	+++	+++

Key:
0 = No effect
++ = Moderate activity
+++ = Marked activity

2. H₂ RECEPTOR ANTAGONISTS (Cimetidine & Ranitidine)

Mechanism of Action

Cimetidine and ranitidine competitively inhibit H_2 receptors.

Clinical Uses

H_2 receptor antagonists inhibit gastric acid secretion. They are effective in the treatment of duodenal and gastric ulcers, hypersecretory states (Zollinger-Ellison syndrome), and reflux esophagitis. By decreasing gastric fluid volume and hydrogen ion content, H_2 blockers reduce the perioperative risk of aspiration pneumonitis. These drugs have no effect on the pH of gastric secretions in the stomach prior to their administration (Table 15–2).

The combination of H_1 and H_2 receptor antagonists provides some protection against drug-induced allergic reactions (eg, chymopapain injection for lumbar disk disease). Although histamine release is not reduced, pretreatment with these agents lessens subsequent hypotension.

Side Effects

Rapid intravenous injection of H_2 receptor antagonists has been rarely associated with hypotension, bradycardia, and cardiac arrest. These adverse cardiovascular effects are more frequent following the administration of cimetidine to critically ill patients. H_2 receptor antagonists change the gastric flora by virtue of their pH effects. The clinical significance of this alteration has yet to be determined. Complications of chronic cimetidine therapy include hepatotoxicity (elevated serum transaminases), interstitial nephritis (elevated serum creatinine), granulocytopenia, and thrombocytopenia. Cimetidine also binds to androgen receptors, occasionally causing gynecomastia and impotence. Finally, cimetidine has been associated with mental status changes ranging from lethargy to sei-

Table 15–2. Pharmacology of aspiration pneumonitis prophylaxis.

Drug	Onset	Duration	Acidity	Volume	LES Tone
Cimetidine (Tagamet)	1–2 hours	4–8 hours	↓↓↓	↓↓	0
Ranitidine (Zantac)	1–2 hours	8–12 hours	↓↓↓	↓↓	0
Antacids (Bictra, Polycitra)	5–10 min	30–60 min	↓↓↓	↑	0
Metoclopramide (Reglan)	IV: 1–3 min PO: 30–60 min[1]	1–2 hours	0	↓↓	↑↑

[1]Oral metoclopramide has a quite variable onset of action and duration of action.
Key:
0 = No effect
↓↓ = Moderate decrease
↓↓↓ = Marked decrease
↑ = Slight increase
↑↑ = Moderate increase
↑↑↑ = Marked increase
LES = Lower esophageal sphincter

zures, particularly in elderly patients. In contrast, ranitidine does not affect androgen receptors and penetrates the blood-brain barrier poorly.

Dosages

As a premedication to reduce the risk of aspiration pneumonitis, cimetidine (300 mg orally, intramuscularly, or intravenously) or ranitidine (150 mg orally; 50 mg intramuscularly or intravenously) should be administered at bedtime and again at least 2 hours before surgery. Because both drugs are eliminated primarily by the kidney, the dosage should be reduced in patients with significant renal dysfunction.

Drug Interactions

Cimetidine reduces hepatic blood flow and binds to the cytochrome P-450 mixed-function oxidases. These effects slow the metabolism of a multitude of drugs, including lidocaine, propranolol, diazepam, theophylline, phenobarbital, warfarin, and phenytoin. Ranitidine also decreases hepatic blood flow, but it is a weak inhibitor of the cytochrome P-450 system, and no significant drug interactions have been demonstrated.

ANTACIDS

Mechanism of Action

Antacids neutralize the acidity of gastric fluid by providing a base (usually hydroxide, carbonate, bicarbonate, citrate, or trisilicate) that reacts with hydrogen ions to form water.

Clinical Uses

Common uses of antacids include the treatment of gastric and duodenal ulcers, reflux esophagitis, and Zollinger-Ellison syndrome. In anesthesiology, antacids provide protection against the harmful effects of aspiration pneumonitis by raising the pH of gastric contents. Unlike H_2 receptor antagonists, antacids have an immediate effect. Unfortunately, they increase intragastric volume. Aspiration of particulate antacids (aluminum or magnesium hydroxide) produces abnormalities in lung function comparable to those that occur following acid aspiration. Nonparticulate antacids (sodium citrate or sodium bicarbonate) are much less damaging to lung alveoli if aspirated. Furthermore, particulate antacids do not mix with gastric contents as well as nonparticulate solutions. Timing is critical, since nonparticulate antacids lose their effectiveness within 30–60 minutes after ingestion.

Dosages

The usual adult dose of a 0.3-M solution of sodium citrate—Bicitra (sodium citrate and citric acid) or Polycitra (sodium citrate, potassium citrate, and citric acid)—is 15–30 mL orally 15–30 minutes prior to induction.

Drug Interactions

Because antacids alter gastric and urinary pH, they change the absorption and elimination of many drugs. The rate of absorption of digoxin, cimetidine, and ranitidine is slowed, while the rate of phenobarbital elimination is quickened.

METOCLOPRAMIDE

Mechanism of Action

Metoclopramide acts peripherally as a cholinomimetic (ie, facilitates acetylcholine transmission at selective muscarinic receptors) and centrally as a dopamine antagonist.

Clinical Uses

By enhancing the stimulatory effects of acetylcholine on intestinal smooth muscle, metoclopramide (1) increases lower esophageal sphincter tone, (2) speeds gastric emptying, and (3) lowers gastric fluid volume. These properties account for its efficacy in the treatment of diabetic gastroparesis, reflux esophagitis, and patients at risk for aspiration pneumonitis. Metoclopramide does not affect the secretion of gastric acid or the pH of gastric fluid.

Metoclopramide produces an antiemetic effect by blocking dopamine receptors in the central nervous system. Its usefulness as an antiemetic during cancer chemotherapy is better documented than its usefulness following general anesthesia.

Side Effects

Rapid intravenous injection may cause abdominal cramping, and metoclopramide is contraindicated in patients with intestinal obstruction or pheochromocytoma. Sedation, nervousness, and extrapyramidal signs from dopamine antagonism are rare and reversible. Nonetheless, metoclopramide is best avoided in patients with Parkinson's disease. Metoclopramide-induced increases in aldosterone and prolactin secretion are probably inconsequential during short-term therapy. Metoclopramide may rarely result in hypotension and dysrhythmias.

Dosages

An adult dose of 10–20 mg of metoclopramide is effective orally, intramuscularly, or intravenously (injected over 5 minutes). Higher doses (1–2 mg/kg) have been used to prevent emesis during chemotherapy. Onset of action is much more rapid following parenteral (3–5 minutes) than oral (30–60 minutes) administration. Because metoclopramide is excreted in the urine, its dose should be decreased in patients with renal dysfunction.

Drug Interactions

Antimuscarinic drugs (eg, atropine, glycopyrrolate) block the gastrointestinal effects of metoclopramide.

Metoclopramide decreases the absorption of orally administered cimetidine. Concurrent use of phenothiazines or butyrophenones (droperidol) increases the likelihood of extrapyramidal side effects.

DOXAPRAM

Mechanism of Action

Doxapram is a central nervous system stimulant. Selective activation of carotid chemoreceptors by low doses of doxapram stimulates hypoxic drive, producing an increase in tidal volume and a slight increase in respiratory rate. At higher doses, the central respiratory centers in the medulla are stimulated.

Clinical Uses

Because doxapram mimics a low PaO_2, it may be useful in patients with chronic obstructive pulmonary disease who are dependent on hypoxic drive yet require supplemental oxygen. Drug-induced respiratory and central nervous system depression, including that seen immediately postoperatively, can be *temporarily* overcome. However, doxapram is not a specific reversal agent and should not replace standard supportive therapy (mechanical ventilation). For example, doxapram will not reverse paralysis due to muscle relaxants, though it may transiently mask respiratory failure. The most common cause of postoperative hypoventilation—airway obstruction—will not be alleviated by doxapram. For these reasons, many anesthesiologists feel that doxapram has limited usefulness.

Side Effects

Stimulation of the central nervous system leads to a variety of possible side effects: mental status changes (confusion, dizziness, seizures), cardiac abnormalities (tachycardia, dysrhythmias, hypertension), and pulmonary dysfunction (wheezing, tachypnea). Vomiting and laryngospasm are of particular concern to the anesthesiologist in the postoperative period. Doxapram should be avoided in patients with a history of epilepsy, cerebrovascular disease, acute head injury, coronary artery disease, hypertension, or bronchial asthma.

Dosages

Bolus intravenous administration (0.5–1 mg/kg) results in transient increases in minute ventilation (onset of action = 1 minute; duration of action = 5–12 minutes). Continuous intravenous infusions (1–3 mg/min) provide longer-lasting effects (maximum dose = 4 mg/kg).

Drug Interactions

The sympathetic stimulation produced by doxapram may exaggerate the cardiovascular effects of monoamine oxidase inhibitors or adrenergic agents. Doxapram should be avoided in patients awakening from halothane anesthesia, since the latter sensitizes the myocardium to catecholamines.

NALOXONE

Mechanism of Action

Naloxone is a competitive antagonist at opioid receptors. Its affinity for μ receptors appears to be much greater than for κ or δ receptors (see Chapter 8). Naloxone has no significant agonist activity.

Clinical Uses

Naloxone reverses the agonist activity associated with endogenous (enkephalins, endorphins) or exogenous opioid compounds. A dramatic example is the reversal of unconsciousness that occurs in a patient with narcotic overdose who has received naloxone. Perioperative respiratory depression caused by overzealous opioid administration is rapidly antagonized (1–2 minutes). Some degree of opioid analgesia can often be spared if the dose of naloxone is limited to the minimum required to maintain adequate ventilation. Low doses of intravenous naloxone reverse the side effects of epidurally administered opioids (Chapter 18) without necessarily reversing the analgesia. The potential efficacy of high-dose naloxone in the treatment of septic shock and focal cerebral ischemia may be related to the release of endorphins during stress.

Side Effects

Abrupt reversal of opioid analgesia can result in sympathetic stimulation due to pain perception (tachycardia, ventricular irritability, hypertension, pulmonary edema), an acute withdrawal syndrome in narcotic dependence, and vomiting. The extent of these side effects is proportionate to the amount of opioid being reversed and the speed of the reversal.

Dosages

In postoperative patients experiencing respiratory depression due to excessive opioid administration, intravenous naloxone (0.4 mg/mL vial diluted to 0.04 mg/mL) can be titrated in increments of 0.5–1 μg/kg every 3–5 minutes until adequate ventilation and alertness are achieved. Intravenous doses in excess of 0.2 mg are rarely indicated. The brief duration of action of intravenous naloxone (30–45 minutes) is due to rapid redistribution from the central nervous system. A more prolonged effect is almost always necessary to prevent recurrence of respiratory depression from longer-acting opiates. Therefore, intramuscular naloxone (twice the required intravenous dose) or a continuous infusion (4–5 μg/kg/h) is recommended. Neonatal respiratory depression resulting from maternal opioid administration is treated with 10 μg/kg, repeated in 2 minutes if necessary. Neonates of opioid-dependent mothers will exhibit withdrawal symptoms if given naloxone. *The primary treatment of respira-*

tory depression is always airway establishment and artificial ventilation.

Drug Interactions

The effect of naloxone on nonopiate anesthetic agents such as nitrous oxide is controversial and probably insignificant. The antihypertensive effect of clonidine may be antagonized by naloxone.

CASE DISCUSSION: MANAGEMENT OF PATIENTS AT RISK FOR ASPIRATION PNEUMONIA

A 58-year-old man is scheduled for elective inguinal hernia repair. His past history reveals a persistent problem with heartburn and passive regurgitation of gastric contents into the pharynx. He has been told by his internist that these symptoms are due to a hiatal hernia.

Why would a history of hiatal hernia concern the anesthesiologist?

Perioperative aspiration of gastric contents (Mendelson's syndrome) is a potentially fatal complication of anesthesia. Hiatal hernia is a predisposing factor for aspiration.

Which patients are predisposed to aspiration?

Patients with altered airway reflexes (eg, drug intoxication, general anesthesia, encephalopathy, neuromuscular disease) or abnormal pharyngeal or esophageal anatomy (eg, hiatal hernia, scleroderma, pregnancy, obesity) are prone to pulmonary aspiration.

Does aspiration consistently result in aspiration pneumonitis?

Not necessarily. The seriousness of the lung damage depends on the volume and composition of the aspirate. Patients are considered to be "at risk" for aspiration pneumonitis if their gastric volume is greater than 25 mL (0.4 mL/kg) *and* their gastric pH is less than 2.5.

Patients who have eaten immediately prior to emergency surgery are obviously "at risk." However, some patients who have fasted for 8 hours or more before elective surgery also meet the "at-risk" criteria. Certain patient populations are especially likely to have large volumes of acidic gastric fluid: outpatients, patients with an acute abdomen, children, diabetics, pregnant women, and obese patients. Furthermore, pain, anxiety, or opioid agonists may delay gastric

emptying. Note that pregnancy and obesity place patients in double jeopardy by increasing the chance of aspiration (increased intra-abdominal pressure and distortion of the lower esophageal sphincter) and the risk of aspiration pneumonitis (increased acidity and volume of gastric contents).

Which drugs lower the risk of aspiration pneumonitis?

H_2 receptor antagonists decrease gastric acid secretion. Although they will not affect gastric contents already in the stomach, further acid production will be inhibited. Both gastric pH and gastric volume are affected. Additionally, ranitidine's long duration of action may provide protection in the recovery room.

Metoclopramide shortens gastric emptying time, increases lower esophageal sphincter tone, and is an antiemetic. It does not affect gastric pH, and it cannot clear large volumes of food in a few hours. Nonetheless, the combination of metoclopramide with ranitidine is a good combination for most "at-risk" patients.

Antacids usually raise gastric fluid pH, but at the same time they increase gastric volume. While antacid administration technically removes a patient from the "at-risk" category, aspiration of a substantial volume of particulate matter will lead to serious physiologic damage. For this reason, clear antacids (eg, sodium citrate) are strongly preferred. In contrast to H_2 antagonists, antacids are immediately effective and alter the acidity of existing gastric contents. Thus, they are useful in emergency situations and in patients who have recently eaten.

Anticholinergic drugs (Chapter 11), particularly glycopyrrolate, decrease gastric secretions if large doses are administered. However, lower esophageal sphincter tone is reduced. Overall, anticholinergic drugs do not reliably reduce the risk of aspiration pneumonitis.

What anesthetic techniques are used in "full stomach" patients?

If the "full stomach" is reversible (eg, recent food intake) and the surgical procedure is elective, the operation should be postponed. If the risk factor is not reversible (eg, hiatal hernia) or the case is emergent, proper anesthetic technique can minimize the risk of aspiration pneumonitis. Regional anesthesia with minimal sedation should be considered in all patients at increased risk for aspiration pneumonitis. If local anesthetic techniques are impractical, the patient's airway must be protected. Delivering anesthesia by mask is definitely contraindicated. As in every anesthetic case, the availability of suction must be confirmed before induction. If there are signs suggesting a difficult airway, intubation should precede induction (see the Case Discussion in Chapter 5). Otherwise, a "rapid-sequence" induction is indicated.

How does a rapid-sequence induction differ from a routine induction?

(1) The patient is *always* preoxygenated prior to induction. Four maximal breaths of oxygen are sufficient to denitrogenate normal lungs. Patients with lung disease require 3–5 minutes of preoxygenation.

(2) Prior "curarization" with a nondepolarizing muscle relaxant may prevent the increase in intra-abdominal pressure that accompanies the fasciculations caused by succinylcholine. However, this step is often omitted since it may decrease lower esophageal sphincter tone.

(3) A wide assortment of blades and endotracheal tubes are prepared in advance. It is prudent to begin with a stylet and an endotracheal tube one-half size smaller than usual to maximize the chances of an easy intubation.

(4) An assistant applies pressure over the cricoid cartilage prior to induction (**Sellick's maneuver**). Because the cricoid cartilage forms an uninterrupted and incompressible ring, pressure over it is transmitted to underlying tissue. The esophagus is collapsed and regurgitated gastric fluid cannot reach the hypopharynx.

(5) No "test dose" of thiopental is given. The induction dose is given as a bolus. Obviously, this dose must be modified if there is any indication that the patient's cardiovascular system is unstable. Other rapidly acting induction agents can be substituted for thiopental (eg, propofol, etomidate, ketamine).

(6) Succinylcholine, 1.5 mg/kg, is administered *immediately* following the thiopental, even if the patient has not yet lost consciousness.

(7) The patient is not artificially ventilated. Once spontaneous efforts have ceased or muscle response to nerve stimulation has disappeared, the patient is rapidly intubated. Cricoid pressure is maintained until the endotracheal tube cuff is inflated and tube position is confirmed.

(8) If the intubation proves difficult, cricoid pressure is maintained and the patient is gently ventilated with oxygen until another intubation attempt can be performed. If intubation is still unsuccessful, spontaneous ventilation should be allowed to return and an awake intubation preformed.

(9) After surgery, the patient should remain intubated until airway reflexes have returned and consciousness has been regained.

What are the relative contraindications to rapid-sequence inductions?

Rapid-sequence inductions are usually associated with increases in intracranial pressure, arterial blood pressure, and heart rate. This technique shares the contraindications of thiopental (eg, hypovolemic shock) and succinylcholine (eg, thermal burns).

Describe the pathophysiology and clinical findings associated with aspiration pneumonitis.

The pathophysiologic changes depend upon the composition of the aspirate. Acid solutions cause atelectasis, alveolar edema, and loss of surfactant. Particulate aspirate will also result in obstruction of small airways and alveolar necrosis. Granulomas may form around food or antacid particles. The earliest physiologic change following aspiration is intrapulmonary shunting, resulting in hypoxia. Other changes may include pulmonary edema, pulmonary hypertension, and hypercapnia.

Wheezing, tachycardia, and tachypnea are common physical findings. Hypotension signals significant fluid shifts into the alveoli and is associated with massive lung injury. Chest roentgenography may not demonstrate diffuse, bilateral infiltrates for several hours after the event. Arterial blood gases reveal hypoxemia, hypercapnia, and respiratory acidosis.

What is the treatment of aspiration pneumonitis?

As soon as regurgitation is suspected, the patient should be placed in a head-down position so that gastric contents drain from the mouth instead of into the trachea. The pharynx and, if possible, the trachea should be thoroughly suctioned. The mainstay of therapy in patients who subsequently become hypoxic is positive-pressure ventilation. Intubation and the institution of positive end-expiratory pressure (PEEP) or continuous positive airway pressure (CPAP) are often required. Bronchoscopy, pulmonary lavage, broad-spectrum antibiotics, and corticosteroids are controversial and rarely indicated.

SUGGESTED READINGS

Garrison JC: Histamine, bradykinin, 5-hydroxytryptamine, and their antagonists. Chapter 23 in: *Goodman and Gilman's The Pharmacological Basis of Therapeutics,* 8th ed. Gilman AG et al (editors). Pergamon, 1990. The effects of histamine H_1 and H_2 receptor antagonism.

Gibbs CP, Modell JH: Management of aspiration pneumonitis. Chapter 40 in: *Anesthesia,* 3rd ed. Miller RD (editor). Churchill Livingstone, 1990. Etiology, pathophysiology, prevention, and treatment.

Hardy J-F: Large volume gastroesophageal reflux: A rationale for risk reduction in the perioperative period. Can J Anaesth 1988;35:162.Includes an evaluation of the patient at risk and techniques of prevention.

McCammon RL: Aspiration pneumonitis prophylaxis and prevention. In: *1988 Review Course Lectures.* International Anesthesia Research Society, *1988.* Overview of clinical considerations.

Smith TC: Opioid reversal and postoperative narcotic analgesia. Chapter 52 in: *Opiates in Anesthesia.* Estrafanous FG (editor). Butterworths, 1984. The disadvantages of pharmacologic reversal of narcotics with opioid antagonists.

Stoelting RK: *Pharmacology and Physiology in Anesthetic Practice.* Lippincott, 1987. Chapter 26 contains a detailed description of antacids and metoclopramide.

Section III
Regional Anesthesia & Pain Management

Spinal, Epidural, & Caudal Blocks   16

*John E. Tetzlaff, MD**

Spinal, epidural, and caudal blocks are all known as **central blocks** and involve injection of local anesthetics onto or immediately adjacent to the spinal cord. Each involves reversible interruption of spinal cord activity, and all have much anatomy and physiology in common. Each block also has unique anatomic, physiologic, and clinical features and specific instrumentation requirements, which will be described individually in this chapter. Applications of central blocks to obstetrics and pediatrics will be presented. A general discussion of the advantages of regional anesthesia versus general anesthesia is presented in this chapter because of the weight of evidence involving spinal and epidural anesthesia and issues such as blood loss, deep venous thrombosis, and postoperative confusion in the elderly. A general discussion of the anatomy of the spinal column is followed by the physiologic responses common to central blocks. Spinal, epidural, and caudal anesthesia are presented individually, highlighting their differences as well as their similarities.

ANATOMY

The structure of the spine confers stability, protection of the spinal cord, and weight-bearing movement in the upright posture. The details of each component—the skeleton, the spinal cord with its coverings and spaces—and the blood supply will be presented here, with emphasis on their relevance to central blocks.

*Staff Anesthesiologist, Department of General Anesthesia, The Cleveland Clinic Foundation, Cleveland, Ohio.

BONY STRUCTURE

The surface anatomy of the back is the key to identification of the underlying anatomy. The spinous process of C2 is felt just below the occipital protuberance. The cervicothoracic junction is identified by the **vertebra prominens,** or spinous process of C7. The thoracic vertebrae are identified by their corresponding ribs. A line drawn between both iliac crests passes between the spinous processes of L4 and L5. In thin individuals, the sacrum is palpable and the sacral hiatus is felt as a diamond-shaped or irregular depression just above or between the gluteal clefts.

The vertebrae are 33 in number, being divided by structural similarity into five regions: cervical, thoracic, lumbar, sacral, and coccygeal. As can be seen in Figure 16–1, the spine is not straight but really a double "C" curve. The cervical and lumbar curves are convex in a ventral direction, whereas the thoracic and sacral curves are convex dorsally. This has practical significance when considering where a solution injected into the cerebrospinal fluid will move if affected by gravity when the patient is prone or supine.

A typical vertebra (Figure 16–2) has structurally similar parts from level to level, and familiarity with its structure facilitates correct needle placement for central block. The structural base of the vertebra is the vertebral body. Adjacent vertebral bodies are held together over the intervening intervertebral disk by strong, fibrous anterior and posterior longitudinal ligaments (Figure 16–3), which maintain the ventral stability of the spine. Posteriorly, a bony and ligamentous network forms the spinal canal and posterior articulation and maintains dorsal stability. Attached directly to the vertebral body dorsally are the paired **pedicles,** which move dorsolaterally to articulate with the **lami-**

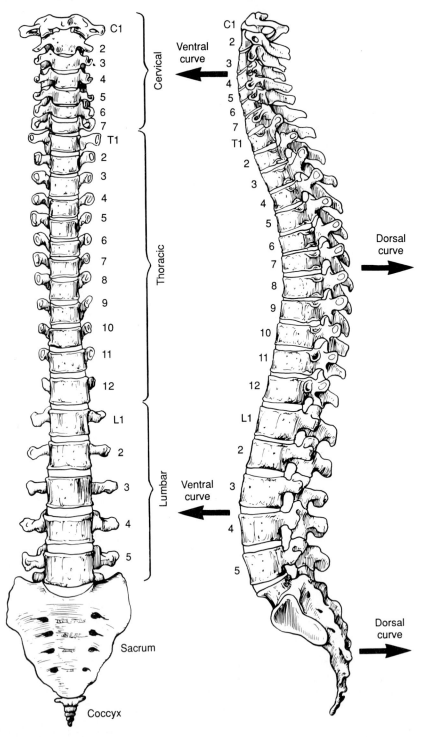

Figure 16–1. The vertebral column. (Reproduced, with permission, from deGroot J, Chusid JG: Correlative Neuroanatomy, 20th ed. Appleton & Lange, 1988.)

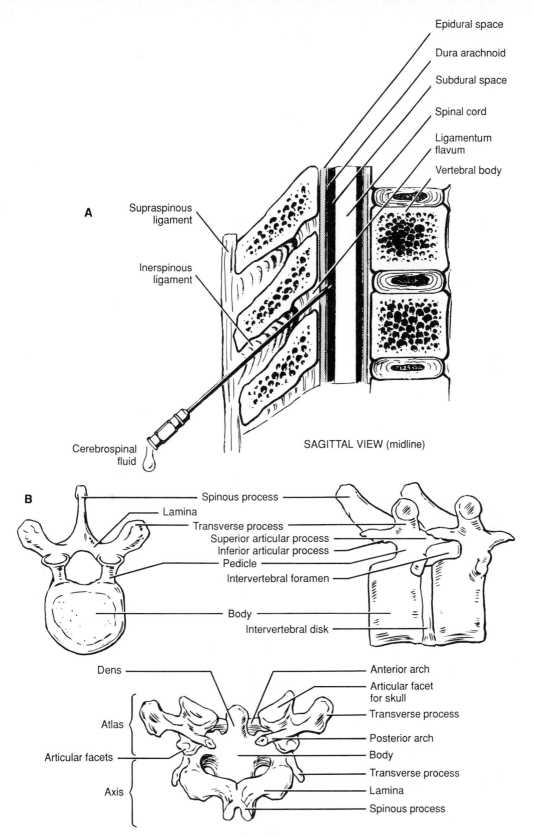

Figure 16–2. *A:* Lumbar vertebrae. *B:* Common features of vertebrae. (Reproduced, with permission, from Katz J: *Atlas of Regional Anesthesia.* Appleton-Century-Crofts, 1985.)

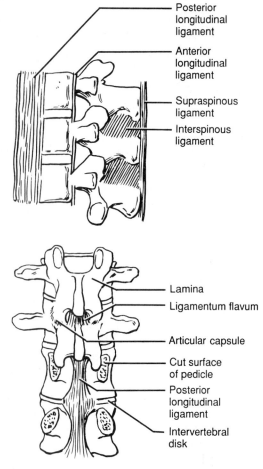

- Posterior longitudinal ligament
- Anterior longitudinal ligament
- Supraspinous ligament
- Interspinous ligament

- Lamina
- Ligamentum flavum

- Articular capsule
- Cut surface of pedicle
- Posterior longitudinal ligament
- Intervertebral disk

Figure 16–3. Ligaments of the spinal column.

nae. The laminae meet and fuse in the midline. The oval space created by the pedicles and laminae forms the **intervertebral foramen.** The confluence of adjacent intervertebral foramina creates the **spinal canal,** in which are housed the spinal cord, its coverings, and its vascular supply. Each pedicle is notched, more so on the inferior surface and less so on the superior surface. This notching from two adjacent pedicles above and below creates the intervertebral foramen, through which exits the corresponding **spinal nerve.** At the junction of the laminae and pedicles are raised areas called **facets** that form the bony component of the synovial joints between posterior elements. With accompanying ligaments, these facets maintain dorsal stability. Just lateral to each facet is the **transverse process,** which accommodates muscular insertions. Dorsal to the posterior midline junction of the laminae is the **spinous process,** which marks the midline in surface anatomy and deep to the surface helps provide for ligamentous insertions that contribute to dorsal stability of the spinal column. The posterior ligaments (Figure 16–3) start with the **supraspinatus,** which

joins adjacent spinous processes dorsally and is most superficial. Next, as one proceeds ventrally, is the **interspinous ligament,** which joins adjacent spinous processes on their horizontal surface. Deepest, as one approaches the spinal canal, is the **ligamentum flavum,** which joins adjacent laminae and is the immediate covering over the **dura mater.** The potential space between ligamentum flavum and dura mater is the **epidural space,** which is confluent laterally with dural sleeves surrounding exiting spinal nerves. This is the anatomic basis for epidural blockade. With a needle, the ligamentum flavum is felt as a firm structure; passage through it conveys a "gritty" sensation, followed by a distinct "pop" and "loss of resistance" as the dense ligament is exited. At this point, any substance (air, liquid) in a connected syringe can be injected easily. The tip of the injecting needle is actually pushing the dura away from ligamentum flavum and creating a negative-pressure epidural space. If no syringe is connected but a drop of saline ("hanging drop") is left in the syringe, the drop will be drawn into the needle. These terms and their significance are discussed later.

Under the adherent **arachnoid membrane** is the spinal cord or its continuation, the **cauda equina,** bathed in cerebrospinal fluid.

Regional differences in vertebral structure are important to central blockade. The **cervical vertebrae** have an extra foramen within their transverse processes for passage of the vertebral artery. In the cervical region, the spinal canal is the widest and the vertebral body the smallest of all spinal regions. The size of the spinal cord and the large muscle groups dictates this. The spinous process is horizontal, and a midline approach is possible with a needle.

The **thoracic vertebrae** are identified by their rib articulations on the transverse process. The facet joints are nearly horizontal, and the spinous processes are more oblique from the horizontal plane and actually overlap. In this region, the midline needle approach is not practical. The paramedian approach avoids the oblique spinous processes and offers the most direct approach to the interlaminar space.

The **lumbar vertebral bodies** are the largest in the spinal column, as are the nearly horizontal spinous processes. The midline approach is easiest at this level, with the interlaminar space being behind the inferior aspect of the superior spinous process. This necessitates a slight cephalad direction in needle placement for the midline approach.

The five **sacral vertebrae** are more or less fused into the sacrum. Dorsal and ventral foramina for nerve exit remain, as does a defect in the roof on the dorsal aspect at the caudal end referred to as the **sacral hiatus.** Penetration of the ligamentous covering of the sacral hiatus places a needle in the epidural space of the sacrum. This is the anatomic basis for **caudal blockade.**

The **coccyx** represents fusion of three or four rudimentary vertebrae and has no anesthetic significance.

THE SPINAL CORD

The spinal cord is that part of the central nervous system within the spinal canal and is the neural structure anesthetized for central blockade. The tissues that surround the cord, including dura mater, fatty tissues, and a venous plexus, are referred to as the **meninges** (Figure 16–4). The outermost area is the **epidural space,** with its veins and fatty connective tissue. The next layer is the **dura mater,** which is a dense, watertight tube that protects the spinal cord, contains the **cerebrospinal fluid,** and is confluent with the intracranial dura, extending distally as far as S2 and farther in children. Spinal nerves exit from an intervertebral foramen at the level of the corresponding vertebral body (Figure 16–5). Because the spinal cord is shorter than the spinal column, as the spinal segments pro-

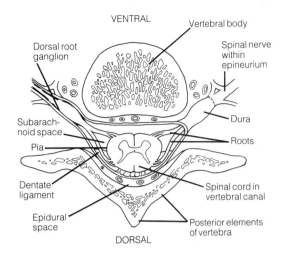

Figure 16–5. Exit of the spinal nerves. (Reproduced, with permission, from deGroot J, Chusid JG: Correlative Neuroanatomy, 20th ed. Appleton & Lange, 1988.)

gress caudally, there is an increasing distance that each nerve must travel to its intervertebral foramen. At the sacral level, this can be 10–12 cm (Figure 16–6). Below L1, the spinal cord is not a single solid structure but has split into terminal branches referred to as the **cauda equina** ("horse's tail") (Figure 16–7) because of the numerous small strands enclosed by dura within cerebrospinal fluid. Because of this change, lumbar puncture is most often performed below L1, since puncture of the intact cord is less likely and the components of the cauda equina will move away from—rather than be impaled by—an advancing needle.

BLOOD SUPPLY

The spinal cord receives its blood supply from two distinct systems, the **anterior spinal artery** and the paired **posterior spinal arteries** (Figure 16–8). The posterior arteries have rich collateral flow and supply the posterior white and gray matter of the cord. The chief origin of the paired posterior spinal arteries is the cerebral arterial system, with collateral contributions from the subclavian, intercostal, lumbar, and sacral arteries. Because of its rich collateral anastomosis, the posterior system is not segmental, and segmental arterial injury is an unlikely cause of cord ischemia in posterior spinal artery distribution. This is not the case for the midline anterior spinal artery, whose branches are segmental, with contributions from branches of the vertebral (high cervical) and three radicular branches: the cervical, thoracic, and radicularis magna of the lumbar region (also known as the **artery of Adamkiewicz**) (Figure 16–9). The ventral cord is supplied by the anterior spinal artery, and a single branch of the aorta (artery of Adamkiewicz) supplies nearly all of the

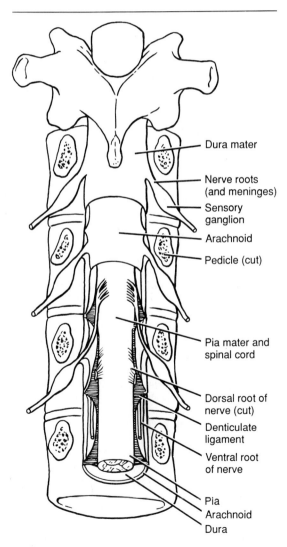

Figure 16–4. The spinal cord.

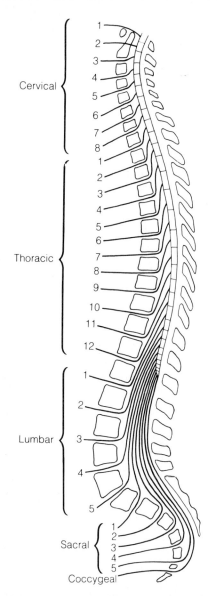

Cervical
1
2
3
4
5
6
7
8

Thoracic
1
2
3
4
5
6
7
8
9
10
11
12

Lumbar
1
2
3
4
5

Sacral
1
2
3
4
5

Coccygeal

Figure 16–6. Course of the spinal nerves. (Reproduced, with permission, from deGroot J, Chusid JG: Correlative Neuroanatomy, 20th ed. Appleton & Lange, 1988.)

flow to the lower thoracic and lumbar segments. Injury to this artery renders this entire segment of cord at risk for ischemia. It is typically unilateral and statistically most often occurs at L1 on the left side.

PHYSIOLOGY

The physiologic response to central blockade is determined by the response of the patient to interruption of afferent and efferent nervous system activity to somatic and visceral structures. The somatic structures are traditionally thought of as sensory and motor, while the visceral structures are more related to the autonomic nervous system. In addition to the physiology of somatic (motor and sensory) blockade, the effect of central blockade on the cardiovascular, pulmonary, renal, gastrointestinal, and endocrine systems will be presented here.

SOMATIC BLOCKADE

Prevention of pain and skeletal muscular movements are the classic objectives of central blockade. In order to discuss the physiology of this end point, the example of a **subarachnoid block for lower abdominal surgery** will be used.

A local anesthetic appropriate for the anticipated duration of the surgery is selected, and after lumbar puncture it is injected into the subarachnoid space. It mixes with cerebrospinal fluid and is exposed to the spinal cord. Spread occurs as a result of a number of factors, including gravity, cerebrospinal fluid pressure, patient position, solution temperature, and others. The local anesthetic becomes less concentrated as it mixes with cerebrospinal fluid, diffuses, and moves into the substance of the central nervous system at the level injected and more proximally. Neural blockade requires penetration of the lipid membrane covering and blockade of the sodium channel within the axoplasm. This occurs at a certain minimum (threshold) concentration referred to as Cm. But nerve fibers are not homogeneous. Similarity exists between fibers that conduct motor, sensory, and sympathetic modalities. There are three main fiber types designated A, B, and C. The A group has four subgroups: alpha, beta, gamma, and delta. The functions of the groups and subgroups are summarized in Table 16–1. Because the site of action at the nerve root has a mixture of these fiber types, the onset of anesthesia is not uniform. Fibers are blocked more easily if they are small and myelinated and less easily if they are large or unmyelinated. This explains why the A γ and B fibers are easily blocked and the large A α and unmyelinated C fibers are hard to block. This causes each fiber type to have a distinct Cm and differential blockade. As diffusion and dilution of the injected agent occurs, the more resistant fibers start to not be completely blocked. The result is that the sympathetic block (judged by temperature sensitivity) may be two segments higher than the sensory block (pain, light touch), which in turn is two segments higher than the motor block. The segments where one mode is blocked and another not blocked are referred to as **zones of differential blockade.** When evaluating the level of a block, it is important to keep in mind which modality is being assessed—ie, temperature (sympathetic), movement (motor), or scratch (sensory)—since the maximum level will be different for each.

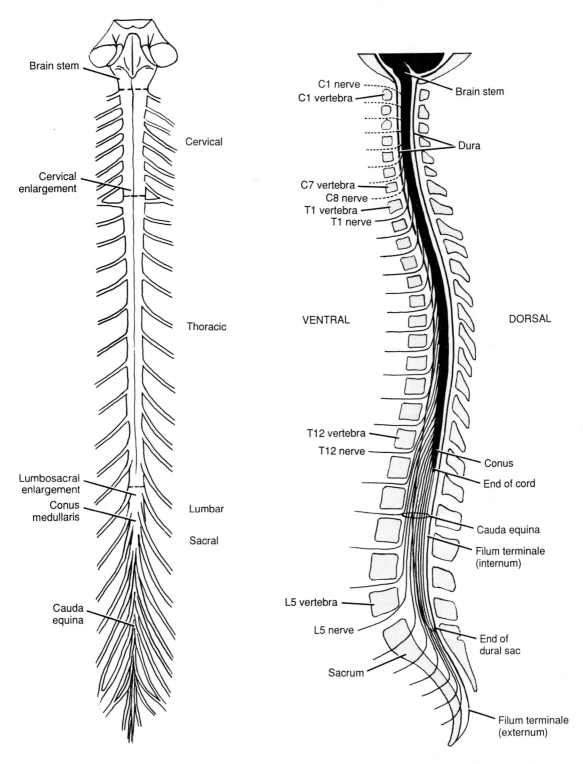

Figure 16–7. Cauda equina. (Reproduced, with permission, from Katz J: *Atlas of Regional Anesthesia*. Appleton-Century-Crofts, 1985.)

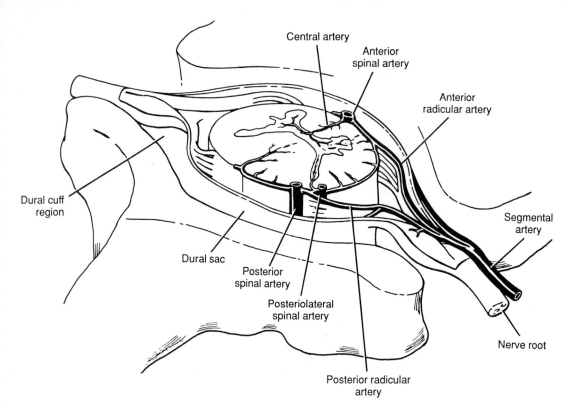

Figure 16–8. Arterial supply to the spinal cord. (Reproduced, with permission, from Katz J: *Atlas of Regional Anesthesia.* Appleton-Century-Crofts, 1985.)

The differential blockade of somatic fibers may lead to clinical management problems. A sense of deep pressure and rough movement is conducted by C fibers, which are difficult to block. Similarly, the motor block achieved may be much lower than the sensory level. Patients may have awareness of pressure and even the ability to move muscle groups, which may be disconcerting to the surgeon or patient. Furthermore, a very anxious patient may interpret any feeling from the surgical site as painful and may be hard to manage for that reason. Advanced warning does a great deal to minimize these problems.

Table 16–1. Nerve fiber classification.

Class	Action	Myelin	Size	C$_m$
A α	Motor	Yes	++++	++++
A β	Light touch, pressure, pain	Yes	+++	+++
A γ	Muscle spindles (proprioception)	Yes	+++	++
A δ	Pain, temperature	Yes	++	+
B	Preganglionic sympathetic fibers	Yes	++	+
C	Pain, pressure	No	+	+++

VISCERAL BLOCKADE

Most of the visceral effects of central blockade are mediated by interruption of autonomic impulses to various organs. The consequences are described by system.

Cardiovascular

Sympathetic denervation results in cardiovascular changes of hemodynamic consequence in proportion to the degree of sympathectomy. The sympathetic chain originates from the lumbar and thoracic spinal cord. The fibers involved in smooth muscle tone of the arterial and venous circulation arise from T5 to L1. The arteries retain most of their tone because of local mediators despite sympathectomy, but the venous circulation does not. The consequence of total sympathectomy is an increase in the volume of the capacitance vessels and a subsequent decrease in venous return to the heart. Without previous fluid administration, hypotension is the consequence. If partial sympathectomy occurs (T8–10 block), there can be physiologic compensation with vasoconstriction, mediated by sympathetic system fibers above the level of the block. This vasoconstriction may even be visible on the skin in fair-skinned individuals. The cardiac accelerator fibers are sympathetic efferents (T1–4), which

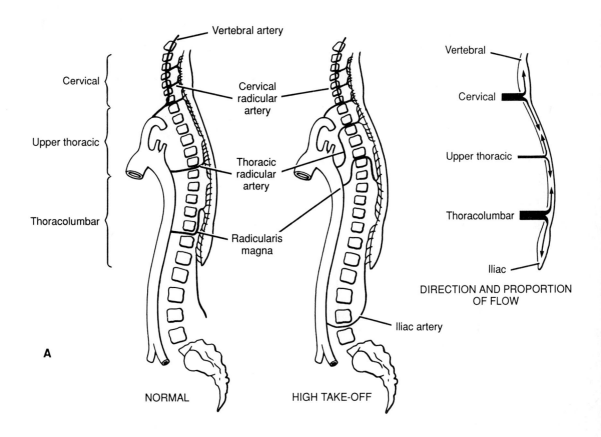

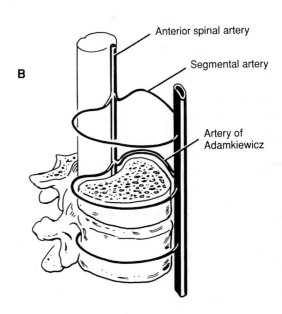

Figure 16–9. Segmental arterial blood supply.

increase heart rate when stimulated. When blocked by high central blockade, unopposed vagal activity leads to bradycardia. Head-down position or fluid administration increases preload, which fills the right atrium and reflexively returns the cardiac output toward normal. Administration of an anticholinergic agent will produce vagolysis and reverse the bradycardia.

The degree of hypotension encountered determines the treatment. The most important target organs are the heart and the brain. The modest decrease in oxygen delivery to the heart is counteracted by the decreased myocardial work and oxygen consumption that result. Afterload is greatly reduced, and the work associated with generating the same cardiac output is reduced as well. This only becomes imbalanced when profound reduction in preload remains uncorrected. The brain is protected during central blockade by cerebrovascular autoregulation, which is mediated by tissue factors in the brain and is unaffected as long as the mean arterial blood pressure remains above 60 mm Hg.

Treatment and prevention of hypotension depend upon understanding its mechanisms. Prevention involves rapid increase in the plasma volume immediately before and during administration of the block. Prehydration with 10–20 mL/kg of crystalloid solution in the healthy patient effectively compensates for the pooling of blood in the venous capacitance vessels from sympathectomy. Avoidance of total sympathetic block and administration of a vasopressor are also preventive. Treatment involves a number of options. Autotransfusion in the head-down position (or with the legs elevated) can augment rapid fluid administration to restore preload. Profound bradycardia is treated with anticholinergics. If these measures fail or if aggressive fluid administration must be avoided, direct and indirect vasopressors can be chosen. Direct vasopressors such as phenylephrine restore venous tone and increase preload. A theoretic disadvantage is the increase in afterload that increases myocardial work. Indirect vasopressors such as ephedrine directly stimulate the heart and replace some of the effects of the sympathetic fibers on cardiac contractility and venous capacitance. In cases of extreme hypotension, epinephrine administration can rapidly restore coronary perfusion before ischemia leads to cardiac arrest.

Pulmonary

The primary influence of central blockade on the pulmonary system has to do with truncal motor blockade. Intercostal muscles are involved in both inspiration and expiration, and anterior abdominal muscles are involved in active expiration. Thoracic level block will impair intercostals at the level injected, and all but the lowest blocks will eliminate active use of abdominal muscles. The diaphragm will remain unaffected, since phrenic nerve blockade is rare even during high cervical block. The reason relates not to exposure of phrenic nerve to local anesthetic but to concentration. Even with total spinal anesthesia, the concentration is well below that capable of blocking A α fibers in the phrenic nerve or the respiratory center in the brainstem. The apnea associated with high central blockade is typically transient and much shorter in duration than the duration of action of the agent—and is most likely related to brainstem ischemia from hypotension.

Even during high thoracic blockade, arterial gas tension should not change in normal patients. Tidal volume, minute ventilation, and maximum inspiratory volume are all maintained by the diaphragm. Maximum breathing capacity and active exhalation are impaired in proportion to the loss of abdominal and intercostal muscle motion. This does not influence ventilation in the normal patient but will affect the patient with obstructive pulmonary disease who is dependent on accessory muscles to actively expire. Loss of the rectus abdominis to stabilize the rib cage and loss of the intercostals to provide general positive expiratory force in these patients can lead to impaired ventilation. The first consequence in the patient with chronic pulmonary disease is subjective dyspnea or exacerbation of existing shortness of breath. This can progress rapidly to a feeling of suffocation and panic despite adequate oxygen saturation and elimination of CO_2. The patient can become difficult to manage intraoperatively. The first objective change is CO_2 retention, which can be followed by acute hypoxia despite supplemental oxygen. Patients with severe restrictive disease or acute bronchospasm who are using accessory muscles to inspire can also be adversely affected by the loss of intercostal and abdominal muscle tone.

In order to retain the respiratory advantages of regional anesthesia in pulmonary patients (avoidance of airway instrumentation, positive pressure, increased ventilation/perfusion mismatch), the motor block should be kept below T 7. In cases where the level must be higher (upper abdominal surgery), a pure regional technique may not be the best choice.

In the postoperative period, if the central block can be maintained for sensory anesthesia without impairing motor function, the patient will be greatly aided by pulmonary toilet. Particularly with epidural analgesia with low-concentration local anesthetics, opioids, or both, the pain from upper abdominal or thoracic incision can be attenuated and the reflexive splinting decreased. This allows effective coughing and deep breathing to clear secretions and avoid atelectasis.

Gastrointestinal

Sympathetic outflow to the intestines originates from T5–L1, decreases peristalsis, maintains tone in sphincters, and opposes the action of the vagus nerve. With sympathectomy, vagal tone dominates and results in a small, contracted gut with active peristalsis, ideally suited to intra-abdominal procedures. Gastric emptying is unaffected, and intraoperative distention of stomach and bowel is less than if general anesthesia were employed.

Liver

Blood flow to the liver decreases in direct proportion to the decrease in mean arterial blood pressure.

The liver extracts more oxygen from the arterial inflow and does not become ischemic. Liver enzymes are unaffected, and liver damage is no more likely to occur than from the same surgery under general anesthesia.

Urinary Tract

Renal blood flow is unaffected by central block due to autoregulation mediated by local tissue factors, except with extreme hypotension. Therefore, urine production is unaffected. Muscle tone in the bladder is eliminated and acute urinary retention is the result during the time when S2–4 remain completely blocked.

Metabolic & Endocrine

Pain and surgery lead to a sympathetic activation that results in a variety of hormonal and metabolic responses. Central block can either temporarily (single-shot) or lastingly (catheter-continuous) alter these responses.

Nociceptive afferent activity stimulates catecholamine release from the adrenal medulla. Increases in blood pressure can have an adverse effect on the myocardial oxygen supply/demand relationship, along with increased gluconeogenesis in the liver. Epidural anesthesia blocks this adrenal response, blocking the hypertension and myocardial stress and preventing hyperglycemia. In obstetric deliveries, the decreased secretion of catecholamines after epidural analgesia for labor results in improved uterine blood flow and an improved acid-base status in the newborn.

SPINAL ANESTHESIA

Injection of local anesthetics into the subarachnoid space produces spinal anesthesia. The history of spinal anesthesia since 1899 and the work of August Bier has been characterized by wide swings in popularity. Surges of acceptance have resulted from technical advances in local anesthetics and needles as well as from research to explain the occurrence of complications and how to eliminate them. Epidemiologic studies by Dripps in the early 1960s established the neurologic safety of spinal anesthesia and gave rise in large part to the current widespread popularity of subarachnoid block.

INDICATIONS

Spinal anesthesia is appropriate for procedures involving the lower extremities, hip, perineum, lower abdomen, and lumbar spine. It can be used for upper abdominal procedures such as cholecystectomy and gastric resection, but very high levels are necessary, and the patients for whom this would be efficacious for

other reasons often do not tolerate T4 sensory levels. The technique also requires a gentle surgeon accustomed to performing major abdominal operations in awake patients, since rough technique causes intolerable discomfort even with a solid block. In these cases, spinal anesthesia can be used in conjunction with light general anesthesia and possibly intrathecal opioids as a balanced anesthetic technique. Some specific indications are discussed in the following paragraphs.

Urologic endoscopic surgery—and, specifically, transurethral resection of the prostate—is a relative indication for central blockade. Preservation of consciousness allows early warning of absorption of irrigation solutions (hypervolemia, hyponatremia) as well as pain from peritoneal stimulation (referred to the shoulder) if the bladder is penetrated. Since many of these patients also have coronary artery disease, they can complain of chest pain if it occurs during operation.

Rectal surgery presents a relative indication for spinal anesthesia. Requiring only sacral anesthesia, rectal surgical procedures are often performed with the patient in the prone position. The physiologic trespass of prone anesthesia is much greater—as are the risks under general anesthesia—than with saddle block spinal anesthesia (explained below). The only exception would be if the block were inadequate or failed by duration; airway management in the prone patient is extremely difficult and risky.

Spinal anesthesia for **repair of hip fracture** in the elderly also has a number of advantages. Low spinal anesthesia is adequate, and the physiologic trespass is small. The awake patient is an effective monitor for angina and central nervous system integrity. Studies have demonstrated decreased blood loss as well as less postoperative confusion and delirium in the geriatric hip fracture population. Decreased thrombogenesis with decreased rates of deep venous thrombosis and pulmonary embolism is also a consideration, but this is better established with epidural anesthesia.

Indications for spinal anesthesia in **obstetrics** are based on its ease of administration, the solid and reliable block achieved, and the low doses of agent that minimize transmission of local anesthetic to the fetus. Saddle block (described later) is used for vaginal delivery, forceps or vacuum extraction, episiotomy repair, and extraction of retained placental fragments. Spinal anesthesia can be used for cesarean section—even under urgent circumstances—as long as blood pressure is aggressively maintained. Prehydration, left uterine displacement, and liberal use of ephedrine prevent the profound hypotension that can compromise the fetus as well as the mother.

Spinal anesthesia has recently been shown to have new applications in **pediatrics.** In the extremely premature infant requiring surgery, the incidence of life-threatening apnea after general anesthesia is alarmingly high. The technical efficacy of neonatal spinal anesthesia has been demonstrated with a dramatic decrease in apnea as long as the infant was not sedated during placement of the block. Several other series have demonstrated the safety and efficacy of spinal anesthesia for inguinal, urologic, and lower extremity procedures in tiny infants.

CONTRAINDICATIONS

There are both absolute and relative contraindications to spinal anesthetics (Table 16–2).

Absolute contraindications include refusal by the patient, skin infection at the lumbar puncture site, bacteremia, hypovolemia, coagulopathy, and increased intracranial pressure. Evaluation of infection and of the patient's volume and clotting status is discussed in the next section.

Relative contraindications are more numerous and harder to evaluate. Issues include existing neuropathy, prior spine surgery, back pain, aspirin use preoperatively, subcutaneous minidose heparin, the uncooperative or emotionally unstable patient, or a resistant surgeon.

PATIENT PREPARATION

To prepare the patient for a spinal anesthetic, informed consent, physical examination, baseline laboratory examinations, and premedication must be considered.

Consent

Patients have many reasons for refusing spinal anesthesia. Prior adverse experience (headache, failed

Table 16–2. Contraindications to central blockade.

Absolute
  Sepsis
  Bacteremia
  Skin infection at injection site
  Hypovolemia
  Coagulopathy
  Therapeutic anticoagulation
  Demyelating central nervous system disease
  Increased intracranial pressure
  Psychosis or dementia
  Lack of consent
Relative
  Peripheral neuropathy
  "Mini-dose" heparin
  Aspirin or other antiplatelet drugs
  Prior lumbar spine surgery
  Chronic back pain
  Certain cardiac lesions
    Idiopathic hypertrophic subaortic stenosis
    Aortic stenosis
  Psychologic or emotional instability
  Uncooperative patients
  Prolonged surgery
  Surgery of uncertain duration
  Surgical team resistance to awake patients

block, painful placement, injury) is hard to argue against. Many patients have heard of disasters associated with spinal anesthesia; often, this "information" amounts to mere gossip and can be easily overborne with a good preoperative visit and reassurance to the effect that current procedures are extremely safe.

Even if the patient is compliant and cooperative when spinal anesthesia is recommended, explanation of the risks and benefits of the procedure is essential for *informed* consent. Risks include pain with lumbar puncture, backache, hypotension, headache, treatable drop in blood pressure, meningitis, nerve injury, and hematoma. Use of lay terms and reassurance about the rarity of the serious risks as well as the treatability of the headache are important.

Physical Examination

In addition to the usual physical examination, a candidate for spinal anesthesia should have a specific evaluation of the lumbar spine. Dermatologic conditions that preclude skin preparation are a contraindication to spinal anesthesia. Kyphoscoliosis or thick layers of adipose tissue should be noted, as should a midline lumbar spine surgical scar. Palpation of lumbar interspaces is valuable as a predictor of the technical ease of spinal anesthesia.

Laboratory Tests

Hematocrit should be measured, since severe anemia will magnify the adverse response to the hypotension that may result from spinal anesthesia. Prothrombin time (PT) and partial thromboplastin time (PTT) are mandatory if any suggestion of coagulation abnormality exists. Even in the absence of clinical bleeding, the bleeding time should be determined in patients who have been taking antiplatelet drugs (aspirin, nonsteroidal anti-inflammatory agents, valproic acid, etc).

Premedication

Many patients who are good candidates for a spinal anesthetic give consent to the procedure but with concern about being awake, hearing things, "being uncomfortable," etc. A good preoperative visit is important to allay these fears, but pharmacologic premedication may establish a basis for a smooth block and intraoperative course.

It is important to obtain informed consent to spinal anesthesia prior to premedication. Once the plan is established, a sedated, calm but not somnolent patient is often the objective. Oral or intramuscular benzodiazepines are good choices. Sometimes, an opioid or opioid-anxiolytic combination given intramuscularly is chosen. Some specific agents and combinations are listed in Table 16–3.

No premedication has any value if it is not administered at the proper time, ie, at the pharmacologically correct interval before the scheduled time of surgery.

Table 16–3. Premedication for central blockade.

Diazepam, 0.1–0.2 mg/kg PO
Midazolam, 1–3 mg IM
Lorezepam, 1–3 mg PO
Diphenhydramine, 0.5–1 mg/kg IM
Pentobarbital, 1–2 mg/kg PO
Morphine, 0.1–0.15 mg/kg IM with hydroxyzine, 1–2 mg/kg
Meperidine, 0.5–1 mg/kg IM with hydroxyzine, 1–2 mg/kg
Chloral hydrate, 10–20 mg/kg PO or PR

EQUIPMENT & SAFETY

General Preparation

A spinal anesthetic must be administered in a space that is fully equipped for patient monitoring, administration of general anesthesia if necessary, and resuscitation afterward. This is mandatory because of the uncommon but not rare complications of spinal anesthesia, including severe hypotension, profound bradycardia, and respiratory insufficiency. The time necessary to obtain equipment and drugs after the onset of one of these complications could make the difference between successful treatment and major morbidity or mortality. Monitoring—to include electrocardiography, blood pressure, auscultation with a precordial stethoscope, and pulse oximetry—will allow early warning of the rare episode of cardiovascular collapse that can occur during spinal anesthesia and allow pharmacologic intervention while cardiac output and arterial circulation remain effective for transport of drugs to their target organs. Minimal requirements for the regional anesthesia cart are listed in Table 17–1.

Needles

Spinal needles are carefully manufactured without surface irregularities and with a tight-fitting removable stylet that completely occludes the needle lumen. A wide variety of sizes with different applications are available, from 16 gauge to 30 gauge. The effect of needle size will be discussed in the section on spinal headache.

Equally diverse are the shapes of the bevel and the tips of the needles. The needles are either sharp or blunt at the tip, with either end-injection or side-injection and either sharp or rounded (blunt) bevel edges. The "standard" is the Quincke-Babcock needle, which has a medium bevel length with sharp edges, a sharp point, and end-injection. Two common alternatives are the Greene and Whitacre needles. The Greene needle has a long bevel with a rounded point and a sharp bevel with end-injection. The Whitacre and other "pencil-point" needles have a rounded bevel, no cutting edges, and side-injection proximal to the bevel. Both blunt needles offer the theoretic advantage of less dural trauma with less subsequent cerebrospinal fluid leaking. This should result in less spinal headache, and clinical studies reward that expectation. The Pitkin needle has a short, sharp bevel and pointed end-

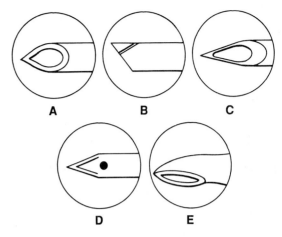

Figure 16–10. Spinal needles. **A:** Quincke-Babcock. **B:** Pitkin. **C:** Greene. **D:** Whitacre. **E:** Tuohy.

injection. It was also designed to minimize spinal headache, but clinical studies do not support the claim. Figure 16–10 shows these needles graphically. The Tuohy needle is an epidural needle that has application in spinal anesthesia for catheter placement for continuous technique.

TECHNIQUE

The procedure begins with establishment of a workable sterile field and identification of anatomic landmarks. The patient is placed in the position decided upon. The iliac crests are palpated. If the thumbs are extended to meet in the midline (size permitting), they will press down in the interspace between L4 and L5 (Figure 16–11). The best interspace palpable is identified and can be marked with fingernail imprint or skin marker. The preparation solution is most often povidone-iodine applied with an abrasive sponge. Preparation starts over the interspace and proceeds in a widening circle outward from this point to the periphery. A sterile field drape is applied, and the povidone-iodine is wiped from the site. It is particularly important to avoid introducing povidone-iodine into the subarachnoid space because of the risk of transverse myelitis. Once the solution is wiped away, the interspace is identified and a position of entry (technique-specific) is chosen. A skin wheal is raised, and the deeper structures are also infiltrated with a longer needle to minimize pain and reflexive movement during needle placement. During deeper infiltration, bony landmarks can be felt and periosteum infiltrated. This minimizes pain and gives the clinician a better three-dimensional idea of how to place the spinal needle into the subarachnoid space. After this, the needle is placed by one of several techniques (see below).

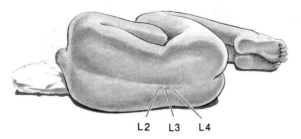

L2 L3 L4

Figure 16–11. Identification of lumbar interspaces. (Reproduced, with permission, from Katz J: *Atlas of Regional Anesthesia.* Appleton-Century-Crofts, 1985.)

Patient Position

A. Sitting Position: This is frequently the easiest position for lumbar puncture. The patient sits on the edge of the operating room bed with legs on a stool, leaning forward with arms crossed. It helps to tell the patient to arch the lower back "like a mad cat." With this maneuver, the skin and deep structures tighten and the natural lumbar spine flexion that results opens the interspaces. Pain from injury (eg, hip fracture) or labor—or uncooperativeness by the patient—limits use of the sitting position. However, this may be the only position in which lumbar puncture can be performed successfully in the morbidly obese.

B. Lateral Decubitus: The patient is placed on the table close to the anesthesiologist, most often with the surgical side of the body down (ie, right side down for right leg surgery). The hips and knees are maximally flexed, and the chest and neck are flexed toward the knees. Patients often understand this if you tell them to assume the position they would be in if they did a "cannonball into the pool." "Assume the fetal position" is another way of asking for what is wanted. This facilitates flexion of the spine, which is essential to open the lumbar interspaces. The lateral decubitus position is useful for patients with hip or leg fracture and for those who consent but cannot cooperate, since an assistant can hold the hips and shoulders and optimally flex the spine. It is useful also for the obstetrics patient who becomes extremely agitated with each contraction.

C. Prone Position: The prone position is often chosen for anorectal surgery. The patient is placed in the surgical position, and lumbar puncture is performed. The advantage is that the patient does not have to be turned, and with hypobaric solution the uphill drift will provide the necessary sacral anesthesia. The disadvantage is the difficulty in verifying correct lumbar puncture, because cerebrospinal fluid will not drip from the needle by gravity but may actually have to be aspirated.

Needle Technique

A. Midline Technique: (Figure 16–12.) The spinous process of the vertebra above and below the level to be used defines the superficial limits of the interspace. Because of the downward angle described by the spinous process in the lumbar region (Figure 16–2A), the skin wheal is raised just below the upper spinous process. The needle is directed so as to pass just under and parallel to this spinous process in the midline, taking into account the slightly cephalad location of the interlaminar space. Smooth passage suggests that the approach has been correct. Superficial contact with bone suggests a spinous process, whereas deeper bone contact is either lamina (on midline) or pedicle (off midline). This information can be used to redirect the needle. Under difficult circumstances, deliberate contact with laminae on both sides can help to identify the midline and facilitate dural puncture. As the needle leaves the subcutaneous tissue and enters the supraspinous and interspinous ligaments, an increase in resistance is felt. Another change occurs as ligamentum flavum is penetrated, and the final change is a decrease in resistance as dura is punctured. With experience, each of the distinct "pops" is felt as needle insertion proceeds, and successful dural puncture is confirmed by withdrawing the stylet to verify free flow of cerebrospinal fluid. The needle is rotated 360 degrees to verify free flow in each quadrant, and the syringe is then connected, cerebrospinal fluid aspirated, and medication injected. Any sharp paresthesia is a warning to reposition the needle. Free flow in each quadrant and successful aspiration before and after injection confirm correct placement. If dural puncture has occurred near the dural sleeve, free flow may not occur in all quadrants, and injection should be withheld. Injecting under these circumstances could result in a poor block or, rarely, could injure the spinal nerve. Aspiration verifies that the needle is still communicating with cerebrospinal fluid after the syringe is connected and has not moved farther in or out.

B. Paramedian Technique: (Figure 16–13.) The paramedian technique is selected when lumbar puncture is difficult, particularly in patients with severe arthritis, kyphoscoliosis, and prior lumbar spine surgery. The approach is off the midline and approaches the interspinous gap lateral to the ligaments.

The midline is identified, and an interspace is chosen. A skin wheal is raised 2 cm lateral to the superior spinous process. The needle is directed 10–15 degrees toward the midline and then advanced. It may help to imagine the needle reaching the midline

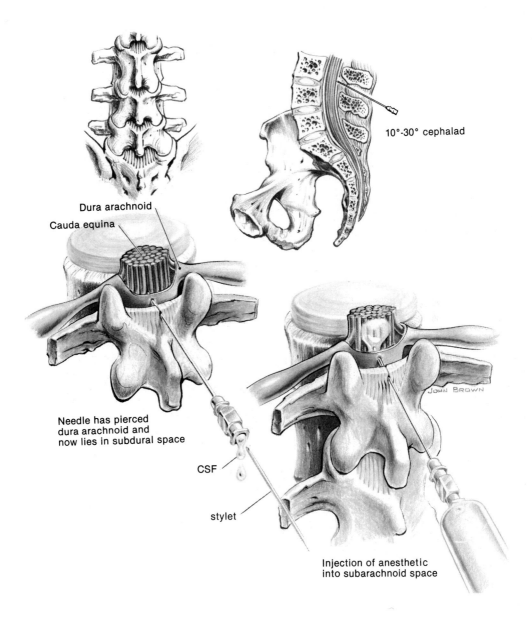

Dura arachnoid

Cauda equina

10°-30° cephalad

Needle has pierced
dura arachnoid and
now lies in subdural space

CSF

stylet

Injection of anesthetic
into subarachnoid space

Figure 16–12. Midline approach lumbar spinal anesthesia. (Reproduced, with permission, from Katz J: *Atlas of Regional Anesthesia.* Appleton-Century-Crofts, 1985.)

4–6 cm below the surface in order to select the angle of approach. The paraspinous muscle mass will be continuous right up to ligamentum flavum, where the last two "pops" (ligamentum flavum and dura) will be encountered just as in the midline approach. With free flow of cerebrospinal fluid, the procedure is then the same as midline.

CONTINUOUS SPINAL ANESTHESIA

Subarachnoid block can be performed in a continuous manner if a catheter is placed in the sub-arachnoid space. Theoretical advantages include lower total dose to achieve surgical anesthesia, gradual onset with less hemodynamic alteration, and prolonged anesthesia made possibly by the ability to reinject the agent and prevent regression of the block during prolonged surgical procedures and recovery.

When first attempted, continuous spinal anesthesia was performed using equipment designed for epidural anesthesia. Limited application resulted from technical difficulty and complications, including excessive post-lumbar puncture cephalalgia and, more ominously, central nervous system injury and infection.

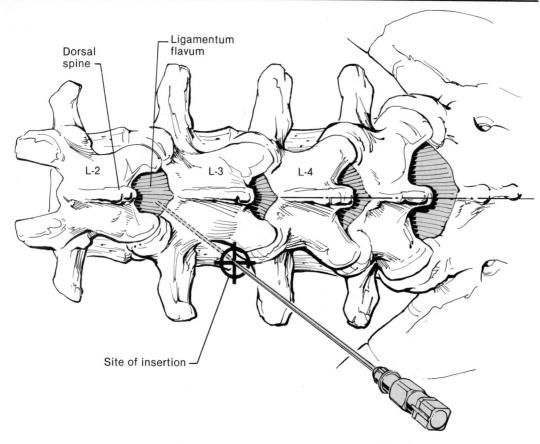

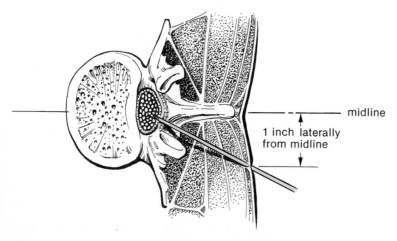

Figure 16–13. Paramedian approach, lumbar spinal anesthesia. (Reproduced, with permission, from Katz J: *Atlas of Regional Anesthesia*. Appleton-Century-Crofts, 1985.)

A resurgence of interest in continuous spinal anesthesia has resulted from refinement of needles and catheters. Twenty-five gauge and smaller needles combined with tiny (32-gauge) catheters have reduced the excessive headache rate even in high-risk groups (young, female). Initial attempts to use these systems can be frustrating, but success is reported to increase dramatically with experience. Limitation of the technique is related to catheter breakage within the subarachnoid space and recent isolated reports of neurologic deficits, specifically those of the cauda equina type. These nerve injuries are thought to have resulted from local high concentrations of the agent near the catheter tip, especially with repeated injection. The ultimate place for continuous spinal anesthesia is still evolving.

FACTORS INFLUENCING SPINAL ANESTHESIA

Lumbar puncture is the first obstacle to spinal anesthesia. Once flow of cerebrospinal fluid is verified, a drug is injected and an anesthetic level achieved. A wide variety of variables determine this outcome and will be presented individually.

Agent

Spinal anesthesia has been attempted with many agents, but only a few remain in common use (Table 16–4).

A. Procaine: Procaine is an ester with a rapid onset and a very short duration of action (45–60 minutes). Some prolongation of the duration can be achieved with added vasoconstrictor. For short procedures, procaine provides a rapid, dense block, and it can be combined with tetracaine for longer procedures. Procaine also lends itself to dilution for differential blockade for diagnosis of pain syndromes. Table 16–4 compares procaine with other spinal agents.

B. Tetracaine: Tetracaine is an ester with an intermediate onset and long duration of action and is the most popular agent for spinal anesthesia. Its duration of action is prolonged by added vasoconstrictors, and it is available in several forms for different uses.

C. Lidocaine: Lidocaine is an amide with a rapid onset and short duration of action which provides a rapid, solid block. The effect of vasoconstrictor is controversial, with some studies showing prolongation of action and others not.

D. Bupivacaine: Bupivacaine is an amide with a slow onset and long duration of action which is unaffected by added vasoconstrictor. While only the glucose-containing solution is available in the USA for spinal anesthesia, in Great Britain and Europe a plain solution is also used for isobaric technique.

Dosage

Another factor that alters the outcome of spinal anesthesia is the dosage of the drug selected. Choice of dose of a given spinal anesthetic agent is determined by a combination of the properties of the agent and the type of surgical procedure to be performed as well as the anticipated duration of surgery. The dose is based on the patient's height, since the height of the spinal column has been shown to be related to the spinal level. It is also based on the patient's age, since the volume of the subarachnoid space as well as the epidural space becomes lower with aging, and the same amount of drug will have more cephalad spread with advancing age. The dose is also determined by the patient's weight, since obesity increases intra-abdominal pressure, causing a decrease in the volume of cerebrospinal fluid and of the epidural space and similarly reflects an increase in the ultimate level of the spinal anesthesia. A further patient factor that influences dosage is pregnancy, since pregnancy increases intra-abdominal pressure and decreases the epidural and subarachnoid space by the associated engorgement of the epidural venous plexus. If the same dose of spinal anesthesia is selected for a pregnant patient as for a nonpregnant patient of the same physique and age, the level will be significantly higher.

A number of factors associated with administration of the block also determine the dose selected. With hyperbaric technique, the posture of the patient during injection and the immediate postinjection period influences the dose. A larger dose administered to a patient immediately placed supine can be associated with a higher block. With hyperbaric technique, the extent of the planned block can also influence the dose. The influence of baricity on outcome is presented later.

Vasoconstrictors

Exogenously administered vasoconstrictors are mixed with local anesthetic solutions to influence the outcome of spinal anesthesia in two ways: prolongation of duration of the block and increase in the intensity of the block (Table 16–4).

Prolongation of spinal anesthesia with vasoconstrictors is an agent-specific phenomenon. The mechanism is thought to involve local vasoconstriction with decreased vascular uptake of the agent. The most commonly used vasoconstrictor is epinephrine, though ephedrine and phenylephrine also have this effect. The classic agent that demonstrates the effect of added epinephrine is tetracaine, since the duration of spinal

Table 16–4. Dosages and actions of commonly used spinal anesthetic agents.

| Drug | Preparation | Doses | | | Duration, Plain (min) | Duration, Epinephrine (min) |
		Perineum, Lower Limbs	Lower Abdomen	T4		
Procaine	10% solution	75 mg	125 mg	200 mg	45	60
Tetracaine	1% solution, dry crystals	6–8 mg	8–14 mg	14–20 mg	90	120–150
Lidocaine	5% in 7.5% glucose	25 mg	50–75 mg	75–100 mg	60	60–90
Bupivacaine	0.75% in 8.25% dextrose; 0.5% plain;[1] 0.75% plain[1]	4–6 mg	8–12 mg	12–20 mg	120–150	120–150

[1]Not available as labeled spinal anesthetic agent in USA.

anesthesia is prolonged by epinephrine by as much as 50%. Spinal anesthesia with procaine is similarly affected—to a lesser degree—by administration of epinephrine, while the duration of bupivacaine is not influenced by the administration of any added vasoconstrictor. Lidocaine gives mixed results, with some studies reporting 30–50% prolongation in duration and others minimal or no prolongation.

The intensity of block is also increased by vasoconstrictors. It is clear from the European literature that with increasing concentration of epinephrine in isobaric bupivacaine, the quality of spinal block is improved. Epinephrine itself may have local anesthetic properties in the subarachnoid space. Furthermore, the increase in intensity of the block may be related to the local vasoconstriction that occurs, allowing tighter binding of the local anesthetic to central nervous system structures and keeping the concentration in the area of the nerves higher during set-up of the block.

Specific Gravity

The specific gravity of the spinal anesthetic solution also influences the outcome of spinal anesthesia. The frame of reference for specific gravity at 37 °C is cerebrospinal fluid, which has a specific gravity of 1.003–1008. Table 16–5 summarizes the specific gravities of the commonly used local anesthetic solutions. The relationship of the specific gravity of the solution to that of cerebrospinal fluid is what alters outcome. If the solution injected into the cerebrospinal fluid has a specific gravity heavier than that of the cerebrospinal fluid (hyperbaric), it will tend to move by gravity to a lower site; if it is lighter (hypobaric), it will tend to move away from the dependent area; and if the agent has a specific gravity identical to or very close to that of cerebrospinal fluid (isobaric), it will stay at about the same level where it is injected.

A. Hyperbaric Technique: Hyperbaric spinal anesthesia is the most widely used. It is most often achieved by mixing the anesthetic agent with dextrose. A number of local anesthetics are formulated in a fixed concentration of dextrose, including bupivacaine solu-

Table 16–5. Specific gravities of some spinal anesthetic agents.[1]

Agent	Specific Gravity
Procaine	
1.5% in water	1.0052
2.5% in D$_5$W	1.0203
Lidocaine	
2% in plain	1.0066
5% in 7.5% dextrose	1.0333
Tetracaine, 0.5% in D$_5$W	1.0203
Bupivacaine	
0.5% in 8.25% dextrose	1.0278
0.5% in water	1.0058

[1]Source: Greene NM: Anesth Analg 19985;64:715.

tion, which is mixed in 8% dextrose, and 5% lidocaine, which is mixed in 7.5% dextrose. Reference to Table 16–5 shows that both of these agents are clearly heavier than cerebrospinal fluid.

The outcome of hyperbaric spinal anesthesia is governed by the posture of the patient during and immediately after the injection and until the agent is fully bound to central nervous system structures. With the patient in the sitting position, the dependent area is the caudal region in most aspects of the subarachnoid space; the agent becomes effective at the level injected, and any spread will tend to go in a caudad direction. This also depends on the posture of the patient not only at the time of injection but for the period after injection up to the time when movement of the agent would no longer be expected. This means in the case of a saddle block that the patient remains sitting for 3–5 minutes, so that only the lower lumbar and sacral nerves will be blocked. In the case of a hyperbaric anesthetic technique that is performed in a sitting position but not intended to be a saddle block, the patient is returned to the supine position immediately after injection. The agent is still not fully protein-bound and will move in a dependent manner and follow the lumbar and thoracic curves of the spinal column. Referring back to our review of anatomy, it is apparent that with the thoracolumbar curve having an apex at T4, full-dose hyperbaric technique will tend to achieve anesthesia at this or at a slightly lower level.

Another application of hyperbaric technique involves injection with the patient in the lateral decubitus position with the extremity to be operated on in a dependent position. Theoretically, if the solution is injected and the patient kept in this position for 3–5 minutes, as in the saddle block technique, the extremity should have a denser, longer-acting block than the nondependent extremity. As a practical matter, however, there may be greater density of block in the lower extremity, but the upper extremity as well as bilateral aspects of the abdomen will become blocked also—ie, the concept of isolated unilateral spinal anesthesia is not borne out by the event.

A number of other factors influence the outcome of the hyperbaric technique. In some cases, after injection, the patient is placed in a head-down position. The legs may be elevated, or the patient may be asked to perform maneuvers that increase intra-abdominal pressure. Some investigators find this to influence the spread upward of hyperbaric anesthesia; others report no such effect. Furthermore, complications associated with hyperbaric technique can also be involved with these factors, such as sudden movement of the lower extremities when spinal anesthetic is moving in a proximal direction, causing the agent to reach a higher level than was planned for. Keeping the patient's neck flexed immediately after injection protects somewhat against progression into the cervical levels by increasing the natural cervical curve, which retards the cephalad movement of hyperbaric spinal anesthesia.

B. Hypobaric Technique: Tetracaine is the most

common agent used for hypobaric technique. A solution of tetracaine mixed in water will have a specific gravity slightly less than that of cerebrospinal fluid and when injected will move away from the dependent area. The classic application of this technique is for colon and rectal surgery, with the patient being placed in the prone position with head slightly lower than hips. After verification of lumbar puncture, the solution is injected and can be expected to move in a nondependent manner away from the head, resulting in anesthesia from the level of injection and caudally to block the sacral dermatomes. This affords the convenience of placing the spinal anesthetic in the position where the surgery will occur and provides a reliable dense block of sacral nerve roots for the usual duration of tetracaine. The solution can be diluted up to approximately 0.3%; with any further dilution, incomplete sensory anesthesia is a risk.

C. Isobaric Technique: Tetracaine, lidocaine, and bupivacaine lend themselves to isobaric anesthetic application. Any of these agents can be mixed in an appropriate concentration and injected either as the commercially prepared plain solutions or diluted with cerebrospinal fluid. The agent most studied in this respect is bupivacaine, which in the 0.5% plain preparation is slightly but insignificantly hypobaric at 37 °C. If this agent is injected in the lumbar area and the patient remains in the seated position for the next 2–3 minutes, the resulting sensory anesthesia is only two to four segments higher than the level where the anesthetic agent is injected. Factors that influence the outcome of this injection include the speed and force of injection, the temperature of the solution, the volume in which the dose is prepared, and the total dose injected. The classic isobaric spinal anesthetic provides a block that is dense in the lower thoracic, lumbar, and sacral areas and is ideally suited to perineal, urologic, and lower extremity surgery. The reliable absence of extension into the upper thoracic levels results in a partial sympathetic block with minimal hemodynamic changes. This makes this technique ideally suited for elderly patients with coexisting disease who sustain injuries to the hip or proximal femur requiring open reduction and internal fixation.

Posture

The position of the patient during injection of local anesthetic and during the onset of block prior to final binding of the agent to central nervous system tissues influences the final level. With the patient in the sitting position, hyperbaric solutions will migrate in a caudad manner and hypobaric solutions in a cephalad manner. With the patient in the supine or lateral position, migration of hypobaric and hyperbaric solutions will be governed by the thoracolumbar curve of the spinal column, with hypobaric solutions moving caudad and hyperbaric solutions moving cephalad. In the lateral decubitus position, the block will be partially ipsilateral.

Theoretically, isobaric solution should not be affected by posture. In addition to the position during injection, movement from this position to a different one will affect the final migration of the local anesthetic to the extent that the agent is unbound at the time the postural change occurs. This is also affected by vasoconstrictors, since epinephrine will induce local vasoconstriction and allow the agent to remain in higher concentration in the area of the spinal cord for a longer period, which means that more movement will occur based on baricity, gravity, and posture for a longer period of time.

Intra-abdominal Pressure

Intra-abdominal pressure has an indirect effect on the final level of injected local anesthetic in the subarachnoid space. This effect is mediated by changes in the contour of the subdural space and the total volume of the cerebrospinal fluid based on transmitted pressure. An example is ascites. In addition to the changes resulting from direct pressure of ascites fluid on the epidural and subarachnoid spaces, the abnormal pattern of venous return causes collateral flow through epidural veins, which expand in size, occupy space, and allow for more proximal spread of an equivalent dose of local anesthetic within the subarachnoid space.

Spinal Curvature

Abnormal curvatures of the spine—specifically, scoliosis and kyphoscoliosis—have an effect on the technical aspects of administration of anesthetic as well as factors that determine the level of spinal anesthesia. The technique of placing the block becomes more difficult because of the rotation and angulation of the vertebral bodies and spinous processes. Finding the midline and the interlaminar space can be difficult, especially in older patients, in whom degenerative changes may complicate the already difficult approach to the midline. Many practitioners find paramedian approaches to lumbar puncture to be easier in patients with severe scoliosis and kyphoscoliosis, especially if there is associated degenerative joint disease. Viewing the anteroposterior and lateral x-rays of the lumbar spine prior to attempting block can overcome some of the technical difficulties by identifying the level where lumbar puncture may be easier. Spinal curvature affects the ultimate level by changing the contour of the subarachnoid space. Severe kyphosis or kyphoscoliosis can be associated with a decreased volume of cerebrospinal fluid, and, with hypobaric technique or rapid injection, a higher than expected level can occur.

Prior Surgery of Spine

Prior spinal surgery, including lumbar laminectomy and lateral fusion of the lumbar spine, is associated with technical difficulties in placing the block and changes in the final level achieved. There may be difficulty in finding the interlaminar space at a level where decompressive laminectomy has been done or where bone graft has been placed for spinal fusion. Approaching the interlaminar space with the paramedian approach can improve the success rate, and the same is true of choosing an interspace cephalad to the upper level of the surgical site. Alterations in the final level of the block as well as incomplete block are related to changes in the contour of the subarachnoid space.

Age

Age of the patient also influences the level of spinal anesthesia achieved. The spinal and epidural spaces are thought to become smaller with advancing age, which makes the distribution of injected local anesthetic greater, with the result that there is more cephalad spread of local anesthetic and that a higher level is achieved with the same dose for patients of the same height. Accordingly, doses are traditionally reduced with advancing age.

Obesity

Obesity is known to interact with spinal anesthesia for two reasons. The first is difficulty in locating the interlaminar space behind a massive amount of soft tissue at the midline in the lumbar area. The spinous processes are frequently not palpable, and a needle longer than the typical 3-inch spinal needle may be necessary. Inability to palpate spinous processes requires generous application of local anesthesia in the skin and occasionally a blind approach to locate the spinous processes followed by an attempt to locate the interlaminar space. The paramedian approach can be very difficult owing to the excessive amount of soft tissue.

Obesity is also associated with increased intra-abdominal pressure resulting from the pannus of the abdomen. This increases the pressure in the epidural space and contributes to cephalad spread of the local anesthetic.

Pregnancy

Pregnancy acts on spinal anesthesia in somewhat the same way as morbid obesity. The gravid uterus causes increased intra-abdominal pressure as well as an increase in volume in the epidural venous plexus, both resulting in smaller and tighter epidural and subarachnoid spaces and correspondingly higher levels of anesthesia. Anesthetic doses are typically reduced by as much as a third in order to achieve the same level as in the nonpregnant patient.

Spread of the Agent

Spread of the local anesthetic into tissues of the central nervous system within the cerebrospinal fluid is determined by a number of factors, including the dose injected, the lipid solubility of the agent, local blood flow, and the surface area exposed to the agent.

The **dose injected** affects distribution of the agent by its relationship to the concentration delivered to any given area. It is obvious that the concentration of the agent will be highest at the level where the agent is injected and lowest at the levels of farthest spread. This is related to diffusion, with subsequent dilution in

cerebrospinal fluid. It is obvious that the more proximal central nervous system structures during the block will have a lower concentration for uptake than areas where the injection occurred, and this will decrease proximal block density.

The **lipid solubility** of the local anesthetic also determines the concentration in central nervous system structures. In spinal anesthesia, local anesthetic is found within the substance of the spinal cord as well as within the nerve roots and dorsal ganglia. It is probably the concentration in the spinal nerves and the dorsal ganglia that accounts for the predominant action of spinal anesthesia, since the concentration found within the substance of the spinal cord itself is too low to have any clinical effect. It stands to reason that at the same concentration and in the same area, a more lipid-soluble agent will have a higher concentration within the substance of the spinal nerves and dorsal ganglia than a less lipid-soluble one. The different sizes of nerve fibers within these structures also play a role, with larger fibers being less easily blocked than the smaller ones at the uppermost level of the block, where the concentration is lowest. This leads to **differential blockade,** with smaller fibers becoming blocked but not larger fibers. In clinical practice, this means there will be sympathectomy at a higher level than the sensory block and a sensory block higher than the motor block. Studies suggest a difference of approximately two spinal levels between these modalities.

Vascularity of the tissue determines movement of local anesthetic once it is injected. If a vasoconstrictor is added, there will be less vascularity and hence greater uptake by central nervous system tissue and a higher concentration of the agent for a longer period of time. Uptake into the substance of the spinal cord represents uptake into an area of high vascularity and a decrease in the concentration in the spinal nerves and dorsal ganglia.

The final factor influencing spread of the agent is the total **surface area exposed.** With hypobaric technique and extension of the block to very high levels, there is exposure over a large area of spinal cord. The total amount of drug in a given central nervous system site will be correspondingly lower and the redistribution and elimination of the agent that much quicker—and the same is true of anesthetic solution that undergoes rapid and direct vascular uptake and does not become involved in binding to central nervous system tissues.

Redistribution

Redistribution of local anesthetics from the subarachnoid space is involved in the termination of spinal anesthesia and is mediated chiefly by redistribution of the agent from the central nervous system via the vascular tree. Redistribution occurs via vascular absorption located both in the epidural space, just outside the dural sleeve, and within the subarachnoid space itself at the arachnoid membrane. Similar to the initial spread of the agent, the rate of redistribution and termination of action of spinal anesthesia is related to the total surface area exposed to the same dose. With the isobaric technique, most of the drug is delivered and is active in a small area, and a given amount of drug will probably have a longer duration at that level than if allowed to spread proximally. Furthermore, duration is likely to be longer if the agent is more lipid-soluble, since removal from the central nervous system will be related to tissue concentration. Vasoconstrictors also affect redistribution of the agent by maintaining an increased vascular tone and by shifting the equilibrium—ie, that between bound and unbound local anesthetic within the substance of the central nervous system—toward remaining in the central nervous system rather than being eliminated by vascular reuptake.

COMPLICATIONS

The incidence of complications is now quite low, in part because of the use of disposable spinal needles and kits. Complications associated with subarachnoid block range from simple problems such as pain with injection, backache, and urinary retention to rare occurrences such as meningitis, transverse myelitis, and anterior spinal cord syndrome. All of these complications will be discussed separately.

Pain on Injection

Despite meticulous attention to placement of the skin wheal and local anesthetic in the deep structures of the back, many patients experience discomfort during spinal needle placement. This is especially true of the patient with an abnormal spine, either from disease, prior surgery, or degenerative joint disease. Even the patient who is warned of this discomfort beforehand may need an opioid analgesic shortly before or during the block.

Backache

Backache may occur as a complication of all lumbar punctures. It is better received by the forewarned patient. As with all needle penetrations of the body into deep structures, there is hyperemia, local tissue irritation, and reflex spasm of muscles. The result is a mild sense of soreness that passes in 10–14 days even with the larger needles used for epidural anesthesia or for continuous spinal anesthesia. It is particularly important to mention this problem in discussing spinal anesthesia as an option with patients who have chronic back pain syndrome. Patients with known herniated disks will have legitimate concerns about whether spinal anesthesia will worsen the pain. While there is no specific evidence that spinal anesthesia exacerbates herniation of a nucleus pulposus, one cannot assure a patient with chronic back pain syndrome that spinal anesthesia will not increase the pain. Any increase in symptoms would probably be brief and not incapacitating, but this again cannot be guaranteed. Particularly in the patient with prior spinal surgery, the technical difficulty of lumbar puncture may be so great that

some reflex muscle spasm and discomfort should be expected from lumbar puncture.

Headache

Spinal headache is related to persistence of the dural puncture, with leakage of cerebrospinal fluid into the surrounding soft tissue leading to a chronic lowering of cerebrospinal fluid pressure. This exerts downward traction on the structures of the central nervous system and on blood vessels that are attached to both the dura and the cranium as well as the brainstem. The result is a headache similar to acute vascular cluster headache. The headache itself is postural in nature, typically begins within 6–12 hours after lumbar puncture, and is worse in the upright position. Other characteristics are its throbbing frontal quality, association with nausea and vomiting, and prompt relief upon resumption of the supine position. It may be that spinal headache typically occurs 6–12 hours postoperatively because this is when the patient first sits up or stands up.

The most obvious factor thought to be associated with post-lumbar puncture cephalalgia is needle size, with spinal headache being more common and more severe as needle size increases. In young patients, lumbar puncture for spinal anesthesia is typically performed with 25- or 26-gauge or even 30-gauge needles. Inadvertent dural puncture during attempted epidural anesthesia is a good example of large-needle lumbar puncture. (The incidence of spinal headache in this situation is influenced by a number of other variables to be discussed later.)

The orientation of the bevel also influences the incidence of spinal headache. The fibers of the dura are arranged in a longitudinal manner, and if the spinal needle enters the dura with the bevel parallel to the fibers, it is thought to separate rather than transect fibers. Needles have been developed specifically for the purpose of creating a less traumatic passage through the dura—examples are the Greene and Whitacre pencil-point needles, which pass through the dura bluntly as opposed to sharply.

Another factor influencing the incidence of spinal headache is the age and sex of the patient, with older patients and male patients having dramatically less spinal headache. Particularly with men over age 50, the incidence of spinal headache should be extremely low. Pregnancy contributes the additional factor of increased intra-abdominal pressure that leads to increased cerebrospinal fluid pressure and leak of cerebrospinal fluid, and the headache syndrome itself is much more common in this patient group.

Conservative treatment of post-lumbar puncture cephalalgia during the first 24 hours involves aggressive hydration, soft diet, stool softeners, abdominal binders, and oral analgesics. If headache persists, the patient can be offered a procedure referred to as the **"epidural blood patch."** This involves identification of the interspace where the lumbar puncture was performed, sterile preparation and draping, and placement of an epidural needle into the epidural space.

With the epidural needle in place, 10–15 mL of the patient's blood is obtained by venipuncture under sterile conditions and injected through the epidural needle until 15 mL has been injected or the patient experiences pressure in the ears. Ninety-five percent of patients have complete relief after the first patch when done 24 hours or more after dural puncture. It is thought to work at the raw surface of the dural tear, serving as a site for deposition of platelets and a subsequent hemostatic plug that closes the dural tear and prevents subsequent leakage of cerebrospinal fluid. If this first procedure does not eliminate the headache, the second attempt has an even higher success rate (approaching 99%). The complications of epidural blood patch are minimal and include pain with placement, backache associated with the dural puncture itself, and lumbar muscle spasm associated with the blood placement. All are typically of short duration and are usually well accepted by the patient whose spinal headache was severe enough to require the intervention.

A new treatment for spinal headache is the use of intravenous caffeine and sodium benzoate. Caffeine is a potent vasoconstrictor, and its presence in the bloodstream prevents traction on the blood vessels and subsequent vascular spasm. Rapid administration of 500 mg of caffeine and sodium benzoate in 1 L of isotonic crystalloid accomplishes two objectives in the treatment of spinal headache: hydration and inhibition of the vascular spasm cycle.

Urinary Retention

Blockade of S2–4 is associated with loss of tone in the bladder, and until tone returns, the reflex to void is inhibited. During this time, overfilling of the bladder can occur, and even after resolution of the blockade voiding may be difficult; this is especially true for the male patient, and in extreme cases can result in a neurogenic bladder requiring intermittent cetheterization. For prolonged central blocks, it is probably wise to insert a bladder catheter and avoid this problem. For other cases where prolonged block is not necessarily planned but evolves during the operation, one should decompress the bladder by catheterization before overfilling occurs. Bladder distention can be associated with hemodynamic alteration, since stimulation of the peritoneum results in hypertension and tachycardia. This can manifest itself clinically as agitation and should be part of the differential diagnosis of postoperative agitation after spinal anesthesia.

Meningitis

The incidence of meningitis after spinal anesthesia has fallen dramatically with the use of disposable needles and trays. The meningitis is of two types. **Chemical (aseptic) meningitis** gives rise to the clinical picture of transverse myelitis and is associated with gross dysfunction at and below the spinal level where it occurs. This was at one time associated with the use of reusable spinal needles which were cleaned in caustic substances. The result was **anterior spinal cord syndrome,** with a motor lesion as well as loss of control of bowel and bladder sphincter mechanisms.

Infectious meningitis from bacterial contamination of the cerebrospinal fluid is less common since the advent of sterile disposable spinal trays. The possibility of meningitis must be considered if meningeal signs occur, especially in the presence of fever or other signs of an infectious process. Early diagnosis and treatment are important to minimize morbidity.

Vascular Injury

Injury to blood vessels in the performance of spinal anesthesia is associated with serious complications, most commonly epidural hematoma due to continued bleeding from the epidural venous plexus. This is reported in patients with coagulopathy or those who have been taking anticoagulants, though it is rare in patients with no apparent risk factors. The clinical picture is of a spinal anesthetic evolving normally and then suddenly progressing toward greater block after some resolution of symptoms. Any spinal anesthetic that does not resolve within a reasonable period should suggest possible epidural hematoma, and aggressive investigation must be considered. Early diagnosis by contrast myolography , contrast-assisted CT scan, or MRI is an indication for decompressive laminectomy, which can preserve function of the central nervous system. The decision whether to perform lumbar puncture on a patient at risk is based on the history and laboratory studies. If the issue is raised, the minimum laboratory evaluation necessary is a platelet count, prothrombin time, partial thromboplastin time, and bleeding time. Abnormality of any of these parameters is a strong contraindication to central blockade. If the procedure is done because of a strong clinical indication or if coagulopathy develops or anticoagulant is administered after the procedure is started, serial evaluation of the patient's neurologic status is essential.

Nerve Injury

During placement of a needle in the subarachnoid space, the needle can come in direct contact with sections of the cauda equina or the nerve roots themselves. The possibility of postoperative nerve injury must be discussed with the patient even though the incidence is thought to be less than 1:10,000 spinal anesthetics. The nerve injuries that do occur tend to consist of persistent paresthesias that resolve without treatment in weeks or months. The incidence of nerve injury that is permanent or long-lasting is less than 1:10,000.

Prevention of devastating neurologic injury depends upon detection of paresthesia with placement of the needle. If the patient complains of paresthesia, questioning must be directed specifically to its character. If the paresthesia persists, needle placement must be changed, and injection must not occur until the paresthesia has resolved or until the needle has been removed and reinserted at a different site. The consequence of injection despite persistence of paresthesia is an unacceptably high probability of intraneural injection with the potential for permanent nerve disruption. Lumbar puncture below L2 should be associated with placement of the needle into the subarachnoid space at the level of the cauda equina, which is less likely to be injured by needle placement. In rare cases of anatomic anomaly, the spinal cord may continue below this level. Contact of the needle directly with the spinal cord will cause severe paresthesia, which mandates removal and replacement of the needle at a lower level.

High Spinal Anesthesia

As the level of sensory anesthesia ascends, the degree of physiologic trespass increases. With high thoracic or cervical levels, severe hypotension, profound bradycardia, and respiratory insufficiency become likely. If profound hypotension persists, hypoperfusion of the medullary respiratory center will lead to apnea. This is the most common presentation of high spinal anesthesia.

A number of factors influence the likelihood of high spinal anesthesia. Total dose injected is a factor, as well as the position of the patient and the baricity of the solution. Sudden increases in intra-abdominal pressure with Valsalva's maneuver, coughing, or lifting the legs immediately after injection may drive the level of a hyperbaric spinal agent cephalad. The subarachnoid block that results from accidental subarachnoid injection during attempted epidural anesthesia can result in a high level because the needle is large and the dose injected may be large.

Treatment of high spinal anesthesia consists first of support of the airway and circulation. When respiratory insufficiency becomes evident, supplemental oxygen is mandatory. If hypoventilation evolves, assisted ventilation with 100% oxygen must be started, along with control of the airway if apnea or unconsciousness ensues. Decreases in heart rate and blood pressure are expected. Rapid administration of intravenous fluid, head-down positioning, and aggressive use of vasopressors are required to stabilize blood pressure. Because it offer mixed central and peripheral support of the blood pressure and cardiac output, ephedrine is often the first agent selected. Phenylephrine can be chosen for its pure α-adrenergic agonist action, constricting the capacitance vessels that have dilated from total sympathectomy. Recent literature suggests that a rapid onset of profound hypotension and hypoperfusion (near cardiac arrest) calls for a stronger vasopressor such as epinephrine. The profound bradycardia is treated with an anticholinergic agent to counteract the unopposed action of vagal parasympathetic tone on the heart after complete block of the sympathetic cardiac accelerators. During the acute crisis, atropine is the anticholinergic most likely to be chosen owing to its rapid onset.

If respiratory and hemodynamic control can be achieved and maintained after high or total spinal anes-

thesia, surgery may proceed. Apnea is often transient, and unconsciousness leaves the patient amnestic without adverse recall. If intubation is required, a small dose of potent inhalational agent will allow toleration of the endotracheal tube.

EPIDURAL ANESTHESIA

Epidural anesthesia is a central block with many applications. Refinements of equipment and technique have made it increasingly popular for a wide variety of surgical, obstetric, and analgesic procedures. Unlike spinal anesthesia, which is an all-or-none block, epidural anesthesia has applications ranging from analgesia with minimal motor block to dense anesthesia with full motor block. These variables can be controlled by choice and concentration of drug and location of the injection. The indications thus include surgical anesthesia, analgesia during the first stage of labor, and prolonged postoperative pain relief after operations on the perineum, hips, and lower extremities. With application of epidural anesthesia to thoracic and cervical regions of the spine, postoperative pain control can be extended for surgical procedures involving the upper abdomen, thorax, and chest.

INDICATIONS

The general indications outlined above for spinal anesthesia apply to epidural anesthesia as well. The additional advantage of epidural anesthesia is its ability to maintain continuous anesthesia after placement of an epidural catheter, thus making the technique suitable for surgical procedures of long duration. This feature of the technique also permits anesthesia to be continued into the postoperative period as analgesia by use of lower concentrations or different agents via the epidural catheter.

Specific Indications

A. Hip and Knee Surgery: Internal fixation of a fractured hip is associated with less intraoperative blood loss when central block anesthesia is used instead of general anesthesia. With epidural anesthesia, the rate of deep venous thrombosis following total hip and knee replacement is lower, which means that pulmonary embolism is less frequent. Epidural anesthesia with continuation into the postoperative period is effective prophylaxis against deep venous thrombosis and pulmonary embolism—a significant advantage since the rate of deep venous thrombosis without prophylaxis following total knee replacement is 30–50% and the leading cause of death in patients undergoing total joint replacement is pulmonary embolism.

B. Lower Extremity Revascularization: Epidural anesthesia has established efficacy for revascularization procedures involving the lower extremities in patients with peripheral vascular disease. Flow studies show that patients with epidural anesthetics have greater distal blood flow during vascular reconstruction of the lower limbs.

C. Obstetric Deliveries: Obstetric patients in difficult labor being managed with epidural anesthetics have babies with better biochemical profiles, an indication of less peripartum stress than when delivery is accomplished without analgesics or with parenteral opioids. Decreased catecholamine levels are thought to be the explanation.

D. Postoperative Management: Low-concentration local anesthetics, opioids, or combinations of these drugs have demonstrated efficacy in the control of postoperative pain and in minimizing the effects of surgery on pulmonary reserve in normal and especially in compromised patients, such as those with chronic obstructive pulmonary disease, morbid obesity, and elderly patients. Postoperative epidural analgesia allows earlier ambulation and better cooperation with physical therapy. Furthermore, minimizing deep venous thrombosis and pulmonary embolism hastens ambulation and shortens the hospital stay.

CONTRAINDICATIONS

Epidural anesthesia shares the contraindications discussed in the section on spinal anesthesia. Further caution is warranted for patients at risk of bleeding into the epidural space. The anesthetic is injected through a 17-gauge needle placed in the epidural space, which has a rich venous plexus without valves, and placement of a large needle in this area imposes a risk of injury to these small blood vessels. The potential for low-grade bleeding is therefore greater than with other venous systems, and the risk must be considered for patients who have been taking antiplatelet drugs or minidose heparin and those undergoing surgical procedures where anticoagulation may be part of the surgical technique. With patients taking medications known to interfere with coagulation, more care is required to verify that hemostatic mechanisms are intact. This includes evaluation of the absolute platelet count, prothrombin time, partial thromboplastin time, and bleeding time. For procedures where anticoagulation is planned or may occur, the epidural needle is placed as atraumatically as possible, and if blood is observed on aspiration, either through the needle or through the epidural catheter, the procedure is usually postponed until the clinician feels secure that full heparinization will not induce bleeding in the closed epidural space, placing the spinal cord in jeopardy.

APPLIED ANATOMY OF THE EPIDURAL SPACE

The boundaries of the epidural space are shown in Figure 16–14. The ventral boundary is the substance of the pedicles of the vertebrae and the periosteum surrounding them as well as the intervertebral foramen. In this small area, the ventral border is the dura. The dorsal border of the epidural space involves the laminae and the articular processes laterally (with the ligaments that connect them), the spinous processes at their bases, and the ligamentum flavum in the interlaminar space. The lateral borders of the epidural space are the pedicles of each vertebral body and the ligamentous coverings of the intervertebral foramina. The superiormost aspect of the epidural space is the foramen magnum, and the most inferior aspect is the sacral hiatus.

Epidural anesthesia is placed at many levels of the spinal column, whereas spinal anesthesia is usually restricted to the lumbar spine. With the nearly horizontal alignment of the lumbar spinous processes, the approach to the lumbar epidural space is most commonly in the midline despite the slight cephalad displacement of the interlaminar space. This is not the case with the thoracic spine, where the short oblique spinous processes make a paramedian approach virtually mandatory. In the cervical region, the large size of the spinal cord requires that needle placement be done with special care, since the cord is immediately beneath the dura and uncontrolled puncture of the dura can result in severe injury to the spinal cord.

The epidural space is filled with loose connective tissue that surrounds the epidural veins and spinal nerve roots and fills the intervertebral foramina. The connective tissue linkage creates resistance to injection in the epidural space and a degree of back pressure with injection of larger volumes. The fat and connective tissue in pediatric patients and in young adults is not as well formed, but with older adults considerable resistance to injection may be encountered.

The epidural venous plexus is concentrated in a ventral and lateral location and very thin in the midline. The veins are valveless and communicate superiorly with intracranial venous sinuses, inferiorly with the sacral plexus, and ventrally with the thoracic and abdominal venae cavae and the azygos system. Any obstruction to venous return involving the vena cava will cause engorgement of the azygos system, with enlargement of the epidural venous system resulting from collateral flow. This occurs in obese or pregnant patients and in those with increased intra-abdominal pressure (eg, due to ascites). The best way to avoid bleeding or placement of needles and catheters directly into veins in the epidural space is to stay as close to the midline as possible on entry into the epidural space. There are no arteries in the epidural space, but the main collateral flow to the anterior spinal artery crosses very close to the lateral borders of the space in the area of the dural cuffs, and epidural needles not in the midline can injure these vessels. Recalling that the lumbar and thoracic regions are supplied segmentally by the frequently unilateral artery of Adamkiewicz (Figure 16–9), the anterior spinal cord is at risk for injury from placement of the epidural needle if the needle is away from the midline.

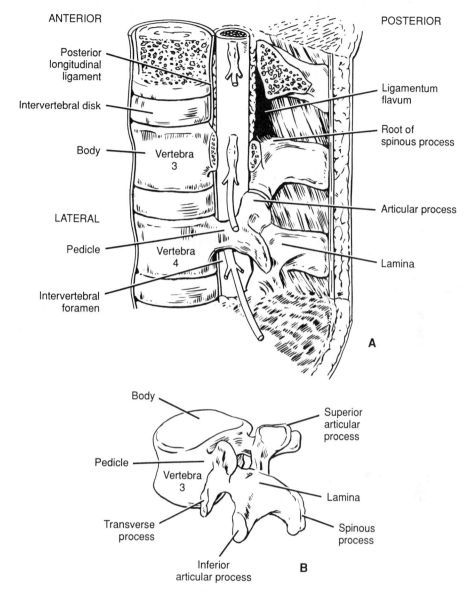

Figure 16–14. Boundaries of the epidural space.

In the lateralmost aspect of the epidural space, the dural cuffs are encountered. In this area, the dura is quite thin and provides access to the cerebrospinal fluid for local anesthetics and forms the basis for epidural anesthesia.

The very large spinal nerves at L5 and S1 are the most difficult nerves to block in the epidural space, and surgical procedures involving the distribution of these nerve roots can be more difficult with epidural anesthesia than with other regional techniques.

Local anesthetics for epidural anesthesia are not injected directly onto nervous tissues but require diffusion from the point of injection. The amount of drug injected is thus considerably greater per spinal segment than it would be for the same number of segments being injected for spinal anesthesia.

APPLIED PHYSIOLOGY FOR EPIDURAL ANESTHESIA

Epidural anesthesia is characterized by physiologic responses similar to those observed with spinal anesthesia, related to the highest level of sympathetic, sensory, and motor blockade. The consequences of sympathetic and motor block are described in the physiology section at the beginning of this chapter; some differences will be described here.

Segmental Blockade

With spinal anesthesia, the effect on sensory, motor, or sympathetic function is uniform from the lowest sacral nerve roots to the highest level blocked. With epidural anesthesia, this may not be the case. Because epidural anesthesia can be performed at any level of the spinal cord and with any concentration of local anesthetic, it is possible to block only a portion of the spinal cord. An example is obstetric epidural analgesia. The needle and catheter is introduced in the midlumbar spine, and enough agent is injected to achieve blockade at and slightly proximal to the level injected. The concentration of the agent is chosen to provide chiefly sympathetic and sensory blockade, with sparing of motor blockade. This is accomplished by selection of a lower concentration of the agent or with bupivacaine, which is known to preserve much motor function at low concentrations. The pain of the first stage of labor is mediated by T10–L1 and is effectively interrupted by a block that covers sensory and sympathetic modalities from the lower thoracic and lumbar regions. This block allows the parturient to be free of pain but still capable of the motor activity called for as labor proceeds from stage 1 to stage 2. If dense sensory and motor blockade of the perineum is required, this segmental block is converted to a more dense sacral and lumbar epidural block by placing the patient in the head-up position and injecting a stronger concentration of the local anesthetic. In the case of bupivacaine, this would be 0.5% as opposed to 0.25% or less, which provides only analgesia with minimal motor block.

Another example of segmental blockade involves the introduction of an epidural catheter and needle in the midthoracic region in order to provide anesthesia or analgesia for an upper abdominal incision, eg, for cholecystectomy. Blockade of sensation from the upper abdomen is achieved with a low dose of local anesthetic. This is possible because the local anesthetic is injected directly into the epidural space at the level where the segments to be blocked originate—as opposed to placing the needle or catheter in the lumbar region and filling the entire epidural space from this level.

Differential Blockade
(Table 16–6)
Some aspects of differential blockade were discussed in the previous paragraphs in reference to agent selection and concentration in order to provide a different quality of block for different purposes. Specific sparing of motor function or specific attempts to achieve dense motor blockade are examples. Strong concentrations of drugs such as 0.75% bupivacaine, 2% lidocaine, or 2% mepivacaine are associated with dense motor blocks, whereas 0.25% bupivacaine, 1% lidocaine, or 1% mepivacaine are associated with sensory block with variable motor block. Each of these concentrations is selected for different indications. Hip surgery is an example where dense motor block would be an advantage, facilitating exposure and placement of endoprosthesis.

TECHNIQUE OF EPIDURAL ANESTHESIA

Safety
An epidural anesthetic must be performed in a working space which is equipped for management of an airway, rapid placement of an endotracheal tube, and full cardiopulmonary resuscitation. The minimal components essential for these procedures are listed in Table 17–1.

At times, epidural anesthesia is instituted in stages. The first stage can be conducted in a nonanesthetizing station involving placement of the epidural needle and catheter without injection of either a test dose or the major portion of the agent for full epidural block. However, even this should be done in an environment where minimum safety precautions are observed, since local anesthetic must be infiltrated into the skin, some pain may be involved, and there is a possibility of allergy or vasovagal response to pain. This is particularly true if the patient is in labor, since hemodynamic or ventilatory embarrassment of the mother rapidly puts both her and the fetus in jeopardy.

Proper verification of what substances are being injected into the epidural space is essential. With epidural catheters now being used for prolonged periods for postoperative pain relief, it is vitally important that catheters be clearly labeled and that nothing be injected that is not properly identified. Every precaution

Table 16–6. Agents for epidural anesthesia.

Agent	Concentration	Onset	Sensory Block	Motor Block
Chloroprocaine	2% 3%	Fast Fast	Analgesic Dense	Mild to moderate Dense
Lidocaine	≥1% 1.5% 2%	Intermediate Intermediate Intermediate	Analgesic Dense Dense	Minimal Mild to moderate Dense
Mepivacaine	1% 2%	Intermediate Intermediate	Analgesic Dense	Minimal Dense
Prilocaine	2% 3%	Fast Fast	Dense Dense	Minimal Dense
Bupivacaine	≥0.25% 0.375–0.5% 0.75%	Slow Slow Slow	Analgesic Dense Dense	Minimal Mild to moderate Moderate to dense

must be taken also to prevent inadvertent injection of contaminated or noxious solutions.

Preparation of the Patient

A. Informed Consent: Consent for epidural anesthesia must be obtained in the same way as for spinal anesthesia. The possibility of inadvertent dural puncture must be mentioned, along with the high incidence of headache if this occurs. However, the relatively low "wet tap" rate ($< 1\%$) in the experienced operator's hands can also be mentioned as well as the fact that if severe post-lumbar puncture cephalalgia occurs, treatment with a very high success rate (epidural blood patch) is available. If the epidural catheter will be left in place for postoperative pain relief— especially if it is placed to be used in conjunction with general anesthesia and designed mainly for postoperative pain relief—this should be mentioned along with the types of monitoring and the quality of the pain relief the patient should expect. If epidural opioids are planned, additional discussion of the possible complications—especially respiratory depression, itching, and urinary retention—should be mentioned along with the types of postoperative follow-up and monitoring that will be used.

B. Preoperative Evaluation: Preoperative evaluation involves the same considerations as those discussed in preparing a patient for spinal anesthesia. However, information about coexisting diseases may make further physical examination or laboratory investigation more important prior to placement of an epidural catheter. An example is the parturient with preeclampsia. Some patients with preeclampsia may have either a decreased platelet count or abnormalities of prothrombin time (PT) and partial thromboplastin time (PTT). These patients are at increased risk for developing a vascular complication associated with placement of an epidural needle or catheter, and this makes the diagnosis of preeclampsia a strong indication for evaluation of the coagulation status.

Certain cardiac valvular lesions such as aortic stenosis and idiopathic hypertrophic subaortic stenosis (IHSS) are associated with poor hemodynamic toleration of sudden drops in systemic vascular resistance. Knowing that these lesions are present allows the anesthesiologist to decide if an epidural anesthetic can be safely administered and determines the speed with which the local anesthetic is injected if an epidural anesthetic is chosen.

Specific details of the planned surgical procedure also influence the choice of epidural anesthesia. Obviously, an epidural anesthetic will be selected for procedures in anatomic regions where the block can be counted on to be reliably solid. This includes the lower extremities, perineum, pelvis, hips, lower abdomen, and even perhaps the upper abdomen. However, epidural anesthesia may not block the largest nerve roots, which makes it less than ideal for procedures in the L5 and S1 dermatomes (around the ankle and foot). Spinal anesthesia may be preferred for procedures in these dermatomes if the procedure is short in duration and regional anesthetic is strongly indicated.

C. Laboratory Assessment: Laboratory assessment for epidural anesthesia is the same as for spinal anesthesia .

D. Premedication: Premedication for epidural anesthesia is virtually identical to that for spinal anesthesia. Because the needle is larger and because the epidural space may be more difficult to find than the subarachnoid space, it may be important to have a patient who is informed, is willing to cooperate, and is adequately premedicated with a good anxiolytic and perhaps an analgesic prior to attempting epidural anesthesia. An uncooperative, agitated patient can be a considerable risk for inadvertent dural puncture and even serious injury to neural structures during conduct of epidural anesthesia.

Equipment

A. The Epidural Needle: (Figure 16–15.) The standard epidural needle is typically 16–18 gauge, 3 inches long, and has a blunt bevel with a gentle curve of 15–30 degrees at the tip. This blunt bevel and curve allow the needle to pass through ligamentum flavum and abut against dura, pushing it away rather than penetrating it. This creates the negative pressure that identifies the epidural space. The most common version of this needle is referred to as a **Tuohy needle,** and

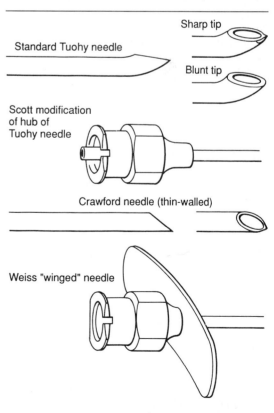

Figure 16–15. Epidural needles.

the curved tip is referred to as a **Huber tip.** The Huber tip is particularly important for performance of the first several epidurals by a beginner, since the incidence of dural puncture without use of the curved tip will be unacceptably high until experience is gained.

Another commonly used epidural needle is the **Crawford needle,** a thin-walled needle with a straight blunt bevel without the curved Huber tip. This needle allows the catheter to pass directly through the end of the needle. In situations where catheter advancement into the epidural space is difficult, this needle may be preferred.

Difficult catheter placement is encountered more frequently in approaches to the epidural spaces which are off the midline. Some of the newer disposable epidural needles have introducer devices set into the hub of the needle that facilitate threading the catheter. The needles that were first manufactured with this modification of the hub were referred to as **Scott needles.**

Other newer disposable epidural needles are manufactured with the Touhy/Huber configuration and contain wings at the junction of the shaft of the needle with the hub, allowing easier control of needle advancement with finger pressure. The original winged needle was referred to as a **Weiss needle**.

Technical Performance of a Block

A. Identification of the Epidural Space: The epidural space is entered after the tip of the needle passes through the ligamentum flavum, indenting the dura and creating negative pressure in the epidural space, which up to that point had been only a potential space. Identification of the precise moment when the needle is advanced into this space decreases the likelihood that the needle will puncture the dura. Methods for identifying this space fall into two broad categories: the "loss of resistance technique" and the "hanging drop" technique.

1. Loss of resistance technique–This is the most common way to identify the epidural space and the easiest way to teach the beginner. It involves direction of the needle through the dermis into the interspinous ligament, which is verified by firm resistance. At this point, the needle introducer is removed and a glass syringe is connected that is filled with air or saline. If the needle tip is correctly buried within the substance of the interspinous ligament, attempted injection will result in a firm feeling and an inability to inject. This signifies that the needle is within the substance of the ligament and can be advanced.

There are two ways of checking the progress of the advancing needle. One involves a two-handed grip on the syringe and needle with continuous firm pressure on the hub as the needle moves forward. As the needle enters the epidural space, the hub advances and the contents of the needle are injected ("loss of resistance" technique). Another approach involves the less cumbersome advancement of the needle a few millimeters at a time, stopping and checking by touching the plunger and confirming that the needle tip is still within the ligament or has moved to where loss of resistance occurs. The latter approach is quicker and more practical but requires some experience to avoid advancing the needle through the epidural space and into the dura without stopping in the correct location. This may be difficult for the beginner, causing a high wet-tap rate.

Whether to inject saline or air with the loss of resistance technique depends on the preference of the practitioner. There have been some reports of air bubbles causing difficulty with incomplete or patchy blocks; however, this probably occurs only with large amounts of air.

2. Hanging drop technique–With this technique, the needle (preferably a wing needle) is placed in the interspinous ligament, the hub is filled with solution—most commonly saline—and 1 drop is allowed to hang from the hub of the needle. As the needle is advanced through the ligamentous structures, the drop does not move; however, on penetration of the ligamentum flavum, with creation of negative pressure in the epidural space, this drop of fluid is drawn into the needle, signifying proper placement in the epidural space. In experienced hands, this is a reliable technique; however, with any tissue obstruction, loss of continuity in the fluid column within the needle will prevent the drop from being drawn into the hub of the needle, so that passage through the epidural space may not be recognized—the first clue to passage through the ligamentum flavum may be the rush of cerebrospinal fluid from dural puncture. As a consequence, the hanging drop technique is usually employed only by more experienced practitioners or is reserved for the paramedian approach to the thoracic epidural space.

B. Level Selected: Three segments of the spinal column where epidural anesthesia is applied are the lumbar, thoracic, and cervical epidural regions. Epidural anesthesia is also performed in the sacral region of the spinal column (caudal anesthesia). The approaches to each of these spaces are described below.

1. Lumbar epidural anesthesia–Lumbar epidural anesthesia may be performed using the midline or paramedian approach, as in spinal anesthesia in the lumbar region.

a. Midline technique–(Figure 16–16.) The patient is positioned, prepped, and draped in a sterile manner, and the interspace at the level of the iliac crest is identified. The interspace easiest to identify is selected, typically at the L3–4 or L4–5 interspace; a skin wheal is raised; and dermal puncture is made with an 18-gauge needle. The epidural needle is introduced through the dermal puncture and advanced slightly cephalad, taking into account the cephalad location of the interlaminar space in reference to the superior spinous process. Once the needle is seated in the midline ligamentous structure, the syringe is connected and firm resistance is identified. It is important that a feeling of being in the ligament is noted at this point, since any equivocal feeling may result in the impression of loss of resistance into a paraspinous muscle area or

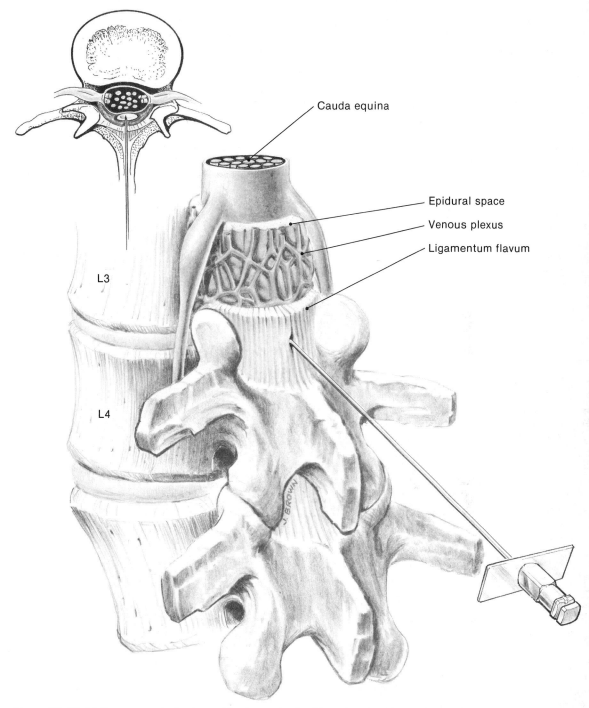

Figure 16–16. Midline approach, lumbar epidural anesthesia. (Reproduced, with permission, from Katz J: *Atlas of Regional Anesthesia.* Appleton-Century-Crofts, 1985.)

fatty deposit, which will result in injection of local anesthetic into a space other than the epidural space and a failed block. Once firm placement of the needle into the ligament is verified, the needle is advanced and the epidural space is identified using the loss of resistance technique described earlier.

b. Paramedian approach–(Figure 16–17.) The paramedian approach is selected in cases where prior surgery or advanced degenerative joint disease contraindicate the midline approach. This is a difficult technique for a beginner, since advancement into firm ligaments with change of resistance upon entering the

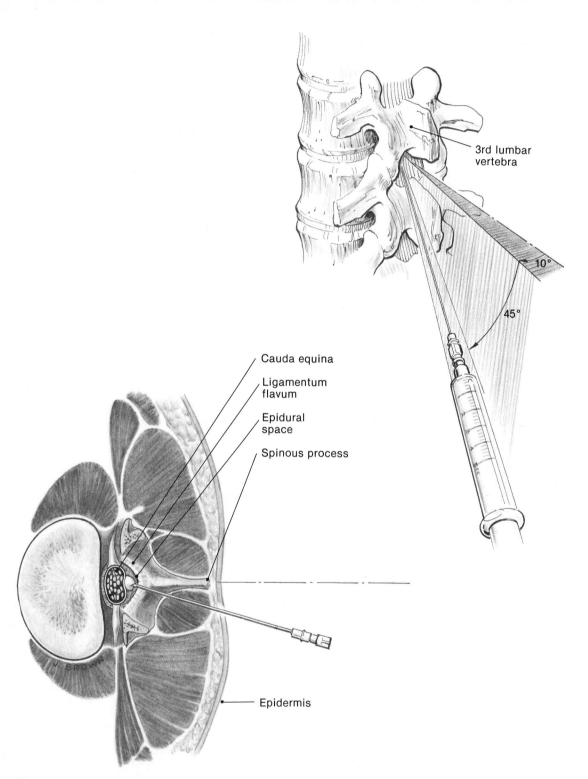

3rd lumbar
vertebra

10°

45°

Cauda equina

Ligamentum
flavum

Epidural
space

Spinous process

Epidermis

Figure 16–17. Paramedian approach, lumbar epidural anesthesia. (Reproduced, with permission, from Katz J: *Atlas of Regional Anesthesia.* Appleton-Century-Crofts, 1985.)

ligamentum flavum does not occur; the needle advances mostly through the paraspinous muscle mass, and resistance is felt only on encountering the ligamentum flavum.

The patient is positioned, prepared, and draped as for the midline approach, and a skin wheal is raised 2–4 cm lateral to the lowest aspect of the superior spinous process. Dermal puncture is made, and the needle is directed toward the midline with the same cephalad deflection used as in the midline approach. The needle is advanced toward the midline in such a way that the midline will be encountered 4–6 cm under the surface. As the dermal structures are penetrated, the syringe is connected to the needle; and as the paraspinous muscle mass is entered, some resistance to injection will be noted. This minimal resistance is verified repeatedly until a sudden increase in resistance is noted when the needle reaches the ligamentum flavum.

In addition to increase in resistance, passage through the ligamentum flavum often transmits a characteristic gritty, coarse sensation. The needle passes through the ligamentum flavum and loss of resistance is encountered, identifying entry into the epidural space. Difficulty with threading a conventional epidural catheter using the curved Touhy needle and the paramedian approach in the lumbar space may be related to the rounded needle tip and the angled approach to the midline, which makes catheter advancement too oblique. For this reason, some practitioners prefer the straight Crawford needle for a paramedian approach to lumbar epidural anesthesia.

2. Thoracic epidural anesthesia–Thoracic epidural anesthesia is more difficult than lumbar epidural anesthesia, and the possibility for injury to the spinal cord is greater. Therefore, it is important that the practitioner be thoroughly familiar with lumbar midline and paramedian approaches to epidural anesthesia prior to attempting thoracic epidural block. Because of the short oblique configuration of the spinous process, thoracic epidural block is typically performed using the paramedian approach, though a midline approach is possible and will be described.

a. Midline approach–(Figure 16–18.) With both approaches to epidural anesthesia, the dermatomes to be anesthetized are typically those at which the needle is introduced. The correct interspace is identified with the patient in a sitting position, prepared and draped in the usual manner. With the upper thoracic segments, the angle of the spinous process is more oblique, and a steep cephalad direction is taken. In the lower thoracic regions, the cephalad approach is still chosen, but it becomes more and more like the cephalad direction used with lumbar epidural anesthesia. The ligaments are identified rapidly and the needle is advanced through the relatively short distance of the supraspinous and interspinous ligaments, and the ligamentum flavum is identified usually no more than 3–4 cm beneath the skin. The sudden loss of resistance

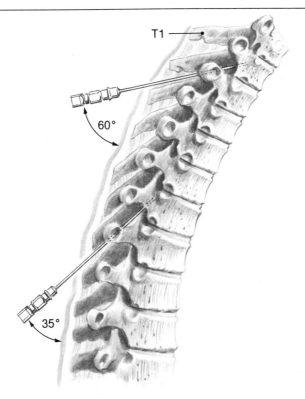

Figure 16–18. Thoracic epidural middle approach. (Reproduced, with permission, from Katz J: *Atlas of Regional Anesthesia.* Appleton-Century-Crofts, 1985.)

identifies the epidural space, and the conduct of epidural anesthesia continues. With all techniques of epidural anesthesia above the lumbar region, the possibility of direct contact with the spinal cord must be considered; during any attempts at identifying the epidural space, if intense, searing pain occurs, the possibility that the epidural needle is in direct contact with the spinal cord must be considered and the needle should be removed and replaced, perhaps at a different level. Figure 16–18 shows the angles of approach by segment for the midline thoracic epidural block.

b. Paramedian approach–(Figure 16–19.) With the paramedian approach, the correct interspace is identified, the back is prepared and draped in the customary manner, and a skin wheal is raised approximately 2 cm lateral to the caudal border of the superior spinous process. In this case, the needle is placed almost perpendicular to the skin with a minimal angle toward the midline of 10–15 degrees and advanced until the lamina or pedicle of the vertebrae is contacted. The needle is pulled back and redirected in a slightly cephalad manner in an attempt to walk off the lamina. When this is accomplished, the tip of the needle should be in contact with ligamentum flavum. The syringe is connected at this point and the needle is advanced, using either loss of resistance or the hanging drop technique to verify proper placement. As with the paramedian approach in the lumbar region, the dis-

tance the needle must be advanced before ligamentum flavum is traversed is quite short, and the epidural space will be entered quite rapidly. The angle of approach is graphically depicted in Figure 16–19.

3. Cervical epidural anesthesia–(Figure 16–20.) Cervical epidural anesthesia is most typically done in the midline with the patient in a sitting position with neck flexed. The correct interspace to be blocked is identified, the area is prepared and draped in the usual manner, and a skin wheal is raised. The epidural needle is inserted in the midline—typically at the interspace between C5 and C6 or between C6 and C7—seated in the spinal ligaments, and advanced into the epidural space using either the loss of resistance or, more often, the hanging drop technique. The advantage of the midline technique and the relatively horizontal alignment of the cervical spine's process are depicted in Figure 16–20.

Strategies for Injection of the Anesthetic Agent

After the needle is placed in the epidural space, there are a number of options for subsequent placement of the full dose of local anesthetic. With many practitioners, the first injection is invariably a test dose (see above). This can be introduced either through the needle or—prior to injecting any local anesthetic—the catheter can be introduced into the epidural space and a

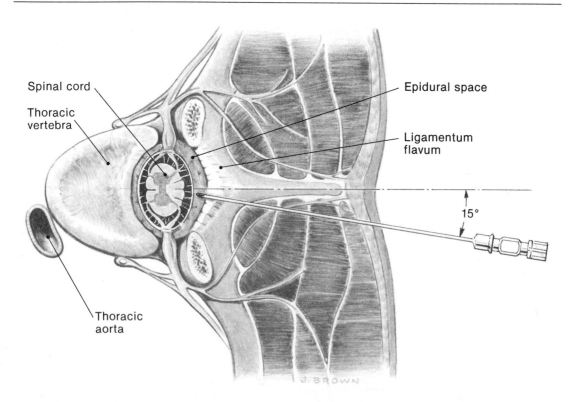

Spinal cord

Thoracic vertebra

Epidural space

Ligamentum flavum

15°

Thoracic aorta

Figure 16–19. Thoracic epidural paramedian approach. (Reproduced, with permission, from Katz J: *Atlas of Regional Anesthesia.* Appleton-Century-Crofts, 1985.)

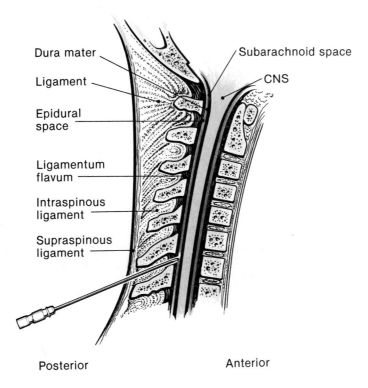

Dura mater

Ligament

Epidural space

Ligamentum flavum

Intraspinous ligament

Supraspinous ligament

Subarachnoid space

CNS

Posterior

Anterior

Figure 16–20. Cervical epidural approach. (Reproduced, with permission, from Katz J: *Atlas of Regional Anesthesia.* Appleton-Century-Crofts, 1985.)

test dose placed through the epidural catheter. It is possible to inject the test dose through the needle and, while waiting for the results, thread the epidural catheter—though many practitioners feel that the epidural catheter must then also receive a test dose injection. Alternatively, after the 3-mL test dose, the full dose of local anesthetic can be injected through the needle in incremental doses and a catheter then placed into the epidural space—or, for short surgical procedures, the needle can be simply removed. A theoretic advantage to injection through the needle prior to placement of the catheter is distention of the epidural space with local anesthetic, which may facilitate placement of the catheter. A theoretic disadvantage is the possibility that the injected anesthetic could prevent correct identification of a paresthesia and perhaps contribute to injury of nervous tissue. Clinical experience has been that either technique is acceptable and associated with a high success rate of catheter placement and a minimal risk to central nervous system structures.

Incremental dosing is an important safety precaution in the conduct of epidural anesthesia. After injection of the test dose, many practitioners feel that one should never inject more than 5 mL at a time and that each injection must be preceded and followed by aspiration to look for cerebrospinal fluid or blood. Limiting the total volume of each injection to 5 mL and allowing a reasonable interval between injections helps ensure that if the subarachnoid space or a blood

vessel is entered, only a small amount will be injected. While 5 mL of a full-strength epidural agent injected directly into the subarachnoid space may be associated with a relatively high subarachnoid block, this is still preferable to accidental injection of the total calculated dose, which would certainly result in a total spinal block of long duration.

Choice of Local Anesthetic

The choice of agent and its concentration are determined by the anticipated duration and the type of surgical procedure and the balanced need for sensory and motor blockade. Table 16–6 lists the agents and concentrations available, with onset times and the quality of sensory and motor block. For example, orthopedic surgery on the lower extremity would require dense sensory anesthesia with moderate to complete (dense) motor blockade.

The use of a catheter permits selection of agents of short or long duration of action. If the single-dose technique is used, agents of either intermediate or long duration are chosen. The orthopedic procedure in our example could be performed using 3% chloroprocaine, which has a fast onset of action and results in dense sensory and motor block; lidocaine or mepivacaine at 1.5% or 2%, either of which has an intermediate onset of action and results in good motor and sensory block; or bupivacaine at 0.5–0.75%, which has a slow onset of action and results in dense sensory anesthesia and varying degrees of motor block. The lower concentrations of bupivacaine are not suitable for procedures requiring dense motor block.

Safety of the agent, the total dose planned, and the practitioner's experience with the agent also enter into the choice of local anesthetic.

FACTORS THAT AFFECT EPIDURAL ANESTHESIA

Dosage

The proper dose for epidural anesthesia is determined by many factors but can be simplified to a range of 1–2 mL of anesthetic for each spinal segment to be anesthetized. This means that if the injection is made at the lumbar epidural space, a large volume is required to achieve motor and sensory block for abdominal surgery. A small amount of agent will be necessary if *analgesia* is the objective and cervical epidural injection is the chosen route. Another factor that influences dosage is the desire for segmental blockade, as in lumbar epidural injection for obstetric analgesia or midthoracic epidural injection for upper abdominal or lower thoracic postoperative analgesia.

The dose selected is always given as a range, since the effect of local anesthetic within the epidural space is not predictable. Furthermore, the size of the epidural space is extremely variable in different patients and changes in composition and size with age.

Local anesthetics in the epidural space are thought to act by two possible mechanisms: (1) by acting directly at the nerve roots and dorsal ganglia outside the dura after diffusion through the intervertebral foramen; or (2) by acting in the subarachnoid space either after diffusion across the dura and meninges or perhaps through the intervertebral foramina via the dural sleeve or epidural lymphatic chain.

The dose of local anesthetic is a function of the volume injected and the concentration of the solution, and the response is not necessarily the same for each dose if volume and concentration are varied. A higher volume of a lower concentration of local anesthetic will result in a higher sensory level with less motor block, whereas a lower volume of higher concentration will result in a lower but denser sensory and motor level. With low concentrations of local anesthetics, the control of motor blockade becomes unimportant, and the volume to be injected is based on the need for sensory level only.

With epidural anesthesia, incremental dosing is possible through the epidural catheter, and the dosage selected can be titrated by serial injection.

Assessment of the success of epidural block should be specific to the anticipated response. Sympathetic block can be assessed by measuring skin temperature, sensory block by pinprick, and motor block by reference to the **Bromage scale,** in which "no block" is defined as full ability to flex the knees and feet, "partial block" as ability to flex the knees and resist gravity with full movement of the feet, "almost complete block" as inability to flex the knees but retained ability to flex the feet, and "complete block" as inability to move the legs or feet.

An important characteristic of each local anesthetic is the time at which redosing must occur to maintain continuous epidural anesthesia. Repeat doses should be injected before the block significantly regresses and the patient experiences pain. This is most easily evaluated by assessing the sensory level. With epidural anesthesia, a characteristic feature of each local anesthetic is its "time to two-segment regression," ie, the time from injection through the time when the maximum sensory level regresses two segments (Table 16–7). When two-segment regression has occurred, one should reinject one-third to one-half the volume of the first dose. Some clinicians will reinject the epidural catheter on a timed interval without clinical assessment, based on their experience with the agent, but because of individual patient variability this may result in either very high or very low block.

Patient Age

The dose required to achieve the same level of anesthesia decreases with age, probably because of the age-related decrease in size or compliance of the epidural space. The same injected dose and volume will have a higher cephalad spread in geriatric patients than in the young adult. Titrating the dose to a desired clinical effect is the best means of adjusting for the variability of epidural anesthesia with advancing age.

Weight & Height

There appears to be minimal correlation between the cephalad spread of epidural anesthesia and weight in adults. A possible exception to this rule is the morbidly obese patient, for whom a reduction of the dose is necessary since in such cases the epidural space is smaller.

The patient's height, however, may have some correlation with cephalad spread. At a patient height of 5 feet, the lower end of the dosage range—1 mL per segment—should be used, with larger volumes approaching 2 mL per segment for taller patients. Complicated calculations have been devised based on height in inches above 5 feet, but the practical approach to dosage with tall patients is probably to give a moderate initial injection followed by clinical assessment and titration via epidural catheter to the desired clinical effect.

Table 16–7. Times to two-segment regression.

Agent	Time Range (min)
Chloroprocaine	50–70
Lidocaine	90–150
Mepivacaine	120–160
Prilocaine	90–130
Bupivacaine	200–260

Posture

The patient's posture during injection was once thought to influence the spread of epidural anesthetic agent because of the effect of gravity or the effect of positioning on the dimensions of the epidural space. Subsequent studies have shown that such differences in response are probably due to variability of the contour of the epidural space itself and not an effect of posture.

For procedures involving the larger L5–S1 and S2 nerve roots, injection of the dose—often through the needle—with the patient in the sitting position may deliver more anesthetic directly to the large nerve roots with a greater likelihood of successful block.

Vasoconstrictors

With epidural anesthesia, the effects of vasoconstrictors are not well defined. In the case of bupivacaine, epinephrine does not affect the time to two-segment regression, whereas in the case of lidocaine and mepivacaine many clinicians feel that the addition of epinephrine does confer a longer duration of action. Since the total dose of local anesthetic required for epidural anesthesia is greater and the possibility of toxicity therefore greater, local vasoconstriction with resulting decreased vascular absorption and lower peak plasma levels are a definite advantage. Local vasoconstriction may also improve the quality of the motor and sensory block.

pH Adjustment of Local Anesthetics

Local anesthetics provided commercially are stored at a pH between 3.5 and 5.5 for chemical stability and bacteriostasis. Being weak bases, they exist chiefly in the ionic form at this pH. While the concentration of the ionic forms favors spread within the epidural space, the onset of block depends on penetration of the lipid nerve cell membranes, and most movement across lipid membranes is by the local anesthetic molecule in the nonionic form. This has led to various modifications of local anesthetic solutions, including carbonation and, more recently, addition of sodium bicarbonate to raise the local anesthetic agent to physiologic pH immediately before injection. This favors the concentration of the nonionic form and may accelerate the onset and perhaps increase the density of the block achieved.

Failure of Epidural Block

Successful epidural blockade depends on many technical factors. Blockade at too low a sensory level can occur if the initial dose is inadequate and if insufficient time is allowed for spread of the anesthetic prior to surgical incision. Even if a slow-onset agent has been selected, if an inadequate level is identified and surgery—for reasons of expediency—is about to commence, a more rapid, shorter-acting agent can be injected through the catheter and the level brought up rapidly with subsequent return to the primary agent.

Segmental sparing is occasionally associated with failure of epidural anesthesia. The anatomy of the epidural space is variable, and some investigators have even demonstrated midline septation of the epidural space. Some practitioners feel that advancement of an epidural catheter farther than 4 cm into the epidural space permits the tip of catheter to migrate from the midline, perhaps into a dural sleeve area, resulting in poor distribution of local anesthetic in the epidural space or unilateral spread based on midline septation. The clinical effect in such cases can sometimes be dealt with by turning the patient to the side where segmental sparing has occurred and reinjecting the catheter. As with low blockade, this anatomic variation should be identified well before the start of surgery. Inadequate motor blockade can also be associated with failure of epidural anesthesia. If this happens, a higher concentration of agent can be used, or one can be selected that has stronger motor block characteristics.

Sacral sparing may also lead to failure of epidural anesthesia, especially for surgery on the lower leg. This has been discussed earlier and is related to the size of the nerve roots. Initial injection in the sitting position is a way of minimizing this problem. If sacral sparing occurs after surgical preparation, elevating the head of the bed and reinjecting the catheter can sometimes achieve deeper block of these large nerve roots. Visceral pain during abdominal surgery is related to stimulation of the peritoneum, and even though the dermatomes involved in lower abdominal surgery are low thoracic, it may be necessary to block the high thoracic region if stimulation of the peritoneum or traction on intra-abdominal structures such as the inguinal ligament or spermatic cord is anticipated.

Several technical factors can be associated with difficulty or failure of epidural anesthesia. **Inadvertent dural puncture** can require withdrawal and repositioning of the needle or an approach at a different level. Occasionally, a wet tap can be converted to subarachnoid anesthesia by injecting an appropriate dose of a spinal anesthetic agent directly into the cerebrospinal fluid or perhaps advancing a catheter through the epidural needle into the subarachnoid space for continuous spinal anesthesia. Similarly, with correct needle placement, the epidural catheter occasionally will be advanced into the subarachnoid space. This is verified by a free flow of cerebrospinal fluid, and the practitioner must then choose between removing the catheter and redoing the epidural or using the catheter for a continuous spinal technique.

A more insidious but rare occurrence is **cannulation of the subdural space.** This is probably related to partial puncture of the dura, with the lumen of the needle not freely in contact with cerebrospinal fluid but with the catheter threading out through the partially occluded tip of the needle and into the subdural space. Cerebrospinal fluid will not be aspirated, but injection of local anesthetic will have a result very different from injection in the epidural space. The consequences of subdural injection of local anesthetics are extremely variable, with reports of very high unilateral blocks and sparing of one modality with complete anesthesia of the other, eg, full sensory anesthesia with no motor block or full motor block with minimal sensory anesthesia. The onset is extremely slow and not appropriate for the volume of local anesthetic injected. Without myelography, the diagnosis is one of exclusion.

Another technical factor associated with failure of epidural block is **cannulation of an epidural vein** by a needle or by the catheter. If cannulation occurs with the needle, it is usually withdrawn and reintroduced into the epidural space. If the catheter freely aspirates blood, it is withdrawn a short distance and injected with saline, and aspiration is repeated. Often the catheter is then no longer within the lumen of the vein. When venous cannulation occurs, an epinephrine-containing test dose is mandatory to verify that local anesthetic is not being injected directly into the venous circulation. If the test dose fails, the catheter must be removed and replaced.

A final cause of failed epidural anesthesia is **false loss of resistance.** In some young adults, the spinal ligaments are quite soft, and resistance to injection is not as distinct as the practitioner has become used to. The practitioner may believe the epidural space has been entered when the needle is in fact within the interspinous ligaments. Injection may then feel not quite as smooth as usual, and no anesthesia will result. An occasional patient may have some cystic degeneration within the substance of the ligament, and entry into this area will be incorrectly perceived as loss of resistance. This will be the case also if the practitioner is considerably off the midline in the midline approach and enters the paraspinous muscles, where minimal resistance will be felt. This too may be appreciated by the practitioner as loss of resistance, and injection of local anesthetic will again result in no anesthesia.

COMPLICATIONS

The types of complications that occur with epidural anesthesia are very similar to those associated with spinal anesthesia (see above). Some differences specific to epidural anesthesia will be presented.

Headache
Because of the large caliber of the needles used for epidural anesthesia, the incidence of headache from dural puncture is quite high, ranging from 40% to 80%. If a wet tap occurs and the epidural catheter is successfully repositioned at a different level, some investigators report as much as a 50% reduction in the ultimate incidence of headache. Injection of saline as a bolus or as a continuous infusion for 24 hours after wet tap also reduces the headache rate. Infusion of 10–15 mL of the patient's own blood through the catheter immediately prior to its removal is a promising technique whose usefulness is not yet established.

Problems With Subsequent Heparinization
If an epidural vein is entered either with the needle or catheter, heparinization should be withheld for a reasonable period of time. In the absence of vascular embarrassment with needle or catheter placement, the incidence of neurologic complications associated with hemorrhage was extremely low in one large series in which patients were subsequently heparinized after placement of an epidural catheter. The key to minimizing these complications is alert observation and monitoring in the postoperative period. Any sudden loss of recovered motor and sensory activity or sphincter tone may be associated with developing epidural hematoma. If postoperative pain control is going to be maintained with an epidural catheter in patients who have been heparinized, one must allow this block to subside periodically and verify that neurologic function is intact.

If a patient with an epidural catheter requires intraoperative anticoagulation that will be maintained into the postoperative period, there may be a problem about how to remove the catheter without placing the central nervous system at risk of injury from bleeding. Consultation with the surgical team may allow brief verified reversal of anticoagulation, removal of the epidural catheter, verification of an intact central nervous system, and then reinstitution of anticoagulation after a reasonable interval.

Infection
Epidural catheters in place for long surgical procedures and postoperative pain relief call for meticulous sterile technique. Sites need to be inspected, dressings changed regularly, and absolute aseptic technique used in preparation of solutions, handling of catheters, and connecting tubing and junctions. Signs of meningitis—nuchal rigidity, fever, and chilling—require urgent diagnostic verification and appropriate treatment to avoid major morbidity.

CAUDAL ANESTHESIA

Caudal anesthesia was actually the first anesthetic approach to the epidural space. The caudal space is the sacral component of the epidural space, and access is through the sacral hiatus, a midline defect of fusion of the caudalmost aspect of the sacrum. This space is not covered by bone but by the dense sacrococcygeal ligament, which is analogous to the supraspinous and interspinous ligaments of the lumbar, thoracic, and cervical spinal levels. It is densely adherent to ligamentum flavum, and the distinct changes in ligament density that one is accustomed to in other approaches to the epidural space do not occur at the sacral level.

INDICATIONS

Caudal anesthesia is indicated for surgical and obstetric procedures that involve the perineum and sacral distributions, such as the anorectal region. Caudal anesthesia is particularly well suited to anal surgery because such operations are performed with the patient in the prone position and because dense sensory anesthesia to the sacral dermatomes can be achieved with limited proximal spread. Historically, caudal anesthesia was used in obstetric practice for anesthesia of the perineum as part of the "double-catheter" technique: A lumbar epidural catheter was placed for segmental epidural analgesia for the first stage of labor and a caudal catheter for segmental analgesia of the perineum for the second stage. This technique has been largely abandoned in favor of the lumbar epidural catheter alone, which is easier to place and better tolerated by the patient.

Caudal anesthesia has increasing application in pediatrics as a means of postoperative pain relief for operations on the lower extremities, perineum, male genitals, and lower abdomen. The procedure is technically easier in children, as the sacral hiatus is easily identified and the sacrococcygeal ligament is less affected by calcification and degenerative joint disease.

CONTRAINDICATIONS

The contraindications for caudal anesthesia are the same as for any central block. Furthermore, because of the proximity to the perianal region, cutaneous or subcutaneous infection must be carefully ruled out; even a suspicion of infection is an absolute contraindication to caudal anesthesia. The presence of sacral decubitus ulcers is also a very strong contraindication to caudal anesthesia, since the risk of injecting bacteria into the central nervous system would be unacceptably high. Morbid obesity represents a relative contraindication because identifying the sacral hiatus and the sacrococcygeal ligament becomes more difficult as the amount of adipose tissue increases.

APPLIED ANATOMY OF CAUDAL ANESTHESIA

The sacrum consists of the fused vertebral bodies and posterior elements of the sacral segments of the spinal column. It articulates on the cephalad side with the lumbar fifth vertebra and on the caudad side with the coccyx. The ventral surface is characterized by segmental foramina on both sides of the midline, which allow passage of the sacral nerves. Posteriorly,

in a similar lateral location, are the dorsal foramina (Figure 16–21). These are smaller than the ventral counterparts and fully closed by overlying muscles. The remnants of spinous processes are identifiable at the first four segments as tubercles, with the area where the tubercle of the fifth segment would be forming the sacral hiatus.

There is great normal variation in the anatomy of the sacrum. Of particular importance to the anesthesiologist is the fact that the sacral hiatus is absent in as many as 5–10% of people, and entry into the caudal epidural canal in these adults is impossible. The sacral hiatus is filled by the sacrococcygeal ligament, which is the structure that a needle being used to perform caudal anesthesia will enter if the sacral hiatus is correctly located. Ventral to the sacrococcygeal ligament is the sacral canal. Within the sacrum, the sacral canal contains the dural sac—which usually terminates at the level of the second sacral segment in adults but occasionally extends lower—as well as the anterior and posterior divisions of the sacral nerves and their dorsal root ganglia enclosed in dural sleeves. There is a rich epidural venous plexus and areolar connective tissue, similar to the lumbar epidural region. Ventral to the sacral canal is the solid body of the sacrum, which is an osseous structure. It can be entered by a needle and contains bone marrow and so represents a route of rapid injection of local anesthetic into the circulation, with the potential for toxic reactions.

APPLIED PHYSIOLOGY OF CAUDAL BLOCKADE

The physiology of caudal blockade is essentially the same as that described for epidural anesthesia in the lumbar region. The extent of the physiologic response to caudal blockade is related to the level achieved, which in turn is related directly to the volume of drug administered. It is possible to create a midthoracic or even a high thoracic anesthetic level from the caudal region by injecting very large volumes of local anesthetic. If this occurs, the physiologic response is indistinguishable from the response to lumbar epidural anesthesia. The extreme variability in caudal anatomy—and specifically the configuration of the sacral canal—makes the performance of high epidural anesthesia from the caudal route extremely variable and rarely used.

CAUDAL ANESTHESIA TECHNIQUE

Safety

Informed consent, preoperative evaluation, physical examination, laboratory investigation, and premedication are all essentially the same as for lumbar epidural anesthesia (see above).

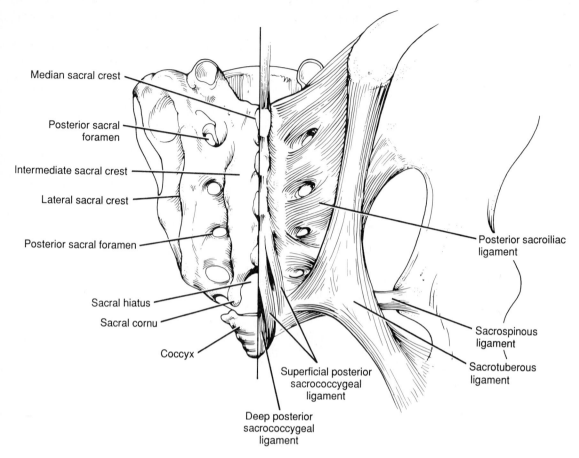

Median sacral crest

Posterior sacral foramen

Intermediate sacral crest

Lateral sacral crest

Posterior sacral foramen

Sacral hiatus

Sacral cornu

Coccyx

Posterior sacroiliac ligament

Sacrospinous ligament

Sacrotuberous ligament

Superficial posterior sacrococcygeal ligament

Deep posterior sacrococcygeal ligament

Figure 16–21. Sacrum, dorsal surface.

Equipment

In contrast to lumbar epidural anesthesia, however, the equipment used for caudal anesthesia is relatively simple. For adult caudal anesthesia, a 1½- to 2-inch, 22-gauge needle is selected; for continuous anesthesia, a 20- or 22-gauge intravenous catheter is placed by the catheter over-needle-approach. A Tuohy epidural needle can be used, but its large size makes successful introduction into the sacral canal more difficult than when smaller needles are used. If a Tuohy needle is successfully placed in the sacral canal, a standard epidural catheter can be threaded.

Conduct of the Block
(Figures 16–16 to 16–22)

The patient is placed prone on a surgical bed flexed in such a way that the patient's head and legs are lower than the hips. Alternatively, the patient can be placed in the lateral decubitus fetal position, with shoulders and knees flexed. This is the only position available for the pregnant patient. The sacral area is prepared with antimicrobial solution, and with sterile technique the practitioner attempts with a finger of the nondominant hand to identify the sacral hiatus. If this is difficult,

placement of the finger in the midline midway between the tip of the coccyx and the level of the posterior superior iliac spine should yield some bony irregularity that suggests an opening. Once the sacral hiatus is identified, a skin wheal is raised and the 20- to 22-gauge 2-inch needle is inserted perpendicular to the skin until the ligament is encountered (noted as an increase in resistance). At this point, the needle is lowered from 90 degrees to an angle of approximately 45 degrees to the surface of the skin and advanced through the ligament. When loss of resistance is perceived, the needle is lowered parallel to the skin and advanced an additional 1–2 cm, ensuring penetration into the caudal epidural space but not to the distal end of the dural sac. At this point, the solution is injected. The volume of solution is based on the knowledge that 1–2 mL per spinal segment is necessary and on the known volume of the sacral canal. At least 12–15 mL appears to be required to adequately fill the sacral canal, taking into account the fairly broad openings of the ventral foramina that allow leakage of solution. Higher doses than necessary are often injected, since the levels achieved are usually not hemodynamically significant and result in successful anesthesia.

This technique is modified only slightly in pedi-

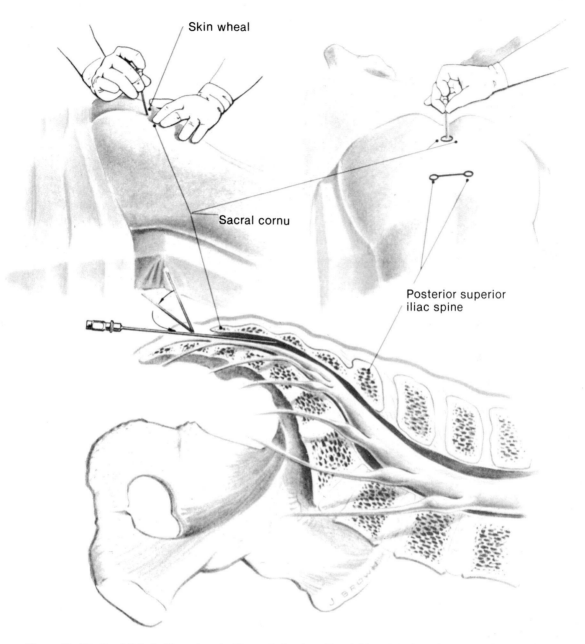

Skin wheal

Sacral cornu

Posterior superior
iliac spine

Figure 16–22. Caudal block. (Reproduced, with permission, from Katz J: *Atlas of Regional Anesthesia.* Appleton-Century-Crofts, 1985.)

atrics. After skin preparation, the sacral hiatus is usually easy to identify and feels like a concave open ("C-shaped") structure. The nondominant hand is placed over the sacral hiatus, pulled just cephalad, and the needle introduced perpendicularly to the skin until the ligament is encountered, dropped to 45 degrees, advanced through the ligament, dropped to parallel, and advanced approximately 1–2 cm into the sacral canal. In pediatrics it is important to avoid penetration deeper or at a steeper angle, since entering the dural sac or the anterior body of the sacrum must be avoided. The sacrum in pediatric patients is less well ossified than in adults, and unplanned injection into that structure may result in high blood levels of anesthetic.

Continuous anesthesia can be achieved with the single-shot technique just described but with an intravenous catheter, injecting the initial dose through the needle and threading the catheter off the needle into the epidural space and securing it in place. If the block is attempted and successfully performed with a Touhy needle, a standard epidural catheter can be advanced into the epidural space and secured in place.

COMPLICATIONS

The complications of caudal block are essentially the same as the those associated with epidural and spinal block (see above). One rare complication of caudal anesthesia in obstetric practice is injury to the fetal head when placing the needle in the caudal epidural space and even injection of local anesthetic directly into the fetal head. Meticulous attention to sterile procedure is important, since infection can have serious consequences.

CASE DISCUSSION: EPIDURAL WET TAP

A 26-year-old female amateur athlete presents to the operating room for repair of an acutely disrupted anterior cruciate ligament. She is otherwise healthy and desires to have a regional anesthetic. Because of her age and sex and the desire to provide continuous postoperative pain relief, an epidural anesthetic is chosen. It is planned to place a lumbar epidural catheter and to induce anesthesia with 2% mepivacaine with epinephrine. The patient is placed in the sitting position, and after appropriate preparation, the 18-gauge Tuohy epidural needle is advanced, using the loss of resistance technique. After a brief perception of loss of resistance, there is free flow of cerebrospinal fluid from the needle.

What is the presumed diagnosis?

It is assumed at this point that the epidural needle has been placed in the subarachnoid space and that the so-called epidural wet tap has occurred.

What is the incidence of wet tap?

In a wide variety of settings, a 1% wet tap rate is considered to be the approximate average. The incidence is higher in teaching institutions and lower as a function of experience.

How should the anesthesiologist proceed at this point?

There are several options. The first is to remove the needle and reinsert it at a different interspace into the epidural space, place a catheter, and proceed as previously planned. The theoretic advantage of this approach rests on several bases. First, studies indicate that placing an epidural catheter subsequent to a wet tap at a different level decreases the subsequent incidence of post-lumbar puncture cephalalgia by as much as 50%. Furthermore, the epidural catheter can be maintained in place and used not only for pain relief but also for infusion of saline, which may also decrease the incidence of post-lumbar puncture

cephalalgia. A theoretic disadvantage is the possibility that through the previous dural puncture, some local anesthetic may become subarachnoid and a response with a higher central block level may result—though clinical experience suggests that this mishap occurs infrequently.

Another alternative is dural puncture to perform spinal anesthesia, injecting an appropriate dose of a spinal anesthetic agent such as bupivacaine or tetracaine in appropriate doses for this patient based on her height and weight and the anticipated surgical procedure. It is important to remember that the needle is large and that after injection the syringe and needle should be kept in place for a few moments so that the considerable back leakage that will occur through the large epidural needle and the large lumbar puncture site will not diminish the effect of the dose of local anesthetic.

The third option is to discontinue the approach to regional anesthesia entirely, though given the patient's preference and the clinical circumstances, there is no reason for electing this alternative.

What is the anticipated outcome of this event?

Given the fact that the patient is a young and female, the probably of severe post-lumbar puncture cephalalgia is quite high. Given the large size of the lumbar puncture, the headache is likely to be profoundly disabling. Conservative measures at the conclusion of the surgical procedure would indicate 24 hours of bed rest, stool softeners to avoid abdominal straining, aggressive intravenous hydration to maintain high cerebrospinal fluid production, and perhaps abdominal binders. The literature reflects a wide diversity of opinions about prevention of the expected high incidence of headaches in this class of patients. One measure advocated involves injection of either a bolus, continuous infusion, or a combination of bolus and continuous infusion of saline through the epidural catheter for as long as 24 hours. The presumption is that the pressure of the injected fluid will counteract leakage of the cerebrospinal fluid through the lumbar puncture site, which is the cause of the headache. Continued leakage of the cerebrospinal fluid is presumed to cause downward traction on the brainstem, and the pain from pulling on blood vessels adherent to the cranial vault is analogous to that experienced with vascular cluster headaches. Another measure that has been described is injection of autologous blood via the epidural catheter, followed by its removal in the immediate postoperative period. A theoretic disadvantage to this approach is that the epidural blood patch is thought to work because of adherence of platelets from fresh autologous blood to the inflamed surface of the punctured dura. It is thought that the cut surface of the dura in a short period of time after the lumbar puncture may not yet have developed a sufficient inflamatory response, and the theoretic success rate of blood patch may not be as high as hoped for. Another approach is to treat conservatively with continued bed rest and, with onset of symptoms, oral or parenteral analgesics. In some cases the headache is benign and self-limited.

What physical signs and symptoms are consistent with post-lumbar puncture cephalalgia?

Headache following lumbar puncture is typically a frontally located postural headache that may be associated with profound nausea, vomiting, disequilibrium, and, rarely, central nervous system long tract signs. The headache improves greatly with resumption of the supine position. With headache after epidural wet tap, the symptoms are often profoundly disabling and rarely allow for scheduled discharge of the patient without treatment. It is often difficult to distinguish post-lumbar puncture cephalalgia of mild intensity from a variety of other common situations. From the obstetric literature, it is apparent that the incidence of mild headache is no greater in the population receiving spinal anesthesia than in the population receiving general anesthesia. This is probably related to the hard operating bed, the stress of labor, and the anticipation of delivery as well as a variety of other mechanical factors. It can sometimes be a challenge to differentiate post-lumbar puncture cephalalgia from headache of myofascial origin. Genuine severe post-lumbar puncture cephalalgia is hard to miss.

If severe headache develops, what is the treatment?

If there is no improvement after 24 hours of conservative therapy, including fluids, bed rest, analgesics, and other supportive measures, one should consider intervention to eliminate the headache. The treatment of choice is the so-called epidural blood patch, which involves placement of an 18-gauge Tuohy epidural needle in the interspace where the wet tap occurred and into the epidural space, followed by injection of 10–20 mL of the patient's own blood obtained under sterile conditions. It is believed that the fresh whole blood forms a clot on the irritated surface of the dura at the site of puncture and in that way allows leakage of cerebrospinal fluid to slow down and eventually stop. The patient is typically brought down to an anesthesia space, an intravenous line is started, and aggressive hydration with non-glucose-containing containing crystaloids is begun. The patient is prepared and draped in the usual manner for an epidural anesthetic, frequently placed in the lateral decubitus rather than the sitting position (of necessity, because of headache pain), and the epidural space is entered carefully at the same level where the wet tap occurred. After the epidural space is identified, a povidone-iodine preparation over the antecubital space is performed, and fresh whole blood is drawn and immediately injected through the epidural needle, which is subsequently removed. The patient is kept supine for varying periods of time while aggressive hydration continues.

The success rate of the epidural blood patch is thought to be as high as 95%, and of the remaining 5% who have presistent headache, a second patch is thought to be successful in as high as 99% of cases.

A newer treatment is with caffeine and sodium benzoate by continuous intravenous infusion for 24 hours. Caffeine is a known vasoconstrictor, and constriction of the irritated blood vessels of the brainstem may be related to the salutary effect of caffeine and sodium benzoate in this situation. This treatment is sometimes chosen before epidural blood patch.

What measures will decrease the rate of epidural wet tap?

Many methods have been described to teach as well as to perform epidural anesthesia, and most are designed to minimize the rate of dural puncture. It is important to ensure that with the loss of resistance technique, the syringe moves freely and that the feeling of increased resistance within the substance of ligaments is easily felt so that when a change occurs it is also rapidly felt. It is important to develop a dexterity that allows the practitioner to feel entry into the ligamentum flavum with its gritty sensation, as this alerts the practitioner to iminent entry into the epidural space. Once in the epidural space, it is important to remember that the needle should not be pushed, twisted, or otherwise adjusted, since the needle tip is firmly against the dura, and any motion will encourage the blunted tip of the needle to core the dura and perhaps penetrate it. It is important also to encourage the patient to avoid deep breathing, coughing, loud talking, or sudden movements. If it is the practitioner's perception that cooperation would not be forthcoming, epidural anesthesia may not be the right choice for that patient.

SUGGESTED READINGS

Cousins MJ, Bridenbaugh PO: *Neuroblockade in Clinical Anesthesia and Management of Pain.* Lippincott, 1988.
Greene NM: *Physiology of Spinal Anesthesia,* 3rd ed. Williams & Wilkins, 1981.

Katz J: *Atlas of Regional Anesthesia.* Appleton-Century-Crofts, 1985.

17   Peripheral Nerve Blocks

*John E. Tetzlaff, MD**

Regional anesthesia for surgery of the extremities is not a new idea. Extremity amputations were performed after surgical exposure of the brachial plexus or femoral-sciatic nerves and application of cocaine before the turn of the century. With the great advances in techniques for general anesthesia during the first half of this century, enthusiasm for regional anesthesia decreased. Its subsequent resurgence in popularity is undoubtedly due to new local anesthetics, improvements in block equipment, and the proliferation of anesthesia residency programs. The gruesome realities of war have reestablished the safety and efficacy of regional anesthesia for combat casualties. Continuous techniques for combined operative anesthesia and postoperative analgesia, new local anesthetics, and the possibility of ultra-long-acting agents present challenges for the 21st century.

It is the purpose of this chapter to discuss peripheral nerve blocks for surgery of the extremities. To do so, preparation of the patient, safety, equipment, and anatomy will be discussed in addition to complications, their diagnosis and treatment, and regional block technique.

PREPARATION OF THE PATIENT

While the surgical procedure and the preference of the surgeon are factors in selecting an anesthetic technique, the suitability, consent, physical status, and preparation of the patient are always the first determinants. Discussion of each of these areas will allow the beginner to determine for each case whether a peripheral block is indicated as a complete anesthetic or part of a combined technique and whether it is likely to be successful and favorably remembered by the patient.

Suitability

Every medical student who spends time with an anesthesiologist who uses a significant amount of regional anesthesia in practice will encounter a patient, apparently a candidate for a block, who is convinced to select a general anesthetic by the experienced regional-

ist. Similarly, every new anesthesia resident can expect to have a case where the block was technically perfect but the anesthetic a disaster. This is where the art of guessing the suitability of a patient for regional anesthesia increases success.

A number of factors make a patient a good candidate for a block. The ability to communicate with the patient is essential. Senility, dementia, or agitation are relative contraindications. Rapid translation should be available when discussing anesthetic options with patients whose language is not English, since frightening sights and sounds not explained can lead to agitation. Cooperation is also required to perform a regional block and to ensure adequate conditions for operation. Inability to remain still due to pain, extremes of age, or psychiatric disease argue against pure regional anesthesia. The need for an unusual surgical position or a long procedure may make even the most motivated patient hard to manage intraoperatively, perhaps even interfering with surgery. The patient's anxiety level must also be considered. Mutilating surgery, diagnostic procedures for cancer, and surgery on the genitals are examples of issues which may be too stressful for some individuals to deal with when awake in the operating room. Sedation can be used, but the extremely anxious patient may respond to pharmacologic anxiolysis with disinhibition and acute psychosis. The patient who is morbidly concerned with death, terrified of sounds in the operating room, or has had to be sedated to near-unconsciousness to gain intravenous access may not be a candidate for a block. The experienced regionalist must always ask the question, "Do I really want to do a block on this patient?" If the answer is no, another anesthetic method should be chosen.

Informed Consent

Attempting to do a block because it is indicated but without consent of the patient is unwise. Careful discussion of the risks and benefits, a description of the technique, forthright comments about the amount of discomfort to be anticipated and the possibility of failure, and what it will be like for the patient during the procedure must precede any block. Premedication must be withheld until this is accomplished. If a complication occurs and this step has been omitted, medicolegal consequences may be magnified.

Some hospitals use surgical consent forms which

*Staff Anesthesiologist, Department of General Anesthesia, The Cleveland Clinic Foundation, Cleveland, Ohio.

the patient signs. Often, this form includes a statement about anesthesia. Some groups have even developed anesthetic consent forms or procedure-specific documents. What is important is not the specific form of the document but rather the honest discussion with the patient, since a signed consent form is not is not legal evidence of consent if the patient does not understand exactly what has been agreed.

Any discussion of regional anesthesia must include general anesthesia. Because it may be impossible to complete the block or because the attempt to achieve anesthesia via block may fail intraoperatively or because of a an unforeseen toxic reaction to the local anesthetic, induction of general anesthesia may be necessary.

Patient's Physical Status

Regional anesthesia does not eliminate the need for a proper preoperative evaluation. Every anesthesiologist has encountered the question, "Can't you just do a block?" from a surgeon in a hurry. To do so is an error in judgment. Coexisting disease may modify block techniques, choice of agent, dosage requirements, or use of exogenous vasoconstrictors. Existing neurologic disease, particularly with neurologic deficits, must be carefully evaluated for risk/benefit ratio. Informed consent discussion with the patient is mandatory for obvious medicolegal reasons. To perform a block on an extremity with an existing deficit may implicate the block in the extent of the deficit postoperatively. Demyelinating neurologic disease is an absolute contraindication to the application of local anesthetics. Coagulopathy or therapeutic anticoagulation may either preclude or greatly exaggerate the risk of regional anesthesia. Coronary artery disease requires careful consideration of the use of catecholamine vasoconstrictors, which are often routinely added to local anesthetics. Hepatic or renal disease has implications for metabolism of local anesthetics and potential toxicity.

Premedication

The essential features of patient preparation have already been covered: an adequate preoperative anesthetic visit and a discussion of risks and benefits of general versus regional anesthesia. Once regional anesthesia has been selected, a few more issues need to be addressed. Premedication can make the difference between an elegant and an awkward anesthetic experience. Regional techniques that require patient cooperation make it important to avoid profound sedation. Large total doses of local anesthetic are safer for the patient who has been premedicated with a benzodiazepine to raise the seizure threshold. A balance must be reached, however. Some anesthesiologists prefer to withhold premedication prior to regional anesthesia—an intentional decision not to raise the seizure threshold. This allows for earliest identification of signs of local anesthetic toxicity. Heavy premedication with benzodiazepines or barbiturates

makes central nervous system toxicity less likely but does obscure early signs.

Some patients will consent to a block but have a reasonable fear of needles. A gentle, anxiolytic premedication is humane, may make the block easier to perform, and may encourage the patient to select a block for another anesthetic in the future.

Equipment & Safety

Since regional blocks take some effort and time to perform, they are often performed outside of the operating room to maximize expedience. Block rooms lend themselves to this objective. Some principles of safety must be applied. The consequences of local anesthetic complications can include apnea, vasomotor collapse, and grand mal seizure activity. Any place where a block is performed must be equipped to deal with these. Table 17–1 lists the contents of a well-equipped regional anesthesia cart.

Employing minimal monitoring standards to perform regional anesthesia can raise interesting arguments. Why the same individual would place five or more monitors to induce general anesthesia yet do a block without monitors is hard to understand. With the risk of apnea, cardiopulmonary collapse, or seizure, early recognition and effortless assessment would

Table 17–1. Contents of regional anesthesia cart.

Pharmaceuticals (regional)
Mepivacaine, 1% and 2%
Lidocaine, 1%, 1.5%, and 2%
Bupivacaine, 0.25%, 0.5%, and 0.75%
Chloroprocaine, 2% and 3%
Tetracaine, 1% liquid (sterile package)
Tetracaine crystals
Epinephrine 1:1000 (sterile package)
Ephedrine, 2.5% or 5% (sterile package)
Phenylephrine, 1% (sterile package)
Dextrose, 10% (sterile)
Pharmaceuticals (resuscitation)
Thiopental sodium
Succinylcholine
Atropine
Ephedrine
Antibiotics
Equipment (resuscitation)
Suction
Ambu bag (or anesthetic circuit)
Masks
Oral airways
Nasal airways
Laryngoscope and blades
Endotracheal tubes
Blood pressure cuff
Pulse oximeter
Equipment (regional)
Needles, B-bevel
Needles, sharp, 18- to 26-gauge
Needles, spinal, 18-, 20-, 22-, and 25-gauge
Needle, pencil-point, Whitacre or other
Needles, epidural
Needles, insulated block
Nerve stimulator, voltage-controlled
Spinal anesthesia trays
Epidural trays

seem prudent. Once the block is complete, the need for monitoring does not decrease. Peak blood levels occur at various times after the block. Numerous reports identify the risk of sudden cardiorespiratory arrest after regional technique, most often central blocks. The use of inferior monitoring standards as determined by anesthetic technique is an invitation to medicolegal complications.

The local anesthetic test dose is another safety issue that stirs controversy. Many anesthesiologists insist that the first injection of local anesthetic for any block be a small increment with epinephrine added, typically 3 mL with 1:200,000 epinephrine (15 μg epinephrine). If this is inadvertently injected into a blood vessel, an adrenergic response should occur 20–30 seconds after injection. The pulse rate should increase 30–40 beats, and the patient often will feel the increase in the strength of contraction of the heart as a palpitation. The effect will be transient, lasting 30–60 seconds. The advantage is a transient hemodynamic alteration that identifies malposition of the injection. Unless the blood vessel happens to flow directly into the cerebral circulation (ie, vertebral artery), central nervous system excitation or total spinal or cardiac depression should not occur. These obvious responses warn the practitioner to reposition the needle prior to further injection. Allied to this technique is incremental injection of local anesthetic. If no more than 5 mL of agent is injected without an interval pause, it is hard to ever achieve a sudden blood or cerebrospinal fluid level of agent that will result in catastrophe. The permanent neurologic deficits associated with massive subarachnoid injection of chloroprocaine following attempted epidural anesthesia involve total doses that would not be possible with a test dose and incremental injection.

Obstetric anesthesiologists worry about the epinephrine-mediated vasoconstriction of the uterine artery leading to fetal hypotension and subsequent distress. This may prevent using epinephrine in the total block dose but usually still allows an epinephrine test dose. Another clinical situation where this decision must be made is the patient with coronary artery disease, who often tolerates increases in heart rate poorly. The risk/benefit decision involves the risk of ischemia from the adrenergic response to epinephrine versus the hemodynamic alteration that could occur if local anesthetic toxicity of the central nervous system were to occur.

GENERAL TECHNIQUES FOR PERIPHERAL NERVE BLOCK

There are many ways to perform peripheral blocks. These include anatomic location, field block, elicita-

tion of paresthesia, perivascular sheath technique, transarterial placement, and use of a nerve stimulator. They have application to some or all of the blocks described later in this chapter and will be presented individually.

CORRECT NEEDLE PLACEMENT

Anatomic Location

Some nerve blocks rely on precise, dependable anatomic relationships. An example is the intercostal block, where a neurovascular bundle is under the interior border of each rib. Striking the lower rib edge and "walking" inferiorly until the needle slips off and advancing the needle 0.5–1 cm farther places the needle very close to the intercostal nerve, and as long as aspiration verifies avoidance of a blood vessel, 5 mL of local anesthetic should produce a block. Digital blocks of the hands and toes and ulnar and median nerve blocks at the wrist are other examples of this technique.

Field Block

Knowing the general location of a nerve allows for deposition of a large volume of agent in several places at that location. This is a field block. A good example is the injection into the body of the coracobrachialis muscle, which is designed to block the musculocutaneous nerve as a supplement to axillary or interscalene brachial plexus block. Superficial cervical and some parts of the ankle block are also examples of field block.

Elicitation of Paresthesia

Placing a needle in direct contact with a nerve will stimulate that nerve. If the nerve has sensory fibers, a paresthesia will result in the corresponding dermatome. This is referred to as elicitation of paresthesia and verifies that the needle tip is proximate to the nerve. Paresthesia will also occur if the needle is within the substance of the nerve, which must be avoided because of the potential for hydrostatic injury to axons during injection. With injection into a perineural location, there is a brief accentuation of paresthesia; with intraneural injection, an intense, searing pain occurs that should signal immediate termination of injection. Intensity is the key to differentiation between accentuation and intraneural injection. If in doubt, *stop!* It has been suggested that intentional elicitation of paresthesia may result in a small but significant increase in nerve injury after axillary block compared to transarterial technique.

Perivascular Sheath Technique

Many nerve bundles are located close to vascular structures, often in a sheath. Use of this relationship is the basis for the perivascular sheath technique. It is helpful to use a needle with a blunt-bevel designed for regional anesthesia. This allows palpation of the changes in tissue planes as the needle is advancing. The thick fascial sheath causes a palpable click as the needle enters this sheath. Once the sheath is entered, if the needle is released, it will often pulsate. The classic model is the axillary perivascular technique. The short, B-bevel needle causes the click (also called "sheath pop") when it is inserted immediately lateral or medial to the area of axillary artery pulsation. The needle is redirected from perpendicular to the skin toward parallel, advanced slightly, and the local anesthetic is then injected. If the sheath is occluded distally, increased proximal spread of the solution is assured. Other examples include the subclavian perivascular block and the femoral "three-in-one" approach to block of the femoral, obturator, and lateral femoral cutaneous nerves.

Transarterial Placement

The brachial plexus is located within a sheath that also includes the axillary artery. If a needle enters this artery and exits a short distance either at the front or back, it will be located within the sheath around the brachial plexus. A small, blunt (B-bevel) needle decreases the likelihood that arterial trauma will occur. Injection in a transarterial location will fill the axillary sheath with local anesthetic. The proximity of the artery demands extra care to verify that injection into the artery does not occur.

Nerve Stimulator

Besides elicitation of paresthesia or pulsation, another way to verify the proximity of a needle to a nerve is to deliver a small electrical stimulus and elicit a motor or sensory evoked response. This can be done with a nerve stimulator with one lead attached to the needle and the other lead grounded elsewhere on the patient. Because the current is delivered to the whole needle and not just the end, localization can be made more precisely by insulating all but the end of the needle. This is referred to as an insulated block needle. Failing this, if the regular needle is inserted to the appropriate motor-evoked response, withdrawn until the response disappears, and then reinserted just until it returns, the response can be assumed to be occurring only from the tip of the needle, where injection will occur.

THE "IMMOBILE NEEDLE"

The "immobile needle" technique was developed by Winnie to increase dexterity with injection. Instead of direct contact between the syringe and the needle, an extension set is inserted into the needle and the syringe is connected to the extension set. The needle can be stabilized against the body once correct placement is obtained, and injection can be performed with the other hand or by an assistant.

REGIONAL BLOCK NEEDLES

A number of needles are specifically designed for performance of blocks. A few will be described.

Blunt-Bevel Needle

The B (blunt-bevel) needle is made to minimize trauma upon direct contact with nerves. The angle of the bevel is increased 20–30 degrees, and the sharpness is decreased. The theory is that a less pointed needle will push nerves as opposed to impaling them. Furthermore, changes in tissue planes are felt more distinctly with this needle, allowing for location of fascial sheaths.

Insulated Needles

Location of nerves by electrical stimulation involves connecting a nerve stimulator to a needle. One lead is attached to the patient as a ground and the other to the needle with an alligator clip, or directly if the needle is manufactured for that function. The current is transmitted to the entire needle, and the point of injection is not necessarily the point of maximum electrical impulse. The insulated needle eliminates this issue by bonding a nonconductor to the needle except for the last millimeter before the bevel. Hence, whatever is being stimulated is also bathed by the injected local anesthetic. Combined with a variable-voltage nerve stimulator, precise location of motor-evoked response at low voltage ensures a high success rate.

The Beaded Needle

The beaded needle is a regional needle designed for use with a nerve stimulator. A flange is welded to the needle, which serves as a gauge of depth and allows attachment of an alligator clip above the bead. This keeps the nonsterile clip away from the sterile needle surface.

UPPER EXTREMITY SOMATIC BLOCKADE

Surgical procedures on the entire upper extremity can be performed by regional block of the brachial plexus or its terminal branches. Techniques will be discussed for blocking this plexus at sites above and below the clavicle, and there will be some discussion of technical difficulties and risks. Also presented will be individual nerve blocks in the upper arm, elbow, wrist, and more distal sites, both as complete anesthesia and as supplements to brachial plexus blockade. The applied anatomy of the brachial plexus will be discussed. Pertinent aspects of this anatomy will be presented with each individual block.

BRACHIAL PLEXUS ANATOMY

The brachial plexus is formed from the anterior primary rami of the fourth through eighth cervical nerves and the first two thoracic nerves (Figure 17–1). The contributions of C4 and T2 are most often minor or absent. As these nerves leave the intervertebral foramina, they converge, forming three distinct trunks behind the anterior and middle scalene muscles (Figure 17–2). Because they are horizontally arranged, they are named superior, middle, and inferior. The superior trunk is predominantly C4–6, the middle trunk is C7, and the inferior trunk is C8–T2, but this is not absolute. This convergence is tightest just medial to the first rib. At the lateral border of the first rib, a division occurs and spatial relationships become horizontal and vertical. Each trunk creates an anterior and posterior division, which—below the clavicle—form the cords of the brachial plexus, named, according to the relationship to the axillary artery, lateral, medial, and posterior. Below the axilla, each cord gives off terminal branches. From its origin up to this point, the plexus is enclosed in a sheath that serves as the basis for many block techniques. A working knowledge of these anatomic arrangements is essential for successful brachial plexus block.

Some further anatomic details are important for successful upper extremity blockade. Some areas of the anterior shoulder are innervated by the superficial cervical plexus (anterior rami C1–4). These rami converge just lateral to their transverse processes, with confluent exit through the platsyma at the posterior border of the sternocleidomastoid muscle (Figure 17–3). This lends itself to field block. The medial brachial cutaneous (C8–T1) and intercostobrachial (T2) nerves innervate the skin of the medial and posterior proximal upper arm (Figure 17–4). Anatomically, they do not lie close to the brachial plexus and must be blocked independently for some shoulder surgery or for distal extremity procedures, where use of a pneumatic tourniquet is planned.

INTERSCALENE BRACHIAL PLEXUS BLOCK

Indications

The interscalene block can be used for any procedure on the upper extremity, including the shoulder, but is used most often with proximal procedures and in cases where the arm cannot be positioned for the axillary approach. The high rate of failure (10–20%) to

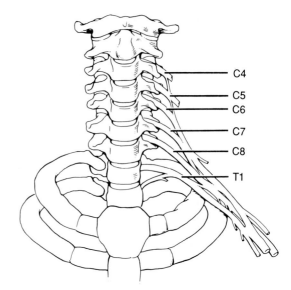

Figure 17–1. Origins of the brachial plexus. (Reproduced, with permission, from Katz J: *Atlas of Regional Anesthesia.* Appleton-Century-Crofts, 1985.)

achieve full block of the ulnar nerve must be kept in mind with hand surgery.

Anatomy

The cervical spinal nerves blend into trunks behind the muscle bellies of the anterior and middle scalene muscles. The interval between these muscles at the level of the cricoid cartilage is an easy place to enter the brachial plexus sheath to elicit a paresthesia or motor-evoked response with a nerve stimulator (Figure 17–5). This can often be located on the surface, where the external jugular vein crosses the level of the cricoid cartilage, and serves as a valuable landmark. The proximity of the stellate ganglion, the phrenic nerve, and the recurrent laryngeal nerve to this location explains their high rate of incidental blockade.

Technique

Palpation of the interscalene groove is the first step in performing this block. The patient is placed supine with the head flat. The head is rotated 30–45 degrees toward the opposite side. At the levels of the cricoid cartilage, the external jugular vein is located. Very often, palpation at this point locates the interscalene groove with no other action necessary. If it does not, the patient is asked to lift the head in this position, and the posterior border of the sternocleidomastoid muscle is identified. With the neck relaxed, the hand is swept laterally, first encountering the groove between the sternocleidomastoid and the anterior scalene muscle, then the anterior scalene muscle itself, and finally the groove between the anterior scalene muscle and the

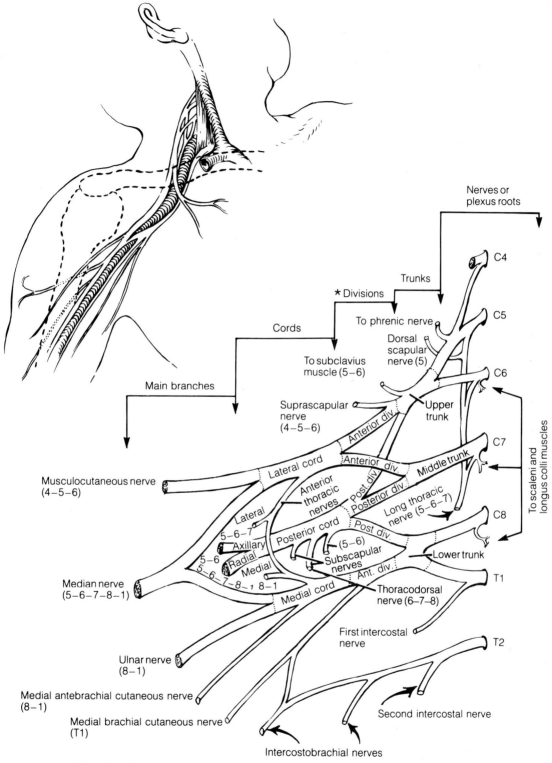

Nerves or plexus roots

C4

Trunks

★ Divisions

To phrenic nerve

C5

Cords

Dorsal scapular nerve (5)

To subclavius muscle (5–6)

C6

Main branches

Suprascapular nerve (4–5–6)

Anterior div.

Upper trunk

Lateral cord

Anterior div.

Middle trunk

C7

Musculocutaneous nerve (4–5–6)

Anterior thoracic nerves

Post. div.

Posterior div.

To scaleni and longus colli muscles

Lateral 5–6–7

Axillary 5–6

Radial 5–6–7–8

Posterior cord

Post div.

Long thoracic nerve (5–6–7)

C8

(5–6)

Subscapular nerves

Medial

Median nerve (5–6–7–8–1)

Medial 8–1

Ant. div.

Lower trunk

Medial cord

Thoracodorsal nerve (6–7–8)

T1

First intercostal nerve

Ulnar nerve (8–1)

T2

Medial antebrachial cutaneous nerve (8–1)

Medial brachial cutaneous nerve (T1)

Second intercostal nerve

Intercostobrachial nerves

★ Splitting of the plexus into anterior and posterior divisions is one of the most significant features in the redistribution of nerve fibers, since it is here that fibers supplying the flexor and extensor groups of muscles of the upper extremity are separated. Similar splitting is noted in the lumbar and sacral plexuses for the supply of muscles of the lower extremity.

Figure 17–2. The brachial plexus. (Reproduced, with permission, from deGroot J, Chusid JG: Correlative Neuroanatomy, 20th ed. Appleton & Lange, 1988.)

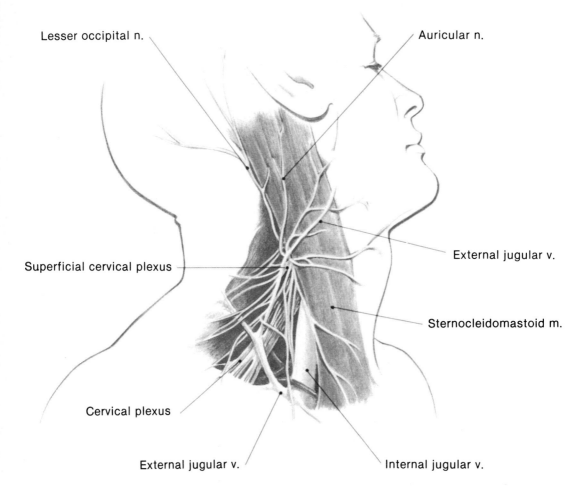

Lesser occipital n.

Auricular n.

Superficial cervical plexus

External jugular v.

Sternocleidomastoid m.

Cervical plexus

External jugular v.

Internal jugular v.

Figure 17–3. Superficial cervical plexus. (Reproduced, with permission, from Katz J: *Atlas of Regional Anesthesia.* Appleton-Century-Crofts, 1985.)

middle scalene muscle. This is much more subtle than the large groove behind the sternocleidomastoid and must be carefully sought. Through a skin wheel, a 25-gauge, ⅝-inch B-bevel needle is introduced (avoiding the external jugular) and directed perpendicularly to the skin, except for a very slight medial and caudal deviation until either paresthesia or a motor-evoked response is elicited. A motor response or paresthesia in the arm must be sought, since stimulation of a high branch of a single nerve root, such as the dorsal scapular, will elicit shoulder and shoulder blade paresthesia when the needle is not correctly in the sheath. The superior trunk (radial, musculocutaneous) is most likely to be stimulated and the presence of such stimulation correlates well with a proximal block. Proximal sheath pressure can facilitate a more distal spread of local anesthetic, but if hand surgery is the objective, the elicitation of a middle or inferior trunk response may be associated with a higher percentage of complete block. This may have to be accomplished lower in the interscalene groove toward the clavicle. Forty milliliters of local anesthetic is injected. Use of a needle less

than 1 inch long minimizes the risk of reaching the vertebral artery or a neural foramen, with resulting morbidity.

Complications

Proximity of the vertebral artery makes intra-arterial injection possible with rapid progression to grand mal seizure after small amounts are injected. Venous injection and rapid absorption in the highly vascular neck can result in less rapid central nervous system excitation phenomena. The neural foramina can be reached, and massive epidural, subarachnoid, or subdural injection can occur. Pneumothorax is possible and more likely with chronic obstructive pulmonary disease owing to the superior displacement of the apex of the lung. Stellate ganglion block results in Horner's sign (myosis, ptosis, anhidrosis) in 30–50% of interscalene blocks. Recurrent laryngeal nerve block (30–50%) leads to hoarseness and weak voice. Phrenic nerve block (30–40%) leads to a feeling of heaviness on the ipsilateral chest and can lead to subjective dyspnea in anxious, unpremedicated patients or patients with se-

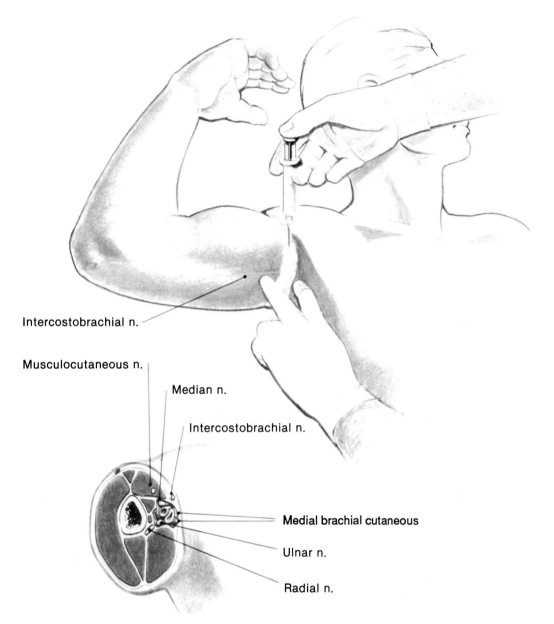

Figure 17–4. Location and block of the intercostobrachial and medial brachial cutaneous nerves. (Reproduced, with permission, from Katz J: *Atlas of Regional Anesthesia.* Appleton-Century-Crofts, 1985.)

vere pulmonary disease. As always, infection and nerve injury are rare but possible.

AXILLARY BLOCK

1. SUPRACLAVICULAR BRACHIAL PLEXUS BLOCK

Indications

The supraclavicular block offers a rapid-onset, dense block of the distal upper extremity. It also offers an arm block with a high distal success rate for hand surgery in patients who cannot circumduct the humerus for approach to the axilla. Enthusiasm for this block is tempered by the relatively high risks of subclavian artery or lung entry with the needle. Pneumothorax may occur in up to 1% of cases, though most are subclinical.

Anatomy

As the trunks are traced laterally, the prevertebral fascia, which invests the anterior and middle scalene muscles as well as the trunks, forms the sheath that surrounds the nerve plexus. As this approaches the

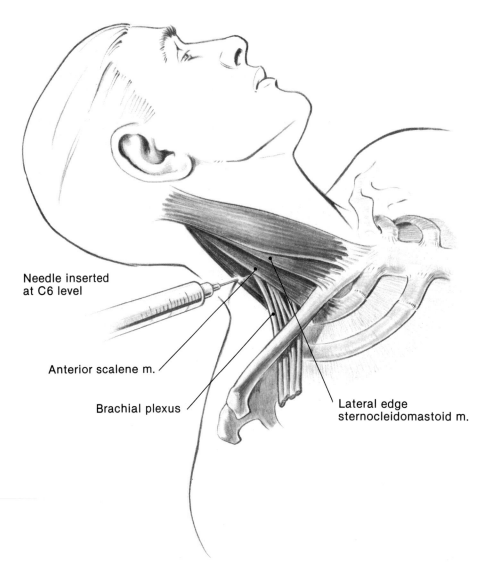

Needle inserted
at C6 level

Anterior scalene m.

Brachial plexus

Lateral edge
sternocleidomastoid m.

Figure 17–5. Block of the brachial plexus in the interscalene groove. (Reproduced, with permission, from Katz J: *Atlas of Regional Anesthesia.* Appleton-Century-Crofts, 1985.)

lateral border of the anterior scalene muscle, it passes between the first rib and clavicle to enter the axilla, with posterior contact with the first rib. The other important relationship is the apex of the subclavian pulse, which lies in the interscalene groove, behind the clavicle. At this point, the trunks are tightly invested in fascia, arranged horizontally on top of the first rib.

Technique
(Figure 17–6)

The patient is positioned supine with the head turned 30–45 degrees to the contralateral side. The midpoint of the clavicle is identified. Palpation of the subclavian artery is attempted by moving off the posterior border of the sternocleidomastoid just above the clavicle and moving over the anterior scalene muscle. The pulse is felt just as the interscalene grove is entered. One finger breadth cephalad, a 22- or 23-gauge 1½-inch B-bevel needle is inserted. It is directed toward the subclavian pulse into the interscalene groove until paresthesia is encountered. If no paresthesia results, the needle is advanced until the first rib is encountered. "Walking the rib" often elicits paresthesia. If the rib is not encountered by 1½ inches or if bright red blood or air is aspirated, the needle is withdrawn and landmarks reevaluated. If air is aspirated, a chest x-ray is mandatory. If the artery is entered, slow withdrawal until just extravascular allows for injection without paresthesia. Twenty-five to 30 mL of local anesthetic is injected.

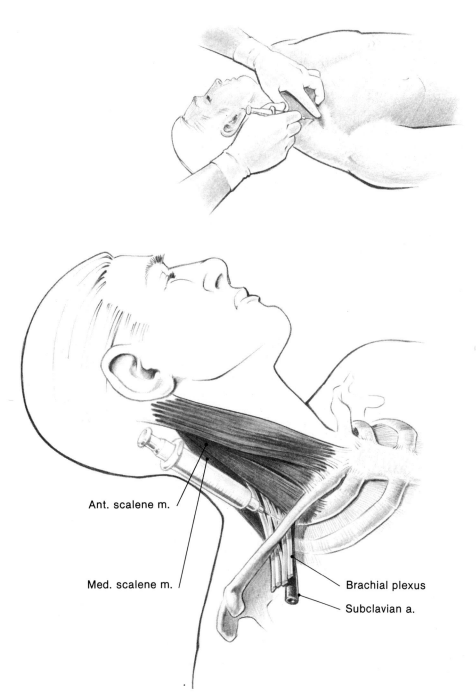

Ant. scalene m.

Med. scalene m.

Brachial plexus

Subclavian a.

Figure 17–6. Supraclavicular block. (Reproduced, with permission, from Katz J: *Atlas of Regional Anesthesia.* Appleton-Century-Crofts, 1985.)

Complications

Pneumothorax and hemothorax are the most common complications of the supraclavicular block. Pneumothorax may be as high as 1%, though clinically significant pneumothorax (> 20%) or tension pneumothorax is are rare. The delayed presentation of these complications makes use of this technique in outpatients questionable.

2. INFRACLAVICULAR BRACHIAL PLEXUS BLOCK

Indications

The indications for the infraclavicular approach to the brachial plexus are the same as the supraclavicular approach, as are the advantages and limitations. If anything, the complication rate is higher.

Anatomy

Performance of this block takes advantage of the tight neural bundle of the brachial plexus in the infraclavicular area, anterior to the coracoid process, before it enters the axilla. At the midpoint of the clavicle, the plexus is $1^{1}/_{2}$–2 inches from the skin surface. It is posterior and lateral to the subclavian artery.

Technique
(Figure 17–7)

The head is positioned in neutral. The mid position of the clavicle is identified, and a skin wheal is raised on the interior surface. A 3-inch 22- or 23-gauge spinal needle is inserted through skin, connected to a syringe, and advanced laterally toward the humeral head. The lateral aspect of the subclavian pulse is also used as an insertion guide. The needle is directed away from the chest wall to avoid the pleura. At 2–$2^{1}/_{2}$ inches, paresthesia will be elicited and 20–25 mL of local anesthetic injected. If air is aspirated at any time, a chest x-ray is mandatory.

Complications

Pneumo-, chylo-, and hemothorax are possible and probably occur at a higher rate than with the supraclavicular approach. Very few clinicians use this block regularly.

3. CLASSIC AXILLARY BRACHIAL PLEXUS BLOCK

Indications

The classic axillary block is the most common peripheral block performed. It has application to any surgical procedure from the mid humerus to the hand. It is technically simple and should have a very low complication rate. Of the approaches to the brachial plexus, the axillary block has the best block rate in the distribution of C7–T1 (ulnar).

Anatomy
(Figure 17–2)

The subclavian artery becomes the axillary artery as it crosses the clavicle. At this same point, each trunk of the brachial plexus gives off an anterior and a posterior division. The anterior divisions of the superior and middle trunks combine to form the lateral cord of the brachial plexus, named for its anatomic relationship to the axillary artery. The posterior divisions of all three trunks form the posterior cord. The anterior division of the inferior trunk forms the medial cord. At the level of the pectoralis minor muscle, the first terminal branches are given off. The terminal branches of each cord should be known by the anesthesiologist to correctly localize a needle during placement and elicitation of paresthesia or motor-evoked response.

Technique
(Figure 17–8)

Axillary block can be accomplished by four different approaches, which all use the location of the axillary pulse as a starting point. Each will be described separately. The patient is positioned supine with the humerus circumducted and the hand behind the head. Care is taken to avoid having the arm lower than the trunk, since forward displacement of the humerus interferes with appreciation of the axillary pulse.

A. Transarterial: The pulse of the axillary artery is identified as proximal as possible—ideally, proximal to the pectoralis ridge. A 25-gauge $^{3}/_{4}$-inch B-bevel needle is inserted until bright red blood is aspirated. The needle is moved forward or withdrawn just until blood aspiration ceases. This is easier to determine with the extension set, "immobile needle" technique. Injection can be performed either posteriorly, anteriorly, or in both locations in relation to the artery. Location is chosen both by the surgical site and the clinician's belief about septation within the sheath. Those that believe the sheath to be anatomically subdivided tend to prefer the double injection technique for surgical procedures which are not in the anatomic distribution of only one cord. Forty milliliters is injected, with distal digital pressure applied to ensure proximal spread in the sheath and improved blockade rate of proximal branches such as the musculocutaneous nerve.

B. Elicitation of Paresthesia: This technique can either be chosen at the outset or can be used if unplanned paresthesia is elicited during any other technique. Knowing the surgical procedure and the sensory distribution, the anesthesiologist selects a paresthesia to be elicited. For example, for fixation of a fifth metacarpal fracture, an ulnar paresthesia should be sought, and in the position for the block a 25-gauge, $^{3}/_{4}$-inch B-bevel needle is inserted just inferior to the pulse (Figure 17–8). The sheath will be encountered first and paresthesia shortly after. Ideal localization occurs when needle movement is ceased just as the paresthesia is encountered. The B-bevel needle de-

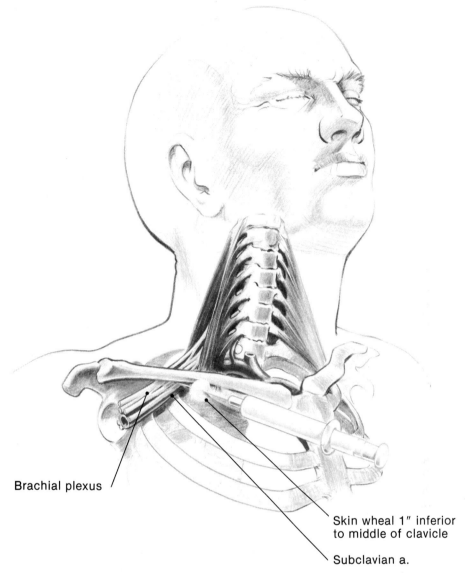

Brachial plexus

Skin wheal 1″ inferior
to middle of clavicle

Subclavian a.

Figure 17–7. Infraclavicular block. (Reproduced, with permission, from Katz J: *Atlas of Regional Anesthesia.* Appleton-Century-Crofts, 1985.)

creases the probability of injecting into the substance of the nerve. With injection, some pressure-induced augmentation of the paresthesia is normal and verifies needle placement. A burning, searing, or excruciating pain signals intraneural injection, which must be stopped immediately to avoid nerve damage. The needle is repositioned, and gentle injection of a small volume verifies needle placement outside the substance of the nerve. Forty milliliters is injected on this paresthesia, with distal pressure applied.

C. Perivascular Injection: The perivascular injection technique can be applied to the axillary brachial plexus block. The B-bevel needle is used to locate the sheath with the needle perpendicular to the skin and

superior to the pulse. Once the needle is inside the sheath, proximity to the artery is verified by disconnecting the needle and observing transmitted pulsation. The needle is then moved to a position almost parallel to the skin, advanced 1–2 cm farther, and fixed. Forty milliliters is injected with distal pressure.

D. Nerve Stimulator: The needle placement in reference to the artery is selected, as with paresthesia block, according to the anatomic distribution to be blocked primarily. For an extensor tendon sheath release of the thumb, the radial nerve is most important, and the correct needle placement is posterior to the artery. Correct placement is verified by a motor-evoked response, which would be evident by thumb

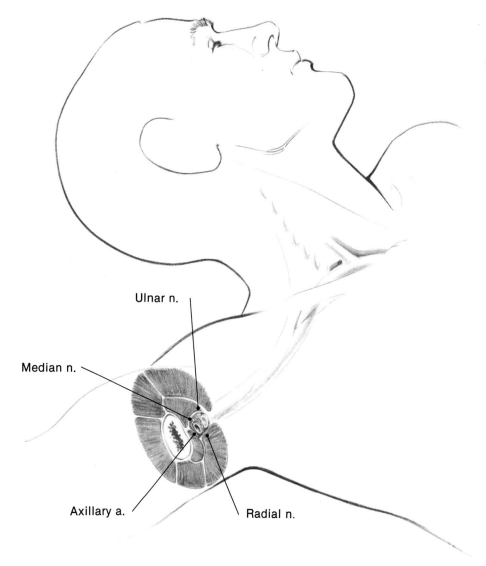

Figure 17–8. Axillary block. Note relationships of nerves to the artery. (Reproduced, with permission, from Katz J: *Atlas of Regional Anesthesia.* Appleton-Century-Crofts, 1985.)

extension. Pulling the needle back until the response ceases and advancing forward until the response just returns more accurately locates the nerve. In addition, a variable voltage nerve stimulator can be used to localize the response at lower and lower currents. Evoked response at 1 mA is highly specific, and at less than 0.5 mA it is nearly 100% successful. With injection, the initial motor response should be briefly exaggerated (augmentation) because the local anesthetic is a hydrochloride salt and a conductor, which increases nerve impulses until conduction block begins. After this brief increase, a rapid decrement (extinction) should occur. Failure to observe augmentation and extinction should suggest malposition of the needle, and

injection should cease to avoid failed block. Forty milliliters is injected with distal pressure.

ISOLATED NERVE BLOCKS

1. INTERCOSTOBRACHIAL & MEDIAL BRACHIAL CUTANEOUS NERVES (Figure 17–4)

Indications

Both the intercostobrachial and the medial brachial nerves are cutaneous nerves that originate in the lower neck and upper thorax and become cutaneous on the medial upper arm. Both must be blocked proximal to the axilla for shoulder surgery with very anterior incisions or for any upper extremity procedure that involves use of a pneumatic tourniquet.

Anatomy

The intercostobrachial nerve derives from the T2 somatic intercostal nerve, and the medial brachial cutaneous nerve derives from C8 and T1. Both become superficial and cutaneous at the pectoral ridge over the humeral head.

Technique
(Figure 17–9)

Both nerves are easily blocked, with the arm circumducted, by means of a linear field injection from the deltoid prominence superiorly to the most inferior aspect of the medial upper arm. Multiple injections can be made with a 1¹/₂-inch, 22- or 23–gauge needle,

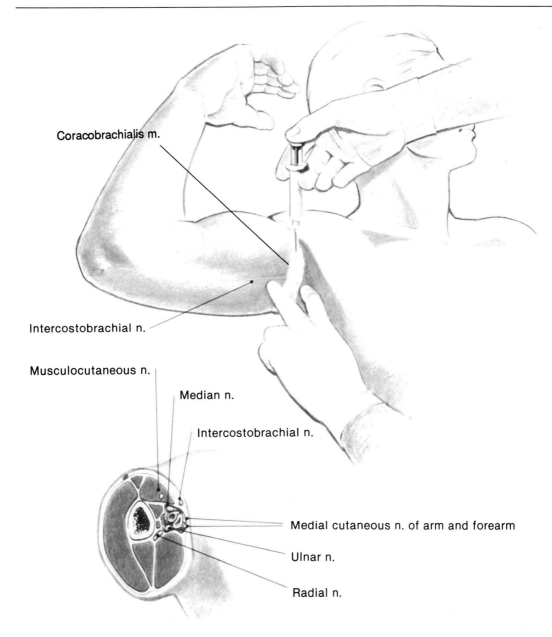

Figure 17–9. Musculocutaneous block: Injection into coracobrachialis. (Reproduced, with permission, from Katz J: *Atlas of Regional Anesthesia.* Appleton-Century-Crofts, 1985.)

with each subsequent needle insertion through a newly numb area. Alternatively, a 3-inch spinal needle can be used for a single puncture. Three to 5 mL of local anesthesia is all that is necessary.

Complications

There are no complications specific to this block.

2. MUSCULOCUTANEOUS NERVE

Indications

The musculocutaneous nerve is the most proximal branch of the brachial plexus involved in surgery of the arm. Because of early branching, distal axillary block techniques often fail to block the musculocutaneous nerve, and supplemental block is necessary for complete motor block of the arm or sensory block in the musculocutaneous distribution of the forearm and wrist.

Anatomy

The musculocutaneous nerve is a branch of the lateral cord proximal to the insertion of the pectoralis minor muscle. It enters the arm by piercing the coracobrachialis. It exits the coracobrachialis and runs ventral to the humerus between the biceps and the brachialis muscles, which it innervates. The terminal sensory limit is cutaneous on the lateral aspect of the forearm and is called the lateral cutaneous nerve of the forearm.

Technique
(Figures 17–9 and 17–10)

Two techniques take advantage of reliable anatomic relationships. The first involves placement of a 22- or 23-gauge $1^{1}/_{2}$-inch needle into the substance of the coracobrachialis through the numb area for intercostobrachialis block (Figure 17–9) and field block infiltration of 5–8 mL of local anesthetic into the belly of the muscle. The alternative approach takes advantage of the relationship of the biceps muscle, the brachial artery, and the nerve on the medial surface of the arm, with the nerve behind the artery. The belly of the biceps is palpated and displaced superiorly, moving the artery away from the nerve, and a 23-gauge $3/_{4}$-inch B-bevel needle is inserted and directed down to periosteum of the humerus and withdrawn a short distance (Figure 17–10). This is performed several times with injection of 1–2 mL for a field block. If paresthesia is elicited, the needle position is altered to avoid intraneural injection.

Complications

Complications result from injection into the axillary or brachial artery or intraneural injection of the nerve.

3. RADIAL NERVE

Indications

Isolated radial nerve block is performed almost invariably as a supplement to incomplete brachial plexus

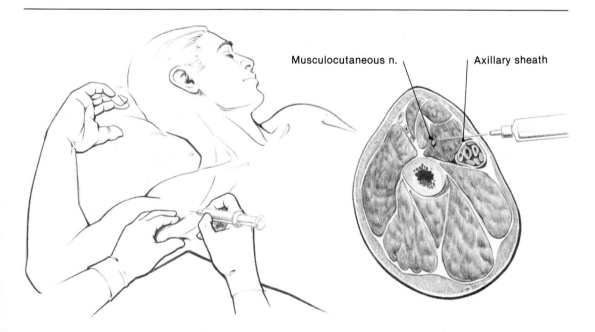

Musculocutaneous n.   Axillary sheath

Figure 17–10. Musculocutaneous block: Injection under biceps muscle. (Reproduced, with permission, from Katz J: *Atlas of Regional Anesthesia.* Appleton-Century-Crofts, 1985.)

block with sparing in the radial distribution. The site for supplemental block depends on the site of surgery and the experience of the clinician.

Anatomy

The radial nerve is a terminal branch of the posterior cord of the brachial plexus. From the axilla, it runs posterior to the humerus, innervating the triceps muscle. It enters the musculospiral groove of the humerus as it moves laterally. Terminal sensory branches include the lateral cutaneous nerve of the arm and the posterior cutaneous nerve of the forearm. After exiting the groove as it approaches the lateral epicondyle, it branches into superficial and deep branches. The deep branch remains close to periosteum and innervates the postaxial extensor group of the forearm. The superficial branch comes close to the dermis and follows the radial artery to innervate the radial aspects of the dorsal wrist and the dorsolateral $3\frac{1}{2}$ digits. The most reliable intervals for isolated block are the musculospiral groove, the radial head, and the site on the lateral distal forearm where the superficial radial nerve crosses from dorsal to volar across the radius (and becomes palpable).

Technique

Three sites are identified.

A. At the Upper Arm: (Figure 17–11.) The radial nerve exits the musculospiral groove between the two heads of the triceps. Palpation of a line between this site and the lateral epicondyle often reveals a palpable nerve. Three to 4 cm proximal to the epicondyle, a 23-gauge B-bevel 3/4-inch needle is inserted toward the nerve or to periosteum and withdrawn 0.5 cm, and 5 mL of local anesthetic is injected. Mild paresthesia is acceptable, but the intense paresthesia of intraneural injection must be avoided. At this level, localization with a nerve stimulator is possible with motor-evoked response of wrist extensors.

B. At the Elbow: (Figure 17–12.) From the antecubital space, the lateral aspect of the biceps tendon is identified at the flexion crease. A 23-gauge $1\frac{1}{2}$-inch B-bevel needle is inserted almost parallel to the forearm. It is directed just superficial to the radial head toward the lateral epicondyle until paresthesia is elicited or periosteum is encountered. With paresthesia, the needle is withdrawn slightly and injection then proceeds as long as intense paresthesia is not encountered. At the periosteum, the needle is withdrawn 1 cm, and 5 mL of local anesthetic is injected. Motor-evoked response can be elicited (wrist extension) with a nerve stimulator.

C. At the Distal Forearm: (Figure 17–13.) At the level of the ulnar styloid, sensory branches to the lateral side of the thumb lie between the radial artery and the flexor carpi radialis tendon. One to 2 milliliters of local anesthetic deposited in this interval, deep to flexor carpi radialis tendon, will block this sensation.

More proximally, dorsal branches are given off. In some individuals, this is palpable as the nerve moves from volar to dorsal. If palpable, 2–3 mL of local anesthetic as a directed field block can be performed. If not palpable, a linear field block at the level of the ulnar styloid from the volar lateral edge of the radius to the mid forearm will interrupt sensation to the dorsoradial $3\frac{1}{2}$ fingers.

Complications

Radial artery injection and intraneural injection

4. MEDIAN NERVE

Indications

Isolated median nerve block is performed almost invariably to supplement a brachial plexus block or as a part of carpal tunnel release done with local anesthesia at the level of the elbow or wrist.

Anatomy

The median nerve results from contribution of the lateral and medial cords of the brachial plexus. It enters the arm and runs medial to the brachial artery. As it enters the antecubital space, it is between the artery and the insertion of the biceps tendon. Just distal to this, it gives off numerous motor branches to wrist and finger flexors and follows the interosseous membrane to the wrist. At the level of the proximal wrist flexion crease, it lies directly behind palmaris longus tendon in the carpal tunnel.

Technique

A. At the Elbow: (Figure 17–14) At the antecubital flexion crease, the biceps insertion is identified medially. The brachial artery is identified. Directly between this artery and tendon, a 23-gauge B-bevel $1\frac{1}{2}$-inch needle is inserted and directed toward the medial epicondyle until paresthesia, a motor-evoked response (wrist flexion), or periosteum is encountered. Withdrawal to 1 cm from periosteum yields a good location. Three to 5 mL is injected—less with paresthesia, more without.

B. At the Wrist: (Figure 17–15) Resisted wrist flexion identifies the palmaris longus tendon. It is marked at the proximal flexion crease. A 25-gauge $\frac{3}{4}$-inch B-bevel needle is inserted deep to the palmaris longus, and 3–5 mL of anesthetic is deposited. Paresthesia should not be specifically elicited.

Complications

Brachial artery injection and intraneural injection are the primary risks.

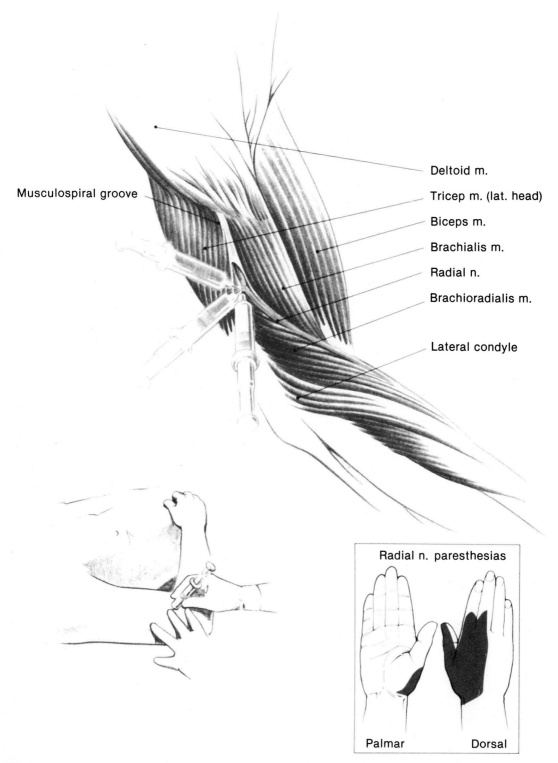

Deltoid m.

Tricep m. (lat. head)

Biceps m.

Brachialis m.

Radial n.

Brachioradialis m.

Lateral condyle

Musculospiral groove

Radial n. paresthesias

Palmar   Dorsal

Figure 17–11. Radial nerve block: Upper arm. (Reproduced, with permission, from Katz J: *Atlas of Regional Anesthesia.* Appleton-Century-Crofts, 1985.)

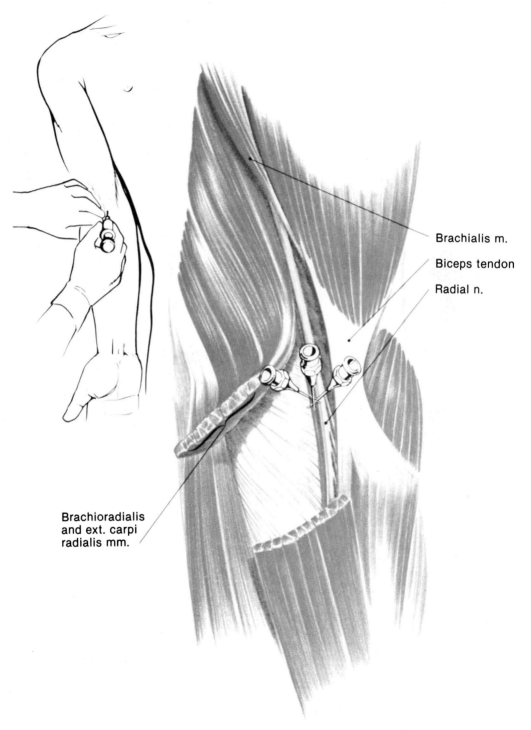

Brachialis m.

Biceps tendon

Radial n.

Brachioradialis
and ext. carpi
radialis mm.

Figure 17–12. Radial nerve block: Antecubital space. (Reproduced, with permission, from Katz J: *Atlas of Regional Anesthesia.* Appleton-Century-Crofts, 1985.)

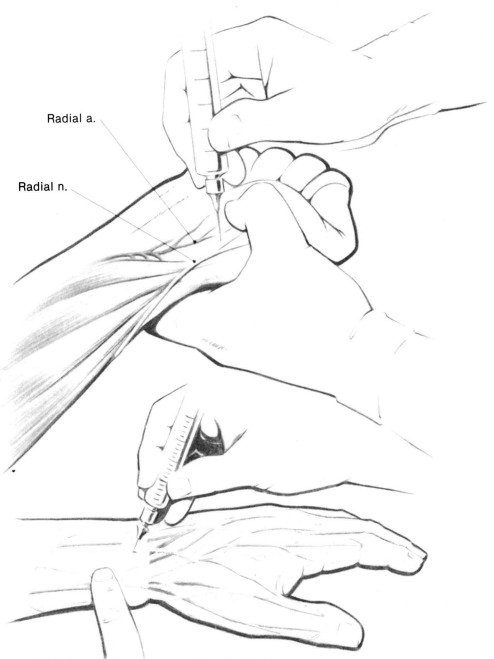

Radial a.

Radial n.

Figure 17–13. Radial nerve block: At the wrist. (Reproduced, with permission, from Katz J: *Atlas of Regional Anesthesia.* Appleton-Century-Crofts, 1985.)

5. ULNAR NERVE

Indications

With the ulnar side of the hand subject to frequent trauma, isolated ulnar nerve block can often serve as the sole anesthetic for a variety of surgical procedures, such as open or closed reduction of fifth metacarpal fracture. Isolated ulnar nerve block is often performed automatically when hand surgery is planned under interscalene block, because of inferior trunk sparing. Obviously, isolated ulnar nerve block can be added to partial axillary block if necessary. The block can be accomplished at the level of the elbow or wrist.

Anatomy

The ulnar nerve leaves the axilla with the axillary artery as the continuation of the medial cord of the

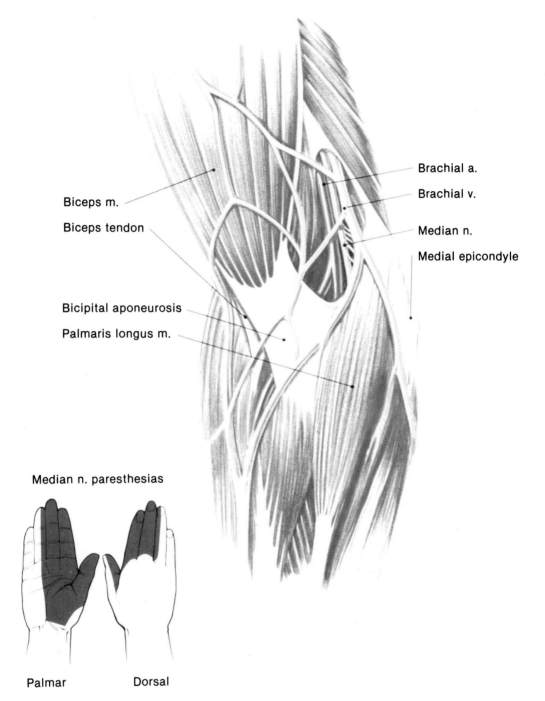

Biceps m.

Biceps tendon

Brachial a.

Brachial v.

Median n.

Medial epicondyle

Bicipital aponeurosis

Palmaris longus m.

Median n. paresthesias

Palmar   Dorsal

Figure 17–14. Median nerve block: Antecubital space. (Reproduced, with permission, from Katz J: *Atlas of Regional Anesthesia*. Appleton-Century-Crofts, 1985.)

brachial plexus and maintains this relationship through the upper arm. At the distal third of the humerus, it moves more medially and passes under the arcuate ligament of the medial epicondyle. Located 2–4 cm proximal to the medial epicondyle, the nerve is frequently palpable. In the distal forearm, the nerve splits into dorsal and palmar terminal branches after having given off muscular branches in the forearm. The final constant relationship in the forearm is the relationship of the nerve to the ulnar artery and flexor carpi ulnaris. In the mid forearm, the nerve lies between the flexor digitorum profundus and the flexor carpi ulnaris. As

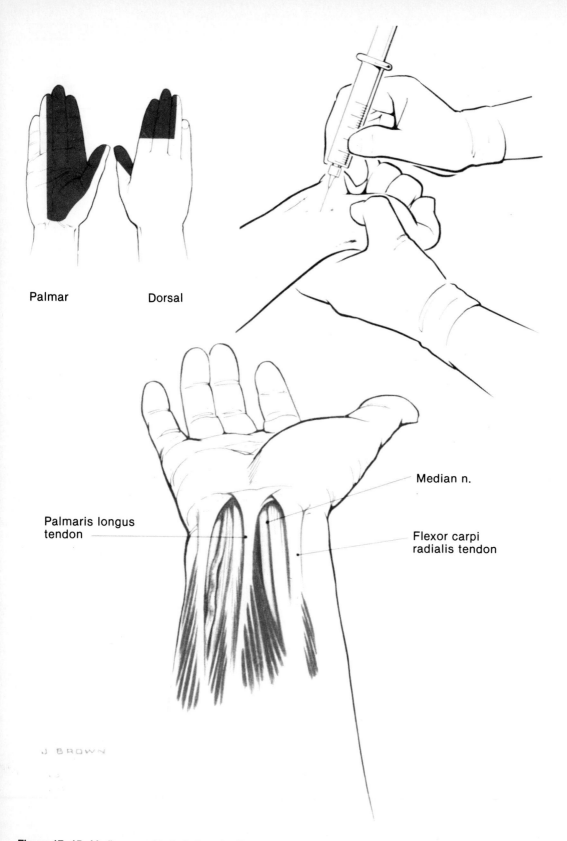

Palmar   Dorsal

Median n.

Palmaris longus
tendon

Flexor carpi
radialis tendon

J BROWN

Figure 17–15. Median nerve block: At the wrist. (Reproduced, with permission, from Katz J: *Atlas of Regional Anesthesia.* Appleton-Century-Crofts, 1985.)

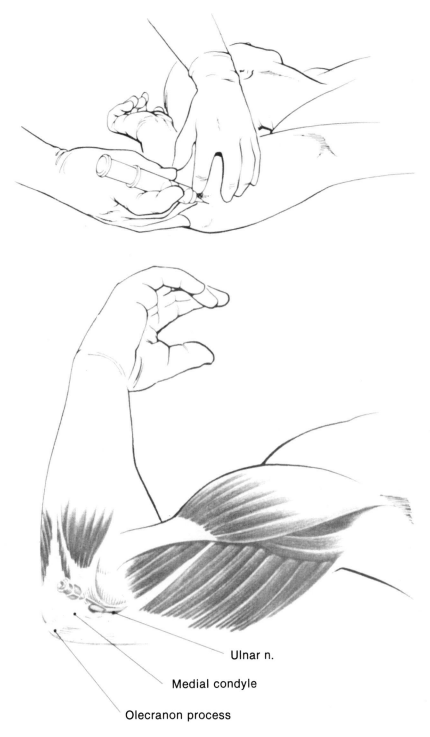

Ulnar n.

Medial condyle

Olecranon process

Figure 17–16. Ulnar nerve block: At the elbow. (Reproduced, with permission, from Katz J: *Atlas of Regional Anesthesia.* Appleton-Century-Crofts, 1985.)

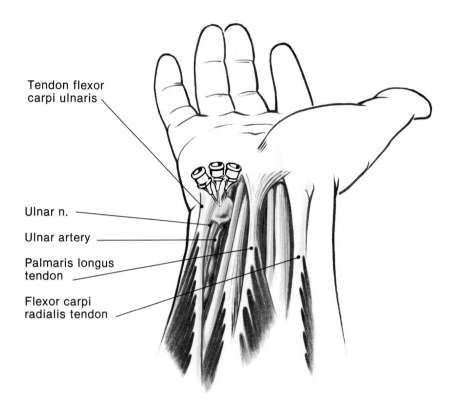

Tendon flexor
carpi ulnaris

Ulnar n.

Ulnar artery

Palmaris longus
tendon

Flexor carpi
radialis tendon

Figure 17–17. Ulnar nerve block: At the wrist. (Reproduced, with permission, from Katz J: *Atlas of Regional Anesthesia.* Appleton-Century-Crofts, 1985.)

Guyton's canal is approached at the wrist, the nerve is immediately lateral to the flexor carpi ulnaris tendon and medial to the artery.

Technique

A.   At the Elbow: (Figure 17–16) A 23-gauge, ³/₄-inch B-bevel needle is selected. The constant location of the nerve within the medial epicondyle is identified, and the nerve is palpated one finger breadth proximal to the arcuate ligament. The needle is inserted until paresthesia or motor-evoked response is elicited (finger movement). Care must be taken to avoid injection during persistent paresthesia, as intraneural injection can result in permanent morbidity.

B.   At the Wrist: (Figure 17–17) A 23-gauge, ¹/₂-inch, B-bevel needle is selected. If the ulnar artery is palpable, it is identified and marked at the proximal wrist flexion crease. Resisted flexion of the wrist identifies the flexor carpi ulnaris tendon, which is marked; the needle is directed just medial to the pulse, or immediately lateral to the flexor carpi ulnaris if no pulse is palpable. At the depth of the tendon or just below, paresthesia is elicited and the needle pulled back slightly. If not, fanwise injection of 3–5 mL will accomplish the block.

Complications

Intraneural injection may occur at the elbow and intraneural or intra-arterial injection at the wrist.

6.   DIGITAL BLOCK

Indications

Digital blocks are indicated for trauma or reconstruction of individual digits as well as in supplementation of partial brachial plexus blockade.

Anatomy

The fingers are supplied by terminal nerve branches which enter the fingers. If the fingers were rectangular, the nerves would enter near the four corners, close to the periosteum of the bone (Figure 17–18).

Technique

In the digital web space, a 25-gauge needle is placed at the base of the finger, and gentle injection of 2–3 mL of anesthetic is performed near periosteum while withdrawing. Entry from the dorsal side is normal, penetrating to near the volar base. Injection continues to the dorsal side. Paresthesia is avoided, as is hydrostatic compression of the tissues. Addition of vasoconstrictors is avoided. Both paresthesia and vasoconstrictors are associated with nerve injury. This is performed on both the radial and the ulnar side of the digit, at the level of the digit, more proximal at the level of the metacarpals.

Complications

Nerve injury is the chief risk of digital block.

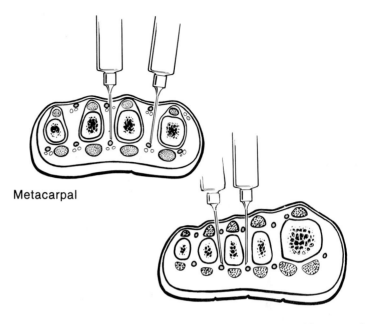

Metacarpal

Metatarsal

Digital

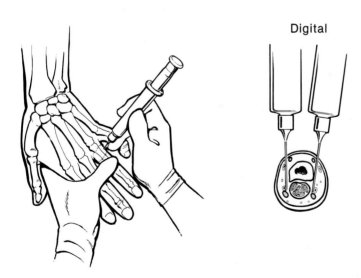

Figure 17–18. Digital block: Hand and foot. (Reproduced, with permission, from Katz J: *Atlas of Regional Anesthesia.* Appleton-Century-Crofts, 1985.)

LOWER EXTREMITY SOMATIC BLOCKADE

Surgery on the lower extremity involves blockade of somatic branches of the lumbar plexus and the sciatic nerve or its terminal branches. "Leg block" can be performed at the level of the hip, the knee, or the ankle.

FEMORAL NERVE

Indications

Femoral nerve block can be performed as a part of "leg block" for any surgical procedure of the lower extremity. It can be performed to relieve the pain of acute femoral fracture for transport or traction placement. It is also used as an intermittent or continuous technique for postoperative pain relief after knee surgery.

Anatomy

The femoral nerve arises from L2–4 within the substance of the psoas muscle. Passing through the psoas compartment, it innervates the iliac muscle and passes ventrally to enter the thigh superficially, lateral to the femoral artery at the level of the inguinal ligament. Distal to this point, motor branches to the quadriceps, sartorius, and pectineus arise as well as numerous sensory branches to the medial and anterior thigh. Rather than being a solid structure at this level, it is more like associated spaghetti strands within a sheath. From just outside the psoas muscle, the nerve is encased in a sheath that is continuous as far as just below inguinal ligament. This allows local anesthetic to be injected distally, to spread proximally, and to block other branches of the lumbar somatic plexus, such as the obturator and lateral femoral cutaneous nerves, provided distal pressure is applied to encourage proximal spread.

Technique

The patient is placed supine (Figure 17–19). The femoral pulse is identified and a 23-gauge, 1-inch B-bevel needle is placed just lateral (1 cm) to the artery. A distinct sheath can be felt, and shortly after, either a paresthesia or a motor-evoked response (movement of quadriceps) is elicited. Twenty milliliters of local anesthetic is injected. If block of the femoral, oburator, and lateral femoral cutaneous nerves are planned, distal pressure is applied and at least 40 mL is injected. This is the "three-in-one" block of Winnie.

Complications

Partial block can result from distal injection due to proximal branching. Intravascular injection is possible, especially if aspiration is too vigorous. Intraneural injection is possible but less likely than other blocks because of the multiple branches of the nerve substance.

OBTURATOR NERVE

Indications

The obturator nerve is blocked for procedures that require muscle relaxation of the adductor muscles of the thigh or surgical procedures including the medial thigh, such as muscle biopsy or adductor release. It is also blocked for procedures where a pneumatic tourniquet is applied to the thigh to facilitate operative dissection distally.

Anatomy

The obturator nerve arises from branches of L2–4 within the substance of the psoas muscle. It emerges medially and moves caudad in the retroperitoneum to the obturator canal. After emerging onto the medial thigh below the inguinal ligament, it becomes sensory to the medial thigh and the hip joint and gives motor branches to the thigh adductor group. The most reliable relationship occurs at the obturator foramen just dorsal to the inferior pubic ramus.

Technique (Figure 17–20)

A 3-inch, 22-gauge spinal needle is inserted through a skin wheal 2 cm lateral and inferior to the pubic symphysis. As the needle is advanced medially toward the interior pubic ramus, small amounts of local anesthetic are injected to decrease patient discomfort. Once periosteum is struck and injected, the needle is "walked off" the inferior ramus until it slips into the obturator foramen. As it does, the needle is advanced 3–4 cm and acquires a lateral and dorsal course. Paresthesia is not sought and rarely encountered. Ten to 20 mL of local anesthetic are injected.

Complications

Failed block and patient discomfort are the most likely untoward events.

LATERAL FEMORAL CUTANEOUS

Indications

The lateral femoral cutaneous nerve block can be used as sole anesthetic for procedures involving the proximal lateral thigh, such as muscle biopsy. It is also blocked for procedures that involve use of a pneumatic tourniquet and is often required for nontourniquet procedures as distal as the knee.

Anatomy

The lateral femoral cutaneous nerve arises from L2 and L3 within the substance of the psoas muscle, and on exiting it proceeds ventrally and laterally to become

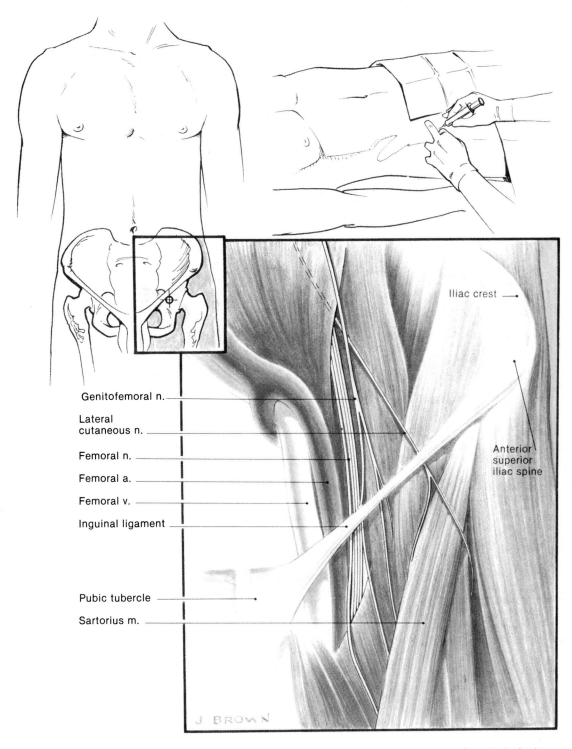

Genitofemoral n.

Lateral
cutaneous n.

Femoral n.

Femoral a.

Femoral v.

Inguinal ligament

Pubic tubercle

Sartorius m.

Iliac crest

Anterior
superior
iliac spine

J. BROWN

Figure 17–19. Femoral nerve block. (Reproduced, with permission, from Katz J: *Atlas of Regional Anesthesia.* Appleton-Century-Crofts, 1985.)

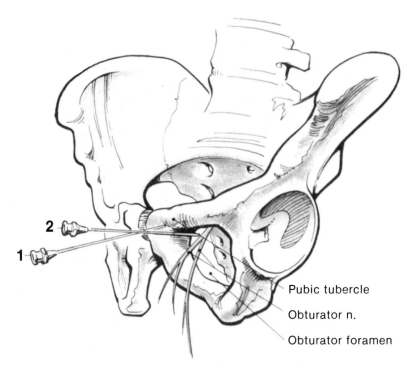

Figure 17–20. Obturator nerve block. (Reproduced, with permission, from Katz J: *Atlas of Regional Anesthesia.* Appleton-Century-Crofts, 1985.)

subcutaneous near the anterior superior iliac spine at the level of the inguinal ligament. The ligament covers the nerve at this level. Distal to this level, it becomes sensory, with branches to the lateral hip and thigh, mostly the proximal two-thirds but often as far as the lateral knee.

Technique
(Figure 17–21)

With the patient supine, the inguinal ligament is palpated and the anterior superior iliac spine identified. One finger breadth medial and inferior to the spine, over the ligament, a skin wheal is raised, and with a 22-gauge 1½-inch needle, the ligamentous fascia is entered. A click is felt, and a decrease of resistance is felt as the needle is directed deeper. Just dorsal to the ligament, 10–15 mL of the local anesthetic is injected in a fanlike manner, including some injected laterally deep to the ligament near the periosteum of the anterior superior iliac spine. Paresthesia may be encountered but is not sought. Severe burning pain with injection requires needle redirection to avoid nerve injury.

Complications

Patient discomfort, failed block, and persistent paresthesia from intraneural injection are the most common untoward sequelae.

SCIATIC NERVE

Indications

The sciatic nerve is blocked for virtually all procedures of the lower extremity and serves as sole anesthetic for cases not involving a tourniquet where there is no overlap with femoral nerve distribution. It may be blocked at the level of the hip or the popliteal fossa or as blocks of its terminal branches at the level of the ankle.

Anatomy

The sciatic nerve forms from branches of L4–S3 at the pelvic brim, leaving the pelvis below the piriformis muscle in the sciatic notch. It passes distally with several constant landmarks. With the leg in neutral position, it lies just dorsal to the superior aspect of the lesser trochanter of the femur (Figure 17–22). This is the basis for the anterior approach. In the lateral position with the hip flexed, it lies midway between the prominence of the greater trochanter and the posterior-superior iliac spine. It splits at various levels into the tibial and common peroneal nerve, and for this reason the block is often performed as proximal as possible.

Technique

A. Anterior Approach: (Figure 17–22) With the patient supine, the femoral artery is identified. Two

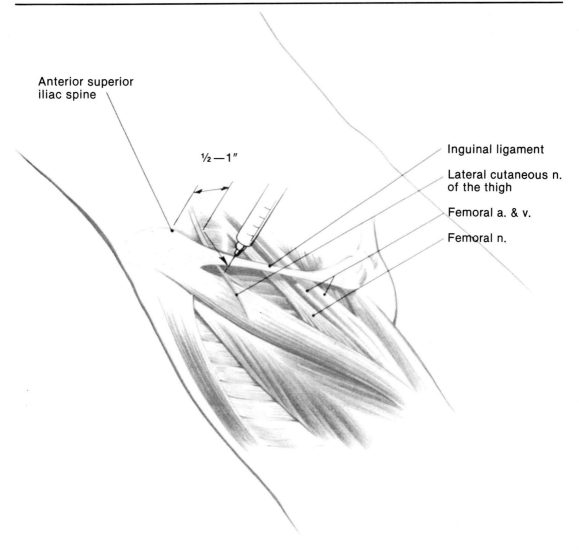

Anterior superior
iliac spine

½ — 1″

Inguinal ligament

Lateral cutaneous n.
of the thigh

Femoral a. & v.

Femoral n.

Figure 17–21. Lateral femoral cutaneous nerve block. (Reproduced, with permission, from Katz J: *Atlas of Regional Anesthesia.* Appleton-Century-Crofts, 1985.)

centimeters medially, a skin wheel is raised. A 22-gauge spinal needle is inserted for injection of local anesthetic for pain relief and directed dorsally until the periosteum of the lesser trochanter is encountered at a depth of 4–6 cm. It is injected, and the needle is "walked" superiorly until step-off occurs. Two to 4 cm farther dorsally, paresthesia or a motor-evoked response (foot dorsiflexion or plantar flexion) is elicited. Twenty milliliters of local anesthetic is injected. This technique is reserved for patients who cannot flex the hip for the traditional, easier, less painful posterior approach.

B. Posterior Approach: (Figure 17–23) The patient is placed in the lateral decubitus position, and the hip and knee are maximally flexed. A line connecting the prominence of the greater trochanter with the posterior superior iliac spine is drawn. At the mid-

point, a 4-cm perpendicular line is drawn caudally. These lines are referred to as Labatt's lines and identify a constant position of the sciatic nerve, in the sciatic notch, proximal to branching. Through a skin wheel, a 22-gauge spinal needle is inserted perpendicular to the skin, and at 4–6 cm from the surface—depending on patient's weight and muscle mass—the nerve can be felt. Confirmatory paresthesia or motor-evoked response (dorsflexion or plantar flexion of the foot) is mandatory. Twenty milliliters of local anesthetic is injected. Searing pain suggests intraneural injection and requires needle redirection.

Complications

Partial block due to injection distal to branching and intraneural injection are the most frequent complications.

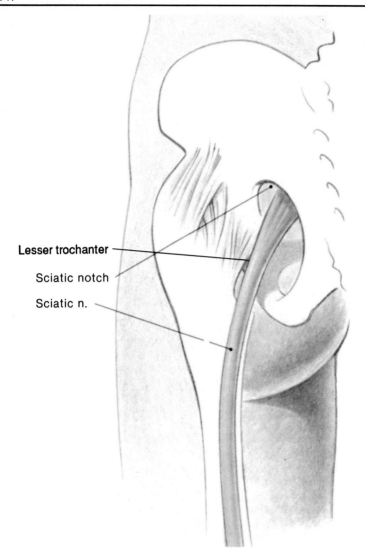

Figure 17–22. Sciatic nerve block: Anterior approach. (Reproduced, with permission, from Katz J: *Atlas of Regional Anesthesia.* Appleton-Century-Crofts, 1985.)

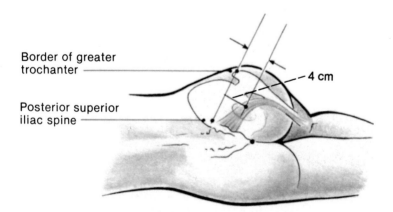

Figure 17–23. Sciatic nerve block: Posterior approach. (Reproduced, with permission, from Katz J: *Atlas of Regional Anesthesia.* Appleton-Century-Crofts, 1985.)

POPLITEAL BLOCK

Indications

Sciatic nerve block in the popliteal fossa is performed for procedures of the foot and ankle, where more proximal block (hip) is not feasible, where no tourniquet or calf tourniquet is adequate. In combination with sural nerve block, it provides complete anesthesia to the foot and ankle.

Anatomy

The sciatic nerve terminates into its branches, the tibial and common peroneal nerves, at the level of the popliteal fossa. The superficial outline of the fossa is formed laterally by the biceps tendon and medially by the semitendinosus tendon. Deep to this, cephalad to the flexion crease, the artery is immediately posterior to the semitendinosus, the vein lateral, and the nerves (within a sheath) just lateral to the vein and medial to the biceps tendon, 4–6 cm deep to the skin.

Technique
(Figure 17–24)

The patient is positioned prone. The outline of the popliteal fossa is identified proximal to the flexion crease of the knee by having the patient flex the knee. If the popliteal artery can be identified, it serves as a landmark. If not, the midline is identified. Two inches proximal to the crease, a skin wheal is raised. A 22-gauge spinal needle is inserted 1 cm lateral to the pulse—or in the midline if the pulse cannot be felt—and advanced 2–4 cm until paresthesia or motor-evoked response (plantar flexion or dorsiflexion of

foot) is elicited. Twenty to 30 mL of local anesthetic is injected.

Complications

Intravascular or intraneural injections are possible.

ANKLE BLOCK

Indications

Ankle block is performed for surgery of the foot, especially in patients too sick to tolerate the hemodynamic fluctuations associated with central block or general anesthesia and potentially less able to tolerate the larger volume of local anesthetic involved in proximal leg block.

Anatomy

Five nerves supply sensation to the foot. The saphenous nerve is a terminal branch of the femoral nerve and the only innervation of the foot not a part of the sciatic system. It supplies superficial sensation to the anteromedial foot and is most constantly located just anterior to the medial malleolus. The deep peroneal nerve runs in the anterior leg as a continuation of the common peroneal nerve, innervates toe extensors, enters the ankle between the flexor hallucis longus and the extensor digitorum longus tendons and provides sensation to the medial half of the dorsal foot, especially the first and second digits. A constant location is just lateral to the flexor hallucis longus at the level of the medial malleolus. The superficial peroneal nerve is also a branch of the common peroneal nerve, which

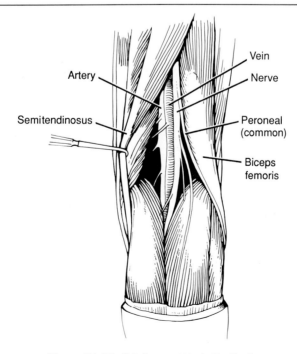

Figure 17–24. Sciatic nerve block: Popliteal.

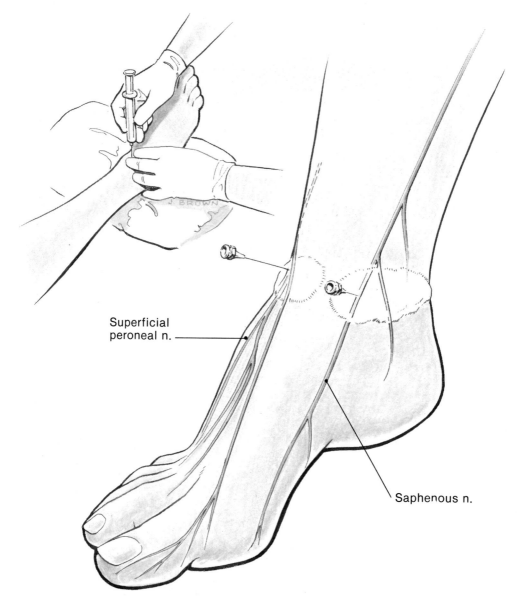

Superficial
peroneal n.

Saphenous n.

Figure 17–25. Ankle block: Saphenous and superficial peroneal nerves. (Reproduced, with permission, from Katz J: *Atlas of Regional Anesthesia.* Appleton-Century-Crofts, 1985.)

descends toward the ankle in the lateral compartment, entering the ankle just lateral to extensor digitorum longus and is cutaneous to the dorsum of the foot as well as all five toes. It is most constantly located lateral to the extensor digitorum longus at the level of the lateral malleolus superficially. The tibial nerve is a direct continuation and enters the foot posterior to the medial malleolus, branching into lateral and medial plantar nerves. It is constantly located behind the posterior tibial artery at the level of the medial malleolus. It is sensory to the heel, the medial sole, and part of the lateral sole of the foot. The sural nerve is the continuation of the posterior tibial nerve and enters the foot

between the Achilles tendon and the lateral malleolus, becoming sensory to the lateral foot. It is most constant superficially between the lateral malleolus and the Achilles tendon.

Technique

The superficial peroneal and saphenous nerves are blocked with subcutaneous infiltration on the dorsal foot—just lateral to the medial malleus for the saphenous and just lateral to the flexor hallucis longus for the superficial peroneal—with 3–5 mL of local anesthetic (Figure 17–25). Through the numb area from saphenous infiltration, a 22-gauge, 1½-inch

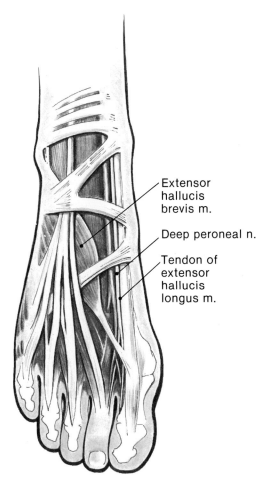

Extensor hallucis brevis m.

Deep peroneal n.

Tendon of extensor hallucis longus m.

Figure 17–26. Ankle block: Deep peroneal nerve. (Reproduced, with permission, from Katz J: *Atlas of Regional Anesthesia.* Appleton-Century-Crofts, 1985.)

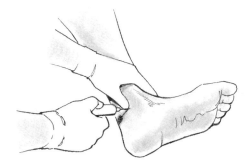

Figure 17–27. Ankle block: Tibial nerve. (Reproduced, with permission, from Katz J: *Atlas of Regional Anesthesia.* Appleton-Century-Crofts, 1985.)

high rate of persistent paresthesia after ankle block. Aggressive injection, especially with high volume, may cause hydrostatic damage to small nerves, especially those within closed ligamentous spaces like the tibial nerve.

needle is inserted just lateral to the extensor digitorum longus tendon in the interval between the flexor hallucis longus and extensor digitorum longus tendons to periosteum or elicitation of paresthesia and 5–8 mL are injected to block the deep peroneal nerve (Figure 17–26). The tibial nerve (Figure 17–27) is blocked posterior to the medial malleolus. The posterior tibial artery is palpated and the needle directed just inferior to the pulse until paresthesia or bone contact is encountered. If paresthesia is encountered, the needle is slightly withdrawn. If periosteum is contacted, the needle is withdrawn 1 cm. The injected volume is 5 mL. The sural nerve (Figure 17–28) is blocked laterally between the lateral malleolus and the Achilles tendon with a deep subcutaneous fan infiltration of 3–5 mL. Epinephrine is usually not added for ankle block due to the number of end arteries and the uncertain vascular supply to the foot in many of the patients.

Complications

In some clinical settings, there is an uncomfortably

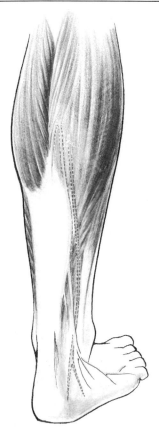

Figure 17–28. Ankle block: Sural nerve. (Reproduced, with permission, from Katz J: *Atlas of Regional Anesthesia.* Appleton-Century-Crofts, 1985.)

DIGITAL BLOCK OF THE FOOT

Because of the similarities, the reader is referred to upper extremity digital block and to Figure 17–18.

TRUNCAL SOMATIC BLOCKADE

CERVICAL PLEXUS
(Figure 17–3)

Indications

The superficial cervical plexus block is performed for unilateral procedures on the neck, such as carotid endarterectomy, and as an adjunct to shoulder surgery under interscalene block, especially with very anterior incisions.

Anatomy

The cervical plexus is formed from the anterior rami of C1–4, which emerge from the platysma muscle posterior to the sternocleidomastoid muscle and becomes cutaneous to the jaw, neck, the occiput posteriorly, and the areas of the chest and shoulder close to the clavicle.

Technique
(Figure 17–3)

The patient is positioned supine with the neck turned, and the posterior border of the sternocleidomastoid is identified. A 22-gauge spinal needle is selected, the sternocleidomastoid is divided into thirds, and at the junction of the upper and middle thirds a skin wheal is raised. The spinal needle is directed cephalad toward the mastoid along the posterior border of the sternocleidomastoid in a subcutaneous plane and injected with 2–3 mL as the needle is withdrawn. Care is made to avoid entering the external jugular vein. As the needle reaches the wheal, it is rotated 180 degrees and directed subcutaneously caudad toward the clavicle along the posterior border of the sternocleidomastoid. A similar amount is injected as the needle is withdrawn.

Complications

Owing to the high level of vascularity of the neck, rapid uptake and intravascular injection are the most common complications.

INTERCOSTAL BLOCKS

Indications

Intercostal blocks are performed for surgical procedures of the chest (breast procedures, tumor excision), in combination with celiac plexus block for upper abdominal surgery, or for pain relief after surgery (eg, cholecystectomy) or trauma (rib fracture).

Anatomy

The intercostal nerves arise from the dorsal and ventral rami of the thoracic spinal nerves. They exit from the spine at the intervertebral foramen and enter a groove on the underside of the corresponding rib, running with the intercostal artery and vein. Branches are given off for sensation in the correct dermatome from the midline dorsally all the way to across the midline ventrally. The constant access relationship is directly underneath the inferior surface of the rib in the midaxillary line.

Technique
(Figure 17–29)

A 22-gauge, $3/4$-inch needle is selected. The patient is placed in the lateral decubitus position, if possible, and the midaxillary line is identified. The correct ribs are identified and marked, and a skin wheal is raised over the caudal border. The needle is inserted, striking the rib, and walked until it steps off the rib inferiorly. It is advanced 1 cm farther. Aspiration confirms that the artery and lung have not been entered, and 3–5 mL is injected.

Complications

Intercostal blocks result in the highest blood levels of local anesthetic per volume injected of any block in the body. Care must be taken to avoid toxic levels of local anesthetic. Intravascular injection is possible.

PARAVERTEBRAL BLOCK

Indications

The paravertebral block is an intercostal block, performed near the midline for posterior cutaneous block or at the upper thoracic segments because of the interference of the scapula and shoulder in access to the intercostal nerve.

Anatomy

See intercostal block. The paravertebral block takes advantage of the constant location of the intercostal nerve just inferior to the transverse process of the spinal segment whose intervertebral foramen it has just exited through.

Technique
(Figure 17–30)

The patient is positioned prone, and a 22-gauge spinal needle with an adjustable bead is selected. The spinous process superior to the level to be blocked identifies the level of the transverse process; 4 cm lateral to this, a skin wheal is raised. The needle is inserted until the transverse process is contacted. The movable bead is moved to the skin to mark the depth of the transverse process. The needle is withdrawn to

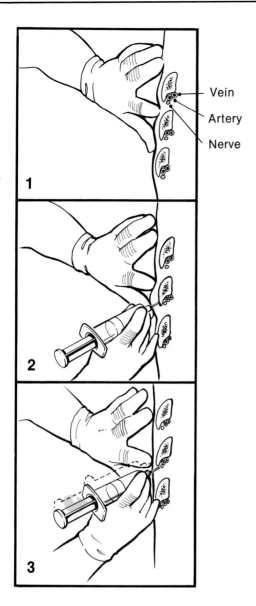

Figure 17–29. Intercostal block. (Reproduced, with permission, from Katz J: *Atlas of Regional Anesthesia.* Appleton-Century-Crofts, 1985.)

subcutaneous tissue and redirected to walk off the inferior edge of the transverse process and advanced to the bead. It is advanced farther, and within 2 cm from this point, paresthesias should be encountered. At the point where paresthesia occurs (or 2 cm of penetration), 5 mL is injected. Under no circumstances should the needle be advanced farther or repetitively moved in and out (seeking to elicit paresthesia), since the risk of pneumothorax is greatly increased by these maneuvers.

Complications

The most common complication of paravertebral block is pneumothorax, related to the number of levels

and the experience of the operator. If air is aspirated, chest x-ray is mandatory. Outpatient procedures utilizing this block should be carefully considered. Intravascular injection and failed block are other possible problems.

INGUINAL BLOCKS

Indications

Ilioinguinal and iliohypogastric blocks are performed as anesthesia for inguinal or genital surgery, such as inguinal herniorrhaphy or orchiopexy or for postoperative pain relief after these operations.

Anatomy

Both nerves arise from T12 and L1. The iliohypogastric splits into two branches prior to becoming cutaneous. The lateral branch is sensory to the lateral aspect of the buttock and hip. The anterior branch becomes superficial just medial to the anterior superior iliac spine, where it sends off a network of branches that innervate the lower abdomen. The ilioinguinal nerve follows the same course and exits peritoneum to enter the inguinal canal, where it provides sensation to the scrotum, penis, medial thigh, or equivalent area of the labia and mons pubis in the female. The constant relationship is the piercing of the inguinal ligament 1 cm medial to the anterior superior iliac spine.

Technique
(Figure 17–31)

A 22-gauge, 3-inch spinal needle is selected. Prior to surgical incision, a point 1 cm medial to the upper aspect of the anterior superior iliac spine is identified and a skin wheal is raised. The needle is inserted perpendicular to the skin until it is just under the fascia, and 8–10 mL of anesthetic is injected fanwise in the method of field block. If the procedure is being done after an inguinal incision has been made or closed, an imaginary line is drawn to the anterior superior iliac spine. From the most lateral aspect of the incision, a 45-degree line toward the midline is imagined, and the needle is inserted along this line for 4–6 cm subcutaneously, and 6-8 mL is injected while withdrawing cephalad and caudal to the incision. The resulting skin distortion and the incision will resemble an arrow (Figure 17–32).

Complications

Both nerves are small, and continued injection after paresthesia persists must be avoided.

PENILE BLOCK

Indications

Penile block is performed for anesthesia during penile surgery or postoperative pain relief afterward.

Identify correct dorsal spine
superior to nerve to be blocked

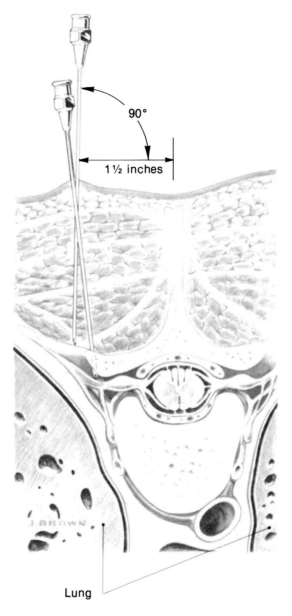

Figure 17–30. Paravertebral block. (Reproduced, with permission, from Katz J: *Atlas of Regional Anesthesia.* Appleton-Century-Crofts, 1985.)

Anatomy

Three nerves contribute to sensation of the penis. The genitofemoral and ilioinguinal nerves contribute to sensation of the base of the penis from the inguinal canal. These nerves become subcutaneous prior to entry onto the dorsal and lateral surfaces of the penis. The principal nerve is the pudendal nerve, which gives off the dorsal nerve of the penis bilaterally. It enters the penis deep to Buck's fascia and divides into dorsal and ventral branches.

Technique
(Figure 17–33)

A fan-shaped field block at the base of the penis, 2–4 cm lateral to the penis on both sides, will accomplish block of these end-sensory nerves without risk of vascular embarrassment of the penis. If more solid block is necessary or if extensive surgery is planned, the dorsal nerve is blocked just lateral to the base of the penis bilaterally with a 23-gauge, ³/₄-inch needle penetrating just through fascia, with 3–5 mL injected,

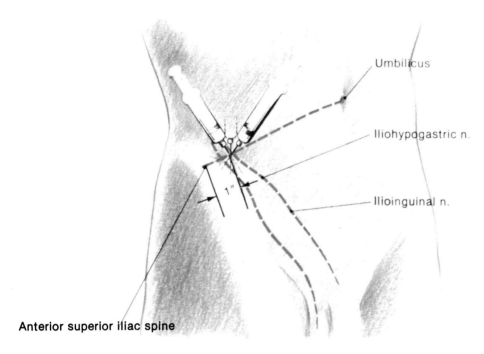

Umbilicus

Iliohypogastric n.

Iliohypogastric n.

1"

Iliohypogastric n.

Iliohypogastric n.

Anterior superior iliac spine

Figure 17–31. Ilioinguinal-iliohypogastric nerve block.

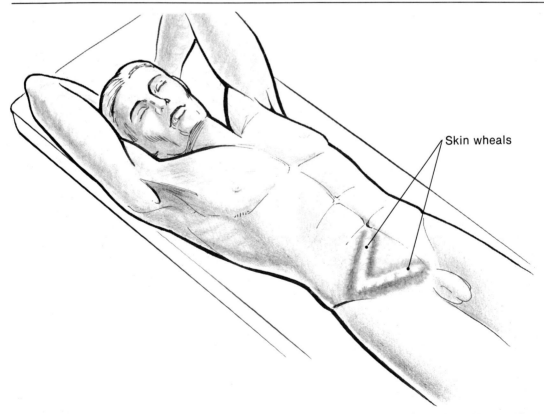

Skin wheals

Figure 17–32. Ilioinginal-iliohypogastric field block. (Reproduced, with permission, from Katz J: *Atlas of Regional Anesthesia.* Appleton-Century-Crofts, 1985.)

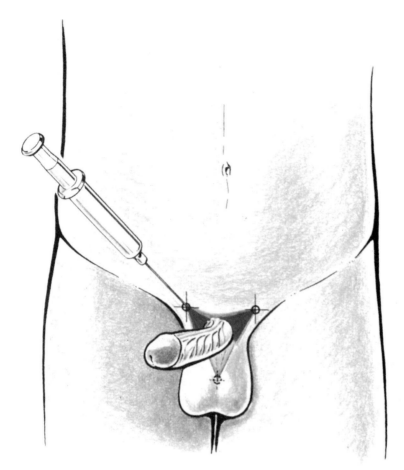

Figure 17–33. Penile block. (Reproduced, with permission, from Katz J: *Atlas of Regional Anesthesia*. Appleton-Century-Crofts, 1985.)

avoiding pressure. Epinephrine or other vasoconstrictors must be avoided because of possible end-artery embarrassment.

Complications

Hemorrhage from trauma to the corpus cavernosum makes this block one that should be done most often by urologists or others with considerable experience if deep injection is necessary. Superficial block for postoperative pain relief is safe and may be done by anyone practicing regional anesthesia.

INTRAVENOUS REGIONAL ANESTHESIA

Intravenous regional anesthesia is a technique that provides solid, dense anesthesia of an extremity for short surgical procedures. With operator experience,

reliability and safety is high and patient satisfaction excellent.

Technique
(Figure 17–34)

An intravenous catheter is placed distally in the extremity. A reliable pneumatic tourniquet with a double bladder and two independent tank and gauge setups is placed on the proximal extremity. The extremity is elevated and exsanguinated by wrapping with an Eschmark elastic bandage and the proximal tourniquet proximal inflated. The Eschmark is removed, and the agent is injected. For the upper extremity, 40–50 mL of 0.5% lidocaine or prilocaine is used. For the lower extremity, 60–75 mL is used. After anesthesia is established, the distal tourniquet is inflated and the proximal one subsequently deflated. At the time limit, the patient will complain of pain from the tourniquet. This can be minimized for brief intervals by switching the tourniquet again, always with inflation first before deflation. With very short procedures, the tourniquet must be left inflated for a total of 20–30 minutes to avoid a rapid intravenous bolus of local anesthetic.

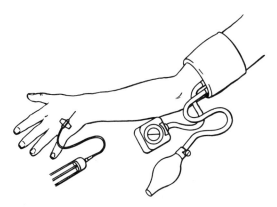

Figure 17–34. Intravenous regional anesthesia.

Deflation with immediate reinflation, repeated several times, also provides a safety margin. The chief complications are patient discomfort and seizure activity.

CASE DISCUSSION: TOTAL SPINAL ANESTHESIA FOLLOWING INJECTION OF ATTEMPTED INTERSCALENE BLOCK

A 32-year-old man with chronic instability of his right shoulder presents to the operating room for capsular advancement for repair of chronic shoulder dislocation. He is otherwise healthy and prefers a regional anesthetic, and an interscalene block with 1.4% mepivacaine with epinephrine 1:200,000 is selected. The interscalene brachial plexus is approached by attempting to elicit paresthesia. A brief paresthesia in the upper arm is encountered; 40 mL of the agent is planned to be injected; and the injection is begun. The patient becomes restless and agitated after approximately 15 mL of the agent are injected. He complains briefly of difficulty with breathing and then becomes apneic and unresponsive.

What is the presumptive diagnosis?

The relationship of this profound change in the patient's status to injection of local anesthetic in the interscalene grove raises the presumption that the change is related to injection into an unintended location. Several nearby structures can contribute to untoward reactions. The proximity of the vertebral artery suggests possible direct interarterial injection of local anesthetic into the brain. However, the prodrome of this event is most typically abrupt onset of grand mal seizure. Other local structures that could be reached behind the interscalene brachial plexus include the epidural, subdural,

and subarachnoid spaces. The rapid timing of apnea and nonresponsiveness after the patient's first complaints makes subarachnoid injection the most likely explanation for this change.

What are the expected hemodynamic responses to this event?

Because massive total spinal anesthesia is the working diagnosis, it should be assumed that total sympathectomy will result rapidly. This will result in a vagally dominated profound bradycardia as well as profound vasodilation of capacitance vessels, with diminished venous return to the heart and profound hypotension being the result. Apnea should be expected for a considerable period of time.

What measures should be taken *immediately*?

Injection of local anesthetic should be stopped. The patient should be placed in Trendelenburg's position, intravenous fluid lines opened as widely as possible, and 100% oxygen by controlled ventilation commenced. It is important to ventilate the patient by mask before proceeding to endotracheal intubation, since oxygenation is the first priority and control of the airway is secondary. If ventilation with 100% oxygen by mask is either very difficult or impossible, rapid intubation of the trachea should be undertaken. It is likely that no muscle relaxant or hypnotic agent will be necessary. Furthermore, the anticipated sympathectomy should be treated. A vagolytic dose of an anticholinergic drug—atropine is the obvious choice—should be injected as well as a vasoactive drug such as ephedrine or phenylephrine (or perhaps both) to counteract the anticipated profound drop in blood pressure. If the bradycardia suddenly becomes profound—especially if cardiac output appears to be severely impaired—rapid switch to epinephrine is probably indicated.

What should be done about the surgical procedure?

Assuming that the airway is secured and that the hemodynamic response to the total spinal anesthesia is rapidly managed and the patient is stable, the conditions of the patient under total spinal anesthetic do not contraindicate proceeding with the planned surgical procedure. The patient will be amnestic and analgesic, and surgical conditions will be ideal. Giving the anticipated duration of mepivacaine in the central nervous system, after a short period of time an amnestic drug such as midazolam should be administered to provide amnesia and lack of intraoperative recall. The anticipated duration of apnea would be consistent with the known duration of action of mepivacaine, ie, slightly greater than that of lidocaine and less than that of bupivacaine with routine spinal anesthesia. However, this may be modified by the large dose that may have entered the subarachnoid space. If there is a doubt about the hemodynamic or central nervous system status of the patient based on the management of the initial events, surgery should be rescheduled for another day.

What factors about the performance of this block may have contributed to this outcome?

During technical performance of the block, a paresthesia was sought as a sign for injection of the local anesthetic in the right location, the interscalene brachial plexus. While a paresthesia was elicited, it was not persistent and was not present at the time of injection. It is possible that the needle elicited a paresthesia and that the anesthesiologist continued to move the needle forward—even very briefly—while the patient reported the paresthesia. With the paresthesia not being persistent, it is possible that the tip of the needle was posterior to the brachial plexus sheath, and this places it in close proximity to the structures mentioned earlier. Insistence on elicitation of paresthesia as well as persistence with brief transient augmentation of the paresthesia on injection will ensure that the needle tip remains within the sheath of the brachial plexus during injection. It may also be that if incremental injection of the local anesthetic were performed, less total mepivacaine would have been injected into the subarachnoid space.

SUGGESTED READINGS

Cousins MJ, Bridenbaugh PO (editors): *Neural Blockade in Clinical Anesthesia and Management of Pain,* 2nd ed. Lippincott, 1988.

Katz J: *Atlas of Regional Anesthesia.* Appleton-Century-Crofts, 1985.

Moore DC: *Regional Block: A Handbook for Use in the Clinical Practice of Medicine and Surgery,* 4th ed. Thomas, 1978.

Prithvi R, Nalte H, Stanton-Hicks M: *Illustrated Manual of Regional Anesthesia.* Springer-Verlag, 1988.

Winnie AP: *Plexus Anesthesia. Perivascular Techniques of Brachial Plexus Block,* vol I. Saunders, 1983.

Pain Management

18

Raymond R. Gaeta, MD,* & William G. Brose, MD†

The role of the anesthesiologist extends beyond the operating room and includes the management of both acute and chronic pain in both the clinic and hospital settings. The anesthesiologist is trained not only in the technical aspects of pain management, such as nerve blocks and spinal catheter placement, but must also utilize diagnostic skills, understanding of pharmacologic principles, and broad medical knowledge in formulating a rational treatment plan for complex pain problems. The coordination of pain management plans by the anesthesiologist is an important role that must incorporate the opinions of varied consultants such as internists, neurologists, neurosurgeons, and other specialists.

Although postoperative pain control accounts for the majority of acute pain management, other acute and chronic disease states will be discussed in this chapter. The discussion of chronic pain will be limited to the areas of oncologic pain and benign pain syndromes, with emphasis on neuropathic and myofascial pain. The text will also discuss some neuroanatomic and physiologic concepts basic to the management of acute and chronic pain.

DEFINITION OF TERMS & REVIEW OF NEUROANATOMY

The International Association for the Study of Pain (IASP) has defined pain as "an unpleasant sensory and emotional experience associated with actual or potential tissue damage, or described in terms of such damage." This definition recognizes the interplay of both physical and psychologic factors of pain and suggests that combined-modality therapy may often be required to treat pain syndromes.

As with any specialty in medicine, agreement about the meanings of various terms and phrases allows greater precision in diagnosis and facilitates communication between consultants. Table 18–1 serves as a brief glossary of several basic terms used in pain management. Two terms—nociceptive and neu-

ropathic pain—will be discussed in the context of basic neuroanatomy.

Multiple stimuli are perceived from skin, somatic structures, joints, and viscera. Nociceptors convert the physical attributes of chemical, thermal, and mechanical stimuli into electrical signals that allow us to perceive noxious stimuli in the environment (Figure 18–1). These events are transduced by free nerve endings in the end organs, and the resultant electrical signals are transmitted via the small myelinated A δ and unmyelinated C fibers. The A δ fibers, both mechanical and thermomechanical, respond to stimuli chiefly in a graded fashion by increasing discharge rates as the stimulus is increased. The unmyelinated C fibers include polymodal nociceptors that respond to chemical, thermal, and mechanical stimuli. These unmyelinated fibers have slower conduction velocities and thus give rise to a dull, slow-onset, burning pain sensation—in contrast to the sharp pinching sensation associated with the faster myelinated A δ fibers.

Neuropathic pain—rather than being a response to environmental events—is related to functional abnormality of the nervous system. Normal nonnoxious stimuli can at times be interpreted as painful by the abnormal nervous system, while at other times pain may be perceived in the absence of any direct stimulus. Neuropathic pain syndromes will be discussed further below in the section on chronic pain.

In both nociceptive and neuropathic pain, signals are transmitted to the spinal cord, where complex interaction occurs (Figure 18–2). The pain fibers enter via the dorsal root and enter Lissauer's tract. They may ascend or descend one or two segments before synapsing in the various laminae of the ipsilateral dorsal horn. Lamina II, also known as the substantia gelatinosa, is of special interest because the site of opiate action is thought to occur within this lamina.

The various neurons that arise from the laminae ascend via multiple nociceptive tracts. The spinothalamic and spinoreticular tracts are significant pain pathways in this system. As the fibers of these neurons ascend, the majority cross the midline to travel in the contralateral portion of the spinal cord. The signals are then transmitted to the brainstem and thalamus and then to the cerebral cortex. Modulation of both ascending and descending signals at these lower brain centers may in part explain the uncoupling of the pain stimulus

*Fellow in Anesthesia, Stanford University Medical Center, Stanford, California.
†Assistant Professor of Anesthesia and Director, Stanford Pain Management Services, Stanford, California.

Table 18–1. Taxonomy of pain.[1]

Allodynia: Pain due to a nonnoxious stimulus to normal skin.
Analgesia: Lack of pain on noxious stimulation.
Dysesthesia: An unpleasant abnormal sensation.
Hypalgesia (hypoalgesia): Diminished sensitivity to noxious stimulation.
Hypesthesia (hypoesthesia): Decreased sensitivity to stimulation.
Hyperalgesia: Increased sensitivity to noxious stimulation.
Hyperesthesia: Increased sensitivity to stimulation.
Hyperpathia: A painful syndrome characterized by delay, overreaction, and aftersensation to a stimulus, especially a repetitive stimulus.

[1]Adapted from: Cousins MJ, Bridenbaugh PO (editors): *Neural Blockade in Clinical Anesthesia and Management of Pain*, 2nd ed. Lippincott, 1988.

and response that occurs in individuals injured in battle or in athletic mishaps.

Despite all we do know about these anatomic tracts, the mechanisms by which modulation and perception of pain occur remain speculative. It is still not possible to define precise "pain pathways," but their future elucidation may give rise to specific treatment options for many acute and chronic pain syndromes.

ACUTE PAIN MANAGEMENT

The management of acute pain has far-reaching consequences beyond a simple decrease in the patient's experience of noxious stimuli. The sympathetic nervous system, neuroendocrine system, and respiratory system are but a few of the physiologic components substantially affected by the pain. Table 18–2 outlines the multiple physiologic responses to pain. *It is the goal of pain management not only to decrease the patient's pain but to return the patient to a more normal physiologic state.*

SYSTEMIC RESPONSES TO PAIN

Sympathetic Nervous System

The sympathetic nervous system—in conjunction with the neuroendocrine system—causes significant changes in cardiovascular homeostasis. The release of catecholamines is associated with increased systemic vascular resistance, tachycardia, and hypertension, with a resultant increase in myocardial oxygen consumption and myocardial work. For patients with marginal myocardial reserve, it is easy to envision clinical situations where myocardial demand exceeds supply, thus leading to further myocardial dysfunction.

Respiratory System

The respiratory system responds to pain in part by decreased movement of the chest wall, leading to reductions in vital capacity and functional residual capacity that may result in atelectasis, decreased clearance of secretions, and lower arterial oxygen tension. These changes occur in patients with normal pulmonary function but can lead to quite significant morbidity in patients with borderline pulmonary function.

Gastrointestinal & Urinary Systems

The gastrointestinal and genitourinary systems are also affected by pain. The increase in adrenergic tone causes increased intestinal secretions with decreased motility and subsequent development of ileus. Nausea, vomiting, and constipation are clinical sequelae. Changes in smooth muscle and sphincter tone in the genitourinary system in response to pain cause urinary retention.

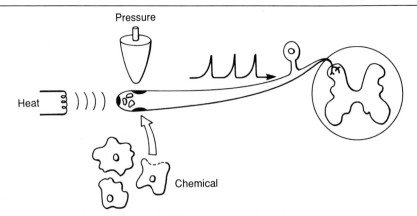

Figure 18–1 Sensitivity range of the C-polymodal nociceptor. Evidence suggests that the terminals are sensitive to direct heat or mechanical distortion. Thus, transduction can occur at the terminal. The terminals are also sensitive to chemicals released from damaged cells. In this manner, any tissue cell can serve as an intermediate in the transduction process. In a sense, all tissue cells are "receptors" for injury. (Reproduced, with permission, from Fields HL: *Pain*. McGraw-Hill, 1987.)

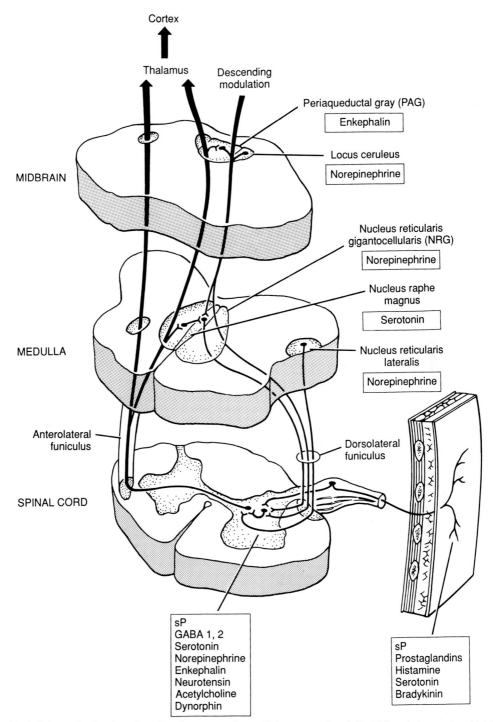

Figure 18–2 Schematic drawing of nociceptive processing outlining ascending (left side) and descending (right side) pathways. Stimulation of nociceptors in the skin surface leads to impulse generation in the primary afferent. Concomitantly with this impulse generation, increased levels of various endogenous algetic agents (substance P, prostaglandins, histamine, serotonin, bradykinin) are detected near the area of stimulation in the periphery. The noxious impulse is conducted to the dorsal horn of the spinal cord, where it is subjected to local factors and descending modulation. The endogenous neurochemical mediators of this interaction at the dorsal horn that have been characterized to date are listed in the figure. Primary nociceptive afferents are relayed to projection neurons in the dorsal horn that ascend in the anterolateral funiculus to end in the thalamus. En route, collaterals of the projection neurons activate the nucleus reticularis gigantocellularis (NRG). Neurons from the NRG project to the thalamus and also activate the periaqueductal gray (PAG) of the midbrain. Enkephalinergic neurons from the PAG and noradrenergic neurons from the NRG activate descending serotonergic neurons of the nucleus raphe magnus (NRM). These fibers join with noradrenergic fibers from the locus ceruleus reticularis lateralis to project descending modulatory impulses to the dorsal horn via the dorsolateral funiculus. (Modified and reproduced, with permission, from Cousins MJ, Bridenbaugh PO: *Neural Blockade in Clinical Anesthesia and Management of Pain,* 2nd ed. Lippincott, 1988.)

Table 18–2. Neuroendocrine and metabolic responses to stress.[1]

Responses	Causes
Endocrine	
Catabolic	Increases in ACTH, cortisol, vasopressin, growth hormone, cAMP, catecholamines, renin, angiotensin II, aldosterone, glucagon
Anabolic	Decreases in insulin, testosterone
Metabolic	
Carbohydrate: Hyperglycemia, glucose intolerance, insulin resistance	Increases in hepatic glycogenolysis (epinephrine, glucagon), gluconeogenesis (growth hormone), cortisol, free fatty acids, epinephrine, glucagon
	Increases in insulin secretion, resistance
Protein: Muscle protein catabolism provides alanine for gluconeogenesis	Increases in cortisol, glucagon (starvation response)
Fat: Lipolysis of tissue fat providing increases in free fatty acids, gluconeogenesis	Increases in catecholamines, glucagon (starvation response)
Water and electrolyte flux	
Retention of H_2O and Na^+ and increased excretion of K^+	Increases in aldosterone, ADH, cortisol, epinephrine
Decreased functional ECF as ECF shifts to vascular and cellular compartments	Increases in catecholamines, ADH, angiotensin II
Cardiovascular	
Venoconstriction (decreased venous capacitance); arteriolar constriction (increased peripheral resistance)	Increases in catecholamines, angiotensin II, ADH
Increased myocardial work	All of the above
Respiratory	
Hypoxemia, hypoventilation, atelectasis	Increased O_2 utilization
Attempt to increase ventilation	Increased CO_2 production

[1]From Cousins MJ, Philips GD (editors): *Acute Pain Management.* Churchill Livingstone, 1986.

Musculoskeletal System

Skeletal muscle also responds to pain with an increase in tone, serving to immobilize an injured area or limb. Although it is a protective mechanism, continued spasm is a source of further pain that may have protracted effects distinct from those associated with the original injury.

POSTOPERATIVE PAIN

Currently, the management of postoperative pain is within the scope of the anesthesiologist's role, particularly in view of the anesthesiologist's familiarity with parenteral and spinal opiates. The consulting anesthesiologist should recommend plans for postoperative management that are individualized for each patient. These suggestions may include choice of agent, route of administration, and the advantages of specific techniques.

1. LOCAL ANESTHETICS

Local anesthetics for postoperative pain relief can be administered by infiltration along the incision line or around the operative site by the surgeon or anesthe-

siologist before the patient leaves the operating room. More specific techniques include nerve blocks—eg, intercostal, brachial plexus, and lower extremity blocks—that can serve larger areas of pain. These techniques allow pain relief of variable duration depending on the agent administered. Incisional infiltration and field blocks are easy and relatively safe methods of achieving some measure of relief and can be administered by the surgeon; specific nerve blocks should be administered by the anesthesiologist in order to reduce the incidence of complications such as pneumothorax, intravascular injection, and intraneural injection of local anesthetic.

Injection of local anesthetics into the **subarachnoid or epidural space** is a specialized technique requiring direct medical supervision perioperatively to detect and treat hypotension, motor blockade, high spinal levels of anesthesia, and local anesthetic toxicity. The duration of analgesia by this technique can be titrated by selecting a longer-acting preparation for single-dose administration or by using a catheter technique to provide continuous delivery of drug. Although both subarachnoid and epidural techniques have been described, the use of epidural local anesthetics may be preferable because of the greater ease of titration.

2. ORAL OPIOIDS

Opioids have long been utilized in the control of postoperative pain. Various routes of administration can be employed. Many patients require very little analgesia, and in those who have resumed oral intake, oral administration may be adequate. Generally, the surgeon will order oral opiates that should be offered to the patient on a regular schedule. The patient may also request medications on an as-needed—"prn"—basis for incidental pain. Codeine and oxycodone may be sufficient in some cases. In patients on restricted oral intake, parenteral opiates may be required.

3. PATIENT-CONTROLLED ANALGESIA

The intramuscular or intravenous injection of opiates such as morphine or meperidine is familiar to most physicians. This technique does provide pain relief but can lead to patient dissatisfaction related to the intermittent nature of drug administration, delays in drug administration, inadequate doses, and long intervals between doses. A technique that minimizes such delays is the use of patient-controlled analgesia, which allows the patient to self-administer intravenous opiates as needed from an apparatus that the physician can preset to deliver a specific dose at a minimal dosing interval. More sophisticated machines can also limit the total dose per hour as an added safety measure. For optimal analgesic management with this apparatus, the patient may need a continuous infusion of drug at nighttime so that sleep is less ap to be disturbed by varying drug levels.

4. SPINAL ANALGESIA

An alternative to intravenous opiates is the technique of spinal administration (epidural or subarachnoid instillation). Opiates can be given as a single dose, as an intermittent bolus, or by continuous infusion into the epidural or subarachnoid space. After administration, the opiate gains access to the substantia gelatinosa in the dorsal horn of the spinal cord.

Candidates for intraspinal opiates are from a spectrum of surgical subspecialties. Postthoracotomy and postlaparotomy patients are excellent candidates because of the effects of pain on the respiratory system, as previously described. Patients who have undergone bladder or radical prostate resection are candidates for similar reasons, even though the operation is in the lower abdomen. Patients who have undergone thoracic or abdominal aneurysm repair can also benefit from this form of pain control. The orthopedic patient may be able to participate more quickly in postoperative rehabilitation after major joint replacement if pain is well managed. In addition to these patients, the postcesarian section, surgical gynecologic, and perhaps the neurosurgical laminectomy patient can benefit from single-dose techniques.

Besides pain relief, patients managed by spinal analgesia derive additional benefit from earlier ambulation, better cooperation with the demands of physical therapy programs, and, more significantly, improvement in respiratory status. With less pain, patients are able to cooperate with deep breathing, incentive spirometry, and pulmonary toilet requirements. These patients would thus be at less risk for postoperative atelectasis, pneumonia, and venous thrombosis.

Preoperative Evaluation & Consent

Candidates for spinal opiates should be screened carefully preoperatively to make certain that the benefits outweigh the risks and that no contraindications fits outweigh the risks and that no contraindications exist. A history of easy bleeding, prolonged bleeding, or aspirin ingestion suggests that a contraindication may exist. Laboratory data may confirm the presence of a coagulopathy or prolongation of the bleeding time. Patients taking anticoagulants such as warfarin or heparin will also have evidence of decreased clotting. If time permits, the coagulopathy can be corrected or the anticoagulant can be reversed so that the spinal technique can be used. Aspirin or other antiplatelet drugs should be discontinued for at least 1 week prior to the procedure. Clearly, in the case of the anticoagulants, reversal should not expose the patient to undue risk of thrombotic events just for the sake of the spinal technique. Other patients may undergo heparinization intraoperatively; however, this is not an absolute contraindication to the spinal technique. The spinal catheter may be placed postoperatively after the heparin has been reversed, or perhaps even placed the day before surgery to allow coagulation to occur. Discussion with the surgeon preoperatively should help formulate a plan.

Other issues regarding the use of spinal analgesia include the presence of infection or tumor at the site of puncture. The presence of systemic infection may be a relative contraindication; however, proved bacteremia with positive blood cultures makes placement of a catheter into the epidural or subarachnoid space an unwarranted risk. Patient consent to the proposed postoperative pain control strategy is an important feature of the consent solicitation procedure. It is implicit in the necessity for informed consent that the anesthesiologist must communicate beforehand with the patient. Many patients are leery of "a needle in the back" and for that reason may not consent to the placement of the epidural or spinal needle while awake. In the course of the preoperative assessment, the anesthesiologist should address these issues and in appropriate cases should offer alternatives that may be more acceptable to the patient.

Intraoperative Management

Once the decision has been made to use a spinal opiate technique for postoperative pain control, the intraoperative anesthetic plan may have to be altered. The doses of parenteral opiates should be reduced to avoid overadministration. Other drugs that can also decrease the level of consciousness postoperatively, such as benzodiazepines, barbiturates, and phenothiazines, should also be given with caution. Moreover, the specific agent and doses should be chosen carefully with regard to the patient's age, clinical status, and type of operation. Reduced dosages are usually appropriate for the elderly or for very ill patients.

The initial dose of opiate can be given before, during, or after the operation depending on the technique selected, the duration of the operation, or the preference of the anesthesiologist. In the case of the patient undergoing cesarian section, it is prudent to withhold the drug until after delivery of the fetus. If a continuous catheter technique is chosen, the opiate can be delivered during the course of anesthesia to allow adequate and stable analgesia upon emergence from anesthesia. One technique is to administer the drug via the epidural catheter approximately 1 hour before the end of surgery. This allows titration of the anesthetic toward the end of the procedure to provide prompt emergence with some pain control already in effect. Various agents can be used for these techniques. Morphine sulfate and hydromorphone are commonly used for both the single-dose and the continuous infusion techniques. Fentanyl also has been advocated for continuous infusion, but its fast onset of action makes it well suited to intermittent boluses via the epidural catheter when analgesia is deemed inadequate by the patient.

Recovery Room Assessment

In the recovery room, after the patient is again communicative, an initial pain assessment can be made. If the patient is comfortable, an infusion of the selected agent can be given via the catheter, with the rate adjusted for the patient's age, operation, and physical condition and the type of operation. In patients who are not comfortable, a fast-onset agent such as fentanyl can be administered. Once the patient is comfortable, a continuous infusion or intermittent bolus regimen may then be initiated. Under some circumstances, the patient may be quite stable but still much too sedated. In such cases, subsequent opiate administration can be delayed until the patient is deemed awake. Further titration of the dosage can be done on the ward according to need.

Respiratory Side Effects
of Spinal Opiates

Detection of side effects requires close observation or clinical monitoring on the ward. The nursing staff should be informed about the potential side effects and instructed in the initial management of the most significant side effect, ie, delayed respiratory depression. Some hospitals require that patients receiving spinal opiates be admitted to the intensive care unit for close observation. However, with adequate nursing supervision and with the aid of monitors, patients may be safely managed on the ward.

Of the side effects that may occur, delayed respiratory depression is the most feared. Opiates delivered into the epidural or subarachnoid space can reach the central nervous system either by absorption into epidural and spinal blood vessels (Figure 18–3)—and thus into the systemic circulation—or by distribution in the cerebrospinal fluid to the central nervous system (Figure 18–4). The problem can be compounded if sedatives or respiratory depressants are given concomitantly. Strategies for detection of respiratory depression include frequent nursing assessments, pulse oximetry, and apnea monitoring. Established protocols will allow the nursing staff to decrease the opiate, discontinue the infusion, or administer the opiate antagonist—naloxone—in response to depressed ventilation. If the patient develops respiratory depression, incremental doses of the antagonist can be given according to the urgency of the clinical situation. Marked respiratory depression should be treated with significant doses of naloxone, but small decreases in respiratory rate or early sedation can be treated with smaller doses of naloxone titrated to effect. In this way the adverse side effects can be treated without entirely reversing the analgesic effects. It must also be remembered that the half-life of naloxone is generally shorter than that of most opiates, so that continuous infusions may be required to allow the opiate concentrations to fall to a therapeutic level.

Other Common Side Effects
of Spinal Opiates

Although delayed respiration is an uncommon event with the lower doses of spinal opiates that are now recommended, other side effects do occur with some frequency. Nausea and vomiting, oversedation, and pruritus represent a significant proportion of reported side effects. Urinary retention from opiates as well as constipation also occur, but these side effects are not unique to the spinal opiate technique. All of the above side effects occur with the administration of opiates by whatever route and can usually be treated without reversing the analgesic effect of the opiate.

Nausea and vomiting can be treated with various agents, including metoclopramide, scopolamine, or small doses of phenothiazines such as droperidol. Care must be taken not to cause undue sedation if scopolamine, droperidol, or combinations of the above are used. Small doses of naloxone or nalbuphine have also been used to reverse some of the side effects without reversing the desired analgesic effects. In the case of **sedation,** the antagonist drugs may be titrated to effect. **Pruritus** does occur with opiate administration; however, the mechanism of pruritus is not solely on the basis of histamine release. Antihistamines such as diphenhydramine or hydroxyzine can cause sedation and do not relieve itching as well as the opiate antagonists. Again, small doses may be sufficient to treat the side effects.

Ileus and **urinary retention** can be precipitated by abdominal operation, the pain, or the opiates used to

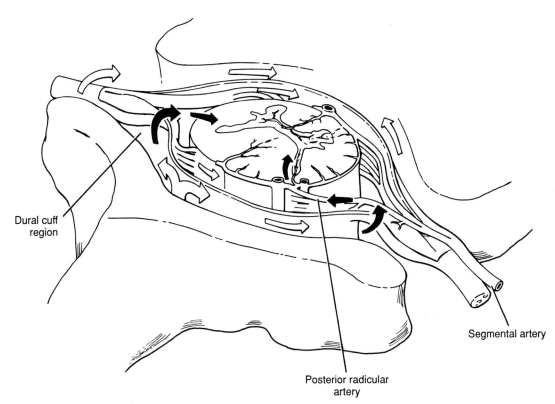

Figure 18–3 Cross section of the spinal cord and epidural space. Opioid spread in epidural space is depicted by white arrows and spread into cerebrospinal fluid and spinal cord by black arrows. In the dural cuff region, the posterior radicular spinal artery is readily accessible to opioid, and this artery directly supplies the dorsal horn region of the spinal cord. (Reproduced, with permission, from Cousins MJ, Bridenbaugh PO:*Neural Blockade in Clinical Anesthesia and Management of Pain,* 2nd ed. Lippincott, 1988.)

relieve the pain. These patients may benefit from the early ambulation afforded by spinal opiates, but other interventions are sometimes required. In patients who have resumed oral intake, laxatives may suffice, while others require enemas for relief. Both urinary retention and ileus may be improved with opiate antagonists or early ambulation, but intermittent catheterization may be required for patients who do not pass urine voluntarily after return to the ward. Continuous bladder drainage by catheter is an alternative. Although urinary retention does occur in some patients, the use of continuous catheterization is not routinely needed and is not necessarily required for the duration of opiate administration.

Sedation & Extubation

Maintenance of normal sleep-wake cycles is important to patient well-being. The goal should be to have the patient sleep at night with little or no residual effects of the sleep medication. Short-acting benzodiazepines, such as intravenous midazolam in small doses, are quite effective. Although other agents such as diphenhydramine, chloral hydrate, and oral benzodiazepines have been used, the ease with which intravenous midazolam is titrated makes it an attractive option. Patients who are mechanically ventilated with expectation of extubation in the near future are handled in somewhat the same way as other patients with regard to respiratory depression and sedation. If the usual criteria for extubation are met, the use of spinal opiates does not preclude extubation.

PAIN ASSOCIATED WITH TRAUMA

Patients suffering traumatic injury such as fractures of the long bones or pelvis may sometimes require consultation by the anesthesiologist. Any of the techniques discussed above may be satisfactory, but the anesthesiologist may be able to recommend combinations of therapy that might be more efficacious. Parenteral opiates have been traditionally used, but the spinal opiate techniques may provide effective relief, particularly for patients with vertebral, rib, pelvis, or lower extremity injury. In combination with nonsteroidal anti-inflammatory agents, patients can be well managed during the convalescent period.

Alternatively, local anesthetics can also be employed by continuous catheter techniques. Catheters can be placed in the epidural or even the brachial

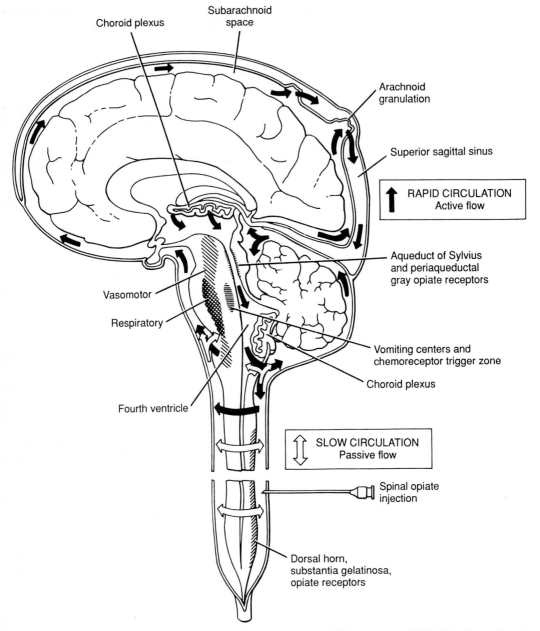

Figure 18–4 Model of circulation of cerebrospinal fluid and spread of opioid in cerebrospinal fluid. After lumbar intrathecal injection, opioid is carried in the passive flow of cerebrospinal fluid over a time course of 3–5 hours. Rapid spread ensues when the opioid mixes with the active flow of the rapid circulation of intracranial cerebrospinal fluid. Spinal and brainstem opioid receptors are shown. The latter are seen to be in close proximity to cardiorespiratory and vomiting control centers. (Reproduced, with permission, from Cousins MJ, Bridenbaugh PO:*Neural Blockade in Clinical Anesthesia and Management of Pain,* 2nd ed. Lippincott, 1988.)

plexus to control pain. Tachyphylaxis may occur with the local anesthetics, limiting their long-term use, but gradual escalation of drug concentrations may allow effective pain control during the early period of acute pain.

PAIN ASSOCIATED WITH MEDICAL DISORDERS

The medical service may seek advice about management of patients with conditions such as pancreatitis, biliary or renal colic, and sickle cell crisis. Recommendations regarding dosage and administration intervals of systemic opiates may be important for management of pain until resolution of the acute problem by medical treatment can be achieved. Strategies to provide more consistent pain relief using patient-controlled analgesia or combination therapy may be helpful. Most medical patients can be managed with the above techniques, and spinal opiates can also be used if no contraindications exist.

CHRONIC PAIN MANAGEMENT

The management of chronic pain is a demanding area in the treatment of pain problems. The spectrum of disease and psychosocial states necessitates a comprehensive approach to patient care that utilizes broad medical knowledge and diagnostic acumen. Consultation with other health care providers in the medical, surgical, psychologic, and physical therapy departments may prove invaluable in structuring a complete management strategy. Consultation may be requested for patients with oncologic pain problems and those with benign pain syndromes. Coordination of these elements is essential for optimal pain management and may best be achieved under the auspices of a pain management clinic.

BENIGN PAIN SYNDROMES

The term "benign pain syndrome" is used to distinguish various forms of chronic pain from syndromes associated with of an oncologic process or its treatment. Chronic pain resulting from "benign" diseases is no less severe or debilitating than that associated with the oncologic syndromes that will discussed below. The same comprehensive approach is utilized in both cases to discern the causes and make decisions about treatment.

The evaluation of a benign pain syndrome begins with the history and physical examination with the intent of identifying the characteristics of the pain and discovering the patient's reaction to it. Evidence of systemic disease must be sought, as it may impact directly on the pain process or in the management of such pain. Certainly, if the process is the result of a previously undetected medical or surgical problem, therapy would be directed toward the primary cause rather than just the symptoms. The quality, location, precipitating factors, and other associated signs are important clues to reaching tentative diagnoses that may have been overlooked by other practitioners. The physician must review the results of laboratory studies

as well as prior treatment successes and failures that can further elucidate the pain problem. Specific information about drug trials, nerve blocks, and physical and psychologic therapies are invaluable to this end. Within the context of the historical assessment, the anesthesiologist should form an independent opinion regarding the patient's psychologic profile by probing the reaction to the chronic pain problem. Although the patient should also be formally evaluated by a psychologist—as will be discussed later—the anesthesiologist has much to gain by assembling a complete, *independent* profile.

The physical examination should support or exclude possible diagnoses as suggested by the history. Besides the cardiorespiratory examination, two areas of special interest are the musculoskeletal and the neurologic examinations. Symptoms referable to these anatomic areas provide valuable data regarding the patient's problem, and the anesthesiologist in the pain clinic setting should be adept at both types of examination. Particular care should be paid to documenting abnormalities in range of motion, muscle tone, and musculoskeletal pain. The neurologic examination should attempt to categorize problems such as central versus peripheral origin of pain, dermatome pain versus specific nerve origin, and nociceptive versus neuropathic pain. Careful documentation is useful in following the clinical course of these patients before, during, and after treatment.

A clinical psychologist with special expertise in pain management should formally evaluate the patient's response to the chronic problem. Depression can be a significant debilitating factor in these patients, and treatment of the depression can be of great assistance. Other patients may not be clinically depressed but may have unhealthy attitudes or behavioral characteristics that perpetuate their problems. Patients may develop symptoms as a means of coping with emotional difficulties, and such cases are best approached from a psychologic basis. The clinical psychologist may also assess the patient's ability to adapt to other modalities for pain management. Suitability for relaxation techniques, biofeedback, and self-hypnosis can be explored.

In addition to the psychologist, the patient should also be seen in the physical and occupational therapy departments to determine if such services might be of benefit. In some cases, physical therapy may be the basis of treatment, with pharmacologic and psychotherapeutic treatment in adjunctive roles.

Other consultants are extremely helpful in evaluation of the patient and in formulation of treatment plans. Other medical and surgical specialties can evaluate problems within their areas of expertise. The radiologist may suggest certain imaging studies to help identify structural problems more efficiently. In difficult cases, all the consultants can be invited to a conference where discussion and interaction can sometimes lead to constructive and comprehensive treatment plans. In cases where patients are seen by various services, coordination of the plans can be facilitated by this approach.

NEUROPATHIC PAIN

Neuropathic pain has been described as a functional abnormality of the nervous system in which the sensation of pain may not be sustained by continued tissue damage. In many cases, the original injury is remote from the site and onset of the neuropathic pain, which can also be far more painful and debilitating than the pain associated with the original insult. Pain of neuropathic origin has several characteristics and intriguing features. As shown in Table 18–3, the burning and electrical qualities of this pain are particularly characteristic. The mechanisms of neuropathic pain are varied. Table 18–4 outlines possible mechanisms.

Of the many types of neuropathic pain syndromes, the **reflex sympathetic dystrophies** are perhaps the most interesting. Although known by various terms, these are treatable disorders in which the pain is sustained by efferent activity in the sympathetic nervous system. This efferent discharge causes vasoconstriction of blood vessels, atrophic changes of the skin, and even bone resorption in the affected areas. Left untreated, this pain can become a chronic disorder that offers few options for long-term treatment success. Early intervention is the key to successful treatment. Sympathetic nerve blocks can effectively block this pain; however, they are best used to facilitate the patient's participation in other resources such as physical therapy, which offers significant chances of success.

Other common types of neuropathic pain are the **deafferentation syndromes,** from nerve avulsion or amputation; and **postherpetic neuralgia (shingles),** from the reactivation of the herpes zoster (varicella zoster) virus. In these cases, the abnormality of the nervous system can lead to quite distressing clinical situations where patients complain bitterly about pain in a limb that has been amputated or injured. These patients, as well as those with postherpetic neuralgia, may have been treated only with opiates by the referring service; however, they certainly could derive significant benefit from evaluation and treatment by a pain management center.

Table 18–3. Clinical features of neuropathic pain.[1]

1. Occurs in the absence of a detectable ongoing tissue-damaging process.
2. Abnormal or unfamiliar unpleasant sensations (dysesthesia), frequently having a burning or "electrical" quality.
3. Delay in onset after precipitating injury.
4. Felt in a region of sensory deficit.
5. Paroxysmal brief shooting or stabbing component.
6. Mild (nonnoxious) stimuli painful (allodynia).
7. Pronounced summation and afterreaction with repetitive stimuli.

[1]From Fields HL: *Pain*. McGraw-Hill, 1987.

Table 18–4. Possible mechanisms of neuropathic pain (with clinical examples).[1]

1. Spontaneous hyperactivity of deafferented spinal transmission neurons (brachial plexus avulsion).
2. Plasticity: development or activation of aberrant inputs to deafferented central pain transmission neurons (stump neuroma, central pain syndromes).
3. Loss of afferent inhibition: nociceptive inputs produce an exaggerated response (entrapment neuropathies, postherpetic neuralgia).
4. Ectopic impulse generation in damaged nociceptive primary afferents: at the regenerating tip, near the dorsal root ganglion, or in demyelinated regions (tic douloureux, diabetic neuropathy).
5. Ephaptic transmission: to primary afferents from motor or sympathetic efferents of from other primary efferents.
6. Sympathetic activation or facilitation of primary afferents (causalgia, reflex sympathetic dystrophy syndrome).
7. Reflex muscle spasm.
8. Epileptic discharge of cortical nociceptive neurons.

[1]From Fields HL: *Pain*. McGraw-Hill, 1987.

MYOFASCIAL PAIN

Myofascial pain related to the musculoskeletal system is quite common. The pain can be continuous, dull, and aching—in contrast to the burning, shooting, electrical pain of neuropathic origin. The patient may report pain in specific muscle groups, and physical examination may identify localized tender spots within these areas. These localized spots are called "trigger points" and are used to help diagnose and treat the myofascial pain syndrome. This syndrome is diagnosed by physical examination with the detection of trigger points. The pain may require treatment, although many cases resolve spontaneously with no sequelae.

TREATMENT OF CHRONIC "BENIGN" PAIN

Treatment of chronic pain syndromes discussed in the preceding paragraphs has involved a multitude of resources. In the case of myofascial pain, trigger point injections with **local anesthetics** may be both diagnostic and therapeutic. **Transcutaneous electrical nerve stimulation (TENS)** has also been effective with management of other chronic pain problems. TENS is accomplished by means of a battery-powered apparatus equipped with controls the patient can use to adjust the pulse and strength of electrical stimulation delivered to the skin via electrodes to provide pain relief on demand.

Nerve blocks with local anesthetics are useful primarily for diagnostic purposes, though they do provide some temporary relief for the patient. Brachial plexus, lumbar sympathetic, celiac plexus, and stellate ganglion blocks are just a few examples of this form of therapy. The local anesthetics can be combined with corticosteroids, as in the case of epidural injection for lower back pain and trigger point injection, to provide immediate pain relief, while the steroids act more slowly to reduce inflammation.

The pharmacologic interventions in chronic pain may combine drugs of various classes to meet the patient's needs. Nonsteroidal agents such as keterolac tromethamine, naproxen, and indomethacin certainly have efficacy in some patients. Other patients benefit from the use of antidepressant agents such as the tricyclics (amitriptyline) or the newer agent fluoxetine. The benefit of these agents is obvious in the depressed chronic pain patient, but some patients with pain of neuropathic origin derive benefit more quickly and at

lower doses than would be expected solely from the antidepressant effects of the drugs.

In the treatment of neuropathic pain, the class of membrane-stabilizing drugs shows promise. Local anesthetics given parenterally provide relief in some of these patients. Agents such as the anticonvulsant carbamazepine and the antiarrhythmic mexiletine share this membrane-stabilizing effect when given orally. Significant and even dramatic results can sometimes be achieved with these drugs. Future research may provide better oral agents for the treatment of neuropathic pain.

The opiates have a role in the treatment of chronic

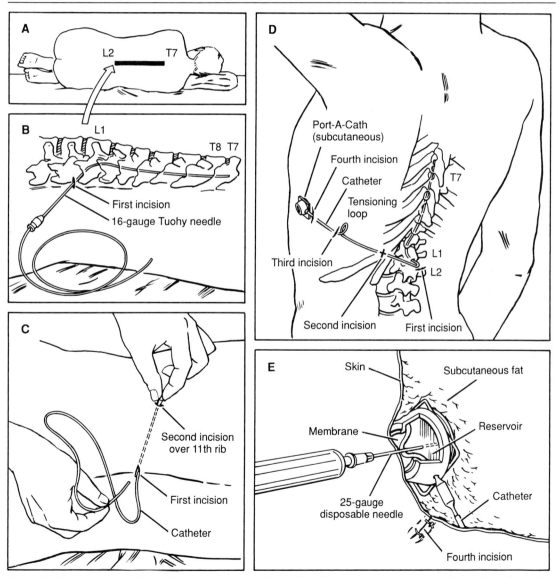

Figure 18–5 Implantation of the epidural portal system. **A:** Position of the patient before implantation. **B:** Insertion of the 16-gauge epidural catheter through a Tuohy needle. **C:** Tunneling technique used to relocate the end of the epidural catheter to the anterior chest wall. **D:** Portal attached to the inserted epidural catheter. **E:** Injection technique and exposed view of the epidural portal. (Reproduced, with permission, from Cousins MJ, Bridenbaugh PO:*Neural Blockade in Clinical Anesthesia and Management of Pain,* 2nd ed. Lippincott, 1988.)

pain despite problems with tolerance and addiction. The opiates can be given orally in long-acting form such as methadone or as part of a "cocktail" that combines agents from various drug classes. The use of spinal opiates, particularly by long-term continuous infusion, may be warranted in some cases. The opiate can be delivered via implanted catheters into the epidural or subarachnoid space (Figure 18–5). Opiates can be injected into the catheter transcutaneously via an implanted subcutaneous portal—or even directly into the catheter by an implanted subcutaneous pump. These more sophisticated methods require coordination and follow-up at a pain management service.

ONCOLOGIC PAIN

The management of patients with oncologic pain is a special aspect of chronic pain management. Historically, patients have been treated with opiates in escalating fashion, culminating in continuous intravenous infusions accompanied by significant sedation. Because the origins of pain in this patient population are multifactorial, this approach is too simplistic. Other factors, including emotional and psychologic ones, have important implications for the patient's care and should be considered when designing a management plan (Figure 18–6).

Tables 18–5 to 18–8 list multiple forms of the mechanisms previously discussed. Nociceptive pain from direct bone invasion by tumor is a prime example. Direct compression of various organs and structures results in a myriad of complaints. Neuropathic pain can result from direct tumor compression or invasion of nervous structures (eg, in the case of genitourinary tumors and the sacral plexus).

Besides pain directly related to the tumor, the treatments required and the patient's overall health status can contribute to the chronic pain process. Neuropathic pain as a result of chemotherapy or radiotherapy has been well described and can be quite devastating to patients otherwise cured of the tumor.

Inactivity and poor health status lead to myofascial syndromes, contractures, and even skin breakdown over bony prominences. In addition, the patient and the family's emotional and psychologic response to cancer can modify the experience of pain and even lead to clinical depression.

Treatment

The treatment plan should consider the multiple causes and treat the various components specifically if possible. The World Health Organization's "stepladder" approach utilizes nonopiates initially with escalation to opiate as required (Figure 18–7). This approach uses **nonsteroidal agents** initially to block prostaglandin synthesis, which is a significant mechanism of pain, particularly in patients with bone involvement. Agents such as the **antidepressant drugs** are also of use as previously described.

At the top of the ladder is the use of **opiates,** which should be given along with adjuvant nonsteroidal agents and antidepressants to provide optimal pain relief without undue sedation. In the terminally ill patient, maintenance of consciousness can be the most important issue for the patient and family. To this end, there are many routes of administration. Oral, sublingual, rectal, and even transdermal opiates are useful first options, particularly for outpatients. Subcutaneous or intravenous patient-controlled analgesia requires more supervision but can still be prescribed for outpatients if assistance is available from motivated family members and home nursing programs.

The use of **spinal opiates** is an alternative. Epidural and subarachnoid opiates offer pain relief with substantially lower total doses of opiate and with less sedation if titrated properly. Catheters can be placed percutaneously or even implanted to provide effective pain relief over prolonged periods. The use of these

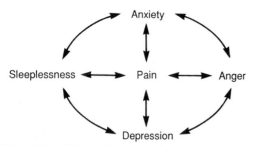

A vicious cycle usually develops:

Figure 18–6 Pain syndromes can be exacerbated by the interplay of multiple psychologic factors. (Reproduced, with permission, from Cousins MJ, Bridenbaugh PO:*Neural Blockade in Clinical Anesthesia and Management of Pain,* 2nd ed. Lippincott, 1988.)

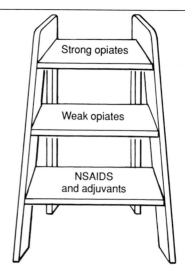

Figure 18–7 The WHO stepladder demonstrates the progression from nonopiates to strong opiates in the management of chronic pain problems

Table 18–5. Pain syndromes in patients with cancer:
Pain directly caused by cancer (primary or metastatic).[1]

Mechanism	Common Sites and Characteristics of Pain
Infiltration of bone by tumor	Dull, constant with or without muscle spasm
Base of skull (jugular foramen, clivus, sphenoid sinus)	Early onset of pain in occiput, vertex, frontal areas, respectively
Vertebral body (subluxation atlas, metastases C7-T1, L1 sacral)	Early onset of pain in neck and skull, neck and shoulders, mid back, lower back, and coccyx, respectively, with or without neurologic deficit.
Metastatic fracture close to nerves	Acute onset of pain and muscle spasm
Infiltration, compression of nerve tissue by tumor	
Peripheral nerve (with or without peripheral and perivascular lymphangitis)	Burning constant pain in area of peripheral sensory loss with or without dysesthesia and hyperalgesia, with or without signs of sympathetic over-activity. See neuropathy definition.
Plexus, eg, lumbar	Radicular pain to anterior thigh and groin (L1-L3) or to leg and foot (L4-S2).
eg, sacral	Dull aching midline perianal pain + sacral sensory loss and fecal and urinary incontinence.
eg, brachial	Radicular pain in shoulder and arm with or without Horner's syndrome (superior pulmonary sulcus or Pancoast tumor).
Meningeal carcinomatosis	Constant headache with or without neck stiffness or low back and buttock pain.
Epidural spinal cord compression (with or without vertebral body infiltration)	Severe neck and back pain locally over involved vertebra, or radicular pain.
Obstruction of hollow viscus, eg, gut, genitourinary tract	Poorly localized, dull, sickening pain, typical visceral pain.
Occlusion of arteries and veins by tumor	Ischemic pain like rest pain (skin) or claudication (muscle) or pain with or without venous engorgement
Stretching of periosteum or fascia, in tissues with tight investment, by tumefaction	Severe localized pain (eg, periosteum) *or* typical visceral pain (eg, ovary)
Inflammation owing to necrosis and infection of tumors (with or without superficial ulceration)	Severe localized pain (eg, perineum), visceral pain (eg, cervix)
Soft tissue infiltration	Localized pain: unsightly and foul-smelling, if ulcerated
Raised intracranial pressure	Severe constant headache, behavorial changes, confusion, etc.

[1]From Cousins MJ, Bridenbaugh PO (editors): *Neural Blockade in Clinical Anesthesia and Management of Pain,* 2nd ed. Lippincott, 1987.

invasive spinal techniques can be complicated by patient factors, of which raised intracranial pressure from mass lesions of the nervous system and coagulopathy are the most significant. In cases of coagulopathy, whether from chemotherapy or from bone marrow or hepatic involvement, the risk-benefit ratio must be weighed carefully. Correction of the coagulopathy with blood products just before the procedures may be helpful.

Utilizing the same catheter techniques, **local anesthetics** can also be administered. Again, close follow-up is required, particularly when local anesthetics cause significant motor blockade, sympathetic blockade, or when high spinal levels are achieved.

Neurolytic blocks can be employed when a specific nerve plexus, dermatome, or nerve root involved in pain transmission can be identified. This technique uses chemicals such as alcohol or phenol to ablate specific nerves. Chemical rhizotomy at the thoracic level can block several dermatomes effectively. The celiac plexus and the sacral plexus are potential sites of blockade in patients with pancreatic or genitourinary tumors. In patients with primarily lower body complaints, a saddle block or even one-sided selective sacral root block can provide pain relief. Because of the significant morbidity associated with the neurolytic blocks—loss of motor and sensory function in previously unaffected regions can result—they should be

Table 18–6. Pain syndromes in patients with cancer:
Pain associated with cancer therapy.[1]

Mechanism	Common Sites and Characteristics of Pain
FOLLOWING SURGERY	
Acute postoperative pain	Wound or referred pain; back or other sites (owing to posture during surgery).
Nerve trauma	Neuralgic pain in area of peripheral nerve or spinal nerve.
Entrapment of nerves in scar tissue	Superficial wound scar hypersensitivity of area supplied by scarred nerves (eg, perineum).
Amputation of limb or other area (eg, breast)	Localized stump pain (neuroma) *or* phantom pain referred to absent region.
FOLLOWING RADIOTHERAPY	
Acute lesions or inflammation of nerves or plexuses; radiation fibrosis of nerves or plexuses	Pain associated with motor and sensory loss, eg, brachial plexus, lumbar plexus distribution; diffuse limb pain, 6 months to many years after radiation with or without lymphedema and local skin changes with or without sensory loss with or without motor loss (difficult to distinguish from tumor recurrence).
Myelopathy of spinal cord	Brown-Séquard's syndrome (ipsilateral sensory and contralateral motor loss) with pain at level of spinal cord damage or referred pain.
Peripheral nerve tumors due to radiation	Painful enlarging mass in area of radiation along line of peripheral nerve or plexus.
FOLLOWING CHEMOTHERAPY	
Vinca akaloid (vincristine > vinblastine)-induced peripheral neuropathy	Burning pain in hands and feet associated with symmetric polyneuropathy.
Steroid pseudorheumatism owing to slow as well as rapid withdrawal of steroid treatment	Diffuse joint and muscle pain with associated tenderness to palpation but no inflammatory signs; pain resolves when steroid reinstituted.
Aseptic necrosis of bone (femoral or humoral head) with chronic steroid therapy	Pain in knee, leg, or shoulder with limitation of movement; bone scan changes delayed after pain onset.
Postherpetic neuralgia, following herpes zoster infection in area of tumor or area of radiotherapy with onset during chemotherapy	Continuous burning pain in area of sensory loss *or* painful dysesthesia *or* intermittent, shocklike pain.

[1]From Cousins MJ, Bridenbaugh PO (editors): *Neural Blockade in Clinical Anesthesia and Management of Pain,* 2nd ed. Lippincott, 1987.

Table 18–7. Pain syndromes in patients with cancer:
Pain unrelated to cancer or cancer therapy.[1]

Mechanism	Common Sites and Characteristics of Pain
Neuropathy (eg, diabetic)	Burning pain in hands, feet
Degenerative disk disease	Back pain with or without radicular pain
Rheumatoid arthritis	Joint pain, on movement
Diffuse osteoporosis	Back pain, limb pain (may be like causalgia)
Posture abnormalities after surgery	Back pain and muscle spasm with or without radicular pain
Myofascial syndromes owing to anxiety	Local pain in muscle with muscle spasm with or without referred pain; trigger areas in muscle
Headache	Typical migraine or tension type

[1]From Cousins MJ, Bridenbaugh PO (editors): *Neural Blockade in Clinical Anesthesia and Management of Pain,* 2nd ed. Lippincott, 1987.

Table 18–8. Pain syndromes in patients with cancer: Pain exacerbated or entirely caused by psychologic factors. (See also Figure 18–6.)

Psychologic Factor	Possible Causes
Anxiety	Sleeplessness Fear of death or of loss of dignity (loss of self-control) Fear of surgical mutilation, uncontrollable pain Fear of the future and of loss of social position and work Confused understanding of disease owing to poor communication Family and financial problems
Depression	Sleeplessness Loss of physical abilities Sense of helplessness Disfigurement Loss of valued social position; financial problems
Anger	Frustration with therapeutic failures Resentment of sickness Irritability caused by pain and general discomfort

utilized after careful consideration of alternatives. Bowel and bladder dysfunction may also ensue. In terminal patients who live beyond the efficacy of the neurolytic block, subsequent development of neuropathic pain can be a severe problem.

CASE SUMMARY: PATIENT WITH ONCOLOGIC PAIN

The patient is a 69-year-old man with metastatic prostate carcinoma who complains of leg, hip, and low back pain. He is currently undergoing radiation therapy, and his pain has been managed with oxycodone with inadequate relief.

What are the characteristics of the patient's pain?

Upon careful questioning, the patient is able to describe three distinct areas of pain, each with its own typical location, quality, severity, and associated findings. He describes the leg pain as a shooting pain down the posterior aspect of his thigh, to his foot. It occurs paroxysmally and is associated with an "electric shock" sensation. When this pain occurs, it is quite severe. There is no particular association with movement.

The second pain is a constant, sharp pain of moderate intensity involving the left hip, exacerbated by movement and worse when lying down or sitting down.

Finally, the patient has back pain, dull in character and worse with movement. The pain is located in the lumbar region, primarily on the right side. There are no associated neurologic findings.

Is the current pain management regimen effective?

The patient is currently undergoing radiation therapy for bony metastases and is receiving hormonal treatment for his prostatic carcinoma. Analgesia has consisted solely of oral opiates, with increasing doses required over the past month. The opiates appear to reduce the pain, but the patient is never pain-free.

Does the physical examination help characterize the return of the pain?

Musculoskeletal examination shows a man standing erect, with normal head and thorax posture. There is some flattening of the normal lumbar lordosis. Range of motion of the neck and thorax is normal, but the patient does have limited rotation of the lumbar spine because of pain. He cannot flex or extend without discomfort. There is some paraspinous spasm on the right in the lumbar region, with trigger points demonstrated in the paraspinous muscles. There is no tenderness in response to palpation of the spinous processes posteriorly.

With the patient now in the right lateral decubitus position, the sciatic notch is quite tender to palpation, with additional radiation of pain into the gluteal region as well as down the posterior aspect of the left leg.

The sensory examination shows intact sensation to temperature and vibration. Light touch over the distribution of the sciatic nerve on the left leg, however, is painful and is described as a tingling sensation. Sensation to light touch is normal on the right leg. The deep tendon reflexes are intact and symmetric, and Babinski's sign is negative.

Review of the CT scan shows no abnormalities in the lumbar spine. There is no evidence of nerve impingement in that region. The pelvis is normal except for an enlarged prostate and a metastatic lesion in the wing of the ilium and also at the sciatic notch.

What are the possible causes of the patient's pain?

The history, physical examination, and radiologic studies suggest that the patient has metastatic lesions to his pelvis, including the sciatic notch, with some impingement of the sciatic nerve. No abnormalities of the lumbar spine were identified.

The patient appears to have nociceptive pain related to the bony metastases as well as neuropathic pain related to sciatic nerve involvement. The findings in the lumbar region suggest a myofascial syndrome related to the patient's inactivity, secondary to pain.

What are the treatment options?

The patient is not well controlled with his oral opiate regimen, and a nonsteroidal anti-inflammatory drug is therefore started after it is determined that there are no contraindications to its use. He is changed from oxycodone to a long-acting morphine preparation. Requests were also sent for a physical therapy evaluation, as well as a psychologic evaluation for feasibility of nonmedical techniques for pain control.

What is the interval follow-up?

The patient returns in 3 weeks after several more radiation treatments as well as initial evaluations by the physical therapy and psychology services. He has begun some physical therapy for his lumbar back pain and has been outfitted with a TENS unit, which seems to help control his pain. The psychologist has begun working with him on relaxation techniques and self-hypnosis, to which the patient seems amenable. The back and hip pain are better, but the patient continues to have paroxysmal shooting pains down the left leg. Because the continued leg pain appears to be of neuropathic origin, a trial of intravenous lidocaine is undertaken after consent is obtained. The patient is kept NPO for 6 hours before the procedure and is placed on appropriate monitors in the clinic. He receives a total dose of 300 mg of lidocaine over one-half hour without evidence of neurologic or cardiovascular compromise. His initial pain score is 70 on a 100 mm visual analog scale, and that is reduced to 0 by the end of the trial period. Based on the clinical response, he was started on an oral membrane stabilizer (mexiletine).

Is this a stable analgesic regimen?

The patient returns in 2 months, with continued left hip and pelvic pain. The shooting pains down the leg have been well controlled with the oral mexiletine. His current situation suggests that he has continuing nociceptive pain, and repeat radiologic study of his pelvis shows progression of the metastatic lesions. The patient's oral opiates have been escalated, with less pain relief. Physical therapy, which had helped with his low back pain initially, is no longer tolerated because of the pain. The patient does, however, continue with self-hypnosis, which allows him to function though with some pain. Earlier in the week, the patient took extra doses of his opiate and found that he became very sleepy and confused. His family states that he is much too difficult to take care of in this condition.

What are the goals of pain management in this situation?

It appears that at this point, oral opiates cannot be increased further because of the side effects. Because

of the advancing nature of the pain, it appears that he would now be a good candidate for spinal opiates. The procedure is discussed with the patient, and informed consent is obtained. The nonsteroidal agent is discontinued for 1 week and the patient is then taken to the operating room, where a lumbar epidural catheter is placed, tunneled, and connected to a subcutaneous pump for the purpose of administering spinal opiates. The patient tolerated the procedure well and was maintained on a constant epidural infusion of morphine. He was not sedated, and his pain was well controlled. He was able to resume the activities of daily life while continuing on mexiletine and nonsteroidal anti-inflammatory drugs. He returned to physical therapy for help with his back pain.

The patient is seen monthly for the next several months to have his pump refilled with opiates. He is still active and in good spirits.

What further options are available to this patient?

Several months later, the patient has a gradual return of his pain, with the left leg being the primary problem. The mexiletine dose is at maximum and can no longer be increased. Discussion with the patient's oncologist reveals that there has been significant progression of the tumor and that his physical status is now deteriorating. By the oncologist's report, the patient has a life expectancy of less than 4 or 5 months. Increases in the spinal opiates do not relieve the pain.

The patient is no longer ambulatory because of the pain, and his life expectancy is now very short. With the increased opiate doses, the patient is sedated and difficult to care for, according to the family. When he is awake, he complains bitterly of his leg pain. Again, the patient is no longer ambulatory, so we would now consider the use of neurolytic blockade. The patient is counseled about the potential side effects of some loss of motor control and perhaps bowel and bladder dysfunction. Because the pain is so severe, the patient wishes to proceed. The patient then has a subarachnoid neurolytic block using phenol. The block is successful, with marked improvement in the pain reports. The block is selective to the left side, with no impairment of motor strength on the right, although there is minor foot drop of the left foot, which is adequately treated with splinting. Bowel and bladder function remain intact.

The patient continues on his nonsteroidal anti-inflammatory drugs as well as his opiates via the implanted pump. He returns home with his family.

The patient eventually succumbs to his prostatic carcinoma, but by family report he was comfortable at the end.

SELECTED READINGS

Bonica JJ: *The Management of Pain*, 2nd ed. Lea & Febiger, 1990.
Cousins MJ, Bridenbaugh PO: *Neural Blockade in Clinical Anesthesia and Management of Pain*, 2nd ed. Lippincott, 1988.

Fields HL: *Pain*. McGraw-Hill, 1987.
Wall P, Melzack R (editors): *Textbook of Pain*, 2nd ed. Churchill Livingstone, 1989.

Section IV
Physiology, Pathophysiology, & Anesthetic Management

Cardiovascular Physiology & Anesthesia

19

Until relatively recently, the effects of anesthetic agents on circulatory physiology were described only in terms of changes in blood pressure and heart rate. The refinement and wider application of newer invasive and noninvasive monitoring techniques (Chapter 6) has provided the physiologic basis for previously observed changes (Chapters 7 and 8). Moreover, recording such physiologic data is no longer limited to research laboratories or specialized centers but is becoming part of routine anesthetic practice. Anesthesiologists must therefore have a thorough understanding of cardiovascular physiology both for its scientific significance in anesthesia and for its practical applications to modern patient management.

The circulatory system consists of the heart, the blood vessels, and the blood. Its function is to provide tissues with oxygen and nutrients and to carry away the by-products of metabolism. The heart propels blood through two vascular systems arranged in series (Figure 19–1). In the pulmonary circulation, blood flows past the alveolar-capillary membrane, takes up oxygen, and eliminates CO_2. In the systemic circulation, oxygenated blood is pumped to metabolizing tissues, and the by-products of metabolism are taken up for elimination by the lungs, kidneys, or liver. This chapter reviews the physiology of the heart and the systemic circulation and the pathophysiology of heart failure. The pulmonary circulation and the physiology of blood and nutrient exchange are discussed in Chapters 22 and 28, respectively.

THE HEART

Although anatomically one organ, the heart can functionally be divided into right and left pumps, each consisting of an atrium and a ventricle. The atria serve both as conduits and as priming pumps, while the ventricles act as the major pumping chambers. The right ventricle receives systemic venous (deoxygenated) blood and pumps it into the pulmonary circulation, while the left ventricle receives pulmonary venous (oxygenated) blood and pumps it into the systemic circulation. Four valves normally ensure unidirectional flow through each chamber (Figure 19–1). The normal pumping action of the heart is the result of a complex series of electrical and mechanical events.

The heart consists of specialized striated muscle in a connective tissue skeleton. Cardiac muscle can be divided into atrial, ventricular, and specialized pacemaker and conducting cells. The self-excitatory nature of cardiac muscle cells and their unique organization allows the heart to function as a highly efficient pump. Serial low-resistance connections (intercalated disks) between individual myocardial cells allow rapid and orderly spread of electrical activity in each pumping chamber. Electrical activity readily spreads from one atrium to another and from one ventricle to another via specialized conduction pathways. The absence of direct connections between the atria and ventricles except through the atrioventricular (AV) node delays conduction and enables atrial contraction to prime the ventricle (see below).

CARDIAC ACTION POTENTIALS

The myocardial cell membrane is normally permeable to K^+ but relatively impermeable to Na^+. A membrane-bound Na^+-K^+ ATPase concentrates K^+ intracellularly in exchange for extrusion of Na^+ out of cells (Chapter 28). Intracellular sodium concentration is kept low, whereas intracellular potassium concentration is kept high relative to the extracellular space. Relative impermeability of the membrane to calcium

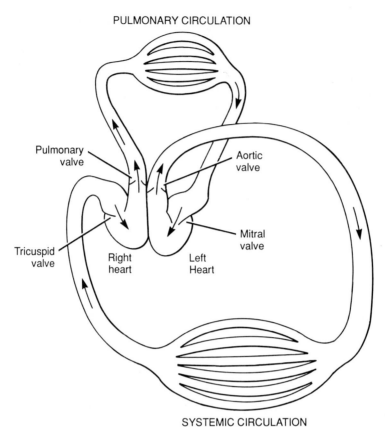

PULMONARY CIRCULATION

Pulmonary valve

Aortic valve

Tricuspid valve

Right heart

Left Heart

Mitral valve

SYSTEMIC CIRCULATION

Figure 19–1. Blood flow in the heart. Note that action of the four valves prevents backward flow of blood.

also maintains a high extracellular to cytoplasmic calcium gradient. Movement of K^+ out of the cell and down its concentration gradient results in a net loss of positive charges from inside the cell. An electrical potential is established across the cell membrane, with the inside of the cell negative with respect to the extracellular environment, because anions do not accompany K^+. Thus, the resting membrane potential represents the balance between two opposing forces: the movement of K^+ down its concentration gradient and the electrical attraction of the negatively charged intracellular space for the positively charged potassium ions.

Normal ventricular cell resting membrane potential is -80 to -90 mV. As with other excitable tissues (nerve and skeletal muscle), when the cell membrane potential becomes less negative and reaches a threshold value, a characteristic action potential (depolarization) develops (Figure 19–2 and Table 19–1). The action potential transiently raises myocardial cell membrane potential to $+20$ mV. In contrast to action potentials in neurons (Chapter 14), the spike in cardiac action potentials is followed by a plateau phase that lasts 0.2–0.3 s. Whereas the action potential for skeletal muscle and nerves is due to abrupt opening of fast sodium channels in the cell membrane, that in cardiac muscle is due to the opening of both fast sodium chan-

nels (the spike) and slower calcium channels (the plateau). Depolarization is also accompanied by a transient decrease in potassium permeability. Subsequent restoration of normal potassium permeability and closure of sodium and calcium channels eventually restores membrane potential to normal.

Following depolarization, the cells are refractory to subsequent normal depolarizing stimuli until phase 4. During phases 1, 2, and early phase 3, another depolarization cannot occur regardless of the stimulus intensity **(absolute refractory period).** However, a supranormal stimulus during the latter part of phase 3 can depolarize the cell membrane and generate another action potential (relative refractory period). In fast-conducting myocardial cells, the refractory period is generally closely correlated with the duration of the action potential. In contrast, the refractory period in slowly conducting myocardial cells can outlast the duration of the action potential.

INITIATION & CONDUCTION OF THE CARDIAC IMPULSE

The cardiac impulse normally originates in the **sinoatrial (SA) node,** a group of specialized pacemaker cells at the junction of the right atrium with the superi-

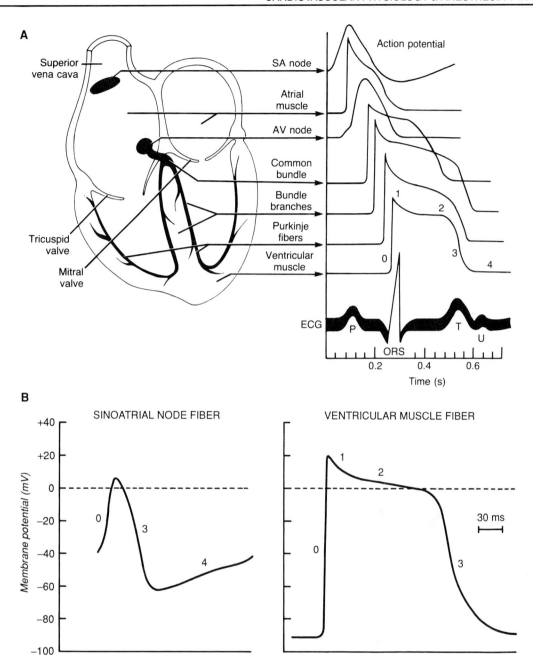

Figure 19–2. Cardiac action potentials. **A:** Note the characteristic action potentials of different parts of the heart. **B:** Pacemaker cells in the SA node lack the same distinct phases as atrial and ventricular muscle cells and display prominent spontaneous diastolic depolarization. See Table 19–1 for an explanation of the different phases of the action potential. (Modified and reproduced, with permission, from Sokolow M, McIlroy M: *Clinical Cardiology,* 5th ed. Appleton & Lange, 1990; originally from Noble MIM: *The Cardiac Cycle.* Blackwell, 1979.)

or vena cava. These cells appear to have an outer membrane that "leaks" sodium (and possibly calcium). The slow influx of sodium results in a less negative, "resting" membrane potential (-50 to -60 mV) and has three important consequences: (1) constant inactivation of fast sodium channels, (2) an action potential with a threshold of -40 mV that is primarily due to

ion movement across the slow calcium channels, and (3) regular spontaneous depolarizations. During each cycle, intracellular "leakage" of sodium causes the cell membrane to become progressively less negative; when threshold potential is reached, calcium channels open, potassium permeability decreases, and an action potential develops. Restoration of normal potassium

Table 19–1. Cardiac action potential.

Phase	Name	Event	Cellular Ion Movement
0	Upstroke	Activation (opening) of fast Na⁺ channels and decreased permeability to K⁺	Na⁺ in
1	Early rapid re-polarization	Inactivation of Na⁺ channel and transient increase in K⁺ permeability	K⁺ out
2	Plateau	Activation of slow Ca²⁺ channels	Ca²⁺ in
3	Final repolarization	Inactivation of Ca²⁺ channels and increased permeability to K⁺	K⁺ out
4	Resting potential or Diastolic re-polarization	Normal permeability restored (atrial and ventricular cells) Intrinsic slow "leakage" of sodium and possibly Ca²⁺ into cells that spontaneously depolarize	K⁺ out Na⁺ in, ?Ca²⁺ in

permeability returns the cells in the SA node to their normal "resting" membrane potential.

The impulse generated at the SA node is normally rapidly conducted across the atria and to the AV node. Specialized atrial fibers speed up conduction both to the left atrium and to the AV node. The **AV node,** which is located in the septal wall of the right atrium just anterior to the opening of the coronary sinus and above the insertion of the septal leaflet of the tricuspid valve, is actually made up of three distinct areas: an upper junctional (AN) region, a middle nodal (N) region, and a lower junctional (NH) region. Although the N region does not possess intrinsic spontaneous activity (automaticity), both junctional areas do. The normally slower rate of spontaneous depolarization in AV junctional areas (40–60 times/min) allows the faster SA node to control heart rate. Any factor that decreases the rate of SA node depolarization or increases the automaticity of AV junctional areas allows them to function as the pacemaker for the heart.

Impulses from the SA node normally reach the AV node after about 0.04 s but leave after another 0.11 s. This delay is the result of the slowly conducting small myocardial fibers within the AV node, which depend on slow calcium channels for propagation of the action potential. In contrast, conduction of the impulse between adjoining cells in the atria and in the ventricles is due primarily to activation and inactivation of the fast sodium channels. The lower fibers of the AV node combine to form the **common bundle of His.** This specialized group of fibers passes into the interventricular septum before dividing into left and right branches to form the complex network of **Purkinje fibers** that depolarizes both ventricles. In sharp contrast to AV nodal tissue, His-Purkinje fibers have the fastest conduction velocities in the heart, resulting in nearly simultaneous depolarization of the entire endocardium of both ventricles (normally within 0.03 s). Spread of the impulse from the endocardium to the epicardium through ventricular muscle requires an additional 0.03 s. Thus, an impulse arising from the SA node normally requires less than 0.2 s to depolarize the entire heart.

Local anesthetics can have important electro-physiologic effects on the heart at blood concentrations generally associated with systemic toxicity. In the case of lidocaine, electrophysiologic effects at low blood concentrations can be therapeutic (Chapter 46). At high blood concentrations, local anesthetics depress conduction by binding to fast sodium channels. The most potent local anesthetics—bupivacaine and to a lesser degree etidocaine—appear to have the greatest effects on the heart, especially on Purkinje fibers and ventricular muscle. Bupivacaine is known to bind inactivated fast sodium channels and dissociates from them slowly. It can cause profound sinus bradycardia and sinus node arrest as well as malignant ventricular arrhythmias.

MECHANISM OF CONTRACTION

Myocardial cells contract as a result of the interaction of two overlapping, rigid contractile proteins, **actin** and **myosin.** These proteins are fixed in position within each cell during both contraction and relaxation. Cell shortening occurs when the two proteins are allowed to fully interact and slide over one another (Figure 19–3). This interaction is normally prevented by two regulatory proteins, **troponin** and **tropomyosin.** The former is attached to actin at regular intervals, while the latter lies within the center of the actin structure. An increase in intracellular calcium concentration (from about 10^{-7} to 10^{-5} mol/L) promotes contraction as calcium ions bind troponin: the resulting conformational change in these regulatory proteins exposes the active sites on actin that allow interaction with myosin bridges (points of overlapping). The active site on myosin functions as a magnesium-dependent ATPase whose activity is enhanced by the increase in intracellular calcium concentration. A series of attachments and disengagements occur as each myosin bridge advances over successive active sites on actin. ATP is consumed during each attachment.

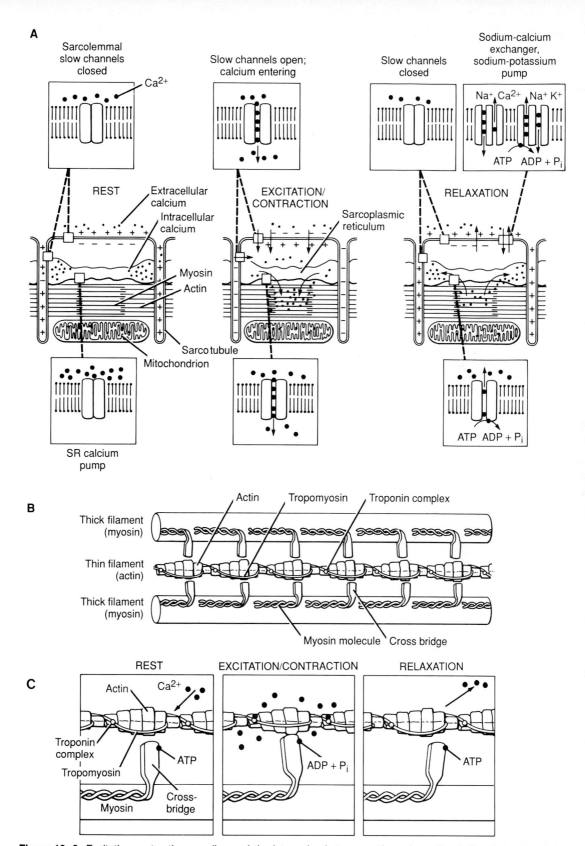

Figure 19–3. Excitation-contraction coupling and the interaction between actin and myosin. **A:** Depolarization of the muscle cell membrane allows entry of calcium into the cell and release of calcium stored in the sarcoplasmic reticulum. **B:** The structure of the actin-myosin complex. **C:** Calcium binds troponin allowing the interaction between actin and myosin. (Modified and reproduced, with permission, from Katz AM, Smith VE: Hosp Pract [Jan] 1985;19:69; and from Braunwald E: The Myocardium: *Failure and Infarction.* HP Publishing Co., 1974.)

Excitation-Contraction Coupling

The quantity of calcium required to initiate contraction exceeds that entering the cell through slow channels during phase 2. The small amount that does enter, however, appears to trigger a release of much larger amounts of calcium stored intracellularly. These stores, which are primarily within cisterns in the sarcoplasmic reticulum and to a lesser extent T tubules, contain bound calcium that is otherwise unavailable. During relaxation, when the slow channels close, intracellular calcium is sequestered again by the sarcoplasmic reticulum. A membrane-bound ATPase actively transports calcium back into the sarcoplasmic reticulum. Thus, relaxation of the heart also normally requires ATP. Other less important mechanisms of relaxation may include (1) an exchange of intracellular calcium for extracellular sodium at the cell membrane (in a 1:2 ratio), and (2) active calcium extrusion by an ATPase in the cell membrane.

The quantity of intracellular Ca^{2+} available, its rate of delivery, and its rate of removal determine, respectively, the maximum tension developed, the rate of contraction, and the rate of relaxation. Sympathetic stimulation increases the force of contraction by raising intracellular calcium concentration via a β_1-adrenergic receptor-mediated increase in intracellular cAMP (Chapter 12). In contrast, factors that depress cardiac contractility unfavorably alter intracellular calcium kinetics. Recent studies suggest that volatile anesthetics depress contractility by decreasing the entry of Ca^{2+} into cells during depolarization, altering the kinetics of its release and uptake into the sarcoplasmic reticulum and decreasing the sensitivity of contractile proteins to calcium. The mechanisms of direct cardiac depression from nitrous oxide and intravenous anesthetics are not well established but presumably involve similar actions.

THE CARDIAC CYCLE

The cardiac cycle can be defined by both electrical and mechanical events (Figure 19–4). Systole refers to contraction, while diastole refers to relaxation. Most diastolic ventricular filling occurs passively before atrial contraction. Contraction of the atria normally contributes 20–30% of ventricular filling. Three waves can generally be identified on atrial pressure tracings (Figure 19–4). The *a* **wave** is due to atrial systole. The *c* **wave** coincides with ventricular contraction and is said to be due to bulging of the atrioventricular valve into the atria. The *v* **wave** is due to the pressure buildup from venous return until the atrioventricular valve opens again. The *x* **descent** is the decline in pressure between the *c* and *v* waves and is said to be due to a pulling down of the atrium by ventricular contraction. Incompetence of the atrioventricular valve on either side of the heart abolishes the *x* descent on that side, resulting in a prominent *cv* wave. The *y* **descent** follows the *v* wave and represents the decline in atrial pressure as the atrioventricular valve opens. The notch in the aortic pressure tracing is referred to as the **incisura** and represents transient backflow of blood into the left ventricle just before aortic valve closure.

DETERMINANTS OF VENTRICULAR PERFORMANCE

Discussions of ventricular function usually refer to the left ventricle, but the same concepts apply to the right ventricle. Although the ventricles are often thought of as functioning separately, their interdependence has recently been appreciated (see below).

Ventricular function is most often equated with **cardiac output,** which can be defined as the volume of blood pumped by the heart per minute. Because the two ventricles function in series, their outputs are normally equal. Cardiac output (CO) is expressed by the following equation:

$$CO = SV \times HR$$

where SV is the **stroke volume** (the volume pumped per one contraction) and HR is heart rate. To compensate for variations in body size, CO is often expressed in terms of total body surface area:

$$CI = \frac{CO}{BSA}$$

where CI is the **cardiac index** and BSA is total body surface area. BSA is usually obtained from nomograms based on height and weight. Normal CI is 2.5–4.2 L/min/m². Note that the normal CI has a wide range and is thus a relatively insensitive measurement of ventricular performance. Abnormalities in CI therefore usually reflect gross ventricular impairment. A more accurate assessment may be obtained if the response of the cardiac output to exercise is evaluated. Under these conditions, failure of the cardiac output to increase and keep up with oxygen consumption is reflected by a falling mixed venous oxygen saturation (Chapter 22). A decrease in mixed venous oxygen saturation in response to increased demand usually reflects inadequate tissue perfusion. Thus, in the absence of hypoxemia or severe anemia, the mixed venous oxygen tension (or saturation) is the best measurement for determining the adequacy of cardiac output (Chapter 22).

1. HEART RATE

Cardiac output is generally directly proportionate to heart rate (Figure 19–5). Heart rate is an intrinsic function of the SA node (spontaneous depolarization) but is modified by autonomic, humeral, and local factors. The normal intrinsic rate of the SA node in young

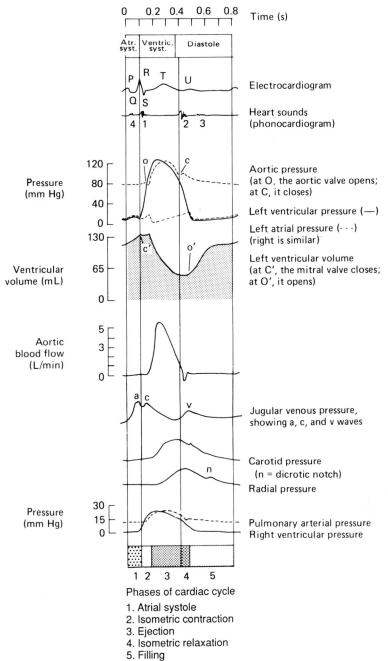

Figure 19–4. The normal cardiac cycle. Note the correspondence between electrical and mechanical events. (Modified and reproduced, with permission, from Ganong WF: *Medical Physiology*, 15th ed. Appleton & Lange, 1991.)

adults is about 90–100 beats/min, but it decreases with age according to the following formula:

**Normal intrinsic heart rate =
118 beats/min − (0.57 × age)**

Enhanced vagal activity slows the heart rate via stimulation of muscarinic cholinergic receptors, while enhanced sympathetic activity increases heart rate via activation of β_1-adrenergic receptors. Sympathetic in-

nervation of the heart originates in the thoracic spinal cord (T1–4) and travels to the heart first through the cervical ganglia and then as the cardiac nerves.

2. STROKE VOLUME

Stroke volume is normally determined by three major factors: **preload, afterload,** and **contractility.** This analysis is analogous to laboratory observations on

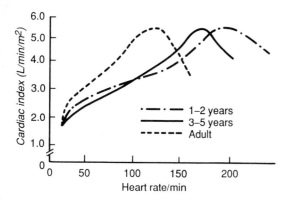

Figure 19–5. The relationship between heart rate and cardiac index. (Reproduced, with permission, from Wetsel RC: *Critical Care: State of the Art 1981.* Society of Critical Care Medicine, 1981.)

Table 19–3. Factors affecting ventricular preload.

Venous return
Blood volume
Distribution of blood volume
Posture
Intrathoracic pressure
Pericardial pressure
Venous tone
Rhythm (atrial contraction)
Heart rate

skeletal muscle preparations. Preload is muscle length prior to contraction, while afterload is the tension against which the muscle has to contract. Contractility is an intrinsic property of the muscle that is related to the force of contraction but independent of both preload and afterload. Since the heart is a three-dimensional multichambered pump, ventricular geometric form as well as valvular dysfunction can also affect stroke volume (Table 19–2).

Preload

Ventricular preload is end-diastolic volume, which is generally dependent on ventricular filling. The relationship between cardiac output and left ventricular end-diastolic volume is known as Starling's law of the heart (Figure 19–6). Note that when heart rate is constant, cardiac output is directly proportionate to preload, until excessive end-diastolic volumes are reached. At that point cardiac output does not appreciably change or may even decrease. Overdistention of either ventricle can lead to excessive dilatation and incompetence of the atrioventricular valves.

A. Determinants of Ventricular Filling: Ventricular filling can be influenced by a variety of factors (Table 19–3), the most important of which is venous return. Because most other factors affecting venous return are usually fixed, venous tone is normally the major determinant of venous return. Increases in metabolic activity enhance venous tone, such that venous return to the heart increases as the volume of venous capacitance vessels decreases. Changes in blood volume and venous tone are important causes of intra-

Table 19–2. Important factors influencing cardiac stroke volume.

Preload
Contractility
Afterload
Wall motion abnormalities
Valvular dysfunction

operative and postoperative changes in ventricular filling and cardiac output. Any factor that alters the normally small venous pressure gradient favoring blood return to the heart also affects cardiac filling. Such factors include changes in intrathoracic pressure (positive-pressure ventilation or thoracotomy), posture (positioning during surgery), and pericardial pressure (pericardial disease).

The most important determinant of right ventricular preload is venous return. In the absence of significant pulmonary or right ventricular dysfunction, venous return is also the major determinant of left ventricular preload. The end-diastolic volumes of both ventricles are normally similar.

Both heart rate and rhythm can also affect ventricular preload. Increases in heart rate are associated with proportionately greater reductions in diastole than systole. Ventricular filling therefore progressively becomes impaired at high heart rates (> 120 beats/min in adults). Absent (atrial fibrillation), ineffective (atrial flutter), or altered timing of atrial contraction (low atrial or junctional rhythms) can also reduce ventricular filling by 20–30%. Because the atrial contribution to ventricular filling is important in maintaining low mean ventricular diastolic pressures, patients with reduced ventricular compliance are most affected by loss of a normally timed atrial systole (see below).

B. Ventricular Compliance: Ventricular end-diastolic volume is difficult to measure clinically. Even newer imaging techniques such as two-dimensional transesophageal echocardiography (TEE), radionuclide imaging, and contrast ventriculography provide only two-dimensional approximations. Left ventricular end-diastolic pressure (LVEDP) can be used as a measure of preload only if the relationship between ventricular volume and pressure (ventricular compliance) is constant. Unfortunately, ventricular compliance is normally nonlinear (Figure 19–7). Moreover, many factors are known to influence ventricular compliance (see below). Nonetheless, measurement of LVEDP or other pressures approximating LVEDP (such as pulmonary capillary wedge pressure) remains the most common means of estimating left ventricular preload (Chapter 6). Central venous pressure can be used as an index of right ventricular preload as well as left ventricular preload in most normal individuals (see above).

Ventricular compliance can decrease as a result of increased wall stiffness or thickening. Common causes

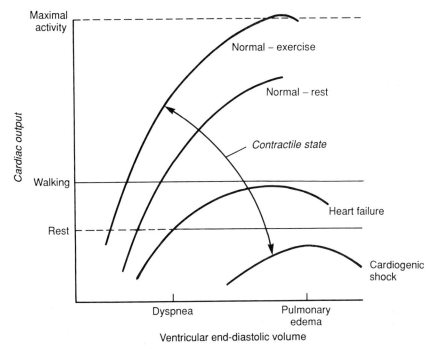

Figure 19–6. Starling's law of the heart.

of decreased compliance include myocardial ischemia, scarring, and hypertrophy. Because of its normally thinner wall, the right ventricle is more compliant than the left. Overfilling or distention of one ventricle—especially when the pericardium is still intact—can decrease the compliance of the other ventricle.

Afterload

Afterload for the intact heart is commonly equated with ventricular wall tension during systole. Wall tension may be thought of as the pressure the ventricle must overcome to reduce its cavity. If the ventricle is

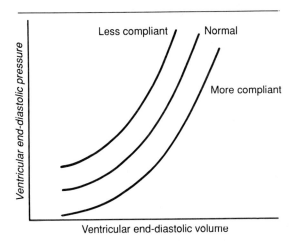

Figure 19–7. Normal and abnormal ventricular compliance.

assumed to be spherical, ventricular wall tension can be expressed by Laplace's law:

$$\text{Circumferential stress} = \frac{P \times R}{2 \times H}$$

where P is intraventricular pressure, R is the ventricular radius, and H is wall thickness. Although the normal ventricle is usually ellipsoidal, this relationship is still useful. The larger the ventricular radius, the greater the wall tension required to develop the same ventricular pressure. Conversely, an increase in wall thickness reduces ventricular wall tension.

Systolic intraventricular pressure is dependent on (1) the force of ventricular contraction, (2) the distensibility of the aorta and its proximal branches, and (3) **systemic vascular resistance (SVR).** Arteriolar tone is the chief determinant of SVR (see below). Because vascular distensibility is generally fixed in any given patient, left ventricular afterload is usually equated clinically with SVR, which is calculated by the following equation:

$$\text{SVR} = 80 \times \frac{\text{MAP} - \text{CVP}}{\text{CO}}$$

where MAP is mean arterial pressure in mm Hg, and CVP is central venous pressure in mm Hg, and CO is cardiac output in L/min. Normal SVR is 900–1500 dyne-sec/cm^{-5}. Systolic blood pressure may be used as an approximation of left ventricular afterload in the absence of chronic changes in the size, shape, or thickness of the ventricular wall or acute changes in systemic vascular resistance.

Right ventricular afterload is mainly dependent on pulmonary vascular resistance and is expressed by the following equation:

$$PVR = 80 \times \frac{PAP - LAP}{CO}$$

where PAP is mean pulmonary artery pressure and LAP is left atrial pressure. In practice, PCWP is usually substituted as an approximation for LAP (Chapter 6). Normal PVR is 50–150 dyne-sec/cm^{-5}.

Cardiac output is inversely related to afterload (Figure 19–8). The right ventricle is more sensitive to changes in afterload than the left ventricle because of the former's thinner wall. Cardiac output in patients with marked right or left ventricular impairment is very sensitive to acute increases in afterload. The latter is especially true in the presence of myocardial depression (as often occurs during anesthesia).

A

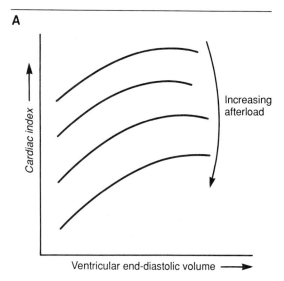

B

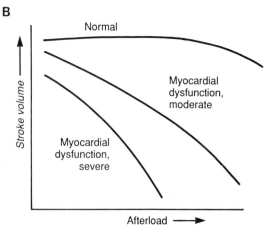

Figure 19–8. The relationship between cardiac output and afterload. A: The effect of increasing afterload on cardiac index. B: Note that patients with myocardial dysfunction become increasingly more sensitive to afterload.

Contractility

Cardiac contractility (**inotropy**) is the intrinsic ability of the myocardium to pump in the absence of changes in preload or afterload. Contractility is related to the rate of myocardial muscle shortening, which is in turn dependent on the intracellular calcium concentration during systole (see above). Experimentally, increases in heart rate can also enhance contractility under some conditions, perhaps due to increased intracellular calcium availability.

Contractility can be altered by neural, humoral, or pharmacologic influences. Sympathetic nervous system activity normally has the most important effect on contractility. Sympathetic fibers innervate atrial and ventricular muscle as well as nodal tissues. In addition to its positive chronotropic effect, norepinephrine release also enhances contractility via β_1 receptor activation. Alpha receptors are also present in the myocardium but appear to have only minor positive inotropic and chronotropic effects. Sympathomimetic drugs and epinephrine secretion from the adrenal glands similarly increase contractility via β_1 receptor activation. Other inotropes also increase intracellular calcium availability during systole but via differing mechanisms. Digoxin increases intracellular calcium indirectly by inhibition of Na^+-K^+ ATPase; the resulting increase in intracellular sodium concentration decreases the normal exchange of intracellular calcium for extracellular sodium. Amrinone increases cAMP levels and secondarily intracellular calcium by inhibiting phosphodiesterase III (the enzyme responsible for degrading cAMP in the heart). Glucagon also enhances contractility by increasing intracellular cAMP levels via activation of a specific nonadrenergic receptor.

Myocardial contractility is depressed by anoxia, depletion of catecholamine stores within the heart, and loss of functioning muscle mass due to ischemia or infarction. Most anesthetics and antiarrhythmic agents are negative inotropes (decrease contractility).

Wall Motion Abnormalities

Regional wall motion abnormalities cause a breakdown of the analogy between the intact heart and skeletal muscle preparations. When the ventricular cavity does not collapse symmetrically or fully, emptying becomes impaired. **Hypokinesis** (decreased contraction), **akinesis** (failure to contract), and **dyskinesis** (paradoxic bulging) during systole reflect increasing degrees of contraction abnormalities. Although contractility may be normal or even enhanced in some areas, abnormalities in other areas of the ventricle can impair emptying and reduce stroke volume. The severity of impairment will depend on the size and number of abnormally contracting areas.

Valvular Dysfunction

Valvular dysfunction can involve any one of the four valves in the heart and can lead to stenosis, incompetence (regurgitation), or both. Stenosis of an atrioventricular (tricuspid or mitral) valve reduces stroke volume primarily by decreasing ventricular preload, while stenosis of a semilunar (pulmonary or aortic) valve reduces stroke volume chiefly by increasing ventricular afterload (Chapter 20). In contrast, valvular incompetence reduces stroke volume without changes in preload, afterload, or contractility and without wall motion abnormalities. The effective stroke volume is reduced by the regurgitant volume with every contraction. When an atrioventricular valve is incompetent, a fraction of the stroke volume flows backward into the atrium during systole. When a semilunar valve is incompetent, a fraction of the stroke volume returns backward into the ventricle during diastole.

ASSESSMENT OF VENTRICULAR FUNCTION

1. VENTRICULAR FUNCTION CURVES

Plotting cardiac output or stroke volume against preload is useful in evaluating pathologic states and understanding drug therapy. Normal right and left ventricular function curves are shown in Figure 19–9. A series of curves can be described for each state of contractility (Figure 19–6).

Ventricular pressure-volume diagrams are also useful because they dissociate contractility from both preload and afterload. Two points are identified on such diagrams: the end-systolic point (ESP) and the end-diastolic point (EDP) (Figure 19–10). For any given contractile state, all ESPs are on the same line—ie, the

relationship between end-systolic volume and end-systolic pressure is fixed.

2. MEASUREMENTS OF CONTRACTILITY

The change in ventricular pressure over time during systole (dP/dt) is defined by the first derivative of the ventricular pressure curve and is often used as a measure of contractility. Contractility is directly proportionate to dP/dt, but accurate measurement of this value requires a high-fidelity ventricular catheter. Although arterial pressure tracings are distorted owing to properties of the vascular tree, the initial rate of rise in pressure (the slope) can serve as a rough approximation; the more proximal the catheter is in the arterial tree, the more accurate the extrapolation will be. The utility of dP/dt is also limited by the fact that it may be affected by preload, afterload, and heart rate. Various correction factors have been used with only limited success.

Ejection Fraction

Ventricular ejection fraction, the fraction of the end-diastolic ventricular volume ejected, is the best clinical measurement of systolic function. Ejection fraction (EF) can be calculated by the following equation:

$$EF = \frac{EDV - ESV}{EDV}$$

where EDV is left ventricular diastolic volume and ESV is end-systolic volume. Normal EF is approximately 0.60 ± 0.10. Measurements can be made preoperatively from cardiac catheterization or intraoperatively from transesophageal echocardiography. Recently developed pulmonary artery catheters with fast-response thermistors allow measurement of the right ventricular ejection fraction. Both ventricles normally have similar ejection fractions.

SYSTEMIC CIRCULATION

The systemic vasculature can be divided functionally into arteries, arterioles, capillaries, and veins. Arteries are the high-pressure conduits that supply the various organs. Arterioles are the small vessels that directly feed and control blood flow through each capillary bed. Capillaries are thin-walled vessels that allow the exchange of nutrients between blood and tissues (Chapter 28). Veins return blood from capillary beds to the heart.

The distribution of blood between the various compartments of the circulatory system is shown in Table 19–4. Note that most of the blood volume is in the

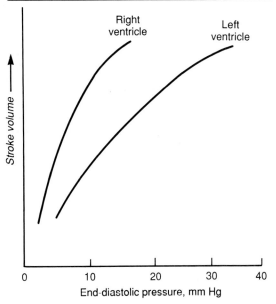

Figure 19–9. Function curves for the left and right ventricles.

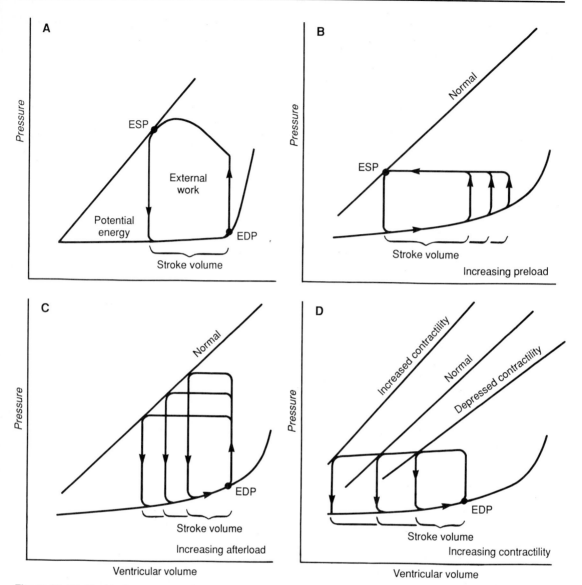

Figure 19–10. Ventricular pressure-volume diagrams. **A:** A single ventricular contraction. Note that stroke volume represents change in volume on the x-axis (difference between end-systolic volume and end-diastolic volume). Note also that the circumscribed area represents external work performed by the ventricle. **B:** Increasing preload with contractility and afterload constant. **C:** Increasing afterload with preload and contractility constant. **D:** Increasing contractility with preload and afterload constant.

systemic circulation—specifically, within systemic veins. Changes in systemic venous tone allows these vessels to function as a reservoir for blood. Following significant blood or fluid losses, a sympathetically mediated increase in venous tone reduces the caliber of these vessels and shifts blood into other parts of the

vascular system. Conversely, venodilatation allows these vessels to accommodate increases in blood volume. Sympathetic control of venous tone is an important determinant of venous return to the heart. Loss of this tone following induction of anesthesia frequently contributes to hypotension.

Table 19–4. Normal distribution of blood volume.

Heart	7%
Pulmonary circulation	9%
Systemic circulation	
Arterial	15%
Capillary	5%
Venous	64%

AUTONOMIC CONTROL OF THE SYSTEMIC VASCULATURE

Although both the sympathetic and parasympathetic systems can exert important influences on the circulation, autonomic control of the vasculature is primarily sympathetic. Sympathetic outflow to the circulation passes out of the spinal cord at all thoracic and the first two lumbar segments. These fibers reach blood vessels via specific autonomic nerves or by traveling along spinal nerves. Sympathetic fibers innervate all parts of the vasculature except for capillaries. Their principal function is to regulate vascular tone. Variation of vascular tone on the arterial side serves to regulate blood pressure and the distribution of blood flow to the various organs. Variations in venous tone alter venous return to the heart.

The vasculature has both sympathetic vasoconstrictor and vasodilator fibers, but the former are more important physiologically in most tissue beds. Sympathetic-induced vasoconstriction (via α_1-adrenergic receptors) can be potent in skeletal muscle, kidneys, gut, and skin; it is least active in the brain and heart. The most important vasodilatory fibers are those to skeletal muscle, which mediate an increase in blood flow (via β_2-adrenergic receptors) in response to exercise. **Vasovagal syncope,** which may occur following intense emotional strain, results from activation of both vagal and sympathetic vasodilator fibers.

Vascular tone and autonomic influences on the heart are controlled by vasomotor centers in the reticular formation of the medulla and lower pons. Distinct vasoconstrictor and vasodilator areas have been identified. Vasoconstriction is mediated by the anterolateral areas of the lower pons and upper medulla. The adrenergic cells in this area distribute fibers widely to the spinal cord. They are also responsible for adrenal secretion of catecholamines as well as enhancing cardiac automaticity and contractility. Vasodilatory areas, which are located in the lower medulla, are also adrenergic but function by projecting inhibitory fibers upward to the vasoconstrictor areas. Vasomotor output is modified by inputs from throughout the central nervous system, including the other areas in the brainstem, hypothalamus, and cerebral cortex. Areas in the posterolateral medulla receive input from both the vagal and the glossopharyngeal nerves and play an important role in mediating a variety of circulatory reflexes (see below). The sympathetic system normally maintains a chronic vasoconstrictor tone on the vasculature. Loss of this tone following induction of anesthesia or sympathectomy frequently contributes to perioperative hypotension.

ARTERIAL BLOOD PRESSURE

Systemic blood flow is pulsatile in large arteries because of the heart's cyclic activity; but by the time blood reaches the systemic capillaries, flow is continuous (laminar). The mean pressure in large arteries, which is normally about 95 mm Hg, falls nearly to zero in the large systemic veins that return blood to the heart (Figure 19–11). The largest pressure drop, nearly 50%, is across the arterioles, which account for the majority of systemic vascular resistance.

Mean arterial blood pressure (MAP) is proportion-

ate to the product of SVR × CO. This is relationship is based on an analogy to Ohm's law as applied to the circulation:

$$MAP - CVP \simeq SVR \times CO$$

Since CVP is normally very small compared to MAP, the former can usually be ignored. From this relationship, it is readily apparent that hypotension is the result of a decrease in SVR, CO, or both: In order to maintain arterial blood pressure, a decrease in one must be compensated by an increase in the other. Mean arterial blood pressure can be measured as the integrated mean of the arterial pressure wave form. Alternatively, MAP may be estimated by the following formula:

$$MAP = \frac{\text{Diastolic blood}}{\text{pressure}} + \frac{\text{Pulse pressure}}{3}$$

where pulse pressure is the difference between systolic and diastolic blood pressure. Arterial pulse pressure is directly related to stroke volume but inversely proportionate to the compliance of the arteriolar tree. Thus, decreases in pulse pressure may be due to a decrease in stroke volume, an increase in systemic vascular resistance, or both.

Transmission of the arterial wave from large arteries to smaller vessels in the periphery is faster than the actual velocity of blood; the wave travels at a rate 15 times the velocity of blood in the aorta. Moreover, reflections of the propagating waves off arterial walls widen pulse pressure before the pulse wave is completely dampened in very small arteries (Figure 19–11).

Control of Arterial Blood Pressure

Arterial blood pressure is regulated by a series of immediate, intermediate, and long-term adjustments involving complex neural, humoral, and renal mechanisms.

A. Immediate Control: Immediate control of blood pressure is primarily the function of autonomic nervous system reflexes. Changes in blood pressure are sensed both centrally, in hypothalamic and brainstem areas, and peripherally by specialized sensors (baroreceptors). Decreases in arterial blood pressure enhance sympathetic tone, increase adrenal secretion of epinephrine, and suppress vagal activity. The resulting systemic vasoconstriction, elevation in heart rate, and enhanced cardiac contractility serve to increase blood pressure. Conversely, hypertension decreases sympathetic outflow and enhances vagal tone.

Peripheral baroreceptors are located at the bifurcation of the common carotid arteries and the aortic arch. Elevations in blood pressure increase baroreceptor discharge, inhibiting systemic vasoconstriction and enhancing vagal tone (**baroreceptor reflex**). Reductions in blood pressure decrease baroreceptor discharge, allowing vasoconstriction and reduction of vagal tone. Carotid baroreceptors send afferent signals to circulatory brainstem centers via Hering's nerve (a branch of

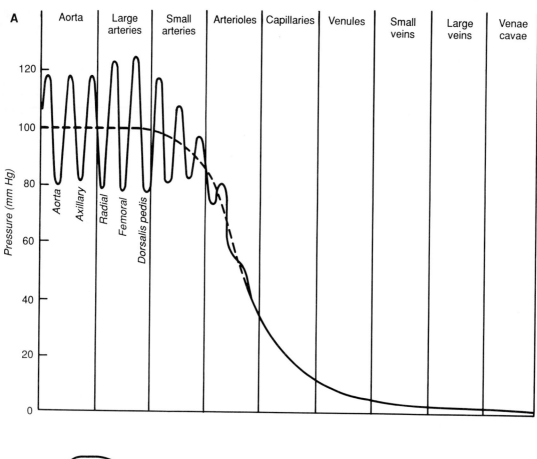

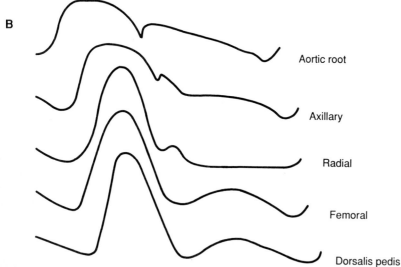

Figure 19–11. Arterial pressure wave forms. *A:* Changes in pressure in the systemic circulation. (Adapted from Guyton AC: *Textbook of Medical Physiology,* 7th ed. Saunders, 1986.) *B:* Note changes in the arterial wave form. (Reproduced, with permission, from Bedford RF: Invasive blood pressure monitoring. In: *Monitoring in Anesthesia and Critical Care Medicine.* Blitt CD (editor). Churchill Livingstone, 1985.)

the glossopharyngeal nerve), while aortic baroreceptor afferents travel along the vagus nerve. Of the two peripheral sensors, the carotid baroreceptor is physiologically more important and is primarily responsi-

ble for minimizing blood pressure changes due to acute events, such as a change in posture. Carotid baroreceptors sense MAP most effectively between pressures of 80 and 160 mm Hg. Adaptation to acute blood pressure changes occurs over the course of 1–2 days, rendering this reflex ineffective for long-term blood pressure control. All volatile anesthetics depress the normal baroreceptor response, but isoflurane appears to have the least effect.

B. Intermediate Control: In the course of a few minutes, sustained decreases in arterial pressure together with enhanced sympathetic outflow activate the renin-angiotensin system (Chapter 31), increase vasopressin secretion, and alter normal capillary fluid exchange (Chapter 28). Both angiotensin II and vasopressin are potent arteriolar vasoconstrictors. Their immediate action is to increase systemic vascular resistance. However, in contrast to angiotensin II formation, moderate to marked hypotension is required for enough vasopressin secretion to produce vasoconstriction (Chapter 28).

Sustained changes in arterial blood pressure can also alter fluid exchange in tissues by their secondary effects on capillary pressures. Hypertension favors interstitial movement of intravascular fluid, while hypotension favors intravascular movement of interstitial fluid. Such compensatory changes in intravascular volume can serve to reduce fluctuations in blood pressure, especially in the absence of adequate renal function (see below).

C. Long-Term Control: Within hours following sustained changes in arterial pressure, the effects of slower renal mechanisms become apparent. By manipulating total body sodium and water balance, the kidneys are capable of restoring blood pressure to normal. Hypotension results in sodium (and water) retention, while hypertension generally increases sodium excretion in normal individuals (Chapter 28)

SYSTEMIC BLOOD FLOW

Most organs regulate their own blood flow according to their metabolic needs in spite of variations in blood pressure. Cardiac output therefore represents the sum of individual blood flows for each organ. The mechanism by which autoregulation occurs remains unclear but probably involves the release of vasodilating substances in response to relative hypoperfusion. Suggested tissue mediators of vasodilation include CO_2, lactic acid, H^+, adenosine, and K^+. Vasodilation also probably occurs in response to a relative deficiency in oxygen tension.

ANATOMY & PHYSIOLOGY OF THE CORONARY CIRCULATION

1. ANATOMY

Myocardial blood supply is derived entirely from the right and left coronary arteries (Figure 19–12). Blood flows from epicardial to endocardial vessels. After perfusing the myocardium, blood returns to the right atrium via the coronary sinus and the anterior cardiac veins. A small amount of blood returns directly into the chambers of the heart via the thebesian veins. The right coronary artery normally supplies the right atrium and ventricle and a variable portion of the posterior left ventricle. The left coronary artery supplies the left atrium and left ventricle (mainly the anterior and lateral walls). The arterial supply to the SA node can be derived from either the right coronary artery (60% of individuals) or the left coronary artery (the remaining 40%). The AV node is supplied by the right coronary artery (90%) or, less frequently, by the circumflex branch of the left coronary artery (10%).

2. DETERMINANTS OF CORONARY PERFUSION

Coronary perfusion is unique in that it is intermittent rather than continuous, like other organs. During contraction, intramyocardial pressures in the left ventricle approach systemic arterial pressure. The force of left ventricular contraction almost completely occludes the intramyocardial part of the coronary arteries; in fact, blood flow may transiently reverse in epicardial vessels. Even during the latter part of diastole, left ventricular pressure eventually exceeds venous (right atrial) pressure. Thus, coronary perfusion pressure is usually determined by the difference between aortic pressure and ventricular pressure, and the left ventricle is perfused almost entirely during diastole. In contrast, the right ventricle is perfused during both systole and diastole (Figure 19–13). Moreover, arterial diastolic pressure is a more important determinant of myocardial blood flow than mean arterial pressure, such that

Coronary perfusion pressure = Arterial diastolic pressure – LVEDP

Decreases in aortic pressure or increases in ventricular end-diastolic pressure can reduce coronary perfusion pressure. Increases in heart rate also decrease coronary perfusion because of the disproportionately greater reduction in diastolic time as heart rate increases (Figure 19–14). Because it is subjected to the greatest intramural pressures during systole, the endocardium tends to be most vulnerable to ischemia during decreases in coronary perfusion pressure.

Control of Coronary Blood Flow

Coronary blood flow normally parallels myocardial metabolic demand. In the average adult male at rest, coronary blood flow is approximately 250 mL/min. The myocardium regulates its own blood flow closely between perfusion pressures of 50 and 120 mm Hg. Beyond this range, blood flow becomes increasingly pressure-dependent.

Under normal conditions, changes in blood flow are entirely due to variations in coronary arterial tone (resistance) in response to metabolic demand. Hypoxia—either directly, or indirectly through the release of

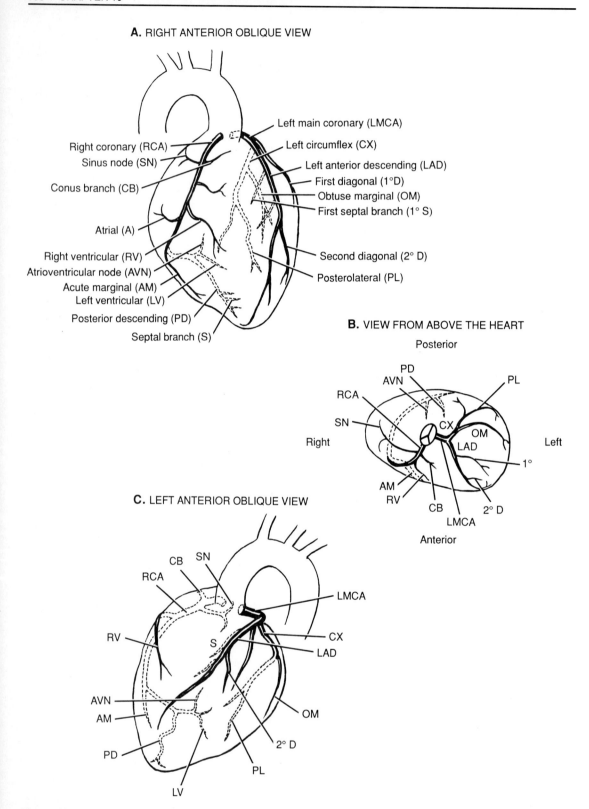

A. RIGHT ANTERIOR OBLIQUE VIEW

Left main coronary (LMCA)
Right coronary (RCA)
Sinus node (SN)
Left circumflex (CX)
Left anterior descending (LAD)
Conus branch (CB)
First diagonal (1°D)
Obtuse marginal (OM)
First septal branch (1° S)
Atrial (A)
Right ventricular (RV)
Atrioventricular node (AVN)
Second diagonal (2° D)
Acute marginal (AM)
Posterolateral (PL)
Left ventricular (LV)
Posterior descending (PD)
Septal branch (S)

B. VIEW FROM ABOVE THE HEART

Posterior

PD
AVN
PL
RCA
SN
CX
OM
Right
LAD
Left
1°
AM
RV
CB
2° D
LMCA

Anterior

C. LEFT ANTERIOR OBLIQUE VIEW

CB SN
RCA
LMCA
RV
CX
S
LAD
AVN
AM
OM
PD
2° D
PL
LV

Figure 19–12. Anatomy of the coronary arteries. **A:** Right anterior oblique view. **B:** View from above. **C:** Left anterior oblique view.

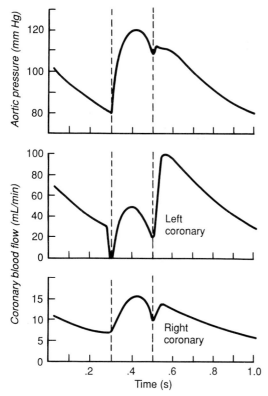

Figure 19–13. Coronary blood flow during the cardiac cycle. (Modified and reproduced, with permission, from Berne RM, Levy MD: *Cardiovascular Physiology,* 2nd ed. Mosby, 1972.)

adenosine—causes coronary vasodilatation. Autonomic influences are generally weak. Both α_1- and β_2-adrenergic receptors are present in the coronary arteries. The α_1 receptors are primarily located on larger epicardial vessels, while β_2 receptors are mainly found on the smaller intramuscular and subendocardial

vessels. Sympathetic stimulation generally increases myocardial blood flow because of an increase in metabolic demand and a predominance of β_2 receptor activation. Parasympathetic effects on the coronary vasculature are generally minor and are weakly vasodilatory.

3. MYOCARDIAL OXYGEN BALANCE

Myocardial oxygen demand is normally the most important determinant of myocardial blood flow. The myocardium normally extracts 65% of the oxygen in arterial blood compared to 25% in most other tissues (Chapter 22). Coronary sinus oxygen saturation is normally 30%. Unlike other tissues, the myocardium therefore cannot compensate for reductions in blood flow by extracting more oxygen from hemoglobin. Any increases in myocardial metabolic demand must be met by an increase in coronary blood flow. Table 19–5 lists the most important determinants of myocardial oxygen demand and supply. Note that the heart rate and, to a lesser extent, ventricular end-diastolic pressure are important determinants of coronary supply as well as demand.

A diastolic-pressure time index (DPTI) has been suggested as a measure of left ventricular blood flow and is expressed by the following equation:

$$\text{DPTI} =$$
Coronary perfusion pressure × Diastolic time

Similarly, a tension-time index (TTI) has been proposed as a measure of oxygen demand:

TTI = Systolic blood pressure × Systolic time

The ratio of the two indices—also called the endocardial viability ratio—can be useful in evaluating oxy-

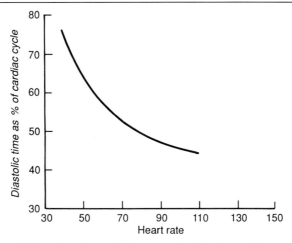

Figure 19–14. The relationship between diastolic time and heart rate.

Table 19–5. Factors affecting myocardial oxygen supply-demand balance.

Supply
  Heart rate
    Diastolic time
  Coronary perfusion pressure
    Aortic diastolic blood pressure
    Ventricular end-diastolic pressure
  Arterial oxygen content
    Arterial oxygen tension
    Hemoglobin concentration
  Coronary vessel diameter
Demand
  Basal requirements
  Heart rate
  Wall tension
    Preload (ventricular radius)
    Afterload
    Contractility

gen supply-demand balance. DPTI/TTI is normally 1 or more. Ratios less than 0.7 are generally associated with subendocardial ischemia.

THE PATHOPHYSIOLOGY OF HEART FAILURE

Heart failure exists when the heart is unable to pump a sufficient amount of blood to meet the body's metabolic requirements. Clinical manifestations usually reflect the effects of the low cardiac output on tissues (fatigue, oxygen debt, or acidosis), the damming-up of blood behind the failing ventricle (systemic or pulmonary venous congestion), or both. The left ventricle is most commonly involved, often with secondary involvement of the right ventricle. Isolated right ventricular failure can occur in the setting of advanced disease of the lung parenchyma or pulmonary vasculature. Left ventricular failure most commonly results from primary myocardial dysfunction (usually from coronary artery disease) but may also result from valvular dysfunction, arrhythmias, or pericardial disease.

Cardiac output is reduced in most forms of heart failure. Inadequate oxygen delivery to tissues is reflected by a low mixed venous oxygen tension and an increase in the arterial-venous oxygen content difference (Chapter 22). In compensated heart failure, the arteriovenous difference may be normal at rest, but it rapidly widens during stress or exercise.

Heart failure is less commonly associated with an elevated cardiac output. This form of heart failure is most commonly seen with sepsis and other hypermetabolic states, which are typically associated with a low SVR.

COMPENSATORY MECHANISMS

Three major compensatory mechanisms are generally present in patients with heart failure: (1) increased preload, (2) increased sympathetic tone, and (3) ventricular hypertrophy. Although these mechanisms can often initially compensate for mild to moderate cardiac dysfunction, with increasing severity of dysfunction they may actually contribute to the cardiac impairment.

Increased Preload

An increase in ventricular size not only reflects an inability to keep up with venous return but also serves to maximize stroke volume by moving the heart up the Starling curve (Figure 19–6). Even when ejection fraction is reduced, an increase in ventricular end-diastolic volume can maintain a normal stroke volume (see above). Worsening venous congestion due to damming-up of blood behind the failing ventricle and excessive ventricular dilatation can rapidly lead to clinical deterioration. Left ventricular failure results in pulmonary vascular congestion and progressive transudation of fluid, first into the pulmonary interstitium and then into alveoli (pulmonary edema). Right ventricular failure leads to systemic venous hypertension, which results in peripheral edema, hepatic congestion and dysfunction, and ascites. Dilatation of the annulus of either atrioventricular valve leads to valvular incompetence, further impairing ventricular output.

Increased Sympathetic Tone

Sympathetic activation increases norepinephrine release from nerve endings in the heart and adrenal secretion of epinephrine into the circulation. Plasma catecholamine levels are generally directly proportionate to the degree of left ventricular dysfunction. Although enhanced sympathetic outflow can initially maintain cardiac output by increasing heart rate and contractility, worsening ventricular function elicits increasing degrees of vasoconstriction in an effort to maintain arterial blood pressure. The associated increase in afterload, however, reduces cardiac output and exacerbates the ventricular failure.

Chronic sympathetic activation in patients with heart failure eventually decreases the response of adrenergic receptors to catecholamines, decreases the number of adrenergic receptors, and reduces cardiac catecholamine stores. Nonetheless, the failing heart becomes increasingly dependent on circulating catecholamines. Abrupt withdrawal in sympathetic outflow or decreases in circulating catecholamine levels, as can occur following induction of anesthesia, may lead to acute cardiac decompensation.

Sympathetic activation tends to redistribute systemic blood flow output away from the skin, gut, kidneys, and skeletal muscle to the heart and brain. Decreased renal perfusion together with activation of the renin-angiotensin-aldosterone axis (Chapter 28) leads to sodium retention and interstitial edema.

Ventricular Hypertrophy

Ventricular hypertrophy can occur with or without dilatation, depending on the type of stress imposed on the ventricle. When the heart is subjected to either pressure or volume overload, the initial response is to increase sarcomere length and optimally overlap actin and myosin. With time, ventricular muscle mass begins to increase in response to the abnormal stress.

In the volume-overloaded ventricle, the problem is an increase in diastolic wall stress. The increase in ventricular muscle mass is only sufficient to compensate for the increase in diameter: the ratio of the ventricular radius to wall thickness is unchanged. Sarcomeres replicate mainly in series, resulting in eccentric hypertrophy. Although ventricular ejection fraction remains depressed, the increase in end-diastolic volume can maintain stroke volume (and cardiac output) normal at rest.

The problem in a pressure-overloaded ventricle is an increase in systolic wall stress. Sarcomeres mainly replicate in parallel, resulting in concentric hypertrophy: hypertrophy is such that the ratio of myocardial wall thickness to ventricular radius increases. As can be seen from Laplace's law (see above), systolic wall stress can then be normalized.

CASE DISCUSSION: A PATIENT WITH A SHORT PR INTERVAL

A 38-year-old man is scheduled for endoscopic sinus surgery following a recent onset of headaches. He gives a history of having passed out at least once during one of these headaches. A preoperative ECG is normal except for a PR interval of 0.116 s with normal P wave morphology.

What is the significance of a short PR interval?

The PR interval, which is measured from the beginning of atrial depolarization (P wave) to the beginning of ventricular depolarization (QRS complex), normally represents the time required for depolarization of both atria, the AV node, and the His-Purkinje system. Although the PR interval can vary with the heart rate, it is normally 0.12–0.2 s in duration. Abnormally short PR intervals can be seen either with low atrial (or upper AV junctional) rhythms or with preexcitation phenomena. The two can usually be differentiated by P wave morphology: With a low atrial rhythm, atrial depolarization is retrograde, resulting in an inverted P wave in leads II, III, and aVF, whereas with preexcitation the P wave is normal during sinus rhythm. If the pacemaker rhythm originates from a lower AV junctional focus, the P wave may be lost in the QRS complex or may follow the QRS.

What is preexcitation?

Preexcitation usually refers to early depolarization of the ventricles by an abnormal conduction pathway in the heart. Rarely, more than one such pathway is present. The most common form of preexcitation is due to the presence of an accessory pathway (bundle of Kent) that connects one of the atria with one of the ventricles. This abnormal connection between the atria and ventricles allows electrical impulses to bypass the AV node (hence the term bypass tract). The ability to conduct impulses along the bypass tract can be quite variable and may be only intermittent or rate-dependent. Bypass tracts may conduct in both directions, retrograde only (ventricle to atrium), or, rarely, anterograde only (atrium to ventricle). The term Wolff-Parkinson-White syndrome is often applied whenever ventricular preexcitation is associated with tachyarrhythmias.

How does preexcitation shorten the PR interval?

In patients with preexcitation, the normal cardiac impulse originating from the SA node is conducted simultaneously through the normal (AV nodal) and anomalous (bypass tract) pathways. Because conduction is more rapid in the anomalous pathway than in the AV nodal pathway, the cardiac impulse rapidly reaches and depolarizes the area of the ventricles where the bypass tract ends. This early depolarization of the ventricle (preexcitation) is reflected by a short PR interval and a slurred initial deflection (delta wave) in the QRS complex. Spread of the anomalous impulse to the rest of the ventricle is delayed because it must be conducted by ordinary ventricular muscle, not by the much faster Purkinje system. The remainder of the ventricle is then depolarized by the normal impulse from the AV node as it "catches up" with the preexcitation front. Although the PR interval is shortened, the resulting QRS is slightly prolonged and represents a fusion complex of normal and abnormal ventricular depolarization.

The PR interval in patients with preexcitation depends on relative conduction times between the AV nodal pathway and the bypass pathway. If conduction through the former is fast, preexcitation (and the delta wave) is less prominent, and QRS will be relatively normal. If conduction is delayed in the AV nodal pathway, preexcitation is more prominent, and more of the ventricle will be depolarized by the abnormally conducted impulse. When the AV nodal pathway is completely blocked, the entire ventricle is depolarized by the bypass pathway, resulting in a very short PR interval, a very prominent delta wave, and a wide, bizarre QRS complex. Other factors that can affect the degree of preexcitation include interatrial conduction time, the distance of the atrial end of the bypass tract from the SA node, and autonomic tone. The PR interval is often normal or only slightly shortened with a left lateral bypass tract (the most common location). Preexcitation may be more apparent at fast heart rates because conduction slows through the AV node with increasing heart rates. Secondary ST segment and T wave changes are also commonly present because of abnormal ventricular repolarization.

What is the significance of preexcitation?

Preexcitation occurs in approximately 0.3% of the general population. An estimated 20–50% of affected individuals develop paroxysmal tachyarrhythmias. Although most patients are otherwise normal, preexcitation can be associated with other cardiac anomalies, including Ebstein's anomaly, mitral valve prolapse, or cardiomyopathies. Depending on its conductive properties, the bypass tract in some patients may predispose to tachyarrhythmias and even sudden death. Tachyarrhythmias include atrioventricular reciprocating tachycardia, atrial fibrillation, and, less commonly, atrial flutter. Ventricular fibrillation can be precipitated by a critically timed premature atrial beat that travels down the bypass tract and catches the ventricle at a vulnerable period (see below). Alternatively, very rapid conduction of impulses into the ventricles by the bypass tract during atrial fibrillation can rapidly lead to myocardial ischemia, hypoperfusion, and hypoxia and culminate in ventricular fibrillation.

Recognition of the preexcitation phenomenon is also important because its QRS morphology on the surface ECG can mimic bundle branch block, right ventricular hypertrophy, ischemia, myocardial infarction, and ventricular tachycardia (during atrial fibrillation).

How do tachyarrhythmias generally develop?

Tachyarrhythmias develop by one of two major mechanisms: (1) abnormal impulse formation or (2) abnormal impulse propagation (reentry). Abnormal impulses result from enhanced or abnormal automaticity or triggered activity. Normally, only cells of the SA node, specialized atrial conduction pathways, AV nodal junctional areas, and His-Purkinje system spontaneously depolarize. Because diastolic repolarization (phase 4) is fastest in the SA node, other areas of automaticity are suppressed. However, enhanced or abnormal automaticity in other areas can usurp pacemaker function from the SA node and lead to tachyarrhythmias. Triggered activity consists of small-amplitude depolarizations that can follow action potentials under some conditions in atrial, ventricular, and His-Purkinje tissue. If these "afterdepolarizations" reach threshold potential, they can result in repetitive sustained electrical activity. Factors that can promote abnormal impulse formation include increased catecholamine levels, electrolyte disorders, ischemia, hypoxia, mechanical stretch, and drug toxicity (especially digoxin).

The most common mechanism for tachyarrhythmias is reentry. Four conditions are necessary to initiate and sustain reentry: (1) two areas in the myocardium that differ in conductivity or refractoriness and that can form a closed electrical loop, (2) unidirectional block in one pathway, (3) slow conduction or sufficient length in the circuit to allow recovery of the conduction block in the first pathway, and (4) excitation of the initially blocked pathway to complete the loop (Figure 19–15). Reentry is usually precipitated by a premature cardiac impulse.

What is the mechanism of reciprocating tachycardia in patients with Wolff-Parkinson-White syndrome?

If the bypass tract is refractory during anterograde conduction of a cardiac impulse (as during a critically timed premature atrial beat) and the impulse is conducted by the AV node, the same impulse can be conducted retrograde from the ventricle back into the atria via the bypass tract. The retrograde impulse can then depolarize the atrium and travel down the AV nodal pathway again, establishing a continuous repetitive circuit (circus movement). The impulse reciprocates between the atria and ventricles and conduction alternates between the AV nodal pathway and the bypass tract. The term "concealed conduction" is often applied because the absence of preexcitation during this arrhythmia results in a normal QRS that lacks a delta wave.

The reciprocating mechanism less commonly involves anterograde conduction through the bypass tract and retrograde conduction through the AV nodal pathway. In such instances, the QRS has a delta wave and is completely abnormal; the arrhythmia can be mistaken for ventricular tachycardia.

How does atrial fibrillation in patients with Wolff-Parkinson-White syndrome differ from the arrhythmia in other patients?

Atrial fibrillation can occur when a cardiac impulse is conducted rapidly retrograde up into the atria (see above) and arrives to find different parts of the atria out of phase in recovery from the impulse. Once atrial fibrillation is established, conduction into the ventricles most commonly occurs through the bypass tract only, and because of the accessory pathway's ability to conduct very rapidly (unlike the AV nodal pathway), the ventricular rate is typically very rapid (180–300 beats/min). The majority of QRS complexes are bizarre, but periodic conduction of an impulse through the AV nodal pathway results in occasional normal-looking QRS complexes. Less commonly, impulses during atrial fibrillation are conducted mainly through the AV nodal pathway (resulting in mainly normal QRS complexes) or through both the bypass tract and the AV nodal pathway (resulting in a mixture of normal, fusion, and bizarre QRS complexes).

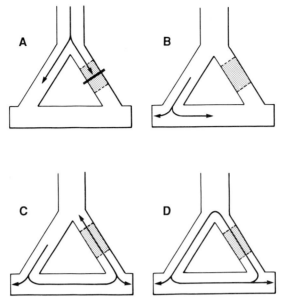

Figure 19–15. The mechanism of reentry. See text for description.

What is the significance of the history of syncope in this patient?

Preoperative evaluation of patients with preexcitation should assess the need for prophylactic perioperative antiarrhythmic therapy or preoperative electrophysiologic studies. Patients with only occasional asymptomatic tachyarrhythmias generally do not require investigation or prophylactic drug therapy. Those with frequent episodes of tachyarrhythmias or arrhythmias associated with significant symptoms require drug therapy and close evaluation. A history of syncope may be ominous because it may indicate the ability to conduct impulses very rapidly through the bypass tract, leading to systemic hypoperfusion and perhaps predisposing to sudden death. This patient should be evaluated preoperatively by a cardiologist for possible electrophysiologic studies and perioperative drug therapy. Such studies can identify the location of the bypass tracts, reasonably predict the potential for malignant arrhythmias by programmed pacing, determine the efficacy of antiarrhythmic therapy, and perhaps even lead to percutaneous catheter or surgical ablation of the bypass tract.

What anesthetic agents can safely be used in patients with preexcitation?

Few data are available comparing the use of different anesthetic agents or techniques in patients with preexcitation. Almost all of the volatile and intravenous agents have been used with equal success. Recommendations are based largely on theoretic consider-

ations. Factors tending to cause sympathetic stimulation and increased cardiac automaticity are undesirable. Premedication with a benzodiazepine helps reduce high sympathetic tone preoperatively. Agents that can increase sympathetic tone such as ketamine and perhaps pancuronium in large boluses should generally be avoided. Anticholinergics should be used cautiously; glycopyrrolate may be preferable to atropine (Chapter 11). Endotracheal intubation should be carried out only after the patient is deeply anesthetized (Chapter 20); pretreatment with a β-adrenergic blocker such as esmolol may be useful. Light anesthesia, hypercapnia, acidosis, and even transient hypoxemia will activate the sympathetic system and are to be avoided. A deep extubation and good postoperative analgesia (without respiratory acidosis) may also help prevent the onset of arrhythmias. When patients with preexcitation are anesthetized for electrophysiologic study and surgical ablation, opioids and benzodiazepines may be the agents least likely to alter conduction characteristics.

How are antiarrhythmic agents selected for tachyarrhythmias?

Most antiarrhythmic agents act by altering myocardial cell conduction (phase 0), repolarization (phase 3), or automaticity (phase 4). Prolongation of repolarization increases the refractoriness of cells. Many antiarrhythmic drugs also exert direct or indirect autonomic effects. Antiarrhythmic agents are generally classified according to mechanism of action or electrophysiologic effects (Table 19–6). Note that some

Table 19–6. Classification of antiarrhythmic agents.

Class	Mechanism of Action	Agents	Intravenous Loading Dose
I	Block fast sodium channels (decrease slope of phase 0)		
Ia	Dissociation intermediate, conduction moderately depressed, repolarization accelerated	Quinidine[1,2] Procainamide Disopyramide[1,3]	NR 10 mg/kg NA
Ib	Dissociation rapid, conduction minimally depressed, repolarization accelerated	Lidocaine Phenytoin Tocainide Mexiletine	1–1.5 mg/kg 5–15 mg/kg NA NA
Ic	Dissociation slow, conduction markedly depressed, no effect on repolarization	Flecainide Encainide	NA NA
II	Block β-adrenergic receptors (decrease automaticity)	Propranolol Esmolol (see also Table 20–7)	1–3 mg 0.5 mg/kg
III	Repolarization prolonged	Amiodarone[4,5] Bretylium[6] Sotalol[7]	5 mg/kg (I) 5–10 mg/kg 1–2 mg/kg (I)
IV	Block slow calcium channels (decrease automaticity and conduction in nodal tissue)	Verapamil (see also Table 20–6)	10–15 mg
Miscellaneous agents		Digoxin Adenosine Moricizine	0.5–0.75 mg 6–12 mg NA

[1]Also blocks muscarinic receptors (vagolytic).
[2]Also blocks α-adrenergic receptors.
[3]Also blocks slow calcium channels.
[4]Also causes noncompetitive α- and β- adrenergic blockade.
[5]Also binds inactivated fast sodium channels.
[6]Transiently releases catecholamine stores in nerve terminals.
[7]Also a weak β-adrenergic receptor blocker.
Key:
  NR = Available but not recommended for intravenous use.
  NA = Not available for intravenous use.
  (I) = Intravenous use is still investigational.

agents have more than one mechanism of action, while others, such as digoxin and adenosine, do not fit this classification very well.

Selection of an antiarrhythmic agent generally depends on whether the arrhythmia is ventricular or supraventricular and whether acute control or chronic therapy is required (Table 19–7). Intravenous agents are usually employed in the acute management of arrhythmias, while oral agents are reserved for chronic therapy. The toxicity of class Ic agents severely limits their use.

Which agents are most useful for tachyarrhythmias in patients with Wolf-Parkinson-White syndrome?

Cardioversion is the treatment of choice in hemodynamically compromised patients. The most useful pharmacologic agents are class Ia drugs, especially procainamide. These agents increase the refractory period and decrease conduction in the accessory pathway. Moreover, class Ia drugs frequently terminate and can suppress the recurrence of atrioventricular reciprocating tachycardia and atrial fibrillation. Beta-adrenergic blocking agents may also be useful, especially in controlling ventricular rate once these rhythms are established. Verapamil and digoxin are contraindicated during atrial fibrillation or flutter in these patients because they can dangerously accelerate the ventricular response: Both agents decrease conduction through the AV node, which favors conduction of impulses down the accessory pathway. The bypass tract is capable of conducting impulses into the ventricles much faster than the AV nodal pathway. Digoxin may also increase the ventricular response by shortening the refractory period and increasing conduction in accessory pathways. Although verapamil can terminate atrioventricular reciprocating tachycardia, its use in this setting may be hazardous because patients can

Table 19–7. Guidelines for the treatment of tachyarrhythmias. (Drugs are listed in general order of preference.)

I. Supraventricular arrhythmias
  A. Paroxysmal supraventricular tachycardia
    1. Acute[1]
      a. Conversion to normal sinus rhythm: adenosine, class IV, II, III,[2] or Ia agent
      b. Control of ventricular rate: digoxin, class IV or II agent
    2. Chronic prophylaxis: class Ia, class II, III,[2] or IV agent
  B. Atrial fibrillation or flutter
    1. Acute[1]
      a. Conversion to normal sinus rhythm: adenosine, class IV, II, III,[2] or Ia agent
      b. Control of ventricular rate: digoxin, class IV or II agent
    2. Chronic
      a. Control of ventricular rate: digoxin, class II, or IV agent
      b. Conversion to normal sinus rhythm[3]
      c. Prophylaxis: class Ia, class II, III,[2] or IV agent
II. Ventricular arrhythmias
  A. Nonsustained ventricular tachycardia
    1. Acute: class Ib, Ia, or III agent
    2. Chronic: class Ia, Ib, Ic, or III agent
  B. Sustained ventricular tachycardia
    1. Acute[1]
    2. Chronic prophylaxis: class II, III, or Ic agent

[1]Cardioversion is the treatment of choice in the presence of hemodynamic compromise.
[2]Specifically refers to amiodarone (note that its use for atrial arrhythmias is not approved by the United States Food and Drug Administration).
[3]Cardioversion usually necessary.

subsequently develop atrial fibrillation or flutter. Moreover, atrial fibrillation may not be readily distinguishable from ventricular tachycardia in these patients if wide QRS tachycardia develops. Procainamide may be preferable to lidocaine in such instances, because the former is generally effective for both arrhythmias.

SUGGESTED READINGS

Ganong WF: *Review of Medical Physiology,* 15th ed. Appleton and Lange, 1991. Contains an excellent review of circulatory physiology.

Goudsouzian N, Karamanian A: *Physiology for the Anesthesiologist,* 2nd ed. Appleton & Lange, 1984. Good chapters on circulatory physiology with some reference to anesthesia.

Guyton AC: *Textbook of Medical Physiology,* 8th ed. Saunders, 1991. The chapters on cardiovascular physiology are one of the highlights of this book.

Stoelting RK: *Pharmacology and Physiology in Anesthetic Practice,* 2nd ed. Lippincott, 1991. Good chapters on circulatory physiology with some reference to anesthesia.

Cardiovascular diseases—especially hypertensive, ischemic, and valvular heart disease—are the medical illnesses most frequently encountered in anesthetic practice and a major cause of perioperative morbidity and mortality. Management of patients with these diseases continues to challenge the ingenuity and resources of the anesthesiologist. The adrenergic response to surgical stimulation and the circulatory effects of anesthetic agents, endotracheal intubation, and positive-pressure ventilation impose additional burdens on an often already compromised cardiovascular system. Most anesthetic agents cause cardiac depression, vasodilatation, or both. Even anesthetics that have no direct circulatory effects may cause apparent circulatory depression in severely compromised patients dependent on chronically enhanced sympathetic activity which, when interrupted by the anesthetic state, can lead to acute circulatory decompensation.

Optimal anesthetic management of patients with cardiovascular disease requires a thorough knowledge of normal cardiac physiology (Chapter 19), the circulatory effects of the various anesthetic agents (Chapters 7–10), and the pathophysiology and treatment of these diseases. The same principles used in treating these diseases preoperatively should be applied intraoperatively. In most instances, the choice of anesthetic agent is not as important as how they are used.

The two most important **preoperative risk factors** are a history of recent (< 6 months) myocardial infarction and evidence of congestive heart failure. Each of these factors has been associated with death rates up to 20–25% and a 14% incidence of life-threatening complications. By identifying patients at greatest risk, appropriate measures may alter the outcome favorably. Indeed, recent studies suggest that a lower complication rate is achieved when invasive monitoring and aggressive hemodynamic interventions (vasodilators or adrenergic blockade) are employed for patients at high risk for cardiac complications.

The most important **intraoperative risk factor** appears to be the operative site, while the least consistent factor is operative time. Although poorly controlled hypertension is not clearly established as a risk factor for postoperative complications, it is frequently associated with wide swings in blood pressure intraoperatively (see below). Interestingly, intraoperative hypertension has been more closely linked to cardiac morbidity than hypotension.

While the superiority of regional anesthesia over general anesthesia for patients with cardiovascular disease seems intuitively obvious, studies supporting this view are lacking. Moreover, the hemodynamic effects of spinal and epidural anesthesia (Chapter 16) may be more detrimental than general anesthesia for some patients (see below).

CARDIAC RISK FACTORS

Cardiovascular complications account for 25–50% of deaths following noncardiac surgery. Perioperative myocardial infarction, pulmonary edema, congestive heart failure, arrhythmias, and thromboembolism are most commonly seen in patients with preexisting cardiovascular disease. The relatively high prevalence of cardiovascular disorders in surgical patients has given rise to attempts to define "cardiac risk" or the likelihood of intraoperative or postoperative fatal or life-threatening cardiac complications (Table 20–1).

HYPERTENSION

PREOPERATIVE CONSIDERATIONS

Hypertension is a leading cause of death and disability in most Western societies and the most frequent preoperative abnormality in surgical patients. Long-standing uncontrolled hypertension accelerates atherosclerosis and hypertensive organ damage. Hypertension is a major risk factor for cardiac, cerebral, renal, and vascular disease. Complications include myocardial infarction, congestive heart failure, stroke, renal

Table 20–1. Preoperative and intraoperative factors associated with cardiac complications following noncardiac surgery.

Preoperative factors
  S_3 gallop
  Elevated jugular venous pressure
  Myocardial infarction within 6 months
  More than five premature ventricular contractions per minute on the preoperative ECG
  A rhythm other than sinus or premature atrial contractions on the preoperative ECG
  Significant aortic stenosis
  Patient age > 70 years
  Emergency surgery
  Poor general condition of the patient
Intraoperative factors
  Intrathoracic, intraperitoneal, or aortic procedures
  Operative time > 3 hours
  Wide hemodynamic variations

failure, peripheral occlusive disease, and aortic dissection.

Definitions

Blood pressure measurements are affected by many variables, including posture, emotional state, recent activity, and drug intake, as well as the equipment and technique used. A diagnosis of hypertension cannot be made by one preoperative reading but requires confirmation by a history of consistently elevated measurements. Preoperative anxiety or pain often produces some degree of hypertension even in normal patients. However, patients with a history of hypertension generally exhibit greater preoperative elevations in blood pressure.

Epidemiologic studies demonstrate a direct continuous correlation between both diastolic and systolic blood pressures and mortality rates. The definition of systemic hypertension is therefore somewhat arbitrary but is generally considered to be a consistently elevated diastolic blood pressure greater than 90–95 mm Hg or a systolic pressure greater than 140–160 mm Hg. Labile (or borderline) hypertension is said to exist when elevated readings are frequent but not consistent. Labile hypertension often precedes sustained hypertension. Accelerated hypertension is defined as a recent, sustained and progressive increase in blood pressure, usually with diastolic blood pressures in excess of 110 mm Hg; renal dysfunction is often present. Malignant hypertension is a true medical emergency characterized by severe hypertension (> 200/140 mm Hg) associated with papilledema and frequently encephalopathy.

Pathophysiology

Hypertension can be either idiopathic (essential) or, less commonly, secondary to other medical conditions such as renal disease, primary hyperaldosteronism, Cushing's syndrome, acromegaly, pheochromocytoma, pregnancy, or estrogen therapy. Essential hypertension accounts for 80–90% of cases and may be associated with an abnormal baseline elevation of cardiac output, systemic vascular resistance (SVR), or both. An evolving pattern is commonly seen over the course of the disease. Initially, cardiac output is elevated but SVR is in the normal range (in reality, it is inappropriately high). As the disease progresses, cardiac output returns to normal but SVR becomes abnormally high. Extracellular fluid volume and plasma renin activity (Chapter 29) may be low, normal, or high.

The mechanisms responsible for the observed changes in hypertensive patients remain elusive but appear to involve abnormal increases in intracellular calcium and perhaps sodium concentrations in vascular smooth muscle, renal tubular cells, or both. The former presumably results in increased arteriolar tone, while the latter impairs renal excretion of sodium. Sympathetic nervous system overactivity and enhanced responses to sympathetic agonists are present in some patients. Overactivity of the renin-angiotensin-aldosterone system (Chapter 29) appears to play an important role in patients with accelerated hypertension.

Long-Term Treatment

The treatment of hypertension in the last few years has deviated from the traditional stepped approach. The latter attempted to control blood pressure by beginning with a diuretic and sequentially adding another class of agents (first a sympatholytic, then a vasodilator, and finally an angiotensin-converting enzyme [ACE] inhibitor) if blood pressure control was inadequate. Single-drug therapy using an adrenergic receptor blocker, calcium channel blocker, or ACE inhibitor now appears to be as effective as the older approach for mild to moderate hypertension but with fewer side effects and therefore better compliance. Familiarity with the names and mechanisms of action of commonly employed antihypertensive agents is mandatory for anesthesiologists (Table 20–2).

Preoperative Management

A recurring question in anesthetic practice is what degree of preoperative hypertension is acceptable for patients scheduled for elective surgery. Except for optimally controlled patients, most hypertensive patients present to the operating room with some degree of hypertension. While data suggest that even moderate degrees of preoperative hypertension (diastolic < 110 mm Hg) are not clearly statistically associated with *postoperative* complications, other data indicate that the untreated or poorly controlled hypertensive patient is more apt to experience *intraoperative* episodes of both marked hypertension and hypotension, myocardial ischemia, or arrhythmias. Intraoperative adjustments in anesthetic depth and use of vasoactive drugs should reduce the incidence of postoperative complications referable to poor control of hypertension preoperatively.

While patients should ideally undergo elective surgery only when rendered normotensive, this approach is not always feasible. Moreover, the decision whether to delay or to proceed with surgery should be individu-

Table 20–2. Oral antihypertensive agents.

Diuretics	
Thiazide type	Hydrochlorothiazide
	Chlorthalidone
Potassium-sparing	Spironolactone
	Triamterine
	Amiloride
Sympatholytics	
Adrenergic receptor blockers	
Beta receptors	Propranolol
	Metoprolol
	Nadolol
	Atenolol
	Timolol
	Acebutolol
	Pindolol
	Carteolol
	Penbutolol
	Betaxolol
Alpha$_1$ receptors	Prazosin
	Doxazocin
	Terazosin
Alpha$_1$ and α_2 receptor	Phenoxybenzamine
Alpha and β receptor	Labetalol
Centrally acting agents	
Alpha$_2$ agonists	Methyldopa
	Clonidine
	Guanabenz
	Guanfacine
	Guanethidine
Postganglionic blocking agents	Guanadrel
	Reserpine
Calcium channel blocking agents	Verapamil
	Nifedipine
	Diltiazem
	Nicardipine
ACE inhibitors	Captopril
	Enalapril
	Lisinopril
Direct vasodilators	Hydralazine
	Minoxidil

Table 20–3. Adverse effects of chronic antihypertensive agents.

Class	Adverse Effects
Diuretics	
Thiazide	Hypokalemia, hyponatremia, hyperglycemia, hyperlipidemia, hyperuricemia
Potassium-sparing	Hyperkalemia
Sympatholytics	
Beta-adrenergic blocking agents	Bradycardia, conduction blockade, myocardial depression, enhanced bronchial tone, sedation
Alpha-adrenergic blocking agents	Postural hypotension
Central α_2 agonists	Postural hypotension, sedation, decreased anesthetic requirements, bradycardia, rebound hypertension, positive Coombs test and hemolytic anemia (methyldopa), hepatitis (methyldopa)
Ganglionic blocking agents	Postural hypotension, diarrhea, salt and fluid retention, depression (reserpine)
Calcium channel blocking agents	Cardiac depression, bradycardia, conduction blockade (verapamil, diltiazem), peripheral edema (nifedipine), enhanced neuromuscular nondepolarizing blockade
Vasodilators	Postural hypotension, reflex tachycardia, fluid retention, systemic lupus erythematosus-like syndrome (hydralazine), pleural or pericardial effusion (minoxidil)
ACE inhibitors	Postural hypotension, renal dysfunction, hyperkalemia, bone marrow depression

alized, based on (1) the severity of the preoperative blood pressure elevation; (2) the likelihood of coexisting myocardial ischemia, ventricular dysfunction, or cerebrovascular or renal complications; and (3) the surgical procedure (whether major surgically induced changes in cardiac preload or afterload are anticipated). In many instances, preoperative hypertension is due to the patient's noncompliance with the drug regimen. With rare exceptions, antihypertensive drug therapy should be continued up to the time of surgery. Surgical procedures on patients with sustained preoperative diastolic blood pressures higher than 110 mm Hg—especially those with evidence of end organ damage—should be delayed until blood pressure is better controlled over the course of several days.

Preoperative Evaluation

A. History: The preoperative history should inquire into the severity and duration of the hypertension, what drug therapy is currently being prescribed, and the presence or absence of hypertensive complications. Symptoms of myocardial ischemia, ventricular

failure, impaired cerebral perfusion, or peripheral vascular disease should be elicited, as well as compliance with the drug regimen. Questions should deal with chest pains, exercise tolerance, shortness of breath (especially at night), dependent edema, postural lightheadedness, syncope, amaurosis, and claudication. Adverse effects of current antihypertensive drug therapy (Table 20–3) should also be identified. Evaluating a history of a previous myocardial infarction or stroke is dealt with below and in Chapter 27, respectively.

B. Physical Examination and Laboratory Evaluation: Ophthalmoscopy is probably the most useful examination in hypertensive patients (other than sphygmomanometry), but unfortunately it is usually not done. Visible changes in the retinal vasculature usually parallel the severity and progression of arteriosclerosis and hypertensive damage in other organs. Other physical findings such as pulmonary rales, a cardiac gallop, or carotid bruit are late findings. Blood pressure should be measured both in the supine and standing positions. Orthostatic changes can be due to volume depletion (Chapter 29), excessive vasodilatation, or sympatholytic drug therapy; preoperative fluid administration can prevent severe hypotension after induction of anesthesia in these patients. Asymptomatic carotid bruits are generally hemodynamically insignificant (Chapter 27).

The ECG is often normal but in patients with a long history of hypertension often shows evidence of ischemia, conduction abnormalities, an old infarction, or left ventricular hypertrophy or strain. A normal ECG does not necessarily exclude coronary artery disease (see below). Similarly, a normal heart size on a chest x-ray does not necessarily exclude ventricular hypertrophy. Positive x-ray findings include a boot-shaped heart, frank cardiomegaly, or pulmonary vascular congestion. Echocardiography is a more sensitive test of cardiac hypertrophy.

Renal function is best evaluated by measurement of serum creatinine and blood urea nitrogen levels (Chapter 32). Serum electrolyte levels should be determined in patients taking diuretics or digoxin or those with renal impairment. Mild to moderate hypokalemia is often seen in patients taking diuretics (3–3.5 meq/L) but usually does not appear to adversely affect outcome. Potassium replacement should probably be undertaken only in symptomatic patients and those who are also taking digoxin (Chapter 28). Hyperkalemia may be encountered in patients taking potassium-sparing diuretics—especially those with impaired renal function (Chapter 29).

Premedication

Premedication reduces preoperative anxiety and is highly desirable in hypertensive patients. Mild to moderate preoperative hypertension often resolves following administration of an anxiolytic agent such as midazolam. Preoperative antihypertensive agents should be continued as close to schedule as possible and can be given with a small sip of water. Central α_2-adrenergic agonists appear to be useful adjuncts for premedicating hypertensive patients. Clonidine, 0.2–0.3 mg, not only augments sedation and decreases the intraoperative anesthetic requirement but also results in greater intra- and postoperative hemodynamic stability. On rare occasions, preoperative clonidine administration has resulted in profound hypotension and bradycardia intraoperatively.

INTRAOPERATIVE MANAGEMENT

Objectives

The overall anesthetic plan for a hypertensive patient is to maintain a stable blood pressure range appropriate for that patient. Patients with labile hypertension or a recent onset of mild hypertension may be treated as normotensive patients. However, those with long-standing or poorly controlled hypertension have altered autoregulation of cerebral blood flow (Chapter 25). Higher than normal mean blood pressures may be required to maintain adequate cerebral blood flow. Because most patients with long-standing hypertension must be assumed to have some element of coronary artery disease and cardiac hypertrophy, excessive blood pressure elevations are also undesirable. Hypertension, especially in association with tachycardia, can precipitate or exacerbate myocardial ischemia, ventricular dysfunction, or both. Arterial blood pressure should generally be kept within 10–20% of preoperative levels. If marked hypertension (> 180/120 mm Hg) is present preoperatively, arterial blood pressure should be maintained in the high normal range (150–140/90–80 mm Hg).

Monitoring

Most hypertensive patients do not require special intraoperative monitors. Direct intra-arterial pressure monitoring should be reserved for patients with wide swings in blood pressure and for those undergoing major surgical procedures associated with rapid or marked changes in cardiac preload or afterload. Electrocardiographic monitoring should focus on detecting signs of ischemia (see below). Urinary output should generally be closely monitored with an indwelling urinary catheter in patients with renal impairment undergoing procedures expected to last more than 2 hours. When invasive hemodynamic monitoring is employed, reduced ventricular compliance (Chapter 19) is often apparent in patients with ventricular hypertrophy; higher pulmonary capillary wedge pressures (12–18 mm Hg) may be required to maintain an adequate left ventricular end-diastolic volume and cardiac output.

Induction

Induction of anesthesia and endotracheal intubation is often a period of hemodynamic instability for hypertensive patients. Regardless of the level of preoperative blood pressure control, many patients with hypertension display an accentuated hypotensive response to induction of anesthesia, followed by an exaggerated hypertensive response to intubation. The hypotensive response at induction may reflect the additive circulatory depressant effects of anesthetic agents and antihypertensive agents (Table 20–3). Many if not most antihypertensive agents and general anesthetics are vasodilators, cardiac depressants, or both. Additionally, many hypertensive patients are volume-depleted preoperatively. Sympatholytic agents also attenuate the normal protective circulatory reflexes (Chapter 19), reducing sympathetic tone and enhancing vagal activity.

Up to 25% of patients are said to exhibit severe hypertension following endotracheal intubation. The duration of laryngoscopy, which bears some relationship to the degree of hypertension, should be as short as possible. Moreover, intubation should generally be performed under deep anesthesia, provided hypotension can be avoided. One of several techniques may be employed before intubation to attenuate the hypertensive response: (1) deepening anesthesia with a potent volatile agent for 10–15 minutes; (2) administering a bolus of a narcotic (fentanyl 2.5–5 μg/kg, alfentanil 15–25 μg/kg, or sufentanil 0.25–0.5 μg/kg); (3) administering lidocaine 1.5 mg/kg (intravenously or intratracheally); (4) β-adrenergic blockade with esmolol 0.3–1.5 mg/kg, propranolol 1–5 mg, or labetalol 10–50 mg; (5) giving nitroprusside 1–2 μg/kg; or (6) topical anesthesia of the airway (Chapter 5). Premedication with clonidine (see above) also appears to be effective in blunting the hypertensive response to intubation.

Choice of Anesthetic Agents

A. Induction Agents: The superiority of any one agent or technique over another has not been clearly established for hypertensive agents. Even following regional anesthesia, hypertensive patients frequently have more exaggerated reductions in blood pressure than normotensive ones. Barbiturates, benzodiazepines, propofol, and etomidate are equally safe for inducing general anesthesia in most hypertensive patients. Ketamine alone is contraindicated for elective procedures because its sympathetic stimulation can precipitate marked hypertension (Chapter 8).

B. Maintenance Agents: Anesthesia may be safely continued with volatile agents (alone or with nitrous oxide), a balanced technique (narcotic + nitrous oxide + muscle relaxant), high doses of opioids, or other totally intravenous techniques. Regardless of the primary maintenance technique, addition of a volatile agent generally allows satisfactory blood pressure control intraoperatively. The vasodilatation and relatively rapid, titratable, and reversible myocardial depression afforded by volatile agents allows titration of their effects against arterial blood pressure. Some clinicians feel that of the opioids, sufentanil may provide the greatest autonomic suppression and control over blood pressure.

C. Muscle Relaxants: With the possible exception of pancuronium, any muscle relaxant can be used routinely. Pancuronium-induced vagal blockade and neural release of catecholamines can exacerbate hypertension in poorly controlled patients. However, when pancuronium is given in small increments slowly, marked increases in heart rate or blood pressure are less likely. Moreover, pancuronium is useful in offsetting excessive vagal tone induced by opioids or surgical manipulations.

D. Vasopressors: Hypertensive patients may display an exaggerated response to both endogenous catecholamines (from intubation or surgical stimulation) and exogenously administered sympathetic agonists. If a vasopressor is necessary to treat excessive hypotension, a small dose of a direct-acting agent such as phenylephrine (25–50 μg) may be preferable to an indirect agent. Nonetheless, small doses of ephedrine (5–10 mg) may be more appropriate when vagal tone is high. Patients taking sympatholytics preoperatively may exhibit a decreased response to ephedrine.

Intraoperative Hypertension

Intraoperative hypertension not responding to an increase in anesthetic depth (especially with a volatile agent) can be treated with a variety of parenteral agents (Table 20–4). Readily reversible causes such as hypoxemia or hypercapnia should always be excluded before initiating antihypertensive therapy. Selection of a hypotensive agent depends on the severity, acuteness, and cause of hypertension, the baseline ventricular function, the heart rate, and the presence of bronchospastic pulmonary disease (Chapter 13). Nitroprusside remains the most rapid and effective agent for the intraoperative treatment of moderate to severe hypertension. Nitroglycerin is less effective but is also useful in treating or preventing myocardial ischemia. Beta-adrenergic blockade alone or as a supplement is a good choice for a patient with good ventricular function and an elevated heart rate but is contraindicated in the presence of bronchospastic disease. Hydralazine provides sustained blood pressure control but may be

Table 20–4. Parenteral agents for the acute treatment of hypertension.

Agent	Dosage Range	Onset	Duration
Nitroprusside	0.5–10 μg/kg/min	30–60 sec	1–5 min
Nitroglycerin	5–100 μg/min	1 min	3–5 min
Esmolol	0.5 mg/kg over 1 min; 50–300 μg/kg/min	1 min	12–20 min
Labetalol	5–20 mg	1–2 min	4–8 hr
Propranolol	1–3 mg	1–2 min	4–6 hr
Trimethaphan	3–4 mg/min	1–3 min	10–30 min
Phentolamine	2.5–5 mg	1–10 min	20–40 min
Diazoxide	1–3 mg/kg slowly	2–10 min	4–6 hr
Hydralazine	5–20 mg	5–20 min	4–8 hr
Nifedipine (sublingual)	10 mg	5–10 min	4 hr
Methyldopa	250–1000 mg	2–3 hr	6–12 hr

associated with reflex tachycardia. The latter is not seen with labetalol because of combined α- and β-adrenergic blockade.

POSTOPERATIVE MANAGEMENT

Postoperative hypertension (Chapter 47) is common and should be anticipated in patients who have poorly controlled hypertension. Close blood pressure monitoring should be continued in the recovery room as well as the early postoperative period. In addition to myocardial ischemia and congestive heart failure, marked sustained elevations in blood pressure can contribute to the formation of wound hematomas and the disruption of vascular suture lines.

Hypertension in the recovery period is often multifactorial and enhanced by respiratory abnormalities, pain, volume overload, or bladder distention (Chapter 47). Contributing causes should be corrected and parenteral antihypertensive agents given, if necessary. Sublingual nifedipine is a useful agent in controlling blood pressure in this setting, particularly if myocardial ischemia is suspected or bronchospasm is present. When the patient resumes oral intake, preoperative medications should be restarted.

ISCHEMIC HEART DISEASE

PREOPERATIVE CONSIDERATIONS

Myocardial ischemia is characterized by a metabolic oxygen demand that exceeds oxygen supply (Chapter 19). Ischemia can therefore result from a marked increase in myocardial metabolic demand, a reduction in myocardial oxygen delivery, or a combination of both. Common causes include severe hypertension or tachycardia (especially in the presence of ventricular hypertrophy); coronary arterial vasospasm or anatomic obstruction; severe hypotension, hypoxemia, or anemia; and severe aortic stenosis or regurgitation.

By far the most common cause of myocardial ischemia is atherosclerosis of the coronary arteries. Coronary artery disease is responsible for well over one-third of all deaths in Western societies and is a major cause of perioperative morbidity and mortality. The overall incidence of coronary artery disease in surgical patients is estimated to be between 5% and 10%. Major risk factors for coronary artery disease include hyperlipidemia, hypertension, diabetes, cigarette smoking, increasing age, male sex, and a positive family history. Other risk factors include obesity, a history of cerebrovascular or peripheral vascular disease, menopause, use of high-estrogen oral contraceptives (in women who smoke), a sedentary life-style, and perhaps a "coronary-prone" behavior pattern. By age 65, the incidence of coronary artery disease is close to 37% for men compared to 18% for women.

Coronary artery disease may be clinically manifested by symptoms of myocardial necrosis (infarction), ischemia (usually angina), arrhythmias (including sudden death), or ventricular dysfunction (congestive heart failure). When symptoms of congestive heart failure predominate, the term **"ischemic cardiomyopathy"** is often used. Three major clinical syndromes are generally recognized: myocardial infarction, unstable angina, and chronic stable angina.

Myocardial Infarction

Myocardial infarction is a serious complication of ischemic heart disease, with an overall mortality rate of 25%. Over half of deaths are estimated to occur within the first hour and are usually due to arrhythmias. With recent advances in interventional cardiology, the hospital mortality rate has been reduced to less than 10–15%. Pump (ventricular) failure is now the leading cause of death in hospitalized patients.

Most myocardial infarctions occur in patients with more than one severely narrowed coronary artery. A transmural infarction occurs in an area distal to a complete occlusion. The occlusion is nearly always due to thrombosis at a stenotic atheromatous plaque. Coronary emboli or severe spasm is less commonly the cause. The size and location of the infarct depend on the distribution of the obstructed vessel and whether collateral vessels have formed. Anterior, apical, and septal infarcts of the left ventricle are usually due to thrombosis in the left anterior descending circulation; lateral and posterior left ventricular infarcts result from occlusions in the left circumflex system, while right ventricular and posterior-inferior left ventricular infarcts are from thrombosis in the right coronary artery. In contrast, subendocardial (nontransmural, or "non-Q wave") infarctions usually occur in the setting of a sustained and severe increased myocardial demand in patients with severe stenosis.

The prognosis following myocardial infarction is generally inversely proportionate to the extent of necrosis. As a result, the current emphasis in management of an evolving myocardial infarction is reperfusion. Thrombolytic therapy with streptokinase or tissue plasminogen activator is most successful within 1–3 hours after the onset of symptoms. Emergency percutaneous transluminal coronary angioplasty or even surgical coronary revascularization may also be performed at some centers for selected patients.

Unstable Angina

This clinical entity is defined as an abrupt increase in severity, frequency (more than three episodes per day) or duration of anginal attacks (crescendo angina), or new onset of angina (within the past 2 months) with minimal activity. Anginal episodes are usually not related to any apparent precipitating factors. The importance of this syndrome is that it usually reflects severe underlying coronary disease and frequently precedes myocardial infarction. Plaque disruption with platelet aggregates or thrombi and vasospasm are frequent pathologic correlates. Patients with unstable angina require admission to a coronary care unit for evaluation and treatment. Anticoagulation is often instituted, and if the ischemia does not resolve with additional medical therapy (see below), the patient is evaluated by coronary angiography for angioplasty or emergent surgical revascularization.

Chronic Stable Angina

Chest pains are most often substernal, exertional, radiate to the neck or arm, and are relieved by rest or nitroglycerin. Variations are common, including epigastric, back, or neck pain or transient shortness of breath due to ventricular dysfunction (anginal equivalent). Nonexertional ischemia and silent (asymptomatic) ischemia are being increasingly recognized as relatively common occurrences. Diabetics are known to have a relatively high incidence of silent ischemia.

Symptoms are generally absent until the atherosclerotic lesions cause 50–75% occlusions in the coronary circulation. When a stenotic segment reaches 70% occlusion, maximum compensatory dilatation is usually present distally: blood flow is usually adequate at rest but becomes inadequate with increased metabolic demand. Extensive collateral blood supply allows some patients to remain relatively asymptomatic in spite of severe disease. Coronary vasospasm is also well established as a cause of transient transmural ischemia in some patients. Ninety percent of vasospastic episodes occur at preexisting stenotic lesions in epicardial vessels. They are often precipitated by a variety of factors, including emotional upset and hyperventilation. Coronary spasm is most often observed in patients who have angina with varying levels of activity or with emotional stress (variable threshold); it is least common with classic exertional (fixed threshold) angina.

The overall prognosis of patients with coronary ar-

tery disease is related to both the number and severity of coronary obstructions as well as ventricular function.

Treatment of Ischemic Heart Disease

The general approach in treating patients with ischemic heart disease is fivefold: (1) correction of coronary risk factors in the hope of slowing disease progression; (2) modification of the patient's life-style so as to eliminate stress and improve exercise tolerance; (3) correction of complicating medical conditions that may exacerbate ischemia, such as anemia, hypoxemia, thyrotoxicosis, fever, infection, or adverse drug effects; (4) pharmacologic manipulation of the myocardial oxygen supply-demand relationship (Chapter 19); and (5) correction of coronary lesions by percutaneous balloon angioplasty or coronary artery bypass surgery. With the exception of the first two, these approaches are of direct relevance to anesthesiologists. The same principles should be applied in the care of these patients in both the operating room and the intensive care unit.

The most commonly used pharmacologic agents are nitrates, calcium channel blockers, and beta-blockers. These drugs also have potent circulatory effects, which are compared in Table 20–5. Any one agent may be employed for mild angina. Calcium channel blockers are the drugs of choice for patients with predominantly vasospastic angina, while β-adrenergic blocking agents are usually used in patients with exertional angina and good ventricular function. Nitrates are good agents for both types of angina.

A. Nitrates: Nitrates relax all vascular smooth muscle but have a much greater effect on venous than arterial vessels. By decreasing venous tone and reducing venous return to the heart (cardiac preload), wall tension and afterload are reduced. All these effects tend to reduce myocardial oxygen demand. The prominent venodilatation makes nitrates excellent agents when congestive heart failure is also present.

Table 20–5. A comparison of antianginal agents.

Effect	Nitrates	Calcium Channel Blockers			β-Blockers
		Verapamil	Nifedipine Nicardipine Nimodipine	Diltiazem	
Preload	↓↓	–	–	–	–/↑
Afterload	↓	↓	↓↓	↓	–
Contractility	–	↓↓	–	↓	↓↓↓
SA node automaticity	↑/–	↓↓	↑/–	↓↓	↓↓↓
AV conduction	–	↓↓↓	–	↓↓	↓↓↓
Vasodilatation Coronary Systemic	↑ ↑↑	↑↑ ↑	↑↑↑ ↑↑	↑↑ ↑	–/↓ –/↓

Key:
↑ = Increases
– = No change
↓ = Decreases

Perhaps equally as important, nitrates dilate the coronary arteries. Even minor degrees of dilatation at stenotic sites may be sufficient to increase blood flow, because flow is inversely related to the fourth power of the radius. Nitrate-induced coronary vasodilation preferentially increases subendocardial blood flow in ischemic areas. This favorable redistribution of coronary blood flow may be in part dependent on the presence of collaterals in the coronary circulation.

Nitrates can be used both for acute ischemia and for prophylaxis against frequent anginal episodes. In contrast to beta-blockers and calcium channel blockers, they do not have a negative inotropic effect—a desirable feature in the presence of ventricular dysfunction. Intravenous nitroglycerin can also be used for controlled hypotensive anesthesia (Chapter 13).

B. Calcium Channel Blockers: The effects of the most commonly used calcium channel blockers are compared in Tables 20–5 and 20–6. This group of agents reduces myocardial oxygen demand by decreasing cardiac afterload and augments oxygen supply by increasing blood flow (coronary vasodilation). Verapamil and diltiazem also reduce demand by slowing the heart rate.

Nifedipine's potent effects on the systemic blood pressure may precipitate hypotension, reflex tachycardia, or both. Its tendency to decrease afterload generally offsets any negative inotropic effect and makes it more suitable than other agents for patients with ventricular dysfunction. In contrast, verapamil and diltiazem have greater effects on cardiac contractility and AV conduction and are therefore contraindicated in patients with ventricular dysfunction, conduction abnormalities, or bradyarrhythmias. Nicardipine and nimodipine generally have the same effects as nifedipine. Nimodipine is also efficacious in preventing cerebral vasospasm following subarachnoid hemorrhage. The latter is presently the only FDA-approved indication for nimodipine.

Calcium channel blockers can have important interactions with anesthetic agents. All agents appear to potentiate both depolarizing and nondepolarizing neuromuscular blockers as well as the circulatory effects of volatile agents. Verapamil may also modestly decrease anesthetic requirements. Both verapamil and diltiazem especially potentiate depression of cardiac contractility and conduction in the AV node by volatile anesthetics. Nifedipine and similar agents especially potentiate systemic vasodilatation by volatile agents.

C. Beta-Adrenergic Blocking Agents: Beta-adrenergic blocking agents decrease myocardial oxygen demand by reducing heart rate and contractility and in some cases afterload (via their antihypertensive effect). Optimal blockade results in a resting heart rate between 50 and 60 beats/min and prevents appreciable increases with exercise (increase < 20 beats/min during exercise). Available agents differ in receptor selectivity, intrinsic sympathomimetic (partial agonist) activity, and membrane stabilizing properties (Table 20–7). The latter, which is often described as a quinidine-like effect (Chapter 19), results in antiarrhythmic activity. Agents with intrinsic sympathomimetic properties are better tolerated by patients with mild to moderate ventricular dysfunction. Nonselective β receptor blockade is contraindicated in patients with significant ventricular dysfunction, conduction abnormalities, or bronchospastic disease. Blockade of β_2-adrenergic receptors also can mask hypoglycemic symptoms in awake diabetic patients, delay metabolic recovery from hypoglycemia, and impair the handling of large potassium loads (Chapter 28). Nonselective blockers can also theoretically intensify coronary vasospasm in some patients and thus may be contraindicated in patients with predominantly vasospastic angina. Cardioselective (β_1 receptor-specific) agents must still be used cautiously in patients with reactive airways, since their selectivity tends to be dose-dependent. Acebutolol may be most useful in patients with bronchospastic airway disease, because it is has both β_1 selectivity and intrinsic sympathomimetic activity.

D. Combination Therapy: Moderate to severe angina frequently requires combination therapy with two or all three classes of agents. Patients with ventricular dysfunction may not tolerate the combined negative inotropic effect of a beta-blocker and a calcium channel blocker together. Similarly, their ad-

Table 20–6. Calcium channel blockers.

Agent	Route	Dosage[1]	Half-Life	Use			
				Angina	Hypertension	Cerebral Vasospasm	SVT
Verapamil	PO	40–240 mg	5 hr	+	+		+
	IV	5–15 mg prn	5 hr	+			+
Nifedipine	PO	30–180 mg	2 hr	+	+		
	SL	10 mg prn	2 hr	+	+		
Diltiazem	PO	30–60 mg	4 hr	+	+		
Nicardipine[2]	PO	60–120 mg	2–4 hr	+	+		
Nimodipine	PO	240 mg	2 hr			+	

[1]Total oral dose per day divided into three doses unless otherwise stated.
[2]Intravenous preparation pending FDA approval.

Table 20–7. A comparison of β-adrenergic blocking agents.

Agent	β₁-Receptor Selectivity	Half-Life	Sympathomimetic	α-Receptor Blockade	Membrane-Stabilizing
Acebutolol	+	2–4 hr	+		+
Atenolol	++	5–9 hr			
Betaxolol	++	14–22 hr			
Esmolol	++	9 min			
Metoprolol	++	3–4 hr			±
Oxprenolol		1–2 hr	+		+
Alprenolol		2–3 hr	+		+
Pindolol		3–4 hr	++		±
Penbutolol		5 hr	+		+
Carteolol		6 hr	+		
Labetalol		4–8 hr		+	±
Propranolol		3–6 hr			++
Timolol		3–5 hr			
Sotalol[1]		5–13 hr			
Nadolol		10–24 hr			

[1]Also possesses unique antiarrhythmic properties.

ditive effect on the AV node may precipitate heart block in susceptible patients. The combination of a long-acting nitrate and nifedipine is generally well tolerated by patients with significant ventricular dysfunction but may cause excessive vasodilation in some patients.

PREOPERATIVE MANAGEMENT

The importance of ischemic heart disease—especially a history of myocardial infarction—as a risk factor for perioperative morbidity and mortality has been discussed above. Numerous investigations have been done to delineate more specific relationships between preoperative electrocardiographic changes, angina, a history of myocardial infarction, angiographic evidence of coronary occlusions, previous coronary artery bypass surgery, and outcome. Most studies confirm that perioperative outcome is related to both disease severity and ventricular function. Patients with extensive (three-vessel or left main) disease, a history of myocardial infarction, or ventricular dysfunction are at greatest risk for cardiac complications. Chronic stable (mild to moderate) angina does not appear to substantially increase perioperative risk.

The most consistent finding relates to the incidence of perioperative myocardial infarction in patients with a previous myocardial infarction (Table 20–8). The risk is the same whether the infarct was transmural or subendocardial. Patients with myocardial infarction less than 6 months previously appear to be at greatest risk. Moreover, the mortality rates reported for such perioperative infarcts are usually over 50%. A history

of prior coronary artery bypass surgery does not appear to increase perioperative risk. More recent but controversial data suggest that the use of invasive hemodynamic monitoring and intraoperative interventions, such as vasodilators and beta-blockers, can substantially reduce the reinfarction rate in patients with a recent (< 6 months) myocardial infarction.

History

The history is of prime importance in patients with ischemic heart disease. Questions should encompass symptoms, current and past treatment, complications, and the results of previous evaluations. This information alone is usually enough to provide some estimate of disease severity and ventricular function.

The most important symptoms to elicit include chest pains, dyspnea, poor exercise tolerance, syncope, or near-syncope. The relationship between symptoms and activity level should be established. Activity should be described in terms of everyday tasks such as walking or climbing stairs. Patients with severe disease may be relatively asymptomatic because of a very sedentary life-style. Characterization of chest pains

Table 20–8. Risk of perioperative myocardial infarction in patients with coronary artery disease.

Patient Group	Infarction Rate
All surgical patients	0.2%
Prior MI (> 6 months previously)	6%
Recent MI (4–6 months previously)	15%
Recent MI (3 months previously)	30%
History of coronary artery bypass surgery	1.2%

may suggest a major role for vasospasm (variable threshold angina). Easy fatigability or shortness of breath suggests compromised ventricular function.

A history of unstable angina or myocardial infarction should establish the time of its occurrence and whether it was complicated by arrhythmias, conduction disturbances, or heart failure. Patients with prior anterior infarctions tend to have more severe disease than those with prior inferior infarctions. Localization of the areas of ischemia is invaluable in deciding which electrocardiographic leads should be monitored intraoperatively. Arrhythmias and conduction abnormalities are more common in patients with previous infarction and those with poor ventricular function.

Physical Examination
& Routine Laboratory Evaluation

Evaluation of patients with coronary artery disease is similar to patients with hypertension (see above); indeed, both diseases are often simultaneously present in the same patient. Laboratory evaluation should also include serum cardiac enzymes in patients who have a history compatible with recent unstable angina who are undergoing emergency procedures. Serum creatine kinase (MB isoenzyme) or lactate dehydrogenase (type 1 isoenzyme) levels are useful in excluding myocardial infarction. Serum digoxin and other antiarrhythmic levels may also be useful in excluding drug toxicity.

The baseline ECG is normal in 25–50% of patients with coronary artery disease but without prior myocardial infarction. Electrocardiographic evidence of ischemia often becomes apparent only during chest pain. The most common baseline abnormalities are nonspecific ST segment and T wave changes. Prior infarction more often than not is manifested by Q waves or loss of R waves in the leads closest to the infarct. First-degree atrioventricular block, bundle branch block, or hemiblock may be present. Persistent ST segment elevation following myocardial infarction is often indicative of a left ventricular aneurysm. A long rate-corrected QT interval ($QT_c > 0.44$ s) may reflect the underlying ischemia, drug toxicity (usually class Ia antiarrhythmic agents, antidepressants, or phenothiazines), electrolyte abnormalities (hypokalemia or hypomagnesemia), autonomic dysfunction, mitral valve prolapse, or, less commonly, a congenital abnormality. Patients with a long QT interval are at risk for developing ventricular arrhythmias—especially polymorphic ventricular tachycardia (torsade de pointes), which can lead to ventricular fibrillation. The long QT interval reflects nonuniform prolongation of ventricular repolarization and predisposes to reentry phenomena (Chapter 19). Elective surgery should be postponed until drug toxicity and electrolyte imbalance are excluded. In contrast to polymorphic ventricular arrhythmias with a normal QT interval, which respond to conventional antiarrhythmics (Chapters 19 and 46), polymorphic tachyarrhythmias with a long QT interval generally respond best to pacing or

magnesium. Patients with congenital prolongation generally respond to β-adrenergic blocking agents.

The chest x-ray is a useful screening test in excluding cardiomegaly or pulmonary vascular congestion secondary to ventricular dysfunction. Rarely, calcification of the coronaries or the aortic valve may be seen.

Holter Monitoring

Continuous ambulatory electrocardiographic (Holter) monitoring is useful in evaluating arrhythmias, antiarrhythmic drug therapy, and the severity and frequency of ischemic episodes. Type II atrioventricular block (see below) or complete heart block necessitates a permanent cardiac pacemaker. Antiarrhythmic therapy is generally indicated in patients with complex ventricular ectopy who have significant left ventricular dysfunction. This includes patients with frequent ($> 6/$min), R-on-T ectopic beats, as well as sustained or nonsustained episodes of ventricular tachycardia. Treatment of ventricular ectopy (with the exception of sustained ventricular tachycardia) in patients with good ventricular function is more controversial because it does not appear to affect survival. Silent (asymptomatic) ischemic episodes are frequent findings in patients with coronary artery disease. Moreover, the occurrence preoperatively of frequent ischemic episodes on Holter monitoring correlates well with intra- and postoperative ischemia.

Specialized Studies

When used as screening tests for the general population, all three currently used noninvasive stress tests (exercise electrocardiography, thallium imaging, and radionuclide angiography) have a low predictability in normal patients but are sufficiently reliable in patients with suspected coronary disease (Bayes theorem). Correct interpretation of these tests preoperatively is important, especially in patients suspected of having coronary artery disease.

A. Exercise Electrocardiography: The utility of this test is limited in patients with baseline ST segment abnormalities and those who are unable to increase their heart rate ($> 85\%$ of maximal predicted) due to fatigue, dyspnea, or drug therapy. Overall sensitivity is 65%, while specificity is 90%. The test is most sensitive (85%) in patients with three-vessel or left main coronary artery disease. A normal test does not necessarily exclude coronary artery disease but suggests that severe disease is not likely. The degree of ST segment depression, its severity and configuration, the time of onset in the test, and the time required for resolution are important findings. Other important findings include changes in blood pressure and the occurrence of arrhythmias. Exercise-induced ventricular ectopy is frequently associated with severe coronary artery disease associated with ventricular dysfunction. The ischemia presumably leads to electrical instability in myocardial cells. Factors associated with severe multivessel disease are listed in Table 20–9.

Table 20–9. Factors associated with severe multivessel disease during exercise electrocardiography.

1. More than 2 mm horizontal or down-sloping ST depression.
2. Persistence of ST depression after exercise for 5 minutes or longer
3. Sustained decrease ($\geq$ 15 mm Hg) in systolic blood pressure for 10 minutes or longer during exercise
4. Failure to reach a maximal heart rate greater than 70% of predicted
5. Frequent or complex ventricular dysrhythmias at a low heart rate

B. Thallium Imaging (Scintigraphy): Thallium studies following exercise or injection of dipyridamole (a coronary vasodilator) have a high sensitivity but only fairly good specificity for detecting coronary artery disease. They are best for detecting two- or three-vessel disease. These scans can locate and quantitate areas of ischemia or scarring and differentiate between the two. Perfusion defects that "fill in" on the redistribution phase represent ischemia, not previous infarction. A dipyridamole-thallium study may be useful in patients with poor conditioning or peripheral vascular disease because it obviates the need for exercise.

C. Radionuclide Angiography: Left ventricular ejection fraction (Chapter 19) and wall motion can be evaluated with this study both at rest and following exercise. When the ejection fraction fails to rise and new wall motion abnormalities are detected following exercise—ie, when both of those criteria are satisfied—this study has nearly 90% specificity and sensitivity for coronary artery disease. Patients with an ejection fraction less than 50% tend to have severe disease and have increased perioperative morbidity.

D. Two-Dimensional Echocardiography: This technique provides information about both regional and global ventricular function. Detectable regional wall motion abnormalities and the derived left ventricular ejection fraction have good correlation with angiographic findings.

E. Coronary Angiography: Coronary angiography remains the "gold standard" in evaluating coronary artery disease and is now associated with an acceptably low complication rate ($<$ 1%). Nonetheless, coronary angiography should be performed only to determine if the patient may benefit from percutaneous transluminal coronary angioplasty or coronary artery bypass grafting prior to noncardiac surgery. The location and severity of occlusions can be defined. Coronary vasospasm may also be observed on angiography. In evaluating fixed stenotic lesions, occlusions greater than 50–75% are generally considered significant. Estimates of percentage of occlusion can be misleading (especially between 40% and 80%) because of large observer variabilities and the assumption that occlusions are concentric when they are often eccentric. The severity of disease is often expressed according to the number of major coronary vessels affected (one-, two-, or three-vessel disease). Significant stenosis of the left main coronary artery is

ominous because it affects almost the entire left ventricle. Moreover, even 50–75% occlusions in the left main artery can be hemodynamically significant.

Ventriculography and measurement of intracardiac pressures also provide important information. The single most important measurement is the ejection fraction. Indicators of significant ventricular dysfunction include an ejection fraction less than 0.5, a left ventricular end-diastolic pressure greater than 18 mm Hg after injection of contrast, a cardiac index less than 2.2 L/min/m^2, and marked or multiple wall motion abnormalities.

Premedication

Allaying fear, anxiety, and pain preoperatively are desirable goals in patients with coronary artery disease. Satisfactory premedication prevents sympathetic activation, which adversely affects the myocardial oxygen supply-demand balance. However, overmedication is equally detrimental and to be avoided because it may result in hypoxemia, respiratory acidosis, and hypotension. A benzodiazepine, alone or in combination with a narcotic, is most commonly used (Chapter 8). Excellent results can also be obtained by a combination of morphine, 0.1–0.15 mg/kg, and scopolamine, 0.2–0.4 mg, intramuscularly. Patients with poor ventricular function and those with coexistent lung disease should receive reduced dosages. All preoperative medications should generally be continued up until the time of surgery. They may be given orally with a small sip of water, intramuscularly, intravenously, sublingually, or transdermally. Sudden withdrawal of antianginal medication perioperatively—especially beta-blockers—can precipitate a sudden increase in ischemic episodes (rebound). Moreover, prophylactic β-adrenergic blockade has been shown to reduce the incidence of intraoperative and postoperative ischemic episodes and appears to be superior to prophylaxis with a calcium channel blocker alone. Many clinicians prophylactically administer nitrates intravenously or transdermally to patients with coronary artery disease in the perioperative period. Although this practice may be theoretically advantageous, its efficacy in patients not previously on long-term nitrate therapy is not well established.

INTRAOPERATIVE MANAGEMENT

The perioperative period is regularly associated with factors and events that can adversely affect the myocardial oxygen demand and supply relationship (Table 20–10). Activation of the sympathetic system plays a major role. Hypertension and enhanced contractility increase myocardial oxygen demand, while tachycardia increases demand and reduces supply (Chapter 19). Although myocardial ischemia is most commonly associated with tachycardia, it may occur even in the absence of any apparent hemodynamic derangement. Sympathetic activation may also play a

Table 20–10. Perioperative factors adversely altering myocardial oxygen supply-demand balance.

Factor	Demand	Supply	Mechanism
Preoperative			
Anxiety	+	−	Sympathetic activation
Pain	+	−	Sympathetic activation
Intraoperative			
Induction agents	−	−	Cardiac depression with or without vasodilation
Intubation	+	−	Sympathetic activation
Maintenance agents	−	−	Cardiac depression with or without vasodilation
Surgical stimulation	+	−	Sympathetic activation
Blood loss	+	−	Sympathetic activation, hypotension
Extubation	+	−	Sympathetic activation
Postoperative			
Pain	+	−	Sympathetic activation
Shivering	+	−	Sympathetic activation, increased preload, marked increase in cardiac output
Complications			
Hypoxemia	+	−	Sympathetic activation, reduced oxygen content
Hypercapnia	+	−	Sympathetic activation
Hypocapnia		−	Possible coronary vasospasm
Acidosis	+	−	Sympathetic activation
Anemia	+	−	Sympathetic activation, reduced oxygen content
Hypovolemia	+	−	Sympathetic activation, hypotension
Fluid overload		−	Sympathetic activation, increased preload

Key:
+ = Increased
− = Decreased

role in precipitating coronary vasospasm in some patients.

Objectives

The overwhelming priority in managing patients with ischemic heart disease is maintaining a favorable myocardial supply-demand relationship. Autonomic-mediated increases in heart rate and blood pressure should be controlled by deep anesthesia or adrenergic blockade, while excessive reductions in coronary perfusion pressure (Chapter 19) or arterial oxygen content are to be avoided. Although exact limits are not predictable, diastolic arterial pressure should generally be maintained at 60 mm Hg or above. Higher diastolic pressures may be preferable in patients with high-grade coronary occlusions. Excessive increases—such as those due to fluid overload—in left ventricular end-diastolic pressure should be avoided because they increase ventricular wall tension (afterload) and can reduce subendocardial perfusion (Chapter 19). Lastly, adequate blood hemoglobin concentrations (> 9–10 mg/dL) and arterial oxygen tensions (> 60 mm Hg) should be maintained.

Monitoring

Intra-arterial pressure monitoring is advisable for all patients with severe coronary artery disease and those with major or multiple cardiac risk factors (Table 20–1). Central venous pressure or pulmonary artery pressure monitoring should be used during prolonged or complicated procedures involving large fluid shifts or blood loss (Chapter 6). Pulmonary artery pressure monitoring is highly desirable for patients with signifi-

cant ventricular dysfunction (ejection fraction < 40–50%). Two-dimensional transesophageal echocardiography (TEE) also provides valuable information, both qualitative and quantitative, on contractility and ventricular chamber size (preload) as well as estimates of cardiac output.

Detection of ischemia intraoperatively is dependent on recognition of electrocardiographic changes, hemodynamic manifestations, or regional wall motion abnormalities on TEE. Doppler TEE also allows detection of the onset of mitral regurgitation due to ischemic papillary muscle dysfunction.

A. Electrocardiography: Early ischemic changes are subtle and can often be overlooked. They involve changes in T wave morphology, including inversion, tenting, or both (Figure 20–1). More obvious ischemia may be seen in the form of progressive ST segment depression. Down-sloping and horizontal ST depression are of greater specificity for ischemia than up-sloping depression. New ST segment elevations are rare during noncardiac surgery and are indicative of severe ischemia, vasospasm, or infarction. Ischemia may also present as an unexplained intraoperative atrial or ventricular arrhythmia or the onset of a new conduction abnormality. The sensitivity of the ECG in detecting ischemia is related to the number of leads monitored. Ideally, at least two leads should be monitored simultaneously. Usually, lead II is monitored for inferior wall ischemia and arrhythmias and V_5 for anterior wall ischemia. An esophageal lead may also be useful in patients with posterior wall ischemia. When only one channel can be monitored, a modified V_5 lead provides the highest sensitivity (Chapter 6).

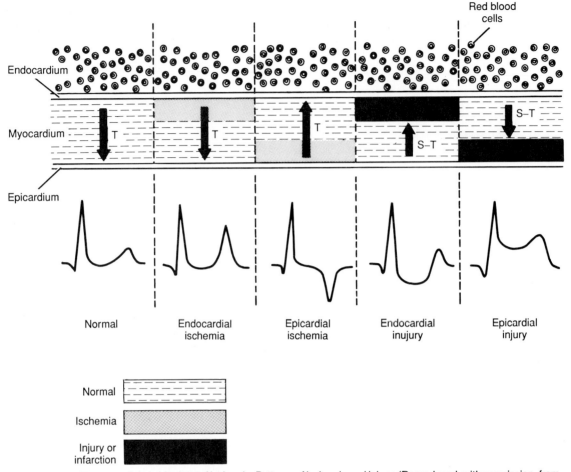

Endocardium

Myocardium

Epicardium

Red blood cells

Normal

Endocardial ischemia

Epicardial ischemia

Endocardial inujury

Epicardial injury

Normal

Ischemia

Injury or infarction

Figure 20–1. Electrocardiographic signs of ischemia. Patterns of ischemia and injury. (Reproduced, with permission, from Schamroth L: *The 12 Lead Electrocardiogram.* Blackwell, 1989.)

B. Hemodynamic Monitoring: The most common hemodynamic abnormalities observed during ischemic episodes are hypertension and tachycardia. They are nearly always the cause rather than the result of ischemia. Hypotension is a late and ominous manifestation. The most sensitive hemodynamic correlates are derived from pulmonary artery pressure monitoring. Ischemia is frequently but not always associated with an abrupt increase in pulmonary capillary wedge pressure. The sudden appearance of a *v* wave on the wedge waveform is usually indicative of acute mitral regurgitation due to ischemic papillary muscle dysfunction or acute left ventricular dilatation.

C. Two-Dimensional Transesophageal Echocardiography: Two-dimensional transesophageal echocardiography can be valuable in detecting new regional wall motion abnormalities. Some studies suggest that detection of a new abnormality is a rapid and more sensitive indicator of myocardial ischemia than electrocardiographic changes. Although the occurrence of new intraoperative abnormalities correlates with postoperative myocardial infarctions in some studies, not all such abnormalities are necessarily is-

chemic. Both regional and global abnormalities can be caused by changes in heart rate, preload, afterload, or drug-induced changes in contractility. Moreover, TEE requires expensive equipment and considerable familiarity with the technique for correct rapid interpretations intraoperatively.

Choice of Anesthesia

A. Regional Anesthesia: Although studies documenting the superiority of regional over general anesthesia are lacking, the former is often a good choice for procedures involving the extremities, the perineum, and possibly the lower abdomen. Precipitous drops in blood pressure following spinal or epidural anesthesia should be rapidly treated with small doses (25–50 μg) of phenylephrine to preserve coronary perfusion pressure until sufficient intravenous fluid can be given. Small doses of ephedrine (5–10 mg) may be preferable in the presence of bradycardia. Marked hypotension can usually be avoided by prior volume loading (Chapter 16). Patients with compensated congestive heart failure usually tolerate the sympathectomy surprising well and may not need preoperative volume loading.

Patchy or incomplete surgical anesthesia or excessive sedation during regional anesthesia defeats the purpose of selecting a regional technique, unnecessarily stresses the patient, and may precipitate myocardial ischemia. Conversion of the regional anesthetic to a general anesthetic is appropriate in such instances and corrects the often associated hypertension, tachycardia, hypoxia, or hypercapnia.

B. General Anesthesia:

1. Induction–The same general principles described for patients with hypertension apply to most patients with ischemic heart disease. Many if not most patients with coronary artery disease have hypertension. The induction technique for patients with moderate to severe coronary artery disease (three-vessel disease, left main disease, or ejection fractions < 50%) requires some modification. The induction should have minimal hemodynamic effects, produce reliable loss of consciousness, and provide sufficient depth of anesthesia to prevent a vasopressor response to intubation (if intubation is required). Regardless of the agent employed, these objectives are most consistently achieved by a slow controlled technique. Induction with small incremental doses of the selected agent usually avoids the precipitous drops in blood pressure that can be seen following a large bolus. Titration of the induction agent—first against loss of consciousness and then to an acceptable decrease in blood pressure—allows for variations in responses between individuals. Moreover, sufficient anesthetic depth for endotracheal intubation can be achieved with less cardiovascular depression than the bolus technique. Administration of a muscle relaxant as soon as the eyelid reflex is lost and controlled ventilation assure generally adequate oxygenation throughout induction. Endotracheal intubation is performed once sufficient anesthetic depth is reached or arterial blood pressure reaches its lowest acceptable limit. Blood pressure, heart rate, and the ECG should be repeatedly assessed with each step during induction.

2. Choice of agents–

a. Induction agents–Selection of a specific agent is not critical in most patients. Barbiturates, etomidate, propofol, benzodiazepines, opioids, and various combinations of these drugs are often used. Ketamine by itself is relatively contraindicated because of its indirect sympathomimetic effects, which can adversely affect the myocardial oxygen demand-supply balance. However, when combined with a benzodiazepine, ketamine does not appreciably increase sympathetic activity and results in relatively stable hemodynamics with minimal myocardial depression. This combination may be most useful in patients with poor ventricular function.

High-dose opioid anesthesia is widely advocated for patients with significant ventricular dysfunction. With the exception of meperidine, opioids alone are associated with minimal or no cardiac depression. In contrast, when they are combined with other intravenous agents (particularly benzodiazepines), significant cardiac depression may result. Apparent cardiac depres-

sion may also occur with "pure" high-dose opioid inductions (Chapter 21), but this more likely represents withdrawal of an elevated baseline sympathetic tone; patients with poor ventricular function often rely on an elevated sympathetic tone to maintain their cardiac output (Chapter 19). Unfortunately, when opioids are used as sole agents, they may not be complete anesthetics because of an unacceptably high incidence of intraoperative awareness (recall) and hypertension (Chapter 21). Moreover, the prolonged respiratory depression following this technique is unsuitable for most noncardiac operations.

Control of the adrenergic response to endotracheal intubation has been discussed in the section on hypertension.

b. Maintenance agents–Patients with good ventricular function are generally managed with volatile agents, while those with depressed ventricular function are usually managed with an opioid-based anesthetic. Those with ejection fractions less than 40–50% are often very sensitive to the depressant effects of the potent volatile agents. Nitrous oxide, especially in the presence of narcotics, can also produce significant cardiac depression.

The effects of each of the three potent volatile agents on the coronary circulation are summarized in Table 20–11. All three have a favorable effect on myocardial oxygen balance, reducing demand more than supply. Isoflurane is the most potent coronary vasodilator. In contrast to the other two agents, isoflurane dilates intramyocardial arteries more than the larger epicardial vessels. This pattern can result in loss of myocardial autoregulation. Some laboratory data and a few clinical reports suggest that isoflurane under certain conditions can cause an intracoronary steal phenomenon that may exacerbate ischemia. Intracoronary steal can occur in an area distal to a high-grade epicardial stenosis which is dependent on nearby collaterals—since vessels supplying the ischemic area are normally maximally dilated, dilatation of intramyocardial vessels in the surrounding normal tissue diverts collateral blood flow away from the ischemic area. In spite of these observations, the clinical significance of these data is highly controversial, and isoflurane remains the most commonly used volatile agent for patients with coronary artery disease.

Detection of intraoperative ischemia should prompt a search for precipitating factors and interventions to

Table 20–11. Effects of the potent volatile agents on the coronary circulation.

Agent	Coronary Dilatation	Coronary Blood Flow	Myocardial Oxygen Demand
Halothane	↑	↓	↓↓
Enflurane	↑↑	↓	↓↓
Isoflurane	↑↑↑	0	↓

Key:
↑ = Increased
↓ = Decreased
0 = No effect

correct it. Oxygenation should be checked and hemodynamic abnormalities (hypotension, hypertension, or tachycardia) corrected. Failure to identify a cause or to reverse the ischemic manifestations may be an indication for starting intravenous nitroglycerin. The latter optimally requires insertion of an arterial line and in some patients (those with moderate to severe ventricular impairment) a pulmonary artery catheter.

c. Muscle relaxants—Lack of significant circulatory side effects generally makes vecuronium, pipecuronium, and doxacurium nearly ideal muscle relaxants for patients with ischemic heart disease. Severe bradycardia has been reported with vecuronium on rare occasions but in nearly all instances has been associated with concomitant administration of a narcotic. Atracurium in doses less than 0.4 mg/kg given slowly also generally has minimal hemodynamic effects. The circulatory effects of succinylcholine are primarily due to stimulation of autonomic ganglia and cardiac muscarinic receptors and can result in variable effects on heart rate and blood pressure (Chapter 9). Its net effect is influenced by preexisting relative sympathetic and parasympathetic tone, premedication with an anticholinergic, and β-adrenergic blockade. Bradycardia may be seen following succinylcholine in patients taking β-adrenergic blocking agents.

When used properly, other muscle relaxants (Chapter 9) can also be safely administered to patients with coronary artery disease. Moreover, their circulatory side effects can be used to balance the side effects of other anesthetic agents—eg, the vagolytic properties of pancuronium can counteract the vagotonic effects of potent narcotics (Chapter 8). The combination of pancuronium with metocurine also results in good hemodynamic stability.

Reversal of muscle paralysis with standard agents does not appear to have any detrimental effects in patients with coronary artery disease. Use of glycopyrrolate instead of atropine may lessen the likelihood of transient tachycardia (Chapter 10).

POSTOPERATIVE MANAGEMENT

Recovery from anesthesia and the immediate postoperative period can continue to stress the myocardium (Table 20–10). The patient should receive supplemental oxygen until adequate oxygenation is established. Shivering often resolves following administration of meperidine, 20–30 mg intravenously, or butorphanol, 1–2 mg intravenously. Postoperative pain should be controlled with generous analgesics or a regional anesthetic technique (Chapter 18). If there is a suspicion of fluid overload or the patient has a history of poor ventricular function, a postoperative chest x-ray is useful. Pulmonary congestion can be rapidly treated with furosemide, 20–40 mg intravenously, or intravenous vasodilator therapy (usually nitroglycerin).

The greatest risk to these patients postoperatively is unrecognized ischemia. The overwhelming majority of perioperative myocardial infarctions occur within the first 3 days following surgery (most commonly after 24–48 hours). The most common presentation is unexplained hypotension. Less than half of patients have chest pain. Other presentations of postoperative myocardial infarction include congestive heart failure, altered mental status, and asymptomatic electrocardiographic findings. Nearly all patients experiencing this complication are over 50 years of age. The diagnosis is usually based on electrocardiographic findings and cardiac enzyme or, less commonly, radionuclide studies.

VALVULAR HEART DISEASE

GENERAL EVALUATION OF PATIENTS WITH VALVULAR HEART DISEASE

Regardless of the lesion or its cause, preoperative evaluation should be primarily concerned with determining the severity of the lesion, its hemodynamic significance, residual ventricular function, and the presence of secondary effects on pulmonary, renal, and hepatic function. Concomitant coronary artery disease should not be overlooked, especially in older patients and those with known risk factors (see above). Myocardial ischemia may also occur in the absence of significant coronary occlusion in patients with severe aortic stenosis or regurgitation.

History

The preanesthetic history should focus on symptoms related to ventricular function and should be correlated with laboratory data. Questions should concern exercise tolerance, fatigability, and pedal edema and shortness of breath—in general (dyspnea), when lying flat (orthopnea), or at night (paroxysmal nocturnal dyspnea). The New York Heart Association functional classification (Table 20–12) is useful for grading the clinical severity of heart failure, comparing patients, and estimating prognosis. Patients should also be questioned about chest pains and neurologic symptoms. Some valvular lesions are associated with thromboembolic phenomena. Prior procedures such as valvulotomy or valve replacement and their effects should also be well documented.

A review of medications should evaluate their efficacy and exclude serious side effects. Commonly used agents include digoxin, diuretics, vasodilators, antiarrhythmics, and anticoagulants. Digoxin is generally most effective for controlling the ventricular rate in patients with atrial fibrillation. The ventricular rate should be less than 80–90 beats/min at rest and should not exceed 120 beats/min with stress or exercise. Signs of digoxin toxicity are primarily cardiac (ar-

Table 20–12. Functional classification of heart disease. (New York Heart Association, 1964.)

Class	Description
I	Asymptomatic
II	Symptoms with moderate activity
III	Symptoms with minimal activity
IV	Symptoms at rest

rhythmias), gastrointestinal (nausea or vomiting), neurologic (confusion), or visual (altered color perception or scotomas). Arrhythmias due to digoxin arise from a combination of enhanced automaticity and decreased conduction in specialized cells in the atria, ventricles, and AV and SA nodes. Preoperative vasodilator therapy may be used to decrease preload or afterload (or both). Excessive vasodilation worsens exercise tolerance and is often first manifested as postural hypotension.

Physical Examination

The most important signs to search for on physical examination are those of congestive heart failure. Left-sided (S_3 gallop or pulmonary rales) as well as right-sided signs (jugular venous distention, hepatojugular reflux, hepatosplenomegaly, or dependent pedal edema) may be present. Auscultatory findings also serve to confirm the valvular dysfunction (Table 20–13), but echocardiographic studies are generally more reliable. Neurologic deficits, which are usually secondary to embolic phenomena, should be documented.

Laboratory Evaluation

In addition to the laboratory studies discussed for patients with hypertension and coronary artery disease, liver function tests (Chapter 34) are useful in patients with severe or chronic right-sided failure to assess hepatic dysfunction secondary to passive hepatic congestion. Arterial blood gases should be measured in patients with significant pulmonary symptoms. Reversal of anticoagulants should be documented with a prothrombin time and partial thromboplastin time prior to surgery.

Electrocardiographic findings are generally nonspecific. They may include T wave or ST segment changes, arrhythmias, conduction abnormalities, or QRS axis deviation reflecting ventricular hypertrophy. A prolonged PR interval may suggest digoxin toxicity. Arrhythmias associated with digoxin toxicity include (in order of decreasing frequency) ventricular ectopy, paroxysmal atrial tachycardia with 2:1 AV block, AV block alone, marked sinus bradycardia, low atrial or AV junctional rhythms, and AV dissociation.

Table 20–13. Effect of diagnostic maneuvers on heart murmurs. (Variable effects have been omitted.)

I. SYSTOLIC MURMURS

Maneuver	PS	TR	HCM	MVP	MR	VSD	AS
Inspiration	↑	↑					
Valsalva	↑		↑	↑			↓
Standing			↑	↑	↓		
Squatting or handgrip			↓	↓	↑	↑	↓
Leg elevation		↑	↓	↓			↑
Transient arterial occlusion					↑	↑	
Amyl nitrite inhalation	↑	↑	↑	↑	↓	↓	↑

II. DIASTOLIC MURMURS

Maneuver	PR	TS	AR	MS
Inspiration	↑	↑		
Valsalva	↑			↓
Squatting or handgrip			↑	↑
Leg elevation		↑		
Transient arterial occlusion			↑	
Amyl nitrite inhalation	↑	↑	↓	↑

Key:
↑ = Increases
↓ = Decreases

Legend:
AR = Aortic regurgitation
AS = Aortic stenosis
HCM = Hypertrophic cardiomyopathy
MR = Mitral regurgitation
MS = Mitral stenosis
MVP = Mitral valve prolapse
PR = Pulmonary regurgitation
PS = Pulmonary stenosis
TR = Tricuspid regurgitation
TS = Tricuspid stenosis
VSD = Ventricular septal defect

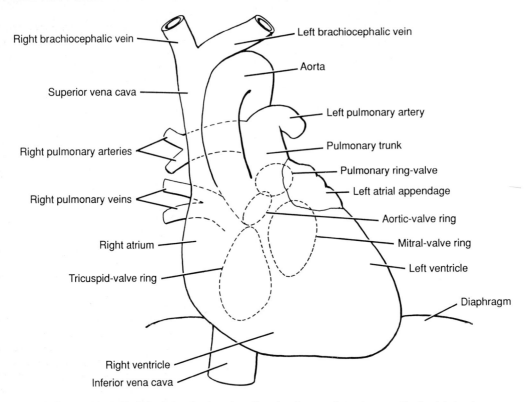

Right brachiocephalic vein

Superior vena cava

Right pulmonary arteries

Right pulmonary veins

Right atrium

Tricuspid-valve ring

Right ventricle

Inferior vena cava

Left brachiocephalic vein

Aorta

Left pulmonary artery

Pulmonary trunk

Pulmonary ring-valve

Left atrial appendage

Aortic-valve ring

Mitral-valve ring

Left ventricle

Diaphragm

Figure 20–2. Radiologic localization of cardiac chambers and structures on the frontal chest x-ray.

The chest x-ray is invaluable in assessing cardiac size and pulmonary vascular congestion. Specific cardiac chamber enlargement may be apparent (Figure 20–2).

Special Studies

Echocardiography, radionuclide angiography, and cardiac catheterization provide important diagnostic and prognostic information about valvular lesions. In many instances, noninvasive studies obviate the need for cardiac catheterization. Information from these studies is best reviewed with a cardiologist. More than one valvular lesion is often found. The following questions must be answered:

(1) Which valvular abnormality is most important hemodynamically?

(2) What is the severity of that lesion?

(3) What degree of ventricular impairment is present?

(4) What is the hemodynamic significance of other identified abnormalities?

(5) Is there any evidence of coronary artery disease?

PREMEDICATION

Premedication with standard dosages of any of the commonly used agents (Chapter 8) is desirable and well tolerated in patients with normal or near-normal ventricular function. In contrast, patients with poor ventricular function tend to be very sensitive to most agents. Premedication dosages should be reduced in proportion to the severity of ventricular impairment. Patients should generally receive their usual medications on the morning of surgery. Supplemental oxygen may be desirable in patients with pulmonary hypertension or underlying pulmonary disease.

ANTIBIOTIC PROPHYLAXIS

The risk of infective endocarditis in patients with valvular heart disease following bacteremic events— including dental, oro- or nasopharyngeal, gastrointestinal, or genitourinary surgery—is well established. Prophylaxis is best accomplished according to the general guidelines of the American Heart Association recommendations (Table 20–14).

SPECIFIC VALVULAR DISORDERS

1. MITRAL STENOSIS

Preoperative Considerations

Mitral stenosis nearly always occurs as a delayed complication of acute rheumatic fever. The stenotic

Table 20–14. Antibiotic prophylaxis against endocarditis.[1] (American Heart Association, 1984.)

I. Dental, oral, nasal, pharyngeal or upper airway procedures
  A. Standard regimen:
    1. Adults:
      a. Penicillin V, 2 g PO 1 hour before and 1 g 6 hours after; or–
      b. Penicillin G, 2 million units IV or IM 0.5 hour before and 1 million units 6 hours after.
    2. Children < 60 lb:
      a. Penicillin V, 1 g PO 1 hour before and 500 mg 6 hours after; or–
      b. Penicillin G, 50,000 units/kg IV or IM 0.5–1 hour before and 25,000 units/kg IV or IM 6 hours after.
  B. Penicillin allergy:
    1. Adults: Erythromycin, 1 g PO 1 hour before and 500 mg 6 hours after.
    2. Children < 60 lb: Erythromycin, 20 mg/kg PO 1 hour before and 10 mg/kg 6 hours after.
  C. High-risk patients:[2]
    1. Adults:
      a. Ampicillin, 2 g IM or IV, plus gentamicin, 1.5 mg/kg IM or IV, 0.5 hour before, and penicillin, 1 g PO 6 hours after; or–
      b. The same combination once 8 hours after.
    2. Children < 60 lb:
      a. Ampicillin, 50 mg/kg IM or IV, plus gentamicin, 2 mg/kg IM or IV, 0.5 hour before, and penicillin, 500 mg PO 6 hours after; or–
      b. The same combination once 8 hours after.
  D. High-risk patients[2] with penicillin allergy:
    1. Adults: Vancomycin, 1 g slowly IV 1 hour before.
    2. Children < 60 lb: Vancomycin, 20 mg/kg slowly IV 1 hour before

II. Genitourinary or gastrointestinal procedures
  A. Standard regimen (high-risk procedures):[2]
    1. Adults: Ampicillin, 2 g IM or IV, plus gentamicin, 1.5 mg/kg IM or IV, 1 hour before, and the same combination once again 8 hours after.
    2. Children < 60 lb: Ampicillin, 50 mg/kg IM or IV, plus gentamicin, 2 mg/kg IM or IV, 1 hour before, and the same combination once again 8 hours after.
  B. Alternative regimen (low-risk procedures):
    1. Adults: Amoxicillin, 3 g PO 1 hour before and 1.5 g 6 hours after.
    2. Children < 60 lb: Amoxicillin, 50 mg/kg PO 1 h before and 25 mg/kg PO 6 hours after.
  C. Penicillin allergy:
    1. Adults: Vancomycin, 1 g slowly IV, plus gentamicin, 1.5 mg/kg IM or IV, 1 hour before, and the same combination 8–12 hours after.
    2. Children < 60 lb: Vancomycin, 20 mg/kg slowly IV, plus gentamicin, 2 mg/kg IM or IV, 1 hour before, and the same combination 8 hours after.

[1]Repeat doses must be modified in the presence of renal impairment.
[2]High risk = prosthetic valve or prior endocarditis.

process is estimated to begin after a minimum of 2 years following the acute disease and results from progressive fusion and calcification of the valve leaflets. Symptoms generally develop after 20–30 years, when the mitral valve orifice is reduced from its normal 4–6 cm^2 opening to less than 2 cm^2.

Pathophysiology

Significant restriction of blood flow through the mitral valve results in a transvalvular pressure gradient that depends on (1) cardiac output, (2) heart rate (diastolic time), and (3) the presence or absence of a normal atrial kick. Increases in either cardiac output or heart rate (decreased diastolic time) necessitate higher flows across the valve and result in higher transvalvular pressure gradients. Similarly, loss of normal atrial systole (which is usually responsible for 20–30% of ventricular filling) necessitates higher diastolic flow across the valve to maintain the same cardiac output. The relationship between cardiac output, valvular area, and the transvalvular gradient can be expressed by the Gorlin equation:

$$\text{Valve area} = \frac{\text{Flow across valve}}{K \times \sqrt{\text{Mean transvalvular gradient}}}$$

where K is a hydraulic pressure constant. When mitral valve flow is expressed as mL/s, pressure as mm Hg, and valve area as cm^2, K = 38.

Mitral valve flow can be derived as follows:

$$\text{Mitral valve flow} = \frac{\text{Cardiac output}}{\text{Diastolic filling pressure} \times \text{Heart rate}}$$

Mitral valve areas below 1 cm^2 are typically associated with transvalvular gradients of 20 mm Hg at rest and dyspnea with minimal exertion and are often referred to as critical mitral stenosis. Patients with valve areas between 1.5 cm^2 and 2.0 cm^2 are generally asymptomatic or have only mild symptoms with exertion. When the mitral valve area is between 1 cm^2 and 1.5 cm^2, most patients are symptomatic with mild to moderate exertion. Although cardiac output may be normal at rest, it fails to increase appropriately during exertion because of decreased left ventricular preload. Left ventricular function is normal in the majority of patients with pure mitral stenosis, but impaired left ventricular function may be encountered in up to 25% of patients and presumably represents residual damage from rheumatic myocarditis or coexistent hypertensive or ischemic heart disease.

Acute elevations in left atrial pressure are rapidly transmitted back to the pulmonary capillaries. When mean pulmonary capillary pressure acutely rises above 25 mm Hg, transudation of capillary fluid results in pulmonary edema. Chronic elevations in pulmonary capillary pressure are partially compensated by increases in pulmonary lymph flow but eventually result in anatomic pulmonary vascular changes leading to irreversible increases in pulmonary vascular resistance and pulmonary hypertension. Reduced lung compliance and a secondary increase in the work of breathing contribute to chronic dyspnea. Right ventricular failure is frequently precipitated by acute or chronic elevations in right ventricular afterload. Marked dilatation of the right ventricle can result in tricuspid or pulmonary valve incompetence.

Embolic events are common in patients with mitral stenosis and atrial fibrillation. Stasis of blood within the enlarged left atrium favors clot formation. Dislodgment of these clots often results in systemic emboli, most commonly to the cerebral circulation. Patients also have an increased incidence of pulmonary emboli, pulmonary infarction, hemoptysis, and recurrent bronchitis. Hemoptysis most commonly results from rupture of pulmonary-bronchial venous communications.

Treatment

The time from onset of symptoms to incapacitation averages 5–10 years. At that stage, most patients die within 2–5 years. Surgical correction (valvuloplasty) is therefore usually undertaken once significant symptoms develop. Recurrent mitral stenosis following valvuloplasty is usually managed with valve replacement. Medical management is primarily supportive and includes limitation of physical activity, sodium restriction, and diuretics. Digoxin is useful only in patients with atrial fibrillation and a rapid ventricular response. Small doses of a β-adrenergic blocking drug may also be useful in controlling heart rate in patients with mild to moderate symptoms. Patients with a history of emboli and those at high risk (age > 40 years and large atrium with chronic atrial fibrillation) are usually anticoagulated. Oral anticoagulants should be stopped 3 days prior to surgery. If the embolic risk is high, heparin is given during that time until 6 hours before surgery and is restarted postoperatively 24–48 hours after surgical bleeding is controlled.

Anesthetic Management

A. Objectives: The principal hemodynamic goals are (1) to maintain a sinus rhythm (if present preoperatively), (2) to avoid tachycardia, (3) to avoid large increases in cardiac output, and (4) to avoid both hypovolemia and fluid overload by judicious fluid therapy .

B. Monitoring: Full hemodynamic monitoring (of direct intra-arterial pressure and pulmonary artery pressure) is generally indicated for all major surgical procedures (especially those associated with large fluid shifts). Overzealous fluid replacement readily precipitates pulmonary edema in patients with severe disease. Pulmonary artery pressures should be monitored closely. Pulmonary capillary wedge pressure measurements in the presence of mitral stenosis reflect the transvalvular gradient and not necessarily left ventricular end-diastolic pressure. Prominent *a* waves and a decreased *y* descent are typically present on the pulmonary capillary wedge pressure waveform in patients who are in sinus rhythm. A prominent *cv* wave on the central venous pressure waveform is usually indicative of secondary tricuspid regurgitation.

C. Choice of Agents: Patients may be very sensitive to the vasodilating effects of spinal and epidural anesthesia. Epidural is preferable to spinal anesthesia because of the more gradual onset of sympathetic blockade. Ketamine alone is generally a poor induction agent for general anesthesia because of its sympathetic stimulation. Similarly, pancuronium-induced tachycardia is to be avoided. In considering whether to use a volatile agent or an opioid, the latter may be a better choice. Volatile agents can produce undesirable vasodilatation or precipitate junctional rhythm with loss of an effective atrial kick. Of the volatile agents, halothane may be the most suitable because it decreases heart rate and is the least vasodilating. Nitrous oxide should be used cautiously, since it can acutely increase pulmonary vascular resistance in some patients.

Intraoperative tachycardia may be controlled by deepening anesthesia with an opioid (excluding meperidine), intravenous esmolol, or digoxin (if the patient is in atrial fibrillation). Verapamil may be less desirable because of the associated vasodilatation. Marked hemodynamic deterioration due to sudden supraventricular tachycardia necessitates cardioversion. Phenylephrine is preferred over ephedrine as a vasopressor because the former lacks β-adrenergic agonist activity. Treatment of acute hypertension or afterload reduction with potent vasodilators should be undertaken only with full hemodynamic monitoring.

2. MITRAL REGURGITATION

Preoperative Considerations

Mitral regurgitation can develop acutely or insidiously as a result of a large number of disorders. Chronic mitral regurgitation is usually the result of rheumatic fever (often with concomitant mitral stenosis), congenital or developmental abnormalities of the valve apparatus, or dilatation, destruction, or calcification of the mitral annulus. Acute mitral regurgitation is usually due to myocardial ischemia or infarction (papillary muscle dysfunction or rupture of a chorda tendinea), infective endocarditis, or chest trauma.

Pathophysiology

The principal derangement is a reduction in forward stroke volume due to backward flow of blood into the left atrium during systole. The left ventricle compensates by dilating and increasing end-diastolic volume. Regurgitation through the mitral valve reduces left ventricular afterload, which often initially enhances contractility. End-systolic volume thus remains normal but eventually increases as the disease progresses. By increasing end-diastolic volume, the volume-overloaded left ventricle can maintain a normal cardiac output even as ejection fraction decreases (Chapter 19). With time, patients with chronic mitral regurgitation eventually develop eccentric left ventricular hypertrophy (Chapter 19) and progressive impairment in contractility as reflected by a decrease in ejection fraction (< 50%).

The regurgitant volume passing through the mitral valve is dependent on (1) the size of the mitral valve orifice (which can vary with ventricular cavity size), (2) the heart rate (systolic time), and (3) the left ventricular-left atrial pressure gradient during systole. The last factor is affected by the relative resistances of the two outflow paths from the left ventricle, namely, systemic vascular resistance and left atrial compliance. Thus, a decrease in systemic vascular resistance or an increase in mean left atrial pressure will reduce the regurgitant volume. Atrial compliance also determines the predominant clinical manifestations. Patients with normal or reduced atrial compliance (acute mitral regurgitation) have mainly pulmonary vascular congestion and edema. Patients with increased atrial compliance (long-standing mitral regurgitation resulting in a large dilated left atrium) primarily show signs of a low cardiac output. Most patients are between the two extremes and exhibit symptoms of both pulmonary congestion and low cardiac output. Patients with a regurgitant fraction less than 30% of the total stroke volume generally have mild symptoms. Regurgitant fractions of 30–60% generally result in moderate symptoms, while fractions greater than 60% are associated with severe disease.

Treatment

Medical treatment includes digoxin, diuretics, and vasodilators. Afterload reduction is beneficial in nearly all patients and may even be lifesaving in patients with acute mitral regurgitation. Reduction of systemic vascular resistance increases forward stroke volume and decreases the regurgitant volume. Surgical treatment is usually reserved for patients with moderate to severe symptoms.

Anesthetic Management

A. Objectives: Anesthetic management should be tailored to the severity of the regurgitation as well as the underlying left ventricular function (see above). Factors that exacerbate the regurgitation, such as slow heart rates (long systole) and acute increases in afterload, should be avoided. Bradycardia can increase the regurgitant volume by increasing left ventricular end-diastolic volume and acutely dilating the mitral annulus. The heart rate should ideally be kept between 80 and 100 beats/min. Acute increases in left ventricular afterload such as following endotracheal intubation and surgical stimulation should be treated rapidly but without excessive myocardial depression. Excessive volume expansion can also worsen the regurgitation by dilating the left ventricle.

B. Monitoring: Monitors are based on the severity of ventricular dysfunction as well as the procedure (see above). Pulmonary artery pressure monitoring is extremely useful in patients with symptomatic disease. Intraoperative afterload reduction with a vasodilator requires full hemodynamic monitoring. Mitral regurgitation may be recognized on the pulmonary artery wedge waveform as a large cv wave and a rapid y descent (Figure 20–3). The height of the cv wave is inversely related to atrial and pulmonary vascular compliance but directly proportionate to pulmonary blood flow and the regurgitant volume. Very large cv waves are often apparent on the pulmonary artery pressure waveform even without wedging the catheter.

C. Choice of Agents: Patients with relatively preserved ventricular function tend to do well with most anesthetic techniques. Spinal and epidural anesthesia are well tolerated provided bradycardia is avoided. Patients with moderate to severe ventricular impairment are often very sensitive to the depressant effects of volatile agents. Opioid-based anesthetics may be more suitable for those patients provided bradycardia is avoided. The selection of pancuronium as muscle relaxant with an opioid-based anesthetic is useful in this regard.

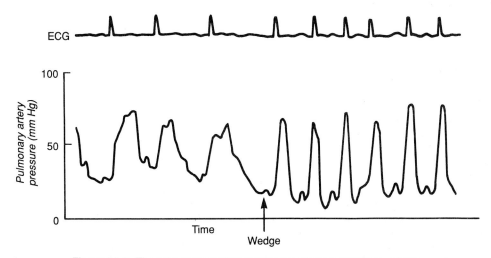

Figure 20-3. The pulmonary capillary wedge waveform in mitral regurgitation.

3. MITRAL VALVE PROLAPSE

Preoperative Considerations

Mitral valve prolapse is characterized by a mid-systolic click with or without a late apical systolic murmur. It is a relatively common abnormality that is present in up to 5% of the general population, being most common in women (up to 15%). The diagnosis is based on auscultatory findings and confirmed by echocardiography, which shows systolic prolapse of mitral valve leaflets into the left atrium. Patients with the murmur often have some element of mitral regurgitation. Pathologically, most patients have redundancy or myxomatous degeneration of the valve leaflets. Most cases of mitral valve prolapse are sporadic or familial, affecting otherwise normal individuals. A high incidence of mitral valve prolapse is found in patients with connective tissue disorders (especially Marfan's syndrome).

The overwhelming majority of patients with mitral valve prolapse are asymptomatic. Manifestations, when they occur, can include chest pains, arrhythmias, embolic events, florid mitral regurgitation, infective endocarditis, and, rarely, sudden death. The diagnosis can made preoperatively by auscultation of the characteristic click but must be confirmed by echocardiography. The prolapse is accentuated by maneuvers that decrease ventricular volume (preload). The ECG is usually normal but in some patients often shows inverted or biphasic T waves or ST segment changes inferiorly. Both atrial and ventricular arrhythmias are common. Although bradyarrhythmias also are reported, paroxysmal supraventricular tachycardia is the most commonly encountered sustained arrhythmia. An increased incidence of abnormal atrioventricular bypass tracts (Chapter 19) is reported in patients with mitral valve prolapse.

Most patients have a normal life span. About 15% develop progressive mitral regurgitation. A smaller percentage develop embolic phenomena or infective endocarditis. Patients with both a click and a systolic murmur appear to be at greater risk for developing complications. Anticoagulation or antiplatelet agents may be used for patients with a history of emboli, while β-adrenergic blocking drugs are commonly employed for arrhythmias.

Anesthetic Management

The management of these patients is based on their clinical course. Most patients are asymptomatic and, except for antibiotic prophylaxis, do not require special care. Patients with a systolic murmur appear to be at greatest risk for infective endocarditis. Ventricular arrhythmias may occur intraoperatively, especially following sympathetic stimulation, and will generally respond to lidocaine or β-adrenergic blocking agents. Relatively deep anesthesia with a volatile agent usually lessens the likelihood of intraoperative arrhythmias. Mitral regurgitation due to prolapse is generally exacerbated by decreases in ventricular size. Thus, hypovolemia and factors that increase ventricular emptying—such as increased sympathetic tone or decreased afterload—should be avoided. Vasopressors with pure α-adrenergic agonist activity (such as phenylephrine) may therefore be preferable to those that are primarily β-adrenergic agonists (ephedrine).

4. AORTIC STENOSIS

Preoperative Considerations

Valvular aortic stenosis is the most common cause of obstruction to left ventricular outflow. Left ventricular outflow obstruction is less commonly due to hypertrophic cardiomyopathy (see below) or, rarely, supravalvular stenosis. Valvular aortic stenosis is nearly always congenital, rheumatic, or degenerative. Abnormalities in the number of cusps (most commonly a bicuspid valve) or their architecture produce turbulence that traumatizes the valve and eventually leads to stenosis. Rheumatic aortic stenosis is rarely isolated but is more commonly associated with aortic regurgitation or mitral valve disease. In the most common degenerative form, calcific aortic stenosis, "wear and tear" results in the build-up of calcium deposits on normal cusps, which prevents them from opening completely.

Pathophysiology

In contrast to acute obstruction of left ventricular outflow, which rapidly dilates the ventricle and reduces stroke volume (Chapter 21), obstruction due to valvular aortic stenosis is nearly always gradual, allowing the ventricle, at least initially, to compensate and maintain stroke volume. Concentric ventricular hypertrophy enables the left ventricle to maintain stroke volume by generating a significant transvalvular gradient and reduce ventricular wall stress (afterload; see Chapter 19). As with mitral stenosis, the transvalvular gradient is proportionate to cardiac output, and the relationship may be expressed by the Gorlin equation as shown on p 325. When aortic valve flow is expressed as mL/s, pressure as mm Hg, and valve area as cm², K = 44.5.

Aortic valve flow can be derived as follows:

$$\text{Aortic valve flow} = \frac{\text{Cardiac output}}{\text{Systolic ejection period} \times \text{Heart rate}}$$

Critical aortic stenosis is said to exist when the aortic valve orifice is reduced to 0.5–0.7 cm² (normal: 2.5–3.5 cm²). With this degree of stenosis, patients generally have a transvalvular gradient of approximately 50 mm Hg at rest (with a normal cardiac output) and are unable to appreciably increase cardiac output. Moreover, further increases in the transvalvular gradient do not appreciably increase stroke volume. Aortic valve areas between 0.7 and 0.9 cm² are generally associated with mild to moderate symptoms. With long-standing aortic stenosis, myocardial contractility progressively deteriorates and further compromises left ventricular function. Most patient with aortic stenosis have a long latency period of 30–60 years (depending on the cause) before significant symptoms develop.

Classically, patients with advanced aortic stenosis have the triad of dyspnea on exertion, angina, and orthostatic or exertional syncope. A prominent feature of aortic stenosis is a decrease in left ventricular compliance due to hypertrophy (Chapter 19). Diastolic stiffness is the result of an increase in ventricular muscle mass or fibrosis. In contrast to left ventricular end-diastolic volume, which remains normal until very late in the disease, left ventricular end-diastolic pressure is elevated early. The decreased diastolic pressure gradient between the left atrium and left ventricle impairs ventricular filling, which becomes quite dependent on a normal atrial contraction. Loss of atrial systole can precipitate congestive heart failure or hypotension in patients with aortic stenosis. Cardiac output may be normal in symptomatic patients at rest but characteristically does not appropriately increase with exertion. Patients may experience angina even in the absence of coronary artery disease. Myocardial oxygen demand is increased because of ventricular hypertrophy, while myocardial oxygen supply is decreased because of marked compression of intramyocardial coronary vessels from high intracavitary systolic pressures (up to 300 mm Hg). Exertional syncope or near-syncope is thought to be due to an inability to tolerate the vasodilation in muscle during exertion. Arrhythmias leading to severe hypoperfusion also probably account for syncope and sudden death in some patients. Calcium emboli may occasionally result in neurologic complications.

Treatment

Once significant symptoms develop, most patients die without surgical treatment within 2–5 years. Percutaneous valvuloplasty has recently been employed successfully in some patients, but its success is short-lived and restenosis usually occurs within 6–12 months.

Anesthetic Management

A. Objectives: Maintenance of a normal sinus rhythm, heart rate, and intravascular volume is critical. Loss of a normally timed atrial systole often leads to rapid deterioration, especially when associated with tachycardia. The combination of the two (atrial fibrillation) seriously impairs ventricular filling and necessitates immediate cardioversion. The reduced ventricular compliance also makes the patient very sensitive to abrupt changes in intravascular volume. Many patients behave as though they have a fixed stroke volume in spite of adequate hydration; under these conditions, cardiac output becomes very rate-dependent. Bradycardia (< 50 beats/min) is therefore poorly tolerated. Heart rates between 60 and 90 beats/min may be optimal in most patients.

B. Monitoring: Close monitoring of the ECG and blood pressure is crucial. Monitoring for ischemia is complicated by baseline ST and T wave abnormalities. Intra-arterial pressure monitoring is desirable in patients with severe aortic stenosis, since many of these patients do not tolerate even brief episodes of hypotension. Pulmonary artery catheterization is also useful, but data should be interpreted carefully; a higher than normal pulmonary capillary wedge pressure is often required to maintain adequate left ventricular end-diastolic volume and cardiac output. Prominent *a* waves are often visible on the pulmonary artery wedge pressure waveform. Vasodilators should generally only be employed when a pulmonary artery catheter is in place, because patients are often very sensitive to these agents.

C. Choice of Agents: Patients with mild to moderate aortic stenosis (generally asymptomatic) may tolerate spinal or epidural anesthesia. However, these techniques should be employed very cautiously because hypotension readily occurs as a result of reductions in preload, afterload, or both. Epidural anesthesia is preferable to spinal anesthesia because of the slower onset of hypotension, which allows more aggressive correction. Spinal and epidural anesthesia are contraindicated in patients with severe aortic stenosis.

The selection of general anesthetic agents is most critical in patients with symptomatic (moderate to severe) aortic stenosis. In these patients, a narcotic-based anesthetic technique generally results in minimal cardiac depression and is therefore preferable. If a volatile agent is used, low concentrations should be employed to avoid excessive myocardial depression, vasodilation, or loss of normal atrial systole. Tachycardia and hypertension, which may precipitate ischemia, should be treated by increasing anesthetic depth. If a β-adrenergic blocking agent is used, esmolol is preferable because of its short half-life. Most patients are extremely sensitive to vasodilators. Moreover, because of an already precarious myocardial oxygen demand-supply balance, they tolerate even mild degrees of hypotension poorly. Hypotension should generally be treated with small doses (25–50 μg) of phenylephrine. Intraoperative supraventricular tachycardias with hemodynamic compromise should be treated with immediate synchronized cardioversion. Frequent ventricular ectopy (which often reflects ischemia) is usually poorly tolerated hemodynamically and should be treated with intravenous lidocaine.

5. HYPERTROPHIC CARDIOMYOPATHY

Preoperative Considerations

Hypertrophic cardiomyopathy can be hereditary (usually with variable penetrance) or may occur sporadically. It has been called by many other names: idiopathic hypertrophic subaortic stenosis, asymmetric septal hypertrophy, hypertrophic obstructive cardiomyopathy, and muscular subaortic stenosis. It is characterized by heterogeneous left ventricular hypertrophy. There is no obvious cause.

Affected patients display diastolic dysfunction that

is reflected by elevated left ventricular end-diastolic pressures in spite of often hyperdynamic ventricular function. The diastolic stiffness is presumably due to the abnormal hypertrophied muscle, which tends to be located in the upper interventricular septum below the aortic valve. In about 25% of patients, the hypertrophy results in dynamic obstruction of left ventricular outflow during systole. Obstruction is the result of the narrowing in subaortic area caused by a systolic anterior motion of the anterior mitral valve leaflet against the hypertrophied septum. In contrast to fixed obstruction (valvular aortic stenosis), the resulting obstruction (and pressure gradient) is dynamic and peaks in mid to late systole. Moreover, the degree of obstruction can vary from beat to beat. Factors that tend to worsen the obstruction include (1) enhanced contractility, (2) decreased ventricular volume, and (3) decreased left ventricular afterload.

Most patients are asymptomatic. Symptomatic patients generally complain of dyspnea on exertion, but there may also be fatigue, syncope, near-syncope, or angina. Symptoms do not necessarily correlate with the presence or severity of dynamic left ventricular outflow obstruction. Sudden death is often the first manifestation in patients under 30 years of age and is the most common cause of death. Both supraventricular and ventricular arrhythmias are common. Patients with obstruction have a characteristic harsh systolic murmur (Table 20–13). The ECG characteristically shows left ventricular hypertrophy and deep, broad Q waves. The diagnosis can be confirmed by echocardiography. Even asymptomatic patients may have myocardial perfusion defects on thallium-201 scans.

Treatment is with β-adrenergic and calcium channel blocking agents. Both agents decrease contractility and can prevent increases in the subaortic pressure gradient in patients with obstruction. Calcium channel blockers may also improve diastolic compliance (relaxation). Amiodarone is generally effective for both supraventricular and ventricular arrhythmias. Nitrates, digoxin, and diuretics are avoided because they can worsen left ventricular obstruction. Surgical myomectomy or myotomy is reserved for patients with moderate to severe symptoms.

Anesthetic Management

Preoperative evaluation of patients with hypertrophic cardiomyopathy should focus on evaluating the potential for significant dynamic obstruction, malignant arrhythmias, and myocardial ischemia. The results of echocardiography (or angiography) and Holter monitoring should ideally be reviewed with a cardiologist. Anesthetic goals should be (1) to minimize sympathetic activation, (2) to expand intravascular volume in order to avoid hypovolemia, and (3) to minimize decreases in left ventricular afterload.

Monitoring requirements should be dictated by the severity of obstruction and the surgical procedure. Full hemodynamic monitoring is generally desirable to guide fluid therapy in the presence of abnormal ventricular compliance. The arterial pressure wave form

in patients with obstruction may be bifid (bisferiens pulse): The initial rapid peak represents early unobstructed ventricular ejection, while the subsequent decrease and second peak are due to dynamic obstruction.

In patients with significant obstruction, some degree of myocardial depression is usually desirable and can be achieved by the use of volatile anesthetic agents, especially halothane and enflurane. Beta-adrenergic agents are also useful in counteracting the effects of sympathetic activation and decreasing obstruction. Regional anesthesia may exacerbate left ventricular outflow obstruction by decreasing both cardiac preload and afterload. Phenylephrine and other pure α-adrenergic agonists are ideal vasopressors in these patients because they do not augment contractility but increase systemic vascular resistance (ventricular afterload).

6. AORTIC REGURGITATION

Preoperative Considerations

Aortic regurgitation usually develops slowly and is progressive (chronic), but it can also develop acutely. Chronic aortic regurgitation may be caused by abnormalities of the aortic valve, the aortic root, or both. Abnormalities in the valve are usually congenital (bicuspid valve) or due to rheumatic fever. Diseases affecting the ascending aorta cause regurgitation by dilating the aortic annulus and include syphilis, annuloaortic ectasia, cystic medial necrosis (with or without Marfan's syndrome), ankylosing spondylitis, rheumatoid and psoriatic arthritis, and a variety of other connective tissue disorders. Acute aortic insufficiency most commonly follows infective endocarditis, trauma, or aortic dissection.

Pathophysiology

Regardless of the cause, aortic regurgitation produces volume overload of the left ventricle. The effective forward stroke volume is reduced because of backward (regurgitant) flow of blood into the left ventricle during diastole. Both systemic arterial diastolic pressure and systemic vascular resistance are typically low. The decrease in cardiac afterload helps facilitate ventricular ejection. Total stroke volume is the sum of the effective stroke volume and the regurgitant volume. The regurgitant volume depends on (1) the heart rate (diastolic time) and (2) the diastolic pressure gradient across the aortic valve (diastolic aortic pressure minus left ventricular end-diastolic pressure). Slow heart rates increase regurgitation because of the associated disproportionate increase in diastolic time (Chapter 19), while increases in diastolic arterial pressure favor regurgitant volume by increasing the pressure gradient for backward flow.

With chronic aortic regurgitation, the left ventricle progressively dilates and undergoes eccentric hypertrophy. The resulting increase in end-diastolic volume maintains an effective stroke volume because end-systolic volume is unchanged. Any increase in the regurgitant volume is compensated by an increase in end-diastolic volume. Left ventricular end-diastolic pressure is usually normal or only slightly elevated, because ventricular compliance initially increases. Eventually, as ventricular function deteriorates, the ejection fraction declines and impaired ventricular emptying is manifested as gradual increases in left ventricular end-diastolic pressure and end-systolic volume.

Sudden incompetence of the aortic valve does not allow compensatory dilatation or hypertrophy of the left ventricle. Effective stroke volume rapidly declines because the normal-sized ventricle is unable to accommodate a sudden large regurgitant volume. The sudden rise in left ventricular end-diastolic pressure is transmitted back to the pulmonary circulation and causes acute pulmonary congestion.

Acute aortic regurgitation typically presents as the sudden onset of pulmonary edema and hypotension, whereas chronic insufficiency usually presents insidiously as congestive heart failure. Symptoms are generally minimal (in the chronic form) when the regurgitant volume remains under 40% of stroke volume but become severe when it exceeds 60%. Angina can occur even in the absence of coronary disease. The myocardial oxygen demand is increased from muscle hypertrophy and dilatation, while myocardial blood supply is reduced by low diastolic pressures in the aorta due to the regurgitation.

Treatment

Most patients with chronic aortic regurgitation remain asymptomatic for 10–20 years. Once significant symptoms develop, the expected survival time is about 5 years. Afterload reduction with arterial vasodilators and angiotensin enzyme inhibitors generally benefits patients with acute or advanced chronic aortic regurgitation. The decrease in arterial blood pressure reduces the diastolic gradient for regurgitation. Early operation is indicated for patients with acute aortic regurgitation because medical management is associated with a high mortality rate. Patients with chronic aortic regurgitation should be operated on before irreversible ventricular dysfunction occurs.

Anesthetic Management

A. Objectives: The heart rate should be maintained toward the upper limits of normal (80–100 beats/min). Bradycardia increases the regurgitant volume, while tachycardia can contribute to myocardial ischemia. Increases in systemic vascular resistance and excessive myocardial depression should also be avoided. The compensatory increase in cardiac preload should be maintained, but overzealous fluid replacement can readily result in pulmonary edema.

B. Monitoring: Full hemodynamic monitoring should generally be employed for all patients with acute aortic regurgitation and those with severe chronic regurgitation. Premature closure of the mitral valve often occurs during acute aortic regurgitation and may cause pulmonary capillary wedge pressure to give a falsely high estimate of left ventricular end-

diastolic pressure. The appearance of a large *cv* wave suggests mitral regurgitation secondary to dilatation of the left ventricle. The arterial pressure wave in patients with aortic regurgitation characteristically has a very wide pulse pressure. A bisferiens pulse (see above) may also be present in some patients and is thought to result from the rapid ejection of a large stroke volume.

C. Choice of Agents: Most patients tolerate spinal and epidural anesthesia provided intravascular volume is maintained. When general anesthesia is required, isoflurane may be ideal because of the associated vasodilatation. A narcotic-based general anesthetic technique is more suitable for patients with depressed ventricular function. Pancuronium is a good choice as a muscle relaxant with the latter technique because it often prevents bradycardia. Intraoperative afterload reduction with nitroprusside optimally requires full hemodynamic monitoring. Ephedrine is generally the preferred vasopressor for the treatment of hypotension. However, small doses of phenylephrine (25–50 μg) can be used when the hypotension is clearly due to excessive vasodilatation. Larger doses of phenylephrine can increase systemic vascular resistance (and arterial diastolic pressure) and may exacerbate the regurgitation.

7. TRICUSPID REGURGITATION

Preoperative Considerations

Tricuspid regurgitation is most commonly due to dilatation of right ventricle from the pulmonary hypertension that usually results from chronic left ventricular failure. Tricuspid regurgitation can also follow infective endocarditis (usually in intravenous drug abusers), rheumatic fever, or chest trauma or may be due to Ebstein's anomaly (downward displacement of the valve due to abnormal attachment of the valve leaflets).

Pathophysiology

Chronic left ventricular failure often leads to sustained increases in pulmonary vascular pressures. The chronic increase in afterload causes the thin-walled right ventricle to progressively dilate, and excessive dilatation of the tricuspid annulus eventually results in regurgitation. An increase in end-diastolic volume allows the right ventricle to compensate for the regurgitant volume and maintain an effective forward flow. Because the right atrium and the vena cava are compliant and usually accommodate the volume overload, mean right atrial and central venous pressures are generally only slightly elevated. Acute or marked elevations in pulmonary artery pressures increase the regurgitant volume and are reflected by an increase in central venous pressure. Moreover, sudden marked increases in right ventricular afterload sharply reduce the effective right ventricular output, reduce left ventricular preload, and can precipitate systemic hypotension.

Chronic venous hypertension leads to passive congestion of the liver and progressive hepatic dysfunction, which can eventually result in cardiac cirrhosis. Severe right ventricular failure with underloading of the left heart may also produce right-to-left shunting through an incompletely closed (or probe-patent) foramen ovale, which can result in marked hypoxemia.

Treatment

Tricuspid regurgitation is generally well tolerated by most patients. Many even tolerate complete surgical excision of the tricuspid valve. The underlying disorder is generally more important than the tricuspid regurgitation itself. Therefore, treatment is aimed at the underlying disease process.

Anesthetic Management

A. Objectives: Hemodynamic goals should be directed primarily toward the underlying disorder. Hypovolemia and factors increasing right ventricular afterload, such as hypoxia and acidosis, should be avoided to maintain effective right ventricular stroke volume and left ventricular preload. Positive end-expiratory pressure and high mean airway pressures are also undesirable during mechanical ventilation because they reduce venous return and increase right ventricular afterload.

B. Monitoring: Monitoring of both central venous and pulmonary artery pressures is useful in these patients. The latter is not always possible, since passage of a pulmonary artery catheter across the tricuspid valve can be difficult because of the regurgitant flow. Central venous pressure is extremely useful in following right ventricular function, while pulmonary artery pressures allow measurement of its afterload and left ventricular preload. Increasing central venous pressures imply worsening right ventricular dysfunction. A prominent *cv* wave is usually present in the central venous pressure waveform. Thermodilution cardiac output measurements are falsely elevated because of the tricuspid regurgitation.

C. Choice of Agents: Anesthetic agents should be selected based on the underlying disorder. Most patients tolerate spinal and epidural anesthesia well. Coagulopathy secondary to hepatic dysfunction should be excluded prior to any regional technique. During general anesthesia, nitrous oxide may exacerbate the pulmonary hypertension and should be administered cautiously if at all.

CASE DISCUSSION: HIP FRACTURE FOLLOWING A FALL IN AN ELDERLY WOMAN

A 71-year-old woman presents for open reduction and internal fixation of a left hip fracture. She gives a history of two episodes of light-headedness several days prior to her fall today. When questioned about her fall, she can only recall standing in her bathroom while brushing her teeth and then awakening on the floor with hip pain. The preoperative ECG shows a sinus rhythm with a PR interval of 220 ms and a right bundle branch block pattern.

Why should the anesthesiologist be concerned about a history of syncope?

A history of syncope in elderly patients should always raise the possibility of arrhythmias and underlying organic heart disease. Although arrhythmias can occur in the absence of organic heart disease, the two are commonly related. Cardiac syncope usually results from an abrupt arrhythmia that suddenly compromises cardiac output and impairs cerebral perfusion. Light-headedness may reflect lesser degrees of cerebral impairment. Both bradyarrhythmias and tachyarrhythmias (Chapter 19) can produce syncope. Table 20–15 lists other causes of cardiac syncope as well as noncardiac causes.

How do bradyarrhythmias commonly arise?

Bradyarrhythmias may arise from either SA node dysfunction or abnormal AV conduction of the cardiac impulse. A delay or block of the impulse can occur anywhere between the SA node and the distal His-Purkinje system (Chapter 19). Reversible abnor-

Table 20–15. Causes of syncope.

Cardiac
  Arrhythmias
    Tachyarrhythmias (usually > 180 beats/min)
    Bradyarrhythmias (usually < 40 beats/min)
  Impairment of left ventricular ejection
    Aortic stenosis
    Hypertrophic cardiomyopathy
    Massive myocardial infarction
    Atrial myxoma
  Impairment of right ventricular output
    Tetralogy of Fallot
    Primary pulmonary hypertension
    Pulmonary embolism
    Pulmonary stenosis
  Biventricular impairment
    Cardiac tamponade
    Massive myocardial infarction
Noncardiac
  Accentuated reflexes
    Vasovagal reflex
    Carotid sinus hypersensitivity
    Neuralgias
  Postural hypotension
    Hypovolemia
    Sympathectomy
    Autonomic dysfunction
  Sustained Valsalva maneuver
  Cerebrovascular disease
  Seizures
  Metabolic
    Hypoxia
    Marked hypocapnia
    Hypoglycemia

malities may be due to abnormal vagal tone, electrolyte abnormalities, drug toxicity, hypothermia, or myocardial ischemia. Irreversible abnormalities, which may initially only be intermittent before they become permanent, reflect either isolated conduction system abnormalities or underlying heart disease (most commonly hypertensive, coronary artery, or valvular heart disease).

What is the pathophysiology of sinus node dysfunction?

Patients with sinus node dysfunction may have a normal baseline 12-lead ECG but have abrupt pauses in SA node activity (sinus arrest) or intermittent block of conduction of the SA impulse to the surrounding tissue (exit block). When pauses are prolonged (> 3 seconds) or the effective ventricular rate is less than 40 beats/min, symptoms are usually present. Patients may experience intermittent dizziness, syncope, confusion, fatigue, or shortness of breath. Symptomatic SA node dysfunction is often referred to as the **sick sinus syndrome.** Sick sinus syndrome is often unmasked by β-adrenergic blocking agents, calcium channel blockers, digoxin, or quinidine. The term **bradycardia-tachycardia syndrome** is often used when patients experience paroxysmal tachyarrhythmias (usually atrial flutter or fibrillation) followed by sinus pauses or bradycardia. The latter probably represents failure of the SA node to recover normal automaticity following suppression by the tachyarrhythmia. The diagnosis must be based on electrocardiographic recordings during symptoms (Holter monitoring) or after provocative tests (carotid baroreceptor stimulation or rapid atrial pacing).

How are atrioventricular conduction abnormalities manifested on the surface 12-lead ECG?

Atrioventricular conduction abnormalities are usually manifested by abnormal ventricular depolarization (bundle branch block), prolongation of the PR interval (first-degree AV block), failure of some atrial impulses to depolarize the ventricles (second-degree AV block), or atrioventricular dissociation (third-degree AV block, also called complete heart block).

What determines the significance of these conduction abnormalities?

The significance of a conduction system abnormality depends on (1) its location, (2) its likelihood for progression to complete heart block, and (3) the likelihood that a more distal pacemaker site will be able to maintain a stable and adequate escape rhythm (> 40 beats/min). The His bundle is normally the lowest area in the conduction system that can maintain a stable rhythm (usually 40–60 beats/min). When conduction fails anywhere above it, a normal His bundle can take over the pacemaker function of the heart and maintain a normal QRS complex unless a distal intraventricular

conduction is present. When the escape rhythm arises farther down in the His-Purkinje system, the rhythm is usually slower (< 40 beats/min), often unstable, and results in a wide QRS complex.

What is the significance of isolated bundle branch block with a normal PR interval?

A conduction delay or block in the right bundle branch results in a typical right bundle branch block (RBBB) QRS pattern on the surface ECG (M-shape or rSR′ in V_1) and may represent a congenital abnormality or underlying organic heart disease. In contrast, a delay or block in the main left bundle branch results in a left bundle branch block (LBBB) QRS pattern (wide R with a delayed upstroke in V_5) and nearly always represents underlying heart disease. The term **hemiblock** is often used if only one of the two fascicles of the left bundle branch are blocked (left anterior or left posterior hemiblock). When the PR interval is normal and in the absence of an acute myocardial infarction, a conduction block in either the left or right bundle rarely leads to complete heart block.

Can the site of AV block always be determined from a 12-lead ECG?

No. A first-degree AV block (PR interval > 200 ms) can reflect abnormal conduction anywhere between the atria and the distal His-Purkinje system. Mobitz type I second-degree AV block, which is characterized by progressive lengthening of the PR interval before a P wave is not conducted (a QRS does not follow the P wave), is usually due to a block in the AV node itself, and progression to third-degree AV block is uncommon.

In patients with Mobitz type II second-degree AV block, atrial impulses are periodically not conducted into the ventricle without progressive prolongation of the PR interval. The conduction block is nearly always in or below the His bundle and frequently progresses to complete (third-degree) AV block, especially following an acute anteroseptal myocardial infarction. The QRS is typically wide.

In patients with third-degree AV block, the atrial rate and ventricular depolarization rates are independent (AV dissociation) because atrial impulses completely fail to reach the ventricles. If the site of the block is in the AV node, a stable His bundle rhythm will result in a normal QRS complex and the ventricular rate will often increase following administration of atropine. If the block involves the His bundle, the origin of the ventricular rhythm is more distal, resulting in wide QRS complexes. A wide QRS complex does not necessarily exclude a normal His bundle, as it may represent a more distal block in one of the bundle branches.

Can AV dissociation occur in the absence of AV block?

Yes. AV dissociation is common during anesthesia with volatile agents in the absence of AV block and results from sinus bradycardia or an accelerated AV junctional rhythm. During isorhythmic dissociation, the atria and ventricles beat independently at nearly the same rate. The P wave often just precedes or follows the QRS complex, and their relationship is generally maintained. In contrast, interference AV dissociation results from a junctional rhythm that is faster than the sinus rate—such that sinus impulses always find the AV node refractory.

How do bifascicular and trifascicular blocks present?

A bifascicular block exists when two of the three major His bundle branches (right, left anterior, or left posterior) are partially or completely blocked. If one fascicle is completely blocked and while the others are only partially blocked, a bundle branch block pattern will be associated with either first-degree or second-degree AV block. If all three are affected, a trifascicular block is said to exist. A delay or partial block in all three fascicles results in either a prolonged PR interval (first-degree AV block) or alternating LBBB and RBBB. Complete block in all three fascicles results in third-degree AV block.

What is the significance of the electrocardiographic findings in this patient?

The electrocardiographic findings (first-degree AV block plus RBBB) suggest a bifascicular block. Extensive disease of the conduction system is likely. Moreover, the patient's syncopal and near-syncopal episodes suggest that she may be at risk for life-threatening bradyarrhythmias (third-degree AV block). Intracardiac electrocardiographic recordings would be necessary to confirm the site of the conduction delay.

How can intracardiac electrocardiographic studies help in localizing conduction abnormalities and determining the need for preoperative pacing?

When a bipolar catheter is placed across the tricuspid valve, electrical activity in the His bundle can be directly recorded. The interval from depolarization of the atrium adjacent to the His bundle to the beginning of depolarization in the His bundle is called the AH interval and is normally 60–125 ms. The AH interval represents conduction time in the AV node. The interval between the beginning of electrical activity in the His bundle and the beginning of ventricular depolarization on the surface ECG is the HV interval and is normally 35–55 ms. The HV interval represents conduction time in the His-Purkinje system. Patients with HV intervals greater than 100 ms are at relatively high risk for developing complete heart block with an inadequate escape rhythm; they should have a permanent pacemaker or at least a temporary pacemaker prior to surgery.

What is appropriate management for this patient?

Cardiologic evaluation is required because of the symptomatic bifascicular block. One of two approaches can be recommended depending on the urgency of the surgery. If the surgery is truly emergent, a temporary transvenous pacing catheter is probably indicated prior to induction of general or regional anesthesia. If the surgery can be postponed 24–48 hours (as with this case), continuous electrocardiographic monitoring, serial 12-lead ECGs, and measurements of cardiac isoenzymes are required to exclude myocardial ischemia or infarction and to try to document electrocardiographic findings during symptoms. Moreover, a brief intracardiac His bundle study can be performed and may be useful in determining the need for a permanent pacemaker. If the HV interval is greater than 100 ms, the patient needs a pacemaker prior to surgery (see above). If the HV interval is normal or 60–100 ms, permanent pacing may not necessarily be indicated, but central (internal jugular) venous access and ready access to pacing equipment are still advisable because of the history of syncope.

What are general perioperative indications for temporary pacing?

Suggested indications include the following: (1) any documented symptomatic bradyarrhythmia; (2) a new bundle branch block, second-degree (type II) AV block, or third-degree AV block associated with myocardial infarction; (3) bifascicular block in a comatose patient (controversial); and (4) refractory supraventricular tachyarrhythmias.

The first three indications generally require ventricular pacing, while the fourth requires atrial pacing electrodes and a programmable rapid atrial pulse generator.

How can temporary cardiac pacing be established?

The most reliable method is generally via a transvenous pacing electrode in the form of a pacing wire or a balloon-tipped pacing catheter. A pacing wire should always be positioned fluoroscopically, but a flow-directed pacing catheter can also be placed in the right ventricle under pressure monitoring. A pacing wire must be used when blood flow has ceased. If the patient has a rhythm, intracardiac electrocardiographic recording showing ST segment elevation when the electrode comes in contact with the right ventricular endocardium confirms placement of either type of electrode. Specially designed pulmonary artery catheters have an extra port for passage of a right ventricular pacing wire. These catheters are especially useful in patients with LBBB, who can develop complete heart block during catheter placement. Transcutaneous pacing is also possible via large stimulating adhesive pads placed on the chest. Lastly, temporary epicardial electrodes can be used following cardiac surgery.

Once positioned, the pacing electrodes are then attached to an electrical pulse generator that periodically delivers an impulse at a set rate and magnitude. Most pacemaker generators can also sense the heart's spontaneous (usually ventricular) electrical activity: when activity is detected, the generator suppresses its next impulse. By altering the generator's sensing threshold, the pacemaker generator can function in a fixed (asynchronous) mode or in a demand mode (by increasing sensitivity). The lowest current through the electrode that can depolarize the myocardium is called the threshold current (usually < 2 mA for transvenous electrodes). A LBBB pattern is observed when the pacing electrode is within the right ventricle, because the right ventricle is depolarized before the left ventricle.

What is AV sequential pacing?

Ventricular pacing often reduces cardiac output because the atrial contribution to ventricular filling is lost. When the AV conducting system is diseased, atrial contraction can still be maintained by sequential stimulation of separate atrial and ventricular electrodes. The "PR interval" can be varied by adjusting the delay between the atrial and ventricular impulses (usually set at 200 ms).

If a pacemaker is placed in this patient, how can its function be evaluated?

If the patient's underlying rhythm is slower than the rate of a demand pacemaker, pacing spikes should be seen on the ECG. The spike rate should be identical to the programmed (permanent pacemaker) or set (temporary) pacemaker rate; a slower rate may indicate a low battery. Every pacing spike should be followed by a QRS complex (100% capture). Moreover, every impulse should be followed by a palpable arterial pulse. If the patient has a temporary pacemaker, the escape rhythm can be established by temporarily slowing the pacing rate or decreasing the current output.

When the patient's heart rate is faster than the set pacemaker rate, pacing spikes should not be observed if the generator is sensing properly. In the latter instance, ventricular capture cannot be evaluated unless the pacemaker rate is increased or the spontaneous heart rate decreases. The latter may be accomplished by transiently increasing vagal tone (Valsalva maneuver or carotid stimulation). Fortunately, when the battery is low, sensing is generally affected before pacing output decreases. A chest x-ray is useful in excluding fracture or displacement of pacing leads. If pacemaker malfunction is suspected, cardiologic consultation is advisable.

What intraoperative conditions may cause the pacemaker to malfunction?

Electrical interference from surgical electrocautery units can be interpreted as myocardial electrical activity and can suppress the pacemaker generator. Problems with electrocautery may be minimized by limiting its use to short bursts, limiting its power output, placing its grounding plate as far from the pacemaker generator as possible, and using bipolar cautery. Moreover, continuous monitoring of an arterial pulse wave (pressure, plethysmogram, or oximetry signal) is mandatory to ensure continuous perfusion during electrocautery. Accentuated myopotentials associated with succinylcholine-induced fasciculations or postoperative shivering can similarly suppress the pacemaker generator.

Hypokalemia can increase the pacing electrodes' threshold for depolarizing the myocardium by hyperpolarizing cells and can result in failure of the pacing impulse to depolarize the ventricle. Myocardial ischemia, infarction, or scarring can also increase the electrode's threshold and cause failure of ventricular capture.

What are appropriate measures if a pacemaker fails intraoperatively?

If a temporary pacemaker fails intraoperatively, the inspired oxygen concentration should be increased to 100%. All connections and the generator battery should be checked. Most units have a battery level indicator and a light that flashes with every impulse. The generator should be set into the asynchronous mode, and the ventricular output should be set on maximum. Failure of a temporary transvenous electrode to capture the ventricle is usually due to displacement of the electrode away from the ventricular endocardium; careful slow advancement of the catheter or wire while pacing often results in capture. Pharmacologic management (atropine, isoproterenol, or epinephrine) may be useful until the problem is resolved. If an adequate arterial blood pressure cannot be maintained with adrenergic agonists, cardiopulmonary resuscitation should be instituted until another pacing electrode (wire) is placed or a new generator box is obtained.

If a permanent pacemaker malfunctions (as with electrocautery), it should generally be converted to an asynchronous mode. Some units will automatically reprogram themselves to the asynchronous mode if malfunction is detected. Other pacemaker units must be reprogrammed by placing either an external magnet or, preferably, a programming device over the generator. The effect of an external magnet on some pacemakers—especially during electrocautery—may be unpredictable and should generally be established preoperatively.

What anesthetic agents are appropriate for patients with pacemakers?

All anesthetic agents have been safely used in patients who already have pacemakers. Even volatile agents appear to have no effect on pacing electrode thresholds. Local anesthesia with light intravenous sedation is usually employed for placement of permanent pacemakers.

SUGGESTED READINGS

Atlee JL: *Perioperative Cardiac Dysrhythmias.* Mosby Year Book, 1989.

Brown DL: *Risk and Outcome in Anesthesia.* Lippincott, 1988. Includes an extensive but concise review of studies examining anesthetic risk and cardiovascular diseases.

Estafanous FG: *Anesthesia and the Heart.* Butterworths, 1989.

Hensley FA, Martin DE: *The Practice of Cardiac Anesthesia.* Little, Brown, 1990.

Kaplan JA: *Cardiac Anesthesia,* 2nd ed. Grune & Stratton, 1987.

Mangano DT: *Preoperative Cardiac Assessment.* Lippincott, 1990.

Stoelting RL, Dierdorf SF, McCammon RL: *Anesthesia and Co-Existing Disease,* 2nd ed. Churchill Livingstone, 1988.

Wood M, Wood AJJ: *Drugs and Anesthesia: Pharmacology for the Anesthesiologist,* 2nd ed. Williams & Wilkins, 1990.

Anesthesia for Cardiovascular Surgery

21

Anesthesia for cardiovascular surgery requires not only a precise understanding of circulatory physiology, pharmacology, and pathophysiology (Chapters 19 and 20) but also thorough familiarity with cardiopulmonary bypass (CPB), myocardial preservation, and surgical techniques. Surgical manipulations often have a profound impact on circulatory function, which means that the anesthesiologist must follow the progress of the surgery intently and anticipate problems associated with each step.

This chapter presents an overview of cardiovascular anesthesia and of the principles, techniques, and physiology of CPB. Because congenital heart disease affects primarily pediatric patients and involves pathophysiology not covered in the previous chapter, that subject is dealt with here. Surgery on the aorta and pericardium presents problems that also require special anesthetic considerations.

CARDIOPULMONARY BYPASS

Cardiopulmonary bypass (CPB) is a technique that diverts venous blood away from the heart, adds oxygen, removes CO_2, and returns the blood to a large artery (usually the aorta). As a result, all blood flow through the heart and most of that through the lungs ceases. When CPB is fully established, the extracorporeal circuit is in series with the systemic circulation and provides both artificial ventilation and perfusion. Unfortunately, this technique is entirely nonphysiologic, since both arterial pressure and blood flow—which is often nonpulsatile—are usually below normal levels. To minimize organ damage during this stressful period, systemic hypothermia (20–28 °C) is usually employed. Topical hypothermia (an ice-slush solution) and cardioplegia (a technique for arresting myocardial electrical activity) are used also to protect the heart.

Operation of the CPB machine is a complex task requiring the uninterrupted attention of a highly specialized technician (perfusionist). Optimal results with CPB can be obtained only by close cooperation and communication between the surgeon, anesthesiologist, and perfusionist.

BASIC CIRCUIT

The CPB machine has five basic components: a venous reservoir, an oxygenator, a heat exchanger, a main pump, and an arterial filter (Figure 21–1). Modern machines employ a single disposable unit with the reservoir, oxygenator, and heat exchanger built in. Most machines also have separate accessory pumps that may be used for blood salvage (cardiotomy suction), venting (draining) the left ventricle, and cardioplegia. Various additional filters, alarms, and in-line pressure, oxygen saturation, and temperature monitors are also typically used.

Prior to use, the CPB circuit must be primed with fluid (1500–2500 mL for adults). A balanced salt solution is generally used, but other components are frequently added, including colloid (albumin or hetastarch), mannitol (for renal protection), heparin, bicarbonate, and potassium (if cardioplegia will not be used). Hemodilution usually occurs at the onset of bypass such that the hematocrit decreases to about 25% in most patients. Blood is used as a priming solution for small pediatric and severely anemic adult patients to prevent severe hemodilution.

Reservoir

The reservoir of the CPB machine receives blood from the patient (usually from the right atrium) via one or two venous cannulas. Blood flows to the reservoir by gravity drainage. Because venous pressure is normally low, the driving force is directly proportionate to the difference in height between the patient and the reservoir but inversely proportionate to the resistance of the cannulas and tubing. Once the machine is primed, a siphon effect is created. Entrainment of air can produce an air lock that may prevent blood flow. The fluid level in the reservoir is critical: if the reservoir is allowed to empty, air can enter the main pump and cause fatal air embolism. A low reservoir level alarm is typically present.

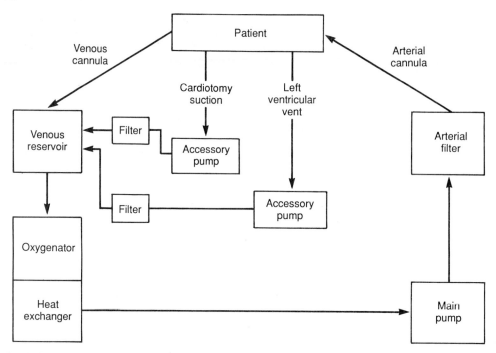

Figure 21–1. The basic design of cardiopulmonary bypass machines. Note that the pump is normally placed after a bubble oxygenator but must be placed before a membrane oxygenator, because the latter type offers greater resistance to blood flow than the bubble type.

Oxygenator

Blood is drained by gravity from the bottom of the venous reservoir into the oxygenator. The two types of oxygenators currently in use—bubble and membrane—differ in the blood-gas interface. At the interface, blood equilibrates with the gas mixture (oxygen) passed through the oxygenator. Carbon dioxide and volatile anesthetics are also frequently added at the oxygenator gas inlet.

A. Bubble Oxygenators: In bubble oxygenators, tiny bubbles (foam) are formed as the in-flowing gas passes through small holes at the base of a blood column. The smaller the bubbles, the larger the surface area for blood to equilibrate with the inflow gases. Bubbles are then removed by passing blood past a defoaming agent (a charged silicone polymer). Oxygenation is dependent on surface area (bubble size and number), oxygen concentration, and transit time of the blood in the oxygenating column. Carbon dioxide elimination is directly proportionate to gas flow and is generally not a problem. Addition of CO_2 gas is often necessary if a normal temperature-corrected arterial CO_2 tension is desired (see below). Bubble oxygenators are generally less expensive than the membrane type and are in wider use. A major disadvantage of bubble oxygenators is trauma to the formed elements in blood, which becomes more significant with longer periods of bypass. For most procedures where CPB is less than 2 hours in duration, the differences between bubble and membrane oxygenators do not appear to be clinically significant.

B. Membrane Oxygenators: The blood-gas interface in a membrane oxygenator is a very thin, gas-permeable silicone membrane. Oxygenation is generally inversely related to the thickness of the blood film in contact with the membrane. As with bubble oxygenators, the final (arterial) CO_2 tension is dependent on total gas flow. Membrane oxygenators are clearly less traumatic to blood and are preferred if a long bypass period is anticipated.

Heat Exchanger

Blood from the oxygenator enters the heat exchanger. The blood is then either cooled or warmed, depending on the temperature of the water flowing through the exchanger. Because gas solubility decreases as blood temperature rises, a filter is built into the unit to catch any bubbles that may form during rewarming.

Main Pump

Modern CPB machines use either an electrically driven double-arm roller or a centrifugal pump to propel blood through the CPB circuit.

A. Roller Pumps: Roller pumps produce flow by compressing large-bore tubing in the main pumping chamber as the heads turn. Subtotal occlusion of the tubing prevents excessive red cell trauma. The constant speed of the rollers pumps blood regardless of resistance encountered and produces continuous non-pulsatile flow. Flow is directly proportionate to the number of revolutions per minute. All roller pumps have a hand crank that can be used in case of electrical power failure.

B. Centrifugal Pumps: Centrifugal pumps consist of a series of cones in a plastic housing. As the cones spin, the blood at the centrally located inlet is propelled to the periphery by the centrifugal forces generated. In contrast to roller pumps, blood flow with centrifugal pumps is pressure-sensitive and must be monitored by an electromagnetic flowmeter. Increases in distal pressure will decrease flow and must be compensated by increasing the pump speed. Because these pumps are nonocclusive, they are less traumatic to blood than roller pumps.

C. Pulsatile Flow: Pulsatile blood flow is possible with some roller pumps. Pulsations can be produced by instantaneous variations in the rate of rotation of the roller heads or by addition of pulsations after flow is generated. Pulsatile flow is not available with centrifugal pumps. Although the matter is controversial, some clinicians feel that pulsatile flow improves tissue perfusion, enhances oxygen extraction, and results in lower systemic vascular resistances during CPB. These observations are supported by experimental studies reporting improved renal and cerebral blood flow during pulsatile perfusion in animals.

Arterial Filter

Particulate matter (thrombi, fat globules, calcium, and tissue debris) enters the CPB circuit with alarming regularity. Although filters are often used at other locations, a final in-line arterial filter (27–40 μm) is mandatory to prevent systemic embolism. Once filtered, the propelled blood returns to the patient, usually via a cannula in the ascending aorta. A normally functioning aortic valve prevents blood from entering the left ventricle.

The filter is always constructed with a (normally clamped) bypass limb in case it becomes clogged or develops high resistance. For the same reason, arterial inflow pressure is measured before the filter. The filter is also designed to trap air, which can be bled out through a built-in stopcock.

Accessory Pumps

A. Cardiotomy Suction: The cardiotomy suction pump aspirates blood from the surgical field during CPB and returns it to the main pump reservoir. A cell-saver suction device may also be used, but that blood is returned to a separate reservoir. At the end of the procedure, the cell-saver blood is centrifuged, washed, and given back to the patient. Excessive suction pressure contributes to red cell trauma. Moreover, excessive use of cell-saver suction (instead of cardiotomy suction) during bypass depletes CPB circuit volume. The high negative pressure of ordinary wall suction produces excessive red cell trauma and precludes blood salvage from that source.

B. Left Ventricular Vent: With time, even after institution of total bypass, blood reaccumulates in the left ventricle as a result of residual pulmonary flow from the bronchial arteries (which arise directly from the aorta or the intercostal arteries) or thebesian vessels (Chapter 19) or as a result of aortic regurgitation. Aortic regurgitation may occur either as a result of surgical manipulation of the heart (functional) or structural valvular abnormalities. Distention of the left ventricle compromises myocardial preservation (see below) and requires decompression (venting). In most centers, this is accomplished by a catheter inserted into the left ventricle via the right superior pulmonary vein and left atrium. Venting is less commonly accomplished through a catheter in the left ventricular apex. The blood aspirated by the vent pump normally passes through a filter and is returned to the venous reservoir.

C. Cardioplegia Pump: Cardioplegia is most often administered via an accessory pump on the CPB machine. This technique allows optimal control over the infusion pressure, rate, and temperature (see below). A separate heat exchanger ensures control of the cardioplegia solution's temperature. Alternatively, cardioplegia may be infused from a cold intravenous fluid bag under pressure.

HYPOTHERMIA

Intentional hypothermia is routinely used following the initiation of CPB. Core body temperature is usually reduced to 20–28 °C. Metabolic oxygen requirements are generally halved with each reduction of 10 °C in body temperature. At the end of the surgical procedure, rewarming via the heat exchanger restores normal body temperature. Profound hypothermia to temperatures of 15–18 °C allows total circulatory arrest for complex repairs for up to 60 minutes. During that time, both the heart and the CPB machine are stopped.

MYOCARDIAL PRESERVATION

Nearly all patients sustain some myocardial damage during cardiac surgery. With proper preservation techniques, however, most of the damage is usually reversible. Although myocardial injury can be related to the anesthetic or surgical technique, it most commonly appears to be related to suboptimal myocardial preservation during CPB. The common denominator in all instances is an imbalance between myocardial oxygen demand and supply, resulting in cell ischemia, injury, or death. Patients at greatest risk are those in functional class IV (New York Heart Association; Table 20–12) or those who have ventricular hypertrophy or severe coronary artery disease. Inadequate myocardial preservation is usually manifested at the end of bypass as a persistently low cardiac output, as myocardial ischemia, or as cardiac arrhythmias.

Aortic cross-clamping during CPB completely abolishes coronary blood flow. While estimates of a safe cross-clamping period are not valid owing to differing vulnerabilities between patients, CPB times longer than 120 minutes are generally considered undesirable. Myocardial ischemia during bypass can also occur before or after cross-clamping. Low arterial pressures, coronary embolism (due to thrombi, platelets, air, fat, or calcium), and excessive surgical manipulation of the heart—causing compression or distortion of the coronary vessels—are all contributory. Areas of myocardium distal to a high-grade coronary obstruction are at greatest risk.

Ischemia causes depletion of high-energy phosphate compounds and an accumulation of intracellular calcium. The latter, through its action on contractile proteins, further depletes energy supplies (Chapter 19). Maintenance of normal cellular integrity and function during CPB depends on reducing energy expenditure and preserving the availability of high-energy phosphate compounds. When coronary blood flow ceases, creatine phosphate and anaerobic metabolism become the principal sources of cellular energy; fatty acid oxidation is impaired. Unfortunately, these energy stores rapidly become depleted, and glycolysis is limited by the progressive acidosis that develops. While measures directed at increasing or replenishing energy substrates in the form of glucose or glutamate infusions are used, the emphasis of myocardial preservation has been on reducing cellular energy requirements to minimal. This is accomplished by systemic (see above) and topical hypothermia (ice slush) and the use of potassium cardioplegia (see below). (Myocardial temperatures of 10–15 °C are usually considered desirable.) The former reduces basal metabolic oxygen consumption, while the latter abolishes the energy expenditure associated with both electrical and mechanical activity.

Ventricular fibrillation and distention are important causes of myocardial damage. Fibrillation can double myocardial oxygen consumption, while distention not only increases oxygen demand but also reduces oxygen supply by interfering with subendocardial blood flow,. Other factors perhaps contributing to myocardial damage include the use of inotropes and excessive administration of calcium.

Potassium Cardioplegia

The most widely used method of arresting myocardial electrical activity is the administration of potassium-rich crystalloid or blood. Following initiation of CPB, induction of hypothermia, and aortic cross-clamping, the coronary circulation is perfused with cold cardioplegia. The resulting increase in extracellular potassium concentration reduces the transmembrane potential (less negative). The latter progressively interferes with the normal sodium current during depolarization, decreasing the rate of rise, amplitude, and conduction velocity of subsequent action potentials (Chapter 19). Eventually, the sodium channels are completely inactivated, action potentials are abolished, and the heart is arrested in diastole. Multiple doses of cold cardioplegia are usually necessary (about every 30 minutes) because of gradual washout of cardioplegia and rewarming of the myocardium.

Washout occurs as a result of persistence of noncollateral coronary blood flow derived from pericardial vessels, which are branches of intercostal arteries. Moreover, multiple-dose cardioplegia may improve myocardial preservation by preventing the excessive build-up of metabolites that inhibit anaerobic metabolism. Preferential warming of the posterior ventricular wall can also occur as a result of direct contact with warmer blood in the descending aorta.

Typical components of potassium cardioplegia are given in Table 21–1. Although the exact composition varies from center to center, the essential elements of cardioplegia are the same. Potassium concentration is kept below 50 meq/L, because higher levels can be associated with a paradoxic increase in myocardial energy requirements and excessive potassium loads. Sodium concentration in cardioplegia is less than that in plasma because ischemia tends to increase intracellular sodium content. A small amount of calcium is needed to maintain cellular integrity, while magnesium appears to control an excessive influx of calcium intracellularly. A buffer—most commonly bicarbonate—is necessary to prevent excessive build-up of acid metabolites; in fact, alkalotic perfusates are reported to produce better myocardial preservation. Alternative buffers include histidine and tromethamine. Other components may include hypertonic agents to control cellular edema (mannitol), glucocorticoids (for its membrane-stabilizing effect), prostacyclin (for its antiplatelet effect), and calcium channel or β-adrenergic blockers (to reduce metabolic demand). Energy substrates may be provided as glucose, glutamate, or aspartate. The question of whether to use crystalloid or blood as a vehicle for achieving cardioplegia remains controversial. Evidence suggests that at least some groups of high-risk patients may do better with blood cardioplegia. Certainly, oxygenated blood cardioplegia has the added benefit of delivering more oxygen than crystalloid cardioplegia.

Because cardioplegia may not reach areas distal to high-grade coronary obstructions (the areas that need it most), many surgeons now also administer cardioplegia retrogradely through the coronary sinus.

Excessive cardioplegia can result in an absence of electrical activity, atrioventricular conduction block, or a poorly contractile heart at the end of bypass. Persistent systemic hyperkalemia may also result. Although calcium administration partially offsets these effects, excessive calcium can enhance myocardial damage. Myocardial performance generally improves with time as the contents of the cardioplegia are cleared from the heart.

Table 21–1. Typical components of cardioplegia solutions.

Potassium	20–40 meq/L
Sodium	100–120 meq/L
Chloride	110–120 meq/L
Calcium	0.7 meq/L
Magnesium	15 meq/L
Glucose	28 mmol/L
Bicarbonate	27 mmol/L

APPROACH TO ANESTHETIC MANAGEMENT OF CARDIAC SURGERY IN ADULTS

The preoperative evaluation and anesthetic management of common cardiovascular diseases are discussed in Chapter 20. The same principles apply whether these patients are undergoing cardiac or noncardiac surgery. An important distinction is that patients undergoing cardiac procedures generally have more advanced disease. The importance of establishing the adequacy of cardiac reserve cannot be overemphasized. This information must be based on exercise (activity) tolerance, measurements of myocardial contractility such as ejection fraction, the severity and location of coronary stenoses, ventricular wall motion abnormalities, cardiac end-diastolic pressures, cardiac output, and valvular gradients (Chapter 20). Fortunately, the surgery improves cardiac function in most patients. Preoperative evaluation should also focus on pulmonary, neurologic, and renal function (Chapters 23, 27, and 32, respectively), since impairment of these organ systems predisposes to postoperative complications.

PREINDUCTION PERIOD

Premedication

The prospect of heart surgery is frightening to most patients. Relatively heavy predication is generally desirable, particularly for patients with coronary artery disease (Chapter 20). Conversely, light premedication is more appropriate in frail patients with valvular disease, who are often physiologically dependent on enhanced sympathetic tone. Habitus, age, and physiologic status should be considered in selecting agents and dosages.

Benzodiazepine sedative-hypnotics (midazolam, 5–10 mg; diazepam, 5–10 mg; or lorazepam, 2–4 mg), alone or in combination with an opioid (morphine, 5–10 mg), are most often used. Alternatively, the time-honored combination of intramuscular morphine, 0.1–0.2 mg/kg, and scopolamine, 0.2–0.4 mg, also provides excellent sedation, analgesia, and amnesia. Dosages should be reduced in patients with poor cardiac reserve and those with underlying pulmonary disease. Supplemental oxygen (2–3 L/min via nasal cannula) is useful in avoiding hypoxemia following premedication.

Preparation

Formulation of a clear anesthetic plan and adequate preparations are essential for cardiac anesthesia. Many patients are critically ill, and there is little time intraoperatively to debate the merits of one technique over another or to search for drugs and equipment. At the same time, the anesthetic plan should not be rigid; if problems are encountered with one technique, the anesthesiologist should be ready to change to another without delay. Organization and meticulous attention to detail are crucial in dealing with intraoperative problems. The anesthesia machine, monitors, infusion pumps, and blood warmer should all be checked before the patient arrives. Drugs—including anesthetic and vasoactive agents—should be immediately available. Ideally, one vasodilator and one inotropic infusion solution should be mixed and ready for use before the start of the procedure.

Venous Access

Cardiac surgery is commonly associated with large and rapid fluid shifts, often with the need for multiple drug infusions. Ideally, two large-bore (16- or 14-gauge) intravenous catheters should be placed. One of these should be in a large central vein, usually the internal jugular vein. The subclavian and external jugular veins are suitable alternatives. Entry into the superior vena cava is not always possible with the latter; nonetheless, it serves as a good site for an extra peripheral intravenous line. Cannulations are usually accomplished while the patient is awake but sedated from premedication. Additional small doses of a narcotic or midazolam may be necessary for central catheterization. Supplemental oxygen via a nasal cannula or a nonrebreathing face mask (together with the use of a pulse oximeter) usually avoids hypoxemia during catheterization.

Multilumen central venous catheters facilitate drug infusion and allow simultaneous measurement of central venous pressures. The side port of the introducer sheath used for a pulmonary catheter can also be used for drug infusions. The catheter site for each intravenous tubing should be clearly marked close to the injection ports. One intravenous port should be dedicated for drug infusions and nothing else and another port for drug boluses. Drug infusions should ideally be given into a central catheter, preferably directly into the catheter or into the injection port closest to the catheter (to minimize dead space).

Blood should be available for immediate transfusion if the patient has already had a midline sternotomy ("redo"); in these cases, the right ventricle may be adherent to the sternum and may be inadvertently entered during the repeat sternotomy.

Monitoring

With few exceptions, most monitors are instituted prior to induction of anesthesia, as this period represents one of the major hemodynamic stresses of the procedure.

A. Electrocardiography: The ECG is continuously monitored with two leads, usually leads II and V_5. Baseline tracings of all leads should be recorded on paper for further reference. The recent advent of monitors with computerized ST segment analysis has improved detection of ischemic episodes.

B. Arterial Blood Pressure: Arterial blood pressure should generally be directly monitored by catheterization of the radial artery in the nondominant hand. The side of a brachial artery cutdown (for cardiac catheterization) should not be used, because doing so is associated with a high incidence of arterial thrombosis and wave distortion. Other useful catheterization sites include the ulnar, brachial, femoral, and axillary arteries. A backup manual or automatic blood pressure cuff should also be in place for comparison with direct measurements.

C. Central Venous and Pulmonary Artery Pressure: Central venous pressure should be monitored in all patients. The decision whether or not to use a pulmonary artery catheter is based on the patient, the procedure, and the preferences of the surgical team. Routine use of a pulmonary artery catheter is controversial. Left ventricular filling pressures may be measured with a left atrial pressure line inserted by the surgeon during bypass. In general, pulmonary artery catheterization should be employed in patients with compromised ventricular function (ejection fraction < 40–50%) or pulmonary hypertension and in those undergoing complicated procedures. The most useful data are pulmonary artery pressures, the wedge pressure, and thermodilution cardiac outputs (Chapter 6). Specialized catheters are also available that provide extra infusion ports, continuous measurements of mixed venous oxygen saturation or right ventricular ejection fraction, or right ventricular pacing. Baseline pressure traces and readings should be obtained and recorded prior to induction.

Pulmonary artery catheters often migrate distally during CPB and may become permanently wedged. Inflation of the balloon under these conditions can rupture a pulmonary artery. When a pulmonary artery catheter is used, it should be routinely pulled back slightly (2–3 cm) during CPB and the balloon subsequently inflated slowly. If the catheter wedges with less than 1.5 mL of air in the balloon, it should be pulled back farther.

D. Urinary Output: Once the patient is asleep, an indwelling urinary catheter is placed to monitor the hourly urinary output. The sudden appearance of red urine may indicate excessive red hemolysis due to CPB or a transfusion reaction.

E. Temperature: Temperature monitors are also usually placed once the patient is anesthetized. Rectal (or bladder), esophageal, and pulmonary artery (blood) temperatures are usually simultaneously monitored.

F. Laboratory Parameters: Intraoperative laboratory monitoring is also important during cardiac surgery. Blood gases, hematocrit, activated clotting time (ACT), and serum potassium measurement capabilities should be immediately available. Glucose and ionized calcium measurements are also useful.

G. Surgical Field: One of the most important intraoperative monitors is that of the surgical field. Once the sternum is opened, lung expansion can be seen through the pleura. When the pericardium is opened, the heart (primarily the right ventricle) is visible, so

that cardiac rhythm, volume, and contractility can often be judged visually. Blood loss and surgical maneuvers must be closely watched and related to changes in hemodynamics and rhythm.

H. Electroencephalography: Computer-processed electroencephalographic recordings can be useful in assessing anesthetic depth during cardiac surgery. The utility of this resource in detecting neurologic insults during CPB, however, is limited by the combined effects of anesthetic agents, hypothermia, and hemodilution. Progressive hypothermia is typically associated with electroencephalographic slowing, burst suppression, and finally an isoelectric recording. Moreover, most strokes during CPB are due to small emboli and are not likely to be detected on the EEG. Artifacts from the CPB roller pump may be seen on the raw EEG but can usually be identified as such by computer processing.

I. Transesophageal Echocardiography (TEE): TEE is a rapidly evolving monitoring modality that can provide valuable information about cardiac anatomy and function during surgery. Two-dimensional TEE can detect regional and global ventricular abnormalities, chamber dimensions, valvular anatomy, and the presence of intracardiac air. Two views are most commonly used during cardiac surgery (Figure 21–2). Doppler color flow imaging during echocardiography further delineates intracardiac blood flow, which allows detection of valvular dysfunction as well as of intracardiac shunts. Colors are usually adjusted so that flow toward the probe is red while flow in the opposite direction is blue. Unfortunately, the cost of these sophisticated monitors limits their widespread use.

Induction

Cardiac operations require general anesthesia, endotracheal intubation, and controlled ventilation. For elective procedures, induction should generally be performed in a slow, smooth, controlled fashion often referred to as a "cardiac induction." The principles are discussed in Chapter 20. Selection of anesthetic agents (see below) is generally less important than the way they are used. It should be emphasized that dose requirements are extremely variable and generally inversely related to ventricular function. Severely compromised patients should be given anesthetic agents slowly and in small increments. A series of challenges may be used to judge when anesthetic depth will allow intubation without a marked vasopressor response or excessive hypotension. Blood pressure and heart rate are continuously evaluated following unconsciousness (loss of the eyelid reflex), insertion of an oral airway, urinary catheterization, insertion of the rectal temperature probe, and finally intubation. A sudden increase in heart rate or blood pressure indicates light anesthesia and the need for more anesthetic prior to the next challenge, while a decrease or no change suggests that the patient is ready for the subsequent stimulus. The muscle relaxant is given as soon as consciousness is lost. Blood pressure reductions greater than 20% gen-

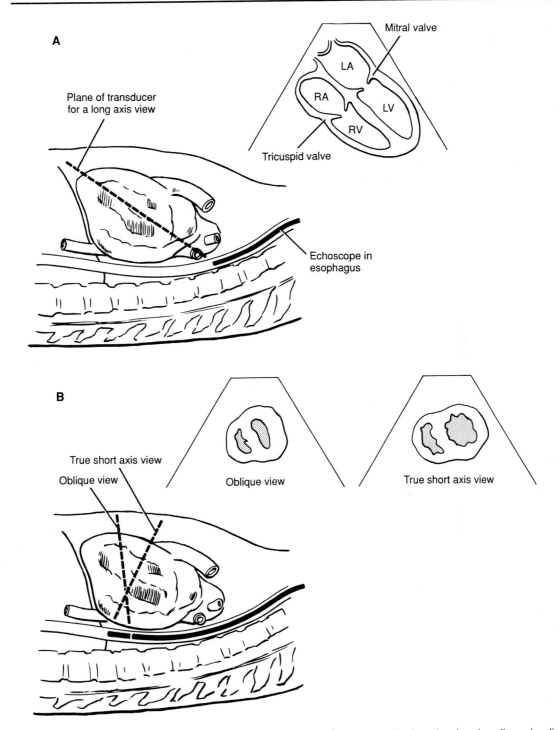

Figure 21–2. The most useful views during transesophageal echocardiography. *A:* The four-chamber view allows visualization of mitral and tricuspid valves and the ventricular septum; all four chamber dimensions can also be evaluated. *B:* The lower short-axis view at the midpapillary level displays myocardium supplied by all three coronary arteries and provides important information on ventricular size and contractility. A good view of the aortic valve can also be obtained from the mid esophagus (not shown).

erally call for administration of a vasopressor (see below).

The period following intubation is often characterized by a gradual decrease in blood pressure resulting from the anesthetized state and a lack of surgical stimulation. Patients are often volume-depleted from preoperative fasting or diuretic therapy and usually respond to fluid boluses. Colloid boluses are in most cases more effective in rapidly expanding intravascular volume than crystalloid boluses (Chapter 29). Small doses of phenylephrine (50–100 μg) or ephedrine (5–10 mg) may be necessary to avoid excessive hypotension. Following intubation and controlled ventilation, hemodynamic measurements are usually repeated; the baseline ACT (normal: < 130 seconds), arterial blood gases, hematocrit, and serum potassium concentration are measured.

Choice of Anesthetic Agents

Although the choice of anesthesia is often thought of as total intravenous versus inhalational, a combination of the two techniques is often used. Total intravenous techniques are generally most suitable for patients with severely compromised ventricular function, while predominantly inhalational techniques are reserved for patients with relatively good ventricular function (ejection fraction 40–50%). In either case, a muscle relaxant must be used to facilitate endotracheal intubation and retraction of the chest and to prevent patient movement and shivering.

A. Inhalation Technique: Inhalational anesthesia is in almost all cases preceded by intravenous induction. Barbiturates, benzodiazepines, opioids, etomidate, propofol, or ketamine, alone or in combination, can be used. Following loss of consciousness, the muscle relaxant is given and a volatile agent is added; its concentration is slowly increased and carefully titrated to the blood pressure. The patient is intubated when anesthetic depth is judged to be sufficient (see above). The major advantage of volatile agents is one's ability to change the anesthetic concentration rapidly. Their principal disadvantage is dose-dependent direct cardiac depression. In spite of reports of its having induced intracoronary steal (Chapter 20), isoflurane remains the most commonly used volatile agent. Nitrous oxide is generally not used because of its tendency to expand any intravascular air bubbles that may form during CPB. When nitrous oxide is used, it should be discontinued 15–20 minutes prior to CPB.

B. Total Intravenous Techniques: High-dose opioid techniques were developed for and continue to be widely used in cardiac anesthesia. The two most commonly used agents, fentanyl and sufentanil, are associated with minimal cardiac depression and relatively stable hemodynamics when given alone. However, when combined with small doses of other intravenous agents, such as benzodiazepines or barbiturates, hypotension due to vasodilation and possibly cardiac depression may be seen. Narcotic-induced bradycardia and muscle rigidity may occur, especially with rapid administration (Chapter 8). A muscle relax-

ant should be given as soon as consciousness is lost to prevent rigidity.

The opioid may be administered in boluses or as a loading dose followed by a continuous infusion. Fentanyl is given as a slow bolus of 25–30 μg/kg for induction and intubation; maintenance anesthesia is provided by additional boluses of 5 μg/kg as needed or by a continuous infusion of 0.3–0.5 μg/kg/min. The total dose of fentanyl used is generally 50–100 μg/kg. The same technique using sufentanil generally employs 5–10 μg/kg for induction and intubation, followed by 1 μg/kg boluses or 0.075 μg/kg/min as a continuous infusion. The total dose of sufentanil is generally 15–25 μg/kg.

High-dose opioid techniques have two major potential disadvantages, ie, failure to control the hypertensive response to stimulation and patient awareness (recall) during surgery. Hypertension is most common in patients with good ventricular function and least likely to occur in those receiving β-adrenergic blockers or those who have marked ventricular dysfunction. Addition of a vasodilator (nitroprusside), a beta-blocker (esmolol), or a volatile agent may be necessary during periods of increased stimulation to prevent hypertension. The likelihood of awareness is diminished by the concomitant use of a benzodiazepine or a low dose of volatile agent.

The combination of ketamine with midazolam (in a 20:1 ratio) for induction and as a complete anesthetic via continuous infusion is also associated with relatively stable hemodynamics and good amnesia.

C. Muscle Relaxants: Unless airway difficulties are expected, intubation is usually performed with a nondepolarizing muscle relaxant. The choice of muscle relaxant is based chiefly on the desired hemodynamic response. Ideally, in most instances, the agent should be devoid of circulatory effects. Vecuronium, doxacurium, and pipecuronium would therefore seem to be good choices. Vecuronium, however, has been reported to markedly enhance opioid-induced bradycardia. Pancuronium may be a better choice with high-dose opioid anaesthesia because of its vagolytic effects. A mixture of pancuronium and metocurine (in a 1:3 ratio) also provides good hemodynamic stability without inducing tachycardia or histamine-mediated hypotension (Chapter 9).

PREBYPASS PERIOD

Following induction and intubation, the anesthetic course is typically characterized by an initial period of minimal stimulation (skin preparation and draping) that is frequently associated with hypotension, followed by discrete periods of intense stimulation that can produce tachycardia and hypertension. These periods of stimulation include the skin incision, sternotomy and sternal retraction, opening the pericardium, and aortic dissection. The anesthetic agent should be adjusted appropriately in anticipation of these events. Accentuated vagal responses resulting in marked bradycardia and hypotension may occur during sternal retraction or opening of the pericardium. This response may be more pronounced in patients who have been taking β-adrenergic blocking agents or verapamil. Deeply anesthetized patients frequently have a progressive decline in cardiac output after the chest is opened. The reduction in cardiac output is probably due to decreased venous return as the normally negative intrathoracic pressure becomes atmospheric. Intravenous fluid administration at least partially reverses this effect.

Myocardial ischemia in the prebypass period is usually (not always) associated with hemodynamic perturbations such as tachycardia, hypertension, or hypotension. Although controversial, prophylactic infusion of nitroglycerin (1–2 µg/kg/min) intraoperatively may reduce the incidence of ischemic episodes.

Cannulation

Cannulation for CPB is a critical time. Aortic cannulation is usually done first because of the hemodynamic problems frequently associated with venous cannulation (see below). Moreover, rapid fluid infusions can be given through the aortic cannula if necessary. The ascending aorta is most often utilized. The small opening of most arterial cannulas produces a jet stream that, if not positioned properly, can cause aortic dissection or preferential flow of blood to the innominate artery during CPB. Reduction of systemic arterial pressure (to 90–100 mm Hg systolic) facilitates placement of the aortic cannula. Bubbles should be completely removed from the arterial cannula, and backflow of blood into the arterial line must be demonstrated before bypass is initiated. Failure to remove all the bubbles results in air emboli, usually into the coronary or cerebral circulations, while failure to enter the aorta properly results in aortic dissection. Some clinicians advocate temporary compression of the carotid arteries during aortic cannulation to decrease the likelihood of reducing cerebral emboli.

One or two venous cannulas are placed in the right atrium, usually through the right atrial appendage. One venous cannula is usually adequate for most coronary artery bypass and aortic valve operations. The single cannula used often has two ports (two-stage) such that when it is properly positioned, one is in the right atrium and the other is in the inferior vena cava.

Separate caval cannulas are used for open heart procedures. Hypotension due to impaired ventricular filling often occurs during manipulation of the venae cavae and the heart. Venous cannulation also frequently precipitates atrial or, less commonly, ventricular arrhythmias. Premature atrial contractions and transient bursts of a supraventricular tachycardia are common. Sustained paroxysmal atrial tachycardia or atrial fibrillation frequently leads to hemodynamic deterioration, which must be treated pharmacologically, electrically, or by immediate anticoagulation and initiation of bypass. Malpositioning of the venous cannulas can interfere with venous return or impede venous drainage from the head and neck (superior vena cava syndrome). Upon initiation of CPB, the former is manifested as poor venous return to the reservoir, while the latter produces edema of the head and neck. Under these circumstances, central venous pressure increases only if the tip of the catheter is high in the vena cava.

Anticoagulation

Anticoagulation must be established prior to CPB to prevent acute disseminated intravascular coagulation and formation of clots in the pump. Moreover, the adequacy of anticoagulation must be confirmed with determination of the ACT. An ACT longer than 400–450 seconds is considered safe at most centers. Heparin, 300–400 units/kg, is usually given while the aortic pursestring sutures are placed during cannulation. Many surgeons prefer to give the heparin themselves directly into the right atrium. If administered by the anesthesiologist, heparin should be given through a central line and the ACT should be measured after 3–5 minutes. Heparin resistance is occasionally encountered; most patients have antithrombin III deficiency and will achieve adequate anticoagulation following infusion of two units of fresh frozen plasma.

BYPASS PERIOD

Initiation

Once the cannulas are properly placed and secured, the ACT is acceptable, and the perfusionist is ready, CPB is initiated. The clamps placed across cannulas during insertion are removed (venous first, then arterial), and the main CPB pump is started. Establishing the adequacy of venous return to the pump reservoir is critical. Normally, the reservoir level rises and CPB pump flow is gradually increased. If venous return is poor, as demonstrated by a decreasing reservoir level, the pump prime will quickly empty and air can enter the pump circuit. The cannulas should be checked for proper placement, forgotten clamps, kinks, or an air lock. Under these circumstances, pump flow should be slowed until the problem is resolved. Adding volume (blood or colloid) to the reservoir may be necessary. With full CPB, the heart should gradually empty; failure to do so or progressive distention implies malpositioning of the venous cannula or aortic regurgitation. In the latter instance, immediate aortic cross-clamping and administration of cardioplegia is necessary.

Flow & Pressure

Systemic arterial pressure is closely monitored as pump flow is gradually increased to 2–2.5 L/min/m². At the onset of CPB, systemic arterial pressure usually decreases abruptly. Initial mean systemic arterial (radial) pressures of 30–40 mm Hg are not unusual. This decrease is usually attributed to abrupt hemodilution, which reduces blood viscosity and effectively lowers systemic vascular resistance. The effect is partially compensated by subsequent hypothermia, which tends to raise blood viscosity again.

Persistent and excessive decreases (< 30 mm Hg) should prompt a search for unrecognized aortic dissection. If dissection is present, CPB must be temporarily stopped until the aorta is recannulated distally. Other possible causes include poor venous return, pump malfunction, or pressure transducer error. Factitious hypertension can occur when the right radial artery is used for monitoring and the aortic cannula is directed preferentially toward the innominate artery.

During CPB, the relationship between pump flow, systemic vascular resistance (SVR), and mean systemic arterial blood pressure may be conceptualized as follows:

Mean arterial pressure = Pump flow × SVR

Consequently, with a constant systemic vascular resistance, mean arterial pressure is proportionate to pump flow. Similarly, at any given pump flow, mean arterial pressure is proportionate to systemic vascular resistance. The general conduct of CPB should be such as to maintain both adequate arterial pressures and blood flows by manipulating pump flow and systemic vascular resistance. Although some controversy still surrounds this issue, most centers strive for blood flows of 2–2.5 L/min/m² (50–60 mL/kg/min) and mean arterial pressures between 50 and 80 mm Hg. Flow requirements are generally proportionate to core body temperature. Evidence also suggests that during moderate hypothermia (20–25 °C), mean blood pressures as low as 30 mm Hg may still provide adequate cerebral blood flow. Systemic vascular resistance can be increased with phenylephrine or methoxamine.

High systemic arterial pressures (> 150 mm Hg) are also deleterious and may promote aortic dissection or cerebral hemorrhage. Generally, when mean arterial pressure exceeds 100 mm Hg, hypertension is said to exist and is treated by decreasing pump flow or adding isoflurane to the oxygenator inflow gas (see below). If the hypertension is refractory to these maneuvers or if pump flow is already low, a vasodilator such as nitroprusside is used.

Monitoring

Additional monitoring objectives during CPB include the pump flow rate, venous reservoir level, arterial inflow line pressure (see above), blood (perfusate) temperature, and in-line oxygen saturation. In-line pH, CO_2 tension, and oxygen tension sensors are also available. Blood gas tensions and pH should be confirmed by direct measurements (see below). In the absence of hypoxemia, low mixed venous oxygen saturations and a progressive metabolic acidosis are indicative of inadequate flow rates.

During bypass, arterial inflow line pressure is nearly always higher than the systemic arterial pressure recorded from a radial artery or even an aortic catheter. The difference in pressure represents the pressure drop across the arterial filter, the arterial tubing, and the narrow opening of the aortic cannula. Nonetheless,

monitoring this pressure is important in detecting problems with an arterial inflow line. Inflow pressures should remain below 300 mm Hg; higher pressures may be indicative of a clogged arterial filter, obstruction of the arterial tubing or cannula, or aortic dissection.

Serial ACT, hematocrit, and potassium measurements are necessary during bypass. The ACT is measured immediately after bypass and every subsequent 20–30 minutes. Cooling generally increases the half-life of heparin and prolongs its effect. A heparin dose-response curve is often used to facilitate calculation of subsequent heparin doses and protamine reversal (Figure 21–3). Although the relationship does not always conform to a linear function, it remains clinically useful. The hematocrit is usually kept between 20% and 25%. Red cell transfusions into the pump reservoir may be necessary. Marked increases in serum potassium concentrations (secondary to cardioplegia) are usually treated with furosemide.

Hypothermia & Cardioplegia

Moderate hypothermia (20–25 °C) is used routinely for most procedures. The lower the temperature, the longer the time necessary for cooling and rewarming. Low temperatures, however, allow lower CPB flows. At a temperature of 20 °C, flows as low as 1.2 L/min/m² may be adequate.

Ventricular fibrillation often occurs as the heart is cooled below 28 °C. Cardioplegia should established immediately, since fibrillation rapidly consumes high-energy phosphates and jeopardizes myocardial preservation (see above). Cardioplegia is achieved by cross-clamping the ascending aorta proximal to the aortic inflow cannula and infusing cardioplegia solution through a small catheter proximal to the cross-clamp; alternatively, it can be given directly into the coronary ostia if the aorta is opened. During aortocoronary bypass grafting, cardioplegia solution may also be given through the graft if the surgeon elects to do the distal anastomosis first. In the presence of severe coronary obstructions, many surgeons will also employ retrograde cardioplegia via a catheter in the coronary sinus (see above).

Ventilation

Ventilation of the lungs is usually continued until adequate pump flows are reached and the heart stops ejecting blood. Following institution of full CPB, ventricular ejection continues briefly until left ventricular volume reaches a critical low level. Discontinuing ventilation prematurely causes any remaining pulmonary blood flow to act as a right-to-left shunt that may promote hypoxemia (Chapter 22). The importance of this mechanism depends on the relative ratio of remaining pulmonary blood flow to pump flow. At some centers, once ventilation is stopped, oxygen flow is continued in the anesthesia circuit with a small amount of PEEP (5 cm H_2O) to prevent postoperative pulmonary dysfunction. Most centers stop all gas flow or

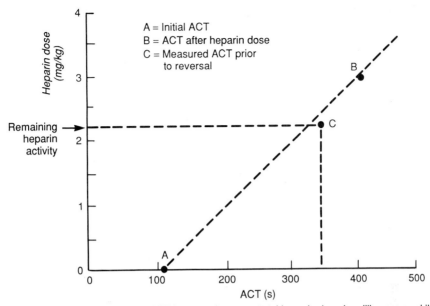

Figure 21–3. Heparin dose-response curve. ACT in seconds versus total heparin dose in milligrams per kilogram.
1. Plot the initial ACT on the *x* axis.
2. Plot the ACT after heparinization.
3. Draw the line that is defined by these two points.
4. If additional anticoagulation is needed, find the desired ACT on that line. The amount of additional heparin needed is the difference on the *y* axis between the present ACT and the desired ACT.
5. If the third point does not lie on the original line, a new line is drawn originating from the baseline ACT and passing midway between the other two points.
6. For reversal of anticoagulation, the protamine dose is based on the remaining heparin activity, which is estimated to be the heparin dose corresponding to the latest ACT on the dose-response line.

continue a low flow of oxygen (1–2 L/min) in the anesthesia circuit. Ventilation is resumed at the conclusion of bypass when the heart begins to eject blood.

Management of Respiratory Gases

Controversy exists about whether to use corrected or uncorrected arterial blood gas tensions during hypothermic CPB. The controversy stems from the fact that the solubility of a gas increases with hypothermia. As a result, although total content does not change (in a closed system), the partial pressure of the gas will decrease as blood temperature drops. The problem is most significant for arterial CO_2 tension because of its effect on arterial pH and cerebral blood flow. Because the plasma bicarbonate concentration does not change, any decrease in arterial CO_2 tension tends to increase pH and make blood alkalotic (by normothermic definitions). Blood with a CO_2 tension of 40 mm Hg and a pH of 7.40 at 37 °C, when cooled to 25 °C will have a CO_2 tension of about 23 mm Hg and a pH of 7.60.

Normally—regardless of the patient's temperature—the blood sample is heated to 37 °C before gas tensions are measured. If the temperature-corrected reading is desired, a table or a program in the blood gas machine can be used to estimate gas tension and pH at the patient's temperature. The practice of temperature-correcting gas tensions and maintaining a "normal"

CO_2 tension of 40 mm Hg and a pH of 7.40 during hypothermia is referred to as "pH-stat management" and has come into question recently. pH-stat management during hypothermic CPB usually requires adding CO_2 to oxygenator gas inflow; in the process, total blood CO_2 content increases. Under these conditions, cerebral blood flow is reported to depend on CO_2 tension and mean arterial blood pressure rather than oxygen consumption (Chapter 25).

The use of uncorrected gas tensions during hypothermia—"α-stat management"—is increasing. The basis of this approach is that preservation of normal protein function depends on maintaining normal intracellular electroneutrality (the balance of charges on proteins). At physiologic pH, these charges are primarily located on the imidazole rings of histidine residues (referred to as α residues). Moreover, as temperature decreases, K_w—the dissociation constant for water—also decreases (pK_w increases). Therefore, at lower temperatures, the electroneutrality of aqueous solutions, where $[H^+] = [OH^-]$, corresponds to a lower $[H^+]$ (a higher pH). Hypothermic "alkalosis" thus does not necessarily reflect $[OH^-] > [H^+]$ but rather an absolute decrease in $[H^+]$. Hypothermic CPB with "α-stat" management usually does not require addition of CO_2 to the oxygenator: the total CO_2 content of blood and electroneutrality are unchanged.

In contrast to "pH-stat" management, "α-stat" appears to preserve cerebral autoregulation of blood flow and may result in improved myocardial preservation. Despite the theoretic and observed differences, comparisons between the two techniques fail to reveal appreciable differences in patient outcome.

Anesthesia

Hypothermia itself is usually anesthetic, but reports of awareness during CPB are common, especially during rewarming. Failure to give anesthetic agents during CPB frequently results in light anesthesia and contributes to awareness. Hypertension often develops and, if muscle paralysis is also allowed to wear off, patient movement may be observed. Additional doses of muscle relaxant and anesthetic agents are necessary during CPB. Low concentrations of a volatile agent (isoflurane) via the oxygenator are frequently employed. The volatile agent, however, should generally be discontinued just prior to termination of bypass to avoid residual myocardial depression. Patients with poor left ventricular function may be very sensitive to the combined residual effects of cardioplegia and a volatile agent. Additional doses of a narcotic or small doses of a benzodiazepine are preferable for these patients. Many clinicians administer a benzodiazepine (midazolam, 5–10 mg intravenously) when rewarming is initiated.

Cerebral Protection

Neurologic complications following CPB may be as high as 40%. Fortunately, in most instances they consist of transient neuropsychiatric dysfunction (ranging from subtle cognitive and intellectual changes to delirium and organic brain syndromes). More serious complications such as strokes are less common. Factors that have been associated with neurologic sequelae include intracardiac (valvular) procedures, advanced age, and preexisting cerebrovascular disease. While embolic phenomena appear responsible for most neurologic deficits, the contribution of cerebral hypoperfusion remains unclear. Although controversial, prophylactic thiopental infusions (completely suppressing electroencephalographic activity) immediately prior to and during bypass have been reported to decrease the incidence and severity of neurologic deficits following intracardiac (open ventricle) procedures but may increase the likelihood of need for inotropic support upon termination of CPB.

TERMINATION OF CPB

Discontinuation of bypass is accomplished by a series of necessary procedures and conditions: (1) rewarming must be completed; (2) air must be evacuated from the heart and any bypass grafts; (3) the aortic cross-clamp must be removed; and (4) lung ventilation must be resumed. The surgeon's decision about when to rewarm is critical; adequate rewarming requires time, but rewarming too soon removes the protective effects of hypothermia. Rapid rewarming often results in large temperature gradients between well-perfused organs and peripheral vasoconstricted tissues; subsequent equilibration decreases core temperature again. Infusion of a vasodilator drug (nitroprusside or nitroglycerin) often speeds the rewarming process and decreases large temperature gradients. Moreover, rapid rewarming can result in formation of gas bubbles in the bloodstream as the solubility of gases rapidly decreases. If the heart fibrillates during rewarming, immediate defibrillation is necessary. Lung inflation facilitates expulsion of (left-sided) intracardiac air by "squeezing" pulmonary vessels and returning blood into the left heart. Transesophageal echocardiography is useful in detecting intracardiac air. Reinflation of the lungs transiently requires higher than normal airway pressure. Overzealous lung expansion can interfere with internal mammary artery grafts.

General guidelines for separation from CPB include the following:

(1) Core body temperature should be at least 37 °C.
(2) A stable rhythm (preferably sinus) must be present. Atrioventricular pacing may be necessary and confers the benefit of a properly timed atrial systole. Persistence of atrioventricular block should prompt measurement of serum potassium concentration. If hyperkalemia is present, it can be treated with calcium, $NaHCO_3$, or glucose and insulin (Chapter 28).
(3) The heart rate must be adequate (generally 80–100 beats/min). Slow heart rates are generally more of a problem than rapid ones and are best treated by pacing. Isoproterenol may be useful in some patients. Supraventricular tachycardias generally require cardioversion.
(4) Laboratory values must be acceptable. Significant acidosis and hyperkalemia should be treated; the hematocrit should be 22–25%.
(5) Adequate ventilation with 100% oxygen must have been resumed.
(6) All monitors must have been recalibrated.

Weaning from CPB

Discontinuation of CPB should be gradual as systemic arterial pressure, ventricular volumes and filling pressures, and cardiac output (if available) are assessed. Central aortic pressure is often measured directly and should be correlated with the radial artery pressure. A reversal of the normal systolic pressure gradient between these two sites is often observed (aortic pressure becomes higher than radial pressure). Central aortic root pressure can also be estimated manually by the surgeon. Ventricular volume and contractility can be estimated visually, while filling pressures are measured directly by central venous, pulmonary artery, or left atrial catheters. Cardiac output is measured by thermodilution. Transesophageal echocardiography can also provide invaluable information about chamber volumes, contractility, and valvular function.

Table 21–2. Hemodynamic subgroups post-CPB.

	Group I Vigorous	Group II Hypovolemia	Group III Pump Failure	Group IV Hyperdynamic
Filling pressure	Low	Low	Normal or high	Low
Blood pressure	Normal	Low	Low or normal	Low
Cardiac output	Normal	Low	Low	High
Systemic vascular resistance	Normal	High	High	Low
Treatment	None	Volume	Inotrope, afterload reduction, IABP	?Vasoconstrictor

Weaning is accomplished by releasing the tapes around the vena cava and progressively clamping the venous return line (tubing). As the beating heart fills, ventricular ejection resumes. Pump flow is gradually decreased as arterial pressure rises. Once the venous line is completely occluded and mean systemic arterial pressure is judged adequate (> 80–90 mm Hg), pump flow is stopped and the patient is evaluated. Most patients fall into one of four groups when coming off bypass (Table 21–2). Patients with good ventricular function are usually quick to develop a good blood pressure and cardiac output and can be separated from CPB immediately. Hyperdynamic patients can also be rapidly weaned; these patients emerge from CPB with a very low systemic vascular resistance, demonstrating good contractility and adequate volume, but have low arterial pressure. The diagnosis is confirmed by measuring cardiac output.

Hypovolemic patients represent a mixed group that includes both patients with normal ventricular function and those with varying degrees of impairment. Those with preserved myocardial function quickly respond to 100-mL aliquots of pump blood infused via the aortic cannula. Blood pressure and cardiac output rise with each bolus, and the increase progressively becomes more sustained. Most of these patients maintain a good blood pressure and cardiac output with a left ventricular filling pressure below 10–15 mm Hg. Ventricular impairment should be suspected in hypovolemic patients whose filling pressures rise during volume infusion without appreciable changes in blood pressure or cardiac output or who require filling pressures above 10–15 mm Hg.

Patients with pump failure emerge from CPB with a sluggish, poorly contracting heart that progressively distends. In such cases, CPB is reinstituted while inotropic therapy is initiated. If systemic vascular resistance is high, afterload reduction with nitroprusside may be tried. The patient should be evaluated for unrecognized ischemia (kinked graft or coronary vasospasm), valvular dysfunction, shunting, or right ventricular failure (the distention is primarily right-sided). Transesophageal echocardiography may facilitate the diagnosis in these cases. If inotropes and afterload reduction fail, intra-aortic balloon counterpulsation (IABCP) is initiated prior to another attempt at weaning the patient. The efficacy of IABCP is critically dependent on proper timing of inflation and deflation of the balloon. The balloon is ideally inflated just after the dicrotic notch to augment diastolic blood pressure and coronary flow. Maximum deflation should be timed just prior to left ventricular ejection to decrease its afterload. Temporary implantable ventricular-assist failure.

Inotropes increase myocardial oxygen demand and should not be used routinely in patients coming off bypass. The routine use of calcium can similarly worsen ischemic injury and may also contribute to coronary spasm (especially in patients who were taking calcium channel blockers preoperatively). Commonly used inotropes and vasopressors are listed in Table 21–3. Dopamine and dobutamine are the most commonly used agents. Dobutamine has wider use because, unlike dopamine, it does not increase filling pressures and is associated with less tachycardia. On the other hand, only dopamine (in low doses) improves renal blood flow (Chapter 12). Amrinone, a selective phosphodiesterase type III inhibitor, is a potent inotrope with significant arterial and venodilator properties. Unlike other inotropes, amrinone may not appreciably increase myocardial oxygen consumption because it does not directly increase heart rate and because it decreases left ventricular afterload. The combination of amrinone and a catecholamine results in synergistic inotropic effects. Clinically, epinephrine is the most potent inotrope and is often effective when others have failed; in lower doses, it has predominantly β agonist activity.

POSTBYPASS PERIOD

During the postbypass period, bleeding is controlled, anticoagulation is reversed, bypass cannulas are removed, and the chest is closed. The surgical team should, however, be ready to resume CPB at any time. Checking for bleeding, especially from the posterior surface of the heart, requires lifting the heart, which can cause severe hypotension. The surgeon should be informed of the extent and duration of the hypotension. Atrial cannulas are removed before the aortic cannula in case the latter must be used to rapidly administer volume to the patient. Most patients need additional blood volume subsequent to termination of bypass. Administration of blood, colloids, and crys-

Table 21–3. Vasopressors and inotropic agents.

Agent	Bolus	Infusion Rate	Action			
			Direct Adrenergic Agonist		Indirect Adrenergic Agonist	Phosphodiesterase Inhibition
			Alpha	Beta		
Epinephrine	2–10 μg	1–2 μg/min	++	++++		
		2–10 μg/min	+++	++++		
		>10 μg/min	++++	+++		
Norepinephrine		2–16 μg/min	++++	+++		
Isoproterenol	1–4 μg	1–5 μg/min		++++		
Dobutamine		2–20 μg/kg/min	+	++++		
Dopamine		2–10 μg/min	+	++	+	
		10–20 μg/kg/min	++	+++	+	
		>20 μg/kg/min	+++	++	+	
Ephedrine	5–25 mg		+	++	+	
Metaraminol	100 μg	40–400 μg/min	+++	++	+	
Phenylephrine	50–200 μg	10–50 μg/min	++++			
Methoxamine	2–10 mg		++++			
Amrinone	0.5–1.5 mg/kg	5–10 μg/kg/min				+

talloid fluid is guided by filling pressures and the post-bypass hematocrit. A final hematocrit of 27–30% is generally desirable. Blood remaining in the CPB reservoir can be transfused via the aortic cannula (if still in place) or processed by a cell saver device and given intravenously. Frequent ventricular ectopy should be treated with lidocaine or procainamide. Ventricular arrhythmias in this setting can rapidly deteriorate into ventricular tachycardia and fibrillation.

Reversal of Anticoagulation

Once hemostasis is judged acceptable and the patient continues to be stable, heparin activity is reversed with protamine. The simplest technique bases the protamine dose on the amount of heparin initially required to produce the desired ACT. Protamine is usually given in a ratio of 1–1.3 mg of protamine per 100 units of heparin. Several alternative dosing techniques of varying sophistication can be used, but all are empiric and should be checked for adequacy by repeating the ACT. Additional protamine doses of 50–100 mg may be necessary. One approach calculates the protamine dose based on the heparin dose-response curve (Figure 21–3).

When given in excess, protamine itself has anticoagulant activity ($1/100$ that of heparin). The latter is the basis of automated protamine titration tests, which can also be used to calculate the protamine dose. Protamine is added in varying quantities to several blood samples. The tube whose protamine concentration best matches heparin activity will clot first. Clotting will be prolonged in tubes containing insufficient protamine as well as those with too much protamine. The protamine dose is then estimated by multiplying the protamine concentration in the tube that clots first by the patient's blood volume.

Protamine administration can result in a number of adverse hemodynamic effects, most of which appear to be either allergic or idiosyncratic reactions. Although protamine given slowly usually has minimal effects, hypotension due to acute systemic vasodilatation or marked pulmonary hypertension may result. Diabetics previously maintained on protamine-containing insulin appear to be at increased risk for allergic reactions.

Persistent Bleeding

Persistent bleeding following bypass often follows long bypass periods (> 2 hours) and in most instances is due to multifactorial causes. Inadequate surgical control of bleeding sites, inadequate reversal of heparin, reheparinization, thrombocytopenia, platelet dysfunction, undiagnosed preoperative hemostatic defects, or newly acquired defects may be responsible. The ACT should return to baseline following protamine; additional protamine doses may be necessary. Reheparinization (heparin rebound) after apparent adequate reversal may be explained by a redistribution either of protamine to peripheral compartments or of peripherally bound heparin to the central compartment. If oozing continues despite adequate surgical hemostasis and the ACT is normal, thrombocytopenia or platelet dysfunction is likely. Both defects are recognized complications of CPB. Platelet transfusion may be necessary to maintain the platelet count above 40,000–60,000/μL. Desmopressin (DDAVP) may be effective in reversing qualitative platelet defects; the role of this agent has not been fully established. Disseminated intravascular coagulation and fibrinolysis may occasionally be encountered; diagnosis should be confirmed with a fibrinogen level, PT, and PTT. Fresh frozen plasma or cryoprecipitate should be given in such cases. Aminocaproic acid, aprotinin, or tranexamic acid may be also be effective in some cases.

Anesthesia

Unless a continuous intravenous infusion technique is used, additional anesthetic agents are necessary following CPB. The selection of agents is often determined by the hemodynamic response of the patient following CPB. Unstable patients usually receive small amounts of a narcotic, while hyperdynamic patients tolerate anesthetic doses of a volatile agent. Hypertension not responding to boluses of a narcotic or the addition of a volatile agent should be treated with nitroprusside.

Even if a volatile agent is used following CPB, a narcotic is usually given to provide sedation during transport to the intensive care unit.

Transportation

Transporting patients from the operating room to the intensive care unit is a hazardous process that is complicated by the possibilities of a complete monitoring blackout, overdosing with or interruption of drug infusions, and hemodynamic instability en route. Portable monitoring equipment, infusion pumps, and a full oxygen cylinder with a self-inflating bag for ventilation should be readied prior to the end of the operation. Minimum monitoring during transportation includes the ECG, arterial blood pressure, and an esophageal stethoscope. A portable pulse oximeter is also desirable, as is an extra pressure channel for central pressures. An endotracheal tube, laryngoscope, succinylcholine, and emergency resuscitation drugs should also accompany the patient. Upon arrival in the ICU, the patient should be attached to the ventilator and breath sounds checked, and an orderly transfer of monitors and infusions (one at a time) should follow. The ICU staff should be given a brief summary of the procedure, intraoperative problems, current drug therapy, and any expected difficulties.

POSTOPERATIVE PERIOD

Depending on the patient, the type of surgery, and local practices, most patients remain on mechanical ventilation for 2–24 hours postoperatively. The emphasis in the first few hours postoperatively should be on maintaining hemodynamic stability and monitoring for excessive postoperative bleeding. Chest tube drainage in the first 2 hours greater than 250–300 mL/h—in the absence of a hemostatic defect—is excessive and often requires surgical reexploration. Drainage subsequently that exceeds 100 mL/h is also worrisome. Intrathoracic bleeding at a site not adequately drained causes cardiac tamponade, which necessitates immediate reopening of the chest.

Hypertension is a common postoperative problem and should generally be treated aggressively so as not to exacerbate bleeding or myocardial ischemia. Nitroprusside is generally the best agent in this setting. Longer-acting agents or beta blockade may be suitable for patients with good ventricular function.

Fluid replacement should be guided by filling pressures. Most patients continue to require volume for several hours following operation. Hypokalemia (due to intraoperative diuretics) often develops and requires potassium replacement.

Extubation should be considered only if the patient is hemodynamically stable and receiving minimal drug infusions and if muscle paralysis has worn off. Caution should be exercised in obese and elderly patients and those with underlying pulmonary disease. Thoracic procedures are typically associated with marked decreases in functional residual capacity and postoperative diaphragmatic dysfunction (Chapter 23). Most patients can be extubated by the following morning.

CONGENITAL HEART DISEASE

OVERVIEW OF CONGENITAL HEART DISEASE

Cardiovascular function in young children differs from that in adults (Chapter 42). The Starling relationship (Chapter 19) plateaus early. Stroke volume is relatively fixed, so that cardiac output is primarily dependent on heart rate. The relatively immature hearts of neonates and infants often tolerate pressure or volume overload poorly. Furthermore, the functions of both ventricles are more interdependent, so that failure of one often precipitates failure of the other (biventricular heart failure). Transition of the neonate from the fetal to the adult circulation is discussed in Chapter 40.

Congenital heart disease encompasses a seemingly endless list of abnormalities. Most are detected in infancy or early childhood and present as cyanosis, congestive heart failure, or both. Cyanosis is most often associated with defects causing abnormal intracardiac communications that allow unoxygenated blood to reach the systemic arterial circulation (right-to-left shunting). Congestive heart failure is most prominent with defects that obstruct the ventricular outflow of either ventricle or markedly increase pulmonary blood flow. The latter is usually due to abnormal intracardiac communications that return oxygenated blood to the right heart (left-to-right shunting). Right-to-left shunting generally decreases pulmonary blood flow, but some complex lesions can increase pulmonary blood flow even in the presence of right-to-left shunting. In many cases, more than one lesion is present; in fact, survival with some anomalies (transposition, total anomalous venous return, or pulmonary atresia) depends on the simultaneous presence of another shunting lesion (patent ductus arteriosus, patent foramen ovale, or ventricular septal defect).

Table 21–4. Classification of congenital heart disease.

Lesions causing outflow obstruction
    Left ventricle:
        Coarctation of the aorta
        Aortic stenosis
    Right ventricle:
        Pulmonary stenosis
Lesions causing left to right shunting
    Ventricular septal defect
    Patent ductus arteriosus
    Atrial septal defect
    Endocardial cushion defect
    Partial anomalous pulmonary venous return
Lesions causing right to left shunting
    With decreased pulmonary blood flow:
        Tetralogy of Fallot
        Pulmonary atresia
        Tricuspid atresia
    With increased pulmonary blood flow:
        Transposition of the great vessels
        Truncus arteriosus
        Single ventricle
        Double outlet right ventricle
        Total anomalous pulmonary venous return
        Hypoplastic left heart

Their complex nature and varying pathophysiology makes classification of these lesions difficult. A commonly used scheme is presented in Table 21–4. For the purpose of anesthetic management, congenital heart defects may be divided into three types of lesions: obstructive lesions, simple shunts, and mixed lesions. Moreover, shunts should be characterized as predominantly right-to-left, left-to-right, or bidirectional.

Obstructive Lesions

The pathophysiology of these lesions in children is similar to that of adult lesions (see Aortic Stenosis, Chapter 20). However, ventricular outflow obstruction differs in children in that it often occurs on the right side of the heart.

Simple Shunts

Simple shunts are isolated abnormal communications between the right and left sides of the heart. Since pressures are normally higher on the left side, blood usually flows across from left to right. As a result, blood flow through the right heart and the lungs increases. Depending on the size and location of the communication, the right ventricle may also be subjected to the higher left-sided pressures, resulting in both pressure and volume overload. Because right ventricular afterload is normally 1/20 that of the left ventricle, even small left-to-right pressure gradients can produce large increases in pulmonary blood flow. The ratio of pulmonary to systemic blood flow can be calculated from oxygen saturation data by the following equation:

$$\dot{Q}_{\text{pulmonary}}/\dot{Q}_{\text{systemic}} = \frac{\text{Systemic arterial saturation} - \text{Mixed Venous saturation}}{\text{Pulmonary venous saturation} - \text{Pulmonary arterial saturation}}$$

A ratio greater than 1 indicates a left-to-right shunt, while a ratio less than 1 indicates a right-to-left shunt. Large increases in pulmonary blood flow produce pulmonary vascular congestion and increase extravascular lung water. The latter interferes with gas exchange, decreases lung compliance, and increases the work of breathing. Distention of the left atrium can also compress the left bronchus, while distention of pulmonary vessels compresses smaller bronchi.

Over the course of several years, chronic increases in pulmonary blood flow produce permanent reactive vascular changes that irreversibly increase pulmonary vascular resistance. Elevation of right ventricular afterload produces hypertrophy and progressively raises right-sided cardiac pressures. With advanced disease, the pressures within the right heart can exceed those within the left heart. Under these conditions, the intracardiac shunt reverses and becomes right-to-left (Eisenmenger's complex).

When the communication is relatively small, blood flow through the shunt is primarily dependent on the size of the communication (restrictive shunt). When the communication is large (nonrestrictive shunt), shunt flow is dependent on the relative balance between pulmonary and systemic vascular resistance. An increase in systemic relative to pulmonary vascular resistance favors left-to-right shunting, while an increase in pulmonary relative to systemic vascular resistance favors right-to-left shunting. Common chamber lesions (single atrium, single ventricle, and truncus arteriosus) represent the extreme form of nonrestrictive shunts; shunt flow with these lesions is bidirectional and totally dependent on relative changes in the ventricular afterloads.

Mixed Lesions

Lesions within this group (also called complex shunts) produce both ventricular outflow obstruction and shunting; the obstruction favors shunt flow toward the unobstructed side. When the obstruction is relatively mild, the amount of shunting is affected by the ratio of systemic to pulmonary vascular resistance, but increasing degrees of obstruction fix the direction and magnitude of the shunt. Tetralogy of Fallot (pulmonary stenosis, ventricular septal defect, overriding aorta, and right ventricular hypertrophy) is the classic example of this type of lesion. Right-to-left shunting across the ventricular septal defect in patients with the tetralogy has both fixed and variable components. The fixed component is determined by the severity of the pulmonary stenosis, while the variable depends on the ratio of pulmonary to systemic vascular resistance as well as dynamic infundibular obstruction. The latter is usually increased by sympathetic tone and is probably responsible for hypercyanotic spells.

Atresia of any one of the cardiac valves represents the extreme form of this group of lesions. Shunting occurs proximal to the atretic valve and is completely fixed; survival depends on another distal shunt (usually the ductus arteriosus), where blood flows in the opposite direction.

GENERAL APPROACH TO ANESTHESIA FOR PEDIATRIC CARDIAC SURGERY

Preoperative Evaluation

The complex nature of these lesions and their operative repair requires close communication between the anesthesiologist, cardiologist, and surgeon. The full hemodynamic significance of the lesion and the surgical plan must be clear preoperatively. Moreover, the patient's condition must be optimized to the maximum extent possible. Congestive heart failure and pulmonary infections should be controlled. Alprostadil (prostaglandin E_1) infusion (0.05 μg/kg/min) is used preoperatively to prevent closure of the ductus arteriosus in patients dependent on ductal flow for survival. Indications for operation include severe hypoxemia, excessive increases in pulmonary blood flow, refractory congestive heart failure, severe left ventricular obstruction, and preservation of ventricular function.

Assessment of disease severity relies on both clinical and laboratory evaluation. Deterioration in infants is manifested by increasing tachypnea, cyanosis, or sweating, especially during feeding. Older children may complain of easy fatigability. Body weight is generally a good indication of overall disease severity. Signs of congestive heart failure include tachycardia, an S_3 gallop, weak pulses, tachypnea, pulmonary rales, bronchospasm, and hepatomegaly. Cyanosis may be noted, but hypoxemia is best assessed by arterial blood gas measurements and the hematocrit. In the absence of iron deficiency, the degree of polycythemia is directly related to the severity and duration of hypoxemia. Clubbing of the fingers is frequently noted in children with cyanotic defects. The evaluation should also search for other congenital abnormalities, which are present in up to 30% of patients with congenital heart disease.

Results of echocardiography, heart catheterization, electrocardiography, and chest x-ray should be reviewed. Laboratory evaluation should include a complete blood count, platelet count, coagulation studies, electrolytes, blood urea nitrogen, and serum creatinine. Ionized calcium and glucose determinations are also useful in neonates and critically ill children.

Preinduction Period

A. Fasting: Fasting requirements vary according to the patient's age (Chapter 42). Patients under 6 months of age should have nothing by mouth for 4 hours prior to surgery. Patients between 6 months and 1 year should be kept NPO for 6 hours. In general, those over 1 year of age may be fasted for 8 hours. A preoperative intravenous infusion that provides maintenance fluid requirements should be used in patients susceptible to dehydration or with severe polycythemia and when excessive delays occur prior to surgery.

B. Premedication: Premedication varies according to age and cardiac and pulmonary reserves. Atropine, 0.02 mg/kg intramuscularly (minimum dose: 0.05 mg), is usually given to all pediatric patients to counteract enhanced vagal tone. Neonates and infants under 6 months of age are given only atropine. Sedation is desirable in older patients, especially with cyanotic lesions (tetralogy of Fallot), as agitation and crying worsen right-to-left shunting. Patients over 6 months of age are usually also given morphine, 0.1 mg/kg, and pentobarbital, 2–4 mg/kg, intramuscularly; scopolamine, 0.01 mg/kg, may be substituted for atropine for enhanced sedation. The pentobarbital should be reduced or omitted in patients with cyanotic lesions or congestive heart failure.

Induction of Anesthesia

A. Hemodynamic Anesthetic Goals:

1. Obstructive lesions–Anesthetic management should strive to avoid hypovolemia, bradycardia, tachycardia, and myocardial depression. The optimal heart rate should be selected according to age (Chapter 42); slow rates decrease cardiac output, while fast rates impair ventricular filling. Some cardiac depression may be desirable in hyperdynamic patients with coarctation of the aorta.

2. Shunts–A favorable ratio of pulmonary to systemic vascular resistance should be maintained in the presence of shunting. For patients with right-to-left shunting, factors known to increase pulmonary vascular resistance such as acidosis, hypercapnia, hypoxia, enhanced sympathetic tone, and high mean airway pressures are avoided; hyperventilation (hypocapnia) with 100% oxygen is usually effective in lowering pulmonary vascular resistance. Specific pulmonary vasodilators are not available; alprostadil (prostaglandin E_1) or nitroglycerin may be tried but often causes systemic hypotension. Systemic vasodilatation also worsens right-to-left shunting and should be avoided; phenylephrine may be used to raise systemic vascular resistance. Conversely, patients with left-to-right shunting benefit from systemic vasodilation and increases in pulmonary vascular resistance, though specific hemodynamic manipulation is generally not attempted.

B. Monitoring: Standard intraoperative monitors are generally used until the patient is anesthetized. Following induction, intra-arterial and central venous pressure monitoring are employed for thoracotomies and all procedures employing CPB. These monitors are usually placed after the patient is anesthetized. Twenty- or 22-gauge catheters are used to catheterize the radial artery; 24-gauge catheters may be more appropriate for small neonates and premature infants. A cutdown may be necessary in some instances. The internal or external jugular veins are generally used for central venous cannulation; if unsuccessful, the central venous catheter may be placed intraoperatively by the surgeon.

C. Venous Access: Venous access is desirable but not always necessary for induction. Agitation and crying are especially undesirable in patients with cyanotic lesions (see above). Intravenous access can be established after induction but before intubation in most patients. Subsequently, at least two intravenous fluid infusions are required; one is typically via a central venous catheter. Extreme caution is necessary to avoid even the smallest air bubbles. Shunting lesions allow the passage of venous air into the arterial circulation; paradoxic embolism can occur through the foramen ovale even in patients without obvious right-to-left shunting (Chapter 26). Aspiration prior to each injection prevents dislodgment of any trapped air at the injection port.

D. Route of Induction: In premature infants and young neonates, the trachea is usually intubated while the patient is awake after adequate preoxygenation. In older patients, inhalational, intravenous, or intramuscular induction is necessary prior to intubation. To a major extent, the effect of premedication and the presence of venous access determine the induction technique. Intubation is facilitated by succinylcholine, 1.5–2 mg/kg, or a nondepolarizing agent (pancuronium, 0.1 mg/kg). Pancuronium's vagolytic effects are especially useful in pediatric patients.

1. Intravenous induction–One may use any of the following for intravenous inductions: thiopental, 3–5 mg/kg; ketamine, 1–2 mg/kg; fentanyl, 25–50 μg/kg; or sufentanil, 5–15 μg/kg. High-dose narcotics are most suitable for very small and critically ill patients when postoperative ventilation is planned. The onset of intravenous agents is more rapid in patients with right-to-left shunting; drug boluses should be given slowly to avoid transiently high arterial blood levels. In contrast, recirculation in patients with large left-to-right shunts dilutes arterial blood concentration and can delay the onset of intravenous agents.

2. Intramuscular induction–Ketamine, 4–10 mg/kg, is most commonly used. Onset of anesthesia is within 5 minutes. Ketamine is a good choice for agitated uncooperative patients as well as patients with decreased cardiac reserve. Its safety with cyanotic lesions is well established. Ketamine does not appear to increase pulmonary vascular resistance in children.

3. Inhalation induction–Halothane is the most commonly used volatile agent. The same technique employed for noncardiac surgery is used (Chapter 42) except that the concentration is increased slowly to avoid excessive cardiac depression. Halothane is most suitable for patients with good cardiac reserve. Its safety in patients with cyanotic heart disease and good cardiac reserve is also established; systemic arterial vasodilation is generally minimal. Halothane induction should not be used in very young patients and those with low cardiac outputs. Nitrous oxide is typically used with inhalation inductions; its concentration should be limited to 50% in patients with cyanotic lesions. Nitrous oxide does not appear to increase pulmonary vascular resistance in pediatric patients. The uptake of inhalation agents, especially less soluble agents such as nitrous oxide, may be slowed in patients with right-to-left shunts; in contrast, no significant effect on uptake is generally observed with left-to-right shunting.

Maintenance Anesthesia

Following induction, narcotics or inhalation anesthetics are used for maintenance. Fentanyl and sufentanil are the most commonly used intravenous agents, while halothane, isoflurane, and nitrous oxide are the most commonly used inhalation agents. The choice of agents should be modified according to the patient's hemodynamic response. Isoflurane may be a more suitable alternative to halothane in some cases. In equianesthetic doses, isoflurane causes less myocardial depression, less slowing of the heart rate, and more vasodilation than halothane. Nitrous oxide can cause cardiac depression in patients with poor cardiac reserve. Moreover, it should probably be discontinued in all patients well before bypass to lessen the likelihood of expansion of intravascular air bubbles (see above).

Cardiopulmonary Bypass

The circuit and technique employed are the same as for adults. Since the smallest circuit volume used is still about 700 mL, blood is used to prime the machine for neonates and infants to prevent excessive hemodilution. CPB may be complicated by intra- and extracardiac shunts and a very compliant arterial system (in very young patients); both tend to lower mean arterial pressure and can impair systemic perfusion. Shunts should be controlled as much as possible at the start of bypass. High flow rates (up to 150 mL/kg/min) may be necessary to ensure adequate perfusion in very young patients. Weaning from CPB is generally not a problem in pediatric patients provided an adequate surgical repair is obtained; primary pump failure is unusual. Difficulty in weaning should prompt the surgeon to check the repair and search for undiagnosed lesions. Intraoperative echocardiography, together with measurement of the pressure and oxygen saturation within the various chambers, usually reveals the problem. Inotropic support may be provided by any of the agents used for adults. Calcium chloride may be useful in critically ill young patients, who often have impaired calcium homeostasis; ionized calcium measurements are invaluable in such cases. Isoproterenol and dobutamine are generally the most useful inotropic agents when pulmonary vascular resistance is elevated.

Hypothermic circulatory arrest. Surgical correction of complex congenital lesions sometimes requires complete circulatory arrest under deep hypothermia. Following institution of CPB, cooling is accomplished by the combination of surface cooling and a cold perfusate. At a core temperature of 15 °C, up to 60 minutes of complete circulatory arrest is generally considered safe. Following the repair, CPB flow is restarted, and rewarming takes place.

Postbypass Period

Because of the large priming volumes used (compared with the patient's blood volume), hemostatic defects from dilution of clotting factors and platelets are commonly seen after CPB in infants; in addition to heparin reversal, administration of fresh frozen plasma and platelets is often necessary.

All patients under 6 months of age should generally remain intubated, as should all other patients undergoing extensive or complicated procedures. Extubation may be considered for older, relatively healthy patients undergoing simple procedures such as closure of a small patent ductus or atrial septal defect or repair of a coarctation.

SURGERY ON THE AORTA

PREOPERATIVE CONSIDERATIONS

Surgery on the aorta represents one of the greatest challenges for anesthesiologists. Regardless of which part of the vessel is involved, the procedure is complicated by the need to cross-clamp the aorta and by the potential for large intraoperative blood losses. Aortic cross-clamping without CPB acutely increases left ventricular afterload and severely compromises organ perfusion distal to the point of occlusion. Severe hypertension, myocardial ischemia, or left ventricular failure may be precipitated. Interruption of blood flow to the spinal cord and kidneys can produce paraplegia and renal failure, respectively. Moreover, emergency aortic surgery is frequently necessary in critically ill patients who are acutely hypovolemic and have a high incidence of coexistent cardiac and pulmonary disease.

Indications for aortic surgery include aortic dissections, aneurysms, occlusive disease, trauma, and coarctation. Lesions of the ascending aorta are those between the aortic valve and the innominate artery, while those of the aortic arch lie between the innominate and left subclavian arteries. Disease distal to the left subclavian artery but above the diaphragm involves the descending thoracic aorta; lesions below the diaphragm involve the abdominal aorta.

SPECIFIC LESIONS OF THE AORTA

Aortic Dissection

Aortic dissection develops either as a result of an intimal tear that allows blood to be forced into the aortic wall (the media) or hemorrhage in the aortic media with extension secondary to disruption of the aortic intima. In either case, a primary degenerative process called medial cystic necrosis is necessary for dissection to occur. Propagation of the dissection is thought to occur as a result of hemodynamic shear forces acting on the intimal tear; indeed, hypertension is a common finding in patients with aortic dissec-

tion. Patients with hereditary connective tissue defects such as Marfan's syndrome and Ehlers-Danlos syndrome eventually develop medial cystic necrosis and are at risk for aortic dissection. Less commonly, dissection occurs from hemorrhage into an atheromatous plaque or at the cannulation site following cardiac surgery.

Dissection along the aortic media may occlude the opening of any artery arising directly from the aorta; may extend into the aortic root, producing incompetence of the aortic valve; or may rupture into the pericardium or pleura, producing cardiac tamponade or hemothorax, respectively. Dissections are most commonly of the proximal type (Daily type A, De Bakey types I and II) involving the ascending aorta. Type II dissections do not extend beyond the innominate artery. Distal dissections (Daily type B, De Bakey type III) originate beyond the left subclavian artery and propagate only distally. Proximal dissections are nearly always treated surgically, while distal dissections may be treated medically. In either case, from the time the diagnosis is suspected, measures to reduce systolic blood pressure (usually to 90–120 mm Hg) and aortic wall stress are initiated. This usually includes intravenous nitroprusside and β-adrenergic blockade (esmolol). The latter is important in reducing the shear forces related to the rate of rise of aortic pressure (dP/dt); dP/dt may actually rise with nitroprusside alone. Alternatively, trimethaphan may be used by itself (Chapter 13).

Aortic Aneurysms

Aneurysms most commonly involve the abdominal aorta but may involve any part of the aorta. The vast majority are due to atherosclerosis. Medial cystic necrosis is also an important cause of thoracic aortic aneurysms. Syphilitic aneurysms characteristically involve the ascending aorta. Dilatation of the aortic root often produces aortic regurgitation. Expanding aneurysms of the upper thoracic aorta can also cause tracheal or bronchial compression or deviation, hemoptysis, and superior vena cava syndrome. Hoarseness and left vocal cord paralysis may be due to compression of the left recurrent laryngeal nerve. Distortion of normal anatomy may also complicate endotracheal or endobronchial intubation or cannulation of the internal jugular and subclavian veins.

The greatest danger from aneurysms is rupture and exsanguination. Acute expansion (due to leaking), manifested as sudden severe pain, may herald rupture. The likelihood of catastrophic rupture is related to size. The data are least equivocal for abdominal aortic aneurysms; rupture occurs in 50% of patients within 1 year when an aneurysm is 6 cm or more in diameter. The normal aorta in adults varies from 2 cm to 3 cm in width (being wider cephalad). Elective resection is generally performed in most patients with aneurysms greater than 4 cm. A prosthetic graft is usually used, and the aneurysm may be completely excised or left in place around the graft. The operative mortality rate is about 2–5% in good-risk patients and exceeds 50% if leaking or rupture has already occurred.

Occlusive Disease of the Aorta

Thromboembolic obliteration of the aorta is most commonly atherosclerotic in origin and occurs at the aortic bifurcation (Leriche's syndrome). Occlusion results from a combination of atherosclerotic plaque and thrombosis. The atherosclerotic process is usually generalized and affects other parts of the arterial system, including the cerebral and coronary arteries (Chapters 20 and 27). Surgical treatment consists of an aortobifemoral bypass with a synthetic graft; proximal thromboendarterectomy may also be necessary.

Aortic Trauma

Aortic trauma may be either penetrating or non-penetrating. Both types of injuries can result in massive hemorrhage and require immediate operation. While penetrating injuries are usually obvious, blunt aortic trauma may be easily overlooked if not suspected and sought. Nonpenetrating aortic trauma typically results from sudden high-speed decelerations resulting from automobile accidents and falls. The injury can vary from a partial tear to a complete aortic transection. Because the aortic arch is relatively fixed while the descending aorta is relatively mobile, the shear forces are greatest and the site of injury is most common just distal to the subclavian artery (aortic isthmus). The most consistent finding is a wide mediastinum on a chest x-ray.

Coarctation of the Aorta

This lesion is usually considered a congenital heart defect. Two types are generally recognized and classified according to the position of the narrowed segment relative to the position of the ductus arteriosus. In the **preductal (infantile) type,** the narrowing occurs proximal to the opening of the ductus. This lesion, which is often associated with other congenital heart defects, is recognized in infancy because of a marked difference in perfusion between the upper and lower halves of the body; the lower body is cyanotic. Perfusion to the upper body is derived from the aorta, while perfusion to the lower half is primarily from the pulmonary artery. **Postductal coarctation** of the aorta may be not recognized until adulthood. The symptoms and hemodynamic significance of the latter lesion depend on the severity of the narrowing and the extent of collateral circulation that develops to the lower body (internal mammary, subscapular, and lateral thoracic to intercostal arteries). Hypertension in the upper body with or without left ventricular failure is usually present.

ANESTHETIC CONSIDERATIONS

Surgery on the Ascending Aorta

Surgery on the ascending aorta routinely employs median sternotomy and cardiopulmonary bypass. The conduct of anesthesia is similar to cardiac operations employing CPB, but the intraoperative course is complicated by aortic regurgitation, long aortic cross-clamp times, and large intraoperative blood losses. Aortic valve replacement and coronary reimplantation are usually necessary. The left radial artery should be used to monitor arterial blood pressure because clamping of the innominate artery may be necessary during the procedure; the femoral and dorsalis pedis arteries are suitable alternatives. A high-dose narcotic technique employing nitroprusside for precise blood pressure control is generally used. Beta-adrenergic blockade (esmolol) should also be employed in the presence of an aortic dissection. Bradycardia worsens aortic regurgitation and should be avoided (Chapter 20). The arterial inflow cannula for CPB is placed in a femoral artery for patients with dissections. In the event that sternotomy may rupture an aneurysm, prior establishment of partial CPB (using the femoral artery and femoral vein) should be considered.

Surgery Involving the Aortic Arch

These procedures are usually performed through a median sternotomy with deep hypothermic circulatory arrest (following institution of CPB). Additional considerations focus on achieving optimal cerebral protection (see above). Hypothermia to 15 °C, thiopental infusion to maintain a flat EEG, and perhaps mannitol (0.5 g/kg) prior to CPB are commonly used. The necessarily long rewarming periods probably contribute to the large intraoperative blood loss commonly observed after CPB.

Surgery Involving the Descending Thoracic Aorta

Surgery limited to the descending thoracic aorta is typically performed through a left thoracotomy without CPB; a thoracoabdominal incision is necessary for lesions that also involve the abdominal aorta. One-lung anesthesia (Chapter 24) greatly facilitates surgical exposure and reduces pulmonary trauma from retractors. Correct positioning of the endobronchial tube may be difficult because of distortion of the anatomy (see above); a flexible pediatric fiberoptic bronchoscope may be invaluable for this purpose.

The aorta must be cross-clamped above and below the lesion. Acute hypertension develops above the clamp, while hypotension results below. Arterial blood pressure should be monitored from the right radial artery, since clamping of the left subclavian artery may be necessary. The sudden increase in left ventricular afterload after application of the aortic clamp may precipitate acute left ventricular failure or myocardial ischemia in patients with underlying ventricular dysfunction or coronary disease. Cardiac output falls while left ventricular end-diastolic pressure and volume rise. The magnitude of these changes is inversely related to ventricular function. Moreover, these effects become less pronounced as the clamp is applied more distally. A nitroprusside infusion is almost always needed to prevent excessive increases in blood pressure and decreases in cardiac output. In patients with good ventricular function, increasing anesthetic depth just prior to cross-clamping may also be helpful.

A major problem in management during these procedures is excessive intraoperative bleeding. A blood scavenging device (cell saver) for autotransfusion is routinely employed. Adequate venous access and intraoperative monitoring are critical. Multiple large-bore (14-gauge) intravenous catheters (preferably with two blood warmers) are mandatory. Pulmonary artery catheterization is invaluable for guiding intraoperative fluid replacement and following cardiac function. The greatest period of hemodynamic instability is the period following release of the aortic cross-clamp ("release hypotension"); the abrupt decrease in afterload together with bleeding and the release of vasodilating acid metabolites from the ischemic lower body can precipitate severe systemic hypotension. Decreasing anesthetic depth, volume loading, and partial or slow release of the cross-clamp are helpful in avoiding severe hypotension. A small dose of a vasopressor may be necessary. Sodium bicarbonate should be used for persistent severe metabolic acidosis (pH < 7.20) in association with hypotension. Calcium chloride may be necessary following massive transfusion of citrated blood products (Chapter 29).

A major complication of clamping the thoracic aorta is spinal cord ischemia and paraplegia. The incidence of transient postoperative deficits and postoperative paraplegia are 11% and 6%, respectively. Higher rates are associated with cross-clamping periods longer than 30 minutes, extensive surgical dissections, and emergency procedures. The classic deficit is that of an anterior spinal artery syndrome with loss of motor function and pinprick sensation but preservation of vibration and proprioception. Anatomic variations in spinal cord blood supply are responsible for the unpredictable occurrence of deficits. The spinal cord receives its blood supply from the vertebral arteries and from the thoracic and abdominal aorta. One anterior and two posterior arteries descend along the cord. Intercostal arteries feed the anterior and posterior arteries in the upper thoracic aorta, while in the lower thoracic and lumbar cord the anterior spinal artery is supplied by the thoracolumbar artery of Adamkiewicz. This artery has a variable origin from the aorta arising between T5 and T8 in 15%, between T9 and T12 in 60%, and between L1 and L2 in 25% of individuals; it nearly always arises on the left side. It may be damaged during surgical dissection or occluded by the aortic cross-clamping. Monitoring somatosensory evoked potentials (Chapters 6 and 25) may be useful in preventing paraplegia, but false-positive and false-negative responses are reported.

Use of a temporary heparin-coated shunt or partial CPB maintains distal perfusion and decreases the incidence of paraplegia, hypertension, and ventricular failure. Partial CPB is generally not used because of frequently massive blood loss following heparinization. A heparin-coated shunt does not require systemic heparinization. It is usually placed proximally in the ascending aorta, left subclavian artery, or left ventricular apex and positioned distally in a common femoral artery. Other measures that may be protective for the spinal cord include mild hypothermia and mannitol. Mannitol's efficacy appears related to its ability to lower cerebrospinal fluid pressure by decreasing its production. Spinal cord perfusion pressure is mean arterial blood pressure minus cerebrospinal fluid pressure; the rise in cerebrospinal fluid pressure following experimental cross-clamping of the aorta may explain how mannitol can increase spinal cord perfusion pressure. The use of nitroprusside to control the hypertensive response to cross-clamping has been implicated as a contributing factor in spinal cord ischemia, since its hypotensive actions also occur distal to the cross-clamp. Excessive blood pressure reduction above the cross-clamp should therefore be avoided to prevent excessive hypotension below it.

An increased incidence of renal failure following aortic surgery is reported with emergency procedures, prolonged cross-clamping periods, prolonged hypotension, and preexisting renal disease. Although controversial, prior infusion of mannitol may decrease the incidence of renal failure.

Surgery on the Abdominal Aorta

Either the transabdominal or the retroperitoneal approach may be used for access to the abdominal aorta. Depending on the location of the lesion, the cross-clamp may be applied to the supraceliac, suprarenal, or infrarenal aorta. Heparinization prior to occlusion is necessary. Intra-arterial blood pressure may be monitored from either upper extremity. In general, the farther distally the clamp is applied, the less the effect on left ventricular afterload. In fact, occlusion of the infrarenal aorta in patients with good ventricular function frequently results in minimal hemodynamic changes. In contrast, release of the clamp frequently produces hypotension; the same techniques to prevent "release hypotension" (see above) should be employed. The large incision and extensive retroperitoneal surgical dissection significantly increase fluid requirements (10–12 mL/kg/h) beyond intraoperative blood loss. Fluid replacement should be guided by central venous or pulmonary artery pressure monitoring, the latter being utilized for all patients with ventricular dysfunction or significant coronary artery disease.

Some centers utilize continuous epidural anesthesia—in addition to general anesthesia—for abdominal aortic surgery. This combined technique decreases the general anesthetic requirement and appears to suppress the release of "stress hormones." It also provides an excellent route for administering postoperative epidural analgesia. Unfortunately, systemic heparinization during surgery introduces the risk of paraplegia secondary to an epidural hematoma. Some studies suggest that if the epidural catheter is carefully placed prior to heparinization, the risk of an epidural hematoma is low.

Postoperative Considerations

All patients undergoing aortic surgery should generally be left intubated and ventilated for 2–24 hours postoperatively. As with cardiac surgery, the initial emphasis in their postoperative care should be in maintaining hemodynamic stability and monitoring for postoperative bleeding. Most patients continue to require a marked increase in maintenance fluids for several hours postoperatively.

PERICARDIAL DISEASE

The parietal pericardium is a fairly stiff fibrous membrane surrounding the heart. It encompasses a relatively fixed intrapericardiac volume that includes the pericardial sac, the pericardial fluid (20–50 mL in adults), the heart, and blood. As a result, the pericardium normally limits acute dilatation of the ventricles and promotes diastolic coupling of the two ventricles (distention of one ventricle interferes with filling of the other). The latter effect is also due to the interventricular septal wall that they share. Moreover, diseases affecting the pericardium or pericardial fluid volume can seriously impair ventricular function.

CARDIAC TAMPONADE

Preoperative Considerations

Cardiac tamponade exists when an increase in pericardial pressure impairs diastolic filling of the heart. Cardiac filling is ultimately related to the diastolic transmural (distending) pressure across each chamber. The transmural pressure across a chamber is the pressure within minus the pericardial pressure. Consequently, any increase in pericardial pressure relative to the pressure within reduces filling. Although pericardial pressure is equally applied to each chamber, the thin-walled atria and the right ventricle appear to be most affected.

Pericardial pressure is normally similar to the pleural pressure (Chapter 22), varying with respiration between −4 and +4 mm Hg. Elevations in pericardial pressure are most commonly due to increases in pericardial fluid volume (as a consequence of effusions or bleeding). The magnitude of the increase depends on the rate of fluid accumulation; sudden increases exceeding 100–200 mL precipitously increase pericardial pressure, while very slow accumulations up to 1000 mL allow the pericardium to stretch with minimal increases in pericardial pressure.

The principal hemodynamic feature of cardiac tamponade is a decrease in cardiac output due to a reduced stroke volume (Chapter 19) with an increase in central venous pressure. In the absence of severe left ventricular dysfunction, equalization of diastolic pressure occurs throughout the heart (RAP = RVEDP = LAP = LVEDP). The central venous pressure wave form (Chapter 19) is characteristic in cardiac tamponade. Impairment of both diastolic filling and atrial emptying abolishes the y descent; the x descent (systolic atrial filling) is normal or even accentuated. Reflex sympathetic activation is a prominent compensatory response in cardiac tamponade. Increases in heart rate and contractility help maintain cardiac output. Arterial vasoconstriction (increased systemic vascular resistance) supports systemic blood pressure, while venoconstriction augments venous return to the heart. Because stroke volume remains relatively fixed, cardiac output becomes primarily dependent on heart rate.

Acute cardiac tamponade usually presents as sudden hypotension, tachycardia, and tachypnea. Physical signs include jugular venous distention, a narrowed arterial pulse pressure, and muffled heart sounds. A prominent pulsus paradoxus (a cyclic inspiratory decrease in systolic blood pressure of more than 10 mm Hg) is typically present. The latter actually represents exaggeration of a normal phenomenon related to inspiratory decreases in intrathoracic pressure. Each decrease augments venous return and increases right ventricular end-diastolic volume (preload) but reduces left ventricular end-diastolic volume. The latter is probably due to right ventricular distention and rightward shift of the interventricular septum. A marked pulsus paradoxus may also be seen with severe airway obstruction and right ventricular infarction. The heart may be normal or enlarged on a chest x-ray. Electrocardiographic signs are generally nonspecific and often limited to decreased voltage in all leads and nonspecific ST segment and T wave abnormalities. Electrical alternans (cyclic alteration in magnitude of the P waves, QRS complex, and T waves) may be seen with large pericardial effusions and is thought to be due to pendular swinging of the heart within the pericardium. Generalized ST segment elevation may also be seen in patients with pericarditis. Echocardiography is invaluable in diagnosing pericardial effusions and cardiac tamponade. Two-dimensional echocardiography is especially accurate in estimating effusion size.

Anesthetic Considerations

Cardiac tamponade requires expeditious evacuation of the pericardial fluid, either surgically or by pericardiocentesis. The latter is associated with a significant risk of lacerating the heart or coronary arteries and of pneumothorax. Traumatic postoperative (following thoracotomy) cardiac tamponade is always treated surgically (thoracotomy), while tamponade due to other causes may be treated by either route. Surgical treatment is also often undertaken for large recurrent pericardial effusions (infectious, malignant, autoimmune, uremic, or radiation-induced) to prevent tamponade. Simple drainage of pericardial fluid may be achieved through a subxiphoid approach, while drainage combined with pericardial biopsy or pericardiectomy uses a left anterior thoracotomy and median sternotomy, respectively.

The anesthetic approach must be tailored to the clinical setting. For the postoperative (still intubated) cardiac patient in extremis, the chest may be reopened immediately in the intensive care unit without the benefit of anesthesia (at least initially). For awake conscious patients undergoing left thoracotomy or median sternotomy, general anesthesia and endotracheal intubation are necessary. Local anesthesia is often used for patients undergoing simple drainage through a subxiphoid approach. Premedication with atropine is often recommended to prevent reflex bradycardia during pericardial manipulation. Small doses of ketamine also provide excellent supplemental analgesia.

Induction of general anesthesia in patients with cardiac tamponade is extremely hazardous and may precipitate cardiac arrest. Pericardiocentesis or subxiphoid drainage under local anesthesia prior to induction is often advisable. Removal of even a small volume of fluid may be sufficient to greatly improve cardiac output and allow safe induction of general anesthesia.

Large-bore intravenous access is mandatory. Monitoring of intra-arterial and central venous pressures is optimal, but placement of these monitors should not delay pericardial drainage if the patient is unstable. The anesthetic technique should maintain a high sympathetic tone until the tamponade is relieved. Cardiac depression, vasodilation, and slowing of the heart rates are to be avoided. Similarly, increases in mean airway pressures can seriously jeopardize venous return. Awake intubation with maintenance of spontaneous ventilation are theoretically desirable, but coughing, straining, hypoxemia, and respiratory acidosis are equally detrimental and should be avoided.

Ketamine is the induction and maintenance agent of choice until the tamponade is relieved. Pancuronium's circulatory effects also make it the muscle relaxant of choice, but succinylcholine can be used initially for intubation. Isoproterenol may be useful as a temporary inotrope and chronotrope. Generous intravenous fluid administration is useful in maintaining venous return and offsetting any vasodilation from the isoproterenol.

CONSTRICTIVE PERICARDITIS

Preoperative Considerations

Constrictive pericarditis may develop as a sequela of acute or recurrent pericarditis. Pathologically, the pericardium is thickened, fibrotic, and often calcified. The parietal pericardium is typically adherent to the heart, often obliterating the pericardial space. The very stiff pericardium limits diastolic filling of the heart; the heart fills only to a fixed volume. In contrast to acute cardiac tamponade, diastolic filling does oc-

cur, but to a limited extent; in fact, filling during early diastole is typically accentuated and manifested by a prominent y descent on the central venous pressure waveform.

Patients with constrictive pericarditis display jugular venous distention, hepatomegaly, and often ascites. In contrast to acute tamponade, constrictive pericarditis prevents respiratory fluctuations in pericardial pressure; venous return to the heart does not increase during inspiration, so a pulsus paradoxus is uncommon. In fact, venous pressure may paradoxically rise during inspiration (Kussmaul's sign). The heart may be large or small on a chest x-ray, which often reveals pericardial calcification. Low QRS voltage and diffuse T wave abnormalities are usually present on the ECG. Atrial fibrillation and conduction blocks may be present.

Anesthetic Considerations

Pericardiectomy is usually reserved for patients with moderate to severe disease. The procedure is usually performed through a median sternotomy. It is complicated by the necessity for extensive manipulations of the heart that interfere with cardiac filling and ejection, induce frequent arrhythmias, and risk cardiac perforation. Cardiopulmonary bypass facilitates management, but the need for heparinization increases blood loss. The pericardium is generally dissected away from the left ventricle first; freeing the right ventricle first has occasionally resulted in pulmonary edema.

Selection of anesthetic agents is generally not as critical as avoiding excessive cardiac depression, vasodilatation, and bradycardia. Cardiac output is generally very rate-dependent. Adequate large-bore intravenous access and direct arterial and central venous pressure monitoring are mandatory. Antiarrhythmic therapy (generally lidocaine) is often necessary. Although cardiac function usually improves immediately following pericardiectomy, some patients display a persistently low cardiac output and require temporary inotropic support postoperatively.

CASE DISCUSSION: A PATIENT WITH A HISTORY OF EXCESSIVE BLEEDING FOLLOWING DENTAL SURGERY

A 55-year-old man is scheduled for resection of a 6-cm abdominal aortic aneurysm. He gives a history of having bled excessively for several days following a dental extraction 10 years earlier. He has not had any other surgery. Laboratory evaluation reveals a platelet count of 225,000/μL, a prothrombin time (PT) of 12.5 s (control = 11.9 s), and a partial thromboplastin time (PTT) of 34 s (control = 29 s).

Do these laboratory values exclude a hemostatic defect?

A bleeding diathesis may exist even in the absence of gross abnormalities on routine laboratory tests. Even if the patient's PTT is considered normal, the history of increased bleeding should alert the clinician to the possibility of a hemostatic defect.

What factors can contribute to excessive bleeding following surgery?

Hemostasis following trauma or surgery is dependent on three major processes: (1) vascular spasm, (2) formation of a platelet plug (primary hemostasis), and (3) coagulation of blood (secondary hemostasis; see Chapter 34). The first two are nearly immediate (seconds), while the last is delayed (minutes). A defect in any of these processes can lead to a bleeding diathesis and increased surgical blood loss. Moreover, severe hemostatic defects can lead to exsanguinating hemorrhage during or following major surgery.

How may a more detailed history and physical examination be helpful in evaluating hemostatic defects?

Although hemostatic defects can be reliably diagnosed only by laboratory tests, a history of excessive bleeding after dental extractions, childbirth, minor surgery, minor trauma, or even during menstruation should suggest a hemostatic defect. Indeed, some hemostatic defects are often not detected by routine testing but require additional specialized tests. A family history of a bleeding diathesis may suggest an inherited coagulation defect but is often absent because the increased bleeding is often minor and goes unnoticed.

Hemostatic defects can often be differentiated by their clinical presentation. Bleeding in patients with primary hemostatic defects usually immediately follows minor trauma, is confined to superficial sites (skin or mucosal surfaces), and often can be controlled by local compression. Pinpoint small hemorrhage from capillaries in the dermis (petechiae) are typically present on examination. Bleeding into subcutaneous tissues (ecchymosis) from small arterioles or venules is also common in patients with platelet disorders. In contrast, bleeding due to secondary hemostatic defects is usually delayed following injury, is typically deep (subcutaneous tissues, joints, body cavities, or muscles), and is often difficult to stop even with compression. Hemorrhages may be palpable as hematomas or may go unnoticed when deeper (retroperitoneal).

Describe the mechanisms involved in primary hemostasis?

Injury to blood vessels normally causes localized spasm as a result of the release of humoral factors (from platelets) as well as local myogenic reflexes. Sympathetic-mediated vasoconstriction is also probably operative in medium-sized vessels. Exposure of circulating platelets to the damaged endothelial surface causes them to undergo a series of changes that result in the formation of a platelet plug. If the break in a vessel is small, the plug itself can often completely stop bleeding. However, if the break is large, coagulation of blood is also necessary to stop the bleeding.

Formation of the platelet plug can be broken down into three stages: (1) adhesion, (2) release of granules, and (3) aggregation. Following injury, circulating platelets immediately adhere to subendothelial collagen via specific glycoprotein receptors. This important interaction is stabilized by a circulating glycoprotein called von Willebrand factor (vWF), which forms additional bridges between subendothelial collagen and platelets. Collagen activates platelets, causing them to release the contents of cytoplasmic granules and to produce thromboxane A_2. This prostaglandin is a potent vasoconstrictor that also promotes platelet aggregation. Platelet granules contain a large number of substances, including adenosine diphosphate (ADP), thromboxane A_2, factor V, vWF, fibrinogen, and fibronectin. The released factors (ADP, fibrinogen, thromboxane A_2) attract and activate additional platelets. The thrombin formed subsequently during the coagulation process is also a potent activator of platelets. Adenosine diphosphate alters platelets' membranes in such a way as to promote platelet aggregation and allow fibrinogen (see Case Discussion in Chapter 34) to attach and stabilize the platelet plug. Normal endothelium produces prostacyclin (PGI_2), which is a vasodilator that inhibits platelet activation and helps to confine the primary hemostatic process to the injured area.

What tests are most helpful in evaluating primary hemostasis?

The most commonly performed tests include a platelet count and a bleeding time. The bleeding time is generally not affected by the platelet count when the latter is greater than $100,000/\mu L$. The normal platelet count is $150,000–450,000/\mu L$. Patients with normally functioning platelets and platelet counts above $100,000/\mu L$ have normal primary hemostasis. When the platelet count is $50,000–100,000/\mu L$, excessive bleeding generally occurs only with severe trauma or extensive surgery. In contrast, patients with platelet counts under $50,000/\mu L$ develop significant bleeding following even minor trauma. When the platelet count is under $20,000/\mu L$, spontaneous bleeding is not unusual. Thrombocytopenia is usually due one of three mechanisms: (1) decreased platelet production, (2) splenic sequestration, or (3) increased destruction. The latter may be due to immune or nonimmune destruction (vasculitis or disseminated intravascular coagulation).

A prolonged bleeding time with a normal platelet count implies a qualitative platelet defect. Although the bleeding time is somewhat dependent on the technique employed, values longer than 10 minutes are generally considered abnormal. Significant intraoperative and postoperative bleeding may be expected when the bleeding time exceeds 15 minutes. Specialized testing is required to diagnose specific platelet functional defects.

What are the most common causes of qualitative platelet defects?

The most common platelet defect is due to inhibition of thromboxane A_2 production by aspirin and nonsteroidal anti-inflammatory drugs (NSAIDs). In contrast to aspirin, which irreversibly acetylates and inactivates cyclooxygenase for the life of the platelet (up to 7 days), enzyme inhibition by NSAIDs is reversible and generally lasts only 24 hours.

The most common inherited bleeding disorder (1:800–1000 patients) is **von Willebrand's disease.** Patients with this disorder produce a defective vWF or low levels of a normal vWF (normal: 5–10 mg/L). Most patients are heterozygous and have relatively mild hemostatic defects that become apparent clinically when they are subjected to major surgery or trauma or following ingestion of aspirin or NSAIDs. In addition to helping link platelets, vWF serves as a carrier for coagulation factor VIII (see Case Discussion in Chapter 34). As a result, patients typically have a prolonged bleeding time, decreased plasma vWF concentration, and decreased factor VIII activity. Acquired forms of von Willebrand's disease may be encountered in patients with some immune disorders and those with tumors that absorb vWF onto their surface.

A bleeding time was obtained on this patient and found to be 18 minutes. Factor VIII activity was found to be 40% and the vWF concentration 3.5 mg/L. A diagnosis of von Willebrand's disease is made.

How should this patient be managed perioperatively?

Treatment with desmopressin (DDAVP) can raise vWF levels in some patients with mild von Willebrand's disease (as well as normal individuals). The drug is usually administered at a dose of 0.3 µg/kg 30 minutes before surgery. Patients who do not respond to desmopressin should receive cryoprecipitate, which is rich in vWF. Prophylactic infusions of cryoprecipitate (usually 10 units) are generally recommended before and immediately after surgery. Cryoprecipitate is often continued twice a day for 2–4 days to guarantee surgical hemostasis. In contrast to patients with von Willebrand's disease, those with other qualitative platelet defects generally require platelet transfusions to correct the hemostatic defect (Chapter 29).

SUGGESTED READINGS

Dinardo JA, Schwartz MJ: *Anesthesia for Cardiac Anesthesia.* Appleton & Lange, 1990.
Ellison N, Jobes DR: *Effective Hemostasis for Cardiac Surgery.* Saunders, 1988.
Gothard JWW, Branthwaite MA: *Anaesthesia for Cardiac Surgery,* 3rd ed. Blackwell, 1987.
Hensley FA, Martin DE: *The Practice of Cardiac Anesthesia.* Little, Brown, 1990.
Kaplan JA: *Cardiac Anesthesia,* 2nd ed. Grune & Stratton, 1987. The standard American text.
Kaplan JA: *Vascular Anesthesia.* Churchill Livingstone, 1991.
Lake CL: *Cardiovascular Anesthesia.* Springer-Verlag, 1985.
Lake CL: *Pediatric Cardiac Anesthesia.* Appleton & Lange, 1987.

Reves JG, Hall KD: *Common Problems in Cardiac Anesthesia.* Year Book, 1987.
Roizen MF: *Anesthesia for Vascular Surgery.* Churchill Livingstone, 1990.
Tarhan S: *Cardiovascular Anesthesia and Postoperative Care,* 2nd ed. Year Book, 1989. Good chapters on pediatric cardiac surgery.
Taylor KM: *Cardiopulmonary Bypass: Principles and Management.* Williams & Wilkins, 1986.
Thomas SJ: *Manual of Cardiac Anesthesia,* 2nd ed. Churchill Livingstone, 1991.
Tinker J: *Cardiopulmonary Bypass.* Saunders, 1989.
Tomlin PJ: *Anesthesia for Vascular Surgery.* Butterworths, 1988.
Yeager MP, Glass DD: *Anesthesiology and Vascular Surgery.* Appleton & Lange, 1990.

Respiratory Physiology & Anesthesia

The importance of pulmonary physiology to anesthetic practice is readily apparent. The most commonly used anesthetics—the inhalation agents—depend on the lungs for uptake and elimination. The most important side effects of both inhalational and intravenous anesthetics are primarily respiratory. Moreover, muscle paralysis, unusual positioning during surgery, and techniques such as one-lung anesthesia and cardiopulmonary bypass profoundly alter normal respiratory physiology.

Much of modern anesthetic practice is based on a thorough understanding of pulmonary physiology and may be considered applied pulmonary physiology. This chapter reviews the basic respiratory concepts necessary for understanding and applying anesthetic techniques. Although the respiratory effects of each of the various anesthetic agents are discussed elsewhere in the book, the overall effects of general anesthesia on lung function are also reviewed here.

CELLULAR RESPIRATION

The principal function of the lungs is to allow gas exchange between venous blood and inspired air. This need arises as a direct result of cellular aerobic metabolism, which creates a constant demand for uptake of oxygen and elimination of CO_2.

AEROBIC METABOLISM

Normally, nearly all human cells derive energy aerobically, ie, by utilizing oxygen. Carbohydrates, fats, and proteins are metabolized to two-carbon fragments (acetyl-CoA) that enter the citric acid cycle within mitochondria (Chapter 34). As the acetyl-CoA is metabolized to CO_2, energy is derived and stored in the reduced form of nicotine adenine dinucleotide (NADH). That energy is subsequently transferred to adenosine triphosphate (ATP) through a process called oxidative phosphorylation. Oxidative phosphorylation

accounts for over 90% of total body oxygen consumption and involves a series of enzyme-mediated (cytochrome) electron transfers that are coupled to ATP formation. In the last step, molecular oxygen is reduced to water.

For glucose, an important cellular fuel, the overall reaction is as follows:

$$C_6H_{12}O_6 + 6O_2 \rightarrow 6CO_2 + 6H_2O + Energy$$

The energy generated is actually stored in a third phosphate bond on adenosine diphosphate (ADP):

$$Energy + ADP + P \rightarrow ATP$$

For every molecule of glucose oxidized, a total of 38 molecules of ATP can be produced. Once formed, the energy stored in ATP can be used for ion pumps, muscle contraction, protein synthesis, or cellular secretion; in the process, the ADP is regenerated:

$$ATP \rightarrow ADP + P + Energy$$

Note: ATP cannot be stored but must be continually formed. A constant supply of metabolic substrates and oxygen is necessary for that purpose.

The ratio of total CO_2 production ($\dot{V}CO_2$) to oxygen consumption ($\dot{V}O_2$) is referred to as the respiratory quotient (RQ) and is generally indicative of the primary type of fuel being utilized. The respiratory quotients for carbohydrates, lipids, and proteins are 1.0, 0.7, and 0.8, respectively. $\dot{V}CO_2$ is normally about 200 mL/min, while $\dot{V}O_2$ is approximately 250 mL/min. Because proteins are generally not used as a primary fuel source, the normal respiratory quotient of 0.8 probably reflects utilization of a combination of both fats and carbohydrates.

ANAEROBIC METABOLISM

Compared to aerobic metabolism, anaerobic metabolism produces a very limited amount of ATP. In the absence of oxygen, ATP can only be produced from the conversion of pyruvate to lactic acid. Since each molecule of glucose yields two pyruvates, a total of

USEFUL FORMULAS

GAS EXCHANGE

Minute ventilation:

$$\dot{V}_{min} = \textbf{Respiratory rate} \times \textbf{Tidal volume}$$

Alveolar ventilation:

$$V_A = \textbf{Respiratory rate} \times (V_T - V_D)$$

Bohr equation:

$$\frac{V_D}{V_T} = \frac{P_ACO_2 - P_ECO_2}{P_ACO_2}$$

Inspired oxygen tension:

$$P_IO_2 = (P_B - P_{H2O}) \times F_IO_2$$

Alveolar oxygen tension:

$$P_AO_2 = P_IO_2 - \frac{P_aCO_2}{R}$$

Arterial oxygen tension:

$$P_aO_2 = 102 - \frac{Age}{3}$$

Blood oxygen content:

$$C = [(0.003\ mL/dL) \times PO_2] + (SO_2 \times Hb \times 1.31\ mL/dL)$$

Venous admixture:

$$\frac{\dot{Q}_s}{\dot{Q}_t} = \frac{Cc'O_2 - CaO_2}{Cc'O_2 - C\bar{v}O_2}$$

Oxygen delivery:

$$\textbf{Oxygen delivery} = CaO_2 \times \dot{Q}_t$$

Fick equation:

$$CaO_2 - C\bar{v}\,O_2 = \frac{\dot{V}O_2}{\dot{Q}_t}$$

PULMONARY MECHANICS

Laminar flow:

$$\textbf{Pressure gradient} = \textbf{Gas flow} \times R_{aw}$$

$$R_{aw} = \frac{8 \times \textbf{Length} \times \textbf{Viscosity of gas}}{\pi \times (\textbf{Radius})^4}$$

Distending pressure:

$$P_{transpulmonary} = P_{alveolar} - P_{intrapleural}$$

$$P_{transthoracic} = P_{atmospheric} - P_{intrapleural}$$

Lung compliance:

$$C_{lung} = \frac{\Delta \textbf{Lung volume}}{\Delta \textbf{Transpulmonary pressure}}$$

Chest compliance:

$$C_{chest} = \frac{\Delta \textbf{Chest volume}}{\Delta \textbf{Transthoracic pressure}}$$

Total compliance:

$$\frac{1}{C_{total}} = \frac{1}{C_{chest\ wall}} + \frac{1}{C_{lung}}$$

NORMAL RESPIRATORY DATA

$V_T = 6\ mL/kg$

$V_D = 2\ mL/kg$

$VC = 60\text{--}70\ mL/kg$

$\dfrac{FEV_1}{FVC} \geq 75\%$

$\dfrac{V_D}{V_T} = 33\%$

$\dot{V}O_2 = 3\text{--}4\ mL/kg/min$ (adults)
$\phantom{\dot{V}O_2 = }6\text{--}8\ mL/kg/min$ (neonates and infants)

$P_aO_2 = 60\text{--}100\ mm\ Hg\ (8\text{--}13\ kPa)$

$P_aCO_2 = 34\text{--}42\ mm\ Hg\ (4.5\text{--}5.5\ kPa)$

$\dfrac{\dot{Q}_s}{\dot{Q}_t} \leq 5\%$

$C_{total} = 100\ mL/cm\ H_2O$

$R_{aw} = 0.5\text{--}2.0\ cm\ H_2O/L/min$

only two ATP molecules is formed per glucose molecule (compared with 38 ATP molecules aerobically). Moreover, the progressive lactic acidosis that develops severely limits the activity of the enzymes involved. When oxygen tension is restored to normal, lactate is reconverted to pyruvate and aerobic metabolism is resumed.

EFFECTS OF ANESTHESIA ON CELL METABOLISM

General anesthesia typically reduces both $\dot{V}O_2$ and $\dot{V}CO_2$ by about 15%. Additional reductions are often seen as a result of hypothermia. The greatest reductions are in cerebral and cardiac oxygen consumption.

FUNCTIONAL ANATOMY OF THE LUNGS

RIB CAGE & MUSCLES OF RESPIRATION

The rib cage contains the two lungs each surrounded by its own pleura. The apex of the chest is small, allowing only for entry of the trachea, esophagus, and blood vessels, while the base is formed by the diaphragm. Contraction of the diaphragm—the principal respiratory muscle—causes the base of the rib cage to descend and its contents (the lungs) to expand. Accessory respiratory muscles can augment lung expansion by their action on the ribs. Each rib (except for the last two) articulates posteriorly with a vertebra and is angulated down as it attaches anteriorly to the sternum; upward and outward rib movement expands the chest.

During normal breathing, the diaphragm (C3–5 innervation) and, to a lesser extent, the external intercostal muscles are responsible for inspiration; expiration is entirely passive. With increasing respiratory effort, the sternocleidomastoid, scalene, and pectoralis muscles are recruited during inspiration. Expiration can also become active and is facilitated by muscles aiding the downward movement of the ribs. These include the abdominal muscles (rectus abdominis, external and internal oblique, and transversus) and perhaps the internal intercostals.

TRACHEOBRONCHIAL TREE

The function of the tracheobronchial tree is to conduct gas flow to the alveoli. Humidification and filtering of inspired air is a function of the upper airway (nose, mouth, and pharynx). Dichotomous division (each branch dividing into two smaller branches), starting with the trachea and ending in alveolar sacs, is estimated to involve 23 generations (Figure 22–1). With each generation (division), the number of airways is approximately doubled. Finally, each alveolar sac contains an average of 17 alveoli. An estimated 300 million alveoli provide an enormous membrane (50–100 m²) for gas exchange in the average adult.

With each successive division, the mucosal epithelium and supporting structures of the airways gradually change. The mucosa makes a gradual transition from ciliated columnar to cuboidal and finally to flat alveolar epithelium. Gas exchange can only occur across the flat epithelium, which begins to appear on respiratory bronchioles (generations 17–19). The wall of the airway gradually loses its cartilaginous support (at the bronchioles) and then its smooth muscle. Loss of cartilaginous support causes the patency of smaller airways to become dependent on radial traction by the elastic recoil of the surrounding tissue; as a corollary, airway diameter becomes dependent on total lung volume (see below).

Cilia on the columnar and cuboidal epithelium normally beat in a synchronized fashion such that mucus (and any associated bacteria or debris) moves up toward the mouth.

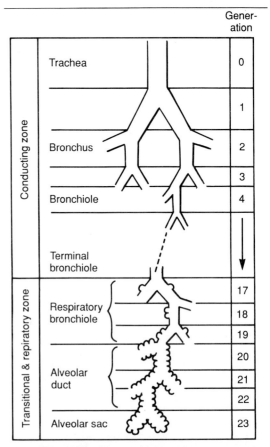

Figure 22–1. Dichotomous division of the airways. (Reproduced, with permission, from Weibel ER: *Morphometry of the Human Lung.* Springer-Verlag, 1963.)

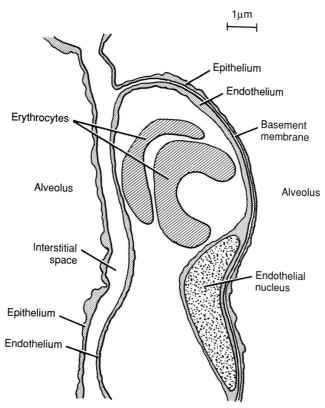

1μm
├──────┤

Epithelium

Endothelium

Erythrocytes

Basement
membrane

Alveolus

Alveolus

Interstitial
space

Endothelial
nucleus

Epithelium

Endothelium

Figure 22–2. The pulmonary interstitial space, with a capillary passing between two alveoli. The capillary is incorporated into the thin (gas-exchanging) side of the alveolus on the right. The interstitial space is incorporated into the thick side of the alveolus on the left. (Redrawn and reproduced, with permission, from Nunn JF: *Applied Respiratory Physiology,* 3rd ed. Butterworths, 1987.)

Alveoli

Alveolar size is a function of both gravity and lung volume. The average diameter of an alveolus is thought to be 0.2 mm. In the upright position, the largest alveoli are at the pulmonary apex, while the smallest tend to be at the base. With inspiration, discrepancies in alveolar size diminish.

Each alveolus is in close contact with a network of pulmonary capillaries. The walls of each alveolus are asymmetrically arranged (Figure 22–2). On one side, the alveolar epithelium and capillary endothelium are separated only by their respective cellular and basement membranes (the thin side); on the other side, the pulmonary interstitial space separates alveolar epithelium from capillary endothelium (the thick side). The pulmonary interstitial space contains mainly elastin, collagen, and perhaps nerve fibers. Gas exchange occurs primarily on the thin side of the alveolocapillary membrane, which is less than 0.4 μm thick. The thick side (1–2 μm) provides structural support for the alveolus.

The respiratory epithelium contains at least two cell types. Type I pneumocytes are flat and form tight (1 nm) junctions. These tight junctions are important in preventing the passage of large oncotically active molecules such as albumin into the alveolus. Type II pneumocytes, which are fewer in number, are round cells that contain prominent cytoplasmic inclusions (lamellar bodies). These inclusions contain surfactant, an important substance necessary for normal pulmonary mechanics (see below). Unlike type I cells, type II pneumocytes are capable of cell division and can produce type I pneumocytes if the latter are destroyed.

PULMONARY CIRCULATION

The lungs are supplied by two circulations, pulmonary and bronchial. The bronchial circulation arises from the left heart and sustains the metabolic needs of the tracheobronchial tree down to the level of the respiratory bronchioles. Below that level, lung tissue is supported by a combination of the alveolar gas and the pulmonary circulation.

The pulmonary circulation normally receives the total output of the right heart via the pulmonary artery, which divides into right and left branches to supply each lung. Deoxygenated blood passes through the pulmonary capillaries, where oxygen is taken up and CO_2 is eliminated. The oxygenated blood is then returned to the left heart by four main pulmonary veins (two from each lung). Although flows through the systemic and pulmonary circulations are equal, the lower pulmonary vascular resistance results in pulmonary vascular pressures one-sixth as great as those in the systemic circulation; as a result, both pulmonary arteries and veins normally have thinner walls with less smooth muscle.

Connections between the bronchial and the pulmonary circulations—and direct communications between pulmonary arterioles and pulmonary venules—are known to exist. The importance of the bronchial circulation in contributing to the normal venous admixture is discussed below. Direct pulmonary arteriovenous communications, bypassing the pulmonary capillaries, are normally insignificant but may become important in certain pathologic states (Chapters 26 and 35).

Pulmonary Capillaries

Pulmonary capillaries are incorporated into the walls of alveoli. The average diameter of these capillaries (about 10 μm) is barely enough to allow passage of a single red cell. Because each capillary network supplies more than one alveolus, blood may pass through several alveoli before reaching the pulmonary veins. Because of the relatively low pressure in the pulmonary circulation, the amount of blood flowing through a given capillary network is affected by both gravity and alveolar size. Large alveoli have a smaller capillary cross-sectional area and consequently increased resistance to blood flow. In the upright position, apical capillaries tend to have reduced flows, while basal capillaries have higher flows.

The pulmonary capillary endothelium has relatively large junctions, 5 nm wide, allowing the passage of large molecules such as albumin. As a result, pulmonary interstitial fluid is relatively rich in albumin. Circulating macrophages and neutrophils are able to pass through the endothelial as well as the smaller alveolar epithelial junctions with relative ease. Pulmonary macrophages are commonly seen in the interstitial space and inside alveoli; they serve to prevent bacterial infection and scavenge foreign particles.

PULMONARY LYMPHATICS

Lymphatic channels in the lung originate in the interstitial spaces of large septa. Because of the large endothelial junctions, pulmonary lymph has a relatively high protein content, and total pulmonary lymph flow is normally as much as 20 mL/min. Large lymphatic vessels travel upward alongside the airways, forming the tracheobronchial chain of lymph nodes. Lymphatic drainage channels from both lungs communicate along the trachea.

MECHANICS OF VENTILATION

BASIC MECHANISM OF BREATHING

Reoxygenation of desaturated blood and elimination of CO_2 result from the periodic exchange of alveolar gas with the fresh gas from the upper airway. This exchange is brought about by small cyclic pressure gradients established within the airways. During spontaneous ventilation, these gradients are secondary to variations in intrathoracic pressure, while during mechanical ventilation they are produced by intermittent positive pressure in the upper airway.

Spontaneous Ventilation

Normal pressure variations during spontaneous breathing are shown in Figure 22–3. The pressure within alveoli is always greater than the surrounding (intrathoracic) pressure unless they are collapsed. Alveolar pressure is normally atmospheric (zero for reference) at end-inspiration and end-expiration. By convention in respiratory physiology, pleural pressure is used as a measure of intrathoracic pressure. Although it may not be entirely correct to refer to the pressure in a potential space, the concept allows the calculation of transpulmonary pressure. Transpulmonary pressure, or $P_{transpulmonary}$, is then defined as follows:

$$P_{transpulmonary} = P_{alveolar} - P_{intrapleural}$$

At end-expiration, intrapleural pressure normally averages about -5 cm H_2O; consequently, transpulmonary pressure is $+5$ cm H_2O.

Diaphragmatic and intercostal muscle activation during inspiration expands the chest and decreases intrapleural pressure to -7.5 cm H_2O. As a result, alveolar pressure also decreases (between -1 and -2 cm H_2O), and an alveolar-upper airway gradient is established; gas flows from the upper airway into alveoli. At end-inspiration (when gas inflow has ceased), alveolar pressure returns to zero, but intrapleural pressure remains decreased; the new transpulmonary pressure ($+7.5$ cm H_2O) sustains lung expansion.

During expiration, diaphragmatic relaxation returns intrapleural pressure to -5 cm H_2O. Now the transpulmonary pressure does not support the new lung volume, and the elastic recoil of the lung causes a reversal of the previous alveolar-upper airway gradient; gas flows out of alveoli, and original lung volume is restored.

Mechanical Ventilation

Most forms of mechanical ventilation intermittently apply positive airway pressure at the upper airway. During inspiration, gas flows into alveoli until alveolar

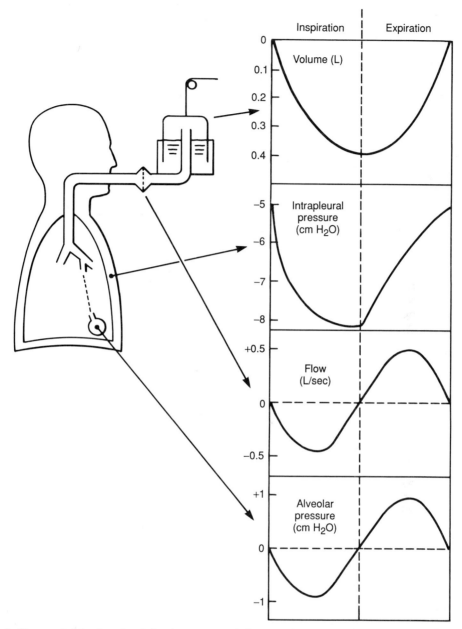

Figure 22–3. Changes in intrapleural and alveolar pressures during normal breathing. Note that at maximal tidal volume, flow is zero and alveolar pressure is atmospheric. (Adapted from West JB: *Respiratory Physiology,* 3rd ed. Williams & Wilkins, 1985.)

pressure reaches that in the upper airway. During the expiratory phase of the ventilator, the positive airway pressure is removed or decreased; the gradient reverses, allowing gas flow out of alveoli.

EFFECT OF ANESTHESIA ON RESPIRATORY PATTERN

Regardless of the agent used, light anesthesia often results in irregular respiratory patterns; breath holding is common. Respirations become regular with deeper levels of anesthesia. Inhalation agents generally produce rapid, shallow respirations, while nitrous-narcotic techniques result in slow, deep respirations.

Interestingly, induction of anesthesia activates expiratory muscles; expiration becomes active. The latter regularly necessitates paralysis during abdominal surgery. Inspiratory muscle activity is also altered; intercostal muscle activity is gradually lost with increasing anesthetic depth. Relative preservation of diaphragmatic function favors abdominal over thoracic chest excursion.

ELASTIC RECOIL

Both the lungs and the chest exhibit elastic properties. The chest has a tendency to expand outward, while the lungs have a tendency to collapse. When the chest is exposed to atmospheric pressure (open pneumothorax), it usually expands about 1 L in adults. In contrast, when the lung is exposed to atmospheric pressure, it collapses completely and all the gas within it is expelled. The recoil properties of the chest are due to structural components that resist deformation and probably include chest wall muscle tone. The elastic recoil of the lungs is due to their high content of elastin fibers and, even more importantly, the surface tension forces acting at the air-fluid interface in alveoli.

Surface Tension Forces

The gas-fluid interface lining alveoli causes them to behave as bubbles. Surface tension forces tend to reduce the area of the interface and favor alveolar collapse. Laplace's law can be used to quantify these forces:

$$Pressure = 2 \times \frac{Surface\ tension}{Radius}$$

The pressure derived from the equation is that within the alveolus. Alveolar collapse is therefore directly proportionate to surface tension but inversely proportionate to alveolar size. Collapse is more likely when surface tension increases or alveolar size decreases. Fortunately, pulmonary surfactant (see above) decreases alveolar surface tension. Moreover, surfactant's ability to lower surface tension is directly proportionate to its concentration within the alveolus. As alveoli become smaller, the surfactant within becomes more concentrated, and surface tension is more effectively reduced. Conversely, when alveoli are overdistended, surfactant becomes less concentrated, and surface tension increases. The net effect is to stabilize alveoli; small alveoli are prevented from getting smaller, while large alveoli are prevented from getting larger.

Compliance

Elastic recoil is usually measured in terms of compliance (C), which is defined as the change in volume divided by the change in distending pressure. Compliance measurements can be obtained for either the chest, the lung, or both together (Figure 22–4). In the supine position, chest wall compliance is reduced because of the weight of the abdominal contents against the diaphragm. Measurements are usually obtained under static conditions, ie, at equilibrium. (Dynamic compliance, which is measured during rhythmic breathing, is also dependent on airway resistance.)

$$C_{lung} = \frac{Change\ in\ lung\ volume}{Change\ in\ transpulmonary\ pressure}$$

Lung compliance is normally 200 mL/cm H_2O.

$$C_{chest} = \frac{Change\ in\ chest\ volume}{Change\ in\ transthoracic\ pressure}$$

where transthoracic pressure = atmospheric pressure − intrapleural pressure.

Normal chest compliance is 200 mL/cm H_2O. Total compliance (lung and chest together) is 100 mL/cm H_2O and is expressed by the following equation:

$$\frac{1}{C_{total}} = \frac{1}{C_{chest\ wall}} + \frac{1}{C_{lung}}$$

LUNG VOLUMES

Lung volumes are important parameters in respiratory physiology and clinical practice (Table 22–1 and Figure 22–5). The sum of all the named lung **volumes** equals the maximal amount the lung can be inflated. Lung **capacities** are clinically useful measurements that represent a combination of two or more volumes.

Functional Residual Capacity

The lung volume at which the inward elastic recoil of the lung equals the outward elastic recoil of the chest is called **functional residual capacity (FRC).** Thus, the elastic properties of both chest and lung define the point from which normal breathing takes place, which is FRC. Factors known to alter the FRC include the following:

(1) Body habitus: FRC is directly proportionate to height. Obesity however can markedly decrease FRC (primarily due to reduced chest compliance).
(2) Sex: FRC is reduced about 10% in females compared to males.
(3) Posture: The decrease in FRC seen in the supine and prone positions is the result of reduced chest compliance as abdominal contents push up against the diaphragm.
(4) Lung disease: Decreased compliance of the lung, chest, or both is characteristic of restrictive pulmonary disorders (Chapter 23), all of which are necessarily associated with a low FRC.

Closing Capacity

As described above (see Functional Anatomy of the Lungs), small airways lacking cartilaginous support are dependent on radial traction by the elastic recoil of surrounding tissue to keep them open; patency of these airways, especially in basal areas of the lung, is highly dependent on lung volume. The volume at which these airways begin to close in dependent parts of the lung is called the **closing capacity.** At lung volumes below closing capacity, alveoli in dependent areas continue to

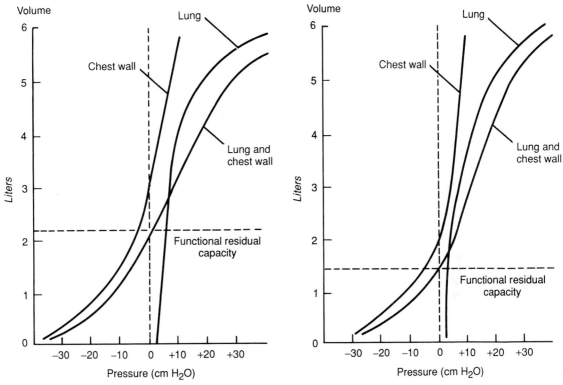

A. UPRIGHT

B. SUPINE

Figure 22–4. The pressure-volume relationship for the chest wall, lung, and both together in the upright **(A)** and supine **(B)** positions. (Modified and reproduced, with permission, from Scurr C, Feldman S: *Scientific Foundations of Anesthesia,* Heinemann, 1982.)

be perfused but are no longer ventilated; intrapulmonary shunting of deoxygenated blood promotes hypoxemia (see below).

Closing capacity is normally well below FRC (Figure 22–6), but it rises steadily with age (Figure 22–7). It is probably responsible for the normal age-related decline in arterial oxygen tension. At an average age of 44 years, closing capacity equals FRC in the supine position; by age 66 years, closing capacity equals or exceeds FRC in the upright position in most individuals.

Vital Capacity

Vital capacity (VC) is the maximal volume of gas that can be exhaled following maximal inspiration. In addition to body habitus, VC is also dependent on respiratory muscle strength and chest-lung compliance. Normal VC is about 60–70 mL/kg.

Table 22–1. Lung volumes and capacities.

Measurement	Definition	Average Adult Values (mL)
Tidal volume (V_T)	Each normal breath	500
Inspiratory reserve volume (IRV)	Maximal additional that can be inspired above V_T	3000
Expiratory reserve volume (ERV)	Maximal volume that can be expired below V_T	1100
Residual volume (RV)	Volume remaining after maximal exhalation	1200
Total lung capacity (TLC)	RV + ERV + V_T + IRV	5800
Functional residual capacity (FRC)	RV + ERV	2300

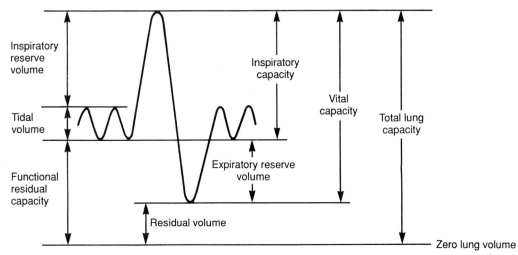

Figure 22–5. Spirogram showing static lung volumes. (Reproduced, with permission, from Nunn JF: *Applied Respiratory Physiology,* 3rd ed. Butterworths, 1987.)

EFFECTS OF ANESTHESIA ON LUNG VOLUMES & COMPLIANCE

Induction of anesthesia consistently produces an additional 15–20% greater reduction in FRC (400 mL in most patients) than that which occurs with the supine position alone. Loss of normal end-expiratory diaphragmatic tone allows the abdominal contents to rise farther up against the diaphragm (Figure 22–8). The higher position of the diaphragm decreases lung volume and reduces both chest and lung compliance. This decrease in FRC is not related to anesthetic depth and may persist for several hours following anesthesia. Head-down (Trendelenburg) position reduces FRC even further as intrathoracic blood volume increases. In contrast, induction of anesthesia in the sitting position appears to have little effect on FRC.

Both FRC and closing capacity are generally reduced to the same extent under anesthesia. Thus, the risk of increased intrapulmonary shunting under anes-

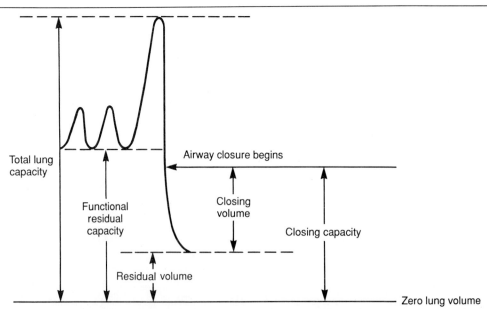

Figure 22–6. The relationship between functional residual capacity, closing volume, and closing capacity. (Reproduced, with permission, from Nunn JF: *Applied Respiratory Physiology,* 3rd ed. Butterworths, 1987.)

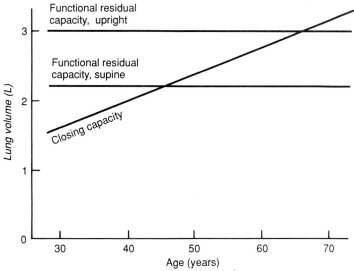

Figure 22–7. The effect of age on closing capacity and FRC. Note that FRC does not change. (Reproduced, with permission, from Nunn JF: *Applied Respiratory Physiology,* 3rd ed. Butterworths, 1987.)

thesia is similar to that in the conscious awake state, being greatest in the elderly, in obese patients, and in those with underlying pulmonary disease.

AIRWAY RESISTANCE

Gas flow in the lung is a mixture of laminar and turbulent flow. Laminar flow may be thought of as consisting of concentric cylinders of gas flowing at different velocities; velocity is highest in the center and decreases as one moves to the periphery. During laminar flow,

$$\text{Flow} = \frac{\text{Pressure gradient}}{R_{aw}}$$

where R_{aw} is airway resistance.

$$R_{aw} = \frac{8 \times \text{Length} \times \text{Viscosity of gas}}{\pi \times (\text{Radius})^4}$$

Turbulent flow is characterized by random movement of the gas molecules down the air passages. Mathematical description of turbulent flow is considerably more complex:

$$\text{Pressure gradient} \approx \text{Flow}^2 \times \frac{\text{Density}}{\text{Radius}^5}$$

Resistance is not constant but increases in proportion to gas flow. Moreover, resistance is directly proportionate to gas density and inversely proportionate to the fifth power of the radius. As a result, turbulent gas flow is extremely sensitive to airway caliber.

Turbulence generally occurs at high gas flows, at sharp angles or branching points, and in response to abrupt changes in airway diameter. Whether turbulent or laminar flow occurs can be predicted by the Reynolds number, which is arrived at by the following equation:

Reynolds number =

$$\text{Linear velocity} \times \text{Diameter} \times \frac{\text{Gas density}}{\text{Gas viscosity}}$$

A low Reynolds number (< 1000) is associated with laminar flow, whereas a high value (> 1500) produces turbulent flow. Laminar flow normally occurs only distal to small bronchioles (< 1 mm). Flow in larger airways is probably turbulent. Of the gases used clinically, only helium has a significantly lower density-to-viscosity ratio so as to be useful clinically during severe turbulent flow (as caused by upper airway obstruction). A helium-oxygen mixture not only is less likely to cause turbulent flow but also reduces airway resistance when turbulent flow is present.

Normal total airway resistance is about 0.5–2 cm $H_2O/L/s$, with the largest contribution coming from medium-sized bronchi (before the seventh generation). Resistance in large bronchi is low because of their large diameters, while resistance in small bronchi is low because of their large total cross-sectional area. At low lung volumes, loss of radial traction increases the contribution of small airways to total resistance; airway resistance becomes inversely proportionate to lung volume (Figure 22–9). Moreover, during forced expiration, reversal of the normal transmural airway pressure can cause collapse of these airways (dynamic airway compression). Two contributing factors are

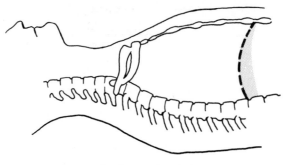

Awake spontaneous

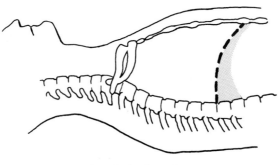

Anesthetized spontaneous

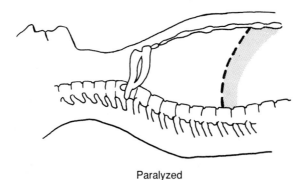

Paralyzed

Figure 22–8. The end-expiratory position of the diaphragm (broken line) in an awake spontaneously ventilating patient, an anesthetized spontaneously ventilating patient, and a paralyzed patient. The shaded area shows diaphragmatic excursion. (Modified and reproduced, with permission, from Froese AB, Bryan AC: Effects of anesthesia and paralysis on diaphragmatic mechanics in man. Anesthesiology 1974;41:242.)

responsible: (1) generation of a positive pleural pressure, and (2) a large pressure drop across intrathoracic airways due to increased airway resistance. The latter is in turn due to high (turbulent) gas flow and the reduced lung volume. The terminal portion of the flow/volume curve is therefore termed effort-independent (Figure 22–10).

Pathologic increases in airway resistance can result from (1) increased bronchial smooth muscle tone, (2) anatomic obstructions within the airway, or (3) external compression.

Forced Vital Capacity

When vital capacity is measured as an exhalation that is as hard and as rapid as possible (Figure 22–11), important information about airway resistance is obtained. The ratio of the volume exhaled in the first second (FEV_1) to the total forced vital capacity (FVC) is proportionate to the degree of airway obstruction. Normally, FEV_1/FVC is 80%. While both FEV_1 and FVC are effort-dependent, forced mid-expiratory flow ($FEF_{25-75\%}$) is effort-independent and may be a more reliable measurement of obstruction.

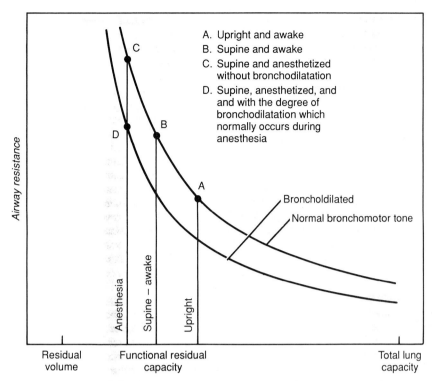

A. Upright and awake
B. Supine and awake
C. Supine and anesthetized without bronchodilatation
D. Supine, anesthetized, and and with the degree of bronchodilatation which normally occurs during anesthesia

Figure 22–9. The relationship between airway resistance and lung volume. (Reproduced, with permission, from Nunn JF: *Applied Respiratory Physiology,* 3rd ed. Butterworths, 1987.)

Effect of Anesthesia on Airway Resistance

The reduction in FRC associated with general anesthesia would be expected to increase airway resistance. However, increases in resistance are not usually observed because of the bronchodilating properties of the volatile inhalational anesthetics. Increased airway resistance is more commonly due to pathologic factors (posterior displacement of the tongue; laryngospasm; bronchoconstriction; or secretions, blood, or tumor in the airway) or equipment problems (small endotracheal tubes or connectors, malfunction of valves, or obstruction of the breathing circuit).

WORK OF BREATHING

Because expiration is normally entirely passive, both the inspiratory and the expiratory work of breathing is performed by the inspiratory muscles (primarily the diaphragm). Three factors must be overcome during ventilation: (1) the elastic recoil of the chest and lung, (2) frictional resistance to gas flow in the airways, and (3) tissue frictional resistance. The last factor is minor and generally ignored.

Respiratory work can be expressed as the product of

volume and pressure (Figure 22–12). During inhalation, both inspiratory airway resistance and pulmonary elastic recoil must be overcome; nearly 50% of the energy expended is stored in the form of pulmonary elastic recoil. During exhalation, the stored potential energy is released and overcomes expiratory airway resistance. Increases in either inspiratory or expiratory resistance are compensated by increased inspiratory muscle effort. When expiratory resistance increases, the normal compensatory response is to increase lung volume such that tidal breathing occurs at an abnormally high FRC. The greater elastic recoil energy stored at a higher lung volume overcomes the added expiratory resistance. Excessive amounts of expiratory resistance also activate expiratory muscles (see above).

Respiratory muscles normally account for only 2% of oxygen consumption but operate at only about 10% efficiency. Ninety percent of the work is dissipated as heat (due to elastic and airflow resistance). In pathologic conditions, muscle efficiency usually progressively decreases with increasing ventilatory effort; moreover, a point is reached where any increase in oxygen uptake (due to augmented ventilation) is consumed by the respiratory muscles themselves.

The work required to overcome elastic resistance increases as tidal volume increases, while the work

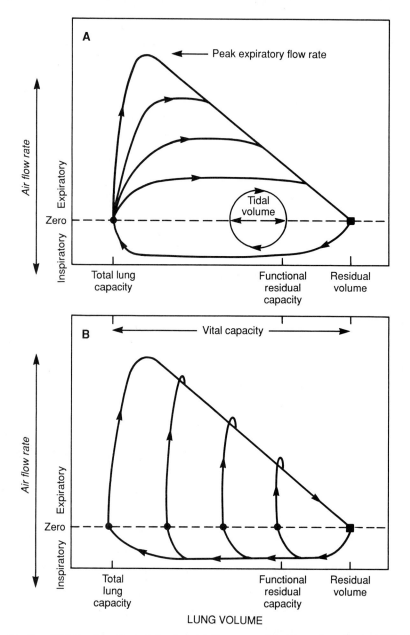

Figure 22–10. Gas flow *(A)* during forced exhalation from total lung capacity with varying effort and *(B)* with maximal effort from different lung volumes. Note that regardless of initial lung volume or effort, terminal expiratory flows are effort-independent. (Reproduced, with permission, from Nunn JF: *Applied Respiratory Physiology,* 3rd ed. Butterworths, 1987.)

required to overcome air flow resistance increases as respiratory rate (and, necessarily, expiratory flow) increases. Faced with either condition, patients minimize the work of breathing by altering respiratory rate and tidal volume (Figure 22–13). Patients with reduced compliance tend to have rapid, shallow respirations, whereas those with increased air flow resistance have a slow, deep breathing pattern.

Effects of Anesthesia on the Work of Breathing

Increases in the work of breathing under anesthesia are most often secondary to reduced lung and chest wall compliance and, less commonly, increases in airway resistance (see above). The problems of increased work of breathing are usually circumvented by controlled mechanical ventilation.

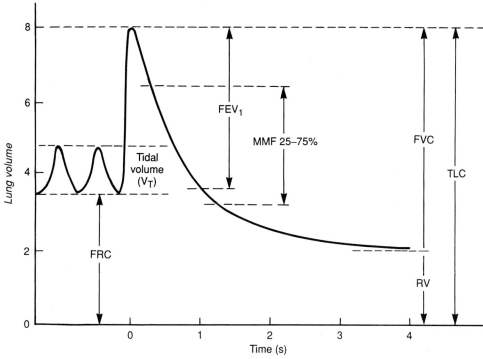

Figure 22–11. The normal forced exhalation curve. $FEF_{25-75\%}$, also called the maximum mid-expiratory flow rate $(MMF_{25-75\%})$, is shown.

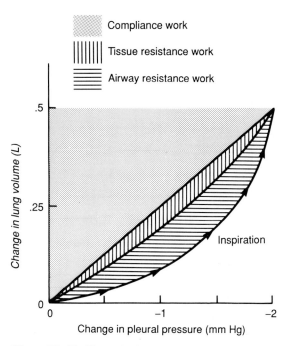

Figure 22–12. The work of breathing and its components during inspiration. (Reproduced, with permission, from Guyton AC: *Textbook of Medical Physiology,* 7th ed. Saunders, 1986.)

VENTILATION/PERFUSION RELATIONSHIPS

VENTILATION

Ventilation is usually measured as the sum of all exhaled gas volumes in 1 minute (minute ventilation, or $\dot{V}_{min}$). If tidal volume is constant,

Minute ventilation = Respiratory rate × Tidal volume

For the average adult at rest, minute ventilation is about 5 L/min.

Not all the inspired gas mixture reaches alveoli; some of it remains in the airways and is exhaled without exchange with alveolar gases. That part of the tidal volume (V_T) not participating in alveolar gas exchange is known as dead space (V_D). Alveolar ventilation ($\dot{V}_A$) is the volume of inspired gases actually taking part in gas exchange in 1 minute.

$$\dot{V}_A = \text{Respiratory rate} \times (V_T - V_D)$$

Dead space is actually composed of gases in nonrespiratory airways (anatomic dead space) as well as in alveoli that are not perfused (alveolar dead space). The sum of the two is referred to as physiologic dead space.

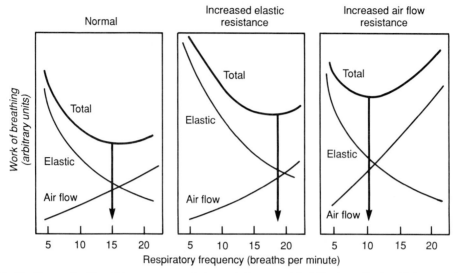

Figure 22–13. The work of breathing versus respiratory rate for normal individuals, patients with increased elastic resistance, and patients with increased airway resistance. (Reproduced, with permission, from Nunn JF: *Applied Respiratory Physiology,* 3rd ed. Butterworths, 19879.)

In the upright position, physiologic dead space is normally about 150 mL for most adults (approximately 2 mL/kg) and is nearly all anatomic. The weight of an individual in pounds is roughly equivalent to dead space in milliliters. Dead space can be affected by a variety of factors (Table 22–2).

Since tidal volume in the average adult is approximately 450 mL (6 mL/kg), V_D/V_T is normally 33%. This ratio may derived by the Bohr equation:

$$V_D/V_T = \frac{P_{A}CO_2 - P_{E}CO_2}{P_{A}CO_2}$$

where $P_{A}CO_2$ is the alveolar CO_2 tension and $P_{E}CO_2$ is the mixed expired CO_2 tension. This equation is useful clinically if arterial CO_2 tension ($P_{a}CO_2$) is used to approximate the alveolar concentration and the CO_2

Table 22–2. Factors affecting dead space.

Factor	Effect
Posture	
Upright	↑
Supine	↓
Position of airway	
Neck extension	↑
Neck flexion	↓
Age	↑
Artificial airway	↓
Positive-pressure ventilation	↑
Drugs	
Anticholinergics	↑
Pulmonary perfusion	
Pulmonary emboli	↑
Hypotension	↑
Lung disease	↑

tension in expired air gases is the average measured over several minutes.

DISTRIBUTION OF VENTILATION

Regardless of body position, alveolar ventilation is unevenly distributed in the lungs. Lower (dependent) areas of the lung tend to be better ventilated than upper areas. This inequality is due to a gravitationally induced gradient in intrapleural pressure and necessarily in transpulmonary pressure (see above). Pleural pressure increases about 1 cm H_2O (becomes less negative) per 3 cm decrease in lung height. This difference places alveoli at different points on the pulmonary compliance curve (Figure 22–14). Because of a higher transpulmonary pressure, alveoli in upper lung areas are near-maximally inflated and relatively noncompliant, and they undergo little more expansion during inspiration. In contrast, the smaller alveoli in dependent areas have a lower transpulmonary pressure, are more compliant, and undergo greater expansion during inspiration.

Airway resistance can also contribute to regional differences in pulmonary ventilation. Final alveolar inspiratory volume is solely dependent on compliance only if inspiratory time is unlimited. In reality, inspiratory time is necessarily limited by the respiratory rate and the time necessary for expiration; consequently, an excessively short inspiratory time will prevent alveoli from reaching the expected change in volume. Moreover, alveolar filling follows an exponential function that is dependent on both compliance and airway resistance. Thus, even with a normal inspiratory time, abnormalities in either compliance or resistance can prevent complete alveolar filling. Regional variations

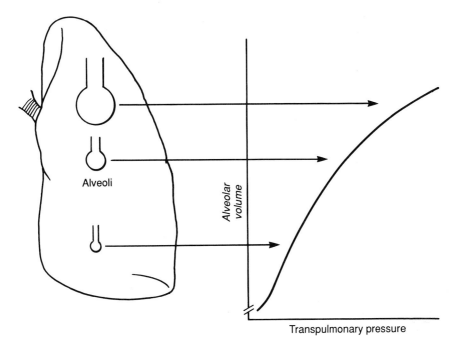

Figure 22–14. The effect of gravity on alveolar compliance in the upright position.

in resistance or compliance not only interfere with alveolar filling but can cause asynchrony in alveolar filling during inspiration (Figure 22–15). Lung inflation can be described mathematically by the time constant, τ. One τ is the time necessary for alveoli to reach 63% of their ultimate change in volume. Ninety-nine percent inflation is completed in $4 \times \tau$. τ = total compliance $\times$ airway resistance.

Variations in time constants within the normal lung can be demonstrated in normal individuals breathing spontaneously during abnormally high respiratory rates. Rapid shallow breathing reverses the normal distribution of ventilation, preferentially favoring upper (nondependent) areas of the lung over lower areas.

PULMONARY PERFUSION

Of the approximately 5 L/min of blood flowing through the lungs, only about 70–100 mL at any one time are within the pulmonary capillaries undergoing gas exchange. At the alveolar-capillary membrane, this small volume forms a 50–100 m² sheet of blood approximately one red cell thick. Moreover, to ensure optimal gas exchange, each capillary perfuses more than one alveolus.

Although capillary volume remains relatively constant, total pulmonary blood volume can vary between 500 mL and 1000 mL. Large increases in either cardiac output or blood volume are tolerated with little change in pressure due to passive dilatation of open vessels and recruitment of collapsed pulmonary vessels. Small increases in pulmonary blood volume normally occur

during cardiac systole and with each normal (spontaneous) inspiration. A shift in posture from supine to erect decreases pulmonary blood volume (up to 27%), whereas Trendelenburg positioning has the opposite effect. Changes in systemic capacitance also influence pulmonary blood volume: systemic venoconstriction shifts blood from the systemic to the pulmonary circulation, whereas vasodilation causes pulmonary to systemic redistribution. In this way, the lung acts a reservoir for the systemic circulation.

Local factors are more important than the autonomic system in influencing pulmonary vascular tone. Hypoxia is a powerful stimulus for pulmonary vasoconstriction (the opposite of its systemic effect). Both arterial and alveolar hypoxia induce vasoconstriction, but the latter is a more powerful stimulus. Hypoxic pulmonary vasoconstriction is an important physiologic mechanism in reducing intrapulmonary shunting and preventing hypoxemia (see below).

Autonomic innervation of the pulmonary vasculature is limited and probably confined to larger arterioles. Both alpha and beta receptors are present. Parasympathetic effects are minimal or nil.

DISTRIBUTION OF PULMONARY PERFUSION

Pulmonary blood flow is also not uniform. Regardless of body position, lower (dependent) portions of the lung receive greater blood flow than upper (nondependent) areas. This pattern is the result of a gravitational gradient of 1 cm H_2O/cm lung height. The nor-

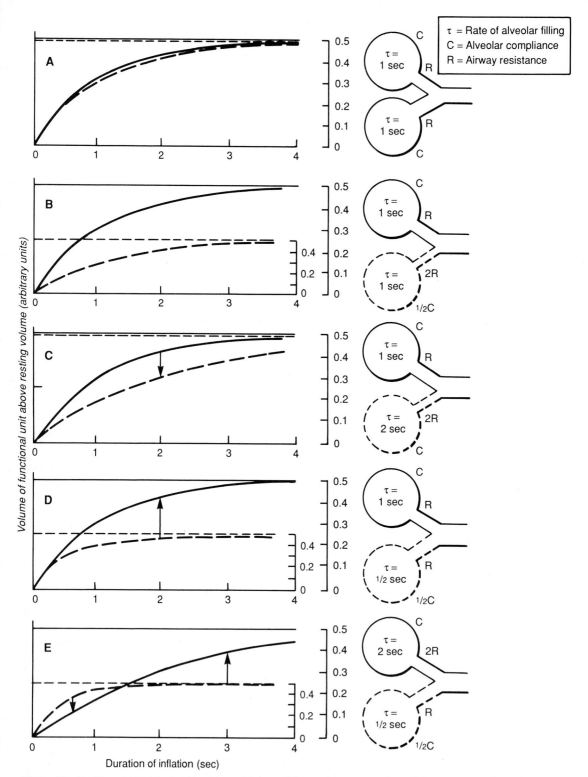

Figure 22–15. The effect of changes in airway resistance (R) and alveolar compliance (C) on the rate of alveolar filling (τ) during a sustained inflation of two alveoli. *A:* Same rate of filling and equal volumes. *B:* Same rate of filling but reduced volume on one side. *C:* Asymmetric filling but ultimately the same volumes. *D:* Same rate of filling but reduced volume on one side. *E:* Asymmetric filling and unequal volumes. (Reproduced, with permission, from Nunn JF: *Applied Respiratory Physiology,* 3rd ed. Butterworths, 1987.)

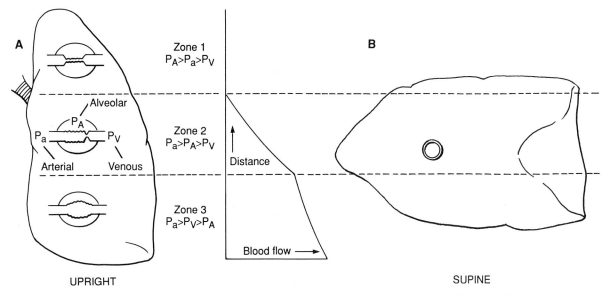

Figure 22–16. The three-zone model of the lung. **A:** Upright position. **B:** Supine position.

mally low pressures in the pulmonary circulation (Chapter 19) allow gravity to exert a significant influence on blood flow.

For simplification, each lung may be divided into three zones, based on alveolar (P_A), arterial (Pa), and venous (Pv) pressures (Figure 22–16). Zone 1 is the upper zone and represents alveolar dead space because alveolar pressure continually occludes the pulmonary arterial capillary. In the middle zone (zone 2), pulmonary capillary flow is intermittent and varies during respiration according to the arterial-alveolar pressure gradient. Pulmonary capillary flow is continuous in zone 3 and is proportionate to the arterial-venous pressure gradient.

VENTILATION/PERFUSION RATIOS

Since alveolar ventilation ($\dot{V}$) is normally about 4 L/min and pulmonary capillary perfusion ($\dot{Q}$) is 5 L/min, the overall $\dot{V}/\dot{Q}$ ratio is 0.8. $\dot{V}/\dot{Q}$ for individual lung units (each alveolus and its capillary) can range from 0 (no ventilation) to infinity (no perfusion); the former constitutes alveolar dead space (zone 1, above), while the latter is referred to as intrapulmonary shunt (Figure 22–17). $\dot{V}/\dot{Q}$ normally ranges between 0.3 and 3.0, with the majority of lung areas being close to 1.0 (Figure 22–18A). Because perfusion increases at a greater rate than ventilation, nondependent (apical) areas tend to have higher $\dot{V}/\dot{Q}$ ratios than dependent (basal) areas (Figure 22–18B).

The importance of $\dot{V}/\dot{Q}$ ratios relates to the efficiency with which lung units resaturate venous blood with oxygen and eliminate CO_2. Pulmonary venous blood (the effluent) from areas with low $\dot{V}/\dot{Q}$ ratios has a low O_2 tension and high CO_2 tension—similar to systemic mixed venous blood. Blood from these units tends to depress arterial oxygen tension and elevate arterial CO_2 tension. Their effect on arterial oxygen tension is much more profound than that on CO_2 tension; in fact, arterial CO_2 tension often decreases owing to a hypoxemia-induced reflex increase in alveolar ventilation (see below). An appreciable compensatory increase in oxygen uptake cannot take place in remaining areas where $\dot{V}/\dot{Q}$ is normal, because pulmonary end-capillary blood is normally already maximally saturated with oxygen (see below).

SHUNT

In pulmonary physiology, "shunting" denotes the process whereby desaturated, mixed venous blood from the right heart returns to the left heart without being resaturated with oxygen in the lungs. The overall effect of shunting is to decrease (dilute) arterial oxygen content. This type of shunt is referred to as right-to-left in cardiac physiology (Chapter 19); in contrast, left-to-right shunts (in the absence of pulmonary congestion) do not produce hypoxemia.

Intrapulmonary shunts are often classified as absolute or relative. Absolute shunt refers to anatomic shunts and lung units where $\dot{V}/\dot{Q}$ is zero. A relative shunt is an area of the lung with a low but finite $\dot{V}/\dot{Q}$ ratio. Clinically, hypoxemia due to a relative shunt can usually be partially corrected by increasing the inspired oxygen concentration, whereas that due to absolute shunts cannot.

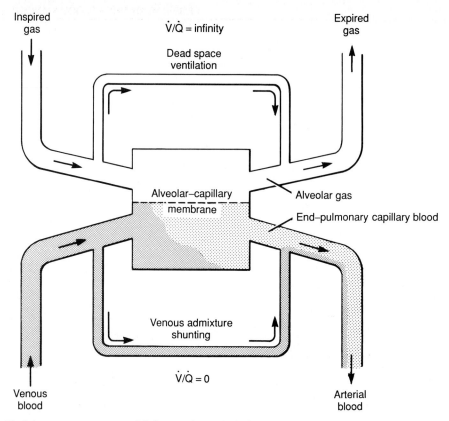

Figure 22–17. A three-compartment model of gas exchange in the lungs, showing dead space ventilation, normal alveolar-capillary exchange, and shunting (venous admixture). (Modified and reproduced, with permission, from Nunn JF: *Applied Respiratory Physiology,* 3rd ed. Butterworths, 1987.)

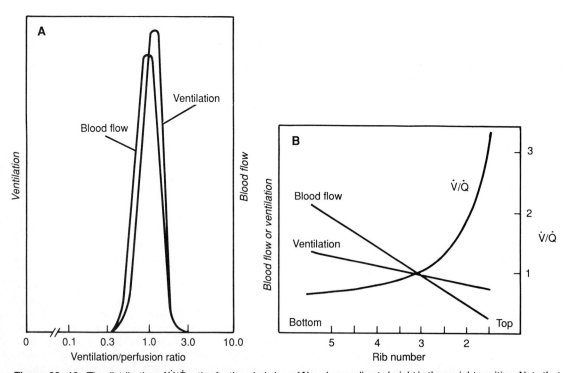

Figure 22–18. The distribution of V̇/Q̇ ratios for the whole lung *(A)* and according to height in the upright position. Note that blood flow increases more rapidly than ventilation in dependent areas. (Reproduced, with permission from West JB: *Ventilation/Blood Flow and Gas Exchange,* 3rd ed. Blackwell, 1977.)

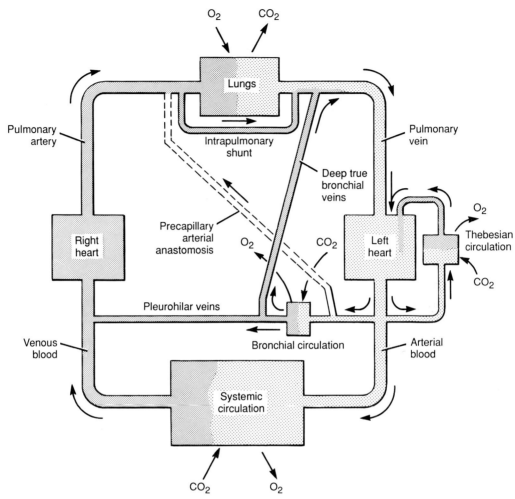

Figure 22–19. Components of the normal venous admixture. (Reproduced, with permission, from Nunn JF: *Applied Respiratory Physiology,* 3rd ed. Butterworths, 1987.)

Venous Admixture

This term refers to a concept rather than an actual physiologic entity. Venous admixture is the amount of mixed venous blood that would have to be mixed with pulmonary end-capillary blood to account for the difference in oxygen tension between arterial and ideal pulmonary end-capillary blood. Ideal pulmonary end-capillary blood is considered to have the same concentrations as alveolar gas. Venous admixture ($\dot{Q}_s$) is usually expressed as a fraction of total cardiac output ($\dot{Q}_t$). The equation for $\dot{Q}_s/\dot{Q}_t$ may be derived by employing the law of conservation of mass for oxygen across the pulmonary bed:

$$\dot{Q}_t \times CaO_2 = (\dot{Q}_s \times C\bar{v}O_2) + (\dot{Q}_c \times Cc'O_2)$$

where

$\dot{Q}_c$ = Blood flow across normally ventilated pulmonary capillaries,

$\dot{Q}_t = \dot{Q}_c + \dot{Q}_s$,

$Cc'O_2$ = Oxygen content of ideal pulmonary end-capillary blood,

CaO_2 = Arterial oxygen content, and

$C\bar{v}O_2$ = mixed venous content.

The simplified equation is—

$$\frac{\dot{Q}_s}{\dot{Q}_t} = \frac{Cc'O_2 - CaO_2}{Cc'O_2 - C\bar{v}O_2}$$

The formula for calculating the oxygen content of blood is given below.

$\dot{Q}_s/\dot{Q}_t$ can be calculated clinically by obtaining mixed venous and arterial blood gas measurements; the former requires a pulmonary artery catheter. The alveolar gas equation is used to derive pulmonary end-capillary oxygen tension. Pulmonary capillary blood can usually be assumed to be 100% saturated for an $FIO_2 > 0.21$.

The calculated venous admixture assumes that all shunting is intrapulmonary and is due to absolute shunts ($\dot{V}/\dot{Q} = 0$). In reality, neither is ever the case; nonetheless, the concept is extremely useful clinically. Normal $\dot{Q}_s/\dot{Q}_t$ is primarily due to (1) communications between deep bronchial veins and pulmonary veins, (2) the thebesian circulation in the heart, and (3) areas of low but finite $\dot{V}/\dot{Q}$ in the lungs (Figure 22–19). "Physiologic shunt" is typically less than 5%.

EFFECTS OF ANESTHESIA ON GAS EXCHANGE

Abnormalities in gas exchange during anesthesia are common. They include increased dead space, hypoventilation (see below), and increased intrapulmonary shunting. Increases in alveolar dead space are most commonly seen during controlled ventilation but may also occur during spontaneous ventilation. General anesthesia commonly increases venous admixture to 5–10%. Elderly patients appear to have the largest increases. Although the physiologic basis of increased shunting is not clear, airway collapse in dependent areas of the lung (see above) is probably responsible. Moreover, inspired oxygen tensions of 30–40% usually prevent hypoxemia, implicating relative shunt. Prolonged administration of high inspired oxygen concentrations ($> 50\%$) may be associated with increases in absolute shunt. In these instances, complete collapse of alveoli with previously low $\dot{V}/\dot{Q}$ ratios is thought to occur once all the oxygen within is taken up (absorption atelectasis). Positive end-expiratory pressure (PEEP) is usually effective in reducing venous admixture and preventing hypoxemia during general anesthesia as long as cardiac output is maintained (Chapter 48).

ALVEOLAR, ARTERIAL, & VENOUS GAS TENSIONS

When dealing with gas mixtures, each gas is considered to contribute separately to total gas pressure, and its partial pressure is directly proportionate to its concentration. Air has an oxygen concentration of approximately 21%; therefore, if the barometric pressure is 760 mm Hg (sea level), the partial pressure of oxygen (PO_2) in air is normally—

$$\textbf{760 mm Hg} \times \textbf{0.21} = \textbf{159.6 mm Hg.}$$

In its general form, the equation may be written as—

$$PO_2 = P_B \times FIO_2$$

where P_B = barometric pressure and
    FIO_2 = the fraction of inspired oxygen.

Two rules of thumb may also be used: (1) partial pressure in millimeters of mercury equals the percentage $\times$ 7; and (2) partial pressure in kilopascals is approximately the same as percentage.

OXYGEN

Alveolar Oxygen Tension

With every breath, the inspired gas mixture is humidified at 37 °C in the upper airway. The inspired tension of oxygen (PIO_2) is therefore reduced by the added water vapor. Water vapor pressure is dependent only on temperature, being 47 mm Hg at 37 °C. In humidified air, the normal partial pressure of oxygen at sea level is—

$$\textbf{(760 − 47)} \times \textbf{0.21} = \textbf{149.3 mm Hg}$$

The general equation is—

$$PIO_2 = (P_B − P_{H_2O}) \times FIO_2$$

where P_{H_2O} = the vapor pressure of water at body temperature.

In alveoli, the inspired gases are mixed with residual alveolar gas from previous breaths, oxygen is taken up, and CO_2 is added. The final alveolar oxygen tension (PAO_2) is therefore dependent on all these factors and can be estimated by the following equation:

$$PAO_2 = PIO_2 − \frac{PaCO_2}{RQ}$$

where $PaCO_2$ = arterial CO_2 tension and
    RQ = respiratory quotient.

RQ is usually not measured and is assumed to be 0.8 at room air, but it is usually assumed to be 1 when an oxygen-enriched mixture is given. Note that large increases in $PaCO_2$ (> 75 mm Hg) readily produce hypoxia ($PAO_2 < 60$ mm Hg) at room air but not at high inspired oxygen concentrations.

A yet simpler method of approximating PAO_2 in millimeters of mercury is to multiply the percent inspired oxygen concentration by 6. Thus, at 40%, PAO_2 is 6 $\times$ 40, or 240 mm Hg.

Pulmonary End-Capillary Oxygen Tension

For all practical purposes, pulmonary end-capillary oxygen tension ($Pc'O_2$) may be considered identical to PAO_2; the PAO_2–$Pc'O_2$ gradient is normally minute. $Pc'O_2$ is dependent on both the rate of oxygen diffusion across the alveolar-capillary membrane and pulmonary capillary blood transit time. The large capil-

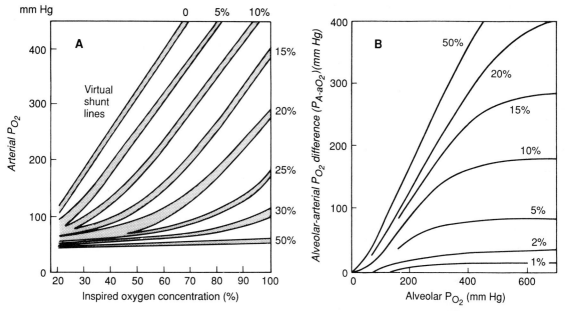

Figure 22–20. Isoshunt curves showing the effect of varying amounts of shunt on PaO_2 *(A)* and the A–a gradient *(B)* for oxygen at different inspired oxygen concentrations and alveolar PO_2, respectively. Note that there is little benefit in increasing inspired oxygen concentration in patients with very large shunts. (Modified and reproduced, with permission, from Nunn JF: *Applied Respiratory Physiology,* 3rd ed. Butterworths, 1987.)

lary surface area in alveoli and the 0.4–0.5 μm thickness of the alveolar-capillary membrane greatly facilitate oxygen diffusion. Additionally, enhanced oxygen binding to hemoglobin at saturations above 80% appears to augment oxygen diffusion (see below). Capillary transit time may be estimated by dividing pulmonary capillary blood volume by cardiac output (pulmonary blood flow); thus, normal capillary transit time is 70 mL ÷ 5000 mL/min, or 0.8 s. Maximum $Pc'O_2$ is usually attained after only 0.3 s, providing a large safety margin.

Oxygen diffusion across the alveolar-capillary membrane is expressed as oxygen diffusing capacity (DLO_2), where DLO_2 = oxygen uptake ÷ (PAO_2 – $Pc'O_2$). Since $Pc'O_2$ cannot be measured accurately, measurement of carbon monoxide diffusion capacity ($DLCO$) is used instead to assess gas transfer across the alveolar-capillary membrane. Carbon monoxide has a very high affinity for hemoglobin; thus, when administered at low concentration, $Pc'CO$ can be considered zero. Therefore, $DLCO$ = carbon monoxide uptake ÷ $PACO$.

Reductions in $DLCO$ imply an impediment in gas transfer across the alveolar-capillary membrane. Such impediments may be due to abnormal $\dot{V}/\dot{Q}$ ratios, excessive destruction of the gas alveolar-capillary membrane, or very short capillary transit times. Abnormalities are accentuated by increases in oxygen consumption and cardiac output, as during exercise.

Arterial Oxygen Tension

PaO_2 cannot be calculated like PAO_2 but must instead be measured. The alveolar to arterial oxygen partial pressure gradient (A–a gradient) is normally less than 15 mm Hg, but it progressively increases with age up to 40 mm Hg. Arterial oxygen tension may be approximated by the following formula (in mm Hg):

$$PaO_2 = 102 - \frac{Age}{3}$$

the range being 60–100 mm Hg (8–13 kPa). Decreases are probably the result of a progressive increase in closing capacity relative to FRC (see above).

The most common cause of hypoxemia is an increased A–a gradient. The A–a gradient for oxygen depends on (1) the amount of right-to-left shunting and (2) mixed venous oxygen tension (see below), which in turn depends on cardiac output, oxygen consumption, and hemoglobin concentration.

The A–a gradient for oxygen is directly proportionate to shunt but inversely proportionate to mixed venous oxygen tension. The effect of each variable on PaO_2 and the A–a gradient can only be determined when the other variables are held constant. Figure 22–20 shows the effect of different degrees of shunting on PaO_2 and the A–a gradient. It should also be noted that the greater the shunt, the less likely that an increase in FIO_2 will prevent hypoxemia.

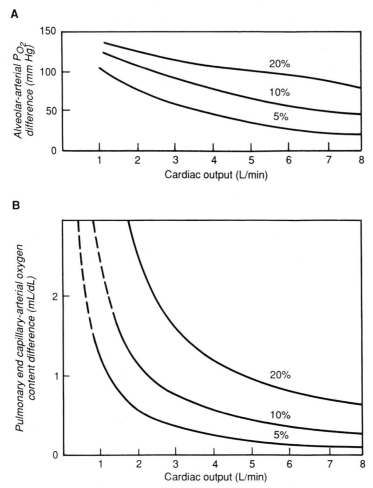

Figure 22–21. The effect of cardiac output on the alveolar-arterial PO_2 difference and pulmonary end-capillary and arterial oxygen content difference with varying degrees of shunting. ($\dot{V}O_2$ = 200 mL/min and PaO_2 = 180 mm Hg.) (Modified and reproduced, with permission, from Nunn JF: *Applied Respiratory Physiology,* 3rd ed. Butterworths, 1987.)

The effect of cardiac output on the A–a gradient (Figure 22–21) is due not only to its secondary effects on mixed venous oxygen tension (Chapter 19) but also to a direct relationship between cardiac output and intrapulmonary shunting. The reduction in intrapulmonary shunting sometimes seen with low cardiac outputs may be secondary to accentuated pulmonary vasoconstriction from a lower mixed venous oxygen tension.

Mixed Venous Oxygen Tension

Normal mixed venous oxygen tension ($P\bar{v}O_2$) is about 40 mm Hg and represents the balance between overall oxygen consumption and oxygen delivery (see below). A true mixed venous blood sample contains venous drainage from the superior vena cava, the inferior vena cava, and the heart; it must therefore be obtained from a pulmonary artery catheter.

CARBON DIOXIDE

Mixed Venous Carbon Dioxide Tension

Normal mixed venous CO_2 tension ($P\bar{v}O_2$) is about 46 mm Hg and is the end result of mixing of blood from tissues of varying metabolic activity. Venous CO_2 tension is lower in tissues with low metabolic activity (skin) but higher in blood from those with relatively high activity (heart).

Alveolar Carbon Dioxide Tension

Alveolar CO_2 tension ($PaCO_2$) represents the balance between total CO_2 production ($\dot{V}CO_2$) and alveolar ventilation (elimination): $PaCO_2 = \dot{V}CO_2 \div \dot{V}A$, where $\dot{V}A$ is alveolar ventilation (Figure 22–22). Clinically, $P\bar{v}CO_2$ is more dependent on alveolar ventilation than $\dot{V}CO_2$, because the latter does not vary

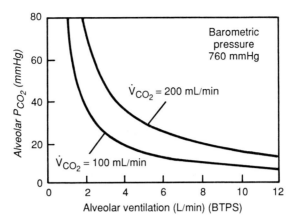

Figure 22–22. The effect of alveolar ventilation on alveolar $PaCO_2$ at two different rates of CO_2 production. (Modified and reproduced, with permission, from Nunn JF: *Applied Respiratory Physiology,* 3rd ed. Butterworths, 1987.)

appreciably under most circumstances. Moreover, the body's large capacity to store CO_2 (see below) buffers acute changes in $\dot{V}CO_2$.

Pulmonary End-Capillary Carbon Dioxide Tension

Pulmonary end-capillary CO_2 tension ($Pc'CO_2$) is virtually identical to $PACO_2$ (for the same reasons discussed in the section about oxygen). A significant gradient is unlikely, especially in view of the fact that the diffusion rate for CO_2 across the alveolar-capillary membrane is 20 times that of oxygen.

Arterial Carbon Dioxide Tension

Arterial CO_2 tension ($PaCO_2$), which is readily measurable, is identical to $Pc'CO_2$ and, necessarily, $PACO_2$. Normal $PaCO_2$ is 38 ± 4 mm Hg (5.1 ± 0.5 kPa); in practice, 40 mm Hg is usually considered normal.

Although low $\dot{V}/\dot{Q}$ ratios tend to increase $PaCO_2$ while high $\dot{V}/\dot{Q}$ ratios tend to decrease it, significant arterial-to-alveolar gradients for CO_2 (in contrast to the PAO_2–PaO_2 gradient) develop only in the presence of marked $\dot{V}/\dot{Q}$ abnormalities. Even moderate to severe disturbances usually fail to appreciably alter arterial CO_2. This observation is at least partly due to a reflex increase in ventilation from concomitant hypoxemia. Moreover, the diffusion capacity for CO_2 ($DLCO_2$) is significantly larger than that for oxygen; the quantity of CO_2 entering alveoli from the pulmonary capillaries is limited only by the total area of the alveolar-capillary membrane and capillary transit time. Even a small increase in the $P\bar{v}CO_2$–$PACO_2$ gradient appreciably increases CO_2 elimination in alveoli with still relatively normal $\dot{V}/\dot{Q}$ ratios.

End-Tidal Carbon Dioxide Tension

Because end-tidal gas normally is primarily alveolar gas and $PACO_2$ is virtually identical to $PaCO_2$, end-

tidal CO_2 tension ($PETCO_2$) is used clinically as an estimate of $PaCO_2$ (Chapter 6). The $PaCO_2$–$PETCO_2$ gradient is normally less than 5 mm Hg and represents dilution of alveolar gas with CO_2-free gas from nonperfused alveoli (alveolar dead space).

TRANSPORT OF RESPIRATORY GASES IN BLOOD

OXYGEN

Oxygen is carried in blood in two forms: (1) dissolved in solution and (2) in reversible association with hemoglobin.

Dissolved Oxygen

The amount of oxygen dissolved in blood can be derived from Henry's law, which states that the concentration of any gas in solution is proportionate to its partial pressure. The mathematical expression is as follows:

Gas concentration $= \alpha \times$ Partial pressure

where $\alpha =$ gas solubility coefficient for a given solution at a given temperature.

The solubility coefficient for oxygen at normal body temperature is 0.003 mL/dL/mmhg. Even with a PaO_2 of 100 mm Hg, the maximum amount of oxygen dissolved in blood is very small (0.3 mL/dL) compared to that bound to hemoglobin (see below).

Hemoglobin

Hemoglobin is a complex large molecule consisting of four heme and four protein subunits. Heme is an iron-porphyrin compound that is an essential part of

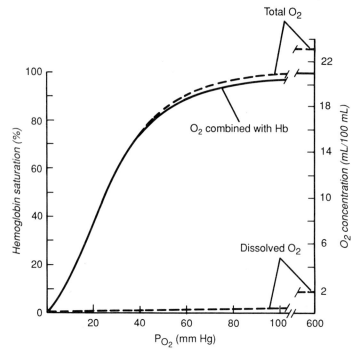

Figure 22–23. The normal adult hemoglobin-oxygen dissociation curve. (Reproduced, with permission, from West JB: *Respiratory Physiology: The Essentials,* 3rd ed. Williams & Wilkins, 1985.)

the oxygen binding sites; only the divalent form (+2 charge) of iron can bind oxygen. The normal hemoglobin molecule (hemoglobin A_1) consists of two alpha and two beta chains (subunits); the four subunits are held together by weak bonds between the amino acid residues. Each gram of hemoglobin can theoretically carry up to 1.39 mL of oxygen.

Hemoglobin Dissociation Curve

Each hemoglobin molecule binds up to four oxygen molecules. The complex interaction between the hemoglobin subunits results in nonlinear (an elongated S shape) binding with oxygen (Figure 22–23). Hemoglobin saturation is the amount of oxygen bound as a percentage of its total oxygen-binding capacity. Four separate chemical reactions are involved in binding each of the four oxygens. The change in molecular conformation induced by the binding of the first three oxygens greatly accelerates binding of the fourth oxygen molecule. The last reaction is responsible for the accelerated binding between 25% and 100% saturation. Near 90% saturation, the decrease in available oxygen receptors flattens the curve until full saturation is reached.

Factors Influencing the Hemoglobin Dissociation Curve

Clinically important factors altering oxygen binding include (1) hydrogen ion concentration, (2) CO_2 tension, (3) temperature, and (4) 2,3-diphosphoglycerate

(2,3-DPG) concentration. Their effect on hemoglobin-oxygen interaction can be expressed by the P_{50}, the oxygen tension at which hemoglobin is 50% saturated (Figure 22–24). Each factor shifts the dissociation curve either to the right (increasing the P_{50}) or to the left (decreasing P_{50}). A rightward shift lowers oxygen affinity, displaces oxygen from hemoglobin, and makes more oxygen available to tissues; a leftward shift increases hemoglobin's affinity for oxygen, reducing its availability to tissues. The normal P_{50} is 26 mm Hg (3.4 kPa).

An increase in blood hydrogen ion concentration reduces oxygen binding to hemoglobin. Because of the shape of the hemoglobin dissociation curve, the effect is more important in venous blood than arterial blood (Figure 22–24); the net result is facilitation of oxygen release to tissue with little impairment in oxygen uptake (unless severe hypoxia is present).

The influence of CO_2 tension on hemoglobin's affinity for oxygen is important physiologically and is known as the Bohr effect. The high CO_2 content of venous capillary blood, by decreasing hemoglobin's affinity for oxygen, facilitates the release of oxygen to tissues; conversely, the lower CO_2 content in pulmonary capillaries increases hemoglobin's affinity for oxygen again, facilitating oxygen uptake from alveoli. Most of the Bohr effect is secondary to the associated rise in hydrogen ion concentration when CO_2 tension increases (Chapter 30).

2,3-DPG, as a by-product of glycolysis (the

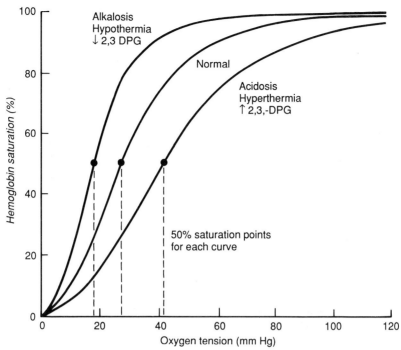

Figure 22–24. The effects of changes in acid-base status, body temperature, and 2,3-DPG concentration on the hemoglobin-oxygen dissociation curve.

Rapoport-Luebering shunt), can accumulate during anaerobic metabolism. Although its effects on hemoglobin under these conditions are theoretically beneficial, its physiologic importance normally appears minor. 2,3-DPG levels may, however, play an important compensatory role in patients with chronic anemia and may significantly affect the oxygen-carrying capacity of blood transfusions (Chapter 29).

Abnormal Hemoglobins

Carbon monoxide, cyanide, nitric acid, and ammonia combine with hemoglobin at oxygen-binding sites, displacing oxygen and shifting the saturation curve to the left. Carbon monoxide is especially potent, having 300 times the affinity of oxygen for hemoglobin. Methemoglobin results when the iron in heme is oxidized to its trivalent form. Nitrates, nitrites, sulfonamides, and other drugs can rarely result in significant methemoglobinemia. Methemoglobin cannot combine with oxygen unless reconverted by the enzyme methemoglobin reductase; methemoglobin also shifts the normal hemoglobin saturation curve to the left. Reduction of methemoglobin to normal hemoglobin is facilitated by reducing agents such as methylene blue or ascorbic acid.

Abnormal hemoglobins can also result from variations in the protein subunit composition. Each variant has its own oxygen saturation characteristics. These include fetal hemoglobin, hemoglobin A_2, and sickle hemoglobin.

Oxygen Content

The total oxygen content of blood is the sum of that in solution plus that carried by hemoglobin. In reality, oxygen binding to hemoglobin never achieves the theoretical maximum (see above) but is closer to 1.31 mL O_2/dL blood. Total oxygen content is expressed by the following equation:

$$\text{Oxygen content} = [(0.003 \text{ mL/dL/mmHg}) \times PO_2] + (SO_2 \times Hb \times 1.31 \text{ mL/g})$$

where Hb is hemoglobin concentration in g/dL blood and SO_2 is hemoglobin saturation at the given PO_2.

Using the above formula and a hemoglobin of 15 g/dL, the normal oxygen content for both arterial and mixed venous blood and the arteriovenous difference can be calculated:

$$CaO_2 = (0.003 \times 100) + (0.975 \times 15 \times 1.31)$$
$$= 19.5 \text{ mL/dL blood}$$

$$C\bar{v}O_2 = (0.003 \times 40) + (0.75 \times 15 \times 1.31)$$
$$= 14.8 \text{ mL/1dL blood}$$

$$(CaO_2 - C\bar{v}O_2) = 4.7 \text{ mL/dL blood.}$$

Oxygen Transport

Oxygen transport is dependent on both respiratory and circulatory function (Chapter 19). Total oxygen delivery (oxygen flux) to tissues is the product of arterial oxygen content and cardiac output: oxygen delivery $= CaO_2 \times \dot{Q}_t$. Note that arterial oxygen content is not only dependent on PaO_2 but on the hemoglobin concentration as well. As a result, deficiencies in oxygen delivery can result from (1) a low PaO_2, (2) a low hemoglobin concentration, or (3) an inadequate cardiac output. Normal oxygen delivery can be calculated as follows: oxygen delivery = 20 mL/dL blood × 5000 mL/min = 1000 mL/min.

The **Fick equation** expresses the relationship between oxygen consumption, oxygen content, and cardiac output:

$$\text{Oxygen consumption} = \dot{V}O_2 = \dot{Q}_t \times (CaO_2 - C\bar{v}O_2)$$

Rearranging the equation:

$$CaO_2 - C\bar{v}O_2 = \frac{\dot{V}O_2}{\dot{Q}_t}$$

Consequently, the arteriovenous difference is a good measure of the overall adequacy of oxygen delivery.

With a normal oxygen consumption of approximately 250 mL/min and a cardiac output of 5000 mL/min, the normal arteriovenous difference by this equation again calculates to be about 5 mL O_2/dL blood. Note that the normal extraction fraction for oxygen, $(CaO_2 - C\bar{v}O_2)/CaO2$, is 5 mL ÷ 20 mL, or 25%; thus, the body normally consumes only 25% of the oxygen carried on hemoglobin. When oxygen demand exceeds supply, the extraction fraction increases above 25%. Conversely, if oxygen supply exceeds demand, the extraction fraction falls below 25%.

Oxygen Stores

The concept of oxygen stores is important in anesthesia. When the normal flux of oxygen is interrupted by apnea, existing oxygen stores are consumed by cellular metabolism; if stores are depleted, hypoxia and eventual cell death follow. Theoretically, normal oxygen stores in adults are estimated to be about 1500 mL. This amount includes the oxygen remaining in the lungs, that bound to hemoglobin (and myoglobin), and that dissolved in body fluids. Unfortunately, hemoglobin's high affinity for oxygen and the very limited quantity of oxygen in solution restrict the availability of these stores. The oxygen contained within the lungs at FRC (initial lung volume during apnea) therefore becomes the most important source of oxygen. Moreover, probably only 80% of that volume is usable.

Apnea in a patient previously breathing room air leaves approximately 480 mL of oxygen in the lungs. (If $FiO_2 = 0.21$ and FRC = 2300 mL, oxygen content = $FiO_2 \times$ FRC). The metabolic activity of tissues rapidly depletes this reservoir (presumably at a rate equivalent to $\dot{V}O_2$); severe hypoxemia usually occurs within 90 seconds. The onset of hypoxemia can be delayed by increasing the FiO_2 prior to the apnea. Following ventilation with 100% O_2, FRC contains about 2300 mL of oxygen; under these conditions,

hypoxemia following apnea is usually delayed for 4–5 minutes. This concept is the basis for preoxygenation prior to induction of anesthesia.

CARBON DIOXIDE

Carbon dioxide is transported in blood in three forms: (1) dissolved in solution, (2) as bicarbonate, and (3) with proteins in the form of carbamino compounds. The sum of all three forms is the total CO_2 content of blood (routinely reported with electrolyte measurements).

Dissolved Carbon Dioxide

Carbon dioxide is more soluble in blood than oxygen, having a solubility coefficient of 0.031 mmol/L/mm Hg.

Bicarbonate

In aqueous solutions, CO_2 slowly combines with water to form bicarbonate, according to the following reaction:

$$H_2O + CO_2 \rightarrow H^+ + HCO_3^-$$

In plasma, less than 1% of the dissolved CO_2 undergoes this reaction. Within red blood cells, however, carbonic anhydrase accelerates the reaction, forming large amounts of bicarbonate. As a result, bicarbonate represents the largest fraction of the CO_2 in blood.

On the venous side of capillaries, CO_2 enters red blood cells and is converted to bicarbonate, which eventually diffuses out of red cells into plasma; chloride ion moves from plasma into red cells to maintain electrical balance. In the pulmonary capillaries, the reverse occurs: CO_2 is eliminated, bicarbonate ions reenter red cells for conversion back to CO_2, and chloride ions move out of red cells into plasma. This sequence is referred to as the chloride shift, or Hamburger shift.

Carbamino Compounds

Carbon dioxide can react with amino groups on proteins as shown by the following equation:

$$R\text{-}NH_2 + CO_2 \rightarrow RNH\text{-}CO_2^- + H^+$$

At physiologic pH, only a small amount of CO_2 is carried in this form. Moreover, most of it is in the form of carboxyhemoglobin. Deoxygenated hemoglobin (deoxyhemoglobin) has an affinity for CO_2 $3\frac{1}{2}$ times that of oxyhemoglobin. As a result, venous blood carries more CO_2 than arterial blood (Haldane effect), the difference being due to greater carbamino-hemoglobin formation in venous blood. PCO_2 normally has little effect on the fraction of CO_2 carried as carbamino-hemoglobin.

Effect of Hemoglobin Buffering on Carbon Dioxide Transport

The buffering action of hemoglobin (Chapter 30) also accounts for part of the Haldane effect. Hemoglobin can act as a buffer at physiologic pH due to its high content of histidine. Moreover, the acid-base behavior of hemoglobin is influenced by its oxygenation state:

$$H^+ + HbO_2 \leftrightarrow HbH^+ + O_2$$

Removal of oxygen from hemoglobin in tissue capillaries causes the hemoglobin molecule to behave more as a base; by taking up hydrogen ions, hemoglobin shifts the CO_2-bicarbonate equilibrium in favor of greater bicarbonate formation:

$$CO_2 + H_2O + HbO_2 \rightarrow HBH^+ + HCO_3^- + O_2$$

As a direct result, deoxyhemoglobin increases the amount of CO_2 that is carried in venous blood as bicarbonate. As CO_2 is taken up from tissue and converted as bicarbonate, the total CO_2 content of blood increases.

In the lungs, the reverse is true. Oxygenation of hemoglobin favors its action as an acid, and the release of hydrogen ions shifts the equilibrium in favor of greater CO_2 formation:

$$O_2 + HCO_3^- + HbH \rightarrow H_2O + CO_2 + HbO_2$$

Bicarbonate concentration decreases as CO_2 is formed and eliminated, so that the total CO_2 content of blood decreases in the lungs.

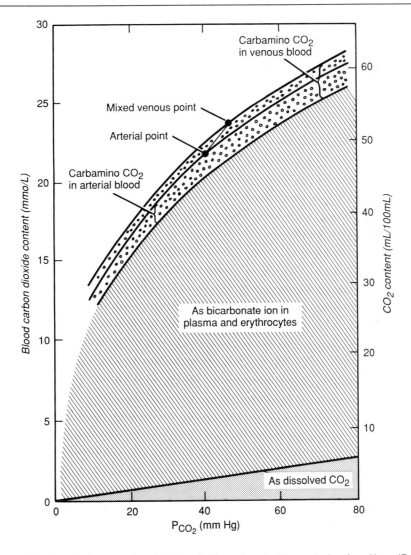

Figure 22–25. The CO_2 dissociation curve for whole blood. (Reproduced, with permission, from Nunn JF: *Applied Respiratory Physiology,* 3rd ed. Butterworths, 1987.)

Carbon Dioxide Dissociation Curve

A CO_2 dissociation curve can be constructed by plotting the total CO_2 content of blood against PCO_2. The contribution of each form of CO_2 can also be quantified (Figure 22–25).

Carbon Dioxide Stores

Carbon dioxide stores in the body are large (approximately 120 L in adults) and primarily in the form of the dissolved CO_2 and bicarbonate. Carbon dioxide stores may be classified as rapidly, intermediately, and slowly equilibrating compartments. Because of the larger capacity of the intermediate and slow compartments, the rate of rise in arterial CO_2 tension is generally slower than its fall following acute changes in ventilation.

CONTROL OF BREATHING

Spontaneous ventilation is the result of rhythmic neural activity in respiratory centers within the brainstem. This activity regulates respiratory muscles to maintain normal tensions of oxygen and CO_2 in the body. The basic neuronal activity is modified by inputs from other areas in the brain as well as various central and peripheral receptors (sensors).

CENTRAL RESPIRATORY CENTERS

The basic respiratory rhythm originates in the medulla. Two medullary groups of neurons are generally recognized: (1) a dorsal respiratory group, which is primarily active during inspiration; and (2) a ventral respiratory group, which is active during expiration. Although not firmly established, the origin of the basic rhythm is due either to intrinsic spontaneous discharge activity in the dorsal group or reciprocating activity between the dorsal and ventral groups. The close association of the dorsal respiratory group of neurons with the tractus solitarius may explain reflex changes in breathing due to vagal or glossopharyngeal nerve stimulation.

Two pontine areas influence the dorsal (inspiratory) medullary center. A lower pontine (apneustic) center is excitatory, while an upper pontine (pneumotaxic) center is inhibitory. The pontine centers appear to fine-tune respiratory rate and rhythm.

CENTRAL SENSORS

The most important of these sensors are chemoreceptors that respond to changes in hydrogen ion concentration. Central chemoreceptors are thought to lie on the anterolateral surface of the medulla and respond primarily to changes in cerebrospinal fluid (CSF) [H^+]. This mechanism is effective in regulating $PaCO_2$, because the blood-brain barrier (Chapter 25) is permeable to dissolved CO_2 but not to bicarbonate ions. Acute changes in $PaCO_2$ but not in arterial [HCO_3^-] are reflected in CSF; thus, a change in CO_2 must result in a change in [H^+]:

$$CO_2 + H_2O \leftrightarrow H^+ + HCO_3^-$$

Increases in $PaCO_2$ elevate CSF hydrogen ion concentration and activate the chemoreceptors. Secondary stimulation of the adjacent respiratory medullary centers increases alveolar ventilation (Figure 22–26) and reduces $PaCO_2$ back to normal. Interestingly, this ventilatory response to hypercapnia appears to be primarily mediated by the external intercostal muscles. Conversely, decreases in CSF hydrogen ion concentration secondary to reductions in $PaCO_2$ reduce alveolar ventilation and elevate $PaCO_2$. Note that the relationship between $PaCO_2$ and minute volume is nearly linear. The $PaCO_2$ at which ventilation is zero (*x*-intercept) is known as the apneic threshold. Spontaneous respirations are typically absent under anesthesia when $PaCO_2$ falls below the apneic threshold. (In the awake state, cortical influences prevent apnea, so apneic thresholds are not ordinarily seen.) In contrast to peripheral chemoreceptors (see below), central chemoreceptor activity is depressed by hypoxia.

PERIPHERAL SENSORS

Peripheral Chemoreceptors

Peripheral chemoreceptors include the carotid bodies (at the bifurcation of the common carotid arteries) and the aortic bodies (surrounding the aortic arch). The carotid bodies are the principal peripheral chemoreceptors in humans and are sensitive to changes sensitive to PaO_2, $PaCO_2$, and pH. They interact with central respiratory centers via the glossopharyngeal nerves, producing reflex increases in alveolar ventilation in response to reductions in PaO_2 or elevations in [H^+] and $PaCO_2$. In contrast to central chemoreceptors, which respond primarily to $PaCO_2$ (really [H^+]), the carotid bodies are most sensitive to PaO_2 (Figure 22–27). Note that receptor activity does not appreciably increase until PaO_2 decreases below 50 mm Hg. Cells of the carotid body (glomus cells) are thought to be primarily dopaminergic neurons. Antidopaminergic drugs (such as phenothiazines), most commonly used anesthetics, and bilateral carotid surgery abolish the peripheral ventilatory response to hypoxemia.

Lung Receptors

Impulses from these receptors are carried centrally by the vagus nerve. Stretch receptors are distributed in

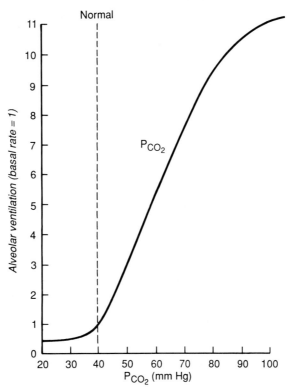

Figure 22–26. The relationship between $PaCO_2$ and minute ventilation. (Reproduced, with permission, from Guyton AC: *Textbook of Medical Physiology,* 7th ed. Saunders, 1986.

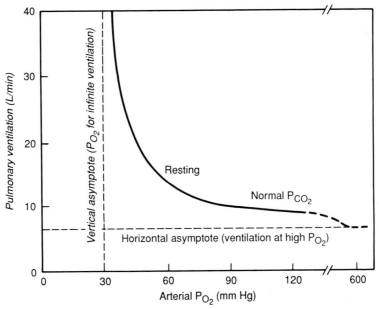

Figure 22–27. The relationship between PaO_2 and minute ventilation. (Reproduced, with permission, from Nunn JF: *Applied Respiratory Physiology,* 3rd ed. Butterworths, 1987.)

the smooth muscle of airways; they are responsible for inhibition of the respiratory rate when the lung is inflated to excessive volumes (Hering-Breuer reflex) and for respiratory stimulation when the lung is deflated (deflation reflex). Stretch receptors normally play a minor role in humans. Irritant receptors in the tracheobronchial mucosa react to noxious gases, smoke, dust, and cold gases; activation produces reflex increases in respiratory rate, bronchoconstriction, and coughing. "J" (juxtacapillary) receptors are located in the interstitial space within alveolar walls; these receptors induce dyspnea in response to expansion of interstitial space volume and various chemical mediators following tissue damage.

Other Receptors

These include various muscle and joint receptors on respiratory muscles and the chest wall. Input from these sources is probably important during exercise and in pathologic conditions associated with decreased lung or chest compliance.

EFFECT OF ANESTHESIA ON THE CONTROL OF BREATHING

The most important effect of most general anesthetics on breathing is a tendency to promote hypoventilation. The mechanism is probably dual: (1) central depression of the chemoreceptor, and (2) depression of external intercostal muscle activity. The magnitude of the hypoventilation is generally proportionate to anesthetic depth. With increasing depth, the slope of the $PaCO_2$/minute ventilation curve decreases and the apneic threshold increases (Figure 22–28). This effect is at least partially reversed by surgical stimulation.

The peripheral response to hypoxemia is even more sensitive to anesthetics than the central CO_2 response and is nearly abolished by even subanesthetic doses of most inhalation agents (including nitrous oxide) and many intravenous agents.

(For the respiratory effects of each individual agent, see Chapters 7 and 8.)

NONRESPIRATORY FUNCTIONS OF THE LUNG

FILTRATION

The unique "in series" position of the pulmonary capillaries within the circulation allows them to act as a filter for debris in the bloodstream. The lungs' high content of heparin and plasminogen activator facilitates the breakdown of entrapped fibrin debris. Although pulmonary capillaries have an average diameter of 7 μm, larger particles have been shown to pass through to the left heart.

RESERVOIR FUNCTION

The role of the pulmonary circulation as a reservoir for the systemic circulation has been discussed above.

METABOLISM

The lungs are metabolically very active organs. In addition to surfactant synthesis, pneumocytes account

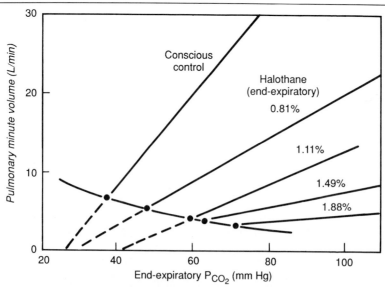

Figure 22–28. The effect of volatile agents (halothane) on the $PaCO_2$-ventilation curve (see text). (Reproduced, with permission, from Nunn JF: *Applied Respiratory Physiology,* 3rd ed. Butterworths, 1987.)

for a major portion of extrahepatic mixed-function oxidation. The pulmonary endothelium is capable of metabolizing most vasoactive compounds, including norepinephrine, serotonin, bradykinin, and a variety of prostaglandins and leukotrienes. In contrast, histamine and epinephrine are generally not metabolized in the lungs. Moreover, the lungs can be a major site of histamine synthesis and release during allergic reactions.

The lungs are also responsible for converting angiotensin I to its physiologically active form, angiotensin II. The enzyme responsible, angiotensin-converting enzyme (ACE), is bound on the surface of the pulmonary endothelium.

CASE DISCUSSION: UNILATERALLY DIMINISHED BREATH SOUNDS DURING GENERAL ANESTHESIA

A 67-year-old man is undergoing colon resection for carcinoma under general anesthesia. He has a history of an old anterior myocardial infarction and compensated congestive heart failure. Arterial and pulmonary artery catheters are placed preoperatively for monitoring during surgery. Following a smooth thiopental-fentanyl induction and an atraumatic intubation with succinylcholine, anesthesia is maintained with 60% nitrous oxide in oxygen, isoflurane, and vecuronium. One-half hour into the operation, the surgeon asks for the Trendelenburg position to facilitate surgical exposure. The pulse oximeter, which had been reading 99% saturation, suddenly drops and remains at 93%. The pulse oximeter's signal strength and waveform are unchanged. Auscultation of the lungs reveals diminished breath sounds over the left lung.

What is the most likely explanation?

Unilaterally diminished breath sounds under anesthesia are most commonly caused by inadvertent placement or migration of the endotracheal tube into one of the two main bronchi. As a result, only one lung is ventilated. Other causes of unilaterally diminished breath sounds (such as pneumothorax, a mucus plug, or atelectasis) are less easily diagnosed but are fortunately less common during anesthesia.

The Trendelenburg (head-down) position typically causes the tip of the endotracheal tube to advance (1–2 cm) relative to the carina. In this case, the tube was apparently placed just above the carina with the patient in the supine position but migrated into the right bronchus when the Trendelenburg position was imposed. The diagnosis is confirmed by drawing the tube back 1–2 cm at a time while the chest is auscultated. Breath sounds will become equal again when the

tip of the tube reenters the trachea. Following initial placement, endotracheal tubes should be routinely checked for correct positioning by auscultating the chest, by ascertaining depth of tube insertion by the markings on the tube (normally 20–22 cm at the teeth for an adult), and by feeling for the cuff in the suprasternal notch.

Are endotracheal tubes just as likely to enter either main bronchus?

In most cases of unintentional endobronchial intubation, the endotracheal tube enters the right bronchus because the latter diverges away from the trachea at a less acute angle than the left bronchus (Chapter 24).

Why did hemoglobin saturation decrease?

Failure to ventilate one lung while it continues to be perfused creates a large intrapulmonary shunt. Venous admixture increases and tends to depress PaO_2 and hemoglobin saturation.

Does a saturation of 93% exclude endobronchial intubation?

No. If both lungs continued to have equal blood flow, venous admixture should have theoretically increased to 50%, resulting in severe hypoxemia and very low hemoglobin saturation. Fortunately, hypoxic pulmonary vasoconstriction is a powerful compensatory response that tends to reduce flow to the hypoxic lung and reduces the expected venous admixture. In fact, if the patient has been receiving a higher inspired oxygen concentration (50–100%), the drop in arterial tension may not be detectable by the pulse oximeter owing to the characteristics of the normal hemoglobin saturation curve. For example, endobronchial intubation in a patient inspiring 50% oxygen might drop PaO_2 from 250 mm Hg to 95 mm Hg; the resulting change in pulse oximeter readings (100–99 to 98–97) may hardly be noticeable.

Arterial and mixed venous blood gas tensions are obtained with the following results:

PaO_2 = 69 mm Hg, $PaCO_2$ = 42 mm Hg, SaO_2x = 93%, PvO_2 = 40 mm Hg, and SvO_2 = 75%. Hemoglobin concentration is 15 g/dL.

What is the calculated venous admixture?

In this case, $Pc'O_2 = PAO_2 = [(760 - 47) \times 0.4] - 42 = 243$ mm Hg.

Therefore, $Cc'O_2 = (15 \times 1.31 \times 1.0) + (243 \times 0.003) = 20.4$ mL/dL.

$CaO_2 = (15 \times 1.31 \times 0.93) + (69 \times 0.003) = 18.5$ mL/dL.

$CvO_2 = (15 \times 1.31 \times 0.75) + (40 \times 0.003) = 14.8$ mL/dL.

$Q_s/Q_t = (20.4 - 18.5)/(20.4 - 14.8) = 32\%$

How does endobronchial intubation affect arterial and end-tidal CO$_2$ tensions?

PaCO$_2$ is typically not appreciably altered as long as the same minute ventilation is maintained (see One-Lung Anesthesia, Chapter 24). P$_{ET}$CO$_2$ also usually does not change as expected.

SUGGESTED READINGS

Goudsouzian N, Karamanian A: *Physiology for the Anesthesiologist,* 2nd ed. Appleton-Century-Crofts, 1984. Good review of respiratory physiology as related to anesthesia.

Nunn JF: *Applied Respiratory Physiology,* 3rd ed. Butterworths, 1987. A classic.

Stoelting RK: *Pharmacology and Physiology in Anesthetic Practice,* 2nd ed. Lippincott, 1991. Contains concise chapters on pulmonary physiology.

West JB: *Respiratory Physiology,* 4th ed. Williams & Wilkins 1984.

Anesthesia for Patients With Respiratory Disease

23

The impact of preexisting pulmonary disease on respiratory function during anesthesia and in the postoperative period is predictable: Greater degrees of preoperative pulmonary impairment are associated with more marked alterations in respiratory function intraoperatively (Chapter 22) and higher rates of pulmonary complications postoperatively. Failure to recognize patients who are at increased risk is a frequent contributory factor. This chapter examines pulmonary risk in general and then reviews the anesthetic approach to patients with the most common types of respiratory disease.

PULMONARY RISK FACTORS

Pulmonary dysfunction is the most common postoperative complication. The incidence of atelectasis, pneumonia, pulmonary embolism, and respiratory failure following surgery varies widely (from 6% to 60%) depending on the patient population studied and the surgical procedures performed. Six risk factors are generally recognized (Table 23–1). With the exception of the operative site and the duration of the procedure, most appear related to the likelihood of preoperative pulmonary dysfunction. The association between smoking and respiratory disease is well established; abnormalities in midexpiratory flow rates are often demonstrable well before symptoms of chronic obstructive lung disease appear. Advancing age is associated with an increasing prevalence of pulmonary disease and an increase in closing capacity even in normal individuals. Obesity decreases functional residual capacity (FRC), increases the work of breathing, and predisposes to deep vein thrombosis.

While the duration of surgery is the least consistent pulmonary risk factor, operative site is a major factor.

Table 23–1. Preoperative pulmonary risk factors.

1. Preexisting pulmonary disease
2. Thoracic or upper abdominal surgery
3. Smoking
4. Obesity
5. Age (>60 years)
6. Prolonged general anesthesia (>3 hours)

Thoracic and upper abdominal surgical procedures can have marked effects on pulmonary function. Operations near the diaphragm often result in diaphragmatic dysfunction and a restrictive ventilatory defect (see below). Upper abdominal procedures consistently decrease FRC (60–70%); the effect is maximal on the first postoperative day and usually lasts 7–10 days. Vertical incisions produce greater impairment than horizontal ones. Rapid shallow breathing with an ineffective cough due to pain (splinting), a decrease in the number of sighs, and impaired mucociliary clearance lead to microatelectasis and loss of lung volume. Intrapulmonary shunting promotes hypoxemia (Chapter 22). Residual anesthetic effects, the recumbent position, sedation from narcotics, abdominal distention, and restrictive dressings may also be contributory. Complete relief of pain with regional anesthesia does not completely correct these abnormalities. Persistent microatelectasis and retention of secretions favor the development of postoperative pneumonia.

While many adverse effects of general anesthesia on pulmonary function are described (Chapter 22), the superiority of regional over general anesthesia for patients with pulmonary impairment is not firmly established.

OBSTRUCTIVE PULMONARY DISEASE

Obstructive lung disease is the most common form of pulmonary dysfunction. The hallmark of these disorders is resistance to airflow. Characteristically, both FEV_1 and the FEV_1/FVC ratio are less than 75% of predicted. Measurement of the midexpiratory flow rate ($FEF_{25-75\%}$; see Chapter 22) is often the only abnormality early in the course of these disorders.

Elevated airway resistance increases the work of breathing and when severe also impairs respiratory gas exchange. The predominance of expiratory airflow resistance results in air trapping; residual and total lung volumes increase. Wheezing is a common finding and represents turbulent air flow. Wheezing may be absent with mild obstruction as well as severe obstruction when airflow has nearly ceased.

1. ASTHMA

Asthma is a common disorder (3–5% of the population). Its hallmark is airway (bronchiolar) hyperreactivity in response to a variety of stimuli. Clinically, asthma is manifested by episodic attacks of dyspnea, cough, and wheezing. Airway obstruction is the result of bronchial smooth muscle constriction, edema, and increased secretions. Classically, the airway obstruction is reversible and can be precipitated by a variety of airborne substances, including pollens, animal danders, dusts, pollutants, and various chemicals. Some patients also develop bronchospasm following ingestion of aspirin, nonsteroidal anti-inflammatory agents, tartrazine, or some yellow dyes. Exercise, emotional excitement, and viral infections also precipitate bronchospasm in many patients.

The term "extrinsic (allergic) asthma" is appropriate when attacks are most often related to environmental exposures; "intrinsic asthma" denotes cases in which attacks usually occur without provocation. Although most patients with extrinsic asthma react positively to various antigens and have elevated IgE levels, this classification is imperfect; many patients show features of both forms. Moreover, overlap with chronic bronchitis (see below) also occurs.

The pathophysiology of asthma involves overactivity of the parasympathetic nervous system and the release of various chemical mediators. The parasympathetic nervous system plays a major role in maintaining normal bronchial tone (Chapter 22). Vagal afferents in the bronchi are sensitive to histamine and multiple noxious stimuli, including cold air, inhaled irritants, and instrumentation (intubation). Reflex vagal activation results in bronchoconstriction, which is mediated by an increase in intracellular cyclic guanosine monophosphate (cGMP). Inhaled substances can also initiate bronchospasm through specific and nonspecific immune mechanisms by degranulating bronchial mast cells. In classic allergic asthma, antigen binding to IgE on the surface of mast cells causes degranulation; bronchoconstriction is the result of the subsequent release of histamine and leukotrienes. The role of prostaglandin D_2 and serotonin, both potent bronchoconstrictors, is uncertain in humans.

Treatment

Drugs used for the treatment of asthma include β-adrenergic agonists, theophylline, anticholinergics, glucocorticoids, and cromolyn; with the exception of the latter, these drugs may be used for the acute or chronic treatment of asthma. Cromolyn sodium, administered via an inhaler, is effective in preventing bronchospasm in most patients with extrinsic asthma and in some with intrinsic asthma. Though devoid of any bronchodilating properties, cromolyn prevents the degranulation of mast cells.

Sympathomimetic agents (Table 23–2) are most commonly given as an aerosol. They produce bron-

Table 23–2. A comparison of commonly used bronchodilators.

Agent	Adrenergic Activity	
	β_1	β_2
Terbutaline	+	+++
Isoproterenol	++++	++
Albuterol	+	++++
Metaproterenol	+	+
Isoetharine	++	+++
Epinephrine	++++	++
Pirbuterol	+	++++
Bitolterol	+	++++

chodilatation via β_2 agonist activity. Activation of β_2-adrenergic receptors on bronchiolar smooth muscle in turn activates adenylyl cyclase; bronchodilatation is the result of formation of intracellular cyclic adenosine monophosphate (cAMP). Use of more selective β_2 agonists such as terbutaline or albuterol decreases the incidence of undesirable β_1 cardiac effects.

Theophylline compounds traditionally are thought to produce bronchodilatation by inhibiting phosphodiesterase, the enzyme responsible for the breakdown of cAMP. Its pulmonary effects appear much more complex and include catecholamine release, blockade of histamine release, and diaphragmatic stimulation. Theophylline has a narrow therapeutic range; therapeutic blood levels should be 10–20 μg/mL.

Anticholinergic agents, through their antimuscarinic action, produce bronchodilatation and may block reflex bronchoconstriction. Ipratropium, a congener of atropine that is given as a metered aerosol, is an effective bronchodilator without appreciable systemic anticholinergic effects.

Because of their anti-inflammatory and membrane-stabilizing effects, potentiation of catecholamines, or both, the glucocorticoids may be used for acute treatment and maintenance of patients with severe asthma. They usually require several hours to become effective. Their principal disadvantage is adrenal suppression with chronic therapy. Beclomethasone, a synthetic steroid used as an inhaled aerosol for maintenance therapy, decreases the incidence of undesirable systemic effects but does not necessarily prevent adrenal suppression.

Preoperative Considerations

The emphasis in evaluating asthmatic patients should be on determining the recent course of the disease and in ascertaining that the patient is in optimal condition. The difference between anesthetizing an asthmatic patient with clearly audible wheezing and one without wheezing preoperatively may be a potentially life-threatening anesthetic experience versus a totally uneventful one. A clinical history is of critical importance. No or minimal dyspnea, wheezing, or cough is optimal. Complete resolution of recent exacerbations should be confirmed by chest auscultation. Patients with frequent or chronic bronchospasm should be receiving therapeutic doses of theophylline, aerosolized bronchodilator treatments, and perhaps glucocorticoids. Pulmonary function testing—particularly expiratory airflow measurements—should be used to confirm clinical impressions. Comparison with previous measurements are invaluable. A chest radiograph may be useful in assessing air trapping; hyperinflation results in a flattened diaphragm, a small-appearing heart, and hyperlucent lung fields.

Asthmatic patients with active bronchospasm presenting for emergency surgery should undergo a period of intensive treatment when possible. Supplemental oxygen, intravenous aminophylline, and aerosolized β_2 agonists can dramatically improve lung function in a few hours. Arterial blood gases may be useful in severe cases. Hypoxemia is common during bronchospasm and is due to increased intrapulmonary shunting. Arterial CO_2 tensions are typically low; even slight hypercapnia is indicative of severe air trapping and may be a sign of impending respiratory failure. An FEV_1 below 25% may also be predictive of respiratory failure.

Some degree of sedation is desirable preoperatively in asthmatic patients presenting for elective surgery—especially those whose disease has an emotional component. Generally, benzodiazepines are the most satisfactory agents for premedication. Anticholinergic agents are not customarily given unless very copious secretions are present or unless ketamine is to be used for induction of anesthesia. In typical intramuscular doses, anticholinergics are not effective in preventing reflex bronchospasm following intubation. The use of an H_2 blocking agent such as cimetidine or ranitidine is theoretically detrimental, since H_2 receptor activation normally produces bronchodilatation; in the event of histamine release, unopposed H_1 activation with H_2 blockade may accentuate bronchoconstriction.

Bronchodilators should be continued up to the time of surgery. Preoperative blood theophylline levels serve three purposes: (1) to ensure optimal bronchodilatation, (2) to detect occult toxicity, and (3) to guide treatment in the event that intraoperative aminophylline is necessary. Patients who have been receiving long-term glucocorticoid therapy should be given supplemental doses to compensate for adrenal suppression. Hydrocortisone (100 mg preoperatively and 100 mg intraoperatively) is most commonly used.

Intraoperative Considerations

The most critical time for asthmatics during anesthesia is during instrumentation of the airway. Regional anesthesia circumvents this problem but does not necessarily eliminate the possibility of bronchospasm. Pain, emotional stress, or stimulation during light general anesthesia can precipitate bronchospasm. Drugs often associated with histamine release (curare,

atracurium, morphine, and meperidine) should be avoided or given very slowly if used. The goal of any general anesthetic is a smooth induction and emergence, with anesthetic depth adjusted to stimulation.

Which induction agent is chosen is not as important as achieving deep anesthesia prior to intubation and surgical stimulation. Thiopental is most commonly used for adults but occasionally can induce bronchospasm due to exaggerated histamine release. Propofol and etomidate are suitable alternatives and in fact are preferred by some clinicians. Ketamine, the only intravenous agent with bronchodilating properties, is a good choice for patients who are also hemodynamically unstable. Ketamine should probably not be used in patients with high theophylline levels, as the combined actions of the two drugs can precipitate seizure activity. Halothane usually provides the smoothest inhalation induction with bronchodilatation in asthmatic children. Enflurane and isoflurane can provide equal bronchodilatation, but the latter must be increased slowly because it exerts a mild irritant effect on the airways.

Prior to intubation, reflex bronchospasm can be blunted by an additional dose of thiopental (1–2 mg/kg), ventilating the patient with 2–3 MAC of a volatile agent for 5 minutes, or intravenous or intratracheal lidocaine (1–2 mg/kg). The latter itself can initiate bronchospasm if an inadequate induction dose of thiopental is used. A large dose of an anticholinergic (atropine, 2 mg, or glycopyrrolate, 1 mg) can also block reflex bronchospasm but causes excessive tachycardia. Although succinylcholine may on occasion induce marked histamine release, it can generally be safely used in most asthmatics. In the absence of capnography, confirmation of correct endotracheal placement by chest auscultation can be difficult in the presence of marked bronchospasm.

Volatile anesthetics are most often employed for maintenance of anesthesia to take advantage of their potent bronchodilating properties. Halothane can sensitize the heart to aminophylline and β-adrenergic agonists administered during anesthesia; for that reason—together with concern over hepatotoxicity—halothane is generally avoided in adults. Ventilation should be controlled with warmed, humidified gases whenever possible. Airflow obstruction during expiration is apparent on capnography as a delayed rise to the end-tidal value (Figure 23–1); the severity of obstruction is generally inversely related to the rate of rise in end-tidal CO_2. Severe bronchospasm is manifested by rising peak inspiratory pressures and incomplete exhalation. Tidal volumes of 12–15 mL/kg with ventilatory rates of 8–10 breaths/min are desirable. Relatively long inspiratory and expiratory times allow more uniform distribution of gas flow and avoid air trapping in the lungs, respectively.

Intraoperative bronchospasm is usually manifested as wheezing and should be treated by increasing the concentration of the volatile agent (deepening the anesthesia). If the wheezing does not resolve, less

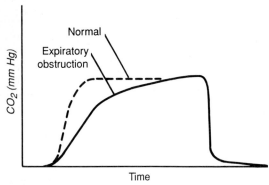

Figure 23–1. Capnograph of a patient with expiratory airway obstruction.

Table 23–3. Syndromes of chronic obstructive lung disease.

Feature	Chronic Bronchitis	Emphysema
Cough	Frequent	With exertion
Sputum	Copious	Scant
Hematocrit	Elevated	Normal
$PaCO_2$ (mm Hg)	Often elevated (>40)	Usually <40 or normal
PaO_2 (mm Hg)	Usually <60	Usually >60
Chest x-ray	Increased lung markings	Hyperinflation
Elastic recoil	Normal	Decreased
Airway resistance	Increased	Normal to slightly increased
Cor pulmonale	Early	Late

common causes of wheezing should always be considered prior to more specific pharmacologic treatment. Obstruction of the endotracheal tube due to kinking, secretions, or an overinflated balloon, endobronchial intubation, pulmonary edema, and pneumothorax can all simulate bronchospasm. Mild bronchospasm may be treated with a β-adrenergic agonist delivered by aerosol into the inspiratory limb of the breathing circuit. (The carrier gas used in available preparations can, however, interfere with mass spectrometer readings.) Moderate to severe bronchospasm should be treated with intravenous aminophylline, subcutaneous terbutaline (0.25 mg), or both. Patients not being given theophylline preparations should receive aminophylline as a 6 mg/kg bolus over 20 minutes followed by 0.5–0.9 mg/kg/h. For patients who have been receiving theophylline preoperatively, a fraction of the normal loading dose (usually one-fourth or one-half) is used depending on the preoperative theophylline level.

At the completion of surgery, the patient should ideally be free of wheezing. Reversal of nondepolarizing muscle relaxants with anticholinesterase agents does not precipitate bronchoconstriction if preceded by the appropriate dose of an anticholinergic (Chapter 10). Deep extubation (before airway reflexes return) prevents bronchospasm on emergence. Lidocaine as a bolus (1–2 mg/kg) or a continuous infusion (1–2 mg/min) may help obtund airway reflexes during emergence.

2. CHRONIC OBSTRUCTIVE LUNG DISEASE

Chronic obstructive lung diseases are the most common pulmonary disorders encountered in anesthetic practice. The prevalence increases with age, is strongly associated with cigarette smoking, and has a male predominance (affecting up to 20% of men). The overwhelming majority of patients are asymptomatic or only mildly symptomatic but on pulmonary function testing show expiratory airflow obstruction. Many cases have an element of reversibility presumably due to bronchospasm (as shown by improvement in response to brochodilator administration). With advancing disease, maldistribution of both ventilation and pulmonary blood flow results in areas of low ventilation/perfusion ratios (intrapulmonary shunt) as well as areas of high ventilation/perfusion ratios (dead space). Traditionally, cases have been classified as chronic bronchitis or emphysema (Table 23–3); however, most patients have features of both.

Chronic Bronchitis

Chronic bronchitis is a clinical diagnosis defined by the presence of a productive cough on most days of 3 consecutive months for at least 2 consecutive years. In addition to cigarette smoking, air pollutants, occupational exposure to dusts, recurrent pulmonary infections, and perhaps familial factors may be responsible. Bronchial mucous gland hypertrophy, inflammation, and edema produce airflow obstruction. Frequent pulmonary infections are common and often associated with bronchospasm. Intrapulmonary shunting is prominent, and hypoxemia is common. Chronic hypoxemia leads to erythrocytosis, pulmonary hypertension, and eventually cor pulmonale (blue bloater syndrome). In the course of disease progression, chronic CO_2 retention gradually develops; the normal ventilatory drive becomes less dependent on arterial CO_2 tension and more on hypoxemia.

Emphysema

Emphysema is a pathologic diagnosis based on irreversible enlargement of the airways distal to terminal bronchioles with destruction of alveolar septa. Mild apical emphysematous changes are often a normal but clinically insignificant consequence of aging. Significant emphysema is nearly always related to cigarette smoking. Less commonly, emphysema at an early age is associated with homozygous α_1-antitrypsin deficiency. Loss of the elastic recoil that normally supports small airways by radial traction allows premature collapse during exhalation (dynamic airway collapse).

Destruction of pulmonary capillaries in the alveolar septa decreases diffusion capacity (for carbon monoxide) and eventually leads to pulmonary hypertension in the terminal stages of the disease. Some patients develop large cystic areas or bullae. Increased dead space ventilation is a prominent feature of emphysema. Arterial oxygen tensions are usually normal or only slightly reduced; CO_2 tension is also typically normal. When dyspneic, patients with emphysema often purse their lips to delay closure of the small airways—which accounts for the term "pink puffers" that is often used.

Treatment

Treatment for chronic obstructive lung disease is primarily supportive. The most important intervention is cessation of smoking. Patients demonstrating a reversible element in airway obstruction ($>$ 15% improvement in FEV_1 following administration of a bronchodilator) should be started on long-term bronchodilator therapy. Even patients who do not show improvement from the bronchodilator may improve clinically with long-term theophylline treatment. Pulmonary infections should be aggressively treated. Exacerbations are often related to bouts of bronchitis; frequent treatment with broad-spectrum antibiotics may be necessary. Hypoxemia should be treated carefully with supplemental oxygen. Careful low-flow oxygen therapy (1–2 L/min) is necessary in patients with CO_2 retention; elevating PaO_2 above 60 mm Hg can abolish the hypoxic respiratory drive and precipitate respiratory failure in some patients. Patients with severe disease and pulmonary hypertension are often started on home oxygen therapy. When cor pulmonale is present, diuretics are used to control peripheral edema; the beneficial effects from digoxin and vasodilators are inconsistent.

Preoperative Considerations

As with asthmatics, these patients should be optimally prepared prior to elective surgical procedures. They should be questioned about recent changes in dyspnea, sputum, and wheezing. Pulmonary function studies, chest radiographs, and blood gas measurements should be reviewed. The presence of bullous changes should be noted. Many patients have concomitant cardiac disease and should also receive a careful cardiovascular evaluation.

In contrast to asthma, only limited improvement in respiratory function may be seen after a short period of intensive preoperative preparation. Nonetheless, preoperative interventions aimed at correcting hypoxemia, relieving bronchospasm, reducing secretions, and treating infections have been shown to decrease the incidence of postoperative pulmonary complications. Patients at greatest risk for complications are those with preoperative pulmonary function measurements less than 50% of predicted. Patients with FEV_1 less than 50% usually have dyspnea on exertion, while those with FEV_1 less than 25% also are dyspneic at rest. The latter finding, in patients with predominantly chronic bronchitis, is also often associated with CO_2 retention and pulmonary hypertension. The possibility of postoperative ventilation in high-risk patients should be discussed with the patient and the surgeon.

Smoking should be discontinued for several weeks or more prior to operation to decrease secretions. Cessation of smoking for as little as 24 hours also has theoretically beneficial effects on oxygen-carrying capacity. Within that time, carbon monoxide levels (half-life of 4–6 hours) and carboxyhemoglobin levels return to normal, shifting the hemoglobin dissociation curve from the left back to normal. Preoperative chest physiotherapy and antibiotics in patients with a change in sputum are beneficial in reducing secretions. Bronchospasm should be treated with therapeutic theophylline levels and aerosolized bronchodilators. Some patients with moderate to severe disease may benefit from a perioperative course of glucocorticoids. Those with malnutrition should receive preoperative nutritional support or supplementation before major surgery. Pulmonary hypertension should be treated by optimizing oxygenation. Perioperative digitalization may be useful in patients with cor pulmonale.

Intraoperative Considerations

Although regional anesthesia is often considered preferable to general anesthesia, high spinal or epidural anesthesia can decrease lung volumes, restrict the use of accessory respiratory muscles, and produce an ineffective cough, leading to retention of secretions. Loss of proprioception from the chest and unusual positioning, such as lithotomy or the lateral decubitus position, often accentuate dyspnea in awake patients.

Preoxygenation prior to induction of general anesthesia prevents the rapid oxygen desaturation often seen in these patients. The selection of anesthetic agents and general intraoperative management are similar to those of asthmatic patients (see above). Unfortunately, the use of bronchodilating anesthetics improves only the reversible component of airflow obstruction bronchospasm; significant expiratory obstruction is still often present under deep anesthesia. Enhanced respiratory depression from anesthetics is often seen with moderate to severe disease. Ventilation should be controlled with large tidal volumes and slow rates to avoid air trapping. Humidified gases should be used if significant bronchospasm is present and for long procedures ($>$ 2 hours). Nitrous oxide should be avoided in patients with large bullae and those known to have pulmonary hypertension. Pneumothorax due to expansion can occur with the former, while further elevations in pulmonary artery pressures may be seen with the latter. Inhibition of hypoxic pulmonary vasoconstriction by inhalation anesthetics is not clinically significant during general anesthesia (Chapter 24).

Measurement of arterial blood gases is desirable for prolonged peripheral, extensive intra-abdominal, and all thoracic procedures. Although pulse oximetry accurately detects significant arterial desaturation, direct measurement of arterial oxygen tensions may be necessary to detect more subtle changes in intrapulmonary shunting. Moreover, only arterial CO_2 measurements should be used to guide ventilation because an increase in the normal arterial to end-tidal CO_2 gradient is often present. Ventilation should be adjusted to maintain a normal arterial pH. Normalization of $PaCO_2$ in patients with preoperative CO_2 retention results in alkalosis (Chapter 30). Hemodynamic monitoring should be dictated by any underlying cardiac dysfunction as well as the extent of the surgery. In patients with pulmonary hypertension, central venous pressure measurements reflect right ventricular function rather than intravascular volume.

At the end of surgery, the timing of extubation should balance the risk of bronchospasm versus pulmonary insufficiency. An awake extubation allows a more accurate assessment of immediate postoperative pulmonary function but risks bronchospasm; deep extubation lessens the risk of reflex bronchospasm but assumes the adequacy of pulmonary function. Patients with an FEV_1 below 50% are most likely to require a period of postoperative ventilation, especially following upper abdominal and thoracic operations. General criteria for extubation are discussed in Chapter 48.

RESTRICTIVE PULMONARY DISEASE

Restrictive pulmonary diseases are characterized by decreased total lung compliance. Lung volumes are typically reduced with relatively normal expiratory flow rates. Although both FEV_1 and FVC are reduced, the FEV_1/FVC ratio is normal. Restrictive pulmonary diseases include many acute and chronic intrinsic (pulmonary) disorders as well as extrinsic (extrapulmonary) disorders involving the pleura, chest wall, diaphragm, or neuromuscular function. Reduced lung compliance increases the work of breathing, resulting in a characteristic rapid shallow breathing pattern. Respiratory gas exchange is usually maintained until the disease process is advanced.

Classification

A. Acute Intrinsic Disorders: Reduced lung compliance in these disorders is primarily due to an increase in extravascular lung water, which is due either to an increase in pulmonary capillary pressure or an increase in pulmonary capillary permeability (Chapter 48). Increased pressure occurs with left ventricular failure and fluid overload, while increased permeability is present with adult respiratory distress syndrome (ARDS). Localized or generalized increases in permeability also occur following aspiration or infectious pneumonitis.

B. Chronic Intrinsic Disorders: There are many causes of these disorders but the end result is the same in all cases, ie, fibrosis of the lung. Causes include diffuse idiopathic pulmonary fibrosis, radiation, drug toxicity (bleomycin and nitrofurantoin), oxygen toxicity, autoimmune diseases, and sarcoidosis.

C. Extrinsic Disorders: These disorders interfere with normal lung expansion. They include pleural effusions, pneumothorax, mediastinal masses, kyphoscoliosis, pectus excavatum, neuromuscular disorders, and increased intra-abdominal pressure due to ascites, pregnancy, or bleeding. Marked obesity also results in a restrictive ventilatory defect (Chapter 36).

Preoperative Considerations

A. Acute Restrictive Pulmonary Disorders: Patients with acute pulmonary disease should be spared elective surgery. Under emergency conditions, oxygenation and ventilation should be optimized to the extent possible. Fluid overload should be treated with diuretics; heart failure also requires vasodilators, administration of an inotrope, or both. Drainage of large pleural effusions should be considered. Similarly, massive abdominal distention may be relieved by drainage of ascites or nasogastric compression. Persistent hypoxemia may require intubation and positive end-expiratory pressure (PEEP). Associated systemic disturbances such as hypotension or infection should be aggressively treated.

B. Chronic Restrictive Pulmonary Disorders: Regardless of the cause, preoperative assessment of chronic restrictive diseases should be based primarily on clinical manifestations. Dyspnea during exertion or at rest necessitates pulmonary function testing. Vital capacities less than 15 mL/kg are indicative of severe dysfunction. The chest radiograph is often helpful in assessing lung volume and the extent of infiltrates or scarring. Hypoxemia is common, but CO_2 retention is indicative of severe disease.

Intraoperative Considerations

A. Acute Restrictive Pulmonary Disorders: Selection of anesthetic agents should be tailored to each patient. Surgical patients with acute pulmonary disorders, such as ARDS, cardiogenic pulmonary edema, or pneumonia, are generally critically ill; anesthetic management should be a continuation of the intensive care they received preoperatively. Anesthesia is most often provided with a combination of intravenous and inhalation agents together with a muscle relaxant. High inspired oxygen concentrations and PEEP may be required. Hemodynamic monitoring is generally advisable.

B. Chronic Restrictive Pulmonary Disorders: Similar to patients with acute disease, intraoperative management in these patients is complicated by a predisposition to hypoxemia and the need to control ventilation to assure optimum oxygenation and ventilation; anesthetic drug selection is not critical. A reduced FRC (and, necessarily, oxygen stores) predisposes these patients to rapid hypoxemia following induction of anesthesia (Chapter 22); accelerated uptake of inhalation anesthetics may also occur. Mechanical ventilation is complicated by high peak airway pressures and an increased risk of pneumothorax. Smaller than normal tidal volumes (8–12 mL/kg) with faster rates (12–16 breaths/min) may be necessary. Ideally, monitoring for hypoxemia with a pulse oximeter should be continued during transport, recovery, and perhaps the early postoperative period.

PULMONARY EMBOLISM

Pulmonary embolism results from the entry of blood clots, fat, tumor cells, air, amniotic fluid, or foreign material into the venous system. Clots from the lower extremities, pelvic veins, or, less commonly, the right atrium or ventricle are usually responsible. Venous stasis or hypercoagulability is often contributory in such cases. Other common risk factors include obesity and estrogen therapy. Fat embolism is discussed in Chapter 48, while air embolism is discussed in Chapter 26.

Embolic occlusions in the pulmonary circulation increase dead space. Localized or generalized reflex bronchoconstriction may also increase areas with low ventilation/perfusion ratios. Pulmonary infarction occurs if the embolus involves a large vessel and collateral blood flow from the bronchial circulation is insufficient for that part of the lung. Pulmonary emboli also acutely increase pulmonary vascular resistance. In previously healthy individuals, occlusion of more than 50% of the pulmonary circulation (massive pulmonary embolism) is necessary before sustained pulmonary hypertension is seen. Patients with preexisting cardiac or pulmonary disease can develop acute pulmonary hypertension with occlusions of lesser magnitude. A sustained increase in right ventricular afterload can precipitate acute right ventricular failure.

Clinical manifestations of pulmonary embolism include acute tachypnea, dyspnea, chest pain, or hemoptysis. Symptoms are often mild and nonspecific unless massive embolism has occurred. Wheezing may be present on auscultation. Arterial blood gas analysis typically shows mild hypoxemia with respiratory alkalosis. The chest x-ray may be normal or may show an area of oligemia, a wedge-shaped density (with an infarct), atelectasis with an elevated diaphragm, or an enlarged proximal pulmonary artery (with acute pulmonary hypertension). Cardiac signs include tachycardia and wide fixed splitting of the second heart sound; hypotension with elevated central venous pressure is usually indicative of right ventricular failure. The ECG may show signs of acute cor pulmonale such as new right axis deviation, right bundle branch block, and tall peaked T waves.

Pulmonary angiography is the most accurate means of diagnosing pulmonary embolism. Radionuclide ventilation/perfusion scans are diagnostic only if a perfusion defect is present in an area with normal ventilation.

Treatment

The best treatment for pulmonary embolism is prevention. Minidose heparin, oral anticoagulation, aspirin, or dextran therapy together with early ambulation can decrease the incidence of postoperative emboli. The use of high elastic stockings and pneumatic compression of the legs may also decrease the incidence of venous thrombosis in the legs but not in the pelvis or the heart.

Systemic anticoagulation prevents the formation of new blood clots or the extension of existing clots. After 1–2 weeks of systemic anticoagulation with heparin, warfarin is started and continued for a variable time (usually 6–12 months). Thrombolytic therapy with tissue plasminogen activator or streptokinase is indicated for patients with massive pulmonary embolism or circulatory collapse. Recent surgery and active bleeding are contraindications to anticoagulation and thrombolytic therapy. In these cases, an inferior vena cava umbrella filter may be placed to prevent recurrent pulmonary emboli. Pulmonary embolectomy may be indicated for patients with massive embolism in whom thrombolytic therapy is contraindicated.

Preoperative Considerations

Patients with acute pulmonary embolism may present to the operating room for placement of a caval umbrella filter or, rarely, for pulmonary embolectomy. In most instances, patients have a history of pulmonary embolism and present for unrelated surgery. In the latter group of patients, the risk of interrupting anticoagulant therapy perioperatively is unknown. If the acute episode is more than 1 year old, the risk of temporarily stopping anticoagulant therapy is probably small. Moreover, except in the case of chronic recurrent pulmonary emboli, pulmonary function has usually returned to normal. The emphasis in the perioperative management of these patients should be in the prevention of new episodes of embolism (see above).

Intraoperative Considerations

Vena cava umbrella filters are usually placed percutaneously under local anesthesia with sedation. Patients may display enhanced sensitivity to the circulatory effects of most anesthetic agents. Decreased venous return during placement of the device can precipitate hypotension.

Although no definite recommendations can be made regarding the choice of anesthesia for patients with a history of pulmonary embolism, recent evidence suggests that regional anesthesia for some procedures (ie, hip surgery) decreases the incidence of postoperative deep venous thrombosis and pulmonary embolism. The use of regional anesthesia is contraindicated in patients with residual anticoagulation or a prolonged bleeding time.

Significant pulmonary embolism is a rare occurrence during anesthesia. Air emboli are common but are often overlooked unless large amounts are entrained (Chapter 26). Thromboembolism may occur intraoperatively during prolonged procedures; a venous thrombus can be dislodged during surgical manipulations in the pelvis. Manipulation of tumors with intravascular extension can similarly produce pulmonary embolism (Chapter 33). Intraoperative pulmonary embolism usually presents as unexplained sudden hypotension, bronchospasm, or both. A decrease in end-tidal CO_2 concentration is also suggestive but not specific. Invasive monitoring may reveal elevated central venous and pulmonary arterial pressures. Treatment is supportive, with intravenous fluids and inotropes.

CASE DISCUSSION: INABILITY TO VENTILATE A PATIENT WITH CHRONIC OBSTRUCTIVE LUNG DISEASE

A 62-year-old man with chronic obstructive pulmonary disease and acute bowel obstruction was brought to the operating room for exploratory laparotomy. A right subclavian central venous catheter was placed preoperatively to guide fluid therapy; some difficulty was apparently encountered, because there are multiple puncture sites on the right neck and subclavian areas. After a smooth rapid-sequence induction with thiopental and succinylcholine, breath sounds were clear and equal bilaterally. Controlled ventilation was initiated, and anesthesia was maintained with a gas mixture of O_2, air, and isoflurane and intravenous vecuronium. Fifteen minutes into the surgery, the pulse oximeter saturation, which had been 97%, rapidly drops below 75%. Peak inspiratory pressures are noted to have increased from 24 to 60 cm H_2O; the spirometer is reading less than 100 mL tidal volume; and the ventilator begins to alarm. The capnograph shows reduced CO_2 exhalation (18 mm Hg) with a reduced up-slope.

What is the first priority?

The first priority should be to maintain adequate oxygenation. The possibility of falsely low pulse oximeter readings should always be considered but is unlikely in this case because of the associated sudden inability to ventilate the patient. The quality of the pulse oximeter trace, signal strength, and its ability to track heart rate usually correlate with the reliability of saturation readings. Clinical signs of hypoxemia are

unreliable; cyanosis is a late finding. Hypoxemia must be assumed to be present until proved otherwise.

Oxygen concentration should immediately be increased to 100% and confirmed by the oxygen analyzer. Mechanical ventilation should be discontinued and the patient ventilated by hand with the anesthesia bag (in the circle system); the latter excludes ventilator malfunction and gives an estimate of the patient-anesthesia circuit compliance. The performance and gas flow characteristics of many anesthesia machine ventilators rapidly deteriorate with high airway pressures; hand ventilation is often more effective in these instances. For very stiff lungs, exchanging the standard 3-L adult anesthesia bag with a less compliant pediatric 1-L bag may be necessary. Even marked hypoventilation with 100% oxygen, in most instances, adequately resaturates venous blood with oxygen (Chapter 22).

After the above steps were undertaken, oxygen saturation increased to 92%, but compliance in the circuit was still poor; peak inspiratory pressures remained higher than 60 cm H_2O.

What is the next step?

The anesthesia circuit and endotracheal tube should be inspected for kinking or blockage. If neither is seen, both lungs are then auscultated with a stethoscope. Bilateral wheezing suggests acute bronchospasm or pulmonary edema. Unilateral breath sounds suggest that the endotracheal tube has advanced too far down and is now endobronchial, or that the patient has developed a pneumothorax. The latter is a strong possibility in this case in view of the apparent difficulty encountered with central venous catheterization. Pneumothorax can also occur with mechanical ventilation alone. Persistence of CO_2 on the capnograph excludes inadvertent extubation.

Breath sounds are barely perceptible bilaterally.

Should a bronchodilator be given?

Not at this point. While severe bronchospasm may result in complete absence of breath sounds without wheezing, occult obstruction of the endotracheal tube or lower trachea by blood or secretions is always a possibility and should be excluded.

Outcome

A suction catheter was passed with some difficulty through the endotracheal tube, and several blood clots were suctioned out. Vigorous suctioning after instillation of saline rapidly improved compliance and returned oxygen saturation to normal. The trachea was apparently traumatized preoperatively during attempts to cannulate the right internal jugular vein. Dislodgment of these clots together with secretions eventually resulted in almost complete obstruction of the endotracheal tube.

SUGGESTED READINGS

Brown DL (editor): *Risk and Outcome in Anesthesia.* Lippincott, 1988.

Cheng EY, Kay J: *Manual of Anesthesia and the Medically Compromised Patient.* Lippincott, 1990.

Katz J, Benumof J, Kadis LB: *Anesthesia and Uncommon Diseases,* 3rd ed. Saunders, 1990.

Nunn JF: *Applied Respiratory Physiology.* Butterworths, 1987. This classic work contains excellent discussions on the pathophysiology of respiratory disorders.

Stoelting RK, Dierdorf SF, McCammon RL: *Anesthesia and Coexisting Disease,* 2nd ed. Churchill Livingstone, 1988.

Vickers MD: *Medicine for Anaesthetists,* 3rd ed. Blackwell, 1989.

24   Anesthesia for Thoracic Surgery

Thoracic surgery presents a unique set of problems for the anesthesiologist. They include the physiologic derangements caused by the lateral decubitus position, the problem of an open pneumothorax, surgical manipulations that may interfere with pulmonary and cardiac function, the risk of massive bleeding, and the necessity for one-lung anesthesia.

PHYSIOLOGY OF THE LATERAL DECUBITUS POSITION

The lateral decubitus position provides optimal access for most operations on the lungs, the pleura, the esophagus, the great vessels, and the thoracic sympathetic chain and vertebrae as well as for many non-thoracic procedures. Unfortunately, this position has the potential to cause major alterations in pulmonary ventilation/perfusion relationships (Chapter 22). Moreover, these derangements are accentuated by induction of anesthesia, initiation of mechanical ventilation, muscle paralysis, and opening the chest. While perfusion continues to favor the dependent (lower) lung, ventilation progressively favors the upper lung. The resulting mismatch markedly increases the risk of hypoxemia.

1.   AWAKE PATIENTS

When an awake supine patient assumes the lateral decubitus position, gravity favors greater blood flow to the dependent (lower) lung while spontaneous ventilation favors greater gas flow to that lung, so that normal ventilation/perfusion matching is thus maintained. Ventilation to the dependent lung is greater than that to the upper lung for two reasons: (1) contraction of the dependent portion the diaphragm is more efficient as a result of its higher position in the chest (from the weight of the abdominal contents); and (2) the dependent lung is on a more favorable part of the compliance curve (Figure 24–1).

2.   ANESTHETIZED, SPONTANEOUSLY BREATHING PATIENTS

Induction of general anesthesia decreases functional residual capacity (Chapter 22). The upper lung moves down to a more favorable part of the compliance curve, while the lower lung moves to a less compliant position (Figure 24–2). As a result, greater ventilation goes to the upper lung. Because perfusion remains greater to the dependent lung, ventilation/perfusion mismatching occurs.

3.   ANESTHETIZED, MECHANICALLY VENTILATED PATIENTS

When the anesthetized patient is started on controlled ventilation, an even greater portion of ventilation goes to the upper lung because the mechanical advantage of the lower portion of the diaphragm is lost. Muscle paralysis accentuates this effect by allowing abdominal contents to rise up farther against the lower diaphragm and impede ventilation of the lower lung.

4.   ANESTHETIZED, MECHANICALLY VENTILATED PATIENTS WITH AN OPEN CHEST

When the chest wall is opened, the upper lung has less restricted movement (its compliance increases). This effect favors yet greater ventilation of the upper lung than its dependent counterpart; perfusion remains unaltered. The potential for severe ventilation/perfusion mismatching and hypoxemia is markedly enhanced.

OPEN PNEUMOTHORAX

The lungs are normally kept expanded by a negative pleural pressure—the net result of the tendency of the lung to collapse and the chest wall to expand. If one side of the chest is opened, the negative pressure is lost and the elastic recoil of the lung on that side tends to collapse it. When the patient is in the lateral decubitus position, spontaneous ventilation with an open pneumothorax results in paradoxic respirations and mediastinal shift, both of which cause progressive hypoxemia and hypercapnia. During general anesthesia, these effects are overcome by the use of controlled positive-pressure ventilation.

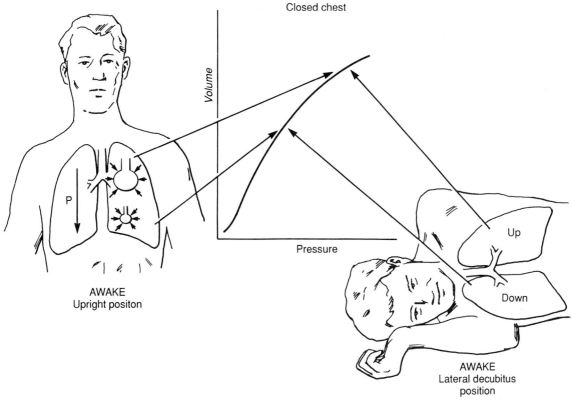

Figure 24–1. The effect of the lateral decubitus position on lung compliance.

1. MEDIASTINAL SHIFT

When the chest is opened on one side, pleural pressure becomes atmospheric on that side but remains negative on the other side. During inspiration, pleural pressure on the dependent side becomes more negative and shifts the mediastinum downward (in the lateral position). During expiration, the mediastinum moves back upward (Figure 24–3). The major effect of a mediastinal shift is to decrease the tidal volume of the dependent lung from compression by the mediastinum. Marked mediastinal shifting may induce shocklike reflex circulatory changes.

2. PARADOXIC RESPIRATION

Spontaneous ventilation in patients with an open pneumothorax results in to-and-fro gas flow between the dependent and nondependent lungs (paradoxic respiration). During inspiration, gas flows from the nondependent lung across the carina to the dependent lung, and the pneumothorax increases. During expiration, the pneumothorax decreases as the gas flow reverses and moves from the dependent to the nondependent (upper) lung (Figure 24–4).

PREOPERATIVE EVALUATION

Preoperative assessment of the patient with pulmonary disease is discussed in detail in Chapter 23. However, it should be emphasized that because smoking is a common risk factor, patients undergoing thoracotomy for a pulmonary malignancy frequently have coexistent chronic obstructive pulmonary disease and coronary artery disease.

Ectopic hormone production by some lung tumors may produce signs and symptoms of Cushing's syndrome, hyperparathyroidism, the syndrome of inappropriate antidiuretic hormone, or the myasthenic (Eaton-Lambert) syndrome. Characteristically, muscle strength increases with repeated effort in the myasthenic syndrome but decreases with myasthenia gravis.

Operative Criteria For Pneumonectomy

Although operability is ultimately a clinical decision, pulmonary function tests are useful preliminary guidelines. The degree of impairment—as measured by routine pulmonary function tests—is directly related to operative risk. Standard preliminary criteria for operability are set forth in Table 24–1. Failure to

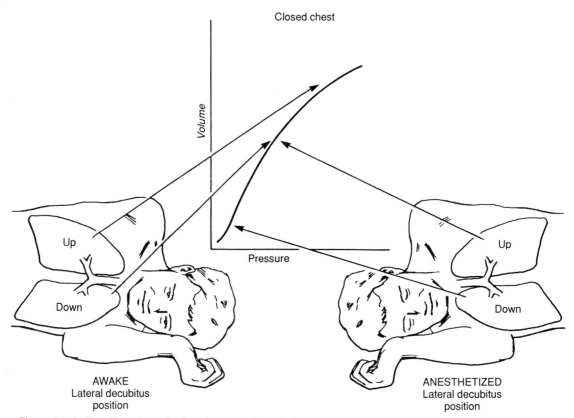

Figure 24–2. The effect of anesthesia on lung compliance in the lateral decubitus position. The upper lung assumes a more favorable position, while the lower lung becomes less compliant.

meet any one of these criteria necessitates split lung function tests if surgery is still contemplated. The criterion for operability is usually then a predicted postoperative FEV_1 greater than 800 mL. The percentage contribution of each lung to total FEV_1 is assumed to be proportionate to the percentage of the total pulmonary blood flow it receives (postoperative FEV_1 = % blood flow $\times$ total FEV_1). Pulmonary blood flow is determined by radioisotopic scanning (^{133}Xe or ^{99m}Tc). Removal of extensively diseased lung (nonventilated but perfused) may not adversely affect pulmonary function and can actually improve oxygena-

tion. If the predicted postoperative FEV_1 is less than 800 mL but resection is still considered, the ability of the remaining pulmonary vasculature to tolerate total blood flow is then tested. The main pulmonary artery on the diseased side is occluded with a balloon catheter; if the mean pulmonary artery pressure rises more than 30–40 mm Hg, the patient is not a candidate for pneumonectomy.

PREOPERATIVE PREPARATION

1. OPTIMIZING MEDICAL STATUS

Patients undergoing thoracic procedures are at increased risk of postoperative pulmonary complications (Chapter 23). Good preoperative preparation has been shown to reduce such complications in high-risk patients. Prophylactic preoperative digitalization is frequently employed in elderly patients but is controversial. Perioperative dysrhythmias (particularly atrial tachycardias) are thought to be the result of surgical manipulation or distention of the right heart following reduction of the pulmonary vasculature. The incidence of dysrhythmias increases with age and with the

Table 24–1. Preoperative laboratory criteria for pneumonectomy.

Test	High-Risk Patients
Arterial blood gas	$PaCO_2 > 45$ mm Hg (on room air)
FEV_1	<2 L
FEV_1/FVC	<50% of predicted
Maximum breathing capacity	<50% of predicted
RV/TLC	<50% of predicted

EXPIRATION

Pneumothorax

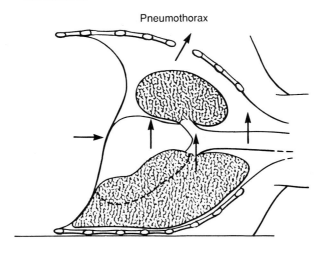

INSPIRATION

Pneumothorax

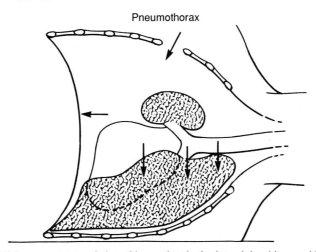

Figure 24–3. Mediastinal shift in a spontaneously breathing patient in the lateral decubitus position. (Reproduced, with permission, from Tarhan S, Moffitt EA: Principles of thoracic anesthesia. Surg Clin North Am 1973;53:813.)

amount of pulmonary resection and is greater with a left than with a right pneumonectomy.

2. PREMEDICATION

Patients with moderate to severe respiratory compromise should receive little or no sedative premedication. Although anticholinergics (atropine, 0.5 mg intramuscularly, or glycopyrrolate, 0.2 mg intramuscularly) can theoretically inspissate secretions and increase dead space, clinically they are useful in reducing copious secretions and vagal reflexes in patients undergoing thoracic procedures.

INTRAOPERATIVE MANAGEMENT

1. MONITORING

Direct arterial pressure monitoring is indicated for one-lung anesthesia (see below), for resections of mediastinal tumors, for procedures on patients with limited pulmonary reserve, and for patients with significant cardiovascular disease. Central venous access with central venous pressure (CVP) monitoring is highly desirable for pneumonectomies and mediastinal tumors. CVP reflects the net effect of venous capacitance, blood volume, and right ventricular function;

EXPIRATION

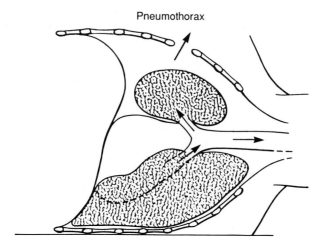

INSPIRATION

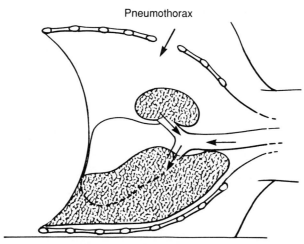

Figure 24–4. Paradoxic respiration in spontaneously breathing patients on their side. (Reproduced, with permission, from Tarhan S, Moffitt EA: Principles of thoracic anesthesia. Surg Clin North Am 1973;53:813.)

consequently, it is only a rough guide to fluid management. Pulmonary artery catheterization is indicated in patients with pulmonary hypertension, cor pulmonale, or left ventricular dysfunction. X-ray localization is mandatory to make certain that the pulmonary artery catheter is not in a lung segment to be resected.

2. CHOICE OF ANESTHESIA

General anesthesia with controlled positive-pressure ventilation is safest; in addition to preventing pulmonary collapse, paradoxic breathing, and a mediastinal shift, it allows control of the operative field to facilitate the surgery.

3. INDUCTION

Following preoxygenation, intravenous barbiturate induction is used for most patients. Intubation is accomplished only after deep anesthesia to prevent reflex bronchospasm and obtund the cardiovascular pressor response. This may be accomplished by incremental doses of barbiturate, narcotic, or both; intravenous or intratracheal lidocaine may also be useful. Deepening anesthesia with a potent inhalational agent is preferable in patients with reactive airways. Use of isoflurane requires slowly increasing its concentration to minimize any irritative effects on the airways. Intubation is facilitated with succinylcholine or a nondepolarizing agent (unless a difficult airway is antici-

Table 24–2. Indications for one-lung anesthesia.

Absolute
    Confine pulmonary infection to one side
    Confine pulmonary bleeding to one side
    Separate ventilation to each lung
        Bronchopulmonary fistula
        Tracheobronchial disruption
        Large lung cyst
    Bronchopleural lavage
Relative
    High priority
        Thoracic aortic aneurysm
        Pneumonectomy
        Upper lobectomy
        Thoracoscopy
    Low priority
        Middle and lower lobectomies
        Sub-segmental resections
        Esophageal surgery

pated). Most thoracotomies can be performed with an ordinary endotracheal tube, but endobronchial techniques for one-lung anesthesia (see below) are useful for certain procedures (Table 24–2).

4. MAINTENANCE OF ANESTHESIA

All anesthetic techniques have been successfully used for thoracic surgery, but the potent halogenated agents (halothane, enflurane, and isoflurane) are preferred by most clinicians. Advantages include (1) potent dose-related bronchodilatation, (2) depression of airway reflexes, (3) the ability to use a high inspired oxygen concentration (F_{IO_2}), (4) the capability for relatively rapid adjustments in anesthetic depth, and (5) minimal effects on hypoxic pulmonary vasoconstriction (see below).

Nitrous oxide (N_2O) is generally not used because of the obligatory decrease in F_{IO_2}. Nitrous oxide can also inhibit hypoxic pulmonary vasoconstriction and exacerbate pulmonary hypertension in some patients. Use of a muscle relaxant during surgery facilitates rib spreading as well as anesthetic management.

5. PATIENT MANAGEMENT

Following induction, intubation, and confirmation of correct endotracheal or endobronchial tube position (see below), additional venous access and monitoring are secured. At least one large-bore intravenous line (14- or 16-gauge) is mandatory for all thoracotomies. Central venous access and a blood warmer are also desirable if excessive blood loss is anticipated.

After venous access and monitoring are secured, the patient is positioned for surgery. Proper positioning is critical for the lateral decubitus position to avoid injuries and to facilitate surgical exposure. The lower arm is flexed while the upper arm is extended in front of the head, pulling the scapula away from the operative field (Figure 24–5). Pillows are placed between the arms and legs, and a towel roll is positioned just beneath the dependent axilla to avoid injury to the brachial plexus; care is taken to avoid pressure on the eyes and the dependent ear.

Maximal anesthesia is required when the ribs are spread. When the chest is opened, venous return decreases as the negative pleural (intrathoracic) pressure is lost. This effect can be reversed with a fluid bolus. Many clinicians tend to restrict fluid administration to some extent during lung resections and favor colloid for fluid boluses. Excessive fluid administration in the lateral decubitus position may promote the lower lung syndrome, ie, gravity-dependent transudation of fluid into the dependent lung, leading to a decrease in functional residual capacity (FRC) and an increase in airway closure. A significant amount of blood is lost in the removed lung during pneumonectomy and must be accounted for in fluid replacement. Sustained vagally mediated reflex bradycardia from surgical manipulations should be treated with intravenous atropine.

During lung resections, the bronchus (or remaining lung tissue) is usually divided with a stapling device. The bronchial stump is then tested for air leak under water by applying 30 cm of positive pressure to the airway. During rib approximation, hand ventilation is helpful in avoiding injury to lung parenchyma from suture needles. Prior to completion of chest closure, all remaining lung segments should be fully expanded

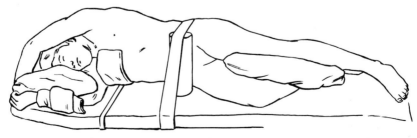

Figure 24–5. Proper positioning for a lateral thoracotomy. (Reproduced, with permission, from Gothard JWW, Branthwaite MA: *Anaesthesia for Thoracic Surgery.* Blackwell 1982.)

manually under direct vision. Controlled ventilation is then resumed and continued until chest tubes are connected to suction. Chest tubes are not needed following a pneumonectomy.

Most patients are extubated early to decrease the risk of pulmonary barotrauma (particularly blowout of a bronchial suture) and infection. Patients with marginal pulmonary reserve should be left intubated until standard extubation criteria are met (Chapter 48).

ONE-LUNG ANESTHESIA

By allowing collapse of the lung on the operative side, one-lung anesthesia greatly improves surgical exposure for many procedures. The technique can also be used to isolate a lung or to facilitate ventilatory management under certain conditions (Table 24–2). Three techniques can be employed: (1) a double-lumen endobronchial tube, (2) a single-lumen endobronchial tube, or (3) a bronchial blocker. Double-lumen tubes are most often used.

1. DOUBLE-LUMEN TUBES

The principal advantages of double-lumen tubes are (1) relative ease of placement, (2) the ability and ease of ventilating either or both lungs, and (3) the ability to suction either lung.

All double-lumen tubes (Table 24–3) share the following characteristics: (1) one lumen that enters either the right or left main bronchus and another that remains in the lower trachea, (2) a preformed curve that allows preferential entry into either bronchus, and (3) separate bronchial and tracheal cuffs. Because of differences in bronchial anatomy on the right and left sides, tubes are designed specifically for the right or left side.

Anatomic Considerations

The adult trachea is 11–12 cm long. It begins at the level of the cricoid cartilage (C6) and bifurcates behind the sternomanubrial joint (T5). Major differences between the right and left main bronchi are as follows: (1) the wider right bronchus diverges away from the trachea at a 25-degree angle, while the left bronchus diverges at a 45-degree angle (Figure 24–6); (2) the right bronchus has upper, middle, and lower lobe

Table 24–3. Types of double-lumen tubes.

Name	Bronchus Intubated	Carinal Hook	Shape of Lumen
Carlens	Left	Yes	Oval
White	Right	Yes	Oval
Bryce-Smith	Right or left	No	Round
Robertshaw	Right or left	No	D-shaped

branches, while the left bronchus divides into only upper and lower lobe branches; and (3) the orifice of the right upper lobe bronchus is 2.5 cm from the carina, while that of the left upper lobe is 5 cm distal to the carina.

Right-sided tubes must have a slit in the bronchial cuff for ventilating the right upper lobe (Figure 24–7). Anatomic variations in the distance between the right upper lobe orifice and the carina can result in difficulties in ventilating that lobe with right-sided tubes. Right-sided tubes were designed for left thoracotomies, while left-sided tubes were designed for right thoracotomies. Many anesthetists, however, use a left-sided tube regardless of the operative side; for left-sided surgery, they withdraw the tube into the trachea prior to clamping of the left main bronchus.

Some older tubes have carinal hooks (eg, Carlens and White), but the risk of laryngeal trauma during placement has caused most clinicians to abandon them. The most widely used double-lumen tube is a disposable version of the Robertshaw tube.

Placement of Double-Lumen Tubes

During placement, laryngoscopy with a curved (MacIntosh) blade often provides better visualization than a straight blade. The double-lumen tube is passed with the distal curvature concave anteriorly and is rotated 90 degrees (toward the side to be intubated) as the tip enters the larynx (Figure 24–8). It is advanced until resistance is felt. Correct tube placement should be established using a preset protocol (Table 24–4). Since displacement may occur when the patient is turned to the lateral decubitus position, tube position should be reconfirmed at that time. Confirmation of correct placement with a flexible bronchoscope is an invaluable aid. Moreover, the bronchoscope may be used for placement: it is passed through the distal lumen and used as a stylet to gently guide the double-lumen tube into proper position.

Table 24–4. Protocol for checking placement of a left-sided double-lumen tube.

1. Inflate the tracheal cuff (5–10 mL of air).
2. Check for bilateral breath sounds. Unilateral breath sounds indicate that the tube is too far down (tracheal opening is endobronchial).
3. Inflate the bronchial cuff (1–2 mL).
4. Clamp the tracheal lumen.
5. Check for unilateral left-sided breath sounds.
   a. Persistence of right-sided breath sounds indicates that the bronchial opening is still in the trachea (tube should be advanced).
   b. Unilateral right-sided breath sounds indicate incorrect entry of the tube into the right bronchus.
6. Unclamp the tracheal lumen and clamp the bronchial lumen.
7. Check for unilateral right breath sounds. Absence or diminution of breath sounds indicates that the tube is still not far enough down and the bronchial cuff is occluding the distal trachea.

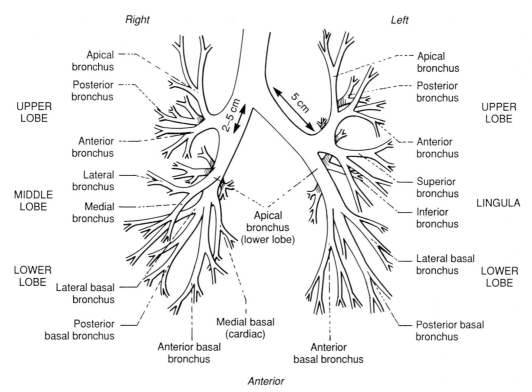

Figure 24–6. Anatomy of the tracheobronchial tree. (Reproduced, with permission, from Gothard JWW, Branthwaite MA: *Anaesthesia for Thoracic Surgery.* Blackwell 1982.)

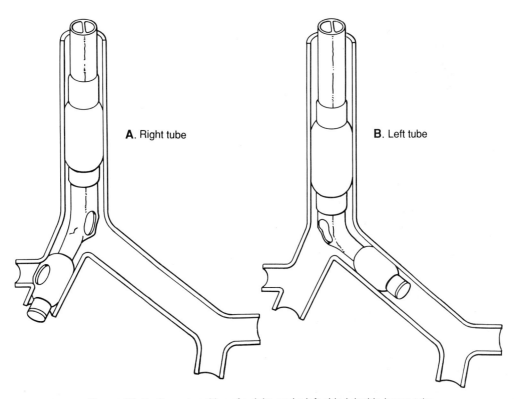

Figure 24–7. Correct position of a right- and a left-sided double-lumen tube.

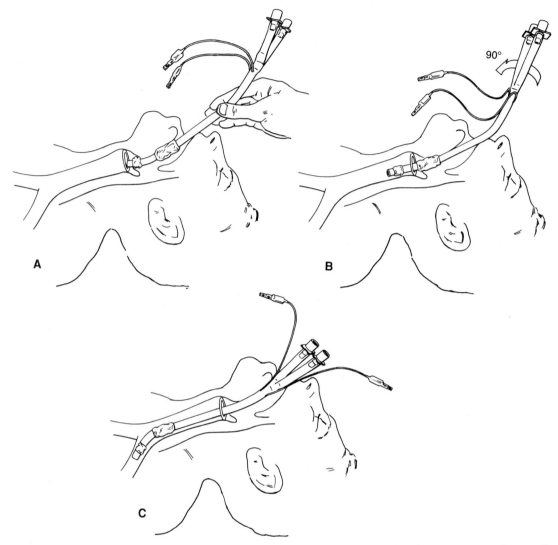

Figure 24–8. Placement of a left-sided double-lumen tube. Note that the tube is turned 90 degrees as soon as it enters the larynx. ***A:*** Initial position. ***B:*** Rotated 90 degrees. ***C:*** Final position.

Complications of Double-Lumen Tubes

Major complications of double-lumen tubes include (1) hypoxemia due to tube malplacement or occlusion, (2) traumatic laryngitis (particularly with a carinal hook), (3) tracheobronchial rupture due to overinflation of the bronchial cuff, and (4) inadvertent suturing of the tube to a bronchus during surgery (detected as difficulty in withdrawing the tube at extubation).

2. SINGLE-LUMEN ENDOBRONCHIAL TUBES

With the exception of the Gordon-Green tube, single-lumen endobronchial tubes are now rarely used. The Gordon-Green tube is a right-sided single-lumen tube that has both tracheal and bronchial cuffs as well as a carinal hook. Inflating the bronchial cuff isolates and allows ventilation of only the right lung. When the bronchial cuff is deflated and the tracheal cuff is inflated, both lungs can be ventilated. When difficulty in ventilating the right upper lobe is encountered with a right double-lumen tube, the Gordon-Green tube is a good alternative for left thoracotomies. A much larger slit in its bronchial cuff (compared to right-sided double-lumen tubes) results in a high success rate for ventilating the right upper lobe. The principal disadvantages of the Gordon-Green tube are the hazards of a carinal hook and the inability to suction the left lung.

3. BRONCHIAL BLOCKERS

Bronchial blockers are inflatable devices that are passed alongside a regular endotracheal tube to selectively occlude a bronchial orifice. Bronchial blockers are rarely used because of the time and skill required for proper placement. They also do not allow suctioning or ventilation of the isolated lung, and they are easily dislodged. Nonetheless, bronchial blockers may be useful for one-lung anesthesia in pediatric patients and for tamponading endobronchial bleeding in some adult patients (see below).

4. PHYSIOLOGY OF ONE-LUNG ANESTHESIA

Intentional collapse of one lung results in perfusion without ventilation on that side and, secondarily, a large intrapulmonary shunt. Mixing of unoxygenated blood from the collapsed lung with the oxygenated blood from the still ventilated lung widens the P_A-a (alveolar-to-arterial) O_2 gradient and can result in hypoxemia. Fortunately, blood flow to the nonventilated lung is decreased by several mechanisms (Chapter 22): (1) hypoxic pulmonary vasoconstriction due to alveolar hypoxia, (2) surgical compression, and (3) increased vascular resistance from the atelectasis.

Factors known to inhibit hypoxic pulmonary vasoconstriction and thus increase intrapulmonary shunting include (1) very high or very low pulmonary artery pressures; (2) hypocapnia; (3) high or low mixed venous PO_2; (4) vasodilators such as nitroglycerin, nitroprusside, and calcium channel blockers; (5) pulmonary infection; and (6) volatile anesthetics (probably not clinically significant).

Factors that decrease blood flow to the ventilated lung can be equally detrimental; by indirectly increasing blood flow to the collapsed lung, they can counteract hypoxic pulmonary vasoconstriction. Such factors include (1) high mean airway pressures in the ventilated lung (from positive end-expiratory pressure, hyperventilation, or high peak inflation pressures); (2) vasoconstrictors (such as dopamine, epinephrine, and phenylephrine), which appear to have a greater effect on normoxic than hypoxic blood vessels; and (3) a low FIO_2, which produces hypoxic pulmonary vasoconstriction in the ventilated lung.

Carbon dioxide elimination is usually not affected by one-lung anesthesia provided minute ventilation is unchanged; arterial CO_2 tension is usually not appreciably altered.

5. MANAGEMENT OF ONE-LUNG VENTILATION

The greatest risk of one-lung anesthesia is hypoxemia. To reduce this risk, the period of one-lung ventilation should be kept to a minimum and 100% oxygen should be used. Adjustments in ventilation are usually not necessary. If peak airway pressures rise excessively (> 30 cm H_2O), tidal volume may be reduced to 8–12 mL/kg and the ventilatory rate increased to maintain the same minute volume. Close monitoring

of the pulse oximeter is mandatory. Periodic arterial blood gas analysis is also necessary to ensure adequate ventilation.

Hypoxemia during one-lung anesthesia requires one or more of the following interventions:

(1) Changing tidal volume and ventilatory rate (variable effect)
(2) Periodic inflation of the collapsed lung with oxygen
(3) Continuous insufflation of oxygen into the collapsed lung
(4) 5–10 cm H_2O of continuous positive airway pressure (CPAP) to the collapsed lung (partial reexpansion of the lung may interfere with the surgery)
(5) 5–10 cm H_2O of PEEP to the ventilated lung (variable effect)
(6) Early ligation of the ipsilateral pulmonary artery (in a pneumonectomy)

ALTERNATIVES TO ONE-LUNG VENTILATION

High-Frequency Ventilation

High-frequency positive-pressure ventilation and high-frequency jet ventilation (Chapter 48) have been used successfully during thoracic procedures as alternatives to one-lung ventilation. A standard endotracheal tube may be used with these techniques. Small tidal volumes (< 2 mL/kg) allow decreased lung excursion to facilitate the surgery but still allow ventilation of both lungs.

Apneic Oxygenation

Ventilation can be stopped for short periods if 100% oxygen is insufflated at a rate greater than oxygen consumption (Chapter 22). Adequate oxygenation is maintained for prolonged periods, but progressive respiratory acidosis limits the use of this technique to 10–20 minutes in most patients. Arterial PCO_2 rises 6 mm Hg in the first minute, followed by a rise of 3–4 mm Hg during each subsequent minute.

POSTOPERATIVE CARE

Hypoxemia and respiratory acidosis are common postoperatively, especially following lateral thoracotomies. These effects are largely due to splinting from pain (Chapter 23). Standard postoperative care should include maintenance of a semiupright (> 30 degrees) position, supplemental oxygen (40–50%), and aggressive pain relief.

1. PAIN RELIEF

Systemic Narcotics

The balance between comfort and respiratory depression in patients with marginal lung function is difficult to achieve with parenteral narcotics alone. These patients benefit from the use of supplemental techniques described below. When parenteral narcotics are used, small intravenous doses are superior to large intramuscular doses. When the patient is awake, patient-controlled analgesia can be initiated (morphine, 2 mg, or meperidine, 10 mg, with a 5- to 10-minute lockout interval).

Intercostal Nerve Block

A long-acting agent such as 0.5% bupivacaine (4–5 mL), injected two levels above and below a lateral thoracotomy incision, typically provides excellent pain relief. These blocks may be done under direct vision intraoperatively or postoperatively. Intercostal blocks have been shown to improve arterial blood gases and pulmonary function tests and shorten the hospital stay. Intraoperative freezing of the intercostal nerves (cryoneurolysis) produces long-lasting anesthesia; nerve regeneration is reported after approximately 1 month.

Epidural Narcotics

Injection of intrathecal or epidural narcotics (morphine, 0.5 mg or 5 mg, respectively) also can provide good pain relief. The lumbar epidural route (through catheter) may be safest and is the preferred route. Good pain relief without autonomic, sensory, or motor blockade typically lasts 6–10 hours. Patients should be monitored carefully for immediate and delayed respiratory depression.

SPECIAL CONSIDERATIONS FOR UNUSUAL PROBLEMS IN PATIENTS UNDERGOING THORACIC PROCEDURES

1. MASSIVE PULMONARY HEMORRHAGE

Patients with pulmonary hemorrhage who have failed medical management may come to surgery for bronchoscopy or lung resection. They represent a group of very high risk patients. The most common cause of death is asphyxia secondary to blood in the airway. In some instances, when the site of bleeding is identified by bronchoscopy preoperatively, a bronchial blocker can be placed to tamponade the bleeding. Premedication should not be given, because patients are usually hypoxic. One-lung anesthesia to protect the other lung is desirable but may not be possible in many patients. Awake intubation in a semiupright position with a large single-lumen tube may be safest.

2. PULMONARY CYSTS & BULLAE

Pulmonary cysts or bullae may be congenital or acquired. Rupture during positive-pressure ventilation can produce a tension pneumothorax. Induction of anesthesia with maintenance of spontaneous ventilation is desirable until the side with the cyst or bullae is isolated with a double-lumen tube or until a chest tube is placed. Nitrous oxide will cause expansion of the air space and is contraindicated in these patients. Rupture may be signaled by sudden hypotension, bronchospasm, or an abrupt rise in peak inflation pressure.

3. BRONCHOPLEURAL FISTULA

Bronchopleural fistulae occur following lung resection (usually pneumonectomy), empyema, or trauma. Most patients come to surgery after conservative treatment with chest tube drainage and antibiotics has failed. Management is complicated by the inability to ventilate the patient with positive pressure (owing to a large air leak), the potential for tension pneumothorax, and, with empyema, the risk of contaminating the other lung.

Intravenous induction with rapid endobronchial intubation is usually safest. A double-lumen tube greatly simplifies anesthetic management by isolating the fistula and providing one-lung anesthesia to the healthy side. Because the air leak is proportionate to the peak airway pressure, high-frequency ventilation with a standard endotracheal tube may also be considered. At the end of the repair, the patient should be extubated if possible.

4. TRACHEAL RESECTION

Tracheal resection is most commonly performed for tracheal stenosis or carcinoma. Little or no premedication is given, since most patients have moderate to severe airway obstruction. Following induction of anesthesia, the patient is intubated with a standard or armored (wire-reinforced) endotracheal tube placed proximal to the lesion. In patients with tracheal stenosis, a small tube can sometimes be passed distal to the site of obstruction.

With high tracheal lesions, the surgeon divides the trachea in the neck and advances a sterile armored tube into the distal trachea for ventilation during the resection. Following resection and completion of the posterior part of the reanastomosis, the armored tube is removed and the original endotracheal tube is advanced distally past the anastomosis (Figure 24–9). Alternatively, high-frequency jet ventilation may be employed during the anastomosis by passing the jet cannula past the obstruction and into the distal trachea (Figure 24–10). Return of spontaneous ventilation and early extubation at the end of the procedure are desirable. Patients should be positioned with the neck flexed immediately postoperatively to minimize tension on the suture line (Figure 24–11).

Management of low tracheal lesions requires thoracotomy and more complicated techniques employing

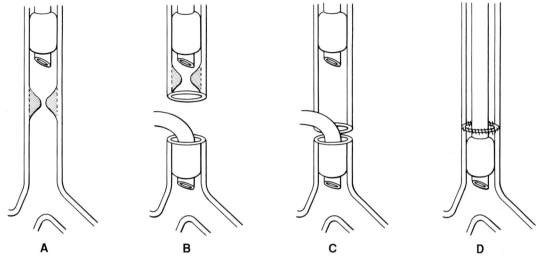

Figure 24–9. Airway management of a high tracheal lesion.

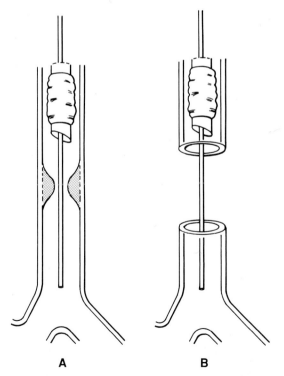

Figure 24–10. Tracheal resection using high-frequency jet ventilation. **A:** Catheter is advanced past obstruction and cuff is deflated when jet ventilation is initiated. **B:** Catheter is advanced distally by surgeon. Jet ventilation can be continued without interruption during resection and reanastomosis.

high-frequency ventilation or even cardiopulmonary bypass.

ANESTHESIA FOR DIAGNOSTIC THORACIC PROCEDURES

1. BRONCHOSCOPY

Topical and local anesthesia for flexible bronchoscopy is discussed in Chapter 5. Rigid bronchoscopy for removal of foreign bodies or tracheal dilatation is usually performed under general anesthesia. These procedures are complicated by the need to share the airway with the surgeon; fortunately, they are often of short duration (5–10 minutes). After a standard intravenous induction, anesthesia is usually maintained with a potent inhalational agent in 100% oxygen and a a short- or intermediate-acting muscle relaxant. One of three techniques can then be used during bronchoscopy: (1) apneic oxygenation with a small catheter alongside the bronchoscope; (2) conventional ventilation through the side arm of a ventilating bronchoscope (when the proximal window of this instrument is opened for suctioning or biopsies, ventilation must be interrupted); or (3) high-frequency ventilation through an injector-type bronchoscope. In the latter instance, a narrow cannula (16- to 18-gauge) in the proximal end of the bronchoscope is used to inject oxygen at high pressures; the Venturi effect created proximally entrains an air-oxygen mixture down the trachea.

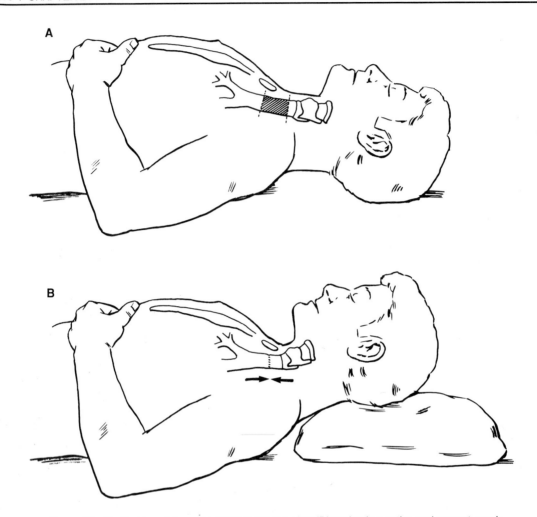

Figure 24–11. Position of the patient before **(A)** and after **(B)** tracheal resection and reanastomosis.

2. MEDIASTINOSCOPY

Mediastinoscopy provides access to the mediastinal lymph nodes and is used to establish either the diagnosis or the resectability of intrathoracic malignancies. Preoperative computerized tomography is essential for evaluating tracheal distortion or compression.

Mediastinoscopy is performed under general endotracheal anesthesia with a muscle relaxant. Venous access with a large-bore intravenous catheter (14- to 16-gauge) is mandatory because of the risk of excessive bleeding and the difficulty in controlling bleeding when it occurs. Because the innominate artery may be compressed during the procedure, blood pressure should be measured in the left arm.

Complications associated with mediastinoscopy include (1) vagally mediated reflex bradycardia from compression of the trachea or the great vessels; (2) excessive hemorrhage (see above); (3) cerebral ischemia from compression of the innominate artery (detected with a plethysmograph or pulse oximeter on the right

hand); (4) pneumothorax (usually presents postoperatively); (5) air embolism (due to 30-degree head elevation, the risk being greatest during spontaneous ventilation); and (6) recurrent laryngeal nerve damage.

CASE DISCUSSION: MEDIASTINAL ADENOPATHY

A 9-year-old boy with mediastinal lymphadenopathy seen on chest a x-ray presents for biopsy of a cervical lymph node.

What are the important preoperative considerations?

(1) Is there any evidence of airway compromise? Tracheal compression may produce dyspnea (proximal

A. NORMAL

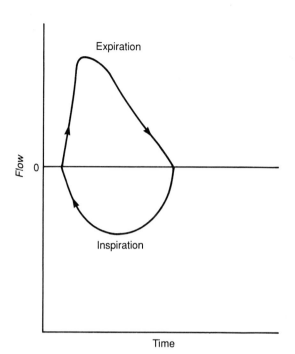

B. VARIABLE EXTRATHORACIC OBSTRUCTION

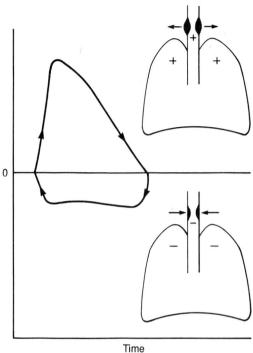

C. VARIABLE INTRATHORACIC OBSTRUCTION

D. FIXED LARGE AIRWAY OBSTRUCTION

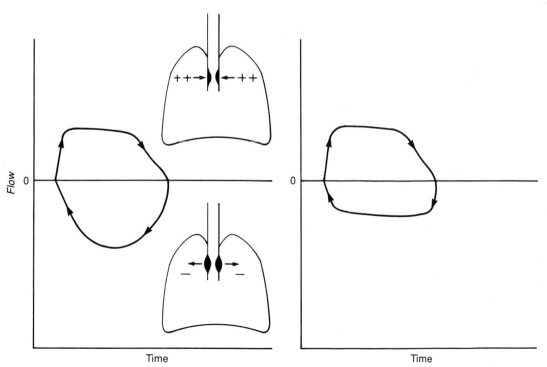

Figure 24–12. Flow volume loops.

obstruction) or a nonproductive cough (distal obstruction). Asymptomatic compression is also common and may only be evident as tracheal deviation on physical or radiographic examinations. A CT scan of the chest provides invaluable information about the presence, location, and severity of airway compression. Flow-volume loops will also detect subtle airway obstruction and provide important information regarding its location and functional importance (Figure 24–12).

(2) Is there any evidence of superior vena cava syndrome? Superior vena cava syndrome is caused by progressive enlargement of a mediastinal mass and resultant compression of the vessel. It can be associated with severe airway obstruction and cardiovascular collapse on induction of general anesthesia.

Caval compression produces venous engorgement and edema of the head, neck, and arms. Direct mechanical compression as well as mucosal edema severely compromise airflow in the trachea. Most patients favor an upright posture, since recumbency worsens the airway obstruction. Cardiac output may be severely depressed owing to impeded venous return from the upper body, direct mechanical compression of the heart, and (with malignancies) pericardial invasion.

What is the anesthetic of choice?

The absence of signs or symptoms of airway compression or superior vena cava syndrome does not preclude potentially life-threatening complications following induction of general anesthesia. Therefore, biopsy of a peripheral node (usually cervical or scalene) under local anesthesia is safest whenever possible. Although establishing a diagnosis is of prime importance, the presence of significant airway compromise or the superior vena cava syndrome may dictate empiric treatment with corticosteroids prior to tissue diagnosis at surgery (cancer is the most common cause). In such instances, the patient can usually safely undergo surgery with general anesthesia once airway compromise and other manifestations of the superior vena cava syndrome are alleviated.

General anesthesia may be indicated (1) for young or uncooperative patients who have no evidence of airway compromise or the superior vena cava syndrome, and (2) for patients requiring thoracotomy who are unresponsive to steroids, radiation, and chemotherapy.

How does the presence of airway obstruction and the superior vena cava syndrome influence management of general anesthesia?

(1) Premedication: Only an anticholinergic should be given. The patient should be wheeled to the operating room in a semiupright position while being given supplemental oxygen.

(2) Monitoring: In addition to standard monitors, an arterial line is mandatory, but it should be placed after induction in young patients. A large-bore intravenous catheter should be placed in a lower extremity, since venous drainage from the upper body may be unreliable.

(3) Airway management: Difficulties with ventilation and intubation should be anticipated. Following preoxygenation, awake intubation with an armored endotracheal tube may be safest in a cooperative patient. Use of a flexible bronchoscope is advantageous in the presence of airway distortion and will define the site and degree of obstruction. *Coughing or straining, however, may precipitate complete airway obstruction,* because the resultant positive pleural pressure increases intrathoracic tracheal compression. Passing the armored tube beyond the area of compression may obviate this problem. Uncooperative patients require induction of general anesthesia prior to intubation.

(4) Induction: The goal should be a smooth induction maintaining spontaneous ventilation and hemodynamic stability. The ability to ventilate the patient with a good airway should be established prior to use of a muscle relaxant. Using 100% oxygen, one of three induction techniques can be used: (a) intravenous ketamine (because it results in greater hemodynamic stability in patients with reduced cardiac output); (b) inhalational induction with a volatile agent; or (c) incremental doses of thiopental or etomidate.

Positive-pressure ventilation can precipitate severe hypotension, and volume loading prior to induction may partly offset impaired ventricular filling secondary to caval obstruction.

(5) Maintenance of anesthesia: The technique selected should be tailored to the patient's hemodynamic status. Following intubation, paralysis prevents coughing or straining.

(6) Extubation: At the end of the procedure, patients should be left intubated until the airway obstruction has resolved, as determined by flexible bronchoscopy or the presence of an air leak around the endotracheal tube when the tracheal cuff is deflated.

SUGGESTED READINGS

Benumof JL: *Anesthesia for Thoracic Surgery.* Saunders, 1987.

Gothard JWW, Branthwaite MA: *Anaesthesia for Thoracic Surgery.* Blackwell, 1982.

Kaplan JA: *Thoracic Anesthesia,* 2nd ed. Churchill Livingstone, 1991.

Marshall BE: *Anesthesia for Thoracic Procedures.* Blackwell, 1987.

Neurophysiology & Anesthesia

25

The anesthetic care of patients with neurosurgical diseases requires a basic understanding of the physiology of the central nervous system. The effects of anesthetic agents on cerebral metabolism, blood flow, cerebrospinal fluid dynamics, and intracranial volume and pressure are often profound. In some instances, these alterations are deleterious, while in others they may actually be beneficial. This chapter reviews important physiologic concepts in anesthetic practice and then discusses the effects of commonly used anesthetics on cerebral physiology. While most of the discussion focuses on the brain, the same concepts also apply, at least qualitatively, to the spinal cord.

CEREBRAL METABOLISM

The brain is normally responsible for 20% of total body oxygen consumption. Most of the oxygen is used in generating ATP to support neuronal electrical activity. The cerebral metabolic rate (CMR) is usually expressed in terms of oxygen consumption ($CMRO_2$), which averages 3–3.5 mL/100 g/min (50 mL/min) in adults. $CMRO_2$ is greatest in the gray matter of the cerebral cortex and generally parallels cortical activity. Because of the relatively high oxygen consumption and the absence of significant oxygen reserves, interruption of cerebral perfusion usually results in unconsciousness within 10 seconds as oxygen tension rapidly drops below 30 mm Hg. If blood flow is not reestablished within minutes (3–8 minutes under most conditions), ATP stores are depleted and irreversible cellular injury begins to occur. The hippocampus and cerebellum appear to be most sensitive to hypoxic injury.

Neuronal cells normally utilize glucose as their primary energy source. Brain glucose consumption is approximately 5 mg/100 g/min, of which over 90% is metabolized aerobically. $CMRO_2$ therefore normally parallels glucose consumption. This relationship does not hold during starvation, when ketone bodies (acetoacetate and β-hydroxybutyrate) also become major energy substrates. Though the brain can also take up and metabolize some lactate, cerebral function is normally dependent on a continuous supply of glucose. Acute sustained hypoglycemia is equally as devastating as hypoxia. Paradoxically, hyperglycemia can exacerbate global hypoxic brain injury by acceler-

ating cerebral acidosis and cellular injury; its effect on focal cerebral ischemia is unclear.

CEREBRAL BLOOD FLOW

Cerebral blood flow (CBF) varies with metabolic activity. It is most commonly measured with a gamma-emitting isotope such as xenon (^{133}Xe). Following systemic injection, detectors placed around the brain measure the rate of radioactive decay, which is directly proportionate to cerebral blood flow. Newer techniques employing positron emission tomography (PET) in conjunction with short-lived isotopes such as ^{11}C and ^{15}O also allow measurement of cerebral metabolic rate (for glucose and oxygen, respectively). Such studies confirm that regional cerebral blood flow (rCBF) parallels metabolic activity and can vary from 10 to 300 mL/100 g/min. For example, motor activity of a limb is associated with a rapid increase in rCBF of the corresponding motor cortex. Similarly, visual activity is associated with an increase in rCBF of the corresponding occipital visual cortex.

Although total cerebral blood flow averages 50 mL/100 g/min, flow in gray matter is about 80 mL/100 g/min while that in white matter is estimated to be 20 mL/100 g/min. Total cerebral blood flow in adults averages 750 mL/min (15–20% of cardiac output). Flow rates below 20–25 mL/100 g/min are usually associated with cerebral impairment, as evidenced by slowing on the EEG. Cerebral blood flow rates between 15 and 20 mL/100 g/min typically produce a flat (isoelectric) EEG, while values below 10 mL/100 g/min are usually associated with irreversible brain damage.

REGULATION OF CEREBRAL BLOOD FLOW

Cerebral Perfusion Pressure

Cerebral perfusion pressure is the difference between mean arterial pressure (MAP) and intracranial pressure (or cerebral venous pressure, whichever is greater). When cerebral venous pressure is significantly greater than intracranial pressure, perfusion pressure becomes the difference between mean arterial pressure and cerebral venous pressure. Because intracranial pressure (ICP) and cerebral venous pressure are normally within a few millimeters of mercury of each other and the former is easier to measure, cerebral perfusion pressure (CPP) is expressed by the equation $CPP = MAP - ICP$. Cerebral perfusion pressure is normally about 100 mm Hg. Moreover, since intracranial pressure is normally less than 10 mm Hg, cerebral perfusion pressure is primarily dependent on mean arterial pressure.

Moderate to severe increases in intracranial pressure (> 30 mm Hg) can significantly compromise cerebral perfusion pressure and cerebral blood flow even in the presence of a normal mean arterial pressure. Patients with cerebral perfusion pressure values less than 50 mm Hg often show slowing on the EEG, while those with a cerebral perfusion pressure between 25 and 40 mm Hg typically have a flat EEG. Sustained perfusion pressures less than 25 mm Hg result in irreversible brain damage.

Autoregulation

Like the heart and kidneys, the brain normally tolerates wide swings in blood pressure with little change in blood flow. The cerebral vasculature rapidly adapts to changes in cerebral perfusion pressure. Decreases in cerebral perfusion pressure result in cerebral vasodilatation, while elevations induce vasoconstriction. In normal individuals, cerebral blood flow remains nearly constant between mean arterial blood pressures of about 60 and 160 mm Hg (Figure 25–1). Beyond these limits, blood flow becomes pressure-dependent. Pressures above 150–160 mm Hg can disrupt the blood-brain barrier (see below) and may result in cerebral edema and hemorrhage.

The cerebral autoregulation curve (Figure 25–1) is shifted to the right in patients with chronic arterial hypertension. Both upper and lower limits are shifted: Flow becomes more pressure-dependent at low "normal" arterial pressures in return for cerebral protection at higher arterial pressures. Studies suggest that long-term antihypertensive therapy can restore cerebral autoregulation limits toward normal.

Both myogenic and metabolic mechanisms have been proposed to explain cerebral autoregulation. The former involves an intrinsic response of smooth muscle cells in cerebral arterioles to changes in mean arterial pressure. The latter theory holds that cerebral metabolic demands determine arteriolar tone. Thus, when tissue demand exceeds blood flow, the release of tissue metabolites causes vasodilation and increases flow. While hydrogen ions were previously thought to mediate this response, other metabolites are probably involved, including adenosine, prostaglandins, and perhaps ionic (electrolyte) concentration gradients.

Extrinsic Mechanisms

The most important extrinsic influences on cerebral blood flow are respiratory gas tensions—particularly $PaCO_2$—and body temperature. Cerebral blood flow is directly proportionate to $PaCO_2$ between tensions of 20 and 80 mm Hg (Figure 25–2). This effect is almost immediate and is thought to be secondary to changes in the pH of cerebrospinal fluid and cerebral tissue. Because ions do not readily cross the blood-brain barrier (see below) but CO_2 does, acute changes in $PaCO_2$ but not HCO_3^- affect cerebral blood flow. Similarly, acute metabolic acidosis has little effect on cerebral blood flow because hydrogen ions (H^+) cannot readily cross the blood-brain barrier. After 24–48 hours, cerebrospinal fluid HCO_3^- concentration adjusts to compensate for the change in $PaCO_2$, so that the effects of hypocapnia and hypercapnia are diminished. Marked hyperventilation ($PaCO_2 < 20$ mm Hg) may result in electroencephalographic changes suggestive of cerebral impairment even in normal individuals.

Only marked changes in PaO_2 alter cerebral blood flow. While hyperoxia may be associated with only minimal decreases (-10%) in cerebral blood flow, severe hypoxemia ($PaO_2 < 50$ mm Hg) profoundly increases cerebral blood flow (Figure 25–2).

Other extrinsic factors affecting cerebral blood flow include body temperature, blood viscosity, and autonomic influences. Cerebral blood flow changes 5–7% per °C. Hypothermia decreases both cerebral metabolic rate and cerebral blood flow, while pyrexia has the reverse effect. Changes in blood viscosity do not appreciably alter cerebral blood flow with hematocrits between 30% and 50%. However, at either extreme, enhancement (with low values during cardiopulmonary bypass) or impairment (with marked polycythemia) may be seen.

Intracranial vessels are innervated by both sympathetic (vasoconstrictive) and parasympathetic (vasodilatory) fibers. The normal physiologic function of this innervation is uncertain but appears to be important in some pathologic states. This is especially true for the innervation of large cerebral vessels by sympathetic fibers originating in the superior cervical sympathetic ganglia. Intense sympathetic stimulation induces marked vasoconstriction in these vessels that can limit cerebral blood flow. Autonomic innervation may also play an important role in cerebral vasospasm following brain injury and stroke.

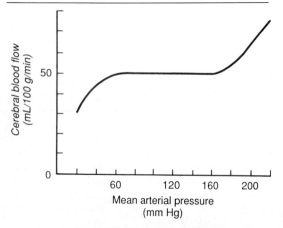

Figure 25–1. Cerebral autoregulation.

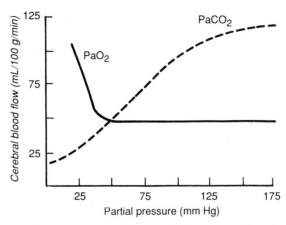

Figure 25–2. The relationship between cerebral blood flow and arterial respiratory gas tensions.

BLOOD-BRAIN BARRIER

Cerebral blood vessels are unique in that the junctions between vascular endothelial cells are nearly fused. The paucity of pores is responsible for what is termed the blood-brain barrier. This lipid barrier allows the passage of lipid-soluble substances but restricts the movement of those that are ionized or have large molecular weights. Thus, the movement of a given substance across the blood-brain barrier is governed simultaneously by its size, charge, lipid solubility, and degree of protein binding in blood. Carbon dioxide, oxygen, and lipid-soluble substances (such as most anesthetics) freely enter the brain, whereas most ions, proteins, and large substances such as mannitol penetrate poorly.

Water moves freely across the blood-brain barrier as a consequence of bulk flow, whereas movement of even small ions is impeded to some extent (the equilibration half-life for sodium is 2–4 hours). As a result, rapid changes in plasma electrolyte concentrations (and, secondarily, osmolality) produce a transient osmotic gradient between plasma and the brain. Acute hypertonicity of plasma results in net movement of water out of the brain, while acute hypotonicity causes a net movement of water into the brain. These effects are short-lived, since equilibration eventually occurs, but when marked they can cause rapid fluid shifts in the brain. Thus, marked abnormalities in serum sodium or glucose concentrations should generally be corrected slowly (Chapter 28). Mannitol, an osmotically active substance that does not normally cross the blood-brain barrier, causes a sustained decrease in brain water content and is often used to decrease brain volume.

The blood-brain barrier may be disrupted by severe hypertension, tumors, trauma, strokes, infection, marked hypercapnia, hypoxia, and sustained seizure activity. Under these conditions, fluid movement across the blood-brain barrier becomes dependent on hydrostatic pressure rather than osmotic gradients.

CEREBROSPINAL FLUID

Cerebrospinal fluid is found in the cerebral ventricles and cisterns and in the subarachnoid space surrounding the brain and spinal cord. Its major function is to protect the central nervous system against trauma.

Most of the cerebrospinal fluid is formed by the choroid plexuses of the cerebral (mainly lateral) ventricles. Smaller amounts are formed directly by their ependymal cell linings and yet smaller quantities from fluid leaking into the perivascular spaces surrounding cerebral vessels (blood-brain barrier leakage). In adults, normal total cerebrospinal fluid production is about 21 mL/h (500 mL/d), yet total cerebrospinal fluid volume is only about 150 mL. Cerebrospinal fluid flows from the lateral ventricles through the interventricular foramina (of Monro) into the third ventricle, through the cerebral aqueduct (of Sylvius) into the fourth ventricle, and through the median aperture of the fourth ventricle (foramen of Magendie) and the lateral aperture of the fourth ventricle (foramina of Luschka) into the cerebellomedullary cistern (cisterna magna) (Figure 25–3). From the cerebellomedullary cistern, cerebrospinal fluid enters the subarachnoid space, circulating around the brain and spinal cord before being absorbed in arachnoid granulations over the cerebral hemispheres.

Cerebrospinal fluid formation involves active secretion of sodium in the choroid plexuses. The resulting fluid is isotonic with plasma despite lower potassium, bicarbonate, and glucose concentrations. Its protein content is limited to the very small amounts that leak into perivascular fluid. Carbonic anhydrase inhibitors (acetazolamide), corticosteroids, spironolactone, furosemide, isoflurane, and vasoconstrictors decrease cerebrospinal fluid production.

Cerebrospinal fluid absorption involves the translocation of fluid from the arachnoid granulations into the cerebral venous sinuses. Smaller amounts are absorbed at nerve root sleeves and by meningeal lymphatics. Although the mechanism remains unclear, ab-

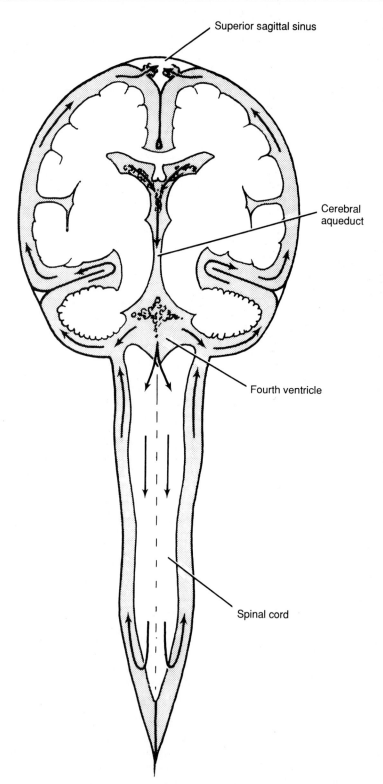

Figure 25–3. The flow of cerebrospinal fluid in the central nervous system. (Reproduced, with permission, from DeGroot J, Chusid JG: *Correlative Neuroanatomy,* 21st ed. Appleton & Lange, 1991.)

sorption appears to be directly proportionate to intracranial pressure and inversely proportionate to cerebral venous pressure. Since the brain and spinal cord lack lymphatics, cerebrospinal fluid absorption is also the principal means by which perivascular and interstitial protein is returned to blood.

INTRACRANIAL PRESSURE

The cranial vault is a rigid structure with a fixed total volume, consisting of brain (80%), blood (12%), and cerebrospinal fluid (8%). Any increase in one component must be offset by an equivalent decrease in another to prevent a rise in intracranial pressure. Intracranial pressure by convention means supratentorial cerebrospinal fluid pressure measured in the lateral ventricles or over the cerebral cortex and is normally 10 mm Hg or less. Minor variations may occur depending on the site measured, but in the lateral recumbent position lumbar cerebrospinal fluid pressure normally approximates supratentorial pressure.

Intracranial compliance is determined by measuring the change in intracranial pressure in response to a change in the intracranial volume. Normally, increases in volume are initially well-compensated (Figure 25–4). However, a point is eventually reached at which further increases produce precipitous rises in intracranial pressure. Major compensatory mechanisms include (1) an initial displacement of cerebrospinal fluid from the cranial to the spinal compartment, (2) an increase in cerebrospinal fluid absorption, (3) a decrease in cerebrospinal fluid production, and (4) a decrease in total cerebral blood volume (primarily venous).

The concept of total intracranial compliance is useful clinically even though compliance probably varies in the different compartments of the brain and is affected by arterial blood pressure and $PaCO_2$. Compliance can be determined in patients with intraventricular catheters by injecting sterile saline. An

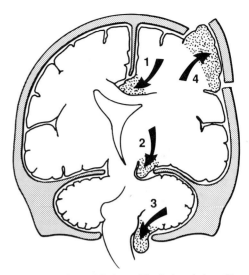

Figure 25–5. Potential sites of brain herniation. (Reproduced, with permission, from Fishman RA: Brain edema. New England J Med 1975;293:706.)

increase in intracranial pressure greater than 4 mm Hg following injection of 1 mL of saline indicates poor compliance. At that point, compensatory mechanisms have been exhausted and cerebral blood flow is progressively compromised as intracranial pressure rises further. Sustained elevations in intracranial pressure can lead to catastrophic herniation of the brain. Herniation may occur at one of four sites (Figure 25–5): (1) the cingulate gyrus under the falx cerebri, (2) the uncinate gyrus through the tentorium cerebelli, (3) the cerebellar tonsils through the foramen magnum, or (4) any area beneath a defect in the skull (transcalvarial).

EFFECT OF ANESTHETIC AGENTS ON CEREBRAL PHYSIOLOGY

Overall, most general anesthetics have favorable effects on the central nervous system. Carbohydrate metabolism decreases, while energy stores in the form of ATP, ADP, and phosphocreatine increase. Determination of the effects of the specific agents are complicated by the concomitant administration of other drugs, surgical stimulation, intracranial compliance, blood pressure, and CO_2 tension. For example, hypocapnia or prior administration of thiopental blunts the increases in cerebral blood flow and intracranial pressure that usually occurs with ketamine and volatile agents.

This section describes the changes generally associated with each drug when given alone. Table 25–1 summarizes and compares the effects of the various anesthetics. The effects of vasoactive agents and muscle relaxants are also discussed.

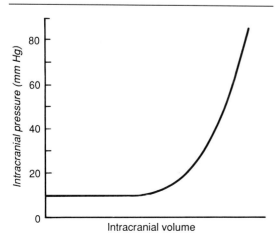

Figure 25–4. Normal intracranial compliance.

Table 25–1. Comparative effects of anesthetic agents on cerebral physiology.

Agent	CMR	CBF	CSF Production	CSF Absorption	CBV	ICP
Halothane	↓↓	↑↑	±	↓	↑↑	↑↑
Enflurance	↓↓	↑	↑	↓	↑↑	↑↑
Isoflurane	↓↓↓	↑	±	↑	↑↑	↑
Nitrous oxide	↓	↑	±	±	±	↑
Barbiturates	↓↓↓	↓↓	±	↑	↓↓	↓↓↓
Etomidate	↓↓↓	↓↓	±	↑	↓↓	↓↓
Propofol	↓↓	↓↓	?	?	↓↓	↓↓
Benzodiazepines	↓	↓	±	↑	↓	↓
Ketamine	±	↑↑	±	↓	↑↑	↑↑
Narcotics	±	±	±	↑	±	±
Lidocaine	↓↓	↓↓	?	?	↓↓	↓↓
Droperidol	±	±	?	?	±	±

Key:
↑ = Increase
↓ = Decrease
± = Little or no change
? = Unknown
Legend:
CMR = Cerebral metabolic rate
CBF = Cerebral blood flow
CSF = Cerebrospinal fluid
CBV = Cerebral blood volume
ICP = Intracranial pressure

1. VOLATILE AGENTS

Cerebral Metabolic Rate

Halothane, enflurane, and isoflurane produce dose-dependent decreases in cerebral metabolic rate. Isoflurane produces the greatest depression (up to 50%), followed by enflurane and then halothane. More-over, isoflurane is the only agent that can produce an isoelectric EEG at clinically useful concentrations (1.5–2 MAC). Enflurane's depression of cerebral metabolic rate is reversed when it precipitates seizure activity on the EEG (see below); in fact, cerebral metabolic rate increases with frank seizure activity.

Cerebral Blood Flow & Volume

Volatile anesthetics increase cerebral blood flow and impair autoregulation in a dose-dependent manner (Figure 25–6). Halothane has the greatest effect on cerebral blood flow; at concentrations greater than 1%, it nearly abolishes cerebral autoregulation. At an equivalent minimum alveolar concentration and blood pressure, halothane increases cerebral blood flow up to 200%, compared with 40% and 20% for enflurane and isoflurane, respectively. The response of the cerebral vasculature to CO_2 is retained with all three volatile agents. Hyperventilation (hypocapnia) can therefore blunt their effects on cerebral blood flow. Hypocapnia is most effective during isoflurane anesthesia.

Increases in cerebral blood volume (10–12%) generally parallel increases in cerebral blood flow, but the relationship is not necessarily linear. Expansion of cerebral blood volume can markedly elevate intracranial pressure in patients with reduced intracranial compliance. Studies indicate that cerebral blood volume increases to the same extent with all three agents, suggesting that each affects cerebral venous capaci-

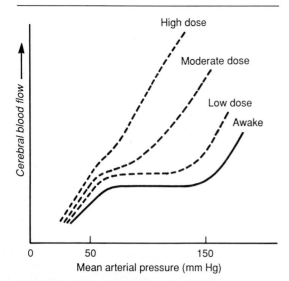

Figure 25–6. Dose-dependent depression of cerebral autoregulation by the volatile anesthetics.

tance to a variable degree. Moreover, these studies demonstrate that hypocapnia effectively blunts the increase in cerebral blood volume only during isoflurane anesthesia.

Cerebrospinal Fluid Dynamics

Volatile anesthetics affect both cerebrospinal fluid formation and absorption. Enflurane is unique in its ability to increase cerebrospinal fluid formation and retard absorption; both effects tend to elevate intracranial pressure in patients with reduced intracranial compliance. Halothane impedes cerebrospinal fluid absorption but only minimally retards formation. Isoflurane, on the other hand, facilitates absorption and is therefore the only volatile agent with favorable effects on cerebrospinal fluid dynamics.

Intracranial Pressure

The net effect of volatile anesthetics on intracranial pressure is the result of immediate changes in cerebral blood volume, delayed alterations on cerebrospinal fluid dynamics, and arterial CO_2 tension (Figure 25–7). Based on these factors, isoflurane appears to be the volatile agent of choice in patients with decreased intracranial compliance.

Luxury Perfusion

Luxury perfusion is the combination of decreased neuronal metabolic demand and increased cerebral blood flow (metabolic supply) associated with volatile anesthetics. These effects may be desirable during induced hypotension and support the use of a volatile agent, particularly isoflurane, for this technique.

Circulatory Steal

In contrast to their potentially beneficial effect during global ischemia (luxury perfusion), a potentially detrimental circulatory steal phenomenon is possible with volatile anesthetics in the setting of focal ischemia. Volatile agents increase blood flow in normal areas of the brain but not in ischemic areas, where arterioles already are maximally vasodilated. This may result in redistribution of blood flow away from ischemic to normal areas.

Seizure Activity

In doses of 1.5–2 MAC, enflurane can cause seizure patterns (spike and wave activity) on the EEG, particularly during hypocapnia. Auditory stimuli are said to precipitate this type of activity. Although spike activity may also occasionally be associated with isoflurane

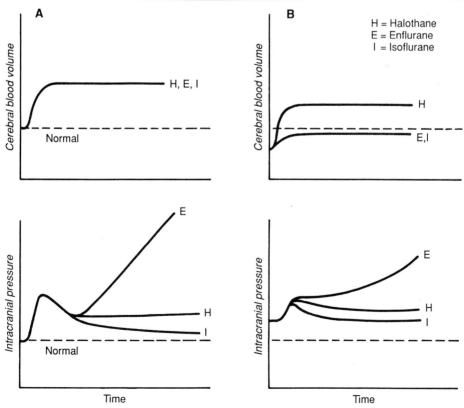

Figure 25–7. Time-related changes in cerebral blood volume and intracranial pressure when volatile agents are administered. **A:** During normocapnia. **B:** Following hyperventilation (hypocapnia).

prior to electrical silence, it does not progress to seizures.

2. NITROUS OXIDE

The effects of nitrous oxide are generally mild and easily overcome by other agents or changes in CO_2 tension. When given alone, however, nitrous oxide can cause mild cerebral vasodilation and increased intracranial pressure.

3. BARBITURATES

Barbiturates have four major actions on the central nervous system: (1) hypnosis, (2) depression of cerebral metabolic rate, (3) reduction of cerebral blood flow due to increased cerebral vascular resistance, and (4) anticonvulsant activity. These properties make barbiturates, especially thiopental, the most commonly used induction agents in neuroanesthesia.

Barbiturates produce dose-dependent decreases in cerebral metabolic rate and cerebral blood flow until the EEG becomes isoelectric. At that point, maximum reductions of nearly 50% are observed. Cerebral metabolic rate is depressed slightly more than cerebral blood flow, such that metabolic supply exceeds metabolic demand (as long as cerebral perfusion pressure is maintained). Because barbiturate-induced cerebral vasoconstriction occurs only in normal areas, these agents tend to redistribute blood flow from normal to ischemic areas in the brain (Robin Hood, or reverse steal, phenomenon). The cerebral vasculature in ischemic areas remains maximally dilated and is unaffected by the barbiturate because of ischemic vasomotor paralysis.

Barbiturates also appear to facilitate cerebrospinal fluid absorption. The resultant reduction in cerebrospinal fluid volume, combined with decreases in cerebral blood flow and cerebral blood volume, make barbiturates highly effective in lowering intracranial pressure. Moreover, even in anesthetic doses, barbiturates do not alter cerebral autoregulation or responsiveness to CO_2. Their anticonvulsant properties are also advantageous in neurosurgical patients who are at increased risk for seizures. The metabolic demand imposed by seizure activity promotes secondary injury in ischemic areas.

Other possible actions of barbiturates include scavenging or suppression of free radical formation and retardation of cerebral edema following ischemic brain injury. All these actions represent the theoretic justification for the controversial use of barbiturates for cerebral protection. Possible indications for the latter include cardiopulmonary bypass, controlled hypotension, head trauma, cardiac arrest, near drowning, Reye's syndrome, and stroke. Studies suggests that barbiturate prophylaxis is more effective in preventing brain injury during focal ischemia than during global ischemia.

4. OTHER INTRAVENOUS ANESTHETICS

Narcotics

Narcotics generally have minimal effects on cerebral blood flow, cerebral metabolic rate, and intracranial pressure, unless $PaCO_2$ rises secondary to respiratory depression. Both autoregulation and CO_2 responsiveness are preserved. Recent studies suggest that not all narcotics have similar effects. Of those commonly used, fentanyl may be the most useful agent in neurosurgical patients. Fentanyl decreases cerebral blood volume and facilitates cerebrospinal fluid absorption, both effects tending to reduce intracranial pressure. Increases in intracranial pressure have been reported in some patients with intracranial tumors following sufentanil administration and to a lesser degree following alfentanil. Moreover, significant decreases in blood pressure adversely affecting cerebral perfusion pressure may be more likely with sufentanil and alfentanil than with fentanyl. Morphine is generally not considered optimal in neuroanesthesia due to poor lipid solubility. The latter results in slow central nervous system penetration and prolonged sedative effects. Potential accumulation of normeperidine and cardiac depression limit the use of meperidine.

Etomidate

Etomidate decreases the cerebral metabolic rate, cerebral blood flow, and intracranial pressure in somewhat the same way as thiopental. Its effect on cerebral metabolic rate is nonuniform, affecting the cortex more than the brainstem. The latter may be responsible for greater hemodynamic stability in unstable patients when compared to barbiturates. Induction with etomidate is associated with a relatively high incidence of myoclonic movements but generally does not result in seizure activity on the EEG. Rare reports of seizures in patients with a history of epilepsy suggest that etomidate is best avoided in those patients.

Propofol

Propofol reduces cerebral blood flow and the cerebral metabolic rate about 30%. Like barbiturates and etomidate, it may be useful in lowering intracranial pressure. Excessive hypotension and cardiac depression, particularly in elderly or unstable patients, compromises cerebral perfusion pressure and is an undesirable feature.

Benzodiazepines

Benzodiazepines lower cerebral blood flow and cerebral metabolic rate but to a lesser extent than barbiturates and etomidate. They also have useful anticonvulsant properties. Midazolam is the benzodiazepine of choice because of its short pharmacokinetic profile.

Midazolam induction frequently causes significant decreases in cerebral perfusion pressure in elderly and unstable patients and may prolong emergence in some instances.

Lidocaine

Intravenous lidocaine decreases the cerebral metabolic rate, cerebral blood flow, and intracranial pressure but to a lesser degree than other agents. Its principal advantage is that it decreases cerebral blood flow (by increasing cerebral vascular resistance) without causing other significant hemodynamic effects. The risks of systemic toxicity and seizures limit the usefulness of repeated dosing.

Droperidol

This agent has little or no effect on cerebral metabolism and minimally reduces blood flow. When used with a narcotic as part of a neuroleptic technique, droperidol may cause undesirable prolonged sedation.

Ketamine

Ketamine is the only intravenous anesthetic that dilates the cerebral vasculature and increases cerebral blood flow (50–60%). Selective activation of certain areas (limbic and reticular) is partially offset by depression of other areas (somatosensory and auditory) such that total cerebral metabolic rate does not change. Cerebral autoregulation and CO_2 responsiveness appear to be preserved. Ketamine also appears to impede cerebrospinal fluid absorption without affecting formation. The increases in cerebral blood flow, cerebral blood volume, and cerebrospinal fluid volume can markedly increase intracranial pressure in patients with decreased intracranial compliance.

5. VASOPRESSORS

With normal autoregulation, vasopressors increase cerebral blood flow only when mean arterial blood pressure is below 50–60 mm Hg or above 150–160 mm Hg. In the absence of autoregulation, vasopressors increase cerebral blood flow by their effect on cerebral perfusion pressure. Under the latter conditions, even pure α-adrenergic agonists increase cerebral blood flow, suggesting little alpha-mediated vasoconstriction in the cerebral circulation. Excessive blood pressure elevations may disrupt the blood-brain barrier.

6. VASODILATORS

In the absence of hypotension, most vasodilators increase cerebral blood flow in a dose-related fashion. The resultant increase in cerebral blood volume can significantly elevate intracranial pressure in patients with decreased intracranial compliance. Of this group of drugs, only trimethaphan and α-adrenergic antagonists have little or no effect on cerebral blood flow and cerebral blood volume.

7. MUSCLE RELAXANTS

Muscle relaxants lack direct action on the brain but can have important secondary effects. Hypertension and histamine-mediated cerebral vasodilation increase intracranial pressure, while systemic hypotension (from histamine release or ganglionic blockade) lower cerebral perfusion pressure. Succinylcholine can increase intracranial pressure, possibly from cerebral vasodilatation, but the increase is generally minimal if an adequate dose of thiopental is given and hyperventilation is initiated at induction. Moreover, a small (defasciculating) dose of a nondepolarizing relaxant, especially metocurine, appears to at least partially blunt the increase. In the majority of instances, increases in intracranial pressure following administration of muscle relaxants are due to a hypertensive response to light anesthesia during subsequent laryngoscopy and intubation. Acute elevations in intracranial pressure will also be seen if hypercapnia or hypoxemia results from prolonged apnea.

ELECTROPHYSIOLOGIC MONITORING

Electrophysiologic monitoring attempts to assess the functional integrity of the central nervous system. The most commonly used monitors for neurosurgical procedures are the EEG and evoked potentials. Proper application of these techniques is critically dependent on monitoring the specific area at risk and recognizing anesthetic-induced changes. Both monitoring modalities are described in Chapter 6.

Electroencephalographic monitoring is most useful for ensuring adequate cerebral perfusion during carotid endarterectomy and controlled hypotension as well as assessing anesthetic depth. Somatosensory evoked potentials test the integrity of the dorsal spinal columns and the sensory cortex and may be useful during resection of spinal tumors, instrumentation of the spine, carotid endarterectomy, and aortic surgery. Brainstem auditory evoked potentials test the integrity of the eighth cranial nerve and the auditory pathways above the pons and are used for surgery in the posterior fossa. Visual evoked potentials may be used to monitor the optic nerve and upper brainstem during resections of large pituitary tumors.

The effects of anesthetic agents on the EEG and evoked potentials are summarized in Tables 25–2 and 25–3. Correct interpretation of changes requires correlation with anesthetic depth- and dose-related changes and with physiologic variables such as blood pressure, body temperature, and respiratory gas ten-

Table 25–2. Electroencephalographic changes during anesthesia.

Activation	Depression
Inhalational agents (sub-anesthetic)	Inhalational agents (1–2 MAC)
Barbiturates (small doses)	Barbiturates (usual doses)
Benzodiazepines (small doses)	Narcotics
Nitrous oxide	Etomidate
Ketamine	Hypocapnia
Mild hypercapnia	Marked hypercapnia
Sensory stimulation	Hypothermia
Hypoxia (early)	Hypoxia (late)
	Ischemia

sions. Electroencephalographic slowing associated with relative hypotension is of greater concern during light anesthesia and intense surgical retraction than during deep anesthesia without stimulation. Regardless of the technique employed, recordings should be bilateral (for comparison) and correlated with the intraoperative course of events.

Electroencephalographic changes can be simplistically described as either activation or depression. Electroencephalographic activation (a shift to predominantly high-frequency and low-voltage activity) is seen with light anesthesia and surgical stimulation, while electroencephalographic depression (a shift to predominantly low-frequency and high-voltage activity) occurs with deep anesthesia or cerebral compromise.

Interpretation of evoked potentials is more compli-

Table 25–3. Effect of anesthetic agents on evoked potentials.

Agent	SSEP		VER		BAER	
	Amp	Lat	Amp	Lat	Amp	Lat
Nitrous oxide	↓		↓	↑	±	±
Halothane	↓	↑			±	↑
Enflurane	↓	↑			±	↑
Barbiturates[1]	±	±	↓	↑	±	±
Narcotics[1]	±	±	±	±	±	±
Etomidate	↑	↑				
Propofol	↓	↑				
Benzodiazepines	±	±				
Isoflurane	↓	↑	↓	↑	±	↑

[1]At very high doses, can increase the latency and decrease the amplitude of SSEP.

Key:
- ↑ = Increase
- ↓ = Decrease
- ± = Little or no effect

Legend:
- SSEP = Somatosensory evoked potentials
- VER = Visual evoked response
- BAER = Brain stem evoked response
- Amp = Amplitude
- Lat = Latency

cated than that of the EEG. Evoked potentials have poststimulus latencies that are described as short, intermediate, and long. Short-latency evoked potentials arise from the nerve stimulated or the brainstem. Intermediate- and long-latency evoked potentials are primarily of cortical origin. In general, short-latency potentials are least affected by anesthetic agents, while long-latency potentials are affected by even subanesthetic levels of most agents. Consequently, only short and intermediate potentials are monitored intraoperatively.

Visual evoked potentials are most affected by anesthetics, while brainstem auditory evoked potentials are least affected. Volatile anesthetics have the greatest effect on evoked potentials, causing dose-dependent decreases in wave amplitude and increases in latencies. To minimize anesthetic-induced changes, some authors recommend limiting isoflurane and enflurane concentrations to 0.5 MAC and halothane to 1 MAC. Nitrous oxide decreases wave amplitude but has no effect on latencies. Intravenous agents in clinical doses generally have minimal effects but in high doses will also decrease amplitude and increase latencies.

CASE DISCUSSION: POSTOPERATIVE HEMIPLEGIA?

A 62-year-old man is undergoing radical neck dissection for a malignant parotid tumor on the right side. Anesthesia is induced with etomidate and maintained with enflurane plus 70% nitrous oxide in oxygen. The tumor was found to extend into the carotid sheath, and during the dissection the carotid artery was injured. The internal carotid artery had to be cross-clamped to control the bleeding and allow repair with a patch graft.

Describe the blood supply of the brain as it relates to this case.

The internal carotid and vertebral arteries from each side supply the majority of blood flow to the brain (Figure 25–8). The internal carotid artery arises at the bifurcation of the common carotid artery in the neck and enters the cranium through the temporal bone. The vertebral artery is a branch of the subclavian artery and ascends through the transverse processes of the cervical vertebrae (starting at C6), entering the skull through the foramen magnum. Anastomotic connections between the contralateral vessels and between the internal carotid and vertebral systems form a complete arterial circuit at the base of the brain (arterial circle of the cerebrum—the circle of Willis). These anastomoses can provide collateral blood flow and protect the brain from ischemia should blood flow cease in one of these vessels proximal to the circle of Willis.

Additional collateral flow may also be available through anastomotic connections between branches of

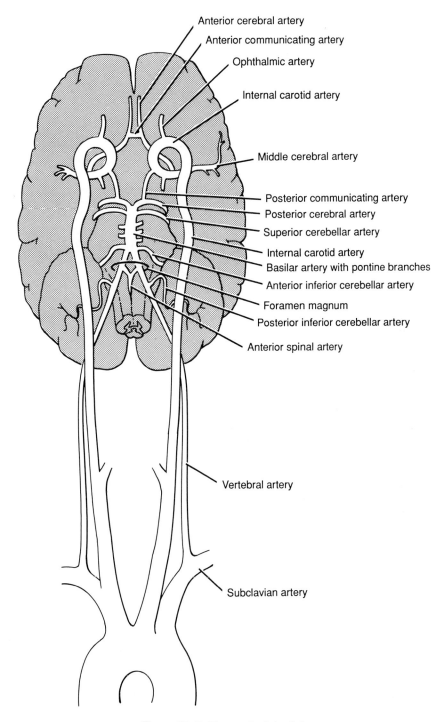

Figure 25–8. The cerebral circulation.

the internal carotid and external carotid arteries. Although the internal carotid artery does not have any major extracranial branches, its ophthalmic branch anastomoses with branches of the facial artery (a tributary of the external carotid artery) in the orbit. Ligation of both internal carotid arteries without neurologic sequelae has been reported in a few patients.

What is the anatomic basis of a hemispheric cerebral infarct occurring in this setting?

The anastomotic vessels completing the circle of Willis (anterior and posterior communicating arteries) are not always well developed. Variations in the size of these vessels are very common, and one or both posterior communicating arteries may be absent. Moreover, the incidence of significant atherosclerotic lesions in the cerebral circulation increases with age (6–8% in patients 60–70 years old). While moderate to severe stenoses or even complete occlusions may be asymptomatic under normal conditions, when cerebral blood flow is compromised these lesions not only predispose to ischemia distally but also limit collateral blood flow to other areas of the brain.

When the surgeon clamps the right internal carotid artery, continued blood flow through the right middle and anterior cerebral arteries (branches of the internal carotid artery) becomes dependent on flow from (1) the left carotid system via the anterior communicating artery, (2) the vertebral-basilar system via the right posterior communicating artery, and (3) anastomoses between the internal and external carotid vessels around the right orbit. The presence of developmental abnormalities or acquired occlusive disease in these vessels would predispose this patient to a cerebral infarct.

What measures, if any, might protect against cerebral ischemia?

Use of a temporary shunt by the surgeon would be highly effective but has its own risks (Chapter 26). Moreover, placement of a shunt in this case may not be technically feasible, or the surgeon may not be prepared to use a shunt.

At least theoretically, manipulation of respiratory gas tensions, arterial blood pressure, and anesthetic agents could also influence the outcome. Hyperventilation vasoconstricts the cerebral vasculature, limiting collateral blood flow, and should therefore be avoided. Hypercapnia may also be detrimental if it induces a cerebral steal phenomena. Consequently, a normal or slightly elevated arterial CO_2 tension is optimal.

The nitrous oxide should be discontinued and the inspired oxygen concentration increased to 100%. Although the resulting increase in dissolved oxygen is small compared to that carried on hemoglobin (Chapter 22), it may theoretically be enough to partially ameliorate ischemia or reduce the amount of infarcted tissue.

Because volatile anesthetics produce cerebral vasodilatation and favor pressure-dependent cerebral blood flow (Figure 25–6), arterial blood pressure should be maintained at normal or slighted high levels.

Consideration should be given to substituting isoflurane for enflurane. In clinically used doses, isoflurane produces less cardiovascular depression and greater depression of CMR (to the point of an isoelectric EEG).

Lastly, prophylaxis with thiopental for cerebral protection may be indicated. While ideally the thiopental should be given until the EEG is isoelectric, it should be given empirically in this setting (500–1500 mg total dose) in small increments (50 mg) to prevent hypotension.

SUGGESTED READINGS

Cucchiara RF, Michenfelder JD: *Clinical Neuroanesthesia.* Churchill Livingstone, 1990.

Frost EAM: *Clinical Anesthesia in Neurosurgery,* 2nd ed. Butterworths, 1991.

Michenfelder JD: *Anesthesia and the Brain.* Churchill Livingstone, 1989.

Nuwer MR: *Evoked Potential Monitoring in the Operating Room.* Raven Press, 1986.

Sperry RJ, Stirt JA, Stone DJ: *Manual of Neuroanesthesia.* BC Decker, 1990.

Weinstein P, Faden A: *Protection of the Brain From Ischemia.* Williams & Wilkins, 1990.

Wood M, Wood JJ: *Drugs and Anesthesia, Pharmacology for Anesthesiologists,* 2nd ed. Williams & Wilkins 1990.

Anesthesia for Neurosurgery

26

Harvey Cushing, one of the founders of neurosurgery, is largely responsible for the development of the anesthesia record. Out of concern for the safety of his patients, he came to emphasize the need to record the surgical patient's pulse, respiratory rate, temperature, and blood pressure intraoperatively. Better understanding of the effects of anesthesia on the central nervous system (Chapter 25) and improvements in anesthetic technique have contributed much to the success of modern neurosurgery. Sophisticated monitoring techniques and better operating conditions under anesthesia have allowed increasingly difficult procedures to be performed on patients previously deemed inoperable.

Standard anesthetic techniques must be modified in the presence of intracranial hypertension and marginal cerebral perfusion. Additionally, many neurosurgical procedures require unusual patient positions—eg. sitting, prone—further complicating management. This chapter applies the principles developed in Chapter 25 to the anesthetic care of neurosurgical patients.

INTRACRANIAL HYPERTENSION

Intracranial hypertension is defined as a sustained increase in intracranial pressure above 15 mm Hg. Uncompensated increases in the tissue or fluid within the rigid cranial vault produce sustained intracranial pressure elevations (Chapter 25). Intracranial hypertension may result from an expanding tissue or fluid mass, interference with normal cerebrospinal fluid absorption, excessive cerebral blood flow, or systemic disturbances promoting brain edema (see below). Multiple factors are often simultaneously present. For example, tumors in the posterior fossa are not only usually associated with some degree of brain edema, but they also readily obstruct cerebrospinal fluid flow by compressing the fourth ventricle (obstructive hydrocephalus).

Although many patients are initially asymptomatic, all eventually develop characteristic symptoms and signs, including headache, nausea, vomiting, papilledema, focal neurologic deficits, and altered consciousness. When intracranial pressure exceeds 30 mm Hg, cerebral blood flow progressively decreases and a vicious cycle is established: ischemia causes brain edema, which in turn increases intracranial pressure, resulting in more ischemia. Unchecked, this cycle continues until the patient succumbs from progressive neurologic damage or catastrophic herniation (Chapter 25).

CEREBRAL EDEMA

Increase in brain water can be produced by several mechanisms. Disruption of the blood-brain barrier (vasogenic edema) is most common and allows the entry of plasma-like fluid into the brain. Increases in blood pressure enhance the formation of this type of edema. Common causes of vasogenic edema include mechanical trauma, inflammatory lesions, brain tumors, hypertension, and infarction. Cerebral edema following metabolic insults, such as hypoxemia or ischemia, results from failure of brain cells to actively extrude sodium and progressive cellular swelling. Interstitial cerebral edema is the result of obstructive hydrocephalus and entry of cerebrospinal fluid into brain interstitium. Lastly, cerebral edema can also be the result of intracellular movement of water secondary to acute decreases in serum osmolality (water intoxication).

Treatment of cerebral edema is ideally directed at the underlying cause. Metabolic disturbances are corrected and operative intervention is undertaken whenever possible. Vasogenic edema—especially that associated with tumors—often responds to corticosteroids (dexamethasone), which appear to promote repair of the blood-brain barrier. Regardless of the cause, fluid restriction, osmotic agents, and loop diuretics are usually effective in temporarily decreasing brain edema and lowering intracranial pressure until more definitive measures can be undertaken. These methods lower intracranial pressure chiefly by removing intracellular water from normal brain tissue.

Mannitol, in doses of 0.25–1.5 g/kg, is especially effective in rapidly decreasing intracranial pressure. Its efficacy is primarily related to its effect on serum osmolality (Chapter 29); a serum osmolality of 300–315 mosm/L is generally considered desirable. Mannitol can transiently decrease blood pressure by virtue of its weak vasodilating properties, but its principal disadvantage is a transient increase in intravascular volume, which can precipitate pulmonary edema in patients with borderline cardiac or renal function. Use of a loop diuretic (furosemide), though less effective and requiring up to 30 minutes, circumvents this problem and may have the additional advantage of directly decreasing cerebrospinal fluid formation. The combined use of mannitol and furosemide may be synergistic but requires close monitoring of the serum potassium concentration (Chapter 28).

CRANIOTOMY FOR PATIENTS WITH MASS LESIONS

PREOPERATIVE MANAGEMENT

Intracranial masses may be congenital, neoplastic (benign, malignant, or metastatic), infectious (abscess or cyst), or vascular (hematoma or malformation). Regardless of the cause, intracranial masses present according to growth rate, location, and intracranial pressure. Slowly growing masses are frequently asymptomatic for long periods, whereas rapidly growing ones usually present acutely. Supratentorial masses typically present as seizures, hemiplegia, or aphasia, while infratentorial masses more commonly present as cerebellar dysfunction (ataxia, nystagmus, and dysarthria) or brainstem compression (cranial nerve palsies, altered consciousness, or abnormal respiration). When intracranial pressure increases, frank signs of intracranial hypertension also develop (see above).

Preanesthetic evaluation should attempt to establish the presence or absence of intracranial hypertension. CT or MRI data should be reviewed for evidence of brain edema, a midline shift greater than 0.5 cm, and ventricular size. Examination should include a neurologic assessment documenting mental status and any existing neurologic deficits. Medications should be reviewed with special reference to corticosteroid, diuretic, and anticonvulsant therapy. Laboratory evaluation should rule out corticosteroid-induced hyperglycemia and electrolyte disturbances due to diuretics or abnormalities in antidiuretic hormone secretion (Chapter 28). Anticonvulsant levels should be checked, especially when seizures are not well controlled.

Premedication

Premedication is best avoided when intracranial hypertension is suspected. Hypercapnia secondary to respiratory depression increases intracranial pressure and may be lethal. Patients with normal intracranial pressure are usually given a benzodiazepine (diazepam orally or midazolam intramuscularly). Corticosteroids

and anticonvulsant therapy should be continued up until the time of surgery.

INTRAOPERATIVE MANAGEMENT

Monitoring

General indications for monitors apply to neurosurgical patients as well, with the exception that intra-arterial pressure monitoring and bladder catheterization are mandatory for most patients undergoing craniotomy. Rapid blood pressure changes during induction, hyperventilation, intubation, positioning, surgical manipulation, and emergence necessitate continuous blood pressure monitoring to ensure optimal cerebral perfusion. Moreover, arterial blood gas measurements are necessary to closely regulate $PaCO_2$. Many neuroanesthesiologists zero the arterial pressure transducer at the level of the head (external auditory meatus)—instead of the right atrium—to facilitate calculation of cerebral perfusion pressure (Chapter 25). End-tidal CO_2 measurements alone cannot be relied upon for precise regulation of ventilation; the arterial to end-tidal CO_2 gradient must be determined (Chapter 6). Central venous access and pressure monitoring should be considered for patients requiring vasoactive drugs. Use of the internal jugular vein for access is somewhat controversial because of the risk of carotid puncture and concern that the catheter might interfere with venous drainage from the brain. Many clinicians avoid this issue by passing a long catheter centrally through the median basilic vein. The external jugular and subclavian veins may be suitable alternatives. A urinary catheter is necessary because of the frequent use of diuretics, the length of most neurosurgical procedures, and its utility in guiding fluid therapy. Neuromuscular function should be monitored on the nonaffected side in patients with hemiparesis (Chapter 27). Monitoring visual evoked potentials may be useful in preventing optic nerve damage during resections of large pituitary tumors. Additional monitors for surgery in the posterior fossa are described below.

Management of patients with intracranial hypertension is greatly facilitated by monitoring intracranial pressure perioperatively. A ventriculostomy or subdural bolt is most commonly employed and is usually placed by the neurosurgeon preoperatively under local anesthesia. Electronic intracranial pressure monitoring is possible utilizing saline-filled tubing with a pressure transducer. The transducer should be zeroed to the same reference level as the arterial pressure transducer (usually the external auditory meatus; see above). A ventriculostomy has the added advantage of allowing removal of cerebrospinal fluid to decrease intracranial pressure.

Induction

Induction of anesthesia and endotracheal intubation are critical periods for patients with compromised intracranial compliance or an already elevated intracranial pressure. Intracranial compliance can be improved by osmotic diuresis, steroids, or removal of cerebrospinal fluid via a ventriculostomy immediately prior to induction. The goal of any technique should be to induce anesthesia and intubate the trachea in a slow, controlled fashion without increasing intracranial pressure or compromising cerebral blood flow. Arterial hypertension during induction increases cerebral blood volume and promotes cerebral edema. Marked or sustained hypertension can lead to marked increases in intracranial pressure that can decrease cerebral perfusion pressure and risk herniation (Chapter 25). Excessive decreases in arterial blood are equally detrimental pressure by compromising cerebral perfusion pressure.

The most common induction technique employs thiopental together with hyperventilation to lower intracranial pressure and blunt the noxious effects of laryngoscopy and intubation. Cooperative patients can be asked to hyperventilate during preoxygenation. All patients are hyperventilated with controlled ventilation once the thiopental is injected. A muscle relaxant is given to facilitate ventilation and prevent straining or coughing, both of which can abruptly increase intracranial pressure. An intravenous narcotic—eg, fentanyl, 5–10 μg/kg—just prior to thiopental blunts the vasopressor response, especially in young patients. Intravenous lidocaine, 1.5–2 mg/kg, following thiopental but prior to intubation, is a suitable alternative in elderly or debilitated patients and does not cause excessive circulatory depression.

The actual induction technique can be varied according to individual patient responses and coexisting diseases. Substitution of etomidate for thiopental may provide even greater protection against circulatory depression. The combination of a small dose of fentanyl, 5 μg/kg, with etomidate, 6–8 mg, is also useful in unstable patients. Conversely, for patients with reactive airways (bronchospastic disease), incremental doses of thiopental together with hyperventilation employing isoflurane may be preferable.

A nondepolarizing muscle relaxant is generally given at induction to facilitate controlled ventilation and tracheal intubation. Vecuronium, pipecuronium, or doxacurium provides the greatest hemodynamic stability (Chapter 9). Succinylcholine may increase intracranial pressure, especially if intubation is attempted prior to the establishment of deep thiopental anesthesia and hyperventilation (Chapter 25). However, prior administration of a small dose of a nondepolarizing relaxant—especially metocurine, 2 mg—appears effective in blunting succinylcholine-induced increases in intracranial pressure.

Hypertension during induction should be treated by deepening the anesthesia with additional thiopental or hyperventilation with low doses (< 1 MAC) of isoflurane. Esmolol and labetalol are also useful in this setting. Because of their effect on cerebral blood volume and intracranial pressure (Chapter 25), vasodilators should generally be avoided until the dura is opened. Transient hypotension should generally be treated with incremental doses of vasopressors (ephedrine or phenylephrine) rather than intravenous fluids.

Positioning

Frontal, temporal, and parieto-occipital craniotomies are performed in the supine position. The head is elevated 15–30 degrees to facilitate venous and cerebrospinal fluid drainage. The head may also be turned to the side to facilitate exposure. Excessive twisting of the neck impedes jugular venous drainage and can increase intracranial pressure. During positioning, the endotracheal tube should be well secured and all breathing circuit connections checked. The risk of unrecognized disconnects may be increased because the operating table is usually turned 90 or 180 degrees away from the anesthesiologist, and both the patient and the breathing circuit are almost completely covered by surgical drapes.

Maintenance of Anesthesia

Anesthesia is usually maintained with a nitrous-narcotic-relaxant technique. Fentanyl may be the most suitable narcotic (Chapter 25). Persistent hypertension requires the use of low-dose (< 1 MAC) isoflurane. Although periods of stimulation are fairly limited, paralysis is important to prevent straining, bucking, or movement. Increased anesthetic requirements can be expected during the most stimulating periods: laryngoscopy-intubation, skin incision, dural opening, periosteal manipulations, and closure.

Hyperventilation should be continued intraoperatively to maintain $PaCO_2$ between 25 and 30 mm Hg. Lower $PaCO_2$ tensions provide little additional benefit and may be associated with cerebral ischemia and impaired oxygen dissociation from hemoglobin. Positive end-expiratory pressure (PEEP) and ventilatory patterns resulting in high mean airway pressures (a high rate with small tidal volumes) should be avoided because of a potentially adverse effect on intracranial pressure by increasing central venous pressure.

Intravenous fluid replacement should be limited to glucose-free isotonic crystalloid (lactated Ringer's or normal saline) or colloid solutions. Hyperglycemia is common in neurosurgical patients (corticosteroid effect) and has been implicated in increasing ischemic brain injury (Chapter 25). While controversy still surrounds the choice between crystalloid and colloid solutions, large amounts of hypotonic crystalloid solutions clearly can worsen brain edema. Colloid solutions should generally be used to restore intravascular volume deficits, while isotonic crystalloid solutions are used for maintenance fluid requirements. Intraoperative fluid replacement should be below calculated maintenance requirements (Chapter 29) for patients with severe brain edema or increased intracranial pressure. Neurosurgical procedures result in minimal redistributive fluid losses but are often associated with "occult" blood loss (underneath surgical drapes or on the floor). Standard guidelines should be used for blood transfusions (Chapter 31).

Emergence

Most patients undergoing craniotomy can be extubated at the end of the procedure as long as intracranial hypertension is no longer present. Patients left intubated should remain sedated, paralyzed, and hyperventilated. Extubation in the operating room requires special handling during emergence. Straining or bucking on the endotracheal tube may precipitate intracranial hemorrhage or worsen cerebral edema. Like induction, emergence must be slow and controlled. After the head dressing is applied and full access to the patient is regained (the table is turned back to its original position at induction), anesthetic gases are discontinued, and the muscle relaxant is reversed. Intravenous lidocaine, 1.5 mg/kg, or a small dose (25–50 mg) of thiopental can be given just before suctioning to suppress coughing prior to extubation. Rapid awakening facilitates immediate neurologic assessment and can generally be expected following a pure nitrous-narcotic technique. Delayed awakening may be seen following a narcotic overdose or prolonged administration of the volatile agent. Narcotic overdosing is manifested by slow respirations (< 12/min) and can be reversed with naloxone in 0.04-mg increments. Most patients are taken to the intensive care unit postoperatively for close monitoring of neurologic function.

SURGERY IN THE POSTERIOR FOSSA

Craniotomy for a mass in the posterior fossa presents a unique set of potential problems: obstructive hydrocephalus, possible injury to vital brainstem centers, unusual positioning, pneumocephalus, postural hypotension, and venous air embolism.

Obstructive Hydrocephalus

Infratentorially located masses can obstruct cerebrospinal fluid flow at the level of the fourth ventricle or the cerebral aqueduct. Even small but critically located lesions can markedly increase intracranial pressure. In such cases, a ventriculostomy is often performed under local anesthesia to decrease intracranial pressure prior to induction of general anesthesia.

Brainstem Injury

Operations in the posterior fossa can injure vital circulatory and respiratory brainstem centers as well as cranial nerves or their nuclei. Such injuries occur as a result of direct surgical trauma, retraction, or ischemia. Damage to respiratory centers is said to be nearly always associated with circulatory changes, so that abrupt changes in blood pressure, heart rate, or rhythm should alert the anesthesiologist to the possibility of such an injury. Communication between the anesthesiologist and the surgeon is critical. Rarely, isolated damage to respiratory centers without premonitory circulatory signs has occurred during operations in the floor of the fourth ventricle; the use of spontaneous ventilation during these procedures has therefore been advocated by some clinicians. At completion of the surgery, brainstem injuries often present as an abnormal respiratory pattern or as an inability to maintain a patent airway following extubation. Monitoring brainstem auditory evoked potentials may be useful in preventing eighth nerve damage during resections of acoustic neuromas as well as other injuries to the brainstem.

Positioning

Although most posterior fossa explorations can be performed with the patient in either the lateral or the prone position, the sitting position is often preferred because the enhanced cerebrospinal fluid and venous drainage facilitates surgical exposure. The lateral position is discussed in Chapter 24, while the prone position is discussed below under spinal surgery.

The patient is actually semirecumbent in the standard sitting position (Figure 26–1); the back is elevated to 60 degrees, while the legs are elevated with the knees flexed to the level of the heart. The latter is important in preventing venous pooling and reducing the risk of venous thromboembolism. The head is fixed in a three-point holder with the neck flexed, while the arms remain at the sides with the hands resting on the lap.

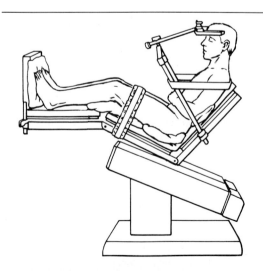

Figure 26–1. The sitting position for craniotomy.

Careful positioning helps avoid injuries. Pressure points such as the elbows, ischial spines, and forehead must be protected with foam padding. Excessive neck flexion has been associated with swelling of the upper airway (due to venous obstruction) and, rarely, quadriplegia (due to compression of the cervical spinal cord). Preexisting cervical spinal stenosis probably predisposes to the latter injury.

Pneumocephalus

The sitting position increases the likelihood of significant pneumocephalus. In this position, air readily enters the subarachnoid space as cerebrospinal fluid is lost during surgery. Because of its potential to increase pneumocephalus (Chapter 7), nitrous oxide should be discontinued well before the dura is closed. Expansion of pneumocephalus following dural closure compresses the brain and may delay or prevent awakening following anesthesia. Indeed, many neuroanesthesiologists advocate not using nitrous oxide altogether for sitting craniotomies (see also below).

Postural Hypotension

Postural hypotension readily occurs in neurosurgical patients because of the intentional volume depletion induced by fluid restriction and diuresis. Moreover, general anesthesia blunts or abolishes the compensatory sympathetic reflexes that are normally active when the body assumes an upright position. Marked hypotension may be observed when patients are placed in the sitting position. Proper positioning (see above) and wrapping the legs with elastic bandages (from the feet to the upper thigh) prior to positioning helps avoid severe hypotension. This measure decreases venous pooling and perhaps the likelihood of venous thrombosis. The use of light anesthesia during positioning helps maintain sympathetic tone. Small doses of a vasopressor, such as ephedrine or phenylephrine, may still be necessary to correct transient hypotension and are preferable to infusion of large amounts of intravenous fluid. Moreover, the hypotension is often followed by hypertension when the pins of the head-holder (Figure 26–1) are applied.

Venous Air Embolism

Venous air embolism can occur when the pressure within an open vein is subatmospheric. These conditions may exist in any position (and during any procedure) whenever the wound is above the level of the heart. The incidence of venous air embolism is highest during sitting craniotomies (20–40%). Low central venous pressures (especially from positioning the legs low) and poor surgical technique are probably contributory.

The physiologic consequences of venous air embolism depend on the volume as well as the rate of air entry and whether the patient has a probe-patent foramen ovale (10% incidence). The latter is important because it can facilitate passage of air into the arterial circulation (paradoxic air embolism). Air bubbles entering the venous system ordinarily lodge in the pulmonary circulation, where their gases eventually diffuse into the alveoli and are exhaled. Small bubbles are well tolerated by most patients. When the amount entrained exceeds the rate of pulmonary clearance, pulmonary artery pressure progressively rises. Eventually, cardiac output decreases in response to increases in right ventricular afterload. Preexisting cardiac or pulmonary disease enhances the effects of venous air embolism; relatively small amounts of air may produce marked hemodynamic changes. Nitrous oxide, by increasing the volume of the entrained air, can markedly accentuate the effects of even small amounts of air. The dose for lethal venous air embolism in animals receiving nitrous oxide anesthesia is one-third to one-half that of control animals. Many clinicians are convinced that nitrous oxide should not be used for surgery on patients in the sitting position. Others continue to use it but in a concentration of 50% instead of 70%, and discontinue it if venous air embolism is detected.

Clinically, signs of venous air embolism are often not apparent until large amounts of air have been entrained. Arterial blood gas values may show only slight increases in $PaCO_2$ as a result of increased pulmonary dead space (areas with normal ventilation but decreased perfusion). Major hemodynamic manifestations such as sudden hypotension can occur well before hypoxemia is noted. Moreover, rapid entrainment of large amounts of air can produce sudden circulatory arrest by obstructing right ventricular outflow (forming an air lock). Paradoxic air embolism can result in a stroke or coronary occlusion, which may only be apparent postoperatively. Paradoxic air emboli are more likely to occur in patients with probe-patent foramen ovale, especially when the normal transatrial (left > right) pressure gradient is reversed. Reversal of this gradient is favored by hypovolemia and perhaps by positive end-expiratory pressure (PEEP). Some studies suggest that a right > left pressure gradient can develop at some time during the cardiac cycle even when the overall mean gradient remains left > right. Transpulmonary passage of venous air into the arterial system has also been demonstrated and suggests that even small bubbles in intravenous infusions should be avoided in all patients.

A. Central Venous Catheterization: Central venous access frequently allows aspiration of entrained air. Many clinicians consider central venous catheterization mandatory for sitting craniotomies. Optimal recovery of air following venous air embolism is probably provided by a multi-orificed catheter positioned high in the atrium. Confirmation of correct positioning is important and is accomplished by intravascular electrocardiography, pressure wave recording, or radiographically.

B. Monitoring for Venous Air Embolism: The most sensitive monitors available should be used. Detecting even small amounts of venous air embolism is important because it allows surgical control of the entry site before additional air is entrained. Currently, the most sensitive intraoperative monitors are transesophageal two-dimensional echocardiography and Doppler probes. These monitors can detect air bubbles as small as 0.25 mL. Transesophageal two-dimensional echocardiography has the added benefits of detecting the size of the bubbles and transatrial passage, as well as evaluating cardiac function. Doppler methods employ a probe over the right atrium (to the right of the sternum and between the third and sixth ribs). Interruption of the regular swishing of the Doppler signal by sporadic roaring sounds indicates venous air embolism. Changes in end-tidal respiratory gas concentrations and in pulmonary artery pressure are less sensitive but important monitors that can also detect venous air embolism before overt clinical signs are present. Venous air embolism causes a sudden decrease in end-tidal CO_2 tension in proportion to the increase in pulmonary dead space; unfortunately, such decreases can also be seen with hemodynamic changes unrelated to venous air embolism. A reappearance (or increase) of nitrogen in expired gases (detected by mass spectrometry) may also be seen with venous air embolism. Mean pulmonary artery pressure increases in direct proportion to the amount of air entrained. Changes in blood pressure and heart sounds (mill wheel murmur) are late manifestations of venous air embolism.

C. Treatment of Venous Air Embolism: Detection of venous air embolism should prompt the following steps:

1. The surgeon should be notified so that the surgical field can be flooded with saline or packed and bone wax applied to the skull edges until the entry site is identified.

2. Nitrous oxide (if used) should be discontinued and 100% oxygen given.

3. The central venous catheter should be aspirated in an attempt to retrieve the entrained air.

4. Intravascular volume infusion should be given to increase central venous pressure.

5. Vasopressors should be given to correct hypotension.

6. Bilateral jugular vein compression, by increasing cerebral venous pressure, may slow air entrainment and help the surgeon identify the source of the embolus. Excessive or prolonged pressure can be detrimental to cerebral perfusion pressure, especially if the carotid arteries are also inadvertently occluded.

7. Some authors advocate PEEP in an effort to increase cerebral venous pressure; however, reversal of the normal transatrial pressure gradient may promote paradoxic embolism (see above).

8. If the above measures fail, the patient should be placed in the left lateral decubitus position with a slight head-down tilt in an attempt to dislodge a possible air lock.

9. Persistent circulatory arrest necessitates the supine position and institution of resuscitation efforts by cardiac compression.

STEREOTACTIC SURGERY

Stereotactic procedures are used for the treatment of involuntary movement disorders, intractable pain, aneurysms, vascular malformations, and epilepsy and in the diagnosis and treatment of deeply situated brain tumors.

These procedures are usually performed under local anesthesia to allow periodic evaluation of the patient. Light neuroleptanalgesia (Chapter 8) is typically used for baseline sedation, while methohexital is given for painful manipulations. Methohexital in small increments (20–30 mg) provides brief periods of hypnosis yet still allows adequate spontaneous ventilation. The ability to rapidly provide controlled ventilation and general anesthesia for emergency craniotomy is mandatory but is complicated by the platform and localizing frame that is attached to the patient's head for the procedure. Although mask ventilation and orotracheal intubation can be readily accomplished in most patients, awake intubation is necessary when the frame cannot be removed in patients with limited access or when a difficult airway is anticipated. Fiberoptic intubation with the patient awake may be safest under these circumstances (Chapter 5).

HEAD TRAUMA

Head injuries are a contributory factor in up to 50% of deaths due to trauma. Most patients with head trauma are young, and many (10–40%) have associated intra-abdominal injuries, long bone fractures, or both. A general discussion of the trauma patient is found in Chapter 39. The significance of a head injury is dependent not only on the extent of the irreversible neuronal damage at the time of injury but also on the occurrence of any secondary insults. These additional insults include (1) systemic factors such as hypoxemia, hypercapnia, or hypotension; (2) formation and expansion of an epidural, subdural, or intracerebral hematoma; and (3) sustained intracranial hypertension. Studies suggest that sustained increases in intracranial pressure of about 60 mm Hg result in irreversible brain edema. Surgical and anesthetic management of these patients is directed at preventing these secondary insults.

PREOPERATIVE MANAGEMENT

Anesthetic care of patients with severe head trauma ideally begins in the emergency department. Measures

Table 26–1. Glasgow Coma Scale.

Category	Score
Eye opening	
Spontaneous	4
To speech	3
To pain	2
Nil	1
Best motor response	
To verbal command	
Obeys	6
To pain	
Localizes	5
Withdraws	4
Decorticate flexion	3
Extensor response	2
Nil	1
Best verbal response	
Oriented	5
Confused conversation	4
Inappropriate words	3
Incomprehensible sounds	2
Nil	1

to ensure the patency of the airway, the adequacy of ventilation and oxygenation, and correction of systemic hypotension should go forward simultaneously with neurologic evaluation. Airway obstruction and hypoventilation are common. Up to 70% of such patients have hypoxemia, which may be complicated by pulmonary contusion, fat emboli, or neurogenic pulmonary edema. The latter is the result of marked systemic and pulmonary hypertension secondary to intense sympathetic nervous system activity. Supplemental oxygen should be given to all patients while the airway and ventilation are evaluated. All patients must be assumed to have a cervical spine injury (10% incidence) until the contrary of that assumption is demonstrated radiographically. Axial traction should be used during airway manipulation to maintain the head in neutral position. Patients with obvious hypoventilation, an absent gag reflex, or a persistent total score below 7 on the Glasgow Coma Scale (Table 26–1) require tracheal intubation and hyperventilation. All other patients should be carefully observed for deterioration. The Glasgow Coma Scale score generally correlates well with the severity of injury and outcome.

Intubation

All patients should be regarded as having a full stomach and should have cricoid pressure applied during ventilation and intubation. Following adequate preoxygenation and hyperventilation by mask, the adverse effects of intubation on intracranial pressure are blunted by prior administration of thiopental, 2–4 mg/kg, and a short-acting muscle relaxant. If the patient is hypotensive (systolic blood pressure

< 100 mm Hg), either a smaller dose of thiopental should be used or etomidate or lidocaine should be substituted. The use of succinylcholine in closed head injury is controversial because of its potential for increasing intracranial pressure and the rare occurrence of hyperkalemia in these patients; vecuronium is a suitable alternative. If a difficult intubation is anticipated, awake intubation, fiberoptic techniques, or tracheostomy may be necessary. Blind nasal intubation is contraindicated in the presence of a basilar skull fracture, which is suggested by cerebrospinal fluid rhinorrhea or otorrhea, hemotympanum, or ecchymosis into periorbital tissues (raccoon sign) or behind the ear (Battle's sign).

Hypotension

Hypotension in the setting of head trauma is nearly always related to other associated injuries (usually intra-abdominal). Bleeding from scalp lacerations may be responsible in children. Hypotension may be seen with spinal cord injuries because of the sympathectomy associated with spinal shock. Correction of the hypotension and control of any bleeding take precedence over radiographic studies and definitive neurosurgical treatment. Fluid resuscitation with primarily colloid solutions and blood may be more advantageous than crystalloid solutions in preventing brain edema; temporary infusion of a vasopressor (dopamine) is often necessary for severe hypotension. Glucose-containing and hypotonic solutions should not be used (see above). The hematocrit should be maintained above 30%. Invasive monitoring of intra-arterial pressure, central venous or pulmonary artery pressure, and intracranial pressure are extremely valuable but should not delay diagnosis and treatment. Dysrhythmias and electrocardiographic abnormalities in the T wave, U wave, ST segment, and QT interval are common following head injuries but are not necessarily associated with cardiac injury.

Diagnostic Studies

The choice between operative and medical management of head trauma is based on radiographic as well as clinical findings. Patients should be stabilized prior to any CT or angiographic studies. Critically ill patients should be closely monitored during such studies. Restless or uncooperative patients may additionally require general anesthesia (see below). Sedation without control of the airway should generally be avoided because of the risk of further increases in intracranial pressure from hypercapnia or hypoxemia. In the event of neurologic deterioration prior to completion of these studies, intravenous mannitol should be considered. If the patient is hemodynamically stable, thiopental may also be given in small incremental doses (50–100 mg) to decrease intracranial pressure and perhaps to provide cerebral protection (Chapter 25). Steroids, even in high doses, do not appear to be of any benefit following head trauma.

INTRAOPERATIVE MANAGEMENT

Operative treatment is usually elected for compound depressed skull fractures, depressed fractures associated with underlying brain injury, and evacuation of epidural, subdural, and some intracerebral hematomas.

Anesthetic management is generally similar to that for other mass lesions associated with intracranial hypertension. Management of the airway is discussed above. Intra-arterial and central venous (or pulmonary artery) pressure monitoring should be established if not already present but should not delay surgical decompression in a rapidly deteriorating patient.

A barbiturate-narcotic-nitrous oxide-muscle relaxant technique is most commonly used. Nitrous oxide should be avoided when air is entrapped within the cranium and during periods of hypotension. Hypotension may occur after induction of anesthesia as a result of the combined effects of vasodilation and hypovolemia and should be treated with α-adrenergic blocking agents (and colloid infusion if necessary). Subsequent hypertension is common with surgical stimulation but may also occur with acute intracranial pressure elevations. The latter is often associated with bradycardia (Cushing phenomenon).

Hypertension is best treated by additional doses of thiopental, hyperventilation, and administration of sub-MAC doses of isoflurane. Excessive hyperventilation should be avoided in trauma patients to avoid excessive decreases in cerebral blood flow. Beta-adrenergic blockade is usually effective in controlling hypertension associated with tachycardia. Cerebral perfusion pressure should be maintained between 70 and 110 mm Hg. Vasodilators should be avoided until the dura is opened. Excessive vagal tone should be treated with atropine.

Disseminated intravascular coagulation may be seen with severe head injuries. Such injuries cause release of large amounts of brain thromboplastin and may also be associated with the adult respiratory distress syndrome (Chapter 48). Disseminated intravascular coagulation should be diagnosed by coagulation tests and treated with fresh-frozen plasma or cryoprecipitate, while adult respiratory distress syndrome may necessitate PEEP. PEEP should only be applied with intracranial pressure monitoring or when the dura is opened. Diabetes insipidus, characterized by copious dilute urine, is frequently seen following injuries to the pituitary stalk. Other likely causes of polyuria should be excluded and the diagnosis confirmed by measurement of urine and serum osmolality prior to treatment with vasopressin (Chapter 28).

The decision whether to extubate the trachea at the conclusion of the surgical procedure depends on the severity of the injury, the presence of concomitant abdominal or thoracic injuries, preexisting illnesses, and the preoperative level of consciousness. Young patients who were conscious preoperatively may be extubated following the removal of a localized lesion, whereas patients with diffuse brain injury should be left intubated. Moreover, persistent intracranial hypertension requires continued paralysis, sedation, hyperventilation, and perhaps a pentobarbital infusion postoperatively.

CRANIOTOMY FOR INTRACRANIAL ANEURYSMS

PREOPERATIVE MANAGEMENT

Patients with intracranial aneurysms can be divided into two groups based on whether rupture (subarachnoid hemorrhage) has occurred.

Unruptured Aneurysms

Patients with unruptured aneurysms typically present with headaches or cranial nerve deficits (from direct nerve impingement). Following diagnosis by CT scanning and angiography, these patients are brought to the operating room for elective clipping or obliteration of the aneurysm. Most patients are in the 40- to 60-year age group and in otherwise good health. Generous premedication is usually desirable.

Ruptured Aneurysms

Ruptured aneurysms present acutely as subarachnoid hemorrhage. If intracranial pressure does not decrease rapidly after the initial sudden increase, death usually follows. Minor bleeding may cause only a mild headache and nuchal rigidity, while massive bleeding produces severe intracranial hypertension and rapid neurologic deterioration. Unfortunately, even minor bleeding in the subarachnoid space appears to predispose to cerebral vasospasm. Vasospasm can result in severe ischemic neurologic deficits and occurs most frequently 3–10 days after rupture.

Neurosurgical management of patients surviving a ruptured aneurysm is complicated by the risks of rebleeding and vasospasm. Early operation to clip the aneurysm is associated with an increased incidence of vasospasm, while delayed clipping increases the likelihood of rebleeding. Most centers favor delayed surgical management, since patients operated on early appear to die from ischemic strokes (vasospasm) instead of rebleeding. The calcium channel antagonists nimodipine and nicardipine appear to be useful in preventing vasospasm and have led to renewed interest in early operation for these patients. Vasospasm, once established, is difficult to treat; the only measures proved to be effective are volume expansion and hypertension. Aminocaproic acid may retard clot fibrinolysis and prevent rebleeding, but it increases the incidence of venous thromboembolism and may contribute to vasospasm. Most surgeons wait until neurologic function improves before undertaking elective clipping. Patients who deteriorate rapidly as a consequence of bleeding are managed in somewhat the same way as patients with head injury and are often followed with intracranial pressure monitoring.

Preanesthetic evaluation should determine whether or not intracranial hypertension is present. Generally, by the time most patients come to surgery, intracranial pressure is normal. A small group of patients, however, may have persistent intracranial pressure elevation. Hydrocephalus develops in these patients as a result of interference with cerebrospinal fluid absorption and is usually evidenced by ventricular enlargement on the CT scan. In addition to neurologic findings, evaluation should include a search for coexisting diseases that may modify the use of elective hypotension intraoperatively (see below). Preexisting hypertension and renal, cardiac, or ischemic cerebrovascular disease are relative contraindications to controlled hypotension. Electrocardiographic abnormalities are commonly seen in patients with subarachnoid hemorrhage but do not necessarily reflect underlying heart disease. Most conscious patients with normal intracranial pressure are sedated following rupture to prevent rebleeding; such sedation should be continued until induction of anesthesia. Patients with persistent intracranial pressure elevation should receive little or no premedication to avoid hypercapnia.

INTRAOPERATIVE MANAGEMENT

Aneurysm surgery can result in exsanguinating hemorrhage as a consequence of rupture or rebleeding. Blood (usually four units) should be available prior to the start of these operations.

Regardless of the anesthetic technique employed, anesthetic management should focus on preventing rupture (or rebleeding) and avoiding factors that promote cerebral ischemia or vasospasm. Intra-arterial and central venous (or pulmonary artery) pressure monitoring are mandatory. Sudden increases in blood pressure with tracheal intubation or surgical stimulation should be avoided. Judicious intravascular volume loading, guided by central venous pressures, allows deep levels of anesthesia without excessive decreases in blood pressure. Because calcium channel blockers cause systemic vasodilatation and reduce systemic vascular resistance, patients receiving these agents preoperatively may be especially prone to hypotension. Hyperventilation is avoided to prevent decreases in cerebral blood flow, especially in patients with vasospasm. Once the dura is opened, mannitol is often given to facilitate surgical exposure and reduce tissue trauma from surgical retraction. Rapid decreases in intracranial pressure prior to dural opening may promote rebleeding by removing a tamponading effect on the aneurysm.

Elective (controlled) hypotension is extremely useful in aneurysm surgery. Decreasing mean arterial blood pressure reduces the transmural tension across the aneurysm, making rupture (or rebleeding) less likely and facilitating surgical clipping. Controlled hypotension can also decrease blood loss and improve surgical visualization in the event of bleeding. The combination of a slightly head-up position with a volatile anesthetic (isoflurane) enhances the effects of any of the commonly used hypotensive agents (Chapter 13). Mean arterial pressure is usually maintained between 60 and 70 mm Hg but may be lowered further for brief periods if necessary. When relative contraindications exist (see above), controlled hypotension (with more conservative limits) may still be used but for brief periods; hypotension is rarely necessary before the dura is opened. Thiopental administration may protect the brain during periods of prolonged or excessive hypotension or vascular occlusion. Rarely, hypothermic circulatory arrest is used for large basilar artery aneurysms.

Most patients should be extubated at the end of surgery. Extubation should be handled similarly to other craniotomies (see above). A rapid awakening allows neurologic evaluation in the operating room prior to transfer to the intensive care unit.

SURGERY FOR ISCHEMIC CEREBROVASCULAR DISEASE

PREOPERATIVE MANAGEMENT

Most patients undergoing procedures to correct cerebrovascular stenosis or occlusion are elderly, hypertensive, and have generalized arteriosclerosis. A significant number are also diabetic. Preoperative evaluation and management should focus on optimizing the patient's clinical status as regards coexisting diseases. Although most postoperative neurologic deficits appear to be related to surgical technique, uncontrolled hypertension preoperatively increases the incidence of new deficits following surgery. Moreover, the most common cause of death following carotid artery surgery is myocardial infarction. Uncontrolled hyperglycemia may also increase morbidity by enhancing ischemic cerebral injury (Chapter 25).

With the possible exception of diuretics, patients should receive their usual medications on schedule until the time of surgery. Blood pressure and the plasma glucose concentration should be well controlled preoperatively. Angina should be stable and controlled, and signs of overt congestive heart failure should be absent. Premedication is tailored to each patient's needs. Alleviation of anxiety to prevent hypertension and tachycardia is desirable. Since most patients are elderly, enhanced sensitivity to premedication should be expected.

INTRAOPERATIVE MANAGEMENT

The emphasis in anesthetic management is on maintaining adequate cerebral perfusion without stressing the heart. Traditionally, this is accomplished by close regulation of arterial blood pressure and avoidance of tachycardia. Intra-arterial pressure monitoring is therefore mandatory. Electrocardiographic monitoring should include the V_5 lead to detect ischemia (Chapter 6). Continuous computerized ST segment analysis is desirable. Additional hemodynamic monitoring should be based primarily on underlying cardiac function (Chapter 6), as these procedures are not usually associated with significant blood loss or fluid shifts. The EEG and somatosensory evoked potentials can be used to indirectly assess cerebral perfusion (Chapter 25). Multiple-channel recording enhances the sensitivity of the EEG.

Carotid surgery may be performed under either local or general anesthesia. Superficial and deep cervical plexus blocks allow the patient to remain awake during surgery, facilitating detection of new neurologic deficits. Unfortunately, with local anesthesia, the airway is not secured, and access to it is nearly impossible once the operation begins. Regardless of the anesthetic technique chosen, mean arterial blood pressure should be maintained at or slightly above the patient's usual range. Intraoperative hypertension usually necessitates the use of an intravenous vasodilator. Nitroglycerin is usually a good choice for mild to moderate hypertension because of its beneficial effects on the coronary circulation. Marked hypertension requires a more potent agent such as nitroprusside (Chapter 13). Beta-adrenergic blockade facilitates management of the hypertension and prevents tachycardia but should be used cautiously (Chapter 12). Pronounced or sustained reflex bradycardia due to manipulation of the carotid baroreceptor should be treated with atropine. Arterial normocapnia should be maintained; hypercapnia may induce intracerebral steal (Chapter 25), while hypocapnia decreases cerebral perfusion.

Heparinization is necessary prior to occlusion of the carotid artery. Electrophysiologic signs of ischemia after carotid cross-clamping dictate the use of a shunt. Ischemic electroencephalographic changes lasting more than 10 minutes may be associated with a new postoperative neurologic deficit. Some surgeons always employ a shunt, but this practice appears to increase the incidence of embolic neurologic deficits. Thiopental administration prior to or shortly after carotid occlusion may provide some degree of cerebral protection.

Although rapid emergence from anesthesia allows immediate neurologic assessment, it also frequently results in hypertension. A vasodilator is often required during emergence. Patients should be observed closely for the possible development of a wound hematoma, which can rapidly compromise the airway.

SURGERY ON THE SPINE

PREOPERATIVE MANAGEMENT

Spinal surgery is most often performed for symptomatic nerve root or cord compression secondary to degenerative disorders. Compression may occur from protrusion of an intervertebral disk or osteophytic bone (spondylosis) into the spinal canal (or an intervertebral foramen). Herniation of an intervertebral disk usually occurs at either the fourth or fifth lumbar or the fifth or sixth cervical levels in patients 30–50 years old. Spondylosis tends to affect the lower cervical spine more than lumbar spine and typically afflicts older patients. Spinal surgery may also be undertaken to correct deformities (scoliosis), decompress the cord, and fixate the spine following spinal trauma or to resect a tumor, a vascular malformation, or an abscess.

Preoperative evaluation should focus on any existing ventilatory impairment and the airway. Anatomic abnormalities and limited neck movements due to disease, traction, or braces complicate airway management and necessitate special techniques (Chapter 5). Neurologic deficits should be documented. Most patients with degenerative disease have considerable pain preoperatively and should be given a narcotic with premedication. Conversely, premedication should be used sparingly in patients with difficult airways or ventilatory impairment.

INTRAOPERATIVE MANAGEMENT

Anesthetic management is complicated primarily by the prone position. Use of the supine position (with head traction) for an anterior approach to the cervical spine facilitates anesthetic management but may be associated with injuries to the trachea, esophagus, recurrent laryngeal nerve, sympathetic chain, carotid artery, or jugular vein. Spinal operations involving multiple levels, fusion, and instrumentation are also complicated by the potential for large intraoperative blood losses. Excessive distraction during spinal instrumentation (Harrington rod or pedicle screw fixation) can additionally injure the spinal cord.

Following induction of anesthesia in the supine position, the patient is turned prone as a single unit (requiring at least four people). Care must be taken to maintain the neck in neutral position. Once in the prone position, the head may be turned to the side (not exceeding the patient's normal range of motion) or can remain face down on a cushioned holder. Extreme caution is necessary to avoid retinal ischemia from pressure on either globe or pressure necrosis of the nose, ears, forehead, breasts (females), or genitalia (males). The chest should rest on parallel rolls (foam) or special supports—if a frame is used—to facilitate ventilation. The arms should be at the sides in a comfortable position with the elbows flexed (avoiding excessive abduction at the shoulder).

Turning the patient prone is a critical period. Monitor disconnects are hard to avoid and are often complicated by hypotension due to blunted postural sympathetic reflexes. Abdominal compression, especially in obese patients, may impede venous return and later contributes to excessive intraoperative blood loss from engorgement of epidural veins. The use of specially designed frames that allow the abdomen to hang free may alleviate these problems.

When significant blood loss is anticipated or the patient has preexisting cardiac disease, intra-arterial and possibly central venous pressure monitoring should be undertaken prior to positioning. In suitable candidates, Elective hypotension or infiltration of the wound with a weak epinephrine solution may decrease intraoperative blood loss. Massive blood loss from aortic or vena caval injury can occur intra- or postoperatively and is often initially occult.

Instrumentation of the spine requires the ability to intraoperatively detect spinal cord injury from excessive distraction. Intraoperative wake-up techniques, employing balanced anesthesia with a short-acting narcotic and muscle relaxant, allow testing of motor function following distraction. Once preservation of motor function is established, the patient is anesthetized again. Monitoring somatosensory evoked potentials may be used alternatively and avoids the problems associated with intraoperative awakening. Unfortunately, somatosensory evoked potentials test only dorsal column function, not motor function. Rare instances have been reported of postoperative neurologic deficits despite preservation of somatosensory evoked potentials intraoperatively. Monitors for motor tract function are currently in the developmental stages.

CASE DISCUSSION: RESECTION OF A PITUITARY TUMOR

A 41-year-old woman presents to the operating room for resection of a 10-mm pituitary tumor. She had complained of amenorrhea and had started noticing some decrease in visual acuity.

What hormones does the pituitary gland normally secrete?

Functionally and anatomically, the pituitary is divided into two parts: anterior and posterior. The latter is part of the neurohypophysis, which also includes the pituitary stalk and the median eminence.

The anterior pituitary is composed of several cell types, each secreting a specific hormone. Anterior pituitary hormones include adrenocorticotropic hormone (ACTH), thyroid-stimulating hormone (TSH), growth hormone (GH), the gonadotropins follicle-stimulating hormone (FSH) and luteinizing hormone (LH), and prolactin (PRL). Secretion of each of these

hormones is regulated by hypothalamic peptides (releasing hormones) that are transported to the adenohypophysis by a capillary portal system. The secretion of FSH, LH, ACTH, TSH, and their respective releasing hormones is also under negative feedback control by the products of their target organs (see below).

The posterior pituitary secretes antidiuretic hormone (ADH; vasopressin) and oxytocin. These hormones are actually formed in supraoptic and paraventricular neurons, respectively, and are transported down axons that terminate in the posterior pituitary. Hypothalamic osmoreceptors and, to a lesser extent, peripheral vascular stretch receptors regulate ADH secretion (Chapter 28).

What is the function of these hormones?

ACTH stimulates the adrenal cortex to secrete glucocorticoids. Unlike mineralocorticoid production, glucocorticoid production is dependent on ACTH secretion. TSH accelerates the synthesis and release of thyroid hormone (thyroxine). Normal thyroid function is dependent on TSH production. The gonadotropins FSH and LH are necessary for normal testosterone production and spermatogenesis in males and cyclic ovarian function in females. Growth hormone promotes tissue growth and increases protein synthesis as well as fatty acid mobilization. Its effects on carbohydrate metabolism are to decrease cellular glucose uptake and utilization and to increase insulin secretion. Prolactin functions to support breast development during pregnancy. Dopamine receptor antagonists are known to increase prolactin secretion.

Through its effect on water permeability in renal collecting ducts, ADH regulates extracellular osmolarity and blood volume (Chapter 29). Oxytocin acts on areolar myoepithelial cells in the milk letdown reflex during suckling and enhances uterine activity during labor.

What factors will determine the surgical approach in this patient?

The pituitary gland is attached to the brain by a stalk and extends downward to lie in the sella turcica of the sphenoid bone. Anteriorly, posteriorly, and inferiorly, it is bordered by bone. Laterally it is bordered by the cavernous sinus, which contains cranial nerves III, IV, V_1, and VI as well as the cavernous portion of the carotid artery. Superiorly, the diaphragma sella, a thick dural reflection, usually tightly encircles the stalk and forms the roof of the sella turcica. In close proximity to the stalk lie the optic nerves and chiasm. In continuity and superior to the stalk lies the hypothalamus.

Generally, tumors under 10 mm in diameter are approached via the transsphenoidal route, while tumors larger than 20 mm in diameter and with significant suprasellar extension are approached via a bifrontal craniotomy. With use of prophylactic antibiotics, morbidity and mortality rates are significantly less with the transsphenoidal approach. With the aid of a microscope, the operation is carried out through an incision in the gingival mucosa beneath the upper lip. The surgeon enters the nasal cavity, dissects through the nasal septum, and finally penetrates the roof of the sphenoid sinus to enter the floor of the sella turcica.

What are the major problems associated with the transsphenoidal approach?

Problems with this approach include the need for mucosal injections of epinephrine-containing solution to reduce bleeding, the accumulation of blood and tissue debris in the pharynx and stomach, the risks of hemorrhage from inadvertent entry into the cavernous sinus or the internal carotid artery, cranial nerve damage, and pituitary hypofunction. Prophylactic glucocorticoid administration is routinely used in most centers. Diabetes insipidus (Chapter 29) develops postoperatively in up to 40% of patients but is usually transient. Less commonly, the diabetes insipidus presents intraoperatively. The supine and slightly head-up position used for this procedure may predispose to venous air embolism.

What type of tumor does this patient have?

Tumors in or around the sella turcica account for 10–15% of intracranial neoplasms. Pituitary adenomas are most common, followed by craniopharyngiomas and then parasellar meningiomas. Primary malignant pituitary and metastatic tumors are rare. Pituitary tumors that secrete hormones (functional tumors) usually present early when they are still relatively small (< 10 mm). Other tumors present late with signs of increased intracranial pressure (headache, nausea and vomiting) or compression of contiguous structures (visual disturbances or pituitary hypofunction). Compression of the optic chiasm classically results in bitemporal hemianopia. Compression of normal pituitary tissue produces progressive endocrine dysfunction. Failure of hormonal secretion usually progresses in the order of gonadotropins, GH, ACTH, and TSH. Diabetes insipidus can also be seen preoperatively. Rarely, hemorrhage into the pituitary results in acute panhypopituitarism (pituitary apoplexy) with signs of a rapidly expanding mass, hemodynamic instability, and hypoglycemia.

This patient has the most common type of secretory adenoma—that producing hyperprolactinemia. Women with this tumor typically have amenorrhea, galactorrhea, or both. Men with prolactin-secreting adenomas may have galactorrhea or infertility but more commonly present with symptoms of an expanding mass.

What other types of secretory hormones are seen?

Adenomas secreting ACTH (Cushing's disease) produce classic manifestations of Cushing's syndrome: truncal obesity, moon facies, abdominal striae, proximal muscle weakness, hypertension, and osteoporosis. Glucose tolerance is typically impaired, but frank diabetes is less common (< 20%). Hirsutism, acne, and amenorrhea are also commonly seen in women.

Adenomas that secrete growth hormone are often large and result in either gigantism (prepubertal patients) or acromegaly (adults). Excessive growth prior to epiphyseal fusion results in massive growth of the entire skeleton. After epiphyseal closure, the abnormal growth is limited to soft tissues and acral parts: hands, feet, nose, and mandible. Patients develop osteoarthritis, which often affects the temporomandibular joint and spine. Glucose tolerance, myopathies, and neuropathies are common. Cardiovascular complications include hypertension, premature coronary disease, and cardiomyopathy in some patients. The most serious anesthetic problem encountered in these patients is difficulty in intubating the trachea.

Are any special monitors required for transsphenoidal surgery?

Monitoring should be carried out in somewhat the same way as for craniotomies. Visual evoked potentials are sometimes employed with large tumors that involve the optic nerves. Special monitoring for venous air embolism—beyond end-tidal CO_2 measurement—is generally not necessary. Venous access with large-bore catheters is desirable in the event of massive hemorrhage.

What modifications, if any, are necessary in the anesthetic technique?

The same principles discussed for craniotomies apply, especially if the patient has evidence of increased intracranial pressure. Intravenous antibiotic prophylaxis and glucocorticoid coverage (hydrocortisone, 100 mg) are usually given prior to induction. Many clinicians avoid nitrous oxide to prevent problems with a postoperative pneumocephalus (see above). Intense muscle paralysis is important to prevent movement while the surgeon is using the microscope. The management of diabetes insipidus is discussed in Chapter 28.

SUGGESTED READINGS

Campkin TV, Turner JM: *Neurosurgical Anaesthesia and Intensive Care,* 2nd ed. Butterworths, 1986.

Cottrell JE: *Anesthesia and Neurosurgery,* 2nd ed. Mosby, 1986.

Cucchiara RF, Michenfelder JD: *Clinical Neuroanesthesia.* Churchill Livingstone 1990.

Frost EAM: *Clinical Anesthesia in Neurosurgery,* 2nd ed. Butterworth-Heinemann, 1991.

Roizen MF: *Anesthesia for Vascular Surgery.* Churchill Livingstone, 1990. Good discussion of cerebrovascular disease.

Sperry RJ, Stirt JA, Stone DJ: *Manual of Neuroanesthesia.* BC Decker, 1989.

Yeager MP, Glass DD: *Anesthesiology & Vascular Surgery.* Appleton & Lange, 1990. Good chapter on cerebrovascular surgery.

Anesthesia for Patients With Neurologic & Psychiatric Diseases

27

Cerebrovascular disease is a major cause of morbidity and death. Patients with a history of stroke, transient ischemic attacks, or asymptomatic extracranial vascular obstructions frequently present to the operating room for unrelated procedures. This chapter discusses a general approach to these patients as well as patients with other common neurologic disorders. Chapter 26 discusses anesthetic management of patients undergoing cerebrovascular surgery.

Nonvascular neurologic diseases and psychiatric disorders are less frequently encountered in surgical patients and are often overlooked. Fortunately, unless increased intracranial pressure is present, special anesthetic techniques are not usually required. Nonetheless, the anesthesiologist must have a basic understanding of the major neurologic and psychiatric disorders and their drug therapy; failure to recognize potentially adverse anesthetic interactions may result in avoidable perioperative morbidity.

CEREBROVASCULAR DISEASE

The incidence of significant cerebrovascular disease in surgical patients is unknown but probably increases with age. Patients with known cerebrovascular disease typically have a history of transient ischemic attacks (TIAs) or stroke. Asymptomatic cervical bruits occur in up to 4% of patients over age 40 but do not necessarily indicate significant carotid artery obstruction. Fewer than 10% of patients with completely asymptomatic bruits have hemodynamically significant carotid artery lesions. Moreover, the absence of a bruit does not exclude significant carotid obstruction.

The risk of postoperative stroke increases with patient age and varies with the type of surgery. The overall risk of stroke following nonneurologic surgery is low. Even in patients with known cerebrovascular disease, the risk is only 0.4–3.3%. An asymptomatic cervical bruit does not appear to increase the risk of

stroke following surgery. Patients undergoing open heart procedures for valvular disease are at highest risk, with an incidence of about 4%. Mortality rates following postoperative stroke have varied widely in different studies (from 0.2% to 50%). Strokes following open heart surgery are usually due to emboli of air, fibrin, or calcium debris. The pathophysiology of postoperative strokes following noncardiac surgery is less clear but may involve severe sustained hypotension or hypertension. Hypotension with severe hypoperfusion can result in intracerebral thrombosis and infarction, while hypertension can result in intracerebral hemorrhage, disruption of the blood-brain barrier, and cerebral edema. The period of time after which a patient may be safely anesthetized following a stroke has not been determined. Most clinicians postpone elective procedures for at least 6 months following a completed stroke.

Patients with TIAs have a history of transient (< 24 hours) impairment and by definition have no residual neurologic impairment. These attacks are thought to be due to emboli of fibrin-platelet aggregates or atheromatous debris from plaques in extracranial vessels. Unilateral visual impairment, numbness or weakness of an extremity, or aphasia is suggestive of carotid disease, while bilateral visual impairment, dizziness, ataxia, dysarthria, bilateral weakness, or amnesia is suggestive of vertebral-basilar disease. Patients with TIAs have a 30–40% chance of developing a thrombotic stroke within 5 years; most (50%) occur within the first year. Patients with TIAs should not undergo any elective surgical procedure without an adequate medical evaluation that generally includes at least noninvasive (Doppler) flow and imaging studies. The presence of an ulcerative plaque or greater than 80% occlusion is generally an indication for carotid endarterectomy.

PREOPERATIVE MANAGEMENT

Preoperative assessment requires careful neurologic and cardiovascular evaluations. The type of stroke, the presence of neurologic deficits, and the extent of residual impairment should be determined. Thrombotic strokes are most common and usually occur in patients with generalized atherosclerosis. Most patients are elderly and have a history of hypertension, diabetes, or both. Coexisting coronary artery disease and renal impairment are common. Embolic strokes are most often associated with mitral valve disease or endocarditis or follow valve replacement. Hemorrhagic strokes are typically due to accelerated hypertension, rupture of a cerebral aneurysm, or both. Many patients, following nonhemorrhagic strokes or TIAs, are placed on long-term warfarin or antiplatelet therapy. The risk of stopping such therapy perioperatively for a few days appears small. Clotting studies and a bleeding time should be used to confirm reversal of their effect prior to operation. Once surgical hemostasis has been achieved (24–48 hours), anticoagulants or aspirin may be resumed postoperatively.

Regardless of the procedure or the type of anesthetic to be administered, blood pressure, angina, congestive heart failure, and hyperglycemia should be under good control preoperatively. With the exception of diuretics and insulin, all patients should receive their usual medications up to the time of surgery. The management of diabetes is discussed in Chapter 36.

INTRAOPERATIVE MANAGEMENT

Although some clinicians feel that regional anesthesia may be safer than general anesthesia for these patients, supporting studies are lacking. No one general technique is clearly superior to another. Because of a leftward shift in cerebral autoregulation (Chapter 25), blood pressure should be maintained at or slightly higher than normal levels. Vasopressors should not be relied upon to maintain blood pressure, as their overuse can precipitate myocardial ischemia. Vasodilators or adrenergic blockade may be necessary during periods of intense stimulation and during emergence. Use of a muscle relaxant facilitates anesthetic management by providing optimal surgical conditions yet allowing appropriate adjustments in anesthetic depth. Wide swings in blood pressure are undesirable and may contribute to postoperative cardiac and cerebral complications.

The use of a paretic or paralyzed extremity for monitoring neuromuscular blockade can result in overdosage. Because resistance to neuromuscular blockade—

Table 27–1. Classification of seizures.

Partial (focal)
Simple
Complex
Partial seizure secondarily generalized
Generalized
Absence (petit mal)
Tonic-clonic (grand mal)
Tonic
Atonic
Myoclonic
Akinetic

as assessed by train-of-four—may be observed in paretic extremities, neuromuscular blockade should be monitored on the nonparetic side. Succinylcholine should probably be avoided in patients with a history of recent stroke and those with extensive muscle wasting because of reports of hyperkalemia in these settings.

SEIZURE DISORDERS

Seizures represent abnormal synchronized electrical activity in the brain. They may be a manifestation of an underlying central nervous system disease, a systemic disorder, or, less commonly, may be idiopathic. On the EEG, seizure activity may be localized to a specific area in the brain or may be generalized. Moreover, initially localized (focal) seizures can subsequently spread, becoming generalized. A simple classification scheme is presented in Table 27–1. Focal seizures (also termed partial) are clinically manifested by motor, sensory, autonomic, or psychic symptoms depending on the cortical area affected. Focal seizures associated with impairment in consciousness are termed complex partial (psychomotor or temporal lobe) seizures. Generalized seizures characteristically produce bilaterally symmetric electrical activity without local onset. They result in abnormal motor activity, loss of consciousness, or both. Generalized activity resulting in isolated and transient lapses in consciousness are termed absence (petit mal) seizures. Other generalized seizures are usually classified according to the type of motor activity. Tonic-clonic (grand mal) seizures are most common and are characterized by a loss of consciousness followed by clonic and then tonic motor activity.

PREOPERATIVE MANAGEMENT

Preoperative evaluation of patients with a seizure disorder should focus on determining the cause and type of seizure activity and what drugs are being given. Seizures in adults are most commonly due to structural brain lesions (head trauma, tumor, or stroke) or metabolic abnormalities (uremia, hypoglycemia, hypocalcemia, or alcohol withdrawal). Idiopathic seizures occur most often in children but may persist into adulthood. Anesthetic evaluation should focus primarily on the underlying disorder and secondarily on the seizures. Management of patients with a mass lesion or increased intracranial pressure is discussed in Chapter 26.

Characterization of the type of seizure is important in detecting such activity perioperatively. Seizures—particularly grand mal seizures—are serious complicating factors in surgical patients and should be

Table 27–2. Commonly used anticonvulsants.[1]

Drug	Half-Life	Dosage[2]	Therapeutic Serum Level
Phenytoin	12–36 h	300–600 mg	10–20 μg/mL
Phenobarbital	80 h	50–200 mg	10–40 μg/mL
Carbamazepine	12–17 h	200–1200 mg	4–10 μg/mL
Primidone	3–12 h	750 mg	5–15 μg/mL
Ethosuximide	30–60 h	250–1500 mg	40–100 μg/mL
Valproic acid	6–16 h	30–60 mg/kg	50–100 μg/mL
Clonazepam	18–30 h	1.5–18 mg	0.02–0.08 μg/mL

[1]Adapted from Katzung BG (editor): *Clinical Pharmacology '88/89.* Appleton & Lange, 1988.
[2]Usual total daily dose for adults.

treated aggressively to prevent musculoskeletal injury, hypoventilation, hypoxemia, and aspiration. Even focal seizures can progress to grand mal seizures. If a seizure occurs, maintaining an open airway and adequate oxygenation take first priority. Intravenous thiopental (50–100 mg), phenytoin (500–1000 mg slowly), or diazepam (5–10 mg) can be used to terminate the seizure.

Most patients with seizure disorders have been receiving anticonvulsants preoperatively (Table 27–2). Drug therapy should be reviewed for efficacy and toxicity. Phenytoin, the most commonly used drug, is effective in all but petit mal seizures. Phenobarbital is less commonly used because of its greater sedating effect. Carbamazepine is usually used for partial seizures. Ethosuximide, valproic acid, trimethadione, and clonazepam are used chiefly for petit mal seizures. Adverse side effects and signs of toxicity should be excluded clinically and by laboratory investigations. Carbamazepine, ethosuximide, valproic acid, and trimethadione may cause bone marrow depression and hepatotoxicity. At toxic levels, most agents cause ataxia, dizziness, confusion, and sedation. Blood levels of anticonvulsants are usually readily available from the hospital laboratory and should be checked in patients with signs of toxicity and those who give a history of recent seizures. Anticonvulsants should ideally be continued throughout the perioperative period to maintain therapeutic levels. Fortunately, most agents have a relatively long half-life, so that a delayed or even a missed dose is often not critical.

INTRAOPERATIVE MANAGEMENT

In selecting anesthetic agents, drugs with possible epileptogenic potential should be avoided. Ketamine and methohexital (in small doses) theoretically can precipitate seizure activity and should be avoided. Theoretically, large doses of atracurium or meperidine may be contraindicated because of the reported epileptogenic potential of their metabolites, laudanosine and normeperidine, respectively. Hepatic microsomal enzyme induction should be expected from preoperative phenobarbital therapy. Enzyme induction may increase dose requirements for intravenous agents and may increase the potential for hepatotoxicity from halothane. The use of enflurane in patients with a seizure disorder is questionable. Enflurane in high concentrations (> 2.5%) and in association with concomitant hypocapnia can precipitate electroencephalographic spike-and-wave patterns resembling seizures even in normal individuals. Phenytoin and carbamazepine may increase dose requirements for nondepolarizing muscle relaxants.

DEGENERATIVE & DEMYELINATING DISEASES

PARKINSON'S DISEASE

Parkinson's disease typically affects patients 50–70 years of age. Also known as paralysis agitans, this slowly progressive disease is characterized by cogwheel rigidity, a resting (pill-rolling) tremor, a fixed facial expression, and festination. Increasing problems with rigidity and tremor eventually result in physical incapacitation, but intellectual function is usually preserved. The disease appears to be related to progressive loss of dopamine in the basal ganglia. This decrease in dopaminergic (inhibitory) activity allows a relative increase in cholinergic (excitatory) influences on the extrapyramidal system. Similar syndromes may be seen following encephalitis, carbon monoxide intoxication, strokes, and metal poisoning and with antipsychotic medications.

Treatment is directed at controlling the symptoms. Anticholinergics may be used for mild disease, but levodopa (a precursor of dopamine) is required for moderate to severe symptoms. Levodopa is used because dopamine does not cross the blood-brain barrier.

Side effects include nausea, vomiting, dyskinesia, cardiac irritability, and orthostatic hypotension. The latter may be due to catecholamine depletion (chronic negative feedback inhibition) and volume depletion perhaps secondary to a natriuretic effect. Preparations combining levodopa with a dopa decarboxylase inhibitor (carbidopa; Sinemet) increase central delivery and allow the use of smaller doses. Bromocriptine, a dopamine agonist, may also be used in some patients. Selegilene, a selective monoamine oxidase B inhibitor, also appears promising in early Parkinson's disease. Unlike nonselective monoamine oxidase inhibitors, it does not cause dangerous potentiation of the effects of catecholamines (see below).

Medication for Parkinson's disease should be continued perioperatively, including the morning of surgery, because the half-life of levodopa is short. Abrupt withdrawal of levodopa can cause worsening of muscle rigidity and may interfere with ventilation. Phenothiazines, butyrophenones (droperidol), and metoclopramide can exacerbate symptoms as a consequence of their antidopaminergic activity and should be avoided. Anticholinergics (atropine) or antihistamines (diphenhydramine) may be used for acute exacerbation of symptoms. Diphenhydramine is especially valuable for premedication and intraoperative sedation in patients with tremor. Induction of anesthesia in patients receiving long-term levodopa therapy may result in either marked hypotension or hypertension. Relative hypovolemia, catecholamine depletion, autonomic instability, and sensitization to catecholamines are probably contributory. Arterial blood pressure should be monitored carefully. Significant hypotension should be treated with small doses of a direct-acting vasopressor such as phenylephrine. Cardiac irritability readily produces dysrhythmias, so halothane, ketamine, and local anesthetic solutions containing epinephrine should be used cautiously if at all. Although the response to muscle relaxants is generally normal, a rare occurrence of hyperkalemia following succinylcholine has been reported. Adequacy of ventilation and airway reflexes should be carefully assessed prior to extubation of patients with moderate to severe disease.

ALZHEIMER'S DISEASE

The prevalence of Alzheimer's disease increases with age to as high as 20% in patients over 80. The disease is characterized by a slow decline in intellectual function (dementia). Loss of recent memory, depression, and emotional lability are common early but often subtle manifestations. Late in the course of the disease, severe extrapyramidal signs, apraxias, and aphasia are often present. Although some degree of brain atrophy is normal with advancing age, patients with Alzheimer's disease usually show marked cortical atrophy with ventricular enlargement, and pathologically their brains characteristically contain neuritic plaques and fibrillary changes. A deficiency of choline acetyltransferase suggests that clinical manifestations are related to impaired cholinergic transmission in the brain.

Treatment is largely supportive. Drugs that increase brain acetylcholine levels, such as physostigmine, may be used for some patients with mild disease.

Anesthetic management of patients with moderate to severe disease is often complicated by disorientation and uncooperativeness. Such patients require repeated reassurance and explanation. Consent must be obtained from the next of kin or a legal guardian if the patient is incapacitated. Because the use of centrally acting drugs must be minimized, premedication is usually not given. Regional anesthesia should be attempted only if the patient is cooperative. Inhalation agents may be preferable for general anesthesia because of their rapid elimination. Centrally acting anticholinergics such as atropine and scopolamine could theoretically contribute to postoperative confusion. Glycopyrrolate, which does not cross the blood-brain barrier, may be the preferred agent when an anticholinergic is required.

MULTIPLE SCLEROSIS

Multiple sclerosis is characterized by demyelination at random and multiple sites in the brain and spinal cord. The disease primarily affects patients between 20 and 40 years of age and typically follows an unpredictable course of frequent attacks and remissions. With time, remissions become less complete, and the disease is progressive and incapacitating. Clinical manifestations depend on the sites affected but frequently include visual disturbances, motor weakness, and paresthesias. Symptoms develop over the course of days and remit over weeks to months. Early diagnosis of exacerbations can often be confirmed by MRI. Remyelination is limited and often fails to occur. Moreover, axonal loss can occur. Changes in neurologic function appear to be related to changes in axonal conduction. Conduction can occur across demyelinated axons but appears to be affected by multiple factors, especially temperature. Increases in body temperature cause exacerbation of symptoms, presumably by decreasing nerve conduction.

Treatment of multiple sclerosis is primarily symptomatic. Diazepam, dantrolene, or baclofen is used to control spasticity; bethanechol is useful for bladder dysfunction and carbamazepine or phenytoin for dysesthesias. ACTH or glucocorticoids may lessen the severity and duration of acute attacks. Immunosuppressants and plasmapheresis may also be effective in some patients.

The effect of stress, anesthesia, and surgery on the course of the disease is controversial. A detrimental effect has been suggested but not substantiated. Overall, the effect of anesthesia is unpredictable. Elective surgery should be avoided during relapse regardless of the anesthetic technique employed. The preoperative consent record should document counseling of the patient to the effect that the stress of surgery and anesthesia might worsen the symptoms. Spinal anesthesia has been reported to cause exacerbation of the disease. Epidural and other regional techniques appear to have no adverse effect, especially in obstetrics. No specific interactions with general anesthetics are generally recognized. Patients with advanced disease may have a labile cardiovascular system due to autonomic dysfunction (see below). In the setting of paresis or paralysis, succinylcholine should be avoided because of the risk of hyperkalemia. Regardless of the anesthetic technique employed, increases in body temperatures should be avoided. Demyelinated fibers are extremely sensitive to increases in temperature; an increase of as little as 0.5 °C may completely block conduction.

AMYOTROPHIC LATERAL SCLEROSIS

Amyotrophic lateral sclerosis is a rapidly progressive disorder of both upper and lower motor neurons. Clinically, patients present in the fifth or sixth decade of life with muscular weakness, atrophy, fasciculation, and spasticity. The disease may initially be asymmetric but over the course of 2–3 years becomes generalized, involving all skeletal and bulbar muscles. Progressive respiratory muscle weakness makes the patient susceptible to aspiration and eventually leads to death from ventilatory failure. Although the heart is unaffected, autonomic dysfunction can be seen.

The primary emphasis in management is judicious respiratory care. As with other patients with lower motor neuron disease, succinylcholine is contraindicated because of the risk of hyperkalemia. Nondepolarizing muscle relaxants should be used sparingly, because patients often display enhanced sensitivity. Adequacy of ventilation should be carefully assessed both intra- and postoperatively; an awake extubation is desirable. Difficulty in weaning patients off of their respirators postoperatively is not uncommon in patients with moderate to advanced disease.

GUILLAIN-BARRÉ SYNDROME

Also known as acute idiopathic polyneuritis, this disorder is characterized by a sudden onset of ascending motor paralysis with variable paresthesias. Bulbar involvement, including respiratory muscle paralysis, is a frequent complication. Pathologically, the disease appears to be an immunologic reaction against the myelin sheath of peripheral nerves. In most instances, the syndrome appears to follow viral respiratory or gastrointestinal infections. Some patients respond to plasmapheresis. The prognosis is good, with most patients recovering completely.

In addition to the respiratory complications, anesthetic management is complicated by lability of the autonomic nervous system. Exaggerated hypo- and hypertensive responses during anesthesia may be seen. As is the case with other lower motor neuron disorders also, succinylcholine should not be used because of the risk of hyperkalemia. The use of regional anesthesia in these patients remains controversial.

AUTONOMIC DYSFUNCTION

Autonomic dysfunction, or dysautonomia, is most consistently manifested as orthostatic hypotension. It may be congenital, familial, or acquired. Patients with dysautonomia also frequently have bladder and bowel dysfunction, decreased sweating, lacrimation and salivation, and sexual impotence.

Congenital or familial dysautonomia occurs most frequently in Jewish children and is usually referred to as Riley-Day syndrome. Patients appear to have an enzyme deficiency in the synthesis of catecholamines. Autonomic dysfunction is prominent and is associated with generalized diminished sensation and emotional lability. Moreover, patients are predisposed to dysautonomic crises triggered by stress and characterized by marked hypertension, tachycardia, diaphoresis, and vomiting. Intravenous diazepam is effective in resolving such episodes.

Acquired autonomic dysfunction can be idiopathic, part of a neurologic disorder (multiple sclerosis, syringomyelia, amyotrophic lateral sclerosis, or spinal cord injury), a complication of a nonneurologic disorder (diabetes, AIDS, or adrenal insufficiency), or drug-induced (alcohol, antihypertensive agents, anesthetics). Degeneration may occur at central or peripheral (or both) components of the autonomic nervous system. Dysautonomia associated with central neurologic signs is referred to as Shy-Drager syndrome. This syndrome is typically characterized by sympathetic and parasympathetic defects as well as cerebellar and extrapyramidal dysfunction.

The major risk in patients with autonomic dysfunction is severe hypotension, compromising cerebral and coronary blood flow. Most patients are chronically hypovolemic. The vasodilatory effects of spinal and epidural anesthesia are poorly tolerated. Similarly, the vasodilatory and cardiac depressant effects of most general anesthetic agents combined with positive airway pressure can be equally deleterious. Continuous intra-arterial blood pressure monitoring is desirable. Hypotension should be treated with fluids and direct-acting vasopressors. The latter are preferable to indirect-acting agents. Enhanced sensitivity to vasopressors due to denervation sensitivity may be observed. Blood loss also is usually poorly tolerated; central venous or pulmonary artery catheterization is invaluable when significant fluid shifts are expected. Body temperature should be monitored closely. Patients with anhidrosis are especially susceptible to hyperpyrexia.

SYRINGOMYELIA

Syringomyelia results in progressive cavitation of the spinal cord. In many cases, obstruction of cerebrospinal fluid outflow from the fourth ventricle appears to be contributory. Increased pressure in the central canal of the spinal cord produces enlargement or diverticulation to the point of cavitation. Syringomyelia typically affects the cervical spine, producing sensory and motor deficits in the upper extremity and, frequently, thoracic scoliosis. Extension upward into the medulla (syringobulbia) leads to cranial nerve deficits. Ventricular-peritoneal shunting and other decompressive procedures have variable success in arresting the disease.

Anesthetic evaluation should focus on defining existing neurologic deficits as well as any pulmonary impairment due to scoliosis. Pulmonary function testing and arterial blood gas analysis may be useful. Autonomic instability should be expected in patients with extensive lesions. Succinylcholine should be avoided when muscle wasting is present because of the risk of hyperkalemia. Adequacy of ventilation and reversal of nondepolarizing muscle relaxants should be closely evaluated prior to extubation.

SPINAL CORD INJURY

Most spinal cord injuries are traumatic and often result in partial or complete transection. Clinical manifestations depend on the level of the transection. Injuries above C3–5 (diaphragmatic innervation) are not compatible with life without ventilatory support. Transections above T1 result in quadriplegia, while those above L4 result in paraplegia. The most common sites of transection are C5–6 and T12–L1. Acute spinal cord transection produces loss of sensation, flaccid paralysis, and loss of spinal reflexes below the level of injury. These findings characterize a period of spinal shock that typically lasts 1–3 weeks. Over the course of a few weeks, spinal reflexes gradually return, together with muscle spasms and signs of sympathetic overactivity.

Overactivity of the sympathetic nervous system is especially prominent with transections above T7 but is unusual with injuries below T10. Interruption of normal descending inhibitory impulses in the cord results in autonomic hyperreflexia. Cutaneous or visceral stimulation below the level of injury can induce intense autonomic reflexes: Sympathetic discharge produces hypertension and vasoconstriction below the transection and a baroreceptor-mediated reflex bradycardia and vasodilatation above the transection. Cardiac dysrhythmias are not unusual.

Anesthetic management depends on the age of the injury. In the early care of acute injuries, the emphasis should be on preventing further spinal cord damage during patient movement, airway manipulation, and positioning. High-dose corticosteroid therapy appears to improve neurologic outcome. The head should be maintained in neutral position with the help of an assistant or should remain in traction during intubation. Awake fiberoptic intubation after topical anesthesia may be safest. Patients with high transections often have impaired airway reflexes and are further predisposed to hypoxemia by a decrease in functional residual capacity. Hypotension and bradycardia are often present prior to induction. Direct arterial pressure monitoring is indicated. Central venous and pulmonary artery pressure monitoring also greatly facilitate management. An intravenous fluid bolus and the use of ketamine for anesthesia may help prevent further decreases in blood pressure; vasopressors may also be required. Succinylcholine can be used safely in the first 24 hours but should not be used thereafter because of the risk of hyperkalemia. The latter can occur within the first week following injury and is due to excessive release of potassium secondary to the proliferation of acetylcholine receptors outside the neuromuscular synaptic cleft. Depolarization of muscle membranes by succinylcholine produces an exaggerated release of potassium extracellularly.

Anesthetic management of patients with nonacute transections is complicated by the possibility of autonomic hyperreflexia in addition to the risk of hyperkalemia. Autonomic hyperreflexia should be expected in patients with lesions above T7 and can be precipitated by surgical manipulations. Regional anesthesia and deep general anesthesia are effective in preventing hyperreflexia. Many clinicians, however, are reluctant to administer spinal and epidural anesthesia in these patients because of the difficulties encountered with determining the anesthetic level, exaggerated hypotension, and technical problems resulting from deformities. Severe hypertension can result in pulmonary edema, myocardial ischemia, or cerebral hemorrhage and should be treated aggressively. Vasodilators and α-adrenergic blocking agents should be readily available. Although the risk of succinylcholine-induced hyperkalemia is reported to decrease 6 months after the injury, nondepolarizing relaxants should still be used in preference. Administration of a small dose of a nondepolarizing relaxant does not reliably prevent hyperkalemia. Body temperature should be monitored carefully, especially in patients with transections above T1, because chronic vasodilatation and loss of normal reflex cutaneous vasoconstriction predispose to hypothermia.

PSYCHIATRIC DISORDERS

DEPRESSION

Depression is a mood disorder characterized by sadness and pessimism. Its cause is multifactorial, but pharmacologic treatment is based on an the presumption that its manifestations are due to a brain deficiency of norepinephrine and perhaps serotonin. Current pharmacologic therapy utilizes three classes of drugs that increase brain levels of these neurotransmitters, namely, tricyclic antidepressants, monoamine oxidase (MAO) inhibitors, and the so-called atypical antidepressants. The mechanisms of action of these drugs result in some potentially serious anesthetic interactions. Electroconvulsive therapy (ECT) is reserved for refractory and severe cases. The use of general anesthesia for ECT is largely responsible for its safety and widespread acceptance.

Tricyclic Antidepressants

These agents are used for the first-line treatment of depression. Less commonly, they are used for chronic pain syndromes. All tricyclic antidepressants work at nerve synapses by blocking neuronal reuptake of catecholamines, serotonin, or both. The most commonly used agents are amitriptyline, imipramine, and doxepin. Most also have significant anticholinergic (antimuscarinic) actions: dry mouth, blurred vision, prolonged gastric emptying, and urinary retention. Cardiac effects include tachycardia, T wave flattening or inversion, and prolongation of the PR, QRS, and QT intervals. Amitriptyline has the most marked anticholinergic effects, while doxepin has the least cardiac effects.

These drugs are generally continued perioperatively. Increased anesthetic requirements, presumably from enhanced brain catecholamine activity, have been reported with these agents. Potentiation of centrally acting anticholinergic agents (atropine and scopolamine) may increase the likelihood of postoperative confusion and delirium. The most important interaction during anesthesia is an exaggerated response to both indirect-acting vasopressors and sympathetic stimulation. Pancuronium, ketamine, and epinephrine-containing local anesthetic solutions should be avoided (especially during halothane anesthesia). Because tricyclics lower the seizure threshold, the use of enflurane may also be questionable. Chronic therapy with tricyclic antidepressants is reported to deplete cardiac catecholamines, theoretically potentiating the cardiac depressant effects of anesthetics. If hypotension occurs, small doses of a direct-acting vasopressor should be used instead of an indirect-acting agent. Amitriptyline's anticholinergic action may occasionally contribute to postoperative delirium.

Monoamine Oxidase (MAO) Inhibitors

Monoamine oxidase inhibitors block the oxidative deamination of naturally occurring amines. At least two MAO isoenzymes (types A and B) with differential substrate selectivities have been identified. Currently available agents that are efficacious for depression are nonselective MAO inhibitors. They include phenelzine, isocarboxazid, and tranylcypromine. Selective MAO-B inhibitors (see above) are not effective in the treatment of depression. Nonselective agents also appear to interfere with many enzymes other than monoamine oxidase. Side effects include orthostatic hypotension, agitation, tremor, seizures, muscle spasms, urinary retention, paresthesias, and jaundice. Their hypotensive effect may be related to the accumulation of false neurotransmitters (octopamine). The most serious sequela is a hypertensive crisis that occurs following ingestion of tyramine-containing foods (cheeses and red wines).

Discontinuing MAO inhibitors at least 2 weeks prior to elective surgery was at one time recommended but is currently a controversial practice. Because these agents (with the exception of tranylcypromine) produce irreversible enzyme inhibition, the 2-week delay allowed sufficient regeneration of new enzyme. Recent studies suggest that patients may be safely anesthetized, at least for electroconvulsive therapy, without this waiting period. Opioids should generally be avoided in patients receiving MAO inhibitors, since rare but serious reactions to narcotics have been reported. Most serious reactions are associated with meperidine, resulting in hyperthermia, seizures, and coma. Similar to the tricyclics, exaggerated responses to vasopressors and sympathetic stimulation should be expected. If a vasopressor is necessary, a direct-acting agent in small doses should be employed.

Atypical Antidepressants

Atypical antidepressants include trazodone, fluoxetine, and clomipramine. Trazodone potentiates the action of serotonin. Fluoxetine selectively blocks neuronal uptake of serotonin, while clomipramine blocks neural uptake of both norepinephrine and serotonin. Clomipramine also appears to be effective in the treatment of obsessive-compulsive disorder. Anesthetic interactions with these agents are not well documented. Trazodone has been associated with an increased incidence of cardiac arrhythmias.

MANIA

Mania is a mood disorder characterized by elation, hyperactivity, and flight of ideas. Manic episodes may alternate with depression in some patients. Mania is thought to be related to excessive norepinephrine activity in the brain. Lithium is the drug of choice for treating acute manic episodes, preventing their recurrence as well as suppressing episodes of depression. Concomitant administration of an antipsychotic (see below) is usually necessary during acute mania.

Lithium's mechanism of action is poorly understood. It has a narrow therapeutic range, with a desirable blood concentration between 0.8 and 1.5 meq/L. Side effects include reversible T wave changes, mild leukocytosis, and on rare occasions hypothyroidism or a vasopressin-resistant diabetes insipidus-like syndrome. Toxic blood concentrations produce sedation, muscle weakness, and slurred speech. Yet higher concentrations result in widening of the QRS complex, atrioventricular block, hypotension, and seizures.

Although lithium is reported to decrease minimum alveolar concentration and prolong the duration of some muscle relaxants, clinically these effects appear to be minor. Nonetheless, neuromuscular function should be closely monitored when muscle relaxants are used. The greatest concern is the possibility of perioperative toxicity. Blood levels should be checked perioperatively. Sodium depletion decreases renal excretion of lithium and can lead to lithium toxicity. Fluid restriction and overdiuresis should be avoided.

SCHIZOPHRENIA

Patients with schizophrenia display disordered thinking, withdrawal, paranoid delusions, and auditory hallucinations. This disorder is thought to be related to an excess of dopaminergic activity in the brain. Antipsychotic drugs remain the only form of treatment for controlling this disease.

The most commonly used antipsychotics include phenothiazines, thioxanthenes, and butyrophenones. All these agents have similar properties with minor variations. Their antipsychotic effect appears to be due to dopamine antagonist activity. Most are sedating and mildly anxiolytic. With the exception of thioridazine, all are potent antiemetics (Chapter 8). Mild α-adrenergic blockade and anticholinergic activity are also observed. Side effects include orthostatic hypotension, acute dystonic reactions, and parkinsonism-like manifestations. T wave flattening, ST segment depression, and prolongation of the PR and QT intervals may be seen, especially in patients taking thioridazine.

Generally, patients whose disease is controlled by antipsychotics present few problems. Continuing antipsychotic medication perioperatively is desirable. Reduced anesthetic requirements may be observed in some patients. Alpha-adrenergic blockade is usually well compensated. Enflurane should probably be avoided, since antipsychotics decrease the seizure threshold.

NEUROLEPTIC MALIGNANT SYNDROME

This syndrome is a rare complication of antipsychotic therapy. In its severe form, the presentation is similar to that of malignant hyperthermia. Muscle rigidity, hyperthermia, rhabdomyolysis, autonomic instability, and altered consciousness are seen. Creatine kinase levels are often high. The mortality rate approaches 20-30%, with deaths occurring primarily as a result of renal failure or dysrhythmias. Treatment with dantrolene appears to be effective. Patients with a history of neuroleptic malignant syndrome should be treated in the same way as those susceptible to malignant hyperthermia (Chapter 42).

SUBSTANCE ABUSE

Behavioral disorders from abuse of psychotropic (mind-altering) substances may involve a socially acceptable drug (alcohol), a medically prescribed drug (diazepam), or an illicit substance (cocaine). Environmental, social, and perhaps genetic factors lead to this type of behavior. A "need" for the substance develops ranging in intensity from a simple desire to a compulsion that consumes the patient's life. Characteristically with chronic abuse, patients develop tolerance to the drug and varying degrees of psychologic and physical dependence. Physical dependence is most often seen with opioids, barbiturates, alcohol, and benzodiazepines. Life-threatening complications primarily due to sympathetic overactivity can develop during abstention. Barbiturate withdrawal is potentially the most lethal and dangerous of the withdrawal syndromes.

Knowledge of a patient's substance abuse preoperatively may prevent adverse drug interactions, predict tolerance to anesthetic agents, and facilitate the recognition of drug withdrawal. The history of substance abuse may be volunteered by the patient (usually only on direct questioning) or deliberately hidden. A high index of suspicion is often required. Sociopathic tendencies are difficult to detect during a short interview. The presence of numerous punctate scars with difficult venous access strongly suggests intravenous drug abuse. Intravenous drug abusers have a relatively high incidence of skin infections, thrombophlebitis, malnutrition, endocarditis, hepatitis B, and HIV infection.

Anesthetic requirements for substance abusers vary depending on whether the drug exposure is acute or chronic (Table 27–3). Elective procedures should be postponed for acutely intoxicated patients and those with signs of withdrawal. When surgery is deemed necessary in patients with physical dependence, perioperative doses of the abused substance should be

Table 27–3. Effect of acute and chronic substance abuse on anesthetic requirements.

Substance	Acute	Chronic
Opioids	↓	↑
Barbiturates	↓	↑
Alcohol	↓	↑
Marihuana	↓	0
Benzodiazepines	↓	↑
Amphetamines	↑ [1]	↓
Cocaine	↑ [1]	0
Phencyclidine	↓	?

[1] Associated with marked sympathetic stimulation.
Key:
↓ = Decreases
↑ = Increases
0 = No effect
? = Unknown

provided or specific agents given to prevent withdrawal. In the case of opioid dependence, any opioid can be used, while for alcohol a benzodiazepine is usually substituted. Tolerance to most anesthetic agents is often seen but is not always predictable. Regional anesthetic techniques should be considered whenever possible. For general anesthesia, a technique primarily relying on a volatile inhalational agent may be preferable so that anesthetic depth can be readily adjusted according to individual need. Narcotics with mixed agonist-antagonist activity should be avoided in opioid-dependent patients because they can precipitate acute withdrawal. Clonidine is a useful adjuvant in treatment of postoperative withdrawal syndromes.

CASE DISCUSSION: ANESTHESIA FOR ELECTROCONVULSIVE THERAPY

A 64-year-old man with depression refractory to drug therapy is scheduled for electroconvulsive therapy (ECT).

How is ECT administered?

The electroconvulsive shock is applied to one or both cerebral hemispheres to induce a seizure. Variables include stimulus pattern, amplitude, and duration. The goal is to produce a therapeutic generalized seizure 30–60 seconds in duration. Electrical stimuli are usually administered until a therapeutic seizure is induced. A good therapeutic effect is generally not achieved until a total of 400–700 seizure seconds have been induced. Since only one treatment is given per day, patients are usually scheduled for a series of treatments, usually 2 or 3 a week. Progressive memory loss often occurs with an increasing number of treatments, especially when electrodes are applied bilaterally.

Why is anesthesia necessary?

When the efficacy of ECT was discovered, enthusiasm was tempered by a relatively high incidence of musculoskeletal injuries. Moreover, when muscle relaxants were used alone, patients sometimes recalled being paralyzed and awake just prior to the shock. The routine use of general anesthesia to ensure amnesia and muscle paralysis to prevent injuries has renewed interest in ECT. The current mortality rate for ECT is estimated to be one death per 10,000 treatments. While some psychiatrists administer the anesthetic, the presence of an anesthesiologist is optimal for airway management and cardiovascular monitoring.

What are the physiologic effects of ECT-induced seizures?

Seizure activity is characteristically associated with an initial parasympathetic discharge followed by a more sustained sympathetic discharge. The initial phase is characterized by bradycardia and increased secretions. Marked bradycardia (< 30 beats/min) and even transient asystole (up to 6 seconds) are occasionally seen. The hypertension and tachycardia that follow are typically sustained for several minutes. Cerebral blood flow, intracranial pressure, intragastric pressure, and intraocular pressure all transiently increase.

Are there any contraindications to ECT?

Absolute contraindications are a recent myocardial infarction (usually < 3 months), a recent stroke (usually < 1 month), and an intracranial mass or increased intracranial pressure from any cause. Relative contraindications include angina, uncontrolled heart failure, significant pulmonary disease, bone fractures, severe osteoporosis, pregnancy, glaucoma, and retinal detachment.

What are the important considerations in selecting anesthetic agents?

Amnesia is required only for the brief period (1–5 minutes) from when the muscle relaxant is given to when a therapeutic seizure has been successfully induced. The seizure itself usually results in a brief period of anterograde amnesia, somnolence, and often confusion. Consequently, only a short-acting induction agent is necessary. Moreover, since most induction agents (barbiturates, etomidate, and propofol) have anticonvulsant properties, small doses must be used. Seizure threshold is increased and seizure duration is decreased by all these agents.

Following adequate preoxygenation, methohexital, 0.5–1 mg/kg, is most commonly employed. Ketamine is generally not used because of an increased incidence of delayed awakening, nausea, and ataxia. Short-acting narcotics such as alfentanil are not given alone because they do not consistently produce amnesia. However, alfentanil (10–25 μg/kg) can be a useful adjunct when very small doses of methohexital (10–20 mg) are required in patients with a high seizure threshold. In very small doses, methohexital may actually enhance seizure activity. Increases in seizure threshold are often observed with each subsequent ECT.

Muscle paralysis is required from the time of electrical stimulation till the end of the seizure. A short-acting agent such as succinylcholine, 0.5–1 mg/kg, is most often selected. Controlled mask ventilation using a self-inflating bag device or an anesthesia circle system is required until spontaneous respirations resume.

Can seizure duration be increased without increasing the electrical stimulus?

Hyperventilation can increase seizure duration and is routinely employed in most centers. Intravenous caffeine 125–250 mg (given slowly) has also been reported to increase seizure duration.

What monitors should be used during ECT?

Monitoring should be similar to that appropriate with the use of any other general anesthetic. Seizure activity is usually monitored by the unprocessed EEG. Seizure activity can also be monitored in an isolated limb: A tourniquet is inflated around one arm prior to injection of succinylcholine, preventing entry of the muscle relaxant and allowing observation of convulsive motor activity in that arm.

How can the adverse hemodynamic effects of the seizure be controlled in patients with limited cardiovascular reserve?

Exaggerated parasympathetic effects should be treated with atropine. In fact, premedication with glycopyrrolate is desirable *in all patients* to prevent both the profuse secretions associated with seizures and to attenuate the bradycardia. Nitroglycerin, nifedipine, and α- and β-adrenergic blockade have all been employed successfully to control sympathetic manifestations. Beta-adrenergic blockade has, however, been reported to decreases the efficacy of ECT.

What if the patient has a pacemaker?

Patients with pacemakers may safely undergo electroconvulsive treatments, but a magnet should be readily available to convert the pacemaker to a fixed mode if necessary.

SUGGESTED READINGS

Alderson JD, Frost EAM: *Spinal Cord Injuries: Anaesthetic and Associated Care.* Butterworths, 1990.

Gilman AG et al (editors): *Goodman and Gilman's The Pharmacological Basis of Therapeutics,* 8th ed. Pergamon, 1990.

Katz J, Benumof JL, Kadis LB: *Anesthesia and Uncommon Diseases,* 3rd ed. Saunders, 1990. Good sections on neurologic disorders and substance abuse.

Stoelting RS, Dierdorf SF, McCammon RL: *Anesthesia and Coexisting Disease,* 2nd ed. Churchill Livingston, 1988. Fairly complete chapters on both neurologic and psychiatric diseases.

Management of Patients With Fluid & Electrolyte Disturbances

28

Fluid and electrolyte disturbances are common in the perioperative period. Large amounts of intravenous fluids are frequently required to correct fluid deficits and compensate for blood loss during surgery. Anesthesiologists must therefore have a clear understanding of normal water and electrolyte physiology. Major disturbances in fluid and electrolyte balance can rapidly alter cardiovascular, neurologic, and neuromuscular functions. This chapter examines the body's fluid compartments and common water and electrolyte derangements, their treatment, and anesthetic implications. Acid-base disorders and intravenous fluid therapy are discussed in subsequent chapters.

NOMENCLATURE OF SOLUTIONS

The system of international units (SI) has still not gained universal acceptance in clinical practice, and many older expressions of concentration remain in common use. Thus, for example, the quantity of a solute in a solution may be expressed in grams, moles, or equivalents. To complicate matters further, the concentration of a solution may be expressed either as quantity of solute per volume of solution or quantity of solute per weight of solvent.

MOLARITY, MOLALITY, & EQUIVALENCY

One **mole** of a substance represents 6.02×10^{23} molecules. The weight of this quantity in grams is commonly referred to as gram-molecular weight. **Molarity** is the standard SI unit of concentration that expresses the number of moles of solute per liter of solution. **Molality** is an alternative term that expresses moles of solute per kilogram of solvent. **Equivalency** is also commonly used for substances that ionize: the number of **equivalents** of an ion in solution is the number of moles multiplied by its charge (valence).

Thus, a 1-molar solution of $MgCl_2$ yields 2 equivalents of magnesium per liter and 2 equivalents of chloride per liter.

OSMOLARITY, OSMOLALITY, & TONICITY

Osmosis is the net movement of water across a semipermeable membrane as a result of a difference in nondiffusible solute concentrations between the two sides. **Osmotic pressure** is the pressure that must be applied to the side with more solute to prevent a net movement of water down its concentration gradient. Since the average kinetic energy of particles in solution is similar regardless of their mass, osmotic pressure is generally dependent only on the number of nondiffusible solute particles. One **osmole** equals 1 mole for nondissociable substances. However, for substances that ionize, each mole results in n osmoles, where n is the number of ionic species produced. Thus, 1 mole of NaCl dissolved in solution produces 2 osmoles. A difference of 1 milliosmole per liter between two solutions results in an osmotic pressure of 19.3 mm Hg. The **osmolarity** of a solution is equal to the number of osmoles per liter of solution, while its **osmolality** equals the number of osmoles per kilogram of solvent. **Tonicity** is a term that is often used interchangeably with osmolarity and osmolality. More correctly, tonicity refers to the effect a solution has on cell volume. An isotonic solution has no effect on cell volume, while hypotonic and hypertonic solutions increase and decrease cell volume, respectively.

FLUID COMPARTMENTS

The average adult male is approximately 60% water by weight. This water is distributed between two major fluid compartments separated by cell membranes: intracellular fluid (ICF) and extracellular fluid (ECF). The latter can be further subdivided into intravascular

Table 28–1. Body fluid compartments (based on an average 70-kg male).

Compartment	Body Weight (%)	Total Body Water (%)	Volume (L)
Intracellular	36	60	25
Extracellular			
Interstitial	19	32	13.5
Intravascular	5	8	3.5
Total	60	100	42

and interstitial compartments. The interstitium includes all fluid that is both outside cells and outside the vascular endothelium. The relative contributions of each compartment to total body water (TBW) and body weight are set forth in Table 28–1.

The volume of fluid (water) within a compartment is determined by its solute composition and concentrations (Table 28–2). Differences in solute concentrations are largely due to the characteristics of the physical barriers that separate compartments (see below). The osmotic forces created by "trapped" solutes govern the distribution of water between compartments and ultimately each compartment's volume.

INTRACELLULAR FLUID

The outer membrane of the cells plays an important role in regulating intracellular volume and composition. A membrane-bound ATP-dependent pump exchanges Na^+ for K^+ in a 3:2 ratio. Because cell membranes are relatively impermeable to sodium and to a lesser extent potassium ions, potassium is concentrated intracellularly while sodium is concentrated extracellularly. As a result, potassium is the most impor-

Table 28–2. The composition of fluid compartments.

	Intracellular	Extracellular	
		Intravascular	Interstitial
Sodium (meq/L)	10	145	142
Potassium (meq/L)	140	4	4
Calcium (meq/L)	<1	3	3
Magnesium (meq/L)	50	2	2
Chloride (meq/L)	4	105	110
Bicarbonate (meq/L)	10	24	28
Phosphorus (meq/L)	75	2	2
Protein (g/dL)	16	7	2

tant determinant of intracellular osmotic pressure, while sodium is the most important determinant of extracellular osmotic pressure.

The impermeability of cell membranes to most proteins results in a high intracellular protein concentration. Because proteins act as nondiffusible solutes (anions), the unequal exchange ratio of 3 Na^+ for 2 K^+ by the cell membrane pump is critical in preventing relative intracellular hyperosmolality. Interference with Na^+-K^+ ATPase activity, as occurs during ischemia or hypoxia, results in progressive swelling of cells.

EXTRACELLULAR FLUID

The principal function of extracellular fluid is to provide cells with nutrients and remove their waste products. Maintenance of a normal extracellular volume—especially the circulating component (intravascular volume)—is critical. For the reasons described above, sodium is quantitatively the most important extracellular cation and the major determinant of extracellular osmotic pressure and volume. Changes in extracellular fluid volume are therefore related to changes in total body sodium content. The latter is a function of sodium intake, renal sodium excretion, and extrarenal sodium losses (see below).

Interstitial Fluid

Very little interstitial fluid is normally in the form of free fluid. Most interstitial water is in chemical association with extracellular proteoglycans, forming a gel. Interstitial fluid pressure is generally thought to be negative (about −5 mm Hg). As interstitial fluid volume increases, interstitial pressure also rises and eventually becomes positive. When the latter occurs, the free fluid in the gel increases rapidly and appears clinically as edema.

Because only small quantities of plasma proteins can normally cross capillary clefts, the protein content of interstitial fluid is relatively low (2 g/dL). Protein entering the interstitial space is returned to the vascular system via the lymphatic system.

Intravascular Fluid

Intravascular fluid, commonly referred to as plasma, is restricted to the intravascular space by the vascular endothelium. Most electrolytes (small ions) freely pass between plasma and the interstitium, resulting in nearly identical electrolyte composition. However, the tight intercellular junctions between adjacent endothelial cells impede the passage of plasma proteins outside the intravascular compartment. As a result, plasma proteins (mainly albumin) are the only osmotically active solutes in fluid exchange between plasma and interstitial fluid.

Increases in extracellular volume are normally proportionately reflected in intravascular and interstitial volume. When interstitial pressure becomes positive,

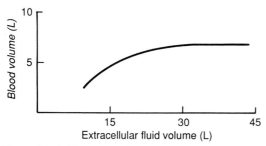

Figure 28–1. The relationship between blood volume and extracellular fluid volume. (Modified and reproduced, with permission, from Guyton AC: *Textbook of Medical Physiology,* 7th ed. Saunders, 1986.)

continued increases in ECF result in expansion of only the interstitial fluid compartment (Figure 28–1). In this way, the interstitial compartment acts as an overflow reservoir for the intravascular compartment. This can be seen clinically in the form of tissue edema.

EXCHANGE BETWEEN FLUID COMPARTMENTS

Diffusion is the random movement of molecules due to their kinetic energy and is responsible for the majority of fluid and solute exchange between compartments. The rate of diffusion of a substance across a membrane depends on (1) the permeability of that substance through that membrane, (2) the concentration difference between the two sides, (3) the pressure difference between either side because pressure imparts greater kinetic energy, and (4) the electrical potential across the membrane for charged substances.

Diffusion Through Cell Membranes

Diffusion between interstitial fluid and intracellular fluid may take place by one of several mechanisms: (1) directly through the lipid bilayer of the cell membrane, (2) through protein channels within the membrane, or (3) by reversible binding to a carrier protein that can traverse the membrane (facilitated diffusion). Oxygen, CO_2, water, and lipid-soluble molecules penetrate the cell membrane directly. Cations such as Na^+, K^+, and Ca^{2+} penetrate the membrane poorly because of the cell transmembrane voltage potential (which is positive to the outside) created by the Na^+-K^+ pump. Therefore, these cations can diffuse only through specific protein channels. Passage through these channels is dependent on membrane voltage and the binding of ligands (such as acetylcholine) to the membrane receptors. Glucose and amino acids diffuse with the help of membrane-bound carrier proteins.

Fluid exchange between the intracellular and interstitial spaces is governed by the osmotic forces created by differences in nondiffusible solute concentrations. Relative changes in osmolality between the intracellu-lar and interstitial compartments result in a net water movement from the hypo-osmolar to the hyperosmolar compartment.

Diffusion Through Capillary Endothelium

Capillary walls are typically 0.5 μm thick, consisting of a single layer of endothelial cells with their basement membrane. Intercellular clefts, 6–7 nm wide, separate each cell from its neighbors. Oxygen, CO_2, water, and lipid-soluble substances can penetrate directly through both sides of the endothelial cell membrane. Only low-molecular-weight water-soluble substances such as sodium, chloride, potassium, and glucose readily cross intercellular clefts. High-molecular-weight substances such as plasma proteins penetrate the endothelial clefts poorly (except in the liver and the lungs, where the clefts are larger).

Fluid exchange across capillaries differs from that across cell membranes in that it is governed by significant differences in hydrostatic pressures in addition to osmotic forces (Figure 28–2). These forces are operative on both arterial and venous ends of capillaries. As a result, there is a tendency for fluid to move out of capillaries at the arterial end and back into capillaries at the venous end. Normally, all but 10% of the fluid filtered is reabsorbed back into capillaries. That which is not reabsorbed (about 2 mL/min) enters interstitial fluid and is then returned by lymphatic flow to the intravascular compartment.

DISORDERS OF WATER BALANCE

The human body at birth is approximately 75% water by weight. By 1 month this value decreases to 65%, and by adulthood to 60% for males and 50% for females. The higher fat content in females decreases water content. For the same reason, obesity and advanced age further decrease water content.

NORMAL WATER BALANCE

The normal adult daily water intake averages 2500 mL, which includes approximately 300 mL as a byproduct of the metabolism of energy substrates. Daily water loss necessarily averages 2500 mL and can roughly be accounted for by 1500 mL in urine, 400 mL in respiratory tract evaporation, 400 mL in skin evaporation, 100 mL in sweat, and 100 mL in feces.

Both ICF and ECF osmolalities are closely regulated in such a way as to maintain a normal water content in tissues. Changes in water content and cell volume can induce serious impairment of function especially in the brain (see below).

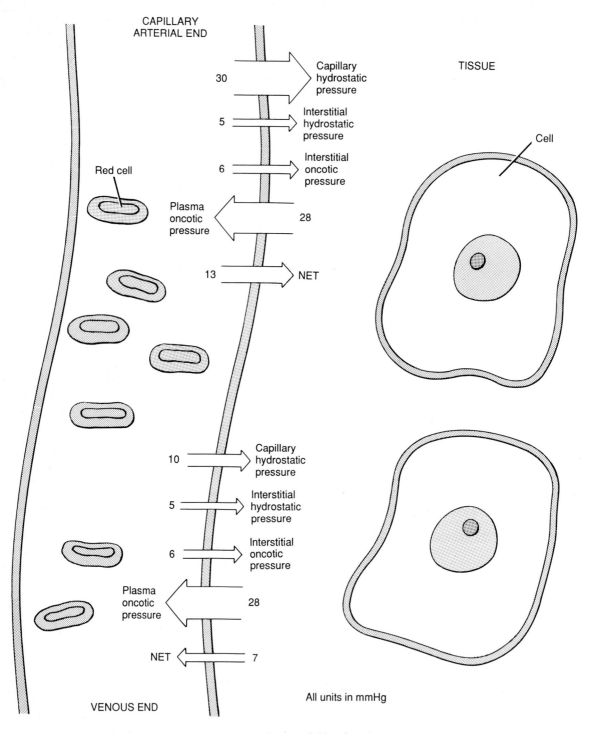

Figure 28–2. Capillary fluid exchange.

RELATIONSHIP BETWEEN PLASMA SODIUM CONCENTRATION, EXTRACELLULAR OSMOLALITY, & INTRACELLULAR OSMOLALITY

The osmolality of ECF is equal to the sum of the concentrations of all dissolved solutes. Because Na^+ together with its anions account for nearly 90% of these solutes, the following approximation is valid:

Plasma osmolality ≈ 2 × Plasma sodium concentration

Moreover, because ICF and ECF are in osmotic equilibrium, plasma sodium concentration generally reflects total body osmolality:

Total body osmolality =
$$\frac{\text{Extracellular solutes + Intracellular solutes}}{\text{TBW}}$$

Since sodium and potassium are the major intra- and extracellular solutes, respectively:

Total body osmolality ≈
$$\frac{(Na^+_{extracellular} \times 2) + (K^+_{intracellular} \times 2)}{\text{TBW}}$$

Combining the two approximations:

$$[Na^+]_{plasma} \approx \frac{Na^+_{extracellular} + K^+_{intracellular}}{\text{TBW}}$$

Using these principles, the effect of isotonic, hypotonic, and hypertonic fluid loads on compartmental water content and plasma osmolality can be calculated (Table 28–3).

In pathologic states, glucose and—to a much lesser extent—urea can contribute significantly to extracellular osmolality. A more accurate approximation of plasma osmolality is therefore given by the following equation:

Plama osmolality (mosm/kg) =
$$[Na^+] \times 2 + \frac{\text{BUN}}{2.8} + \frac{\text{Glucose}}{18}$$

where $[Na^+]$ is expressed as meq/L and BUN and glucose as mg/dL. Urea is an ineffective osmole because it readily permeates cell membranes and is therefore frequently omitted from this calculation:

Effective plasma osmolality $= [Na^+] \times 2 + \dfrac{\text{Glucose}}{18}$

Plasma osmolality normally varies between 280 and 290 mosm/kg. A discrepancy between the measured and calculated osmolality is referred to as an **osmolal gap.** Significant osmolal gaps are indicative of a high concentration of an abnormal osmotically active molecule in plasma such as ethanol, mannitol, methanol,

ethylene glycol, or isopropyl alcohol. Osmolal gaps may also be seen in patients with chronic renal failure (attributed to retention of small solutes), patients with ketoacidosis (due to a high concentration of ketone bodies), and those receiving large amounts of glycine (as during transurethral resection of the prostate). Lastly, osmolal gaps may also be present in patients with marked hyperlipidemia or hyperproteinemia. In such instances, the protein or lipid part of plasma contributes significantly to plasma volume; although plasma $[Na^+]$ is decreased, $[Na^+]$ in the water phase of plasma (true plasma osmolality) remains normal.

CONTROL OF PLASMA OSMOLALITY

Plasma osmolality is closely regulated by osmoreceptors in the hypothalamus. These specialized neurons control the secretion of antidiuretic hormone (ADH) and the thirst mechanism. Plasma osmolality is therefore maintained within relatively narrow limits by varying both water intake and water excretion.

Secretion of Antidiuretic Hormone

Specialized neurons in the supraoptic nuclei of the hypothalamus are very sensitive to changes in extracellular osmolality. When ECF osmolality increases, these cells shrink and release ADH (arginine vasopressin) from the posterior pituitary. Antidiuretic hormone markedly increases water reabsorption in renal collecting tubules (Chapter 31), which tends to reduce plasma osmolality to normal again. Conversely, a decrease in extracellular osmolality causes osmoreceptors to swell and suppresses the release of ADH. Decreased ADH secretion allows a water diuresis, which tends to increase osmolality to normal. With complete suppression of ADH secretion, the kidneys can excrete up to 10–20 L of water per day.

Nonosmotic Release of ADH

The carotid baroreceptors and possibly atrial stretch receptors can also stimulate ADH release following a 5–10% decrease in blood volume (see below). Other nonosmotic stimuli include pain, emotional stress, and hypoxia.

Thirst

Osmoreceptors in the lateral preoptic area of the hypothalamus are also very sensitive to changes in extracellular osmolality. Activation of these neurons by increases in ECF osmolality induces thirst and causes the individual to drink water. Conversely, hypo-osmolality suppresses thirst.

Thirst is the major defense mechanism against hyperosmolality and hypernatremia, because it is the only mechanism that increases water intake. Unfortunately, the thirst mechanism is only operative in conscious individuals who are capable of drinking.

Table 28–3. Effect of different fluid loads on extracellular and intracellular water contents.[1]

A. Normal

Total body solute = 280 mosm/kg × 42 kg = 11,760 mosm
Intracellular solute = 280 mosm/kg × 25 kg = 7000 mosm
Extracellular solute = 280 mosm/kg × 17 kg = 4760 mosm
Extracellular sodium concentration = 280 ÷ 2 = 140 meq/L

	Intracellular	Extracellular
Osmolality	280	280
Volume (L)	25	17
Net water gain	0	0

B. Isotonic load: 2 L of isotonic saline (NaCl)

Total body solute = 280 mosm/kg × 44 kg = 12,320 mosm
Intracellular solute = 280 mosm/kg × 25 kg = 7000 mosm
Extracellular solute = 280 mosm/kg × 19 kg = 5320 mosm

	Intracellular	Extracellular
Osmolality	280	280
Volume	25	19
Net water gain	0	2

Net effect: Fluid remains in extracellular compartment.

C. Free water (hypotonic) load: 2 L water

New body water = 42 + 2 = 44 kg
New body osmolality = 11,760 mosm ÷ 44 kg = 267 mosm/kg
New extracellular volume = 7000 mosm ÷ 267 mosm/kg = 26.2 kg
New extracellular sodium concentration = 267 ÷ 2 = 133 meq/L

	Intracellular	Extracellular
Osmolality	267.0	267.0
Volume	26.2	17.8
Net water gain	+1.2	+0.8

Net effect: Fluid distributes between both compartments.

D. Hypertonic load: 600 meq NaCl (no water)

Total body solute = 11,760 + 600 = 12,360 mosm/kg
New body osmolality = 12,360 mosm/kg ÷ 42 kg = 294 mosm
New extracellular solute = 600 + 4760 = 5360 mosm
New extracellular volume = 5360 mosm ÷ 294 mosm/kg = 18.2 kg
New intracellular volume = 42 − 18.2 = 23.8 kg
New extracellular sodium concentration = 294 ÷ 2 = 147 meq/L

	Intracellular	Extracellular
Osmolality	294.0	294.0
Volume	23.8	18.2
Net water gain	−1.2	+1.2

Net effect: An intracellular to extracellular movement of water.

[1]Based on a 70-kg adult male.

HYPEROSMOLALITY & HYPERNATREMIA

Hyperosmolality occurs whenever total body solute content increases relative to TBW and is usually but not always associated with hypernatremia ($[Na^+] > 145$ meq/L). Hyperosmolality without hypernatremia may be seen during marked hyperglycemia or following the accumulation of abnormal osmotically active substances in plasma (see above). In the latter two instances, plasma sodium concentration may actually decrease as water is drawn from the intracellular to the extracellular compartment. For every 100 mg/dL increase in plasma glucose concentration, plasma sodium decreases approximately 1.6 meq/L.

Hypernatremia is nearly always the result of either a loss of water in excess of sodium (hypotonic fluid loss) or the retention of large quantities of sodium. Even when renal concentrating ability is impaired, thirst is normally highly effective in preventing hypernatremia. Hypernatremia is therefore most commonly seen in debilitated patients who are unable to drink, the very aged, the very young, and patients with altered consciousness. Patients with hypernatremia may have a low, normal, or high total body sodium content (Table 28–4).

Hypernatremia & Low Total Body Sodium Content

These patients have lost both sodium and water, but the water loss is in excess of the sodium loss. Hypotonic losses can be renal (osmotic diuresis) or extrarenal (diarrhea or sweat). In either case, patients usually manifest signs of hypovolemia (Chapter 29). Urinary sodium concentration is generally greater than 20 meq/L with renal losses and less than 10 meq/L with extrarenal losses.

Table 28–4. Causes of hypernatremia.

Low total body sodium content
Loss of water and sodium (water > sodium)
  Renal (urinary osmolality < 800 mosm/kg)
    Osmotic diuresis
      Hyperglycemia
      Manitol
  Extrarenal (urinary osmolality > 800 mosm/kg)
    Gastrointestinal
      Osmotic diarrheas
    Insensible
      Sweat
Normal total body sodium content
Loss of water
  Renal (urinary osmolality variable)
    Diabetes insipidus
      Central
      Nephrogenic
    Essential hypernatremia (reset osmoreceptors)
  Extrarenal (urinary osmolality > 800 mosm/kg)
    Burns
    Increased respiratory losses
Increased total body sodium content[1]
Massive salt ingestion
Hypertonic saline
$NaHCO_3$ therapy
Primary hyperaldosteronism
Cushing's syndrome

[1]Urinary osmolality may be either isotonic or hypertonic.

Hypernatremia & Normal Total Body Sodium Content

This group of patients generally manifests signs of water loss without overt hypovolemia unless the water loss is massive. Total body sodium content is generally normal. Nearly pure water losses can occur via the skin, respiratory tract, or kidneys. The most common cause of hypernatremia with a normal total body sodium content is diabetes insipidus (in conscious individuals). Diabetes insipidus is characterized by marked impairment in renal concentrating ability that is due either to decreased ADH secretion (central diabetes insipidus) or failure of the renal tubules to respond normally to circulating ADH (nephrogenic diabetes insipidus). Rarely, "essential hypernatremia" may be encountered in patients with central nervous system disorders. These patients appear to have reset osmoreceptors that function at a higher baseline osmolality.

A. Central Diabetes Insipidus: Lesions in or around the hypothalamus and the pituitary stalk frequently produce diabetes insipidus. Transient diabetes insipidus is also commonly seen following neurosurgical procedures and head trauma (Chapter 26). The diagnosis is suggested by a history of polydipsia, polyuria (often > 6 L/d), and the absence of hyperglycemia or compulsive water drinking behavior. In the perioperative setting, the diagnosis of diabetes insipidus is suggested by marked polyuria without glycosuria and a urinary osmolality lower than plasma osmolality. The absence of thirst in unconscious individuals leads to marked water losses and can rapidly produce hypovolemia. The diagnosis of central diabetes insipidus is

confirmed by an increase in urinary osmolality following the administration of exogenous ADH. Aqueous vasopressin is the treatment of choice for acute central diabetes insipidus. Vasopressin in oil is longer-lasting but is more likely to cause water intoxication. Desmopressin (DDAVP), a synthetic analogue of ADH with a 12- to 24-hour duration of action, is available as an intranasal preparation that can be used both in the ambulatory and perioperative settings.

B. Nephrogenic Diabetes Insipidus: Nephrogenic diabetes insipidus can be congenital but is more commonly secondary to other disorders. These include chronic renal disease, certain electrolyte disorders (hypokalemia and hypercalcemia), side effects of some drugs (amphotericin B, lithium, methoxyflurane, demeclocycline), and a variety of other disorders (sickle cell disease, hyperproteinemias). ADH secretion in these patients is normal, but the kidneys fail to respond to ADH. Urinary concentrating ability is therefore impaired. The diagnosis is confirmed by failure of the kidneys to produce a hypertonic urine following the administration of exogenous ADH. Treatment is generally directed at the underlying illness and ensuring an adequate fluid intake.

Hypernatremia & Increased Total Body Sodium Content

This condition most commonly results from the administration of large quantities of hypertonic saline solutions (3% NaCl or 7.5% $NaHCO_3$). Patients with primary hyperaldosteronism and Cushing's syndrome may also have small elevations in serum sodium concentration along with signs of increased sodium retention.

Clinical Features of Hypernatremia

Neurologic manifestations predominate in patients with hypernatremia and are generally thought to be due to cellular dehydration. Restlessness, lethargy, and hyperreflexia can progress to seizures, coma, and ultimately death. Symptoms correlate more closely with the rate of movement of water out of brain cells than with the absolute level of hypernatremia. Rapid decreases in brain volume can rupture cerebral veins and result in focal intracerebral or subarachnoid hemorrhages. Seizures and serious neurologic damage are common, especially in children with acute hypernatremia when plasma $[Na^+]$ exceeds 158 meq/L. Chronic hypernatremia is generally better tolerated than the acute form. After 24–48 hours, intracellular osmolality begins to rise as a result of increases in intracellular inositol and amino acid (glutamine and taurine) concentrations. As intracellular solute concentration increases, neuronal water content slowly returns to normal.

Treatment of Hypernatremia

The treatment of hypernatremia is aimed at restoring plasma osmolality back to normal as well as correcting the underlying problem. **Water deficits** should gener-

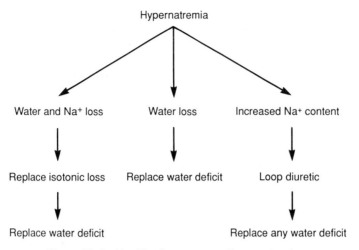

Figure 28–3. Algorithm for treatment of hypernatremia.

ally be corrected over 48 hours with a hypotonic solution such as 5% dextrose in water (see below). Abnormalities in extracellular volume must also be corrected (Figure 28–3). Hypernatremic patients with decreased total body sodium should be given isotonic fluids to restore plasma volume to normal *prior to treatment with a hypotonic solution.* Hypernatremic patients with increased total body sodium should be treated with a loop diuretic along with intravenous 5% dextrose in water. The treatment of diabetes insipidus is discussed above.

Rapid correction of hypernatremia can result in seizures, brain edema, permanent neurologic damage, and even death. Serial serum osmolalities should be obtained during treatment. In general, plasma sodium concentration should not be decreased faster than 1 meq/L/h.

Example: A 70-kg-man is found to have a plasma [Na$^+$] of 160 meq/L. What is his water deficit?

If one assumes that the hyponatremia is from water loss only, then total body osmoles are unchanged. Thus, assuming he had a normal [Na$^+$] of 140 meq/L and a TBW content that is 60% of body weight–

Normal TBW × 140 = Present TBW × Plasma [Na$^+$], or 70 × 0.6 × 140 = Present TBW × 160

Solving the equation–

Present TBW = 36.7 L
Water deficit = Normal TBW − Present TBW, or (70 × 0.6) − 36.7 = 5.3 L

To replace this deficit over 48 hours, one would give 5% dextrose in water intravenously, 5300 mL over 48 hours, or 110 mL/h.

Note that this method ignores any coexisting isotonic fluid deficits, which if present should be replaced with an isotonic solution.

Anesthetic Considerations

Hypernatremia increases the minimum alveolar concentration for inhalational anesthetics in animal studies, but its clinical significance is more closely related to the associated fluid deficits. Hypovolemia accentuates any vasodilation or cardiac depression from anesthetic agents and predisposes to hypotension and hypoperfusion of tissues. Decreases in the volume of distribution for drugs necessitate dose reductions for most intravenous agents, while decreases in cardiac output enhance the uptake of inhalation anesthetics.

Elective surgery should be postponed in patients with significant hypernatremia (> 150 meq/L) until the cause is established and fluid deficits are corrected. Both water and isotonic fluid deficits should be completely corrected prior to surgery.

HYPO-OSMOLALITY & HYPONATREMIA

Hypo-osmolality is nearly always associated with hyponatremia ([Na$^+$] < 135 meq/L). Table 28–5 lists rare instances in which hyponatremia does not necessarily reflect hypo-osmolality (pseudohyponatremia). Routine measurement of plasma osmolality in hypo-

Table 28–5. Causes of pseudohyponatremia.[1]

Hyponatremia with a normal plasma osmolality
Asymptomatic
Marked hyperlipidemia
Marked hyperproteinemia
Symptomatic
Marked glycine absorption during transurethral surgery
Hyponatremia with an elevated plasma osmolality
Hyperglycemia
Administration of mannitol

[1]Adapted from Rose RD: *Clinical Physiology of Acid-Base and Electrolyte Disorders,* 3rd ed. McGraw-Hill, 1989.

Table 28–6. Classification of hyponatremia.

Decreased total sodium content
  Renal
    Diuretics
    Mineralocorticoid deficiency
    Salt-losing nephropathies
    Osmotic diuresis (glucose, mannitol)
    Renal tubular acidosis
  Extrarenal
    Vomiting
    Diarrhea
    "Third-spacing"
Normal total sodium content
  Syndrome of inappropriate antidiuretic hormone
  Glucocorticoid deficiency
  Hypothyroidism
  Drug-induced
    Chlorpropamide
    Cyclophosphamide
    Vincristine
    Carbamezapine
Increased total sodium content
  Congestive heart failure
  Cirrhosis
  Nephrotic syndrome
  Renal failure

natremic patients rapidly excludes pseudohyponatremia.

Hyponatremia invariably reflects water retention from either an absolute increase in TBW or a loss of sodium in excess of water. The kidneys' normal capacity to produce dilute urine with an osmolality as low as 40 mosm/kg (specific gravity 1.001) allows them to excrete over 10 L of free water per day if necessary. Because of this tremendous reserve, hyponatremia is nearly always the result of a defect in urinary diluting capacity (urinary osmolality > 100 mosm/kg or specific gravity > 1.003). Rare instances of hyponatremia without an abnormality in renal diluting capacity (urinary osmolality < 100 mosm/kg) are generally attributed to primary polydipsia or "reset" osmoreceptors; the latter two conditions can be differentiated by water restriction.

Clinically, hyponatremia is best classified according to total body sodium content (Table 28–6).

Hyponatremia & Low Total Body Sodium

Progressive losses of both sodium and water eventually lead to extracellular volume depletion. As the intravascular volume deficit reaches 5–10%, nonosmotic ADH secretion is activated (see above). With further volume depletion, the stimuli for nonosmotic ADH release overcome any hyponatremia-induced suppression of ADH. *Preservation of circulatory volume takes place at the expense of plasma osmolarity.*

Fluid losses resulting in hyponatremia may be renal or extrarenal in origin. Renal losses are most commonly related to thiazide diuretics and result in a urinary [Na+] greater than 20 meq/L. Extrarenal losses are typically gastrointestinal and usually produce a

urine [Na+] of less than 10 meq/L. A major exception to the latter is hyponatremia due to vomiting, which can result in a urinary [Na+] greater than 20 meq/L. In those instances, bicarbonaturia from the associated metabolic alkalosis (Chapter 30) obligates concomitant excretion of Na+ with HCO_3^- to maintain electrical neutrality in the urine; urinary chloride concentration, however, is usually less than 10 meq/L.

Hyponatremia & Increased Total Body Sodium

Edematous disorders are characterized by an increase in both total body sodium and TBW. When the increase in water exceeds that in sodium, hyponatremia occurs. Edematous disorders include congestive heart failure, cirrhosis, renal failure, and nephrotic syndrome. Hyponatremia in these settings results from progressive impairment of renal free water excretion and generally parallels underlying disease severity. Pathophysiologic mechanisms include nonosmotic ADH release and decreased delivery of fluid to the distal diluting segment in nephrons (Chapter 31). The "effective" circulating blood volume is reduced (see below).

Hyponatremia With Normal Total Body Sodium

Hyponatremia in the absence of edema or hypovolemia may be seen with glucocorticoid insufficiency, hypothyroidism, drug therapy (chlorpropamide and cyclophosphamide), and the syndrome of inappropriate antidiuretic hormone secretion (SIADH). The latter diagnosis requires exclusion of other causes of hyponatremia and the absence of hypovolemia, edema, and adrenal, renal, or thyroid disease. A variety of malignant tumors, pulmonary diseases, and central nervous system disorders are commonly associated with SIADH. In most such instances, plasma ADH concentration is not elevated but is inadequately suppressed relative to the degree of hypo-osmolality in plasma.

Clinical Manifestations of Hyponatremia

Symptoms of hyponatremia are primarily neurologic and due to an increase in intracellular water. Their severity is generally related to the rapidity with which extracellular hypo-osmolality develops. Patients with mild to moderate hyponatremia ([Na+] > 125 meq/L) are frequently asymptomatic. Early symptoms are typically nonspecific and may include anorexia, nausea, and weakness. Progressive cerebral edema, however, results in lethargy, confusion, seizures, coma, and finally death. Serious manifestations are generally associated with plasma sodium concentrations less than 120 meq/L.

Patients with slowly developing or chronic hyponatremia are generally less symptomatic. A gradual compensatory loss of intracellular solutes (primarily

Na$^+$, K$^+$, and amino acids) appears to restore cell volume to normal. Neurologic symptoms in patients with chronic hyponatremia may be related more closely to changes in cell membrane potential (due to a low extracellular [Na$^+$]) than to changes in cell volume.

Treatment of Hyponatremia

As with hypernatremia, the treatment of hyponatremia (Figure 28–4) is directed at correcting both the underlying disorder as well as the plasma [Na$^+$]. Isotonic saline (Chapter 29) is generally the treatment of choice for hyponatremic patients with decreased total body sodium content. Once the extracellular fluid deficit is corrected, spontaneous water diuresis returns plasma [Na$^+$] to normal. Conversely, water restriction is the primary treatment modality for hyponatremic patients with normal or increased total body sodium. More specific treatments such as hormonal replacement in patients with adrenal or thyroid hypofunction and measures aimed at improving cardiac output in patients with heart failure (Chapter 20) may also be indicated. Demeclocycline, a drug that antagonizes ADH activity at the renal tubules, has proved to be a useful adjunct to water restriction in the treatment of patients with SIADH.

Acute symptomatic hyponatremia requires prompt treatment. In such instances, correction of plasma [Na$^+$] to 130 meq/L is usually sufficient to alleviate symptoms. The amount of NaCl necessary to raise plasma [Na$^+$] to the desired value ([Na$^+$]$_d$), the **Na$^+$ deficit,** can be estimated by the following formula:

$$\text{Na}^+ \text{ deficit} = \text{TBW} \times (\text{Desired [Na}^+] - \text{Present [Na}^+])$$

Very rapid correction of hyponatremia has been associated with demyelinating lesions in the pons, resulting in serious permanent neurologic sequelae. The rapidity with which hyponatremia is corrected should be tailored to the severity of symptoms. The following correction rates have been suggested: for mild symp-

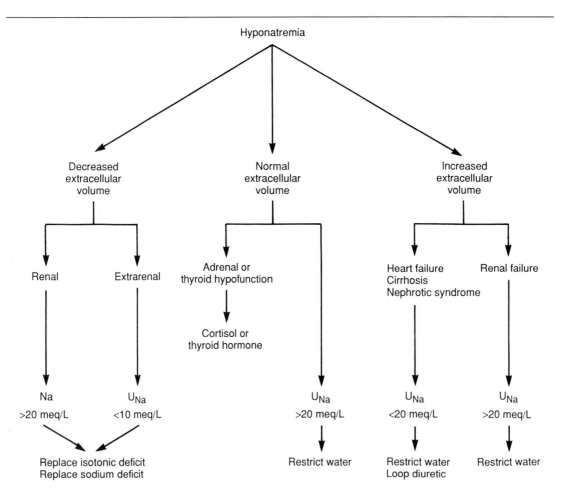

U$_{Na}$ = Urinary sodium concentration

Figure 28–4. Algorithm for treatment of hyponatremia.

toms, 0.5 meq/L/h or less; for moderate symptoms, 1 meq/L/h or less; and for severe symptoms, 1.5 meq/L/h or less.

Example: An 80-kg woman is lethargic and is found to have a plasma $[Na^+]$ of 118 meq/L. How much NaCl must be given to raise her plasma $[Na^+]$ to 130 meq/L?

$$Na^+ \text{ deficit} = TBW \times (130 - 118)$$

TBW is approximately 50% of body weight in females:

$$Na^+ \text{ deficit} = 80 \times 0.5 \times (130 - 118) = 480 \text{ meq}$$

Since normal (isotonic) saline contains 154 meq/L, the patient should receive 480 meq ÷ 154 meq/L, or 3.12 L of normal saline. For a correction rate of 0.5 meq/L/h, this amount of saline should be given over 24 hours (130 mL/h).

Note that this calculation does not take into account any coexisting isotonic fluid deficits, which, if present, should also be replaced.

Rapid correction of hyponatremia can be achieved by giving a loop diuretic to induce water diuresis while replacing urinary sodium losses with isotonic saline. Even more rapid corrections can be achieved with intravenous hypertonic saline (3% NaCl). Hypertonic saline may be indicated in markedly symptomatic patients with a plasma $[Na^+]$ less than 110 meq/L, but it should be given cautiously since it can precipitate pulmonary edema, especially in patients with increased body sodium content.

Anesthetic Considerations

Hyponatremia is often a manifestation of a serious underlying disorder and requires careful evaluation preoperatively. Plasma sodium concentrations above 130 meq/L are generally considered safe for patients undergoing general anesthesia. Plasma $[Na^+]$ should be corrected above 130 meq/L for all elective procedures, even in the absence of symptoms. Lower concentrations may result in significant cerebral edema that can be manifested intraoperatively as a decrease in minimum alveolar concentration or postoperatively as agitation, confusion, or somnolence. Patients undergoing transurethral resection of the prostate can absorb significant amounts of water from irrigation fluids (as much as 20 mL/min) and are at high risk for rapid development of profound acute water intoxication (Chapter 33).

DISORDERS OF SODIUM BALANCE

Extracellular fluid volume is directly proportionate to total body sodium content. Variations in ECF vol-

ume are due to changes in total body sodium content. A positive sodium balance increases ECF volume, while a negative sodium balance decreases ECF volume. It is important to reemphasize that *extracellular (plasma) sodium concentration is more indicative of water balance than total body sodium content* (see above).

NORMAL SODIUM BALANCE

Net sodium balance is equal to total sodium intake (adults average 170 meq/d) minus both renal sodium excretion and extrarenal sodium losses. (One gram of sodium yields 43 meq of sodium ions, whereas 1 g of sodium chloride yields 17 meq of sodium ions.) The kidneys' ability to vary urinary sodium excretion from less than 1 meq/L to more than 100 meq/L allows them to play a critical role in sodium balance (Chapter 31).

REGULATION OF SODIUM BALANCE & EXTRACELLULAR FLUID VOLUME

Because of the relationship between ECF volume and total body sodium content, regulation of one is intimately tied to the other. This regulation is achieved via sensors (see below) that detect changes in the most important component of ECF, namely, the "effective" intravascular volume. The latter correlates more closely with the rate of perfusion in renal capillaries than with measurable intravascular fluid (plasma) volume. Indeed, with edematous disorders (heart failure, cirrhosis, and renal failure), "effective" intravascular volume can be independent of the measurable plasma volume, ECF volume, and even cardiac output.

Extracellular fluid volume and total body sodium content are ultimately controlled by appropriate adjustments in renal sodium excretion. In the absence of renal disease, diuretic therapy, and selective renal ischemia, urinary sodium concentration reflects "effective" intravascular volume. A low urine sodium concentration (< 10 meq/L) is therefore generally indicative of a low "effective" intravascular fluid volume and reflects secondary retention of sodium by the kidneys.

Control Mechanisms

The multiple mechanisms involved in regulating ECF volume and sodium balance normally complement one another but can function completely independently of one another. In addition to altering renal sodium excretion, some mechanisms also produce more rapid compensatory hemodynamic responses when "effective" intravascular volume is reduced (Chapter 19).

A. Sensors of Volume: The principal volume receptors in the body are really baroreceptors. Since blood pressure is the product of cardiac output and systemic vascular resistance (Chapter 19), significant changes in intravascular volume (preload) not only affect cardiac output but also transiently affect arterial blood pressure. Thus, the baroreceptors at the carotid sinus and afferent renal arterioles (juxtaglomerular apparatus) indirectly function as sensors of intravascular volume. Changes in blood pressure at the carotid sinus modulate sympathetic nervous system activity and nonosmotic ADH secretion, while changes at the afferent renal afferent arterioles modulate the renin-angiotensin-aldosterone system. Stretch receptors in both atria are also known to sense changes in intravascular volume; the degree of atrial distention modulates the release of atrial natriuretic hormone (see below) and ADH.

B. Effectors of Volume Change: Regardless of the mechanism, effectors of volume change ultimately alter urinary sodium excretion. Decreases in "effective" intravascular volume decrease urinary sodium excretion, while increases in the "effective" intravascular volume increase urinary sodium excretion. These mechanisms include the following:

1. Renin-angiotensin-aldosterone—Aldosterone secretion enhances sodium reabsorption in the distal nephron (Chapter 31) and is a major determinant of urinary sodium excretion. Angiotensin II also has some direct effect by enhancing sodium reabsorption in the proximal renal tubules.

2. Atrial natriuretic peptide (ANP)—This peptide is normally released from both right and left atrial cells following atrial distention. Atrial natriuretic peptide appears to have two major actions: arterial vasodilatation and increased urinary sodium and water excretion in the renal collecting tubules. Afferent arteriolar dilatation and efferent arteriolar constriction may also increase GFR. Other reported effects include the inhibition of both renin and aldosterone secretion and antagonism of ADH.

3. Pressure natriuresis—Even small elevations of blood pressure can result in a relatively large increase in urinary sodium excretion. Pressure diuresis appears to be independent of any known humorally or neurally mediated mechanism.

4. Sympathetic nervous system activity—Enhanced sympathetic activity increases sodium reabsorption in the proximal renal tubules, resulting in sodium retention, and mediates renal vasoconstriction, which reduces renal blood flow (Chapter 31). Conversely, stimulation of left atrial stretch receptors results in decreases in renal sympathetic tone and increases renal blood flow (cardiorenal reflex) and, potentially, glomerular filtration.

5. Glomerular filtration rate and plasma sodium concentration—The amount of sodium filtered in the kidneys is directly proportionate to the product of the GFR and plasma sodium concentration. Since GFR is generally directly proportionate to intravascular volume, intravascular volume expansion can increase sodium excretion. Conversely, intravascular volume depletion decreases sodium excretion.

6. Tubuloglomerular balance—Despite wide variations in the amount of sodium filtered in nephrons, sodium reabsorption in the proximal renal tubules is normally controlled within narrow limits. Factors considered to be responsible for tubuloglomerular balance include the rate of renal tubular flow and changes in peritubular capillary hydrostatic and oncotic pressures. Altered sodium reabsorption in the proximal tubules can have a marked effect on renal sodium excretion.

7. Antidiuretic hormone—Although ADH secretion has little effect on sodium excretion, nonosmotic secretion of this hormone (see above) can play an important part in maintaining extracellular volume with moderate to severe decreases in the "effective" intravascular volume.

Extracellular Osmoregulation Versus Volume Regulation

Osmoregulation serves to protect the normal ratio of solutes to water, whereas extracellular volume regulation serves to preserve absolute solute and water content. Differences between the two mechanisms are highlighted in Table 28–7. As noted previously, volume regulation generally takes precedence over osmoregulation.

Anesthetic Implications

Problems related to altered sodium balance are due to its manifestations as well as the underlying disorder. Disorders of sodium balance present either as hypovolemia (sodium deficit) or hypervolemia (sodium excess). Both disturbances require correction prior to elective surgical procedures. Cardiac, liver, and renal function should also be carefully evaluated in the presence of sodium excess (generally manifested as tissue edema).

Hypovolemic patients are sensitive to the vasodilating and negative inotropic effects of the volatile anesthetics, barbiturates, and agents associated with histamine release (morphine, meperidine, curare, atracurium). Dosage requirements for other drugs must also be reduced to compensate for decreases in their volume of distribution. Hypovolemic patients are especially sensitive to the sympathetic blockade of spinal and epidural anesthesia. If an anesthetic must be administered prior to complete correction of the hypovolemia, ketamine may be the induction agent of choice for general anesthesia; etomidate may be a suitable alternative.

Hypervolemia should generally be corrected preoperatively with diuretics. Abnormalities in cardiac, renal, and hepatic function should also be corrected whenever possible. The major hazard of increases in extracellular volume is impaired gas exchange due to pulmonary interstitial edema, alveolar edema, or large collections of pleural or ascitic fluid.

Table 28–7. Osmoregulation versus volume regulation.[1]

	Volume Regulation	Osmoregulation
Purpose	Control extracellular volume	Control extracellular osmolality
Mechanism	Vary renal Na^+ excretion	Vary water intake Vary renal water excretion
Sensors	Afferent renal arterioles Carotid baroreceptors Atrial stretch receptors	Hypothalamic osmoreceptors
Effectors	Renin-angiotensin-aldosterone Sympathetic nervous system Tubuloglomerular balance Renal pressure natriuresis Atrial natriuretic peptide Antidiuretic hormone	Thirst Antidiuretic hormone

[1]Adapted from Rose BD: *Clinical Physiology of Acid-Base and Electrolyte Disorders,* 3rd ed. McGraw-Hill, 1989.

DISORDERS OF POTASSIUM BALANCE

Potassium plays a major role in the electrophysiology of cell membranes (Chapter 19) as well as carbohydrate and protein synthesis (see below). The resting cell membrane potential is normally dependent on the ratio of intracellular to extracellular potassium concentrations. Intracellular potassium concentration is estimated to be 140 meq/L, while extracellular potassium concentration is normally about 4 meq/L. Although the regulation of intracellular $[K^+]$ is poorly understood, extracellular $[K^+]$ generally reflects the balance between potassium intake and excretion.

Under some conditions (see below), a redistribution of K^+ between the ECF and ICF compartments can result in marked changes in extracellular $[K^+]$ without a change in total body potassium content.

NORMAL POTASSIUM BALANCE

Dietary potassium intake averages 80 meq/d in adults (range, 40–140 meq/d), and about 70 meq of that amount is normally excreted in urine and 10 meq is lost through the gastrointestinal tract.

Renal excretion of potassium can vary from as little as 5 meq/L to over 100 meq/L. Nearly all the potassium filtered in glomeruli is normally reabsorbed in the proximal tubule and the loop of Henle. The potassium excreted in urine is the result of distal tubular secretion. Potassium secretion in the distal tubules is coupled to aldosterone-mediated reabsorption of sodium (Chapter 31).

REGULATION OF EXTRACELLULAR POTASSIUM CONCENTRATION

The major determinants of urinary potassium excretion are extracellular $[K^+]$ and aldosterone secretion. Urinary potassium excretion generally parallels its extracellular concentration. Extracellular $[K^+]$ is a major determinant of aldosterone secretion from the adrenal gland. Hyperkalemia stimulates aldosterone secretion, while hypokalemia suppresses aldosterone secretion. Renal tubular flow in the distal nephron may also be an important determinant of potassium secretion. High tubular flow rates (as during osmotic diuresis; Chapter 31) increase potassium secretion by keeping the capillary to renal tubular gradient for potassium secretion high. Conversely, slow tubular flow rates increase $[K^+]$ in tubular fluid and decrease the gradient for K^+ secretion.

INTERCOMPARTMENTAL SHIFTS OF POTASSIUM

Intercompartmental shifts of potassium are known to occur following changes in extracellular pH (Chapter 30), circulating insulin levels, circulating catecholamine activity, plasma osmolality, and possibly hypothermia. Exercise can also transiently increase plasma $[K^+]$ as a result of the release of K^+ by muscle cells; the increase in plasma $[K^+]$ (0.3–2 meq/L) is proportionate to the intensity and duration of muscle activity. Intercompartmental potassium shifts are also thought to be responsible for changes in plasma $[K^+]$ in syndromes of periodic paralysis (Chapter 37).

Changes in extracellular hydrogen ion concentration (pH) directly affect extracellular $[K^+]$. During acidosis, extracellular hydrogen ions enter cells, displacing intracellular potassium ions (Chapter 30); the movement of potassium ions out of cells maintains electrical balance but increases extracellular and plasma $[K^+]$. Conversely, during alkalosis, extracellular potassium ions move into cells to balance the movement of hydrogen ions out of cells; as a result, plasma $[K^+]$ decreases. Although the relationship can be quite variable, a useful rule of thumb is that plasma potassium concentration changes approximately 0.6 meq/L per 0.1 unit change in arterial pH.

Changes in circulating insulin levels can directly alter plasma $[K^+]$. Insulin enhances the activity of membrane-bound Na^+-K^+ ATPase, increasing cellular uptake of potassium in the liver and in skeletal muscle. In fact, insulin secretion may play an important role in the basal control of plasma potassium concentration and facilitates the handling of increased potassium loads.

Sympathetic stimulation also increases intracellular uptake of potassium by enhancing Na^+-K^+ ATPase activity. This effect is primarily mediated through activation of β_2-adrenergic receptors. Plasma $[K^+]$ often decreases following the administration of β_2-adrenergic agonists as a result of uptake of potassium by muscle and the liver. Moreover, β-adrenergic blockade can impair the handling of a potassium load in some patients.

Acute increases in plasma osmolality are reported to increase plasma $[K^+]$ (about 0.6 meq/L per 10 mosm/L). In such instances, the movement of water out of cells (down its osmotic gradient) is accompanied by movement of K^+ out of cells. The latter may be the result of "solvent drag" or the increase in intracellular $[K^+]$ that follows cellular dehydration.

Hypothermia has been reported to lower plasma $[K^+]$ as a result of cellular uptake. Rewarming reverses this shift and may result in transient hyperkalemia if potassium was given during the hypothermia.

HYPOKALEMIA

Hypokalemia is defined as plasma $[K^+]$ less than 3.5 meq/L and can occur as a result of (1) an intercompartmental shift of K^+ (see above), (2) increased potassium loss, or (3) an inadequate potassium intake (Table 28–8). Plasma potassium concentration typically correlates poorly with the total potassium deficit. A decrease in plasma $[K^+]$ from 4 meq/L to 3 meq/L usually represents a 100- to 200-meq deficit, while a plasma $[K^+]$ below 3 meq/L can represent a deficit anywhere between 200 meq and 400 meq.

Hypokalemia Due to the Intracellular Movement of Potassium

Hypokalemia due to the intracellular movement of potassium occurs with alkalosis, insulin therapy, β_2-adrenergic agonists, hypothermia, and during attacks of hypokalemic periodic paralysis (see above).

Table 28–8. Causes of hypokalemia.

Intercompartmental potassium shifts
  Alkalosis
  Insulin administration
  β_2-Adrenergic agonists
  Periodic paralysis
  Hypothermia
  Treatment of megaloblastic anemia
  Transfusion of frozen red cells
Increased potassium losses
  Renal
    Diuretics
    Increased mineralocorticoid activity
      Primary hyperaldosteronism
      Secondary hyperaldosteronism
        Edematous disorders
        Renovascular hypertension
        Renin-secreting tumor
      Mineralocorticoid tumor
      Chronic licorice ingestion
      Bartter's syndrome
      Congenital adrenal hyperplasia
        11β-Hydroxylase deficiency
        17α-Hydroxylase deficiency
      Glucocorticoid excess
    Renal tubular acidosis
    Ketoacidosis
    Salt-wasting nephropathies
    Administration of sodium with nonreabsorbable anions
      Sodium penicillins (carbenicillin)
    Hypomagnesemia
    Amphotericin B therapy
    Urinary diversion with a long ileal loop
  Extrarenal
    Gastrointestinal
      Diarrhea
      Laxative abuse
      Vomiting
      Fistula
      Urinary diversion with a ureterosigmoidostomy
    Sweat
    Dialysis
Decreased potassium intake

Hypokalemia may also be seen following transfusion of frozen red cells; these cells lose potassium in the preservation process and take up potassium following reinfusion. Cellular K^+ uptake by red blood cells (and platelets) also accounts for the hypokalemia seen in patients recently treated with folate or vitamin B_{12} for megaloblastic anemia.

Hypokalemia Due to Increased Potassium Losses

Increased potassium losses are nearly always either renal or gastrointestinal. Renal wasting of potassium is most commonly the result of a diuresis or enhanced mineralocorticoid activity. Other renal causes include hypomagnesemia (see below), renal tubular acidosis (Chapter 30), ketoacidosis, salt-wasting nephropathies, and some drug therapies (carbenicillin and amphotericin B). Increased gastrointestinal loss of potassium is most commonly due to vomiting, nasogastric suctioning, or diarrhea. Other gastrointestinal causes include fistulae, laxative abuse, villous adenomas, and pancreatic tumors secreting vasoactive intestinal peptide.

Chronic increased sweat formation occasionally causes hypokalemia, especially when potassium intake is limited. Dialysis with a low-potassium-containing dialysate solution can also cause hypokalemia. Uremic patients may actually have a total body potassium deficit (primarily intracellular) despite a normal or even high plasma concentration; the absence of hypokalemia in these instances is probably due to an intercompartmental shift from the acidosis. Dialysis in these patients unmasks the total body potassium deficit and often results in hypokalemia.

A urinary $[K^+]$ less than 20 meq/L is generally indicative of increased extrarenal losses, while concentrations greater than 20 meq/L suggest renal wasting of K^+.

Hypokalemia Due to Decreased Potassium Intake

Because of the kidney's ability to decrease urinary potassium excretion to as low as 5–20 meq/L, marked reductions in potassium intake are required to produce hypokalemia. Low potassium intakes, however, often accentuate the effects of increased potassium losses.

Effects of Hypokalemia

Hypokalemia can produce widespread organ dysfunction (Table 28–9). Most patients are asymptomatic until plasma $[K^+]$ falls below 3 meq/L. Cardiovascular effects are most prominent and include an abnormal ECG, dysrhythmias, decreased cardiac contractility, and a labile arterial blood pressure due to autonomic dysfunction. Chronic hypokalemia has also

Table 28–9. Effects of hypokalemia.[1]

Cardiovascular
  Electrocardiographic changes
  Dysrhythmias
  Myocardial dysfunction
  Myocardial fibrosis
  Orthostatic hypotension
Neuromuscular
  Skeletal muscle weakness
  Tetany
  Rhabdomyolysis
  Ileus
Renal
  Polyuria (nephrogenic DI)
  Increased ammonia production
  Increased bicarbonate reabsorption
  Increased Na^+ retention
  Tubulointerstitial nephropathy (fibrosis)
Hormonal
  Decreased insulin secretion
  Decreased growth hormone secretion
  Decreased aldosterone secretion
Metabolic
  Negative nitrogen balance
  Encephalopathy in patients with liver disease

[1] Adapted from Schrier RW (editor): *Renal and Electrolyte Disorders,* 3rd ed. Little, Brown, 1986.

been reported to cause myocardial fibrosis. Electrocardiographic manifestations include T wave flattening, an increasingly prominent U wave, ST segment depression, increased P wave amplitude, and prolongation of the PR interval (Figure 28–5). Increased myocardial cell automaticity and delayed repolarization promote both atrial and ventricular dysrhythmias.

Neuromuscular effects of hypokalemia include skeletal muscle weakness, ileus, muscle cramping, tetany, and, rarely, rhabdomyolysis. Renal dysfunction is also common and typically includes impaired concentrating ability (resistance to ADH, resulting in polyuria), sodium retention, increased bicarbonate reabsorption often resulting in alkalosis, and increased production of ammonia resulting in impairment of urinary acidification. Increased ammonia production represents intracellular acidosis; hydrogen ions move intracellularly to compensate for intracellular potassium losses. The resulting metabolic alkalosis, together with increased ammonia production, can precipitate encephalopathy in patients with advanced liver disease. Chronic hypokalemia has been associated with renal fibrosis (tubulointerstitial nephropathy).

Hypokalemia can impair insulin secretion and perhaps antagonizes its peripheral effects, often leading to hyperglycemia even in nondiabetic individuals. Altered protein metabolism during chronic hypokalemia has also been reported to produce a negative nitrogen balance.

Treatment of Hypokalemia

The treatment of hypokalemia depends on the presence and severity of any associated organ dysfunction. Significant electrocardiographic changes such as ST segment changes or dysrhythmias mandate continuous electrocardiographic monitoring, especially during intravenous K^+ replacement. Digoxin therapy—as well as the hypokalemia itself—sensitizes the heart to changes in potassium ion concentration. Muscle strength should also be periodically assessed in patients with weakness.

Oral replacement with potassium chloride solutions is generally safest (60–80 meq/d). Replacement of the potassium deficit usually requires several days. Intravenous replacement should be reserved for patients with serious cardiac manifestations or muscle weakness. The goal of intravenous therapy is to remove the patient from immediate danger and not necessarily to correct the entire potassium deficit. Peripheral intravenous replacement should not exceed 8 meq/h because of the irritative effect of potassium on peripheral veins. Dextrose-containing solutions should generally be avoided, because the resulting hyperglycemia and secondary insulin secretion may actually lower plasma $[K^+]$ even further. Faster intravenous replacement (10–20 meq/h) requires a central venous catheter and close electrocardiographic monitoring. Higher replacement rates may be safest through a femoral catheter, because very high localized K^+ concentrations may occur within the heart with standard central ven-

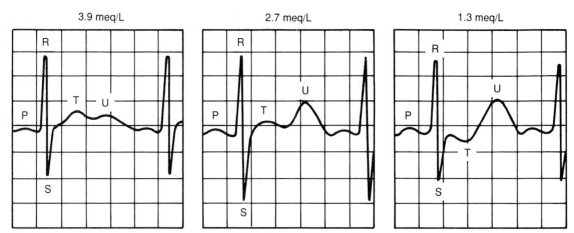

Figure 28–5. Electrocardiographic effects of hypokalemia. Note progressive flattening of the T wave, an increasingly prominent U wave, increased amplitude of the P wave, prolongation of the PR interval, and ST segment depression.

ous catheters. Intravenous replacement should generally not exceed 240 meq/d.

Potassium chloride is the preferred potassium salt when a metabolic alkalosis is also present because it also corrects the chloride deficit. Potassium bicarbonate or equivalent (K^+ acetate or K^+ citrate) is preferable for patients with metabolic acidosis. Potassium phosphate is a suitable alternative with concomitant hypophosphatemia (diabetic ketoacidosis).

Anesthetic Considerations

Hypokalemia is a common preoperative finding. This decision to proceed with elective surgery is often arbitrarily based on lower limits somewhere between 3 and 3.5 meq/L. The decision, however, should be based also on the rate at which the hypokalemia developed as well as the presence or absence of secondary organ dysfunction. In general, chronic mild hypokalemia (3–3.5 meq/L) without electrocardiographic changes does not appear to substantially increase anesthetic risk. The latter may not apply to patients receiving digoxin, who may be at increased risk of developing digoxin toxicity from the hypokalemia; plasma $[K^+]$ values above 4 meq/L are desirable in such patients.

The intraoperative management of hypokalemia requires vigilant electrocardiographic monitoring. Intravenous potassium should be given if atrial or ventricular dysrhythmias develop. Glucose-free intravenous solutions should be used and hyperventilation avoided to prevent further decreases in plasma $[K^+]$. Increased sensitivity to muscle relaxants may be seen in some patients. Dosages of muscle relaxants should therefore be reduced 25–50%, and a nerve stimulator should be used to follow the degree of paralysis and the adequacy of reversal.

HYPERKALEMIA

Hyperkalemia exists when plasma $[K^+]$ exceeds 5.5 meq/L. Hyperkalemia rarely occurs in normal in-

dividuals because of the kidney's tremendous capacity to excrete potassium. When potassium intake is increased slowly, the kidneys can excrete as much as 500 meq of K^+ per day. The sympathetic system and insulin secretion also appear to play important roles in preventing acute increases in plasma $[K^+]$ following potassium loads.

Hyperkalemia can result from (1) an intercompartmental shift of potassium ions, (2) decreased urinary excretion of potassium, or, rarely, (3) an increased potassium intake (Table 28–10). Hyperkalemia can also be spurious. Falsely elevated plasma potassium levels may be measured if the red cells hemolyze in a blood specimen (most commonly due to prolonged application of a tourniquet while obtaining a venous sample). In vitro release of potassium from white cells in a blood specimen can also falsely increase the measured plasma $[K^+]$ when the leukocyte count exceeds $70,000/\mu L$. A similar release of potassium from platelets occurs when the platelet count exceeds $1,000,000/\mu L$.

Hyperkalemia Due to Extracellular Movement of Potassium

Movement of K^+ out of cells can be seen with succinylcholine administration, acidosis, cell lysis following chemotherapy, rhabdomyolysis, hyperosmolality, digitalis overdoses, arginine hydrochloride administration, β_2-adrenergic blockade, and during episodes of hyperkalemic periodic paralysis. The average increase in plasma $[K^+]$ of 0.5 meq/L following succinylcholine can be exaggerated following large burns or severe muscle trauma and in patients with spinal cord injuries (Chapter 9). Beta$_2$-adrenergic blockade accentuates the increase in plasma $[K^+]$ that occurs following exercise. Digitalis inhibits Na^+-K^+ ATPase in cell membranes; digitalis overdose has been reported to cause hyperkalemia in some patients. Arginine hydrochloride, which is used to treat metabolic alkalosis, can cause hyperkalemia as the cationic arginine ions enter cells and potassium ions move out to maintain electroneutrality.

Table 28–10. Causes of hyperkalemia.

Pseudohyperkalemia
  In vitro red cell hemolysis
  Marked leukocytosis
  Marked thrombocytosis
Intercompartmental shifts
  Acidosis
  Hypertonicity
  Tissue breakdown
  Rhabdomyolysis
  Severe exercise
  β_2-Adrenergic blockade
  Periodic paralysis
  Succinylcholine
  Digitalis overdose
  Arginine HCl
Decreased renal potassium excretion
  Renal failure
  Decreased mineralocorticoid activity
    Primary adrenal insufficiency
      Addison's disease
      Bilateral adrenalectomies
    Congenital adrenal hyperplasia
      21-Hydroxylase enzyme deficiency
    Hyporeninemic hypoaldosteronism
    Acquired immunodeficiency syndrome
    Competitive potassium-sparing diuretics
      Spironolactone
    ACE inhibitors
    Cyclosporine
    Nonsteroidal anti-inflammatory drugs
    Heparin
  Isolated decreased potassium secretion in distal nephron
    Pseudohypoaldosteronism
    Noncompetitive potassium-sparing diuretics
      Amiloride
      Triamterine
    Sickle cell disease
    Renal allograft
    Systemic lupus erythematosus
    Urinary obstruction
Increased potassium intake
  Transfusion of old whole blood
  Salt substitutes
  Potassium penicillin

Hyperkalemia Due to Decreased Renal Excretion of Potassium

Decreased renal excretion of potassium can result from (1) marked reductions in glomerular filtration, (2) decreased aldosterone activity, or (3) a defect in potassium secretion in the distal nephron.

Glomerular filtration rates less than 5 mL/min are nearly always associated with hyperkalemia. Patients with lesser degrees of renal impairment can also readily develop hyperkalemia when faced with increased potassium loads (dietary, catabolic, or iatrogenic).

Decreased aldosterone activity can result from a primary defect in adrenal hormone synthesis or a defect in the renin-aldosterone system. Patients with primary adrenal insufficiency (Addison's disease) and those with isolated 21-hydroxylase adrenal enzyme deficiency have marked impairment of aldosterone synthesis. Patients with the syndrome of isolated hypoaldosteronism (also called hyporeninemic hypoaldosteronism, or type IV renal tubular acidosis) are usually diabetics with some degree of renal impairment; they appear to

have an impaired ability to increase aldosterone secretion in response to hyperkalemia. Although usually asymptomatic, these patients develop hyperkalemia with increased potassium intakes or when given potassium-sparing diuretics. They also often have varying degrees of Na^+ wasting and a hyperchloremic metabolic acidosis. Similar findings have been reported in some patients with AIDS.

Drugs interfering with the renin-aldosterone system have the potential to cause hyperkalemia, especially in the presence of any degree of renal impairment. Nonsteroidal anti-inflammatory agents (with the possible exception of sulindac) inhibit prostaglandin-mediated renin release. Angiotensin-converting enzyme (ACE) inhibitors interfere with angiotensin II-mediated release of aldosterone. Large doses of heparin can interfere with aldosterone secretion. The potassium-sparing diuretic spironolactone directly antagonizes aldosterone activity at the kidneys. The mechanism for cyclosporine-induced hyporeninemic hypoaldosteronism is not clear.

Decreased renal excretion of potassium can also occur as a result of an intrinsic or acquired defect in the distal nephron's ability to secrete potassium. Such defects may occur even in the presence of normal renal function and are characteristically unresponsive to mineralocorticoid therapy. The kidneys of patients with pseudohypoaldosteronism display an intrinsic resistance to aldosterone. Acquired defects have been associated with systemic lupus erythematosus, sickle cell anemia, obstructive uropathies, and cyclosporine nephropathy in transplanted kidneys.

Hyperkalemia Due to Increased Potassium Intake

Increased potassium loads rarely cause hyperkalemia in normal individuals unless large amounts are given rapidly and intravenously. Hyperkalemia, however, may be seen when potassium intake is increased in patients receiving β_2-adrenergic blockers or those with renal impairment or insulin deficiency. Unrecognized sources of potassium include potassium penicillin, sodium substitutes (primarily potassium salts), and transfusion of old whole blood. The plasma $[K^+]$ in a unit of whole blood can be increased by as much as 30 meq/L after 21 days of storage. The risk of hyperkalemia from multiple transfusions is reduced by minimizing the volume of plasma given through the use of packed red blood cell transfusions.

Effects of Hyperkalemia

The most important effects of hyperkalemia are on skeletal and cardiac muscle. Skeletal muscle weakness is generally not seen until plasma $[K^+]$ is greater than 8 meq/L. The weakness is due to sustained spontaneous depolarization of the muscle membrane (similar to succinylcholine), eventually resulting in ascending paralysis. Cardiac manifestations (Figure 28–6) are usually consistently present when plasma $[K^+]$ is greater than 7 meq/L. Electrocardiographic changes characteristically progress (in order) from symmetrically

3.6 meq/L　　　　　　6.8 meq/L　　　　　　8.4 meq/L

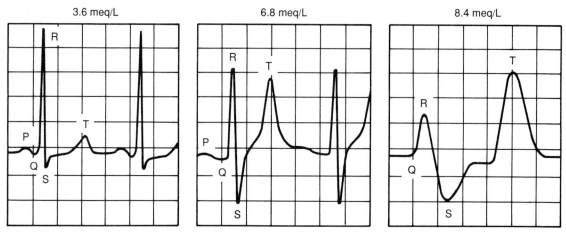

Figure 28–6. Electrocardiographic effect of hyperkalemia. Electrocardiographic changes characteristically progress from symmetrically peaked T waves, often with a shortened QT interval, to widening of the QRS complex, prolongation of the PR interval, loss of the P wave, loss of R wave amplitude, and ST segment depression (occasionally elevation)—to an ECG that resembles a sine wave—before final progression into ventricular fibrillation or asystole.

peaked T waves (often with a shortened QT interval) → widening of the QRS complex → prolongation of the PR interval → loss of the P wave → loss of R wave amplitude → ST segment depression (occasionally elevation) → an ECG that resembles a sine wave— before progression to ventricular fibrillation and asystole. Contractility appears to be relatively well preserved. Hypocalcemia, hyponatremia, and acidosis accentuate the cardiac effects of hyperkalemia.

Treatment of Hyperkalemia

Because of its lethal potential, hyperkalemia exceeding 6 meq/L should always be treated. Treatment is directed at reversing cardiac manifestations, skeletal muscle weakness, and restoration of plasma [K$^+$] to normal. The number of treatment modalities employed (see below) depends on the severity of manifestations as well as the cause of hyperkalemia. Hyperkalemia associated with hypoaldosteronism can be treated with mineralocorticoid replacement. Drugs contributing to hyperkalemia should be discontinued and sources of increased potassium intake reduced or stopped.

Calcium (5–10 mL of 10% calcium gluconate or 3–5 mL of 10% calcium chloride) partially antagonizes the cardiac effects of hyperkalemia and is useful in patients with marked hyperkalemia. Its effects are rapid but unfortunately short-lived. Care must be exercised in patients taking digoxin, since calcium potentiates digoxin toxicity.

When metabolic acidosis is present, intravenous sodium bicarbonate (usually 45 meq) will promote cellular uptake of potassium and can decrease plasma [K$^+$] within 15 minutes. An intravenous infusion of glucose and insulin (25 g of glucose per 10 units of insulin) may be more effective than NaHCO$_3$ in promoting cellular uptake of potassium and lowering plasma [K$^+$], but it takes up to 1 hour for peak effect to occur.

For patients with some renal function, furosemide is a useful adjunct in increasing urinary excretion of po-

tassium. In the absence of renal function, elimination of excess potassium can only be accomplished with nonabsorbable cation exchange resins such as oral or rectal sodium polystyrene sulfonate (Kayexalate). Each gram of resin binds up to 1 meq of K$^+$ and releases 1.5 meq of Na$^+$.

Dialysis is indicated in symptomatic patients with severe or refractory hyperkalemia. Hemodialysis is faster and more effective than peritoneal dialysis in decreasing plasma [K$^+$]. Maximal potassium removal with hemodialysis approaches 50 meq/h, compared with 10–15 meq/h for peritoneal dialysis.

Anesthetic Considerations

Elective surgery should not be undertaken in patients with hyperkalemia. Anesthetic management of hyperkalemic surgical patients is directed at both lowering the plasma potassium concentration and preventing any further increases. The ECG should be carefully monitored. Succinylcholine is contraindicated, as is the use of any potassium-containing intravenous solutions such as lactated Ringer's injection. The avoidance of metabolic or respiratory acidosis is critical to prevent further increases in plasma [K$^+$]. Ventilation should be controlled under general anesthesia; mild hyperventilation may even be desirable. Lastly, neuromuscular function should be monitored closely, since hyperkalemia can accentuate the effects of muscle relaxants.

DISORDERS OF CALCIUM BALANCE

Calcium ions are involved in nearly all essential biologic functions, including muscle contraction, the release of neurotransmitters and hormones, blood coagulation, and bone metabolism. It is not surprising that abnormalities in calcium balance can result in profound physiologic derangements.

NORMAL CALCIUM BALANCE

Calcium intake in adults averages 600–800 mg/d. Intestinal absorption of calcium occurs primarily in the small bowel but is quite variable. Up to 80% of the daily calcium intake is normally lost in feces.

The kidneys are responsible for calcium excretion. Renal calcium excretion averages 100 mg/d but can be varied from as low as 50 mg/d to over 300 mg/d. Normally, 98% of the filterable calcium is reabsorbed. Calcium reabsorption parallels that of sodium in the proximal renal tubules and the ascending loop of Henle. In the distal tubules, however, calcium reabsorption is dependent on parathyroid hormone secretion, while sodium reabsorption is dependent on aldosterone secretion. Increased parathyroid hormone levels enhance distal calcium reabsorption and decrease urinary calcium excretion.

Plasma Calcium Concentration

The normal plasma calcium concentration is 8.5–10.5 mg/dL (2.1–2.6 mmol/L). Approximately, 50% is in the free ionized form, 40% is protein-bound (mainly to albumin), and 10% is complexed with anions such as citrate and amino acids. It is the free ionized calcium concentration ($[Ca^{2+}]$) that is physiologically most important. Plasma $[Ca^{2+}]$ is normally 4.5–5 mg/dL (2.2–2.5 meq/L or 1.1–1.25 mmol/L). Changes in plasma albumin concentration affect total but not ionized calcium concentrations: for each increase or decrease of 1 g/dL in albumin, the total plasma calcium concentration increases or decreases approximately 0.8 mg/dL, respectively.

Changes in plasma pH directly affect the degree of protein binding and thus ionized calcium concentration. Ionized calcium increases approximately 0.16 mg/dL for each decrease of 0.1 unit in plasma pH and decreases by the same amount for each 0.1 unit increase in pH.

Regulation of Extracellular Ionized Calcium Concentration

Ninety-nine percent of total body calcium is contained within bone; of that amount, only 0.5–1% is exchangeable with extracellular calcium. Extracellular $[Ca^{2+}]$ is closely regulated by three hormones: parathyroid hormone, vitamin D, and calcitonin. These hormones act primarily on bone, the distal renal tubules, and the small bowel.

PTH is the most important regulator of plasma $[Ca^{2+}]$. Decreases in plasma $[Ca^{2+}]$ stimulate PTH secretion, while increases in plasma $[Ca^{2+}]$ inhibit PTH secretion. The calcemic effect of parathyroid hormone is due to (1) mobilization of calcium from bone, (2) enhancement of calcium reabsorption in the distal

renal tubules, and (3) an indirect increase in intestinal absorption of calcium via acceleration of 1,25-dihydroxycholecalciferol synthesis in the kidneys (see below).

Vitamin D exists in several forms in the body, but 1,25-dihydroxycholecalciferol has the most important biologic activity. It is the product of the metabolic conversion of (primarily endogenous) cholecalciferol, first by the liver to 25-cholecalciferol and then by the kidneys to 1,25-dihydroxycholecalciferol. The latter transformation is enhanced by secretion of parathyroid hormone as well as hypophosphatemia. Vitamin D augments intestinal absorption of calcium, facilitates the action of parathyroid hormone on bone, and appears to augment renal reabsorption of calcium in the distal tubules.

Calcitonin is a polypeptide hormone that is secreted by parafollicular cells in the thyroid gland. Its secretion is stimulated by hypercalcemia and inhibited by hypocalcemia. Calcitonin inhibits bone reabsorption and increases urinary calcium excretion.

HYPERCALCEMIA

Hypercalcemia can occur as a result of a variety of disorders (Table 28–11). In primary hyperparathyroidism, parathyroid hormone secretion is increased and independent of $[Ca^{2+}]$. In contrast, in secondary hyperparathyroidism (chronic renal failure or malabsorption), the elevated parathyroid hormone levels are in response to chronic hypocalcemia (Chapter 32). Prolonged secondary hyperparathyroidism, however, can occasionally result in autonomous secretion of PTH, resulting in a normal or elevated $[Ca^{2+}]$ (tertiary hyperparathyroidism).

Patients with cancer can present with hypercalcemia whether or not bone metastases are present. Direct bony destruction or secretion of humoral mediators of hypercalcemia (PTH-like substances, osteoclast factors, or prostaglandins) is probably responsible in most patients. Hypercalcemia due to increased turnover of calcium from bone can also be encountered in patients

Table 28–11. Causes of hypercalcemia.

Hyperparathyroidism
Primary
Tertiary
Malignancy
Excessive vitamin D intake
Excessive vitamin A intake
Paget's disease of bone
Granulomatous disorders
Sarcoidosis
Tuberculosis
Chronic immobilization
Milk-alkali syndrome
Hyperthyroidism
Adrenal insufficiency
Drug-induced
Thiazide diuretics
Lithium

with benign conditions such as Paget's disease and chronic immobilization. Increased gastrointestinal absorption of calcium can lead to hypercalcemia in patients with the milk-alkali syndrome (marked increase in calcium intake), hypervitaminosis D, or granulomatous diseases (enhanced sensitivity to vitamin D). The mechanisms responsible for other causes of hypercalcemia are poorly understood.

Effects of Hypercalcemia

Hypercalcemia often produces anorexia, nausea, vomiting, weakness, and polyuria. Ataxia, irritability, lethargy, or confusion can rapidly progress to coma. Hypertension is often present initially before hypovolemia supervenes. Electrocardiographic signs include a shortened ST segment and a shortened QT interval. Hypercalcemia increases cardiac sensitivity to digitalis. Pancreatitis, peptic ulcer disease, and renal failure can also complicate hypercalcemia.

Treatment of Hypercalcemia

Symptomatic hypercalcemia requires rapid treatment. The most effective treatment is establishment of a brisk diuresis (urinary output 200–300 mL/h) with an intravenous saline infusion and a loop diuretic to accelerate calcium excretion. Dialysis may be necessary in the presence of renal or cardiac failure. Additional treatment depends on the cause and may include glucocorticoids, calcitonin, plicamycin (mithramycin), or phosphates.

Anesthetic Considerations

Hypercalcemia is a medical emergency and should be corrected, if possible, prior to administration of any anesthetic. Ionized calcium levels should be monitored closely. If surgery must be performed, saline diuresis should be continued intraoperatively with great care to avoid hypovolemia; central venous or pulmonary artery pressure monitoring may be advisable for patients with decreased cardiac reserve. Serial measurements of $[K^+]$ and $[Mg^{2+}]$ are helpful in detecting iatrogenic hypokalemia and hypomagnesemia. Responses to anesthetic agents are not predictable. Ventilation should be controlled under general anesthesia. Acidosis should be avoided so as not to raise plasma $[Ca^{2+}]$ any further.

HYPOCALCEMIA

Hypocalcemia should be diagnosed only on the basis of the plasma ionized calcium concentration. When direct measurements of plasma $[Ca^{2+}]$ are not available, the total calcium concentration must be corrected for decreases in plasma albumin concentration (see above). The causes of hypocalcemia are listed in Table 28–12.

Hypocalcemia due to hypoparathyroidism is a relatively common cause of symptomatic hypocalcemia. Hypoparathyroidism may be surgical, idiopathic, part of multiple endocrine defects (most often with adrenal

Table 28–12. Causes of hypocalcemia.

Hypoparathyroidism
  Surgical
  Idiopathic
  Infiltrative disease
  Hypomagnesemia
  Sepsis
  Burns
Pseudohypoparathyroidism
Vitamin D deficiency
  Nutritional
  Malabsorption
    Postsurgical (gastrectomy, short bowel)
    Inflammatory bowel disease
    Chronic pancreatitis
    Biliary cirrhosis
  Altered vitamin D metabolism
    Inherited defects
    Renal insufficiency
    Hepatic failure
    Drug induced (phenobarbital, phenytoin)
Hyperphosphatemia
Precipitation of calcium
  Pancreatitis
  Rhabdomyolysis
  Fat embolism
Chelation of calcium
  Multiple transfusions
    Liver disease
    Renal disease
    Hypothermia
  Rapid infusion of large amounts of albumin

insufficiency), or associated with hypomagnesemia. Magnesium deficiency is postulated to impair the secretion of PTH and antagonize its effects on bone. Hypocalcemia during sepsis is also thought to be due to suppression of parathyroid hormone release. Hyperphosphatemia (see below) is also a relatively common cause of hypocalcemia, especially in patients with chronic renal failure. Hypocalcemia due to vitamin D deficiency may be the result of a markedly reduced intake (nutritional), vitamin D malabsorption, or abnormal vitamin D metabolism.

Chelation of calcium ions with the citrate ions in blood preservatives is an important cause of perioperative hypocalcemia; similar transient decreases in $[Ca^{2+}]$ are also theoretically possible following rapid infusions of large volumes of albumin. Hypocalcemia following acute pancreatitis is thought to be due to precipitation of calcium with fats (soaps) following the release of lipolytic enzymes and fat necrosis; hypocalcemia following fat embolism may have a similar basis. Precipitation of calcium (in injured muscle) may also be seen following rhabdomyolysis.

Less common causes of hypocalcemia include calcitonin-secreting medullary carcinomas of the thyroid, osteoblastic metastatic disease (breast and prostate cancer), and pseudohypoparathyroidism (familial unresponsiveness to parathyroid hormone).

Effects of Hypocalcemia

Manifestations include paresthesias, confusion, laryngeal stridor (laryngospasm), carpopedal spasm

(Trousseau's sign), masseter spasm (Chvostek's sign), and seizures. Biliary colic and bronchospasm have also been described. Cardiac irritability can lead to dysrhythmias. Decreased cardiac contractility may result in heart failure, hypotension, or both. Decreased responsiveness to digitalis and β-adrenergic agonists have also been reported. Electrocardiographic signs include prolongation of the QT interval. The severity of electrocardiographic manifestations does not necessarily correlate with the degree of hypocalcemia.

Treatment of Hypocalcemia

Symptomatic hypocalcemia is a medical emergency and should be treated immediately with intravenous calcium chloride (3–5 mL of a 10% solution) or calcium gluconate (10–20 mL of a 10% solution). (Ten milliliters of 10% $CaCl_2$ contains 272 mg of Ca^{2+}, whereas 10 mL of 10% calcium gluconate contains only 93 mg of Ca^{2+}). To avoid precipitation, intravenous calcium should not be given with bicarbonate- or phosphate-containing solutions. Serial ionized calcium measurements are mandatory. Repeat boluses or a continuous infusion (Ca^{2+} 1–2 mg/kg/h) may be necessary. Plasma magnesium concentration should be checked to exclude hypomagnesemia. In chronic hypocalcemia, oral calcium ($CaCO_3$) and vitamin D replacement are usually necessary. Treatment for hyperphosphatemia is discussed below.

Anesthetic Considerations

Hypocalcemia should be corrected preoperatively. Serial ionized calcium levels should be monitored intraoperatively in patients with a history of hypocalcemia. Alkalosis should be avoided to prevent further decreases in $[Ca^{2+}]$. Intravenous calcium may be necessary following rapid transfusions of citrated blood products or large volumes of albumin solutions (Chapter 29). Potentiation of the negative inotropic effects of barbiturates and volatile anesthetics should be expected. Responses to muscle relaxants are inconsistent and require close monitoring with a nerve stimulator.

DISORDERS OF PHOSPHORUS BALANCE

Phosphorus is an important intracellular constituent. Its presence is required for the synthesis of (1) the phospholipids and phosphoproteins in cell membranes and intracellular organelles, (2) the phosphonucleotides involved in protein synthesis and reproduction, and (3) ATP used for the storage of energy.

NORMAL PHOSPHORUS BALANCE

Phosphorus intake averages 800–1500 mg/d in adults. About 80% of that amount is normally ab-sorbed in the proximal small bowel. The kidneys are the major route for phosphorus excretion and are responsible for regulating total body phosphorus content. Urinary excretion of phosphorus depends on both intake and plasma concentration. Parathyroid hormone secretion can augment urinary phosphorus excretion by inhibiting its proximal tubular reabsorption. The latter effect may be offset by PTH-induced release of phosphate from bone.

Plasma Phosphorus Concentration

Plasma phosphorus exists in both organic and inorganic forms. Organic phosphorus is mainly in the form of phospholipids. Of the inorganic phosphorus fraction, 80% is filterable in the kidneys, while 20% is protein-bound. The majority of inorganic phosphorus is in the form of $H_2PO_4^-$ and HPO_4^{2-}. By convention, plasma phosphorus is measured as milligrams of elemental phosphorus. Normal plasma phosphorus concentration is 2.5–4.5 mg/dL (0.8–1.45 mmol/L) in adults and up to 6 mg/dL in children. Plasma phosphorus concentration is usually measured during fasting, because a recent carbohydrate intake transiently decreases the plasma phosphorus concentration. Plasma phosphorus concentration has important effects on vitamin D formation. Hypophosphatemia increases vitamin D production, while hyperphosphatemia depresses it. The latter plays an important role in the genesis of secondary hyperparathyroidism in patients with chronic renal failure (Chapter 32).

HYPERPHOSPHATEMIA

Hyperphosphatemia may be seen with increased phosphorus intakes (abuse of phosphate laxatives or excessive potassium phosphate administration), decreased phosphorus excretion (renal insufficiency), or massive cell lysis (following chemotherapy for lymphoma or leukemia).

Effects of Hyperphosphatemia

Although hyperphosphatemia itself does not appear to be directly responsible for any functional disturbances, its secondary effect on plasma $[Ca^{2+}]$ can be important. Marked hyperphosphatemia is thought to lower plasma $[Ca^{2+}]$ by precipitation and deposition of calcium phosphate in bone and soft tissues.

Treatment of Hyperphosphatemia

Hyperphosphatemia is generally treated with phosphate-binding antacids such as aluminum hydroxide or aluminum carbonate.

Anesthetic Considerations

While specific interactions between hyperphosphatemia and anesthesia are generally not described, renal function should be carefully evaluated (Chapter 32). Secondary hypocalcemia should also be excluded.

HYPOPHOSPHATEMIA

Hypophosphatemia is usually the result of either a negative phosphorus balance or cellular uptake of extracellular phosphorus (an intercompartmental shift). Intercompartmental shifts of phosphorus can occur during alkalosis and following carbohydrate ingestion or insulin administration. Large doses of aluminum- or magnesium-containing antacids, severe burns, inadequate phosphorus supplementation during hyperalimentation, diabetic ketoacidosis, alcohol withdrawal, and prolonged respiratory alkalosis can all produce a negative phosphorus balance and lead to severe hypophosphatemia. In contrast to respiratory alkalosis, metabolic alkalosis rarely leads to severe hypophosphatemia.

Effects of Hypophosphatemia

Mild to moderate hypophosphatemia (1.5–2.5 mg/dL) is generally asymptomatic. In contrast, severe hypophosphatemia (< 1.5 mg/dL) is often associated with widespread organ dysfunction. Cardiomyopathy, a decreased 2,3-diphosphoglycerate level leading to impaired oxygen delivery, hemolysis, impaired leukocyte function, platelet dysfunction, encephalopathy, skeletal muscle myopathy, respiratory failure, rhabdomyolysis, metabolic acidosis, and hepatic dysfunction have all been associated with severe hypophosphatemia.

Treatment of Hypophosphatemia

Because of the risk of hypocalcemia and metastatic calcification, oral phosphorus replacement is preferable to parenteral replacement. Potassium or sodium phosphate (2–5 mg of elemental phosphorus per kilogram, or 15–45 mmol slowly over 6–12 hours) is generally used for intravenous correction of severe symptomatic hypophosphatemia.

Anesthetic Considerations

Anesthetic management of patients with hypophosphatemia requires familiarity with its complications (see above). Hyperglycemia and respiratory alkalosis should be avoided to prevent further decreases in plasma phosphorus concentration. Neuromuscular function must be monitored carefully when muscle relaxants are given. Some patients with severe hypophosphatemia may require mechanical ventilation postoperatively.

DISORDERS OF MAGNESIUM BALANCE

Magnesium is an important intracellular cation that functions as a cofactor in many enzyme pathways.

Only 2% of total body magnesium stores are in the ECF compartment; the remainder is distributed between bone (67%), muscle (20%), and other tissues (11%).

NORMAL MAGNESIUM BALANCE

Magnesium intake averages 20–30 meq/d (240–370 mg/d) in adults. Of that amount, only 30–40% is absorbed, mainly in the distal small bowel. Renal excretion is the primary route for elimination, averaging 6–12 meq/d. Nearly all magnesium reabsorption occurs in the thick ascending limb of the loop of Henle. Factors known to increase magnesium reabsorption in the kidneys include hypomagnesemia, parathyroid hormone, hypocalcemia, ECF depletion, and metabolic alkalosis. Factors known to increase renal excretion include hypermagnesemia, acute volume expansion, hypercalcemia, ketoacidosis, diuretics, phosphate depletion, and alcohol ingestion.

Plasma Magnesium Concentration

Plasma [Mg^{2+}] is closely regulated between 1.5 and 2.1 meq/L (0.7–1 mmol/L). Although the exact mechanisms involved remain unclear, they involve interaction of the gastrointestinal tract (absorption), bone (storage), and the kidneys (excretion).

HYPERMAGNESEMIA

Increases in plasma [Mg^{2+}] are nearly always due to excessive intake (magnesium-containing antacids or laxatives), renal impairment (GFR < 30 mL/min), or both. Iatrogenic hypermagnesemia can also occur during magnesium sulfate therapy for gestational hypertension. Less common causes include adrenal insufficiency, hypothyroidism, and lithium administration.

Effects of Hypermagnesemia

Symptomatic hypermagnesemia typically presents with neurologic, neuromuscular, or cardiac manifestations. Hyporeflexia, sedation, and skeletal muscle weakness are characteristic features. Hypermagnesemia appears to impair the release of acetylcholine and decreases motor end-plate sensitivity to acetylcholine in muscle. Vasodilatation and myocardial depression can lead to hypotension. Electrocardiographic signs are inconsistent but often include prolongation of the PR interval and widening of the QRS complex. Marked hypermagnesemia can lead to respiratory arrest.

Treatment of Hypermagnesemia

All sources of magnesium intake (most often antacids) should be stopped. Intravenous calcium (1 g calcium gluconate) can temporarily antagonize most of the effects of hypermagnesemia. A loop diuretic along with an infusion of 0.5-normal saline in 5%

dextrose enhances urinary magnesium excretion. Diuresis with normal saline is generally not recommended to lessen the likelihood of iatrogenic hypocalcemia, because the latter potentiates the effects of hypermagnesemia. Dialysis may be necessary in patients with marked renal impairment.

Anesthetic Considerations

Hypermagnesemia requires close monitoring of the ECG, blood pressure, and neuromuscular function. Potentiation of the vasodilating and negative inotropic properties of anesthetics should be expected. Dosages of muscle relaxants should be reduced by 25–50%. A urinary catheter is required when a diuretic and saline infusions are used to enhance magnesium excretion (see above). Serial measurements of $[Ca^{2+}]$ and $[Mg^{2+}]$ may be useful.

HYPOMAGNESEMIA

Hypomagnesemia is a common and frequently overlooked problem, especially in critically ill patients. Deficiencies of magnesium are generally the result of inadequate intake, reduced gastrointestinal absorption, or increased renal excretion (Table 28–13).

Effects of Hypomagnesemia

Most patients with hypomagnesemia are asymptomatic, but weakness, fasciculation, paresthesias, confusion, ataxia, and seizures may be encountered. Cardiac manifestations include electrical irritability and potentiation of digoxin toxicity. Prolongation of the PR and QT intervals may also be present. Hypomagnesemia is frequently associated with both hypocalcemia (impaired parathyroid hormone secretion) and hypokalemia (due to renal K^+ wasting). The effects of concomitant hypocalcemia often predominate (see above).

Treatment of Hypomagnesemia

Asymptomatic hypomagnesemia can be treated orally (magnesium oxide) or intramuscularly (magnesium sulfate). Serious manifestations such as seizures should be treated with intravenous magnesium sulfate, 1–2 g (8–16 meq) given slowly over 15 minutes.

Anesthetic Considerations

Although no specific anesthetic interactions are described, coexistent electrolyte disturbances such as hypocalcemia and hypokalemia are often present and should be corrected prior to surgery (see above). Isolated hypomagnesemia should also be corrected prior to elective procedures because of its potential for causing cardiac dysrhythmias.

CASE DISCUSSION: ELECTROLYTE ABNORMALITIES FOLLOWING URINARY DIVERSION

A 70-year-old man with carcinoma of the bladder presents for radical cystectomy and ileal loop urinary diversion. He weighs 70 kg and has a 20-year history of hypertension. Preoperative laboratory measurements revealed normal plasma electrolyte concentrations and a BUN of 20 mg/dL with a serum creatinine of 1.5 mg/dL. The operation lasts 4 hours and is performed under uncomplicated general anesthesia. The estimated blood loss is 900 mL. Fluid replacement consists of 3500 mL of lactated Ringer's injection and 750 mL of 5% albumin.

One hour after admission to the recovery room, the patient is awake, his blood pressure is 130/70 mm Hg, and he appears to be breathing well (18 breaths/min, $FiO_2 = 0.4$). Urinary output has been only 20 mL in the last hour. Laboratory measurements are as follows: Hb 10.4 g/dL, plasma Na^+ 133 meq/L, K^+ 3.8 meq/L, Cl^- 104 meq/L, total CO_2 20 mmol/L, PaO_2 156 mm Hg, arterial blood pH 7.29, $PaCO_2$ 38 mm Hg, and calculated HCO_3^- 18 meq/L.

What is the most likely explanation for the hyponatremia?

Multiple factors tend to promote hyponatremia postoperatively, including nonosmotic ADH secretion (surgical stress, hypovolemia, and pain), large evap-

Table 28–13. Causes of hypomagnesemia.

Inadequate intake
Nutritional
    Prolonged fasting
Hyperalimentation
Reduced gastrointestinal absorption
Malabsorption syndromes
Small bowel or biliary fistulas
Prolonged nasogastric suctioning
Severe diarrhea
Increased renal losses
Diuresis
    Sodium load
    Hyperglycemia
    Diuretics (osmotic and loop diuretics)
    Hypercalciuria
Diabetic ketoacidosis
Hyperparathyroidism
Hyperaldosteronism
Hypophosphatemia
Drugs
    Cisplatin
    Aminoglycosides
    Amphotericin B
    Alcohol
Postobstructive diuresis
Multifactorial
Chronic alcoholism
Protein-calorie malnutrition
Hyperthyroidism
Pancreatitis
Burns

orative and functional fluid losses (tissue sequestration), and the administration of hypotonic intravenous fluids. Hyponatremia is especially common postoperatively in patients who have received relatively large amounts of lactated Ringer's injection (130 meq/L); the postoperative plasma [Na$^+$] generally approaches 130 meq/L in such patients. (Fluid replacement in this patient was appropriate considering basic maintenance requirements, blood loss, and the additional fluid losses usually associated with this type of surgery; see Chapter 29.)

Why is the patient hyperchloremic and acidotic (normal arterial blood pH is 7.35–7.45)?

Operations for supravesical urinary diversion utilize a segment of bowel (ileum, ileocecal segment, jejunum, or sigmoid colon) that is made to function as a conduit or reservoir. The simplest and most common procedure utilizes an isolated loop of ileum as a conduit: The proximal end is anastomosed to the ureters, and the distal end is brought through the skin, forming a stoma.

Whenever urine comes in contact with bowel mucosa, the potential for significant fluid and electrolyte exchange exists. The ileum actively absorbs chloride in exchange for bicarbonate and sodium in exchange for potassium or hydrogen ions. When chloride absorption exceeds sodium absorption, plasma chloride concentration increases while plasma bicarbonate concentration decreases—a hyperchloremic metabolic is established. Hypokalemia can also result if significant amounts of Na$^+$ are exchanged for K$^+$. Potassium losses through the conduit are increased by high urinary sodium concentrations. Moreover, a potassium deficit may be present—even in the absence of hypokalemia—because movement of K$^+$ out of cells (secondary to the acidosis) can prevent an appreciable decrease in extracellular plasma [K$^+$].

Are there any factors that tend to increase the likelihood of hyperchloremic metabolic acidosis following urinary diversion?

The longer the urine is in contact with bowel, the greater the chance that hyperchloremia and acidosis will occur. Mechanical problems such as poor emptying or redundancy of a conduit—along with hypovolemia—thus predispose to hyperchloremic metabolic acidosis. Preexisting renal impairment also appears to be a major risk factor and probably represents an inability to compensate for the excessive bicarbonate losses.

What treatment, if any, is required for this patient?

The ileal loop should be irrigated with saline—through the indwelling catheter or stent—to exclude partial obstruction and ensure free drainage of urine. Hypovolemia should be considered and treated based on central venous pressure measurements or the response to a fluid challenge (Chapter 29). A mild to moderate systemic acidosis (arterial pH $>$ 7.25) is generally well tolerated by most patients. Moreover, hyperchloremic metabolic acidosis following ileal conduits is often transient and usually due to urinary stasis. Persistent or more severe acidosis requires treatment with sodium bicarbonate. Potassium replacement may also be required if hypokalemia is present.

Are electrolyte abnormalities seen with other types of urinary diversion?

Procedures employing bowel as a conduit (ileal or colonic) are less likely to result in a hyperchloremic metabolic acidosis than those where bowel functions as a reservoir. The incidence of hyperchloremic metabolic acidosis approaches 80% following ureterosigmoidostomies. In contrast, newer techniques for continent reservoirs such as the Kock pouch and Indiana pouch appear to be associated with a very low incidence of electrolyte abnormalities postoperatively.

SUGGESTED READINGS

Cogan MG: Fluid and Electrolytes: *Physiology and Pathology.* Appleton & Lange, 1991.

Drop LJ: Ionized calcium, the heart, and hemodynamic function. Anesth Analg 1985;64:432. A comprehensive review of ionized calcium measurement.

Maxwell MH, Kleeman CR: *Clinical Disorders of Fluid and Electrolyte Metabolism,* 4th ed. McGraw-Hill, 1987. An encyclopedic reference.

Rose BD: *Clinical Physiology of Acid-Base Disorders,* 3rd ed. McGraw-Hill, 1989.

Schrier RW (editor): *Renal and Electrolyte Disorders,* 3rd ed. Little, Brown , 1986. Although some chapters are a bit long, overall this book is excellent. It combines basic science, medical physiology, and clinical practice admirably.

Fluid Management & Transfusion

Rational perioperative fluid management requires an understanding of normal fluid and electrolyte balance (Chapter 28). All patients except those undergoing the most minor surgical procedures require venous access and intravenous fluid therapy. Some require transfusion of blood or blood components. Maintenance of a normal intravascular volume is highly desirable in the perioperative period. The anesthesiologist should be able to assess intravascular volume accurately and replace any fluid or electrolyte deficits and ongoing losses. Errors in fluid replacement or transfusion may result in considerable morbidity or even death.

EVALUATION OF INTRAVASCULAR VOLUME

Because measurements of fluid compartment volumes are not readily available, clinical evaluation of intravascular volume must be relied upon. Intravascular volume can be assessed using physical or laboratory examinations or with the aid of sophisticated hemodynamic monitoring techniques. Regardless of the method employed, serial evaluations are necessary to confirm initial impressions and guide fluid therapy. Moreover, modalities should complement one another, because all parameters are indirect, nonspecific measures of volume; reliance on any one parameter may be erroneous and is therefore hazardous.

PHYSICAL EXAMINATION

Physical examination is most reliable preoperatively. Skin turgor, the hydration of mucous membranes, palpation of a peripheral pulse, the resting heart rate and blood pressure and their (orthostatic) changes from the supine to sitting positions, and urinary flow rate are all invaluable as clues to hypovolemia (Table 29–1). Unfortunately, many drugs used during anesthesia, as well as the physiologic effects of surgical stress, alter these signs and render them unreliable even in the immediate postoperative period. Intraoperatively, the fullness of a peripheral pulse (radial or dorsalis pedis), urinary flow rate, and indirect signs such as the response of blood pressure to vasodilating or negatively inotropic anesthetics are most often used.

Pitting edema—presacral in the bedridden patient or pretibial in the ambulatory patient—and increased urinary flow are signs of hypervolemia in patients with normal cardiac, hepatic, and renal function. Late signs of hypervolemia include tachycardia, pulmonary rales, wheezing, cyanosis, and pink, frothy respiratory secretions.

LABORATORY EVALUATION

Several laboratory measurements may be used as indices of intravascular volume. These include serial hematocrits, arterial blood pH, urinary specific gravity, urinary sodium concentration, serum sodium, and the serum creatinine to blood urea nitrogen (BUN) ratio. Because these measurements are affected by many other variables and results are often delayed, they are only indirect indices of intravascular volume and usually cannot be relied upon intraoperatively. Laboratory signs of dehydration include a rising hematocrit, a progressive metabolic acidosis, a urinary specific gravity greater than 1.010, a urinary sodium less than 20 meq/L, hypernatremia, and a BUN/creatinine ratio greater than 10:1. Evidence of volume overload is not consistently present with these measurements; only radiographic signs of increased vascular and interstitial markings or frank pulmonary edema are reliable.

HEMODYNAMIC MEASUREMENTS

Hemodynamic monitoring is discussed in Chapter 6. Central venous pressure monitoring is indicated in patients with normal cardiac and pulmonary function when volume status is difficult to assess by other means or when rapid or major alterations are expected. Central venous pressure readings must be interpreted in light of the clinical setting. Low values (< 5 mm Hg) may be normal unless associated with other signs of hypovolemia. Moreover, the response to a fluid bolus (250 mL) is equally as important: a small elevation (1–2 mm Hg) indicates the need for more fluid,

Table 29–1. Signs of fluid loss (hypovolemia).

Sign	Fluid Loss (Expressed as Percentage of Body Weight)		
	5%	10%	15%
Mucous membranes	Dry	Very dry	Parched
Sensorium	Normal	Lethargic	Obtunded
Orthostatic changes in pulse or blood pressure	Mild	Present	Marked
Urinary flow rate	Mildly decreased	Decreased	Markedly decreased
Pulse rate	Normal or increased	Increased	Markedly increased
Blood pressure	Normal	Mildly decreased	Decreased

whereas a large increase (> 5 mm Hg) suggests the need for a slower rate of administration and a reevaluation of volume status. Central venous pressure readings greater than 12 mm Hg are elevated and imply hypervolemia in the absence of right ventricular dysfunction, increased intrathoracic pressure, or restrictive pericardial disease.

Pulmonary artery pressure monitoring is necessary if central venous pressures do not correlate with the clinical assessment or if the patient has primary or secondary right ventricular dysfunction; the latter is usually due to pulmonary or left ventricular disease. Pulmonary capillary wedge pressure (PCWP) readings of less than 5 mm Hg indicate hypovolemia in the presence of confirmatory clinical signs; however, values less than 15 mm Hg may be associated with relative hypovolemia in patients with poor ventricular compliance. PCWP measurements greater than 20 mm Hg are elevated and generally imply left ventricular volume overload. The presence of mitral valve disease (especially stenosis), severe aortic stenosis, or a left atrial myxoma or thrombus alters the normal relationship between PCWP and end-diastolic ventricular volume (Chapters 6, 19, 20, and 21). Increased thoracic and pulmonary airway pressures also introduce errors; consequently, all pressure measurements should always be obtained at end-expiration and interpreted in the context of the clinical setting.

Newer techniques of measuring ventricular volumes with transesophageal two-dimensional echocardiography or by radioisotopes are more accurate but are not widely available.

INTRAVENOUS FLUIDS

Intravenous fluid therapy may consist of infusions of crystalloids, colloids, or a combination of both. Crystalloid solutions are aqueous solutions of low-molecular-weight ions (salts) with or without glucose, whereas colloid solutions also contain high-molecular-weight substances such as proteins or large glucose polymers. Theoretically, colloid solutions maintain plasma colloid oncotic pressure (Chapter 28) and for the most part remain intravascular, whereas crystalloid solutions rapidly equilibrate with and distribute throughout the entire extracellular fluid space.

Controversy continues regarding the use of colloid versus crystalloid fluids for surgical patients. Proponents of colloids argue that by maintaining plasma oncotic pressure, colloids are more effective in restoring normal intravascular volume and cardiac output. Crystalloid proponents, on the other hand, maintain that the crystalloid solutions are equally as effective when given in sufficient amounts and that colloids may actually have detrimental effects in patients with increased pulmonary capillary permeability. They theorize that in those patients, leakage of the colloid into the pulmonary interstitium favors the formation of pulmonary edema fluid by increasing interstitial colloid osmotic pressure. While many studies are available to support or refute either position, several generalizations can reasonably be made:

(1) Crystalloids, when given in sufficient amounts, can be just as effective as colloids in restoring intravascular volume.
(2) Replacing an intravascular volume deficit with crystalloids generally requires 3–4 times the volume needed when using colloids.
(3) Most surgical patients have an extracellular fluid deficit that exceeds the intravascular deficit.
(4) Severe intravascular fluid deficits can be more rapidly corrected using colloid solutions.

CRYSTALLOID SOLUTIONS

A wide variety of solutions are available (Table 29–2). Solutions are chosen according to the type of fluid loss being replaced. Losses primarily due to water loss are replaced with hypotonic solutions, also called maintenance-type solutions. Losses that involve both water and electrolyte deficits are replaced with isotonic electrolyte solutions, also called replacement-type solutions. Glucose is provided in some solutions to maintain tonicity or to prevent ketosis due to fasting.

Table 29–2. Composition of crystalloid solutions.

Solution	Tonicity (mosm/L)	Na+ (meq/L)	Cl− (meq/L)	K+ (meq/L)	Ca²+ (meq/L)	Glucose (g/L)	Lactate (meq/L)
5% dextrose in water (D₅W)	Hypo (253)					50	
Normal saline (NS)	Iso (308)	154	154				
D₅ ¼NS	Iso (330)	38.5	38.5			50	
D₅ ½NS	Hyper (407)	77	77			50	
D₅NS	Hyper (561)	154	154			50	
Lactated Ringer's injection (LR)	Iso (273)	130	109	4	3		28
D₅LR	Hyper (525)	130	109	4	3	50	28

Since most intraoperative fluid losses are isotonic, replacement-type solutions are generally used. The most commonly used solution is lactated Ringer's injection. Although it is slightly hypotonic, providing approximately 100 mL of free water per liter and tending to lower serum sodium to 130 meq/L, lactated Ringer's appears to be the most physiologic solution when large volumes are necessary. The lactate in this solution is converted by the liver into bicarbonate. When given in large volumes, normal saline produces a dilutional hyperchloremic acidosis because of its high chloride content (154 meq/L): plasma bicarbonate concentration decreases as chloride concentration increases (Chapters 28 and 30). Normal saline is the preferred solution for hypochloremic metabolic acidosis and for diluting packed red blood cells prior to transfusion. Five percent dextrose in water (D₅W) is used for replacement of pure water deficits and as a maintenance fluid for patients on sodium restriction. Hypertonic 3% saline is employed in therapy of severe symptomatic hyponatremia (Chapter 28). Some authors have advocated the use of hypertonic 3–7.5% saline solutions for the resuscitation of patients in hypovolemic shock (Chapter 39).

COLLOID SOLUTIONS

The osmotic activity of the high-molecular-weight substances in colloids tends to maintain these solutions intravascularly. While the intravascular half-life of a crystalloid solution is 20–30 minutes, most colloid solutions have intravascular half-lives between 3 and 6 hours. The substantial cost and occasional complications associated with colloids tend to limit their use. Generally accepted indications for colloids include (1) fluid resuscitation in patients with severe intravascular fluid deficits (eg, hemorrhagic shock) prior to the arrival of blood for transfusion, and (2) fluid resuscitation in the presence of severe hypoalbuminemia or

conditions associated with large protein losses such as burns.

Many clinicians also use colloid solutions in conjunction with crystalloids when fluid replacement needs exceed 3–4 L prior to transfusion.

Several colloid solutions are generally available. All are derived from either plasma proteins or synthetic glucose polymers and are supplied in isotonic electrolyte solutions.

Blood-derived colloids include albumin (5% and 25% solutions) and plasma protein fraction (5%). Both are heated at 60 °C for at least 10 hours to minimize the risk of transmitting hepatitis and other virally transmitted diseases. Plasma protein fraction contains alpha and beta globulins in addition to albumin and has occasionally resulted in hypotensive reactions. These reactions are allergic in nature and may involve activators of prekallikrein.

Synthetic colloids include dextrose starches and gelatins. Gelatins are associated with histamine-mediated allergic reactions and are not available in the United States. Dextran is available as dextran 70 (Macrodex) and dextran 40 (Rheomacrodex), which have average molecular weights of 70,000 and 40,000, respectively. Although dextran 70 is a better volume expander than dextran 40, the latter also improves blood flow through the microcirculation, presumably by decreasing viscosity. Antiplatelet effects are also described for dextrans. Infusions exceeding 20 mL/kg/d can interfere with blood typing, may prolong bleeding time (with dextran 40), and have been associated with renal failure. Dextrans can also be antigenic, and both mild and severe anaphylactoid allergic reactions are described.

Hetastarch (hydroxyethyl starch) is available as a 6% solution with an average molecular weight of 450,000. It is highly effective as a plasma expander and less expensive than albumin. Hetastarch is nonantigenic, and anaphylactoid reactions are rare. Coagulation studies and bleeding times are generally not significantly affected after infusions of 1–2 L.

PERIOPERATIVE FLUID THERAPY

Perioperative fluid therapy includes replacement of normal losses (maintenance requirements), preexisting fluid deficits, and surgical wound losses including blood loss.

NORMAL MAINTENANCE REQUIREMENTS

In the absence of oral intake, fluid and electrolyte deficits can rapidly develop as a result of continued urine formation, gastrointestinal secretions, sweating, and insensible losses from the skin and respiratory tract. Normal maintenance requirements can be estimated from Table 29–3. Because these losses are normally hypotonic (more water than electrolytes), solutions such as D_5 $\frac{1}{4}$NS and D_5 $\frac{1}{2}$NS are appropriate.

PREEXISTING DEFICITS

Patients presenting for surgery after an overnight fast without any fluid intake will have a preexisting deficit proportionate to the duration of the fast. The deficit can be estimated by multiplying the normal maintenance rate by the length of the fast. For the average 70-kg man fasting for 8 hours, this amounts to (40 + 20 + 50) mL/h × 8 hours, or 880 mL. (In reality, this deficit will be somewhat less as a result of renal conservation.)

Abnormal fluid losses frequently contribute to preoperative deficits. Preoperative bleeding, vomiting, diuresis, or diarrhea is often contributory. Occult losses (really redistribution; see below) due to fluid sequestration by traumatized or infected tissues or ascites can also be substantial. Increased insensible losses due to hyperventilation, fever, and sweating are often overlooked.

Ideally, all deficits should be replaced preoperatively in all patients. The fluids used should be similar in composition to the fluids lost (Table 29–4).

Table 29–3. Estimating maintenance fluid requirements.

Weight	Rate
For the first 10 kg	4 mL/kg/h
For the next 10–20 kg	Add 2 mL/kg/h
For each kg above 20 kg	Add 1 mL/kg/h

Example: What are the maintenance fluid requirements for a 25-kg child?
Answer: 40 + 20 + 5 = 65 mL/h

Table 29–4. Electrolyte content of body fluids.

Fluid	Na+ (meq/L)	K+ (meq/L)	Cl− (meq/L)	HCO₃− (meq/L)
Sweat	30–50	5	45–55	
Saliva	2–40	10–30	6–30	30
Gastric juice High acidity Low acidity	10–30 70–140	5–40 5–40	80–150 55–95	5–25
Pancreatic secretions	115–180	5	55–95	60–110
Biliary secretions	130–160	5	90–120	30–40
Ileal fluid	40–135	5–30	20–90	20–30
Diarrheal stool	20–160	10–40	30–120	30–50

SURGICAL FLUID LOSSES

Blood Losses

One of the most important tasks of the anesthesiologist is to continually monitor and estimate blood loss. While estimates are complicated by occult bleeding into the wound or under the surgical drapes, accuracy is important to guide fluid therapy and transfusions.

The most commonly used method for estimating blood loss is measurement of blood in the surgical suction container and visually estimating the blood on surgical sponges and laparotomy pads ("laps"). A fully soaked sponge (4 × 4) is said to hold 10 mL of blood, whereas a soaked "lap" holds 100–150 mL. More accurate estimates are obtained if sponges and "laps" are weighed before and after use (particularly during pediatric procedures). Use of irrigating solutions complicates estimates, but their use should be noted and some attempt made to compensate for them. Serial hematocrits or hemoglobin concentrations reflect the ratio of blood cells to plasma, not necessarily blood loss; moreover, rapid fluid shifts and intravenous replacement affect measurements. Hematocrits may be useful during long procedures or when estimates are difficult.

Other Fluid Losses

Many surgical procedures are associated with obligatory losses of fluids other than blood. Such losses are due mainly to evaporation and internal redistribution of body fluids. Evaporative losses are most apparent with large wounds and directly proportionate to the surface area exposed and the duration of the surgical procedure.

Internal redistribution of fluids—often called "third spacing"—can cause massive fluid shifts and severe intravascular depletion. Traumatized, inflamed, or infected tissue (as occurs with burns, extensive injuries, surgical dissections, or peritonitis) can sequester large amounts of fluid in its interstitial space and can translocate fluid across serosal surfaces (ascites) or into bowel lumen. The result is an obligatory increase in a nonfunctional component of the extracellular compartment, as this fluid does not readily equilibrate with the rest of the compartments. This fluid shift cannot be prevented by fluid restriction and is at the expense of both the functional extracellular and the intracellular fluid compartments. Cellular dysfunction as a result of hypoxia can produce an increase of the intracellular fluid volume, also at the expense of the functional extracellular compartment (Chapter 28).

INTRAOPERATIVE FLUID REPLACEMENT

Intraoperative fluid therapy should include supplying basic fluid requirements and replacing residual preoperative deficits as well as intraoperative losses (blood, fluid redistribution, and evaporation). Selection of the type of intravenous solution depends upon the surgical procedure and the expected blood loss. For procedures involving minimal blood loss and fluid shifts, maintenance solutions can be used. For all other procedures, lactated Ringer's injection is generally used even for maintenance requirements. The first liter is often given with glucose (D_5LR) to prevent ketosis.

Replacing Blood Loss

Ideally, blood loss should be replaced with crystalloid or colloid solutions to maintain intravascular volume (normovolemia) until the danger of anemia outweighs the risks of transfusion. At that point, further blood loss is replaced with transfusions of red blood cells to maintain hemoglobin concentration (or hematocrit) at that level. For most patients, that point corresponds to a hemoglobin between 7 and 10 g/dL (or a hematocrit of 21–30%). Below a hemoglobin concentration of 7 g/dL, the resting cardiac output has to increase greatly to maintain a normal oxygen delivery (Chapter 22). A level of 10 g/dL is generally used for elderly patients and those with significant cardiac or pulmonary disease. Higher limits are also used if continuing rapid blood loss is expected.

In practice, most clinicians give lactated Ringer's injection in approximately 3–4 times the volume of the blood lost (or in a 1:1 ratio when using colloids) until the transfusion point is reached. At that time, blood is replaced unit for unit as it is lost, either with whole blood or reconstituted packed red blood cells (one unit of whole blood is approximately 500 mL).

Table 29–5. Average blood volumes.

Age	Blood Volume
Neonates Premature Full-term	 95 mL/kg 85 mL/kg
Infants	80 mL/kg
Adults Men Women	 75 mL/kg 65 mL/kg

The transfusion point can be determined preoperatively from the hematocrit and by estimating blood volume (Table 29–5). Patients with a normal hematocrit should generally be transfused only after losses greater than 10–20% of their blood volume. The exact point is based on the patient's medical condition and the surgical procedure. The amount of blood loss necessary for the hematocrit to fall to 30% can be calculated as follows:

(1) Estimate blood volume from Table 29–5.
(2) Estimate the red cell volume at the preoperative hematocrit ($RBCV_{preop}$).
(3) Estimate red cell volume at a hematocrit of 30% ($RBCV_{30\%}$), assuming normal blood volume is maintained.
(4) Calculate the red cell volume lost when the hematocrit is 30%; $RBCV_{lost} = RBCV_{preop} - RBCV_{30\%}$.
(5) Allowable blood loss = $RBVC_{lost} \times 3$.

Example: An 85-kg woman has a preoperative hematocrit of 35%. How much blood loss will decrease her hematocrit to 30%?

Estimated blood volume = 65 mL/kg × 85 kg = 5525 mL
$RBCV_{35\%}$ = 5525 × 35% = 1934 mL.
$RBCV_{30\%}$ = 5525 × 30% = 1657 mL.
Red cell loss at 30% = 1934 − 1657 = 277 mL.
Allowable blood loss = 3 × 277 mL = 831 mL.

Therefore, transfusion should be considered when this patient's blood loss exceeds 800 mL.

Other useful guidelines commonly used are as follows: (1) one unit of red blood cells will increase hemoglobin 1 g/dL and the hematocrit 2–3% (in adults); and (2) a 10 mL/kg transfusion of red blood cells will increase hemoglobin concentration by 3 g/dL.

Replacing Redistributive & Evaporative Losses

Since these losses are primarily related to wound size and the extent of surgical dissections and manipulations, procedures can be classified according to the degree of tissue trauma. These additional fluid losses can be replaced according to Table 29–6, based on whether tissue trauma is minimal, moderate, or severe. These values are only guidelines, and actual needs vary considerably from patient to patient.

Table 29–6. Redistributive and evaporative surgical fluid losses.

Degree of Tissue Trauma	Additional Fluid Requirement
Minimal (eg, herniorrhapy)	0–2 mL/kg/h
Moderate (eg, cholecystectomy)	2–4 mL/kg/h
Severe (eg, bowel resection)	4–8 mL/kg/h

TRANSFUSION

BLOOD GROUPS & COMPATIBILITY TESTING

1. BLOOD GROUPS

Human red cell membranes are estimated to contain at least 300 different antigenic determinants. At least 20 separate blood group antigen systems are known; the expression of each is under genetic control from a separate chromosomal locus. Fortunately, only the ABO and the Rh systems are important in the majority of blood transfusions. Individuals often produce antibodies (alloantibodies) to the alleles they lack within each system. Such antibodies are responsible for the most serious reactions to transfusions. Antibodies may occur "naturally" or in response to sensitization from a previous transfusion or pregnancy.

The ABO System

Simplistically, the chromosomal locus for this system produces three alleles: A, B, and O. Each represents an enzyme that modifies a cell surface glycoprotein, producing a different antigen. (Actually, the O enzyme is functionally silent and there are two variants of A: A_1 and A_2.) Almost all individuals not having A or B "naturally" produce antibodies against those antigens (Table 29–7) within the first year of life. The H antigen is functionally related to the ABO system but is produced by a different chromosomal locus. Absence of the H antigen (hh genotype, also called the Bombay phenotype) prevents expression of the A or B genes; these very rare individuals will have anti-A and anti-B antibodies regardless of their ABO genotype.

The Rh System

The genetics of the Rh gene is complicated, probably involving three chromosomal loci with a total of six alleles. For simplicity, only the presence or absence of the most common and most immunogenic allele, the D antigen, is considered. Individuals lacking this allele are called Rh-negative and usually develop antibodies against the D antigen only after exposure in the course of a previous (Rh-positive) transfusion or pregnancy (an Rh-negative mother delivering an Rh-positive baby).

Other Systems

Other systems include the Lewis, P, I, MNSs, Kidd, Duffy, Lutheran, Xg, Sid, Cartright, York, Chido, and Rodgers antigens. Fortunately, with a few exceptions, alloantibodies against these systems rarely cause serious hemolytic reactions.

2. COMPATIBILITY TESTING

The purpose of such testing is to predict and to prevent antigen-antibody reactions as a result of red blood cell transfusions. Donor and recipient blood are typed and checked for the presence of adverse antibodies.

ABO-Rh Testing

The most severe transfusion reactions are due to ABO incompatibility; naturally acquired antibodies can react against the absent (foreign) antigens, activate complement, and result in intravascular hemolysis. The patient's red cells are tested with serum known to have antibodies against A and against B to determine blood type. Because of the almost universal prevalence of natural ABO antibodies, confirmation of blood type is then made by testing the patient's serum against red cells with known antigen type.

The patient's red cells are also tested with anti-D antibodies to determine Rh. If the subject is Rh-negative, the presence of anti-D antibody is checked by mixing his serum against Rh-positive red cells. The probability of developing anti-D antibodies after a single exposure to the Rh antigen is 50–70%.

Crossmatching

A crossmatch mimics the transfusion: donor cells are mixed with recipient serum. A reliable test requires at least 45 minutes to complete. Crossmatching serves three functions: (1) it confirms ABO and Rh typing (in less than 5 minutes), (2) it detects antibodies to the other blood group systems, and (3) it detects antibodies in low titers or those that do not agglutinate easily. The latter two require at least 45 minutes.

Antibody Screen

The purpose of this test is to detect in the serum the presence of the antibodies that are most commonly associated with non-ABO hemolytic reactions. The test (also known as the indirect Coombs test) requires 45 minutes and involves mixing the subject's serum with red cells of known antigenic composition; if specific antibodies are present, they will coat the red cell membrane, and addition of an anti-globulin antibody results in red cell agglutination. Screens are routinely done on all donor blood and may be done for a potential recipient instead of a crossmatch (below).

Table 29–7. ABO blood grouping.

Type	Naturally Occurring Antibodies in Serum	Incidence[1]
A	anti-B	45%
B	anti-A	8%
AB	—	4%
O	anti-A, anti-B	43%

[1] Rates are based on individuals of western European ancestry.

Type & Crossmatch
Versus Type & Screen

The incidence of a serious hemolytic reaction after transfusion of an ABO- and Rh-compatible transfusion with a negative screen but without a crossmatch is less than 1%. Crossmatching, however, assures optimal safety and detects the presence of less common antibodies not usually tested for in a screen. Because of the time involved and the practice of reserving crossmatched units for a specific patient, crossmatches are now performed only for elective surgical procedures where the probability of transfusion is high.

Maximum Surgical Blood
Ordering Schedule

Most hospitals compile a list of their most commonly performed operations and the maximum number of units that can be crossmatched preoperatively. Such practices prevent needless excessive crossmatching of blood. Lists are usually based on each institution's own experience. A crossmatch-to-transfusion ratio less than 2.5:1 is considered acceptable. Only a type and screen is performed if the incidence of transfusion for a procedure is less than 10%. If transfusion is required, a crossmatch is performed. Allowances are typically made for anemic patients and those with coagulation disorders.

EMERGENCY TRANSFUSIONS

When a patient is exsanguinating, the need to transfuse arises prior to completion of a crossmatch, screen, or even blood typing. If the patient's blood type is known, an abbreviated crossmatch, requiring less than 5 minutes, will confirm ABO compatibility. If the recipient's blood type is not known with certainty and transfusion must be started before determination, type O Rh-negative blood may be used. In these instances, packed red blood cells should be used instead of whole blood to minimize the transfer of anti-A and anti-B antibodies. These antibodies can react with the recipient's own red cells (if A or B antigens are present) or with type-specific red blood cells transfused subsequently; as a result, once type O Rh-negative whole blood is used, further transfusions should be type O Rh-negative until anti-A and anti-B titers are determined in the patient's serum.

BLOOD BANK PRACTICES

Donors are screened to exclude medical conditions that might adversely affect the recipient. The hematocrit is determined, and if it is normal the blood is typed, screened for antibodies, and tested for hepatitis B, hepatitis C, syphilis, and HIV. Recently, some blood banks have also begun to test for the human T cell lymphotropic viruses I and II (HTLV-I and HTLV-II; see below).

Once blood is collected, a preservative-anticoagulant solution is added. The most commonly used solution is CPD-A, which contains citrate as an anticoagulant (by binding calcium), phosphate as a buffer, dextrose as a red cell energy source, and adenine as a precursor for ATP synthesis. CPD-A preserved blood can be stored for 35 days, after which the viability of the red cells rapidly decreases. A unit of whole blood plus preservative is typically 450–500 mL.

Almost all units collected are separated into their component parts, namely, red blood cells, platelets, and plasma. When centrifuged, one unit of whole blood yields 250 mL of packed red blood cells (hematocrit 70%); following the addition of more saline preservative, the volume of a unit of packed red cells often reaches 350 mL. Red cells are stored at 1–6 °C.

The supernatant is centrifuged to yield platelets and plasma. The unit of platelets obtained generally contains 50–70 mL of plasma and can be stored at 20–24 °C for 5 days. The remaining plasma supernatant is further processed and frozen to yield fresh frozen plasma. Cryoprecipitate and factor concentrates (such as factor VIII) can also be prepared from the plasma supernatant. One unit of blood yields 200 mL of plasma, which is frozen for storage; once thawed, it must be transfused within 24 hours.

INTRAOPERATIVE TRANSFUSION
PRACTICES

Whole Blood

Whole blood is indicated for acute blood loss in the setting of hypovolemic shock. It is also probably indicated for transfusions in surgical procedures with an expected blood loss of greater than 1500 mL. Slower rates of hemorrhage should be managed with packed red blood cells. Although whole blood contains plasma and therefore also provides more effective volume resuscitation, a rapid decrease in platelet viability and factor V and factor VIII activity occurs with storage. Concomitant platelet or fresh frozen plasma transfusions may be necessary.

Packed Red Blood Cells

Most blood transfusions should be given as packed red blood cells, since doing so allows optimal utilization of blood bank resources. Packed red blood cells are ideal for patients requiring red cells but not volume replacement (eg, anemic patients in compensated congestive heart failure). Most surgical patients, however, do require volume as well as red blood cells; consequently, the packed red cells are reconstituted with an isotonic solution, preferably normal saline. In addition to providing volume, the added saline decreases viscosity and facilitates rapid transfusion. Lactated Ringer's injection should not be used because the calcium in it may reverse the anticoagulant effects of the citrate preservative.

Prior to transfusion, each unit should be carefully

checked against the blood bank slip and the recipient's identity bracelet. The transfusion tubing should contain a 170-μm filter to trap any clots or debris; use of smaller filters (20–40 μm) is probably not necessary except for prevention of febrile transfusion reactions in sensitized patients (see below). All blood for intraoperative transfusion should be warmed to 37 °C during infusion; failure to do so can result in profound hypothermia. The additive effects of hypothermia and the typically low levels of 2,3-diphosphoglycerate in stored blood can cause a marked leftward shift of the hemoglobin-oxygen dissociation curve (Chapter 22) and, at least theoretically, promote tissue hypoxia.

Fresh Frozen Plasma (FFP)

Fresh frozen plasma contains all plasma proteins, including all clotting factors. Transfusions of FFP are indicated in the treatment of isolated factor deficiencies, the reversal of warfarin therapy, and the correction of coagulopathy associated with liver disease. Each unit of FFP generally increases the level of each clotting factor by 2–3% in adults. Fresh frozen plasma may also be used in patients who have received massive blood transfusions (see below) and continue to bleed following platelet transfusions. Patients with antithrombin III deficiency or thrombotic thrombocytopenic purpura also benefit from FFP transfusions.

Each unit of FFP carries the same infectious risk as a unit of whole blood. Additionally, occasional patients may become sensitized to plasma proteins. ABO-compatible units should generally be given but are not mandatory. As with red cells, FFP should be warmed to 37 °C prior to transfusion.

Platelets

Platelet transfusions should be given to patients with thrombocytopenia or dysfunctional platelets in the presence of bleeding. Prophylactic platelet transfusions are also indicated in patients with platelet counts below 10,000–20,000/μL because of an increased risk of spontaneous hemorrhage.

Platelet counts less than 50,000/μL are associated with increased blood loss during surgery. Thrombocytopenic patients about to undergo surgery or invasive procedures should receive prophylactic platelet transfusions preoperatively: The platelet count should be increased to 100,000/μL. Each unit of platelets should be expected to increase the count by 5,000–10,000/μL. Lesser increases can be expected in patients with a history of prior platelet transfusions. Platelet dysfunction can also increase surgical bleeding even when the platelet count is normal and can be diagnosed preoperatively with a bleeding time. Platelet transfusions may also be indicated in patients with dysfunctional platelets and increased surgical bleeding.

ABO-compatible platelet transfusions are desirable but not necessary. Transfused platelets generally survive only 1–7 days following transfusion. ABO com-

patibility may increase platelet survival. Rh sensitization can occur in Rh-negative recipients owing to the presence of a few red cells in Rh-positive platelet units. Moreover, anti-A or anti-B antibodies in the 70 mL of plasma in each platelet unit can cause a hemolytic reaction against the recipient's red cells when a large number of ABO-incompatible platelet units are given. Administration of Rh immunoglobulin to Rh-negative individuals can protect against Rh sensitization following Rh-positive platelet transfusions. Patients who develop antibodies against HLA or specific platelet antigens require HLA compatible or single donor units.

Granulocyte Transfusions

Granulocyte transfusions, prepared by leukapheresis, may be indicated in neutropenic patients with bacterial infections not responding to antibiotics. Transfused granulocytes have a very short circulatory life span, so that daily transfusion of 10–30 × 10^9 granulocytes are usually required. Irradiation of these units decreases the incidence of graft-versus-host reactions, pulmonary endothelial damage, and other problems associated with transfusion of leukocytes (see below).

COMPLICATIONS OF BLOOD TRANSFUSION

IMMUNE COMPLICATIONS

Immune complications following blood transfusions are primarily due to sensitization of the recipient to donor red cells, white cells, platelets, or plasma proteins. Less commonly, the transfused cells or serum may mount an immune response against the recipient.

1. HEMOLYTIC REACTIONS

Hemolytic reactions usually involve specific destruction of the transfused red blood cells by the recipient's antibodies. Less commonly, hemolysis of a recipient's red blood cells occurs as a result of the transfusion of red cell antibodies. Incompatible units of platelet concentrates, FFP, clotting factor concentrates, or cryoprecipitate may contain small amounts of plasma with anti-A or anti-B (or both) alloantibodies. Transfusions of large volumes of such units can lead to intravascular hemolysis. Hemolytic reactions are commonly classified as either acute (intravascular) or delayed (extravascular).

Acute Hemolytic Reactions

Acute intravascular hemolysis is usually due to ABO blood incompatibility and is reported with frequencies of approximately 1:25,000–6000 transfusions. These reaction are often severe. The risk of a fatal hemolytic reaction is about 1:500,000–100,000 transfusions. In awake patients, symptoms include chills, fever, nausea, and chest and flank pain. In anesthetized patients, the reaction is manifested by a rise in temperature, unexplained tachycardia, hypotension, hemoglobinuria, and diffuse oozing in the surgical field. Disseminated intravascular coagulation, shock, and renal shutdown can develop rapidly. The severity of a reaction often depends on how much incompatible blood has been given. If the volume of the incompatible blood given is less than 5% of total blood volume, the reaction is usually not severe.

Management of hemolytic reactions can be summarized as follows:

(1) Once a hemolytic reaction is suspected, the transfusion should be stopped immediately.
(2) The unit should be rechecked against the blood slip and the patient's identity bracelet.
(3) Blood should be drawn to identify hemoglobin in plasma, to repeat compatibility testing, and to obtain coagulation studies and a platelet count.
(4) A urinary catheter should be inserted, and the urine should be checked for hemoglobin.
(5) Osmotic diuresis should be initiated with mannitol and intravenous fluids.
(6) Low-dose dopamine may help preserve renal blood flow and support blood pressure.
(7) In the presence of rapid blood loss, platelets and FFP are indicated.

Delayed Hemolytic Reactions

This type of hemolytic reaction—also called extravascular hemolysis—is generally mild and is caused by antibodies to non-D antigens of the Rh system or to foreign alleles in other systems such as the Kell, Duffy, or Kidd antigens. Following an ABO and Rh D-compatible transfusion, patients have a 1–1.6% chance of forming antibodies directed against foreign antigens in these other systems. By the time significant amounts of these antibodies have formed (weeks to months), the transfused red cells have been cleared from the circulation. Moreover, the titer of these antibodies subsequently decreases and may become undetectable. However, reexposure to the same foreign antigen during a subsequent red cell transfusion triggers an anamnestic antibody response against the foreign antigen. The hemolytic reaction is therefore typically delayed 2–21 days after transfusion, and symptoms are generally mild, consisting of malaise, jaundice, and fever. The patient's hematocrit typically fails to rise in spite of the transfusion and the absence of bleeding. The serum unconjugated bilirubin increases as a result of hemoglobin breakdown.

Diagnosis of delayed antibody-mediated hemolytic reactions may be facilitated by the antiglobulin (Coombs) test. The direct Coombs test detects the presence of antibodies on the membrane of red cells. In this setting, however, this test cannot distinguish between recipient antibodies coated on donor red cells versus donor antibodies coated on recipient red cells. The latter requires a more detailed reexamination of pretransfusion specimens from both the patient and the donor.

The treatment of delayed hemolytic reactions is primarily supportive. The frequency of delayed hemolytic transfusion reactions is estimated to be approximately 1:2500–1500 transfusions. Pregnancy (exposure to fetal red cells) can also be responsible for the formation of alloantibodies to red cells in women.

2. NONHEMOLYTIC IMMUNE REACTIONS

Nonhemolytic immune reactions are due to sensitization of the recipient to the donor's white cells, platelets, or plasma proteins.

Febrile Reactions

White cell or platelet sensitization is typically manifested as a febrile reaction. Such reactions are relatively common (1–3% of transfusion episodes) and are characterized by an increase in temperature without evidence of hemolysis. Patients with a history of febrile reactions should receive white cell-poor red cell transfusions only. Red cell transfusions can be made leukocyte-poor by washing, centrifugation, filtration, or freeze-thaw techniques. Use of a 20- to 40-μm filter will trap most of the white cell and platelet contaminants.

Urticarial Reactions

Urticarial reactions are usually characterized by erythema, hives, and itching without fever. They are relatively common (1% of transfusions) and are thought to be due to sensitization of the patient to transfused plasma proteins. The use of packed red blood cells instead of whole blood lessens the likelihood of urticaria-type reactions. Urticarial reactions can be treated with antihistaminic drugs (H_1 and perhaps H_2 blockers).

Anaphylactic Reactions

Anaphylactic reactions are rare (approximately 1:150,000 transfusions). These severe reactions may occur after only a few milliliters of blood have been given, typically in IgA-deficient patients with anti-IgA antibodies who receive IgA-containing blood transfusions. The prevalence of IgA deficiency is estimated to be 1:800–600 in the general population. Such reactions call for treatment with epinephrine, fluids, and corticosteroids. Patients with IgA deficiency should receive thoroughly washed packed red cells, deglycerolized frozen red cells, or IgA free blood units.

Noncardiogenic Pulmonary Edema

The adult respiratory distress syndrome (ARDS) is a rare complication of blood transfusion (< 1:10,000). It is thought to be due to transfusion of antileukocyte antibodies that interact with and cause the patient's white cells to aggregate in the pulmonary circulation. Damage to the alveolocapillary membrane triggers the syndrome. Alternatively, transfused white cells interact with leukoagglutinins in the patient. Treatment of ARDS is discussed in Chapter 48.

Graft-Versus-Host Disease

This type of reaction may be seen in immune-compromised patients. Cellular blood products contain lymphocytes capable of mounting an immune response against the compromised (recipient) host. Irradiation (1500–3000 cGy) of red cell, granulocyte, and platelet transfusions effectively inactivates lymphocytes without altering the efficacy of such transfusions.

Posttransfusion Purpura

Profound thrombocytopenia can rarely occur following blood transfusions and is due to the development of platelet alloantibodies. The platelet count typically drops precipitously 1 week after transfusion. Plasmapheresis is generally recommended.

Immune Suppression

Transfusion of leukocyte-containing blood products appears to be immunosuppressive. This is most clear in renal transplant recipients, in whom preoperative blood transfusions appear to improve graft survival.

NONIMMUNE COMPLICATIONS

1. COMPLICATIONS OF MASSIVE BLOOD TRANSFUSION

Massive transfusion is generally defined as the need to transfuse one to two times the patient's blood volume. For most adult patients, that is the equivalent of 10–20 units.

Coagulopathy

The most common cause of bleeding following massive blood transfusion is dilutional thrombocytopenia. Dilution of the coagulation factors is unusual in previously normal patients. Coagulation studies and platelet counts, if readily available, ideally should guide platelet and FFP transfusion. Viscoelastic analysis of whole blood clotting (thromboelastography and Sonoclot analysis) may also be useful.

Citrate Toxicity

Calcium binding by the citrate preservative can theoretically become significant following transfusion of large volumes of blood or blood products. Clinically significant hypocalcemia, causing cardiac depression, does not occur in most normal patients unless the transfusion rate exceeds one unit every 5 minutes. Because

citrate metabolism is primarily hepatic, patients with hepatic disease or dysfunction (and possibly hypothermic patients) may require calcium infusion during massive transfusion (Chapter 28).

Hypothermia

Massive blood transfusion is an absolute indication for warming all blood products and intravenous fluids to normal body temperature. Hypothermia can hamper cardiac resuscitation. Ventricular dysrhythmias progressing to fibrillation often occur at temperatures close to 30 °C.

Acid-Base Balance

The most common abnormality after massive blood transfusion is metabolic alkalosis. Once normal perfusion is restored, any metabolic acidosis resolves, and a progressive metabolic alkalosis supervenes as citrate and lactate contained in transfusions and resuscitation fluids are converted to bicarbonate by the liver.

Serum Potassium Concentration

The extracellular concentration of potassium in stored blood steadily increases with time. Although hyperkalemia can occur following rapid transfusion of old blood units, hypokalemia is more common. The amount of extracellular potassium transfused with each unit is typically less than 4 meq per unit. Hypokalemia is usually associated with metabolic alkalosis and is the result of the uptake of potassium by cells (Chapters 28 and 30).

2. INFECTION

Viruses

A. Hepatitis: Until recently, the overall incidence of hepatitis following blood transfusion was 7–10%. Ninety percent of these cases were said to be due to non-A, non-B hepatitis. The hepatitis C virus was recently identified and found to be responsible for at least 80–90% of cases of "non-A, non-B hepatitis." Seventy-five percent of patients with posttransfusion hepatitis C were anicteric, and up to 50% went on to develop chronic active hepatitis. Moreover, of this latter group, 10–20% developed cirrhosis. The routine testing of donor units for antibodies against hepatitis C is expected to markedly reduce the incidence of transfusion-related hepatitis and its associated morbidity. The current risk of hepatitis C infection is estimated to be between 1:5000 and 1:150 transfusions.

B. Acquired Immune Deficiency Syndrome (AIDS): The virus responsible for this disease, human immunodeficiency virus (HIV-1), is transmissible by blood transfusion. All blood is tested for the presence of anti-HIV-1 antibody, the only current marker for infectivity. Unfortunately, because of an estimated 6- to 8-week period required to develop the antibody after donor infection, infectious units can go undetected. The current rate of transmission of the HIV virus by transfusion is estimated to be 1:100,000–40,000 transfusions.

C. Other Viral Infections: Cytomegalovirus (CMV) and Epstein-Barr virus (EBV) usually cause asymptomatic or mild systemic illness. Unfortunately, some individuals become asymptomatic infectious carriers; the white cells in blood units from such donors are capable of transmitting either virus. Immunocompromised and immunosuppressed patients (eg, premature infants and organ transplant recipients) are particularly susceptible to severe CMV infections through transfusions. Such patients should only receive CMV-negative units. Human T cell lymphotropic viruses I and II are leukemia and lymphoma viruses that have been reported to be transmitted by blood transfusion. Parvovirus transmission has been reported following transfusion of coagulation factor concentrates and implicated as causing aplastic anemia.

Parasites

Parasitic diseases reported to be transmitted by transfusion include malaria, toxoplasmosis, and Chagas' disease. Fortunately, such cases are very rare.

Bacteria

Both gram-positive and gram-negative bacteria can rarely contaminate blood transfusions and transmit disease. To avoid the possibility of significant bacterial contamination, blood products should be administered over a period shorter than 4 hours. Specific bacterial diseases transmitted by blood transfusions from donors include syphilis, brucellosis, salmonellosis, yersiniosis, and various rickettsioses.

ALTERNATIVE STRATEGIES FOR MANAGEMENT OF BLOOD LOSS DURING SURGERY

AUTOLOGOUS TRANSFUSIONS

Patients undergoing elective surgical procedures with a high probability for transfusion can donate their own blood for use during that surgery. Collection is usually started 4–5 weeks prior to the procedure. The patient is allowed to donate a unit as long as the hematocrit is at least 34% or hemoglobin at least 11 g/dL. A minimum of 72 hours is required between donations to make certain that plasma volume returns to normal. With iron supplementation, four units can usually be collected prior to the operation. Recent studies suggest that autologous blood transfusions do not adversely affect survival in patients undergoing operations for cancer.

BLOOD SALVAGE & REINFUSION

This technique is used widely during cardiac and major reconstructive vascular surgery. The shed blood is aspirated intraoperatively together with an anticoagulant (heparin) into a reservoir. After a sufficient amount of blood is collected, the red blood cells are concentrated and washed to remove debris and anticoagulant and then reinfused into the patient. The concentrates obtained usually have hematocrits of 50–60%. To be used effectively, this technique requires blood losses greater than 1000–1500 mL. Contraindications include septic contamination of the wound and perhaps malignancy, though concerns about the possibility of reinfusing malignant cells via this technique may be not justified (see above). Newer, simpler systems allow reinfusion of shed blood without centrifugation.

HEMODILUTION

Hemodilution relies on the premise that if the concentration of red blood cells is decreased, total red cell loss is reduced when large amounts of blood are shed. Blood is typically removed just prior to surgery and is replaced with crystalloid and colloids such that the patient remains normovolemic but has a hematocrit of 21–25%. The removed blood is then given back to the patient during or after the surgery as transfusion is needed.

DONOR-DIRECTED TRANSFUSIONS

Patients can request donated blood from family members or friends known to be ABO-compatible. Most blood banks generally require donation at least 3 days prior to surgery to process the donated blood and confirm compatibility. Studies comparing the safety of donor-directed units to that of random donor units have not found any difference.

CASE DISCUSSION: A PATIENT WITH SICKLE CELL DISEASE

A 24-year-old black woman with sickle cell anemia presents with abdominal pain and is scheduled for cholecystectomy.

What is sickle cell anemia?

Sickle cell anemia is a hereditary hemolytic anemia resulting from the formation of an abnormal hemoglobin (Hb S). Hb S differs structurally from the normal adult hemoglobin (Hb A) only in the substitution of valine for glutamic acid at the sixth position of the beta chain (Chapter 22). Functionally, sickle hemoglobin has less affinity for oxygen (P-50 = 31 mm Hg) as well as decreased solubility. Upon deoxygenation, Hb S readily polymerizes and precipitates inside red blood cells, causing them to sickle. Patients produce variable amounts (2–20%) of fetal hemoglobin (Hb F). It is likely that cells with large amounts of Hb F are somewhat protected from sickling. The continuous formation and destruction of irreversibly sickled cells leads to anemia. Hematocrits are typically 18–30% due to extravascular hemolysis. Red cell survival is reduced to 10–15 days, compared with up to 120 days in normal individuals.

What is the difference between sickle cell anemia and sickle cell trait?

When the genetic defect for adult hemoglobin is on both the maternally and paternally derived chromosomes (No. 11), the patient is homozygous for Hb S and has sickle cell anemia (Hb SS). When only one chromosome has the sickle gene, the patient is heterozygous and has sickle cell trait (Hb AS). Patients with sickle trait produce variable amounts of Hb A (55–60%) and Hb S (35–40%). Unlike those with Hb SS, they are generally not anemic, are asymptomatic, and have a normal life span. Sickling occurs only under extreme hypoxemia or in low-flow states. Sickling is especially apt to occur in the renal medulla; indeed, many patients with sickle trait have impaired renal concentrating ability. Some patients with Hb AS have been reported to have renal medullary, splenic, and pulmonary infarcts.

What is the prevalence of sickle cell gene in black Americans?

Sickle cell anemia is primarily a disease of blacks of Central African ancestry. Approximately 0.2–0.5% of black Americans are homozygous for the sickle gene, while approximately 8–10% are heterozygous. Sickle cell anemia is less commonly found in patients of Mediterranean ancestry.

What is the pathophysiology of sickle cell anemia?

Conditions favoring the formation of deoxyhemoglobin—eg, hypoxemia, acidosis, intracellular hypertonicity or dehydration, increased 2,3-DPG levels, or increased temperature—can precipitate sickling in patients with Hb SS. Hypothermia may also be detrimental because of the associated vasoconstriction (see below). Intracellular polymerization of Hb S distorts red cells, makes them less pliable and "more sticky," and increases blood viscosity. Sickling may initially be reversible but eventually becomes irreversible in some cells. Formation of red cell aggregates in capillaries can obstruct the microcirculation in tissues. A vicious cycle is established where circulatory stasis leads to localized hypoxia, which causes more sickling.

Table 29–8. Manifestations of sickle cell anemia.

Neurologic
 Stroke
 Subarachnoid hemorrhage
 Coma
 Seizures
Ocular
 Vitreous hemorrhage
 Retinal infarcts
 Proliferative retinopathy
 Retinal detachment
Pulmonary
 Increased intrapulmonary shunting
 Pleuritis
 Recurrent pulmonary infections
 Pulmonary infarcts
Cardiovascular
 Congestive heart failure
 Cor pulmonale
 Pericarditis
 Myocardial infarction
Gastrointestinal
 Cholelithiasis (pigmented stones)
 Cholecystitis
 Hepatic infarcts
 Hepatic abscesses
 Hepatic fibrosis
Hematologic
 Anemia
 Aplastic anemia
 Recurrent infections
 Splenic infarcts
 Splenic sequestration
 Functional asplenia
Genitourinary
 Hematuria
 Renal papillary necrosis
 Impaired renal concentrating ability (isosthenuria)
 Nephrotic syndrome
 Renal insufficiency
 Renal failure
 Priapism
Skeletal
 Synovitis
 Arthritis
 Aseptic necrosis of femoral head
 Small bone infarcts in hands and feet (dactylitis)
 Biconcave ("fishmouth") vertebrae
 Osteomyelitis
Skin
 Chronic ulcers

How do patients with sickle cell anemia usually present?

Patients with Hb SS generally first develop symptoms in infancy, when levels of fetal hemoglobin (Hb F) decline appreciably. The disease is characterized both by acute episodic crises and by chronic and progressive features (Table 29–8). Children display retarded growth and have recurrent infections. Recurrent splenic infarction leads to splenic atrophy and functional asplenism by adolescence. Patients usually die from recurrent infections or renal failure. Crises are often precipitated by infection, cold weather, dehydration, or other forms of stress. Crises may be divided into three types:

(1) Vaso-occlusive crises: Depending on the vessels involved, these acute episodes can result in micro- or macroinfarctions. Most painful crises are thought to be due to microinfarcts in the various tissues. Clinically, they present as acute abdominal, chest, back, or joint pain. Differentiation between surgical and nonsurgical causes of abdominal pain is difficult. Most patients form pigmented gallstones by adulthood, and many present with acute cholecystitis. Vaso-occlusive phenomena in larger vessels can produce thromboses resulting in splenic, cerebral, pulmonary, hepatic, renal, and, less commonly, myocardial infarctions.

(2) Aplastic crisis: Profound anemia (Hb 2–3 g/dL) can rapidly occur when red cell production in the bone marrow is exhausted or suppressed. Infections and folate deficiency may play a major role. Some patients also develop leukopenia.

(3) Splenic sequestration crisis: Sudden pooling of blood in the spleen can occur in infants and young children and can cause life-threatening hypotension. The mechanism is thought to be partial or complete occlusion of venous drainage from the spleen.

How is sickle cell anemia diagnosed?

Red blood cells from patients with sickle cell anemia readily sickle following addition of an oxygen-consuming reagent (metabisulfite) or a hypertonic ionic solution (solubility test). Confirmation requires hemoglobin electrophoresis.

What is the optimal way to prepare patients with sickle cell anemia for surgery?

Optimal preoperative preparation is desirable for all patients undergoing surgery: Patients should be well-hydrated, infections should be controlled, and the hemoglobin concentration should be at an acceptable level. Preoperative transfusion therapy must be individualized to the patient and to the surgical procedure. Most authors advocate partial exchange transfusions before major surgical procedures. Unlike simple transfusions, exchange transfusions decrease blood viscosity. They also increase oxygen-carrying capacity and decrease the likelihood of sickling. The goal of such transfusions is generally to achieve a hematocrit of 35–40% with 40–50% normal hemoglobin (Hb A_1). Although the benefits of exchange transfusions for patients undergoing anesthesia have yet to be demonstrated, exchange transfusions clearly help patients experiencing a crisis.

Are there any special intraoperative considerations?

Conditions that might promote hemoglobin desaturation or low-flow states should be avoided. Every effort must be made to avoid hypo- and hyperthermia, acidosis, and even mild degrees of hypoxemia, hypo-

tension, or hypovolemia. Generous hydration and a relatively high (> 50%) inspired oxygen tension are desirable. The major compensatory mechanism in these patients is an increased cardiac output, which should be maintained intraoperatively. Central venous pressure monitoring or pulmonary artery pressure with mixed venous oxygen saturation monitoring may be useful in some patients. Mild alkalosis may help avoid sickling, but even moderate degrees of respiratory alkalosis may have an adverse effect on cerebral blood flow. Many clinicians will also avoid the use of tourniquets. Studies are not available to support or reject the use of any one regional or general anesthetic technique.

Are there any special postoperative considerations?

The same principles applied intraoperatively hold for the postoperative period. Most perioperative deaths occur in the postoperative period. Hypoxemia and pulmonary complications appear to be major risk factors. Supplemental oxygen, optimal pain control, pulmonary physiotherapy, and early ambulation are desirable to avoid such complications.

What is the pathophysiology of thalassemia?

Thalassemia is a hereditary defect in the production of one or more of the normal subunits of hemoglobin. Patients with thalassemia may be able to produce normal Hb A but have reduced amounts of alpha or beta chain production (Table 29–9). The severity of this defect depends on the subunit affected and the degree with which hemoglobin production is affected. Symptoms may be absent or severe. Patients with α-thalassemia produce reduced amounts of α-subunit, while patients with β-thalassemia produce reduced amounts of the β-subunit. The formation of hemoglobins with abnormal subunit composition can alter the red cell membrane and lead to variable degrees of hemolysis as well as ineffective hematopoiesis. The latter can result

Table 29–9. Classification of thalassemias.[1]

	α/β Production Ratio	Clinical Severity
Normal	1	0
α-Thalassemias		
Silent	0.9	0
α-Thalassemia trait	0.7	0
Hemoblobin H disease	0.3	++
Hydrops fetalis	0	++++
β-Thalassemias		
β-Thalassemia trait (thalassemia minor)	2	0 to +
β-Thalassemia intermedia	3 to ∞	++ to +++
β-Thalassemia major (Cooley's anemia)	3 to ∞	++++

[1]Adapted from Bunn HF in: *Harrison's Principles of Internal Medicine,* 12th ed. McGraw-Hill, 1991.

in hypertrophy of the bone marrow and often an abnormal skeleton. Maxillary hypertrophy may make intubation difficult. Thalassemias are most common in patients of Southeast Asian, African, Mediterranean, and Indian ancestry.

What is the significance of sickle cell anemia and thalassemia in the same patient?

The combination of Hb S and thalassemia, most commonly sickle β-thalassemia, has a quite variable and unpredictable effect on disease severity. In general, the combination tends to be milder in black patients than in those of Mediterranean ancestry.

What is hemoglobin C disease?

Substitution of lysine for glutamic acid at position 6 on the beta subunit results in hemoglobin C (Hb C). Approximately 0.05% of black Americans carry the gene for Hb C. Patients homozygous for Hb C generally have only a mild hemolytic anemia and splenomegaly. They rarely develop significant complications. The tendency for Hb C to crystallize in hypertonic environments is probably responsible for the hemolysis and characteristically produces target cells on the peripheral blood smear.

What is the significance of the genotype Hb SC?

Nearly 0.1% of black Americans are simultaneously heterozygous for both Hb S and Hb C (Hb SC). These patients generally have a mild to moderate hemolytic anemia. Some patients occasionally have painful crises, splenic infarcts, and hepatic dysfunction. Eye manifestations similar to those associated with Hb SS disease are especially prominent. Females with Hb SC have a high rate of complications during the third trimester of pregnancy and delivery.

What is the hematologic significance of glucose-6-phosphate dehydrogenase deficiency?

Red blood cells are normally well protected against oxidizing agents. The sulfhydryl groups on hemoglobin are protected by reduced glutathione. The latter is regenerated by NADPH (reduced nicotinamide adenine dinucleotide phosphate), which itself is regenerated by glucose metabolism in the hexose monophosphate shunt. Glucose-6-phosphate dehydrogenase (G6PD) is a critical enzyme in this pathway. A defect in this pathway results in an inadequate amount of

Table 29–10. Drugs to avoid in patients with G6PD deficiency.

Drugs that may cause hemolysis
Sulfonamides
Antimalarial drugs
Nitrofurantoin
Nalidixic acid
Aminosalicylic acid
Phenacetin
Acetanilid
Vitamin K
Probenecid
Methylene blue
Quinine[1]
Quinidine[1]
Chloramphenicol[1]
Other drugs[2]
Prilocaine
Nitroprusside

[1]May be safe in patients with the A⁻ variant.
[2]Should be avoided because of their potential to cause methemoglobinemia.

reduced glutathione, which can potentially result in the oxidation and precipitation of hemoglobin in red cells (seen as Heinz bodies) and hemolysis.

Abnormalities in G6PD are relatively common. Nearly 250 variants are described. Depending on the functional significance of the enzyme abnormality, clinical manifestations can be quite variable. Up to 15% of black American males have the common clinically significant A⁻ variant. A second variant is common in individuals of eastern Mediterranean ancestry, and a third in individuals of Chinese ancestry. Because the locus for the enzyme is on the X chromosome, abnormalities are X-linked traits, with males being primarily affected. As red blood cells age, G6PD activity normally decreases. Consequently, aging red cells are most susceptible to oxidation. This decay is markedly accelerated in patients with the Mediterranean variant but only moderately so in patients with the A⁻ variant. Most patients are typically not anemic but can develop hemolysis following oxidant stresses such as viral and bacterial infections or ingestions of some drugs (Table 29–10). Hemolysis can also be precipitated by metabolic acidosis. Hemolytic episodes can present with hemoglobinuria and hypotension. They are generally self-limited because only the older population of cells is destroyed. Mediterranean variants may be associated with some degree of chronic hemolytic anemia, and some patients are exquisitely sensitive to fava beans.

Treatment is primarily preventive. Measures aimed at preserving renal function (see above) are indicated in patients who develop hemoglobinuria.

SUGGESTED READINGS

Boutrous AR et al: Comparison of hemodynamic, pulmonary, and renal effects of use of three types of fluids after major surgical procedures on the abdominal aorta. Crit Care Med 1979;7:9.

Rossi E, Simon TL, Moss GS: *Principles of Transfusion Medicine.* Williams & Wilkins 1990.

Shires T, Williams J, Brown F: Acute changes in extracellular fluid associated with major surgical procedures. Ann Surg 1961;154:803.

Shoemaker WC, Hauser CJ: Critique of crystalloid versus colloid in shock lung. Crit Care Med 1979;7:117.

Skillman JJ, Smith DE, Zarins CD: Randomized trial of albumin vs. electrolyte solutions during abdominal aortic operations. Surgery 1975;78:291.

Virgilio RW et al: Crystalloid versus colloid resuscitation: Is one better? Surgery 1979;85:129.

[The foregoing are the most commonly referenced articles in the "crystalloid versus colloid" controversy.]

Petz LD: *Clinical Practice of Transfusion Medicine.* Churchill Livingstone, 1989.

Questions and Answers About Transfusions. American Society of Anesthesiologists. ASA Press, 1987.

Stehling LC: Recent advances in transfusion therapy. Adv Anesth 1987;4:213.

Stoelting RK, Dierdorf SF, McCammon RL: *Anesthesia and Co-Existing Disease,* 2nd ed. Churchill Livingstone, 1988. Contains a good discussion of transfusion therapy and hemoglobinopathies.

30

Acid-Base Balance

Most biochemical reactions in the body are dependent on maintenance of a physiologic hydrogen ion concentration. Because changes in hydrogen ion concentration can produce widespread organ dysfunction, it is closely regulated in body fluids.

This regulation—often referred to as acid-base balance—is of prime importance to anesthesiologists. Changes in ventilation and perfusion are common during anesthesia and can rapidly alter acid-base balance. A thorough understanding of acid-base disturbances, their physiologic effects, and treatment is thus essential for proper anesthetic management.

This chapter examines acid-base physiology, common disturbances, and their anesthetic implications. Clinical measurements of blood gases and their use in interpreting acid-base disorders are also discussed.

DEFINITIONS: ACID-BASE CHEMISTRY

Hydrogen Ion Concentration & pH

In any aqueous solution, water molecules reversibly dissociate into hydrogen and hydroxide ions:

$$H_2O \leftrightarrow H^+ + OH^-$$

This process is described by the dissociation constant, K_w:

$$K_w = [H^+][HO^-] = 10^{-14}$$

The concentration of water is omitted from the denominator of this expression because it does not vary appreciably and is already included in the constant. Therefore, if one is given $[H^+]$ or $[OH^-]$, the concentration of the other ion can be readily calculated.

Example: If $[H^+] = 10^{-8}$ nmol/L, then $[OH^-] = 10^{-14} \div 10^{-8} = 10^{-6}$ nmol/L.

Arterial $[H^+]$ is normally 40 nmol/L, or 40×10^{-9} mol/L. Hydrogen ion concentration is more commonly expressed as pH, because dealing with numbers of this order of magnitude is awkward. The pH of a solution is defined as the negative logarithm (base 10) of $[H^+]$ (Figure 30–1). Normal arterial pH is therefore $-\log(40 \times 10^{-9}) = 7.40$

Acids & Bases

Clinically, an acid is usually defined as a chemical species that can act as a proton (H^+) donor, while a base is a species that can act as a proton acceptor (Brönsted-Lowry definitions). The acidity of an aqueous solution therefore reflects its $[H^+]$. A strong acid is a substance that readily and almost irreversibly gives up an H^+ and increases $[H^+]$, while a strong base avidly binds H^+ and decreases $[H^+]$. In contrast, weak acids reversibly donate H^+, while weak bases reversibly bind H^+; both tend to have less of an effect on $[H^+]$. Most biologic compounds are either weak acids or weak bases.

For a solution containing the weak acid HA, where—

$$HA \leftrightarrow H^+ + A^-$$

a dissociation constant, K, can be defined as follows:

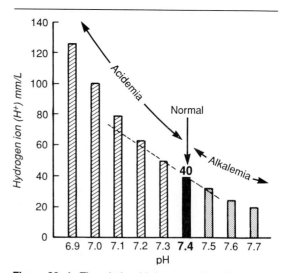

Figure 30–1. The relationship between pH and [H$^+$]. Note that between a pH of 7.10 and 7.50, the relationship between pH and [H$^+$] is nearly linear. (Reproduced, with permission, from Narins RG, Emmett M: Simple and Mixed Acid-base Disorders: A Practical Approach. Medicine 1980;59:161.)

$$K = \frac{[H^+][A^-]}{[HA]}, \text{ or } [H^+] = K \frac{[HA]}{[A^-]}$$

The negative logarithmic form of the latter equation is called the Henderson-Hasselbalch equation:

$$pH = pK + \log \frac{[A^-]}{[HA]}$$

From this equation, it is apparent that the pH of this solution is related to the ratio of the dissociated anion to the undissociated acid.

Conjugate Pairs & Buffers

When the weak acid HA is in solution, HA can act as an acid by donating an H^+, while A^- can act as a base by taking up H^+. A^- is therefore often referred to as the conjugate base of HA. A similar concept can be applied for weak bases. Consider the weak base B, where–

$$B + H^+ \leftrightarrow BH^+$$

BH^+ is therefore the conjugate acid of B.

A buffer is a solution that contains a weak acid and its conjugate base or a weak base and its conjugate acid (conjugate pairs). Buffers minimize any change in $[H^+]$ by readily accepting or giving up hydrogen ions. From the Henderson-Hasselbalch equation, it is readily apparent that buffers are most efficient in minimizing changes in the $[H^+]$ of a solution (ie, $[A^-]$ = $[HA]$) when $pH = pK$. Moreover, the conjugate pair must be present in significant quantities in solution to act as an effective buffer.

DEFINITIONS: CLINICAL DISORDERS

A clear understanding of acid-base disorders and compensatory physiologic responses requires precise terminology (Table 30–1). The suffix -osis is used here to denote any pathologic process that alters arterial pH. Thus, any disorder that tends to lower pH is an **acidosis,** while one tending to increase pH is termed an **alkalosis.** If the disorder primarily affects $[HCO_3^-]$, it is termed **metabolic.** If the disorder primarily affects

Table 30–1. Defining acid-base disorders.

Disorder	Primary Change	Compensatory Response
Respiratory Acidosis Alkalosis	↑ $PaCO_2$ ↓ $PaCO_2$	↑ HCO_3^- ↓ HCO_3^-
Metabolic Acidosis Alkalosis	↓ HCO_3^- ↑ HCO_3^-	↓ $PaCO_2$ ↑ $PaCO_2$

$PaCO_2$, it is termed **respiratory.** Secondary compensatory responses (see below) should be referred to as just that and not as an "-osis."

When only one pathologic process occurs by itself, the acid-base disorder is considered to be simple. The presence of two or more primary processes comprises a mixed acid-base disorder.

The suffix **-emia** is used to denote the net effect of all primary processes and compensatory physiologic responses (see below) on arterial blood pH. Since arterial blood pH is normally 7.36–7.44 in adults, the term **acidemia** signifies a pH < 7.35 while **alkalemia** signifies a pH > 7.45.

COMPENSATORY MECHANISMS

Physiologic responses to changes in $[H^+]$ are characterized by three phases: (1) immediate chemical buffering, (2) respiratory compensation (whenever possible), and (3) a slower but more effective renal compensatory response that may nearly normalize arterial pH even if the pathologic process is still present.

BODY BUFFERS

Physiologically important buffers in humans include the bicarbonate (H_2CO_3/HCO_3^-), hemoglobin (HbH/Hb^-), other intracellular proteins (HPr/Pr^-), phosphate ($H_2PO_4^-/HPO_4^{2-}$), and ammonium (NH_3/NH_4^+) buffers. The effectiveness of these buffers in the various fluid compartments is related to their concentration (Chapter 28). Bicarbonate is the most important buffer in the extracellular fluid compartment. Hemoglobin, though restricted inside red blood cells, also functions as an important buffer in blood. Other proteins probably play a major role in buffering the intracellular fluid compartment. Phosphate and ammonium ions are important buffers in urine.

Buffering of the extracellular compartment can also be accomplished by the exchange of extracellular H^+ for Na^+ and Ca^{2+} ions from bone and by the exchange of extracellular H^+ for intracellular K^+ (Chapter 28).

The Bicarbonate Buffer

Although in the strictest sense the bicarbonate buffer consists of H_2CO_3 and HCO_3^-, CO_2 tension ($PaCO_2$) may be substituted for H_2CO_3, since:

$$H_2O + CO_2 \leftrightarrow H_2CO_3 \leftrightarrow H^+ + HCO_3^-$$

This hydration of CO_2 is catalyzed by carbonic anhydrase. If adjustments are made in the dissociation constant for the bicarbonate buffer and if the solubility coefficient for CO_2 (0.03 mmol/L) is taken into consideration, the Henderson-Hasselbalch equation for bicarbonate can be written as follows:

$$pH = pK' + \log \frac{[HCO_3^-]}{0.03 \times PaCO_2}$$

where $pK' = 6.1$.

Note that its pK' is not close to the normal arterial pH of 7.40, which means that bicarbonate would not be expected to be an efficient extracellular buffer (see above). The bicarbonate system is important for two reasons: First, bicarbonate (HCO_3^-) is present in relatively high concentrations in extracellular fluid. Second—and more importantly—$PaCO_2$ and plasma $[HCO_3^-]$ are closely regulated by the lungs and the kidneys, respectively. The ability of the lungs and kidneys to alter the $[HCO_3^-]/PaCO_2$ ratio allows them to exert important influences on arterial pH.

A simplified and more practical derivation of the Henderson-Hasselbalch equation for the bicarbonate buffer is as follows:

$$[H^+] = 24 \times \frac{PaCO_2}{[HCO_3^-]}$$

Because pH can be readily converted to $[H^+]$ (Table 30–2), this equation is very useful clinically. Note that below 7.40, $[H^+]$ increases 1.25 nmol/L for each 0.01 decrease in pH; above 7.40, $[H^+]$ decreases 0.8 nmol/L for each 0.01 increase in pH.

Example: If arterial pH = 7.28 and $PaCO_2 = 24$ mmol/L, what should the plasma $[HCO_3^-]$ be?

$$[H^+] = 40 + [(40 - 28) \times 1.25] = 55 \text{ nmol/L}$$

Therefore,

$$55 = 24 \times \frac{24}{[HCO_3^-]}, \text{ and } [HCO_3^-] =$$

$$\frac{(24 \times 24)}{55} = 10.5 \text{ mmol/L}$$

It should be emphasized that *the bicarbonate buffer is effective against metabolic but not respiratory acid-base disturbances.* If 3 mmol/L of a strong nonvolatile

Table 30–2. The relationship between pH and $[H^+]$.

pH	$[H^+]$
6.80	158 neq/L
6.90	126 neq/L
7.00	100 neq/L
7.10	79 neq/L
7.20	63 neq/L
7.30	50 neq/L
7.40	40 neq/L
7.50	32 neq/L
7.60	25 neq/L
7.70	20 neq/L

acid such as HCl is added to extracellular fluid, the following takes place:

$$\underset{H^+}{\overset{3 \text{ mmol/L}}{}} + \underset{HCO_3^-}{\overset{24 \text{ mmol/L}}{}} \rightarrow H_2CO_3 \rightarrow H_2O +$$

$$\underset{CO_2}{\overset{3 \text{ mmol/L}}{}} + \underset{HCO_3^-}{\overset{21 \text{ mmol/L}}{}}$$

Note that HCO_3^- reacts with H^+ to produce CO_2. Moreover, the CO_2 generated is normally eliminated by the lungs such that $PaCO_2$ is unchanged. Consequently, $[H^+] = 24 \times 40 \div 21 = 45.7$ nmol/L and pH = 7.34. Furthermore, the decrease in $[HCO_3^-]$ reflects the amount of nonvolatile acid added.

In contrast, an increase in CO_2 tension (volatile acid) has a minimal effect on $[HCO_3^-]$. If, for example, $PaCO_2$ increases from 40 to 80 mm Hg, the dissolved CO_2 only increases from 1.2 mmol/L to 2.2 mmol/L. Moreover, the equilibrium constant for the hydration of CO_2 is such that an increase of this magnitude minimally drives the reaction to the left:

$$H_2O + CO_2 \leftrightarrow H_2CO_3 \leftrightarrow H^+ + HCO_3^-$$

If the valid assumption that $[HCO3-]$ does not appreciably change is made, then–

$$[H^+] = \frac{24 \times 80}{24} = 80 \text{ nmol/L and pH} = 7.10$$

In this example, $[H^+]$ increases by 40 nmol/L, and since HCO_3^- is produced in a 1:1 ratio with H^+, $[HCO_3^-]$ also increases by 40 nmol/L. Thus, extracellular $[HCO_3^-]$ increases negligibly, from 24 mmol/L to 24.000040 mmol/L. Therefore, the bicarbonate buffer is not effective against increases in $PaCO_2$, and changes in $[HCO_3^-]$ are not indicative of the severity of respiratory acidosis.

Hemoglobin as a Buffer

Quantitatively, hemoglobin functions as the most important noncarbonic buffer in extracellular fluid. Hemoglobin is a complex molecule with multiple buffering sites. The principal buffering sites are histidine moieties with a pK of approximately 6.8. Simplistically, hemoglobin may be thought of as existing in red blood cells in an equilibrium as a weak acid (HHb) with its potassium salt (KHb). *In contrast to the bicarbonate buffer, hemoglobin is capable of buffering both carbonic (CO_2) and noncarbonic (nonvolatile) acids:*

$$H^+ + KHb \leftrightarrow HHb + K^+$$
$$\text{and } H_2CO_3 + KHb \leftrightarrow HHb + HCO_3^-$$

PULMONARY COMPENSATION

The reflex changes in alveolar ventilation responsible for pulmonary compensation of $PaCO_2$ are mediated by chemoreceptors within the brain stem (Chapter 22). These receptors respond to changes in cerebrospinal spinal fluid pH. Pulmonary compensatory responses are important in defending against marked changes in pH during metabolic disturbances.

Pulmonary Compensation During Metabolic Acidosis

Decreases in arterial blood pH stimulate medullary respiratory centers, increasing alveolar ventilation, lowering $PaCO_2$, and tending to restore arterial pH towards normal. The pulmonary response to lower $PaCO_2$ occurs rapidly but may not reach a predictably steady state until 12–24 hours; pH is never completely restored to normal. *$PaCO_2$ normally decreases 1–1.5 mm Hg below 40 mm Hg for every 1 mmol/L decrease in plasma $[HCO_3^-]$.*

Pulmonary Compensation During Metabolic Alkalosis

Increases in arterial blood pH depress respiratory centers, resulting in relative alveolar hypoventilation, which tends to elevate $PaCO_2$ and restore arterial pH toward normal. The pulmonary response to metabolic alkalosis is generally less predictable than that to metabolic acidosis. Hypoxemia, as a result of progressive hypoventilation, eventually activates oxygen-sensitive chemoreceptors (Chapter 22) that stimulate ventilation and limit the pulmonary compensatory response. Consequently, $PaCO_2$ usually does not rise above 55 mm Hg in response to metabolic alkalosis. As a general rule, *$PaCO_2$ can be expected to increase 0.25–1 mm Hg for each 1 mmol/L increase in $[HCO_3^-]$.*

RENAL COMPENSATION

The kidneys' ability to control the amount of HCO_3^- reabsorbed from filtered tubular fluid, form new HCO_3^-, and eliminate H^+ in the form of titratable acids and ammonium ions (Chapter 31) allows them to exert a major influence on pH during both metabolic and respiratory acid-base disturbances.

Renal Compensation During Acidosis

The renal response to acidemia is threefold: (1) increased reabsorption of the filtered HCO_3^-, (2) increased excretion of titratable acids, and (3) increased ammonia production.

Although these mechanisms are probably activated immediately, their effects are generally not appreciable for 12–24 hours and may not be maximal for up to 5 days.

A. Increased Reabsorption of HCO_3^-: Bicarbonate reabsorption is shown in Figure 30–2. Briefly, CO_2 within renal tubular cells combines with water in the presence of carbonic anhydrase. The carbonic acid (H_2CO_3) formed rapidly dissociates into H^+ and

HCO_3^-. Bicarbonate ion then enters the bloodstream while the H^+ is secreted into the renal tubule, where it reacts with filtered HCO_3^- to form H_2CO_3. Carbonic anhydrase associated with the luminal brush border catalyzes the dissociation of H_2CO_3 into CO_2 and H_2O. The CO_2 thus formed can diffuse back into the renal tubular cell to replace the CO_2 originally consumed. The proximal tubules normally reabsorb 80–90% of the filtered bicarbonate load, while the distal tubules are responsible for the remaining 10–20%. Unlike the proximal H^+ pump, the H^+ pump in the distal tubule is capable of generating steep H^+ gradients between tubular fluid and tubular cells and can result in a urinary pH as low as 4.4 (compared to a pH of 7.40 in plasma).

B. Increased Excretion of Titratable Acids: When most of the HCO_3^- in tubular fluid is reclaimed, the H^+ secreted into the tubular lumen can combine with HPO_4^{2-} to form $H_2PO_4^-$ (Figure 30–3). The latter is also not readily reabsorbed because of its charge and is eliminated in urine. The net result is that H^+ is excreted from the body as $H_2PO_4^-$, and HCO_3^- is generated in the process and can enter the bloodstream. With a pK of 6.8, the $H_2PO_4^-/HPO_4^{2-}$ pair is normally an ideal urinary buffer. However, when urinary pH approaches 4.4, all the phosphate reaching the distal tubule is in the $H_2PO_4^-$ form; HPO_4^{2-} ions are no longer available for eliminating H^+.

C. Increased Formation of Ammonia: After complete reabsorption of HCO_3^- and consumption of the phosphate buffer, NH_3/NH_4^+ becomes the most important urinary buffer. Deamination of glutamine within the mitochondria of proximal tubular cells is the principal source of NH_3 production in the kidneys. Acidemia markedly increases renal NH_3 production. The ammonia formed is then able to passively cross the cell's luminal membrane, enter tubular fluid, and react with H^+ to form NH_4^+. Unlike NH_3, NH_4^+ cannot readily penetrate the luminal membrane and is therefore trapped within the tubules. Thus, excretion of NH_4^+ in urine effectively eliminates H^+.

Renal Compensation During Alkalosis

The tremendous amount of HCO_3^- normally filtered and subsequently reabsorbed allows the kidneys to rapidly excrete large amounts of bicarbonate if necessary (Chapter 28). As a result, the kidneys are highly effective in protecting against metabolic alkalosis. *Metabolic alkalosis therefore generally occurs only in association with concomitant sodium deficiency or mineralocorticoid excess.* Sodium depletion decreases extracellular fluid volume and enhances Na^+ reabsorption in the proximal tubule (Chapter 28): Increased H^+ secretion in exchange for augmented Na^+ reabsorption favors continued HCO_3^- formation even in the face of metabolic alkalosis. Similarly, increased mineralocorticoid activity augments aldosterone-mediated Na^+ reabsorption in exchange for H^+ secretion in the distal tubules (Chapter 28). The resulting increase in HCO_3^-

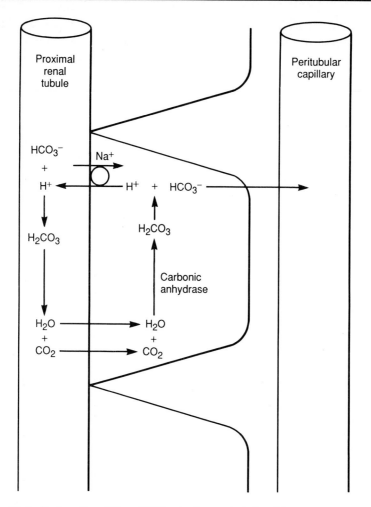

Figure 30–2. Reclamation of filtered HCO_3^- by the renal tubules. CA = carbonic anhydrase.

formation can initiate or propagate metabolic alkalosis. Metabolic alkalosis is commonly associated with increased mineralocorticoid activity even in the absence of sodium depletion (Chapters 28 and 36).

ACIDOSIS

PHYSIOLOGIC EFFECTS OF ACIDEMIA

The overall effects of acidemia represent the balance between its direct effects and sympathoadrenal activation. With worsening acidosis (pH < 7.20), direct depressant effects predominate. Direct myocardial and smooth muscle depression reduces cardiac contractility and peripheral vascular resistance, resulting in progressive hypotension (Chapter 19). Severe acidosis can lead to tissue hypoxia despite a rightward shift in hemoglobin affinity for oxygen (Chapter 22). Both cardiac and vascular smooth muscle become less responsive to endogenous and exogenous catecholamines, and the threshold for ventricular fibrillation is decreased. Progressive hyperkalemia as a result of the movement of K^+ out of cells in exchange for extracellular H^+ (Chapter 28) is also potentially lethal. Plasma $[K^+]$ increases approximately 0.6 meq/L for each 0.10 decrease in pH.

RESPIRATORY ACIDOSIS

Respiratory acidosis is defined as a primary increase in $PaCO_2$. This increase drives the reaction $H_2O + CO_2 \leftrightarrow H_2CO_3 \leftrightarrow H^+ + HCO_3^-$ to the right, leading to an increase in $[H^+]$ and a fall in arterial pH. For the reasons described above, $[HCO_3^-]$ is minimally affected.

$PaCO_2$ represents the balance between CO_2 production and CO_2 elimination (Chapter 22):

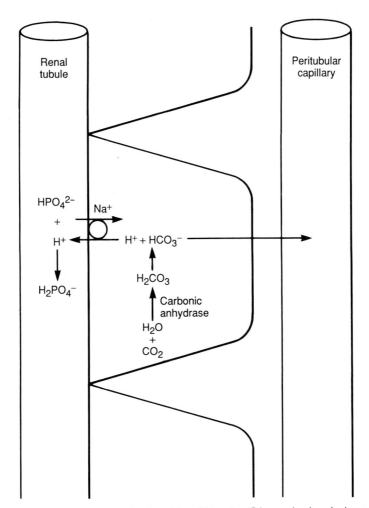

Figure 30–3. Formation of a titratable acid in urine. CA = carbonic anhydrase.

$$PaCO_2 \approx \frac{CO_2 \text{ production}}{\text{Alveolar ventilation}}$$

Carbon dioxide production is a by-product of fat and carbohydrate metabolism. Muscle activity, body temperature, and thyroid hormone activity can all have major influences on CO_2 production. Because CO_2 production does not appreciably vary under most circumstances, respiratory acidosis is usually the result of alveolar hypoventilation (Table 30–3). However, in patients with a limited capacity to increase alveolar ventilation, increased CO_2 production can precipitate respiratory acidosis.

Acute Respiratory Acidosis

The compensatory response to acute (6–12 hours) elevations in $PaCO_2$ is limited. Buffering is primarily provided by hemoglobin and the exchange of extracellular H^+ for Na^+ and K^+ from bone and the intracellular fluid compartment (see above). The renal response to retain more bicarbonate is still very limited. As a result, *plasma [HCO_3^-] increases only about 1 mmol/L for each 10 mm Hg increase in $PaCO_2$ above 40 mm Hg.*

Chronic Respiratory Acidosis

"Full" renal compensation characterizes chronic respiratory acidosis. As stated above, renal compensation is appreciable only after 12–24 hours and may not peak until 3–5 days. During that time, the sustained increase in $PaCO_2$ has been present long enough to permit maximal renal compensation. *During chronic respiratory acidosis, plasma [HCO_3^-] increases approximately 4 mmol/L for each 10 mm Hg increase in $PaCO_2$ above 40 mm Hg.*

Treatment of Respiratory Acidosis

The treatment of respiratory acidosis is to reverse the imbalance between CO_2 production and alveolar ventilation. In most instances, this is accomplished by increasing alveolar ventilation. Measures aimed at reducing CO_2 production (eg, dantrolene, muscle paralysis, antithyroid medication, or reduced carbohydrate intake) are useful only in specific instances (malignant

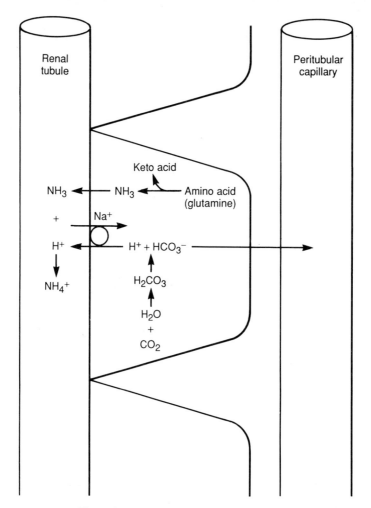

Figure 30–4. Formation of ammonia in urine.

hyperthermia, status epilepticus, thyroid storm, and parenteral nutrition, respectively). Temporizing measures aimed at improving alveolar ventilation include bronchodilatation, reversal of narcosis, administration of a respiratory stimulant (doxapram), or improving lung compliance (diuresis). Moderate to severe acidosis (pH < 7.20), CO_2 narcosis, and impending respiratory muscle fatigue are indications for mechanical ventilation (Chapter 48). An increased inspired oxygen concentration is also usually necessary, since coexistent hypoxemia is common. Intravenous $NaHCO_3$ is rarely necessary unless marked acidosis (pH < 7.1) is present and is associated with cardiovascular collapse. Sodium bicarbonate therapy will transiently increase $PaCO_2$:

$$H^+ + HCO_3^- \rightarrow CO_2 + H_2O$$

Patients with a baseline chronic respiratory acidosis require special consideration (Chapter 23). When such patients develop acute ventilatory failure, the goal of therapy should be to return $PaCO_2$ to the patient's "normal" baseline. Normalizing the patient's $PaCO_2$ to 40 mm Hg will result in metabolic alkalosis (see below). Oxygen therapy must also be carefully controlled, because the respiratory drive in these patients becomes dependent on hypoxemia not $PaCO_2$; "normalization" of PaO_2 or relative hyperoxia can precipitate severe hypoventilation.

METABOLIC ACIDOSIS

Metabolic acidosis is defined as a primary decrease in $[HCO_3^-]$. Pathologic processes can initiate metabolic acidosis by one of three mechanisms: (1) consumption of HCO_3^- by a strong nonvolatile acid, (2) renal or gastrointestinal wasting of bicarbonate, or (3) rapid dilution of the extracellular fluid compartment with a bicarbonate-free fluid.

A fall in plasma $[HCO_3^-]$ without a proportionate reduction in $PaCO_2$ decreases arterial pH. The pulmo-

Table 30–3. Causes of respiratory acidosis.

Alveolar hypoventilation
  Central nervous system depression
    Drug-induced
    Sleep disorders
    Pickwickian syndrome
    Cerebral ischemia
    Cerebral trauma
  Neuromuscular disorders
    Myopathies
    Neuropathies
  Chest wall abnormalities
    Flail chest
    Kyphoscoliosis
  Pleural abnormalities
    Pneumothorax
    Pleural effusion
  Airway obstruction
    Upper airway
      Foreign body
      Tumor
      Laryngospasm
      Sleep disorders
    Lower airway
      Severe asthma
      Chronic obstructive airway disease
      Tumor
  Parenchymal lung disease
    Pulmonary edema
      Cardiogenic
      Noncardiogenic
    Pulmonary emboli
    Pneumonia
    Aspiration
    Interstitial lung disease
  Ventilator malfunction
Increased CO_2 production
  Large carbohydrate loads (enteral or parenteral nutrition)
  Malignant hyperthermia
  Intense shivering
  Prolonged seizure activity
  Thyroid storm
  Extensive thermal injury (burns)

Table 30–4. Causes of metabolic acidosis.

Increased anion gap
  Increased production of endogenous nonvolatile acids
    Renal failure
      Acute
      Chronic
    Ketoacidosis
      Diabetic
      Starvation
    Lactic acidosis
    Mixed
      Nonketotic hyperosmolar coma
      Alcoholic
    Inborn errors of metabolism
  Ingestion of toxin
    Salicylate
    Methanol
    Ethylene Glycol
    Paraldehyde
    Toluene
    Sulfur
  Rhabdomyolysis
Normal anion gap (hyperchloremic)
  Increased gastrointestinal losses of HCO_3^-
    Diarrhea
    Anion exchange resins
    Ingestion of $CaCl_2$, $MgCl_2$
    Fistulae (pancreatic, biliary, or small bowel)
    Ureterosigmoidostomy or obstructed ileal loop
  Increased renal losses of HCO_3^-
    Renal tubular acidosis
    Carbonic anhydrase inhibitors
    Hypoaldosteronism
  Dilutional
    Large amounts of bicarbonate-free fluids
  Total parenteral nutrition
  Increased intake of chloride-containing acids
    Ammonium chloride
    Lysine hydrochloride
    Arginine hydrochloride

nary compensatory response in a simple metabolic acidosis (see above) characteristically never reduces $PaCO_2$ to a level that completely normalizes pH.

Table 30–4 lists disorders that can cause metabolic acidosis. Note that differential diagnosis of metabolic acidosis is facilitated by calculation of the anion gap.

The Anion Gap

The anion gap in plasma is most commonly defined as the difference between the major measured cations and the major measured anions:

Anion gap = Major plasma cations − Major plasma anions,

or

Anion gap = $[Na^+]$ − $([Cl^-]$ + $[HCO_3^-])$

Using normal values,

Anion gap = 140 − (104 + 24) = 12 meq/L
(normal range = 9–15 meq/L)

In reality, an anion gap cannot exist because electroneutrality must be maintained in the body; the sum of all anions must equal the sum of all cations. Therefore,

Anion gap = Unmeasured anions − Unmeasured cations

"Unmeasured cations" include K^+, Ca^{2+}, and Mg^{2+}, while "unmeasured anions" include phosphates, sulfates, and all organic anions (including plasma proteins). Some clinicians include plasma $[K^+]$ in the calculation. Plasma albumin normally accounts for the largest fraction of the anion gap (about 11 meq/L). Any process that increases "unmeasured anions" or decreases "unmeasured cations" will increase the anion gap. Conversely, any process that decreases "unmeasured anions" or increases "unmeasured cations" will decrease the anion gap.

High Anion Gap Metabolic Acidosis

Metabolic acidosis with a high anion gap is characterized by an increase in relatively strong nonvolatile acids. These acids dissociate into H^+ and their respective anions; the H^+ consumes HCO_3^- to produce CO_2, while their anions (conjugate bases) accumulate and take the place of HCO_3^- in extracellular fluid (hence the anion gap increases). Nonvolatile acids can be endogenously produced or ingested.

A. Failure to Excrete Endogenous Nonvolatile Acids: Approximately 1 meq/kg/d of sulfuric acid, phosphoric acid, and incompletely oxidized organic acids are normally produced by the metabolism of dietary and endogenous proteins. These acids are normally eliminated by the kidneys in urine. Glomerular filtration rates below 20 mL/min (renal failure) typically result in progressive metabolic acidosis from the accumulation of these acids.

B. Increased Endogenous Nonvolatile Acid Production: Severe tissue hypoxia following hypoxemia, hypoperfusion (ischemia), or inability to utilize oxygen (cyanide poisoning) can result in lactic acidosis. Lactic acid is the end product of the anaerobic metabolism of glucose (glycolysis) and can rapidly accumulate under these conditions. Lactate levels can be readily measured and are normally 0.3–1.3 mmol/L. An absolute or relative lack of insulin can result in hyperglycemia and progressive ketoacidosis from accumulation of β-hydroxybutyric and acetoacetic acids. Ketoacidosis may also be seen following starvation and alcoholic binges. The pathophysiology of the acidosis often associated with severe alcoholic intoxication and nonketotic hyperosmolar coma is often complex and may represent a build-up of lactic, keto, or other unknown acids. Some inborn errors of metabolism, such as maple syrup urine disease, methylmalonic aciduria, propionic acidemia, and isovaleric acidemia, produce a high anion gap metabolic acidosis as a result of accumulation of abnormal amino acids.

C. Ingestion of Exogenous Nonvolatile Acids: Ingestion of large amounts of salicylates frequently results in metabolic acidosis. Salicylic acid as well as other acid intermediates rapidly accumulate and produce a high anion gap acidosis. Because salicylates also produce direct respiratory stimulation, most adults develop mixed metabolic acidosis with superimposed respiratory alkalosis (see below). Ingestion of methanol (methyl alcohol) frequently produces acidosis and visual disturbances (retinitis). Symptoms are typically delayed until the slow oxidation of methanol by alcohol dehydrogenase produces formic acid, which is highly toxic to the retina. The high anion gap represents the accumulation of many organic acids, including acetic acid. The toxicity of ethylene glycol is also the result of the action of alcohol dehydrogenase to produce glycolic acid. Glycolic acid, the principal cause of the acidosis, is further metabolized to form oxalic acid, which can be deposited in the renal tubules and result in renal failure.

Normal Anion Gap Metabolic Acidosis

Metabolic acidosis associated with a normal anion gap is typically characterized by hyperchloremia. Plasma $[Cl^-]$ increases to take the place of the HCO_3^- ions lost. Hyperchloremic metabolic acidosis is most commonly due to abnormal gastrointestinal or renal losses of HCO_3^-.

A. Increased Gastrointestinal Loss of HCO_3^-: Diarrhea is the most common cause of hyperchloremic acidosis. Diarrheal fluid contains 20–50 mmol/L of HCO_3^-. Small bowel, biliary, and pancreatic fluids are all rich in HCO_3^-. Loss of large volumes of these fluids can lead to a hyperchloremic metabolic acidosis. Patients with ureterosigmoidostomies and those with ileal loops that are too long or become partially obstructed frequently develop hyperchloremic metabolic acidosis (Chapter 28). The ingestion of chloride-containing anion exchange resins (cholestyramine) or large amounts of calcium or magnesium chloride can result in increased absorption of chloride and loss of bicarbonate ions to the resin or in the formation of insoluble salts within the intestines, respectively.

B. Increased Renal Loss of HCO_3^-: Renal wasting of HCO_3^- can occur as a result of failure to reabsorb filtered HCO_3^- or to secrete adequate amounts of H^+ in the form of titratable acid or ammonium ion. These defects are encountered in patients taking carbonic anhydrase inhibitors such as acetazolamide and those with renal tubular acidosis.

Renal tubular acidosis comprises a group of nonazotemic defects of H^+ secretion by the renal tubules, resulting in a urinary pH that is too high for the systemic acidemia. They may be due to a primary renal defect or secondary to a systemic disorder. The site of the H^+-secreting defect may be in the distal (type 1) or proximal (type 2) renal tubule. Hyporeninemic hypoaldosteronism is commonly referred to as type 4 renal tubular acidosis (Chapter 28). With distal renal tubular acidosis, the defect occurs at a site after most of the filtered HCO_3^- has been reclaimed. As a result, there is a failure to acidify the urine, so that net acid excretion is less than daily net acid production. This disorder is frequently associated with hypokalemia, demineralization of bone, nephrolithiasis, and nephrocalcinosis. Alkali ($NaHCO_3$) therapy with 1–3 mmol/kg/d is usually sufficient to reverse those side effects. With the less common proximal renal tubular acidosis, defective H^+ secretion in the proximal tubule results in massive wasting of HCO_3^-. Concomitant defects in tubular reabsorption of other substances such as glucose, amino acids, or phosphates are common. The hyperchloremic acidosis results in volume depletion and hypokalemia. Treatment involves giving alkali (as much as 10–25 mmol/kg/d) and potassium supplements.

C. Other Causes of Hyperchloremic Acidosis: A dilutional hyperchloremic acidosis can occur when extracellular volume is rapidly expanded with a bicarbonate-free fluid such as normal saline. Amino acid infusions (parenteral hyperalimentation) contain organic cations in excess of organic anions and can produce hyperchloremic metabolic acidosis because chloride is commonly used as the anion for the cationic amino acids. Lastly, the administration of large quantities of chloride-containing acids such as ammonium chloride or arginine hydrochloride can cause hyperchloremic metabolic acidosis.

Treatment of Metabolic Acidosis

Several general measures can be undertaken to control the severity of acidemia until the underlying processes is corrected. Any respiratory component of the acidemia should be corrected. Respiration should be controlled if necessary; a $PaCO_2$ in the low 30s may be desirable to partially return pH towards normal. If arterial blood pH remains below 7.20, alkali therapy in the form of $NaHCO_3$ (usually a 7.5% solution) should be given. $PaCO_2$ may transiently rise as HCO_3^- is consumed by acids (emphasizing the need to control ventilation in severe acidemia). The amount of $NaHCO_3$ given is decided empirically as a fixed dose (1 meq/kg) or is derived from the base excess and the calculated bicarbonate space (see below). In either case, serial blood gas measurements are mandatory to avoid complications (namely, overshoot alkalosis and sodium overload) and to guide further therapy. Raising arterial pH to 7.20–7.30 is usually sufficient to overcome the adverse physiologic effects of the acidemia. Profound or refractory acidemia may necessitate acute hemodialysis with a bicarbonate dialysate.

Specific therapy for diabetic ketoacidosis includes replacement of the existing fluid deficit (as a result of a hyperglycemic osmotic diuresis) as well as insulin, potassium, phosphate, and perhaps magnesium replacement. The treatment of lactic acidosis should be directed first at restoring adequate oxygenation and tissue perfusion. Alkalinization of the urine with $NaHCO_3$ to a pH greater than 7.0 increases elimination of salicylate following salicylate poisoning. Ethanol infusions are indicated following methanol or ethylene glycol intoxication. Ethanol competes for the alcohol dehydrogenase and slows down the formation of formic acid from methanol and from glycolic and oxalic acids, respectively.

A. Base Excess: The base excess value is derived graphically or electronically from a nomogram originally developed by Siggaard-Andersen (Figure 30–5). Conceptually, it is the amount of acid or base that must be added to return blood pH to 7.40 and $PaCO_2$ to 40 mm Hg at full O_2 saturation and 37 °C. Unlike plasma $[HCO_3^-]$ calculation, base excess takes into account noncarbonic (hemoglobin) buffering in the blood. A positive base excess is indicative of metabolic alkalosis, while a negative base excess is indicative of metabolic acidosis.

B. Bicarbonate Space: This space is defined as the volume that HCO_3^- will distribute to when given intravenously. While this theoretically should equal the extracellular fluid space (approximately 25% of body weight), in reality it ranges anywhere between 25% and 60% of body weight depending on the severity and duration of the acidosis. This variation is at least partly related to the amount of intracellular buffering that has taken place.

Example: Calculate the amount of $NaHCO_3$ necessary to correct a base excess (BE) of -10 meq/L for a 70-kg man with an estimated HCO_3^- space of 30%:

$NaHCO_3$ = BE × 30% × Body weight
$NaHCO_3$ = -10 meq/L × 30% × 70 kg × 1 L/kg = 210 meq

In practice, only 50% of the calculated dose (105 meq) is usually given, after which another blood gas is measured.

ANESTHETIC CONSIDERATIONS IN PATIENTS WITH ACIDOSIS

Acidemia can potentiate the depressant effects of most sedatives and anesthetic agents on the central nervous and circulatory systems. Since most opioids are weak bases, acidosis can increase the fraction of the drug in the nonionized form and facilitate penetration of the opioid into the brain. Increased sedation and depression of airway reflexes may predispose to pulmonary aspiration. The circulatory depressant effects of both volatile and intravenous anesthetics can also be exaggerated. Moreover, any agent that rapidly decreases sympathetic tone can potentially allow unopposed circulatory depression in the setting of acidosis. Halothane is more arrhythmogenic in the presence of acidosis. Succinylcholine should generally be avoided in acidotic patients with hyperkalemia to prevent further increases in plasma $[K^+]$. Lastly, respiratory—but not metabolic—acidosis augments nondepolarizing neuromuscular blockade and may prevent its antagonism by reversal agents.

ALKALOSIS

PHYSIOLOGIC EFFECTS OF ALKALOSIS

Alkalosis increases the affinity of hemoglobin for oxygen and shifts the oxygen dissociation curve to the left, making it more difficult to give up oxygen to tissues (Chapter 22). Movement of H^+ out of cells in exchange for the movement of extracellular K^+ into cells can produce hypokalemia (Chapter 28). Alkalosis increases the number of anionic binding sites for Ca^{2+} on plasma proteins and can therefore decrease ionized plasma $[Ca^{2+}]$, leading to circulatory depression and neuromuscular irritability (Chapter 28). Respiratory alkalosis reduces cerebral blood flow (Chapter 25), increases systemic vascular resistance, and may precipitate coronary vasospasm (Chapter 19). In the lungs, respiratory alkalosis increases bronchial

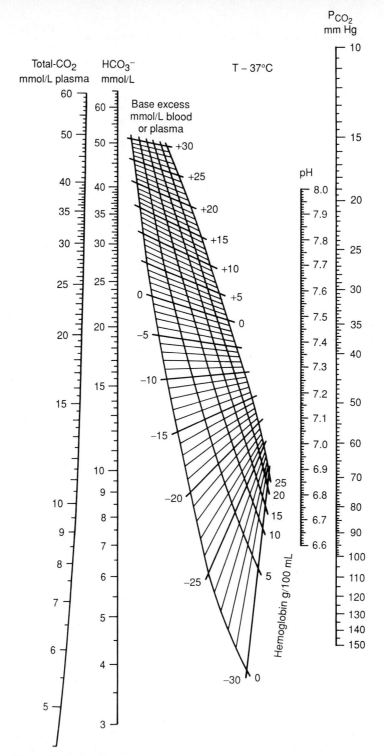

Figure 30–5. The Siggaard-Andersen nomogram for calculating base excess.

smooth muscle tone (bronchoconstriction) but decreases pulmonary vascular resistance (Chapter 22).

RESPIRATORY ALKALOSIS

Respiratory alkalosis is defined as a primary decrease in PaCO₂. The mechanism is usually an inap-

propriate increase in alveolar ventilation relative to CO_2 production. Table 30–5 lists the most common causes of respiratory alkalosis. *Plasma [HCO₃⁻] usually decreases 2 mmol/L for each 10 mm Hg acute decrease in PaCO₂ below 40 mm Hg*. The distinction between acute and chronic respiratory alkalosis is not always made, because the compensatory response to chronic respiratory alkalosis is quite variable: *Plasma*

Table 30–5. Causes of respiratory alkalosis.

Central stimulation
  Pain
  Anxiety
  Ischemia
  Stroke
  Tumor
  Infection
  Fever
  Drug-induced
    Salicylates
    Progesterone (pregnancy)
    Analeptics (doxapram)
Peripheral stimulation
  Hypoxemia
  High altitude
  Pulmonary disease
    Congestive heart failure
    Noncardiogenic pulmonary edema
    Asthma
    Pulmonary emboli
  Severe anemia
Unknown mechanism
  Sepsis
  Metabolic encephalopathies
Iatrogenic
  Ventilator-induced

Table 30–6. Causes of metabolic alkalosis.

Chloride-sensitive
  Gastrointestinal
    Vomiting
    Gastric drainage
    Chloride diarrhea
    Villous adenoma
  Renal
    Diuretics
    Posthypercapnic
    Low chloride intake
  Sweat
    Cystic fibrosis
Chloride-resistant
  Increased mineralocorticoid activity
    Primary hyperaldosteronism
    Edematous disorders (secondary hyperaldosteronism)
    Cushing's syndrome
    Licorice ingestion
    Bartter's syndrome
  Severe hypokalemia
Miscellaneous
  Massive blood transfusion
  Acetate-containing colloid solutions (Plasmanate)
  Alkaline administration with renal insufficiency
    Alkali therapy
    Combined antacid and cation exchange resin therapy
  Hypercalcemia
    Milk-alkali syndrome
    Bone metastases
  Sodium penicillins
  Glucose feeding after starvation

$[HCO_3^-]$ decreases 2–5 mmol/L for each 10 mm Hg decrease in $PaCO_2$ below 40 mm Hg.

Treatment of Respiratory Alkalosis

Correction of the underlying process is the only treatment for the hyperventilation. For severe alkalemia (arterial pH > 7.55), intravenous hydrochloric acid or ammonium chloride may be necessary (see below).

METABOLIC ALKALOSIS

Metabolic alkalosis is defined as a primary increase in plasma $[HCO_3^-]$. Most cases of metabolic alkalosis can be divided into (1) those associated with NaCl deficiency and ECF depletion, often described as chloride-sensitive; and (2) those associated with enhanced mineralocorticoid activity, commonly referred to as chloride-resistant (Table 30–6).

Chloride-Sensitive Metabolic Alkalosis

Extracellular fluid depletion causes the renal tubules to avidly reabsorb Na$^+$. Because not enough Cl$^-$ is available to accompany all the Na$^+$ ions reabsorbed, increased H$^+$ secretion must take place to maintain electroneutrality. In effect, HCO_3^- ions that might otherwise have been excreted are reabsorbed, resulting in metabolic alkalosis. Physiologically, maintenance of extracellular fluid volume is therefore given priority over acid-base balance. Because secretion of K$^+$ ion can also maintain electroneutrality, potassium secretion is also enhanced. Moreover, hypokalemia augments H$^+$ secretion (and HCO_3^- reabsorption) and will also propagate metabolic alkalosis. Indeed, severe hy-

pokalemia alone can cause alkalosis. Urinary chloride concentrations during a chloride-sensitive metabolic alkalosis are characteristically low (< 10 mmol/L).

Diuretic therapy is the most common cause of chloride-sensitive metabolic alkalosis. Diuretics such as furosemide, ethacrynic acid, and thiazides increase Na$^+$, Cl$^-$, and K$^+$ excretion, resulting in NaCl depletion, hypokalemia, and usually mild metabolic alkalosis. Loss of gastric fluid is also a common cause of chloride-sensitive metabolic alkalosis. Gastric secretions contain 25–100 mmol/L of H$^+$, 40–160 mmol/L of Na$^+$, about 15 mmol/L of K$^+$, and approximately 200 mmol/L of Cl$^-$. Vomiting or continuous loss of gastric fluid by gastric drainage (nasogastric suctioning) can result in marked metabolic alkalosis, extracellular volume depletion, and hypokalemia. Rapid normalization of $PaCO_2$ after plasma $[HCO_3^-]$ has risen in chronic respiratory acidosis results in metabolic alkalosis (posthypercapnic alkalosis; see above). Infants being fed formulas containing Na$^+$ without chloride readily develop metabolic alkalosis because of the increased H$^+$ (or K$^+$) secretion that must accompany sodium absorption.

Chloride-Resistant Metabolic Alkalosis

Increased mineralocorticoid activity commonly results in metabolic alkalosis even when it is not associated with extracellular volume depletion. Inappropriate (unregulated) increases in mineralocorticoid activity cause sodium retention and expansion of extracellular fluid volume. Decreased sodium reabsorption in the proximal renal tubule results in a large sodium load at the distal tubule. Increased H^+ and K^+ secretion takes place to balance enhanced mineralocorticoid-mediated sodium reabsorption, resulting in metabolic alkalosis and hypokalemia. Urinary chloride concentrations are typically greater than 20 mmol/L in such cases.

Other Causes of Metabolic Alkalosis

Metabolic alkalosis is rarely encountered in patients given even large doses of $NaHCO_3$ unless renal excretion of HCO_3^- is impaired. The administration of large amounts of blood products and some plasma protein-containing colloid solution frequently results in metabolic alkalosis. The citrate and acetate contained in these fluids is converted by the liver into HCO_3^-. Patients receiving high doses of sodium penicillin (especially carbenicillin) can develop metabolic alkalosis. Because penicillins act as nonabsorbable anions in the renal tubules, increased H^+ (or K^+) secretion must accompany sodium absorption. For reasons that are not clear, hypercalcemia due to nonparathyroid causes (milk-alkali syndrome and bone metastases) is also often associated with metabolic alkalosis. The pathophysiology of alkalosis following refeeding is also unknown.

Treatment of Metabolic Alkalosis

As with other acid-base disorders, correction of metabolic alkalosis is never complete until the underlying disorder is treated. When ventilation is controlled, any respiratory component contributing to alkalemia should be corrected by decreasing minute ventilation to normalize $PaCO_2$. The treatment of choice for chloride-sensitive metabolic alkalosis is intravenous saline (NaCl) administration and potassium (KCl) replacement. Cimetidine or ranitidine therapy is useful when excessive loss of gastric fluid is a factor. Acetazolamide may also be useful in edematous patients. Alkalosis associated with primary increases in mineralocorticoid activity readily responds to aldosterone antagonists (spironolactone). When arterial blood pH is greater than 7.60, intravenous hydrochloric acid (0.1 mol/L), ammonium chloride (0.1 mol/L), arginine hydrochloride, or hemodialysis should be considered.

ANESTHETIC CONSIDERATIONS IN PATIENTS WITH ALKALEMIA

Respiratory alkalosis appears to prolong the duration of opioid-induced respiratory depression; this effect may be due to increased protein binding of opioids. Cerebral ischemia can occur from marked reduction in cerebral blood flow during respiratory alkalosis, especially during hypotension. The combination of alkalemia and hypokalemia can precipitate severe atrial and ventricular dysrhythmia. Potentiation of nondepolarizing neuromuscular blockade is reported with alkalemia but may be more directly related to concomitant hypokalemia.

DIAGNOSIS OF ACID-BASE DISORDERS

Interpretation of acid-base status from analysis of blood gases requires a systematic approach. A recommended approach follows (Figure 30–6):

(1) Look at arterial pH: Is acidemia or alkalemia present?
(2) Look at $PaCO_2$: Is the change in $PaCO_2$ consistent with a respiratory component?
(3) If the change $PaCO_2$ does not explain the change in arterial pH, does the change in $[HCO_3^-]$ indicate a metabolic component?
(4) Make a tentative diagnosis (Table 30–1).
(5) Compare the change in $[HCO_3^-]$ with the change in $PaCO_2$. Does a compensatory response exist (Table 30–7)? Because arterial pH is related to the ratio of $PaCO_2$ to $[HCO_3^-]$, both pulmonary and renal compensatory mechanisms are *always* such that $PaCO_2$ and $[HCO_3^-]$ change in the same direction. A change in opposite directions implies a mixed acid-base disorder. Arterial pH generally changes 0.08 unit for every 10 mm Hg change in $PaCO_2$ during simple respiratory disturbances and 0.15 unit for every 10 mmol/L change in $[HCO_3^-]$ during a simple metabolic disturbance.
(6) If the compensatory response is more or less than expected, by definition a mixed acid-base disorder exists.

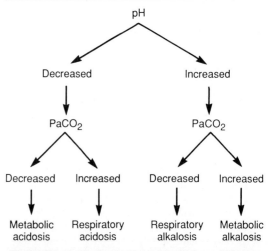

Figure 30–6. Diagnosis of simple acid-base disorders.

Table 30–7. Normal compensatory responses in acid-base disturbances.

Disturbance	Response	Expected Change
Respiratory acidosis		
Acute	↑ [HCO₃⁻]	1 meq/L/10 mm Hg increase in PaCO₂
Chronic	↑ [HCO₃⁻]	4 meq/L/10 mm Hg increase in PaCO₂
Respiratory alkalosis		
Acute	↓ [HCO₃⁻]	2 meq/L/10 mm Hg increase in PaCO₂
Chronic	↓ [HCO₃⁻]	2–5 meq/L/10 mm Hg increase in PaCO₂
Metabolic acidosis	↓ PaCO₂	1–1.5 × the decrease in [HCO₃⁻]
Metabolic alkalosis	↑ PaCO₂	0.25–1 × the increase in [HCO₃⁻]

(7) Calculate the anion gap in the case of metabolic acidosis.

(8) Measure urinary chloride concentration in the case of metabolic alkalosis.

MEASUREMENT OF BLOOD GAS TENSIONS & pH

Values obtained by routine blood gas measurement include oxygen and carbon dioxide tensions (PO_2 and PCO_2), pH, [HCO_3^-], base excess, and the percent oxygen saturation of hemoglobin. As a rule, only PO_2, PCO_2, and pH are directly measured. [HCO_3^-] is derived using the Henderson-Hasselbalch equation, base excess from the Siggaard-Andersen nomogram, and oxygen saturation from the hemoglobin dissociation curve. Oxygen saturation is often measured directly with an oximeter. Some machines also measure hemoglobin concentration.

Sample Source & Collection

Arterial blood samples are most commonly utilized clinically, though capillary or venous blood can be used if its limitations are recognized. Oxygen tension in venous blood (normally 40 mm Hg) reflects tissue extraction, not pulmonary function. Venous PCO_2 is usually 4–6 mm Hg higher than $PaCO_2$. Consequently, venous blood pH is usually 0.05 unit lower than arterial blood pH. Despite these limitations, venous blood is often useful in determining acid-base status. Capillary blood represents a mixture of arterial and venous blood, and the values obtained reflect that. Samples are usually collected in heparin-coated syringes and should be analyzed as soon as possible. Air bubbles should be eliminated, and the sample should be capped and placed on ice to prevent significant uptake of gas from blood cells or loss of gases to the atmosphere. Although heparin is highly acidic, excessive amounts of heparin in the sample syringe usually lower pH only minimally but decrease PCO_2 in direct

proportion to the percent dilution and have a variable effect on PO_2.

Temperature Correction

Changes in temperature directly affect measurements of PCO_2, PO_2, and, indirectly, pH. Decreases in temperature lower the partial pressure of a gas in solution—even though the total gas content does not change—because gas solubility is inversely proportionate to temperature. Both PCO_2 and PO_2 therefore decrease during hypothermia, but pH increases because temperature does not appreciably alter [HCO_3^-]: $PaCO_2$ decreases, but [HCO_3^-] is unchanged. Since blood gas tensions and pH are always measured at 37 °C, controversy exists over whether to correct the measured values to the patient's actual temperature. "Normal" values at temperatures other than 37 °C are not known. Many clinicians use the measurements at 37 °C directly regardless of the patient's actual temperature (Chapter 21).

pH MEASUREMENT

When a metal is placed in solution with its salt, the tendency of the metal to ionize into the solution leaves the metal with a negative charge. If two different metals (electrodes) and their salts are separated by a porous partition (allowing transfer of charge), the tendency for one metal to go into solution more than the other results in an electromotive force between the two electrodes. For pH measurements, a silver/silver chloride electrode and a mercury/mercurous chloride (calomel) electrode are most commonly used. The silver electrode is in contact with the test solution through pH-sensitive glass. The calomel electrode interfaces with the test solution through a potassium chloride solution and a porous plug (Figure 30–7). The electromotive force developed between the two electrodes is proportionate to [H^+].

CARBON DIOXIDE MEASUREMENT

Modification of the pH electrode system allows measurement of PCO_2. In this system (the Severinghaus electrode), the two electrodes are separated by sodium bicarbonate solution. The test sample is in contact with the bicarbonate solution through a thin Teflon membrane that allows CO_2 to equilibrate between the test sample and the bicarbonate solution (Figure 30–8). The pH of the bicarbonate solution consequently reflects the PCO_2 of the test solution.

OXYGEN MEASUREMENT

PO_2 is most commonly measured polarographically using the Clark electrode. In this system, platinum communicates with a silver/silver chloride electrode

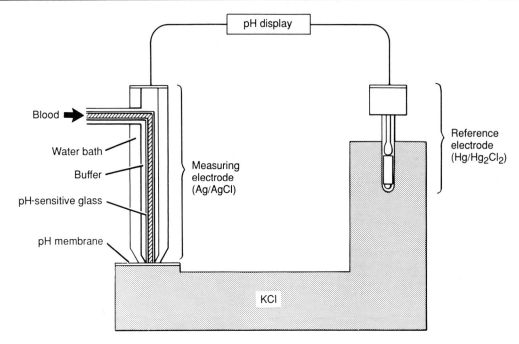

Figure 30–7. The pH electrode. (Modified and reproduced, with permission, from Shapiro BA, Harrison RA, Walton JR: *Clinical Application of Blood Gases,* 3rd ed. Year Book, 1982.)

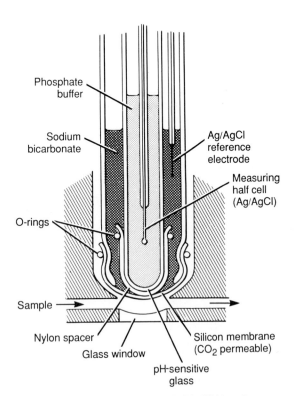

Figure 30–8. The CO_2 electrode. (Modified and reproduced, with permission, from Shapiro BA, Harrison RA, Walton JR: *Clinical Application of Blood Gases,* 3rd ed. Year Book, 1982.)

through an electrolyte solution (NaCl and KCl). The test sample is separated from the electrolyte solution by a membrane allowing oxygen to diffuse freely (Figure 30–9). When a negative voltage is applied to the platinum electrode, the electrical current that flows between the two electrodes is directly related to PO_2.

CASE DISCUSSION: A COMPLEX ACID-BASE DISTURBANCE

A 1-month-old male infant with an anorectal malformation undergoes anoplasty. Postoperatively, he is found to be in congestive heart failure resulting from coarctation of the aorta. He is noted to have tachypnea, decreased urine output, poor peripheral perfusion, hepatomegaly, and cardiomegaly. Following endotracheal intubation, the infant is placed on a ventilator and is allowed to breath spontaneously (intermittent mandatory ventilation 20 breaths/min, $FIO_2 = 1.0$). Initial arterial blood gas, hemoglobin, and electrolyte measurements are as follows:

$PaCO_2 = 11$ mm Hg
pH = 7.47
$PaO_2 = 209$ mm Hg
Calculated $[HCO_3^-] = 7.7$ mmol/L
Base excess $= -14.6$ mmol/L

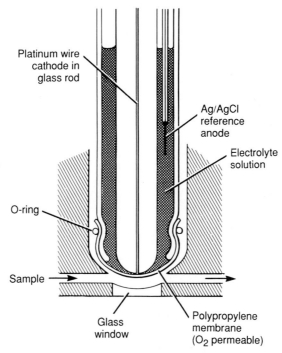

Figure 30–9. The O_2 electrode. (Modified and reproduced, with permission, from Ledingham IM, MacDonald AM, Douglas IHS: Monitoring of ventilation. In: *Textbook of Critical Care.* Shoemaker WC, Thompson WL, Holbrook PR [editors]. Saunders, 1984.)

Hb = 9.5 g/dL
$[Na^+]$ = 135 meq/L
$[Cl^-]$ = 95 meq/L
$[K^+]$ = 5.5 meq/L
$[\text{Total } CO_2]$ = 8 meq/L

Note that the [total CO_2] normally measured with electrolytes includes both plasma $[HCO_3^-]$ and dissolved CO_2 in plasma.

What is the acid-base disturbance?

Using the approach described above, the patient clearly has an alkalosis (pH > 7.45), which is at least partly respiratory in origin ($PaCO_2$ < 40 mm Hg). Since $PaCO_2$ has decreased by nearly 30 mm Hg, we would expect $[HCO_3^-]$ to be (40 − 10) ÷ 10 × 2 mmol/L below 24 mmol/L, or 18 mmol/L. In fact, the patient's $[HCO_3^-]$ is nearly 10 mmol/L less than that! The patient therefore also has a mixed acid-base disturbance: primary respiratory alkalosis *and* primary metabolic acidosis. Note that the difference between the calculated $[HCO_3^-]$ and the $[HCO_3^-]$ expected for a pure respiratory alkalosis roughly corresponds to the base excess. The latter is larger because of the low hemoglobin concentration.

What are the probable causes of these disturbances?

The respiratory alkalosis is probably due to conges-tive heart failure, while the metabolic acidosis is prob-

ably due to lactic acidosis secondary to poor perfusion. The latter is suggested by the calculated anion gap:

Anion gap = 135 − (95 + 8) = 32 meq/L

The lactate level was in fact measured and found to be elevated at 14.4 mmol/L. It is probable that fluid over-load precipitated the congestive heart failure.

What treatment is indicated?

Treatment should be directed at the primary process, ie, the congestive heart failure. The patient was treated with digoxin and furosemide. The hemoglobin con-centration is low for this infant's age (normal, 14–16 g/L), so transfusion following diuresis is also prob-ably indicated.

Following diuresis, the patient's tachypnea has im-proved, but perfusion still appears to be poor. Repeat laboratory measurements are as follows ($FiO_2 = 0.5$):

$PaCO_2$ = 23 mm Hg
pH = 7.52
PaO_2 = 136 mm Hg
Calculated $[HCO^{3-}]$ = 18 mmol/L
Base excess = −3.0 mmol/L
Hb = 10.3 g/dL
$[Na^+]$ = 137 meq/L
$[Cl^-]$ = 92 meq/L
$[K^+]$ = 3.9 meq/L
$[\text{Total } CO_2]$ = 18.5 meq/L

What is the acid-base disturbance?

Respiratory alkalosis is still present, while the base excess appears to have improved. Note that hemoglobin concentration has increased slightly, but $[K^+]$ has decreased as a result of the diuresis. With the new $PaCO_2$, the expected $[HCO_3^-]$ should be $(40 - 23) \div 10 \times 2$ below 24 mmol/L, or 20.6 mmol/L. Therefore, the patient still has metabolic acidosis because the calculated $[HCO_3^-]$ is 2 mmol/L less. Note again that this difference is close to the given base deficit. Note also that the anion gap is still high:

$$\text{Anion gap} = 137 - (92 + 18) = 27$$

Moreover, the repeat lactate measurement is now 13.2 mmol/L.

The high anion gap and lactate level explain why the patient is still not doing well and indicate that a new process is masking the severity of the metabolic acidosis (which is essentially unchanged).

Given the clinical course, it is likely that the patient now has a triple acid-base disorder: respiratory alkalosis, metabolic acidosis, and now metabolic alkalosis. The latter is probably due to hypovolemia from excessive diuresis (chloride-sensitive metabolic alkalosis). Note also that the metabolic alkalosis is nearly equal in magnitude to the metabolic acidosis.

The patient was subsequently given packed red blood cells in saline, and within 24 hours all three disorders began to improve:

$PaCO_2$ = 35 mm Hg
pH = 7.51
PaO_2 = 124 mm Hg
Calculated $[HCO^{3-}]$ = 26.8 mmol/L
Base excess = +5.0 mmol/L
Hb = 15 g/dL
$[Na^+]$ = 136 meq/L
$[Cl^-]$ = 91 meq/L
$[K^+]$ = 3.2 meq/L
[Total CO_2] = 27 meq/L
Lactate = 2.7 mmol/L

Outcome

Note that the respiratory alkalosis and the metabolic acidosis have now resolved, and the metabolic alkalosis is now most prominent.

Intravenous KCl replacement and a small amount of saline were judiciously given, followed by complete resolution of metabolic alkalosis. The patient subsequently underwent surgical correction of the coarctation.

SUGGESTED READINGS

Blitt CD: *Monitoring in Anesthesia and Critical Care Medicine,* 2nd ed. Churchill Livingstone, 1990.

Narins RG, Emmett M: Simple and mixed acid-base disorders: A practical approach. Medicine 1980;59:161. An outstanding review of complicated acid-base problems.

Oh MS, Carroll HJ: The anion gap. N Engl J Med 1977;207:814. An excellent review of the anion gap.

Rose BD: *Clinical Physiology of Acid-Base and Electrolyte Disorders,* 3rd ed. McGraw-Hill, 1989.

Schrier RW: *Renal and Electrolytes Disorders.* Little, Brown, 1986. Includes two excellent chapters on acid-base balance.

Shapiro BA: *Clinical Application of Blood Gases,* 4th ed. Mosby Year Book, 1989.

Tinker JH: *Cardiopulmonary Bypass: Current Concepts and Controversies.* Saunders, 1989. Contains an excellent discussion of temperature correction of blood gas measurements.

Renal Physiology & Anesthesia

31

The kidneys play a vital role in regulating the volume and composition of body fluids, eliminating toxins, and elaborating hormones such as renin, erythropoietin, and the active form of vitamin D. Discussions of intraoperative electrolyte, fluid, and acid-base therapies call upon a basic understanding of renal physiology. Moreover, surgery and anesthesia can have important effects on renal function. Failure to take these effects into consideration could result in serious errors in patient management. Fluid overload, hypovolemia, and postoperative renal failure are major causes of postoperative morbidity and mortality.

Diuretics are an important class of drugs that are frequently employed in the perioperative period. Preoperative diuretic therapy is common in patients with hypertension and with cardiac, hepatic, and renal disease. Diuretics are also used intraoperatively, particularly during neurosurgical, cardiac, major vascular, ophthalmic, and urologic procedures. Familiarity with the various types of diuretics, their mechanisms of action, side effects, and potential anesthetic interactions is therefore essential.

THE NEPHRON

Each kidney is made up of approximately 1 million functional units called nephrons. Anatomically, a nephron consists of a tortuous tubule with at least six very specialized segments. At its proximal end (Bowman's capsule), an ultrafiltrate of blood is formed, and as this fluid passes through the nephron, its volume and composition are modified by both the reabsorption and the secretion of solutes. The final product is eliminated as urine.

The six major anatomic and functional divisions of the nephron include (1) the glomerular capillaries, (2) the proximal convoluted tubule, (3) the loop of Henle, (4) the distal renal tubule, (5) the collecting tubule, and (6) the juxtaglomerular apparatus (Figure 31–1 and Table 31–1).

The Glomerular Capillaries

The glomerulus is composed of tufts of capillaries that jut into Bowman's capsule, providing a large surface area for the filtration of blood. Blood flow is provided by a single **afferent arteriole** and is drained by a single **efferent arteriole** (see below). Endothelial cells in glomeruli are separated from the epithelial cells of Bowman's capsule only by their fused basement membranes. The endothelial cells are perforated with relatively large fenestrae (500–1000 nm), but the epithelial cells interdigitate tightly with one another, leaving relatively small slits (70–100 nm). The two cell types with their basement membranes provide an effective filtration barrier for cells and large-molecular-weight substances. This barrier appears to have multiple anionic sites that give it a net negative charge which favors the filtration of cations but somewhat hinders filtration of anions.

Glomerular filtration pressure (about 60 mm Hg) is normally about 60% of mean arterial pressure and is opposed by both plasma oncotic pressure (about 25 mm Hg) and renal interstitial pressure (about 10 mm Hg). Both afferent and efferent arteriolar tone are important determinants of filtration pressure: Filtration pressure is directly proportionate to efferent arteriolar tone but inversely proportionate to afferent arteriolar tone. Approximately 20% of plasma is normally filtered as blood passes through the glomerulus.

The Proximal Tubule

Sixty-five to 75 percent of the ultrafiltrate formed in Bowman's capsule is normally reabsorbed isotonically (proportionate amounts of water and sodium) in the proximal renal tubules (Figure 31–2). The major function of the proximal tubule is Na^+ reabsorption. Sodium is actively transported out of proximal tubular cells at their capillary side by membrane-bound Na^+-K^+ ATPase (Figure 31–3). The resulting low intracellular concentration of Na^+ allows passive movement of Na^+ down its gradient from tubular fluid into epithelial cells.

Sodium reabsorption is coupled with the reabsorption of other solutes and the secretion of H^+ (Figure 31–3). Specific carrier proteins use the low concentration of Na^+ inside cells to transport phosphate,

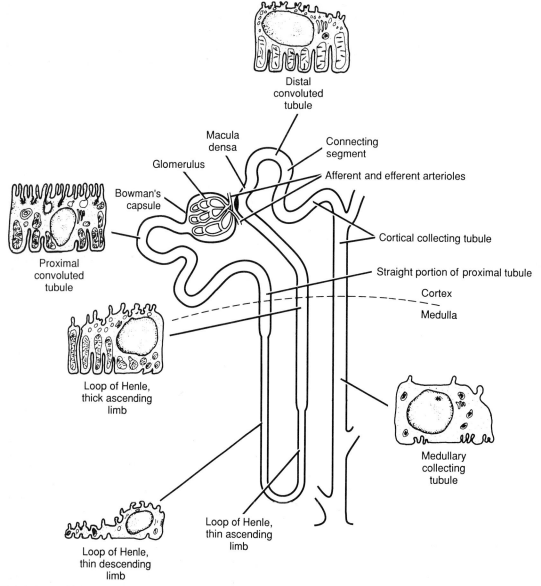

Figure 31–1. Major anatomic divisions of the nephron. (Modified and reproduced, with permission, from Ganong WF: *Review of Medical Physiology,* 14th ed. Appleton & Lange, 1989.)

glucose, and amino acids. The net loss of intracellular positive charges, due to Na^+-K^+ ATPase activity (exchanging $3Na^+$ for $2K^+$), favors the absorption of other cations (K^+, Ca^{2+}, and Mg^{2+}). Thus, the Na^+-K^+ ATPase at the basolateral side of the renal cells provides the energy for the reabsorption of most solutes. Sodium reabsorption at the luminal membrane is also coupled with countertransport (secretion) of H^+. The latter mechanism is responsible for reabsorption of 90% of the filtered bicarbonate ions (Figure 30–2). Unlike other solutes, chloride can traverse the tight junctions between adjacent tubular epithelial cells. As a result, chloride reabsorption is generally passive and follows its concentration gradient. Active chloride reabsorption may also take place as a result of a K^+-Cl^- cotransporter that extrudes both ions at the capillary side of the cell membrane (Figure 31–3).

The proximal tubules are capable of secreting organic cations and anions. Organic cations such as creatinine, cimetidine, and quinidine may share the same pump mechanism and thus can interfere with the excretion of one another. Organic anions such as urate,

Table 31–1. Functional divisions of a nephron.[1]

Segment	Function
Glomerulus	Ultrafiltration of blood
Proximal tubule	Reabsorption Sodium chloride Water Bicarbonate Glucose, protein, amino acids Potassium, magnesium, calcium Phosphates,[2] uric acid, urea Secretion Organic anions Organic cations Ammonia production
Loop of Henle	Reabsorption Sodium, chloride Water Potassium, calcium, magnesium Countercurrent multiplier
Distal tubule	Reabsorption Sodium,[3] chloride Water Potassium Calcium[4] Bicarbonate Secretion Hydrogen ion[3] Potassium[3] Calcium
Collecting tubule	Reabsorption Sodium,[3,6] chloride Water[5,6] Potassium Bicarbonate Secretion Potassium[3] Hydrogen ion[3] Ammonia production
Juxtaglomerular apparatus	Secretion of renin

[1] Adapted from Rose BD: *Clinical Physiology of Acid-Base and Electrolyte Disorders,* 3rd ed. McGraw-Hill, 1989.
[2] Inhibited by parathyroid hormone.
[3] At least partly aldosterone-mediated.
[4] Augmented by parathyroid hormone.
[5] Antidiuretic hormone-mediated.
[6] Inhibited by atrial natriuretic peptide.

keto acids, penicillins, cephalosporins, diuretics, salicylates, and most x-ray dyes also appear to share common secretory mechanisms. Both pumps probably play a major role in the elimination of many circulating toxins.

The Loop of Henle

The loop of Henle consists of descending and ascending portions. The thin descending segment is a continuation of the proximal tubule and descends from the renal cortex into the renal medulla. In the medulla, it acutely turns back upon itself and rises back upward toward the cortex as the ascending portion. The ascending portion consists of functionally distinct thin and thick segments (Figure 31–1). Cortical nephrons have relatively short loops of Henle, while those near the medulla (juxtamedullary nephrons) loop deeply into the medulla. Cortical nephrons outnumber juxtamedullary nephrons approximately 7:1. The loop of Henle is responsible for maintaining a hypertonic medullary interstitium and indirectly provides the collecting tubules with the ability to concentrate urine (see below).

Only 25–35% of the ultrafiltrate formed in Bowman's capsule normally reaches the loop of Henle. This part of the nephron usually reabsorbs 15–20% of the filtered sodium load. With the exception of the ascending thick segment, solute and water reabsorption in the loop of Henle is passive and follows concentration and osmotic gradients, respectively. However, in the ascending thick segment, active Na^+ reabsorption is due to Na^+-K^+ ATPase activity on the capillary side of epithelial cells. In contrast to what takes place in proximal tubular cells, Na^+ reabsorption in this part of the nephron is directly coupled to both K^+ and Cl^- reabsorption (Figure 31–4). Moreover, $[Cl^-]$ in tubular fluid appears to be the rate-limiting factor.

Unlike the descending limb and the thin ascending limb, the thick part of the ascending limb is impermeable to water. As a result, tubular fluid flowing out of the loop of Henle is hypotonic (100–200 mosm/L) and the interstitium surrounding the loop of Henle is therefore hypertonic. A countercurrent multiplier mechanism is established such that both the tubular fluid and medullary interstitium become increasingly hypertonic with increasing depth into the medulla (Figure 31–5). Urea also reaches high concentrations in the medulla and contributes substantially to its hypertonicity (below).

The thick ascending loop of Henle is also an important site for calcium and magnesium reabsorption. Parathyroid hormone may augment calcium reabsorption at this site.

The Distal Tubule

The distal tubule receives hypotonic fluid from the loop of Henle and is normally responsible for only minor modifications. Sodium reabsorption in the distal tubule normally accounts for only about 5% of the filtered sodium load. As in other parts of the nephron, the energy is derived from Na^+-K^+ ATPase activity on the capillary side, but on the luminal side Na^+ is reabsorbed by a Na^+-Cl^- carrier. Sodium reabsorption in this segment is directly proportionate to Na^+ delivery. Aldosterone-mediated Na^+ reabsorption is known to occur in the late distal tubule (connecting segment) as well as the collecting tubules (see below). The distal tubule is the major site of parathyroid hormone- and vitamin D-mediated calcium reabsorption.

The Collecting Tubule

The collecting tubule can be divided into cortical and medullary portions. Together they normally ac-

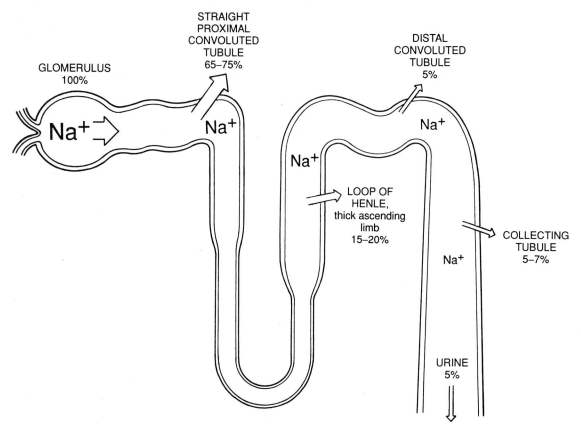

Figure 31–2. Sodium reabsorption in the nephron. Numbers represent the percentage of the filtered sodium load reabsorbed at each site. (Modified and reproduced, with permission, from Cogan MG: *Fluid and Electrolytes: Physiology and Pathophysiology.* Appleton & Lange, 1991.)

count for the reabsorption of 5–7% of the filtered sodium load.

A. The Cortical Collecting Tubule: The cortical portion of the collecting tubule is a continuation of the distal tubule and appears to be the principal site of aldosterone-mediated Na^+ reabsorption. At this site, Na^+ reabsorption is electrogenic—ie, Cl^- must be also be reabsorbed or K^+ (or H^+) must be secreted to maintain electroneutrality. Increases in intracellular $[K^+]$ favor K^+ secretion. Aldosterone enhances Na^+-K^+ ATPase activity in this part of the nephron by increasing the number of open K^+ and Na^+ channels in the luminal membrane. A K^+-absorbing ATPase pump may also be present. Although the role of atrial natriuretic peptide is not entirely clear (Chapter 28), it appears to decrease Na^+ reabsorption in the collecting tubules.

B. The Medullary Collecting Tubule: The medullary collecting tubule courses down from the cortex through the hypertonic medulla before joining collecting tubules from other nephrons to form a single ureter in each kidney. This part of the collecting tubule is the principal site of action for antidiuretic hormone (ADH). The permeability of its luminal membrane to water is entirely dependent of the presence of ADH

(Chapter 28). Dehydration increases ADH secretion, rendering the luminal membrane permeable to water. As a result, water is osmotically drawn out of the tubular fluid passing through the medulla, and a concentrated urine (up to 1000–1200 mosm/L) is produced. Conversely, adequate hydration suppresses ADH secretion; the fluid in the collecting tubules therefore passes through the medulla unchanged and remains hypotonic (100–200 mosm/L).

C. Hydrogen Ion Secretion: Both cortical and medullary collecting tubules contain a H^+-secreting ATPase on their luminal membrane. This pump is responsible for reabsorption of HCO_3^- in the distal nephron and plays a major role in acid-base balance (Chapter 30). The hydrogen ions secreted are excreted in urine in the form of titratable acids (phosphates) and ammonium ions. Acidemia and aldosterone secretion enhance H^+ secretion at this site.

D. Role of the Collecting Tubule in Maintaining a Hypertonic Medulla: Differential permeability for urea between the cortical and medullary collecting tubules partly accounts for the contribution of urea to the hypertonicity of the renal medulla. Cortical collecting tubules are freely permeable to urea, whereas medullary collecting tubules are normally imperme-

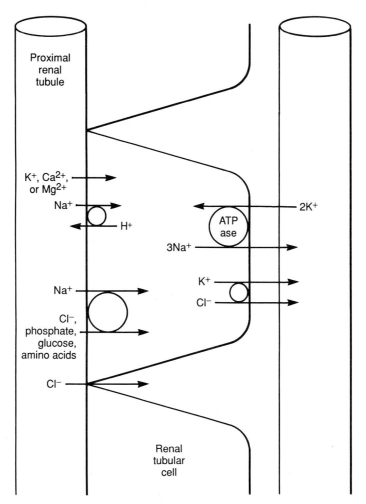

Figure 31–3. Reabsorption of solutes in proximal tubules. Note that Na$^+$-K$^+$ ATPase supplies the energy for reabsorption of most solutes by maintaining a low intracellular concentration of sodium.

able. However, in the presence of ADH, the innermost part of the medullary collecting tubules becomes moderately permeable to urea. Thus, when ADH is secreted, water moves out of the collecting tubules and the urea becomes highly concentrated. Urea can then diffuse out deeply into the medullary interstitium, increasing its tonicity.

The Juxtaglomerular Apparatus

This small organ within each nephron consists of a specialized segment of the afferent arteriole, containing **juxtaglomerular cells** within its wall, and a closely associated segment of the early distal tubule, the **macula densa** (Figure 31–6). Juxtaglomerular cells contain the enzyme renin and are innervated by the sympathetic nervous system. Release of renin is dependent on (1) β_1-adrenergic sympathetic stimulation, (2) changes in afferent arteriolar wall pressure (Chapter 28), and (3) changes in chloride flow past the macula densa. Renin released into the bloodstream

acts on angiotensinogen, a protein synthesized by the liver, to form angiotensin I. This inert decapeptide is then rapidly converted, primarily in the lungs, by angiotensin-converting enzyme (ACE) to form angiotensin II. Angiotensin II plays a major role in blood pressure regulation (Chapter 19) and aldosterone secretion (Chapter 28).

THE RENAL CIRCULATION

Renal function is intimately related to renal blood flow. In fact, the kidneys are the only organs for which oxygen consumption is determined by blood flow; the reverse is true in other organs. The combined blood flow through both kidneys normally accounts for 20–

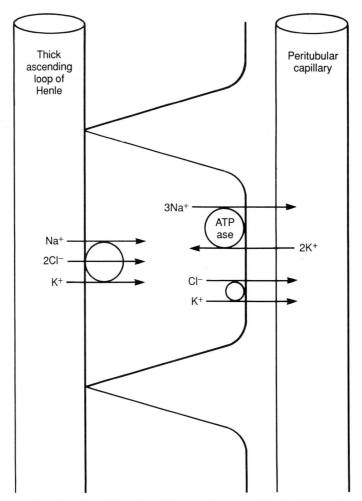

Figure 31–4. Sodium and chloride reabsorption in the thick ascending loop of Henle. All four sites on the luminal carrier protein must be occupied for transport to occur. The rate-limiting factor appears to be chloride concentration in tubular fluid.

25% of total cardiac output. In most individuals, each kidney is supplied by a single renal artery arising from the aorta. The renal artery then divides at the renal pelvis into interlobar arteries, which in turn give rise to arcuate arteries at the junction between renal cortex and medulla (Figure 31–7). Arcuate arteries further divide into interlobular branches that eventually supply each nephron via a single afferent arteriole. Blood from each glomerulus is drained via a single efferent arteriole and then travels alongside adjacent renal tubules in a second (peritubular) system of capillaries. In contrast to the glomerular capillaries, which favor filtration, peritubular capillaries are primarily "reabsorptive." Venules draining the second capillary plexus finally return blood to the inferior vena cava via a single renal vein on each side.

CONTROL OF RENAL BLOOD FLOW & GLOMERULAR FILTRATION

Clearance

The concept of clearance is frequently used in measurements of renal blood flow (RBF) and the glomerular filtration rate (GFR). The renal clearance of a substance is defined as the volume of blood that is completely cleared of that substance per unit of time (usually per minute).

Renal Blood Flow

Renal plasma flow (RPF) is most commonly measured by p-aminohippurate (PAH) clearance. PAH at low plasma concentrations can be assumed to be completely cleared from plasma by filtration and secretion in one passage through the kidneys. Consequently–

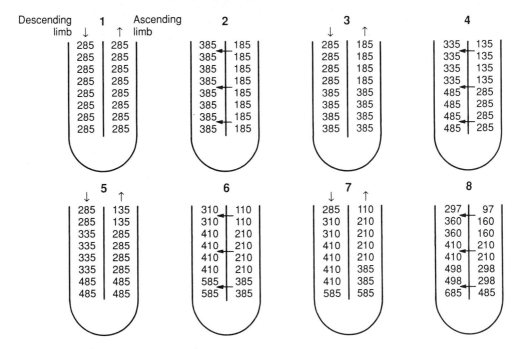

Figure 31–5. The countercurrent multiplier mechanism. This mechanism is dependent on differential permeability and transport characteristics between the descending and ascending limbs. The descending limb and the thin ascending limb are permeable to water, Na⁺, Cl⁻, and urea. The thick ascending limb is impermeable to water and urea, actively reabsorbs Na⁺ and Cl⁻, and therefore can generate an osmotic gradient. This figure depicts from "time zero" a progressive 200 mosm/kg gradient between the descending and ascending limbs. Note that as urine flows, the gradient remains unchanged but the osmolality progressively increases at the bottom of the loop. (Adapted from Pitts RF: *Physiology of the Kidney and Body Fluids,* 3rd ed. Year Book, 1974.)

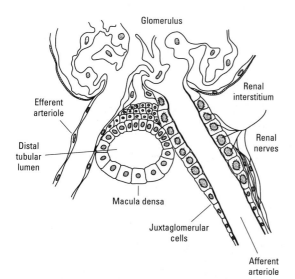

Figure 31–6. The juxtaglomerular apparatus. (Modified and reproduced, with permission, from Ganong WF: *Review of Medical Physiology,* 14th ed. Appleton & Lange, 1989.)

$$RPF = \text{Clearance of PAH} = \frac{[PAH]_{urine}}{[PAH]_{plasma}} \times \text{Urine flow}$$

where $[PAH]_U$ = urinary concentration of PAH and $[PAH]_P$ = plasma PAH concentration.

If the hematocrit is known, then–

$$RBF = \frac{RPF}{1 - \text{Hematocrit}}$$

Renal plasma flow and RBF are normally about 660 mL/min and 1200 mL/min, respectively. More sophisticated inert gas washout measurement techniques show that the majority of renal blood flow normally goes to the cortex and that blood flow progressively decreases inside the medulla toward the renal hilum.

A. Control of Renal Blood Flow: Regulation of renal blood flow represents a complex interplay between intrinsic autoregulation, tubuloglomerular balance, and hormonal and neuronal influences.

1. Intrinsic regulation–Autoregulation of renal blood flow normally occurs between mean arterial

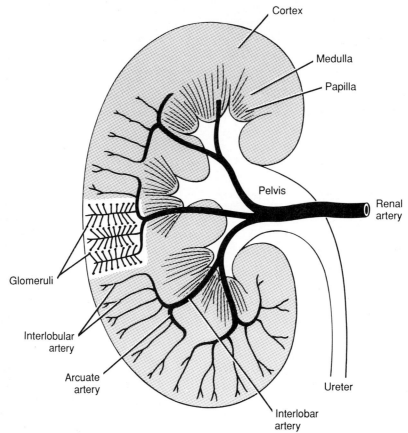

Figure 31–7. The renal circulation. (Modified and reproduced, with permission, from Leaf A, Cotran RS: *Renal Pathophysiology.* Oxford Univ Press, 1976.)

blood pressures of 80 and 180 mm Hg. Although the exact mechanism is not known, it is thought to be an intrinsic myogenic response of the afferent arterioles to changes in blood pressure. Within these limits, RBF (and GFR) can be kept relatively constant by afferent arteriolar vasoconstriction or vasodilation. Outside the autoregulation limits, RBF becomes pressure-dependent. Glomerular filtration generally ceases when mean systemic arterial pressure is less than 40–50 mm Hg.

2. Tubuloglomerular feedback–Changes in renal tubular flow rates affect GFR: Increases in tubular flow tend to reduce GFR, while decreases in flow tend to favor increases in GFR. Tubuloglomerular feedback probably plays an important role in maintaining GFR constant over a wide range of perfusion pressures. Although the mechanism is poorly understood, the macula densa appears to be responsible for tubuloglomerular feedback by inducing reflex changes in afferent arteriolar tone and possibly glomerular capillary permeability. Angiotensin II probably plays only a passive role in this mechanism.

3. Hormonal regulation–Increases in afferent arteriolar pressure stimulate renin release and formation of angiotensin II (see above). Angiotensin II

causes generalized arterial vasoconstriction and secondarily reduces RBF. Because angiotensin preferentially constricts the efferent arteriole more than the afferent arteriole, the GFR tends to be relatively preserved. This relative preservation of GFR appears to be at least partly mediated by angiotensin-induced prostaglandin synthesis and is blocked by inhibitors of prostaglandin synthesis such as nonsteroidal anti-inflammatory drugs. In contrast, adrenal catecholamines (epinephrine and norepinephrine) directly and preferentially increase afferent arteriolar tone, but marked decreases in GFR are minimized indirectly through activation of renin release and angiotensin II formation.

4. Neuronal regulation–Sympathetic outflow from the spinal cord at T_4–L_1 reaches the kidneys via the celiac and renal plexuses. Sympathetic nerves innervate the juxtaglomerular apparatus as well as the renal vasculature. This innervation is probably responsible for stress-induced reductions in RBF (below).

B. Redistribution of Renal Blood Flow: Redistribution of renal blood flow, from cortical nephrons with short loops of Henle to larger juxtamedullary nephrons with long loops, is known to occur under certain conditions. Sympathetic stimulation, increased levels of catecholamines and angiotensin II, and heart failure can cause redistribution of renal blood flow to the medulla. Although the significance of this redistribution remains controversial, it appears to be associated with sodium retention.

Glomerular Filtration Rate

The glomerular filtration rate is normally about 20% of RPF. Clearance of inulin, a fructose polysaccharide which is completely filtered but is neither secreted nor reabsorbed, is a good measure of GFR. Normal values for GFR are about 125 mL/min in men and 100 mL/min in women. Though less accurate than inulin clearance, **creatinine clearance** is a much more practical and widespread measurement of GFR. Creatinine clearance tends to overestimate GFR because some creatinine is normally secreted by renal tubules. Creatinine is a product of phosphocreatine breakdown in muscle. Creatinine clearance is calculated as follows:

$$\text{Creatinine clearance} = \frac{[\text{Creatinine}]_{urine} \times \text{Urinary flow}}{[\text{Creatinine}]_{plasma}}$$

where $[\text{creatinine}]_U$ = creatinine concentration in urine and $[\text{creatinine}]_P$ = creatinine concentration in plasma.

The ratio of GFR to RPF is called the filtration fraction (FF) and is normally 20%. GFR is dependent on the relative tones of both the afferent and efferent arterioles (see above). Afferent arteriolar dilatation or efferent arteriolar vasoconstriction can increase the FF and maintain GFR, even when RPF decreases. Afferent arteriolar tone appears to be responsible for maintaining GFR nearly constant over a wide range of blood pressures.

EFFECTS OF ANESTHESIA ON RENAL FUNCTION

Clinical studies attempting to define the effects of anesthetic agents on renal function are complicated by difficulties in differentiating between direct and indirect effects and often fail to control many important variables. These variables include the type of surgical procedure, fluid administration, and preexisting cardiac and renal function. Several conclusions, however, can be stated:

(1) Reversible decreases in RBF, GFR, urinary flow, and sodium excretion occur during both regional and general anesthesia.
(2) Changes are generally less marked during regional anesthesia.

(3) Most of these changes are indirect and are mediated by autonomic and hormonal influences.
(4) These effects can be at least partially overcome by maintenance of an adequate intravascular volume and a normal blood pressure.
(5) Only a few anesthetics (methoxyflurane and, theoretically, enflurane) in high doses can cause specific renal toxicity.

INDIRECT EFFECTS

Cardiovascular Effects

Most inhalation and intravenous anesthetics cause some degree of cardiac depression or vasodilatation and therefore are capable of decreasing arterial blood pressure. The sympathetic blockade associated with regional anesthesia (spinal or epidural) can similarly cause hypotension as a result of increased venous capacitance and arterial vasodilatation. Decreases in blood pressure below the limits of autoregulation can therefore be expected to reduce RBF, GFR, urinary flow, and sodium excretion. Intravenous fluid administration often at least partially reverses the hypotension and ameliorates its effects on renal function.

Neural Effects

Sympathetic activation commonly occurs in the perioperative period as a result of light anesthesia, intense surgical stimulation, tissue trauma, or anesthetic-induced circulatory depression. Sympathetic overactivity increases renal vascular resistance and activates various hormonal systems (see below). Both effects tend to reduce RBF, GFR, and urinary output.

Endocrine Effects

Endocrine changes during anesthesia generally reflect a stress response that may be induced by surgical stimulation, circulatory depression, hypoxia, or acidosis. Increases in catecholamines (epinephrine and norepinephrine), renin, angiotensin II, aldosterone, ADH, adrenocorticotropic hormone, and cortisol are common. Catecholamines, ADH, and angiotensin II all reduce RBF by inducing renal arterial constriction. Aldosterone enhances sodium reabsorption in the distal tubule and collecting tubule, resulting in sodium retention and expansion of the extracellular fluid compartment (Chapter 28). Nonosmotic release of ADH also favors water retention and, if marked, may result in hyponatremia (Chapter 28). The endocrine response to surgery and anesthesia is probably at least partly responsible for the transient postoperative fluid retention that is seen in many patients.

DIRECT EFFECTS

The direct effects of anesthetics on renal function are minor compared to the secondary effects described above.

Volatile Agents

Halothane, enflurane, and isoflurane have been reported to decrease renal vascular resistance. Studies of their effect on autoregulation have had conflicting results. In some animal studies, halothane appears to depress sodium reabsorption.

Nephrotoxicity. Methoxyflurane has been associated with a syndrome of polyuric renal failure. Its nephrotoxicity is dose-related and due to the release of fluoride ions from its metabolic degradation. Plasma fluoride concentrations greater than 50 μmol/L have been associated with renal toxicity that is characterized by a defect in urinary concentrating ability. Methoxyflurane doses greater than 1 MAC for 2 hours are associated with a high incidence of renal impairment. Fluoride production is negligible from halothane and isoflurane metabolism but can become significant following the prolonged administration of enflurane. Since fluoride excretion is dependent on GFR, patients with preexisting renal impairment may be more susceptible to this syndrome. High plasma fluoride concentrations following prolonged enflurane anesthesia may also occur in obese patients and those receiving isoniazid therapy, but an increased incidence of renal dysfunction has not been reported.

Intravenous Agents

Studies on narcotics and barbiturates generally show minor effects when these agents are used alone. In the presence of nitrous oxide, the agents can produce effects similar to those observed with volatile agents. Ketamine is reported to minimally affect renal function and to preserve renal function during hemorrhagic hypovolemia. Agents with α-adrenergic blocking activity such as droperidol may prevent catecholamine-induced redistribution of renal blood flow.

DIURETICS

Diuretics increase urinary output by decreasing the reabsorption of Na^+ and water. They are most commonly classified according to their principal site of action. Unfortunately, many diuretics have more than one mechanism of action, so the classification system is imperfect; only major mechanisms will be reviewed here.

Because nearly all diuretics are highly protein-bound and only the free drug can be filtered and enter the renal tubule, most diuretics require secretion by the proximal tubule (usually via the organic anion pump) to exert their action. Impaired delivery into the renal tubules may account for resistance to diuretics in patients with impaired renal function.

GLOMERULAR (FILTRATION) DIURETICS

These agents can increase GFR by increasing cardiac output. Most drugs in this category are not usually classified as diuretics because they have other major actions. These "diuretics" include methylxanthines (aminophylline), cardiac glycosides (digitalis), inotropes (dopamine and dobutamine), and saline infusions. Methylxanthines may also have some direct actions on the renal tubules.

PROXIMAL TUBULAR DIURETICS

1. OSMOTIC DIURETICS (Mannitol)

The osmotically active diuretics (Chapter 28) are filtered at the glomerulus and undergo limited or no reabsorption in the proximal tubule. Their presence in the proximal tubule limits the passive water reabsorption that normally follows active sodium reabsorption. Although their major effect is to increase water excretion, in large doses they will increase electrolyte (sodium and potassium) excretion. The same mechanism also impairs water and solute reabsorption in the loop of Henle.

Mannitol is the most commonly used osmotic diuretic. It is a six-carbon sugar that normally undergoes little or no reabsorption. In addition to its diuretic effect, it also appears to increase renal blood flow. The latter can wash out some of the medullary hypertonicity and interfere with renal concentrating ability.

Uses

A. Prophylaxis Against Acute Renal Failure in High-Risk Patients: This group includes patients with massive trauma, major hemolytic reactions, rhabdomyolysis, and severe jaundice as well as those undergoing cardiac or aortic operations. Its efficacy in these instances may be related to (1) dilution of nephrotoxic substances within the renal tubules, (2) prevention of sludging and obstruction within the tubules, (3) maintenance of renal blood flow, and perhaps (4) reduction of cellular swelling and preservation of cellular architecture.

B. Evaluation of Acute Oliguria: Mannitol in the presence of hypovolemia will augment urinary output. In contrast, it will have little effect in the presence of severe glomerular or tubular injury.

C. Conversion of Oliguric Renal Failure to Nonoliguric Renal Failure: Although this indication is controversial, the lower mortality rate associated with nonoliguric renal failure still prompts many clinicians to use mannitol in that setting.

D. Acute Reduction of Intracranial Pressure and Cerebral Edema: See Chapter 26.

E. Acute Reduction of Intraocular Pressure in the Perioperative Period: See Chapter 38.

Intravenous Dosage

Mannitol, 0.25–1 g/kg.

Complications

Mannitol solutions are hypertonic and acutely raise plasma and extracellular osmolality. A rapid intra- to extracellular shift of water can transiently increase intravascular volume and precipitate cardiac decompensation and pulmonary edema in patients with limited cardiac reserve. Transient hyponatremia and reductions in hemoglobin concentration are also common and represent acute hemodilution due to rapid movement of water out of cells (Chapter 28). If fluid and electrolyte losses are not replaced following large doses, mannitol can result in hypovolemia, hypokalemia, and hypernatremia.

2. CARBONIC ANHYDRASE INHIBITORS

Carbonic anhydrase inhibitors such as acetazolamide interfere with proximal secretion of H^+ and consequently HCO_3^- reabsorption (Chapter 30). Their effect on the enzyme in the distal tubule is limited. They increase Na^+ excretion because they interfere with the exchange of Na^+ for H^+ in proximal tubules (Figure 31–4). Reabsorption of both Na^+ and HCO_3^- at more distal sites in the nephron tends to limit their diuretic effect.

Uses

A. Correction of Metabolic Alkalosis in Edematous Patients: Carbonic anhydrase inhibitors often potentiate the effects of other diuretics.

B. Alkalinization of Urine: Alkalinization enhances urinary excretion of weakly acidic compounds such as uric acid.

C. Reduction of Intraocular Pressure: Inhibition of carbonic anhydrase in the ciliary processes reduces the formation of aqueous humor and, secondarily, intraocular pressure. This is a common indication during ophthalmic surgery.

Intravenous Dosage

Acetazolamide, 250–500 mg.

Complications

Because their effects are limited by the distal nephron, carbonic anhydrase inhibitors generally produce only a mild hyperchloremic metabolic acidosis (Chapter 30). Hypokalemia can occur following acute administration. Large doses of acetazolamide have been reported to cause drowsiness, paresthesias, and confusion. Alkalinization of the urine can interfere with the excretion of amine drugs such as quinidine.

3. LOOP DIURETICS

The loop diuretics include furosemide, bumetanide, and ethacrynic acid. All loop diuretics inhibit Na^+ and Cl^- reabsorption in the thick ascending limb. Sodium reabsorption at that site requires that all four sites on the $Na^+-K^+-2Cl^-$ luminal carrier protein be occupied. Loop diuretics compete with Cl^- for its binding site on the carrier protein (Figure 31–4). With a maximal effect, they can lead to excretion of 15–20% of the filtered sodium load. Both urinary concentrating and urinary diluting capacities are impaired. The large amounts of Na^+ and Cl^- presented to the distal nephron overwhelm its limited reabsorptive capability. The resulting urine remains hypotonic. The reason for the latter is not clear but may relate to rapid urinary flow rates that prevent equilibration with the hypertonic renal medulla or interference with the action of ADH on the collecting tubules. A marked increase in diuresis may occur when loop diuretic are combined with thiazides, especially metolazone.

Some studies suggest that furosemide increases renal blood flow and can reverse the redistribution of blood flow from the cortex to the medulla.

Loop diuretics increase urinary calcium and magnesium excretion. Ethacrynic acid is the only diuretic (other than mannitol and filtration diuretics) that is not a sulfonamide derivative, and it may for that reason be the diuretic of choice in patients allergic to sulfonamide drugs.

Uses

A. Edematous States (Sodium Overload): These disorders include heart failure, cirrhosis, the nephrotic syndrome, and renal insufficiency. When given intravenously, these agents can rapidly reverse cardiac and pulmonary manifestations.

B. Hypertension: Loop diuretics may be used as adjuncts to other hypotensive agents, particularly when thiazides (below) are ineffective.

C. Evaluation of Acute Oliguria: The response to a small dose (10–20 mg) of furosemide may be useful in differentiating between oliguria due to hypovolemia and oliguria due to redistribution of renal blood flow to juxtamedullary nephrons. Little or no response is seen with hypovolemia, whereas resumption of normal urine output occurs with the latter.

D. Conversion of Oliguric Renal Failure to Nonoliguric Renal Failure: Use of these drugs in this setting is as controversial as with mannitol. Moreover, mannitol may be more effective.

E. Treatment of hypercalcemia.

F. Rapid correction of hyponatremia (Chapter 28).

Intravenous Dosages

Furosemide, 20–100 mg; bumetanide, 0.5–1 mg; ethacrynic acid, 50–100 mg.

Complications

Increased delivery of Na^+ to the distal and collecting tubules increases K^+ and H^+ secretion at those sites and can result in hypokalemia and metabolic alkalosis. Marked Na^+ losses will also lead to hypovolemia and prerenal azotemia (Chapter 48); secondary hyperaldosteronism often accentuates the hypokalemia and metabolic alkalosis. Hypercalciuria can result in stone formation and occasionally hypocalcemia. Hypomagnesemia may be seen in patients receiving long-term therapy. Hyperuricemia is thought to be due to increased urate reabsorption and competitive inhibition of urate secretion in the proximal tubule. Reversible hearing loss has been reported with both furosemide and ethacrynic acid.

DISTAL TUBULAR DIURETICS

1. THIAZIDE-TYPE DIURETICS

This group of agents includes thiazides, chlorthalidone, metolazone, and indapamide. These diuretics act at the "cortical diluting segment"—that part of the nephron between the thick ascending limb of the loop of Henle and the site of aldosterone-mediated sodium reabsorption in the distal tubule. Inhibition of sodium reabsorption at this segment impairs urinary diluting but not concentrating ability. The thiazide diuretics compete for the Cl^- site on the luminal Na^+-Cl^- carrier protein. When given alone, thiazide-type diuretics increase Na^+ excretion to only 3–5% of the filtered load because of enhanced compensatory Na^+ reabsorption in the collecting tubules. They also have some carbonic anhydrase inhibiting activity in the proximal tubule. The latter is normally masked by sodium reabsorption in the loop of Henle but is probably responsible for the often marked ("high ceiling") diuresis seen when thiazides are combined with loop diuretics.

In contrast to their effects on sodium excretion, thiazide-type diuretics augment Ca^{2+} reabsorption in the distal tubule.

Indapamide has some vasodilating properties and is the only thiazide-type diuretic with significant hepatic elimination.

Uses

A. Hypertension: Thiazides are often selected as first-line agents in the treatment of hypertension (Chapter 20).

B. Edematous Disorders (Sodium Overload): These agents are exclusively used as oral agents for mild to moderate sodium overload.

C. Hypercalciuria: Thiazide diuretics are often used in patients with hypercalciuria who form renal stones.

D. Nephrogenic Diabetes Insipidus: The efficacy of these agents in this disorder is due to their ability to impair diluting capacity and increase urine osmolality.

Intravenous Dosages

These agents are only given orally.

Complications

Though quantitatively less so than loop diuretics, increased delivery of sodium to the collecting tubules still results in enhanced K^+ secretion and frequently hypokalemia. Enhanced H^+ secretion can result in metabolic alkalosis. Impairment of renal diluting capacity may produce hyponatremia in some patients. Hyperuricemia, hyperglycemia, hypercalcemia, and hyperlipidemia may also be seen.

COLLECTING TUBULE DIURETICS

Diuretics inhibiting Na^+ reabsorption in the collecting tubules can maximally excrete only 1–2% of the filtered Na^+ load. Because of their generally favorable effect on potassium balance, these agents are also known as potassium-sparing diuretics. These weak agents are usually employed in conjunction with other more potent diuretics for their potassium-sparing effect.

1. ALDOSTERONE ANTAGONISTS (Spironolactone)

Spironolactone is a direct aldosterone receptor antagonist in collecting tubules. Its action to inhibit K^+ secretion in exchange for Na^+ reabsorption is therefore dependent on the presence of aldosterone. As a result, spironolactone is only effective in patients with hyperaldosteronism. Spironolactone also has some antiandrogenic properties.

Uses

A. Primary and Secondary Hyperaldosteronism: Spironolactone is most commonly used as an adjuvant in the treatment of refractory edematous states associated with secondary hyperaldosteronism (Chapter 28). It is especially effective in patients with advanced liver disease.

B. Hirsutism: This less common indication relies on spironolactone's antiandrogenic properties.

Intravenous Dosage

Spironolactone is only given orally.

Complications

Spironolactone can result in hyperkalemia in patients with high potassium intakes or renal insufficiency and those receiving beta-blockers or ACE inhibitors. Metabolic acidosis may also be seen. Other side effects include diarrhea, lethargy, ataxia, gynecomastia, and sexual dysfunction.

2. NONCOMPETITIVE POTASSIUM-SPARING DIURETICS

Triamterene and amiloride are not dependent on aldosterone activity in the collecting tubule. They inhibit Na^+ reabsorption and K^+ secretion by decreasing the number of open sodium channels in the luminal membrane of collecting tubules. Amiloride may also inhibit Na^+-K^+ ATPase activity in the collecting tubule.

Uses
A. Hypertension: These agents are often combined with thiazides to prevent hypokalemia.
B. Congestive Heart Failure: They are often added to more potent (loop) diuretics in patients with marked potassium wasting.

Intravenous Dosages
These agents are only given orally.

Complications
Amiloride and triamterine can cause hyperkalemia and metabolic acidosis similar to those which occur with spironolactone (see above). Both can also cause nausea, vomiting, and diarrhea. Amiloride is generally associated with fewer side effects, but paresthesias, depression, muscle weakness, and cramping may occasionally be seen. Triamterene on rare occasions has resulted in renal stones and is potentially nephrotoxic, especially when combined with nonsteroidal anti-inflammatory agents.

CASE DISCUSSION: INTRAOPERATIVE OLIGURIA

A 58-year-old woman is undergoing radical hysterectomy under general anesthesia. She was in good health prior to the diagnosis of uterine carcinoma. An indwelling urinary catheter is placed following induction of general anesthesia. Total urinary output was 60 mL for the first 2 hours of surgery. After the third hour of surgery, only 5 mL of urine is noted in the drainage reservoir.

Should the anesthesiologist be concerned?
Decreases in urinary output during anesthesia are very common. Although decreases may be expected owing to the physiologic effects of surgery and anesthesia (above), a urinary output of less than 20 mL/h in adults generally requires evaluation.

What issues should be addressed?
The following questions should be answered:

(1) Is there a problem with the urinary catheter and drainage system?
(2) Are hemodynamic parameters compatible with adequate renal function?
(3) Could the decrease in urine output be directly related to surgical manipulations?

1. How can the urinary catheter and drainage system be evaluated intraoperatively?
Incorrect catheter placement is not uncommon and should be suspected if there has been total absence of urine flow since the time of catheter insertion. The catheter may be inadvertently placed and inflated in the urethra in men or the vagina in women. Catheter displacement, kinking, obstruction, or disconnection from the reservoir tubing can all present with features similar to this case, with complete or near-complete cessation of urinary flow. The diagnosis of such mechanical problems requires retracing and inspecting the path of urine (often under the surgical drapes) from the catheter to the collection reservoir. Obstruction of the catheter can be confirmed by inability to irrigate the bladder with saline through the catheter.

2. What hemodynamic parameters should be evaluated?
Decreased urinary output during surgery is most commonly due to hemodynamic changes. In most instances, a decrease in intravascular volume (hypovolemia), cardiac output, or mean arterial blood pressure is responsible. Redistribution of renal blood flow from the renal cortex to the medulla may also play a role.

Intravascular volume depletion can rapidly develop when intravenous fluid replacements do not match intraoperative blood loss, insensible fluid losses, and sequestration of fluid by traumatized tissues (thirdspacing). Oliguria requires careful assessment of intravascular volume to exclude hypovolemia (Chapter 29). An increase in urinary output following an intravenous fluid bolus is highly suggestive of hypovolemia. In contrast, oliguria in patients with a history of congestive heart failure may require inotropes, vasodilators, or diuretics. Central venous or pulmonary artery pressure monitoring is useful in patients with underlying cardiac, renal, or advanced hepatic disease as well as in patients experiencing extensive blood loss (Chapter 6).

When mean arterial blood pressure drops below the lower limit of renal autoregulation (= 80 mm Hg), urinary flow may become blood pressure-dependent. The latter may be especially true in patients with chronic systemic hypertension, in whom renal autoregulation occurs at higher mean arterial blood pressures. Reductions in anesthetic depth, intravenous fluid boluses, or the administration of a vasopressor may increase blood pressure and urinary output in such instances.

Occasionally, otherwise normal patients may exhibit decreased urinary output in spite of normal intravascular volume, cardiac output, and mean arterial blood pressure. A small dose of a loop diuretic (furosemide, 5–10 mg) usually restores normal urinary flow in such instances.

3. How can surgical manipulations influence urinary output?

In addition to the neuroendocrine response to surgery, mechanical factors related to the surgery itself can alter urinary output. This is especially true during pelvic surgery, when compression of the bladder by retractors, unintentional cystotomy, and ligation or severing of one or both ureters can dramatically affect urinary output. Retractor compression combined with a head-down (Trendelenburg) position commonly impedes emptying of the bladder. Excessive pressure on the bladder will often produce hematuria. When mechanical problems with the urinary catheter drainage system and hemodynamic factors are excluded (see above), a surgical explanation should be sought. The surgeon should be notified so that the position of retractors can be checked, the ureters identified, and their path retraced in the operative area. Intravenous methylene blue or indigo carmine—both dyes that are excreted in urine—is useful in identifying the site of an unintentional cystotomy or the end of a severed ureter. Note that the appearance of the dye in the urinary drainage reservoir does not exclude unilateral ligation of one ureter. Methylene blue and, to a much lesser extent, indigo carmine can transiently give falsely low pulse oximeter readings (Chapter 6).

Outcome

After the integrity of the urinary catheter and drainage system was checked, 2 L of lactated Ringer's injection along with 250 mL of 5% albumin and 10 mg of furosemide were administered intravenously but failed to increase urinary output. Indigo carmine was given intravenously, and the proximal end of a severed left ureter was subsequently identified. A urologist was called, and the ureter was reanastomosed.

SUGGESTED READINGS

Bastron RD, Deutsch S: *Anesthesia and the Kidney.* Grune & Stratton, 1976.

Cogan MG: *Fluid and Electrolytes: Physiology and Pathophysiology.* Appleton & Lange, 1991.

Rose BD: *Clinical Physiology of Acid-Base and Electrolyte Disorders,* 3rd ed. McGraw-Hill, 1989.

Sladen N: Effect of anesthesia and surgery on renal function. Crit Care Clin 1987;3:373. One of the few recent reviews on the topic.

Anesthesia for Patients With Renal Disease

32

Diseases affecting the kidneys are often sorted into syndromes based on common clinical and laboratory findings: nephrotic syndrome, acute renal failure, chronic renal failure, nephritis, nephrolithiasis, and urinary tract obstruction and infection. The anesthetic care of patients with these syndromes is facilitated by grouping patients according to the status of their preoperative renal function rather than by syndrome. This chapter examines the basis for this approach and the anesthetic considerations applicable within each group. Renal physiology and the effects of anesthesia on renal function are discussed in Chapter 31.

EVALUATING RENAL FUNCTION

Accurate assessment of renal function relies heavily on laboratory determinations (Table 32–1). Renal impairment can be due to glomerular dysfunction, tubular dysfunction, or obstruction of the urinary tract. Because abnormalities of glomerular function cause the greatest derangements and are most readily detectable, the most useful laboratory tests are those related to the glomerular filtration rate (GFR; see Chapter 31).

Table 32–1. Grouping of patients according to glomerular function.

	Creatinine Clearance (mL/min)
Normal	100–120
Decreased renal reserve	60–100
Mild renal impairment	40–60
Moderate renal insufficiency	25–40
Renal failure	<25
End-stage renal disease[1]	<10

[1] This term applies only to patients with chronic renal failure.

BLOOD UREA NITROGEN (BUN)

The primary source of urea in the body is the liver. During protein catabolism, ammonia is produced from the deamination of amino acids. Hepatic conversion of ammonia to urea prevents the build-up of toxic ammonia levels:

$$2NH_3 + CO_2 \rightarrow H_2N-CO-NH_2 + H_2O$$

Blood urea nitrogen (BUN) is therefore directly related to protein catabolism and inversely related to glomerular filtration. As a result, BUN is not a reliable indicator of the glomerular filtration rate (GFR) unless protein catabolism is normal and constant. Renal handling of urea is discussed in Chapter 31.

The normal BUN concentration is 10–20 mg/dL. Lower values can be seen during starvation, whereas elevations are usually due to decreases in GFR or increases in protein catabolism. The latter may be due to a high catabolic state (trauma or sepsis), degradation of blood either in the gastrointestinal tract or in a large hematoma, or a high-protein diet. BUN concentrations greater than 50 mg/dL are generally associated with renal impairment.

SERUM CREATININE

Creatine is a product of muscle metabolism that is nonenzymatically converted to creatinine. Creatinine is then filtered (and to a minor extent secreted) but not reabsorbed in the kidneys (Chapter 31). Serum creatinine concentration is therefore directly related to body muscle mass but inversely related to glomerular filtration (Figure 32–1). Because body muscle mass is usually fairly constant, serum creatinine measurements are generally reliable indices of GFR. The normal serum creatinine concentration is 0.8–1.3 mg/dL in men and 0.6–1 mg/dL in women. Note from Figure 32–1 that each doubling of the serum creatinine represents a 50% reduction in GFR. Large meat meals, cimetidine therapy, and increases in acetoacetate (as during ketoacidosis) can increase serum creatinine

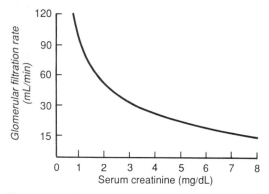

Figure 32–1. The relationship between the serum creatinine concentration and the glomerular filtration rate.

measurements without a change in GFR. Meat meals increase the creatinine load, while high acetoacetate concentrations interfere with the most common laboratory method for measuring creatinine. Cimetidine appears to inhibit creatinine secretion by the renal tubules.

GFR declines with increasing age in most individuals (5% per decade after age 20), but because muscle mass also declines the serum creatinine remains relatively normal. Thus, in elderly patients small increases in serum creatinine may represent large changes in GFR. Using age and lean body weight (in kg), GFR can be estimated by the following formula:

Creatinine clearance =

$$\frac{(140 - \textbf{Age}) \times \textbf{Lean body weight}}{72 \times \textbf{Plasma creatinine}}$$

For women, this equation must be multiplied by 0.85 to compensate for a smaller muscle mass.

The serum creatinine concentration requires 48–72 hours to equilibrate at a new level following acute changes in GFR.

BUN:CREATININE RATIO

Low renal tubular flow rates enhance urea reabsorption but do not affect creatinine handling. As a result, the BUN to serum creatinine ratio increases above 10:1. Decreases in tubular flow can be caused by decreased renal perfusion or obstruction of the urinary tract. BUN:creatinine ratios greater than 10:1 are therefore seen in volume depletion and in edematous disorders associated with decreased tubular flow (eg, heart failure, cirrhosis, nephrotic syndrome) as well as in obstructive uropathies. Increases in protein catabolism can also increase this ratio (see above).

CREATININE CLEARANCE

As discussed in Chapter 31, creatinine clearance measurements are the most accurate method available for clinically assessing overall renal function (really GFR). Although measurements are usually performed over 24 hours, 2-hour creatinine clearance determinations are reasonably accurate and easier to perform. Mild renal impairment generally results in creatinine clearances of 40–60 mL/min. Clearances between 25 and 40 mL/min produce moderate renal dysfunction and nearly always cause symptoms. Creatinine clearances less than 25 mL/min are indicative of overt renal failure.

URINALYSIS

Urinalysis continues to be the most common test routinely performed for evaluating renal function. Although its utility for that purpose is justifiably questionable, urinalysis can be helpful in identifying some disorders of renal tubular dysfunction as well as some nonrenal disturbances. A routine urinalysis typically includes pH, specific gravity, detection and quantification of glucose, protein, and bilirubin content, and microscopic examination of the urinary sediment. Urinary pH is helpful only when arterial pH is also known. A urinary pH greater than 7.0 in the presence of systemic acidosis is suggestive of renal tubular acidosis. Specific gravity is related to urinary osmolality. A specific gravity greater than 1.018 after an overnight fast is indicative of adequate renal concentrating ability. A lower specific gravity in the presence of hyperosmolality in plasma is consistent with diabetes insipidus.

Glycosuria is the result either of a low tubular threshold for glucose (normally 180 mg/dL) or of hyperglycemia. Proteinuria detected by routine urinalysis should be evaluated by means of 24-hour urine collection. Urinary protein excretions greater than 150 mg/d are significant. Elevated levels of bilirubin in the urine are seen with biliary obstruction.

Microscopic analysis of the urinary sediment detects the presence of red or white blood cells, bacteria, casts, and crystals. Red cells may be indicative of bleeding due to tumor, stones, infection, coagulopathy, or trauma. White cells and bacteria are generally associated with infection. Disease processes at the level of the nephron produce tubular casts. Crystals may be indicative of abnormalities in oxalic acid, uric acid, or cystine metabolism.

ALTERED RENAL FUNCTION & THE EFFECTS OF ANESTHETIC AGENTS

Most drugs commonly employed during anesthesia are at least partly dependent on renal excretion for elimination. In the presence of renal impairment, dosage modifications may be required to prevent accumulation of the drug or active metabolites. Moreover, the systemic effects of azotemia can potentiate the pharmacologic actions of many of these agents. This latter observation may be due to decreased protein binding of the drug, greater brain penetration due to some breach of the blood-brain barrier, or a synergistic effect with the toxins retained in renal failure (see below).

INTRAVENOUS AGENTS

Barbiturates

Patients with renal disease often exhibit increased sensitivity to barbiturates during induction, even though pharmacokinetic profiles appear to be unchanged. The mechanism appears to be an increase in free circulating barbiturate as a result of decreased protein binding. Acidosis may also favor a more rapid entry of these agents into the brain by increasing the nonionized fraction of the drug (Chapter 25).

Ketamine

Ketamine pharmacokinetics are minimally altered by renal disease. Some active hepatic metabolites are dependent on renal excretion and can potentially accumulate in renal failure. Ketamine's secondary hypertensive effect is undesirable in hypertensive renal patients.

Propofol & Etomidate

The pharmacokinetics of both propofol and etomidate are not significantly affected by impaired renal function. Decreased protein binding of etomidate in patients with hypoalbuminemia may enhance its pharmacologic effects.

Benzodiazepines

These drugs undergo hepatic metabolism and conjugation prior to elimination in urine. Because most are highly protein-bound, increased sensitivity may be seen in patients with hypoalbuminemia. Diazepam should be used cautiously in the presence of renal impairment because of a potential for the accumulation of active metabolites.

Narcotics

Most narcotics currently in use in anesthetic management (morphine, meperidine, fentanyl, sufentanil, and alfentanil) are inactivated by the liver; some of these metabolites are then excreted in urine. With the exception of morphine and meperidine, significant accumulation of active metabolites generally does not occur with these agents. The accumulation of morphine and meperidine metabolites has been reported to prolong respiratory depression in some patients with renal failure. Increased levels of normeperidine, a metabolite of meperidine, have also been associated with seizures. The pharmacokinetics of the most commonly used opioid agonist-antagonists (butorphanol, nalbuphine, and buprenorphine) are unaffected by renal failure.

Anticholinergic Agents

In doses used for premedication, atropine and glycopyrrolate can generally be used safely in patients with renal impairment. However, because up to 50% of these drugs and their active metabolites are normally excreted in urine, the potential for accumulation exists following repeated doses. Scopolamine is less dependent on renal excretion, but its central nervous system effects can be enhanced by azotemia.

Phenothiazines, H₂ Blockers, & Related Agents

Most phenothiazines such as promethazine are metabolized to inactive compounds by the liver. Although pharmacokinetic profiles are not appreciably altered by renal impairment, potentiation of their central depressant effects by azotemia can also occur. Their antiemetic actions are particularly useful in the setting of preoperative nausea. Droperidol may be partly dependent on the kidneys for excretion. Although accumulation may be seen following large doses in patients with renal impairment, relatively small doses of droperidol (< 2.5 mg) are usually used clinically. All H_2 receptor blockers are very dependent on renal excretion. Metoclopramide is partly excreted unchanged in urine and will accumulate in renal failure.

INHALATIONAL AGENTS

Volatile Agents

Volatile anesthetic agents are nearly ideal for patients with renal dysfunction because of their lack of dependence on the kidneys for elimination, their ability to control blood pressure, and generally minimal effects on renal blood flow (Chapter 31). Although patients with mild to moderate renal impairment do not exhibit altered uptake or distribution, accelerated induction and emergence may be seen in severely anemic patients (Hb < 5 g/dL) with chronic renal failure; this observation may be explained by a decrease in the blood:gas partition coefficient or a decrease in minimum alveolar concentration (Chapter 7). Because of its potential nephrotoxicity, methoxyflurane is the only volatile agent that should not be used (Chapters 7 and 31). Enflurane is also generally a poor choice for patients with renal disease undergoing long procedures because of a similar potential for fluoride accumulation.

Nitrous Oxide

Many clinicians omit or limit the use of nitrous oxide to 50% in patients with renal failure in an attempt to increase arterial oxygen content in spite of anemia. This rationale may only be justified in severely anemic patients (Hb < 7 g/dL), in whom even a small increase in the dissolved oxygen content may represent a significant percentage of the arterial to venous oxygen difference (Chapter 22).

MUSCLE RELAXANTS

Succinylcholine

Succinylcholine can be safely used in the presence of renal failure provided the serum potassium concentration is known to be less than 5 meq/L at the time of induction. When the serum potassium is higher or is in doubt, a nondepolarizing muscle relaxant should be used instead. Although decreased pseudocholinesterase levels have been reported in a few uremic patients following dialysis, significant prolongation of neuromuscular blockade is rarely seen.

Atracurium & Mivacurium

Mivacurium is minimally dependent on the kidneys for elimination. Atracurium is degraded in plasma by enzymatic ester hydrolysis and nonenzymatic Hofmann elimination. These agents may be the drugs of choice for muscle relaxation of short and intermediate duration, respectively, in patients with renal failure.

Vecuronium

The elimination of this relaxant is primarily hepatic, but up to 10–20% of the drug is eliminated in urine. The effects of large doses of vecuronium (> 0.1 mg/kg) are only modestly prolonged in patients with renal insufficiency.

Curare

Elimination of curare is dependent on both renal and biliary excretion; 40–60% of a dose of curare is normally excreted in urine. Increasingly prolonged effects are observed following repeated doses in patients with significant renal impairment. Smaller doses and longer dosing intervals are therefore required for maintenance of optimal muscle relaxation.

Pancuronium, Pipecuronium, Alcuronium, & Doxacurium

All these agents are primarily dependent on renal excretion (60–90%). Although pancuronium is metabolized by the liver into less active intermediates, its elimination half-life is still primarily dependent on renal excretion (60–80%). Neuromuscular function should be closely monitored if these agents are used in patients with abnormal renal function.

Metocurine, Gallamine, & Decamethonium

All three agents are almost entirely dependent on renal excretion for elimination and should generally be avoided in patients with impaired renal function.

Reversal Agents

Renal excretion is the principal route of elimination for edrophonium, neostigmine, and pyridostigmine.

The half-lives of these agents in patients with renal impairment are therefore prolonged at least as much as any of the above relaxants. Problems with inadequate reversal of neuromuscular blockade are usually related to other factors (Chapter 9).

ANESTHESIA FOR PATIENTS WITH RENAL FAILURE

PREOPERATIVE CONSIDERATIONS

Acute Renal Failure

Acute renal failure is a rapid deterioration in renal function that results in retention of nitrogenous waste products (azotemia). These substances, many of which behave as toxins, are by-products of protein and amino acid metabolism. They include urea, guanidine compounds (including creatine and creatinine), urates, aliphatic amines, and various peptides and metabolites of aromatic amino acids.

Azotemia can be divided into prerenal, renal, and postrenal types depending on its causes (Chapter 48). **Prerenal azotemia** results from an acute decrease in renal perfusion. **Renal azotemia** is usually due to intrinsic renal disease, renal ischemia, or nephrotoxins. **Postrenal azotemia** is the result of urinary tract obstruction or disruption. Both prerenal and postrenal azotemia are readily reversible in their initial stages but with time progress to renal azotemia. Most adult patients with renal failure develop oliguria. Nonoliguric patients (those with urinary outputs > 400 mL/d) continue to form urine that is qualitatively poor; these patients tend to have greater preservation of GFR. Although glomerular filtration and tubular function are impaired in both cases, abnormalities tend to be less severe in nonoliguric renal failure.

The course of acute renal failure varies widely, but the oliguria typically lasts for 2 weeks and is followed by a diuretic phase marked by a progressive increase in urine output. This diuretic phase often results in very large urinary outputs and is usually absent in nonoliguric renal failure. Urinary function improves over the course of several weeks but may not return to normal for up to 1 year. A more complete discussion of acute renal failure is found in Chapter 48.

Chronic Renal Failure

This syndrome is characterized by a progressive and irreversible decline in renal function over the course of at least 3–6 months. The most common causes are hypertensive nephrosclerosis, diabetic nephropathy, chronic glomerulonephritis, and polycystic renal disease.

The full manifestations of this syndrome (Table 32–2)—often referred to as **uremia**—are seen only after the GFR decreases below 25 mL/min. Patients with

Table 32–2. Manifestations of uremia.

Neurologic
  Peripheral neuropathy
  Autonomic neuropathy
  Muscle twitching
  Encephalopathy
    Asterexis
    Myoclonus
    Lethargy
    Confusion
    Seizures
    Coma
Cardiovascular
  Fluid overload
  Congestive heart failure
  Hypertension
  Pericarditis
  Arrhythmias
  Conduction blocks
  Vascular calcification
  Accelerated atherosclerosis
Pulmonary
  Hyperventilation
  Interstitial edema
  Alveolar edema
  Pleural effusion
Gastrointestinal
  Anorexia
  Nausea and vomiting
  Delayed gastric emptying
  Hyperacidity
  Mucosal ulcerations
  Hemorrhage
  Dynamic ileus
Metabolic
  Metabolic acidosis
  Hyperkalemia
  Hyponatremia
  Hypermagnesemia
  Hyperphosphatemia
  Hypocalcemia
  Hyperuricemia
  Hypoalbuminemia
Hematologic
  Anemia
  Platelet dysfunction
  Leukocyte dysfunction
Endocrine
  Glucose intolerance
  Secondary hyperparathyroidism
  Hypertriglyceridemia
Skeletal
  Osteodystrophy
  Periarticular calcification
Skin
  Hyperpigmentation
  Ecchymosis
  Pruritus

Table 32–3. Complications of dialysis.

Neurologic
  Disequilibrium syndrome
  Dementia
Cardiovascular
  Intravascular volume depletion
  Hypotension
  Arrhythmias
Pulmonary
  Hypoxemia
Gastrointestinal
  Ascites
Hematologic
  Anemia
  Transient neutropenia
  Residual anticoagulation
  Hypocomplementemia
Metabolic
  Hypokalemia
  Large protein losses
Skeletal
  Osteomalacia
  Arthropathy
  Myopathy
Infectious
  Peritonitis
  Transfusion-related hepatitis

clearances below 10 mL/min (often said to have end-stage renal disease) are dependent on dialysis for survival until successfully transplanted. Dialysis may take the form of intermittent hemodialysis employing an arteriovenous fistula or continuous peritoneal dialysis via an implanted catheter.

The generalized effects of uremia can usually be controlled by dialysis. Unfortunately, with time some uremic complications can become refractory. Moreover, some complications are directly related to the dialysis itself (Table 32–3). Hypotension, neutropenia, hypoxemia, and the disequilibrium syndrome are generally transient and resolve within hours after dialysis. Factors contributing to hypotension during dialysis include the vasodilating effects of acetate dialysate solutions, autonomic neuropathy, and rapid removal of fluid. The interaction of white cells with cellophane-derived dialysis membranes can result in neutropenia and leukocyte-mediated pulmonary dysfunction leading to hypoxemia. **Disequilibrium syndrome** is characterized by transient neurologic symptoms that appear to be related to a more rapid lowering of extracellular osmolality than intracellular osmolality.

Manifestations of Renal Failure

A. Metabolic: Patients with overt renal failure typically develop multiple metabolic abnormalities, including hyperkalemia, hyperphosphatemia, hypocalcemia, hypermagnesemia, hyperuricemia, and hypoalbuminemia. Water and sodium retention can result in worsening hyponatremia and extracellular fluid overload, respectively. Failure to excrete nonvolatile acids produces a high anion gap metabolic acidosis (Chapter 30).

Hyperkalemia is the most lethal of these abnormalities because of its effect on the heart (Chapter 28). It is usually present in patients with creatinine clearances of less than 5 mL/min, but it can develop rapidly in patients with higher clearances when challenged with large potassium loads (trauma, hemolysis, infections, or potassium administration).

Patients with renal failure also rapidly lose tissue proteins and readily develop hypoalbuminemia. Anorexia, protein restriction, and dialysis (especially peritoneal dialysis) are contributory.

B. Hematologic: Anemia is nearly always

present when the creatinine clearance is below 30 mL/min. Hemoglobin concentrations are generally 6–8 g/dL. Decreased erythropoietin production, decreased red cell production, and decreased cell survival are thought to be responsible. Additional factors include gastrointestinal blood loss, hemodilution, and bone marrow suppression from recurrent infections. Even with transfusions, hemoglobin concentrations greater than 9 g/dL are often difficult to maintain. Erythropoietin administration appears to partially correct the anemia. Increased levels of 2,3-diphosphoglycerate develop in response to the decrease in oxygen-carrying capacity. 2,3-DPG facilitates the unloading of oxygen from hemoglobin (Chapter 22). The metabolic acidosis (see above) also favors a rightward shift in the hemoglobin-oxygen dissociation curve. In the absence of symptomatic heart disease, most patients tolerate the anemia remarkably well.

Both platelet and white cell function are impaired in patients with renal failure. Clinically, this is manifested as a prolonged bleeding time and increased susceptibility to infections, respectively. Most patients have decreased platelet factor III activity. Patients recently hemodialyzed may also have residual anticoagulant effects from heparin.

C. Cardiovascular: Cardiac output has to increase in renal failure to maintain oxygen delivery in the face of a decrease in oxygen-carrying capacity. Sodium retention and abnormalities in the renin-angiotensin system result in systemic arterial hypertension. Left ventricular hypertrophy is a common finding in chronic renal failure. The extracellular fluid overload from sodium retention—together with the increased demand imposed by anemia and hypertension—make these patients especially prone to congestive heart failure and pulmonary edema. Conduction blocks are not uncommon and may be due to deposition of calcium in the conduction system. Arrhythmias are common and may be in part related to the metabolic abnormalities. Uremic pericarditis may develop in some patients; patients may be asymptomatic, may present with chest pain, or may develop cardiac tamponade. Patients with chronic renal failure also characteristically develop accelerated peripheral vascular and coronary artery disease.

Intravascular volume depletion may occur during the diuretic phase of acute renal failure if fluid replacement is inadequate. Hypovolemia also develops if too much fluid is removed during dialysis.

D. Pulmonary: Without dialysis or bicarbonate therapy, patients may be dependent on an increase in minute ventilation to compensate for the metabolic acidosis (Chapter 30). Pulmonary extravascular water is often increased in the form of interstitial edema, resulting in a widening of the alveolar to arterial oxygen gradient and predisposing to hypoxemia. Increased permeability of the alveolar-capillary membrane in some patients can result in pulmonary edema even with normal pulmonary capillary pressures; a characteristic picture resembling "butterfly wings" may be seen on the chest x-ray.

E. Endocrine: Abnormal glucose tolerance is characteristic of renal failure and is thought to be due to peripheral resistance to insulin; patients therefore often handle large glucose loads poorly. Secondary hyperparathyroidism in patients with chronic renal failure can produce metabolic bone disease, which may predispose to fractures. Abnormalities in lipid metabolism frequently lead to hypertriglyceridemia and probably contribute to accelerated atherosclerosis. Increases in the circulating levels of proteins and polypeptides normally degraded in the kidneys are often seen; these include parathyroid hormone, insulin, glucagon, growth hormone, luteinizing hormone, and prolactin.

F. Gastrointestinal: Anorexia, nausea, vomiting, and adynamic ileus are commonly associated with azotemia. Hypersecretion of gastric acid increases the incidence of peptic ulceration and gastrointestinal hemorrhage, which occurs in 10–30% of patients. Delayed gastric emptying secondary to autonomic neuropathy can predispose to aspiration perioperatively. Patients with chronic renal failure also have a high incidence of viral hepatitis (types B and C), often followed by residual hepatic dysfunction.

G. Neurologic: Asterixis, lethargy, confusion, seizures, and coma are manifestations of uremic encephalopathy. Symptoms generally correlate with the degree of azotemia. Autonomic and peripheral neuropathies are common in patients with chronic renal failure. Peripheral neuropathies are typically sensory and involve the distal lower extremities.

Preoperative Evaluation

The generalized effects of azotemia mandate a thorough evaluation of patients in renal failure. Most patients with acute renal failure requiring surgery are critically ill. Their renal failure is frequently associated with a postoperative complication or trauma. Patients with acute renal failure also tend to have accelerated protein breakdown. Optimal perioperative management is dependent on preoperative dialysis. Hemodialysis is more effective than peritoneal dialysis and can be readily accomplished via a temporary subclavian or femoral dialysis catheter. The need for dialysis in nonoliguric patients should be assessed on an individual basis. Indications for dialysis are listed in Table 32–4.

Patients with chronic renal failure most commonly present to the operating room for creation or revision of an arteriovenous fistula under local or regional anes-

Table 32–4. Indications for dialysis.

Fluid overload
Hyperkalemia
Severe acidosis
Metabolic encephalopathy
Pericarditis
Coagulopathy
Refractory gastrointestinal symptoms
Drug toxicity

thesia. Regardless of the procedure or the anesthetic employed, complete evaluation is required to make certain that they are in optimal medical condition—all reversible manifestations (Table 32–2) of uremia should be controlled. Preoperative dialysis on the day of surgery or on the previous day is usually necessary.

Physical and laboratory evaluation should focus on both cardiac and respiratory functions. Signs of fluid overload or hypovolemia should be sought (Chapter 29). Intravascular volume depletion often results from overzealous dialysis. A comparison of the patient's current weight with previous pre- and postdialysis weights may be helpful. Hemodynamic data, if available, and a chest x-ray are invaluable in confirming

Table 32–5. Drugs with a potential for significant accumulation in patients with renal impairment.

Muscle relaxants
Metocurine
Gallamine
Decamethonium
Pancuronium
Pipecurium
Doxacurium
Alcuronium
Anticholinergics
Atropine
Glycopyrrolate
Metoclopramide
H$_2$ receptor antagonists
Cimetidine
Ranitidine
Digitalis
Diuretics
Calcium channel antagonists
Nifedipine
Diltiazem
β-Adrenergic blockers
Propranolol
Nadolol
Pindolol
Atenolol
Antihypertensives
Clonidine
Methyldopa
Captopril
Enalapril
Lisinopril
Hydralazine
Nitroprusside (thiocyanate)
Antiarrhythmics
Procainamide
Disopyramide
Bretylium
Tocainide
Encainide (genetically determined)
Bronchodilators
Terbutaline
Psychiatric
Lithium
Antibiotics
Penicillins
Cephalosporins
Aminoglycosides
Tetracycline
Anticonvulsants
Carbamazepine
Ethosuximide
Primidone

clinical impressions. Arterial blood gas analysis is also useful in detecting hypoxemia and evaluating acid-base status. The ECG should be examined carefully for signs of hyperkalemia or hypocalcemia (Chapter 28) as well as ischemia, conduction blocks, and ventricular hypertrophy. Echocardiography should be employed in patients suspected of having a pericardial effusion; a friction rub may not be audible on auscultation.

Preoperative red blood cell transfusions should generally be given only to severely anemic patients (hemoglobin < 6–7 g/dL) or when significant intraoperative blood loss is expected. A bleeding time and coagulation studies are advisable, especially if regional anesthesia is being considered. Serum electrolyte, BUN, and creatinine measurements are necessary to assess the adequacy of dialysis. Glucose measurements are helpful in evaluating the potential need for perioperative insulin therapy.

Preoperative drug therapy should be carefully reviewed for drugs with significant renal elimination (Table 32–5). Dosage adjustments and measurements of blood levels (when available) are necessary to prevent drug toxicity.

Premedication

Alert patients who are relatively stable can be given reduced doses of a narcotic (Table 8–6) or a benzodiazepine (Table 8–3). Promethazine, 12.5–25 mg intramuscularly, is a useful adjunct for additional sedation and for its antiemetic properties. Aspiration prophylaxis with an H$_2$ blocker may be indicated in patients with nausea, vomiting, or gastrointestinal bleeding (Chapter 15). Metoclopramide, 10 mg orally or slowly intravenously, may also be useful in accelerating gastric emptying, preventing nausea, and decreasing the risk of aspiration. Preoperative medications—especially antihypertensive agents—should be continued till the time of surgery (Chapter 20). The management of diabetic patients is discussed in Chapter 36.

INTRAOPERATIVE CONSIDERATIONS

Monitoring

The surgical procedure as well as the patient's general medical condition dictate monitoring requirements. To prevent clotting, blood pressure should not be measured in an arm with an arteriovenous fistula. Intra-arterial, central venous, and pulmonary artery monitoring are often indicated, especially for patients undergoing procedures associated with major fluid shifts (Chapter 6); intravascular volume is often difficult to assess based on clinical signs alone. Direct intra-arterial blood pressure monitoring may also be indicated in poorly controlled hypertensive patients regardless of the procedure. Aggressive invasive monitoring may be indicated especially in diabetic patients with advanced renal disease undergoing major surgery; this group of patients may have up to ten times the perioperative morbidity of diabetics without renal disease. The latter probably reflects the high incidence of advanced cardiovascular complications in the first group.

Induction

Patients with nausea, vomiting, or gastrointestinal bleeding should undergo rapid-sequence induction with cricoid pressure (Chapter 15). The barbiturate dose should be reduced (thiopental, 2–3 mg/kg) in debilitated or critically ill patients. Etomidate, 0.2–0.4 mg/kg, is a suitable alternative. Induction with small increments of a barbiturate (such as thiopental, 50 mg) is preferable to a bolus dose in patients not at high risk for aspiration. A narcotic, beta-blocker (esmolol), or lidocaine may be used to blunt the hypertensive response to intubation (Chapter 20). Succinylcholine, 1.5 mg/kg, can be used for endotracheal intubation if the serum potassium is less than 5 meq/L. Atracurium (0.4 mg/kg) and mivacurium (0.15 mg/kg) may be the muscle relaxants of choice for intubating hyperkalemic patients. Atracurium in this dosage generally causes little histamine release (Chapter 9). Vecuronium, 0.1 mg/kg, may be a suitable alternative, but some prolongation of its effects should be expected.

Maintenance

The ideal maintenance technique should be able to control hypertension with minimal effects on cardiac output, because an increase in cardiac output is the principal compensatory mechanism for anemia. Isoflurane, nitrous oxide, fentanyl, sufentanil, alfentanil, and morphine are generally regarded as satisfactory maintenance agents. Isoflurane is the preferred volatile agent because it has the least effect on cardiac output (Chapter 7). Nitrous oxide should be used cautiously in patients with poor ventricular function and should probably not be used in patients with very low hemoglobin concentrations (< 7 g/dL) to allow the administration of 100% oxygen (see above). Meperidine may not be a good choice because of the accumulation of normeperidine (see above). Morphine may be used, but some prolongation of its effects may be encountered.

Controlled ventilation is safest for patients with renal failure. Spontaneous ventilation under anesthesia can result in respiratory acidosis that may exacerbate preexisting acidemia, leading to potentially severe circulatory depression and dangerous increases in serum potassium concentration (Chapter 30). Respiratory alkalosis may also be detrimental because it shifts the hemoglobin dissociation curve to the left (Chapter 22), can exacerbate preexisting hypocalcemia (Chapter 28), and may reduce cerebral blood flow (Chapter 25).

Fluid Therapy

Superficial operations involving minimal tissue trauma require replacement of only insensible fluid losses with 5% dextrose in water. Procedures associated with major fluid losses or shifts require isotonic crystalloids, colloids, or both (Chapter 29). Lactated Ringer's injection is best avoided in hyperkalemic patients when large volumes of fluid may be required, because it contains potassium (4 meq/L); normal saline may be used instead. Glucose-free solutions should generally be used because of the glucose intolerance associated with uremia. Blood loss should generally be replaced with packed red blood cells. Blood transfusion either has no effect or may be beneficial for patients in renal failure who are renal transplant candidates; such transfusion may decrease the likelihood of rejection following renal transplantation in some patients.

ANESTHESIA FOR PATIENTS WITH MILD TO MODERATE RENAL IMPAIRMENT

PREOPERATIVE CONSIDERATIONS

The kidneys normally exhibit a large reserve in function. GFR, as determined by creatinine clearance, can decrease from 120 to 60 mL/min without any clinically perceptible change in renal function. Even patients with creatinine clearances of 40–60 mL/min usually are asymptomatic. These patients have only mild renal impairment but may still be thought of as having decreased renal reserve. The emphasis in the care of these patients should be on preserving remaining renal function.

When creatinine clearance reaches 25–40 mL/min, renal impairment is moderate, and patients can be said to have renal insufficiency: Significant azotemia is always present, and hypertension and anemia are common. Correct anesthetic management of this group of patients is as critical as management of those with frank renal failure. The latter is especially true during procedures associated with a relatively high incidence of postoperative renal failure, such as cardiac and aortic reconstructive surgery. Intravascular volume depletion, sepsis, obstructive jaundice, crush injuries, recent contrast dye injections, and aminoglycoside or nonsteroidal anti-inflammatory drug therapy are additional major risk factors for an acute deterioration in renal function. Hypovolemia appears to be an especially important factor in the development of acute postoperative renal failure. Because the mortality rate of postoperative renal failure is as high as 50–60%, the emphasis in management of these patients is on prevention. The increased perioperative risk associated with the combination of advanced renal disease and diabetes has already been alluded to (see above).

Prophylaxis against renal failure with solute diuresis

appears to be effective and indicated in high-risk patients undergoing cardiac, major aortic reconstructive, and possibly other surgical procedures. Mannitol (0.5 g/kg) is generally employed and should be started prior to or at the time of induction (Chapter 31). Intravenous fluids should be given concomitantly to prevent intravascular volume depletion. Intravenous infusions of low-dose dopamine may also be beneficial by increasing renal blood flow via activation of vasodilatory dopaminergic receptors in the renal vasculature.

INTRAOPERATIVE CONSIDERATIONS

Monitoring

Standard monitors are used for procedures involving minimal fluid losses. For operations associated with significant blood or fluid losses, monitoring hourly urinary output and intravascular volume is critical (Chapter 29). Although an adequate urinary output does not ensure preservation of renal function, urinary outputs greater than 0.5 mL/kg/h are generally desirable. Intra-arterial pressure monitoring is also desirable if rapid changes in blood pressure may be encountered, such as in poorly controlled hypertensive patients and in those undergoing procedures associated with abrupt changes in cardiac preload or afterload.

Induction

Selection of an induction agent is not as critical as ensuring an adequate intravascular volume prior to induction. Induction of anesthesia in patients with renal insufficiency frequently results in hypotension when hypovolemia is present. Unless a vasopressor is given, the hypotension typically resolves only following intubation or surgical stimulation. Renal perfusion, which may already be compromised by the hypovolemia, deteriorates further, first as a result of hypotension and then from sympathetically or pharmacologically mediated renal vasoconstriction. If sustained, the decrease in renal perfusion could contribute to postoperative renal impairment. Preoperative hydration usually prevents this sequence of events.

Maintenance

All maintenance agents are acceptable with the possible exception of methoxyflurane. Although enflurane can be used safely for short procedures, it is best avoided in patients with renal insufficiency because of the availability of other satisfactory agents. Deterioration in renal function during this period may be due to any adverse hemodynamic effects of surgery (hemorrhage) or anesthesia (cardiac depression or hypotension), indirect hormonal effects (sympathoadrenal activation or ADH secretion), or positive-pressure ventilation (impeded venous return; see Chapter 31). These effects are almost completely reversible when sufficient intravenous fluids are given to maintain a normal or slightly expanded intravascular volume. The

administration of predominantly α-adrenergic vasopressors (phenylephrine, methoxamine, and norepinephrine) may also be detrimental. Once mean arterial blood pressure, cardiac output, and intravascular volume are adequate, a low-dose dopamine infusion (2–5 μg/kg/min) can be used in patients with marginal urine output in an attempt to preserve renal blood flow and renal function.

Fluid Therapy

As discussed above, judicious fluid administration is critical in managing patients with decreased renal reserve or renal insufficiency. Concern over fluid overload is justified, but problems are rarely encountered in patients with normal urinary outputs if rational guidelines and appropriate monitors are employed (Chapter 29). Indeed, the consequences of excessive fluid overload—namely, pulmonary congestion or edema—are easier to treat than those of acute renal failure.

CASE DISCUSSION: A PATIENT WITH UNCONTROLLED HYPERTENSION

A 59-year-old man with a recent onset of hypertension is scheduled for reconstruction of a stenotic left renal artery. His preoperative blood pressure is 180/110 mm Hg.

What is the cause of this man's hypertension?

Renovascular hypertension is one of few surgically correctable forms of hypertension. Others include coarctation of the aorta, pheochromocytoma, Cushing's disease, and primary hyperaldosteronism.

Most studies suggest that renovascular hypertension accounts for 2–5% of all cases of hypertension. It characteristically presents either as a relatively sudden onset of hypertension in individuals below age 35 or above age 55 years. Renal artery stenosis can also be responsible for the development of accelerated or malignant hypertension in previously hypertensive individuals of any age.

What is the pathophysiology of the hypertension?

Unilateral or bilateral stenosis of the renal artery decreases the perfusion pressure to the kidneys distal to the obstruction. Activation of the juxtaglomerular apparatus and release of renin increases circulating levels of angiotensin II and aldosterone, resulting in peripheral vascular constriction and sodium retention, respectively (Chapter 31). The resulting systemic arterial hypertension is often marked.

In nearly two-thirds of patients, the stenosis is due to

an atheromatous plaque in proximal renal artery. These patients are typically men over the age of 55 years. In the remaining third, the stenosis is more distal and due to malformations of the arterial wall, commonly referred to as fibromuscular hyperplasia (or dysplasia). This latter lesion most commonly presents in women below the age of 35 years. In 30–50% of patients with renovascular hypertension, bilateral renal artery stenosis is present. Less common causes of stenosis include dissecting aneurysms, emboli, polyarteritis nodosa, radiation, trauma, extrinsic compression from retroperitoneal fibrosis or tumors, and hypoplasia of the renal arteries.

What clinical manifestations other than hypertension may be present?

Signs of secondary hyperaldosteronism can be prominent. These include sodium retention in the form of edema, a metabolic alkalosis, and hypokalemia. The latter can cause muscle weakness, polyuria, and even tetany.

How is the diagnosis made?

The diagnosis is suggested by the clinical presentation (see above). A midabdominal bruit may also be present, but the diagnosis requires laboratory and radiographic confirmation. The captopril test is a good screening test; it relies on the observation that administration of an angiotensin-converting enzyme inhibitor to these patients greatly increases plasma renin activity. If the test is positive, digital subtraction angiography is used to demonstrate the stenosis. If the latter is not available, a rapid-sequence intravenous pyelogram can suggest the diagnosis when appearance of the dye is delayed on the affected side. Renal arteriography is often used to confirm the anatomic defect preoperatively.

Which patients are most likely to benefit from surgery?

The functional significance of the lesion is evaluated by selective catheterization of both renal veins and measurement of plasma renin activity in blood from each kidney. Plasma renin activity is typically elevated on the stenotic side. Patients with renal artery stenosis with a plasma renin activity ratio on the two sides greater than 1.5:1 have a greater than 90% cure rate following surgery. Administration of an angiotensin-converting enzyme inhibitor greatly magnifies the difference in renal vein plasma renin activity between the two sides. If the stenosis is bilateral, the split plasma renin activity ratios may be less than 1.5:1, yet the patient may still benefit from surgery.

Should this patient undergo the procedure given his present blood pressure?

The current emphasis in the treatment of renovascular stenosis is surgical because of the propensity for progressive loss of renal function with medical treatment alone. Nonetheless, optimal medical therapy is important in preparing these patients for surgery. When compared with well-controlled patients, those with poorly controlled hypertension have a high incidence of problems intraoperatively: marked hypertension, hypotension, myocardial ischemia, and arrhythmias (Chapter 20). Ideally, arterial blood pressure should be well controlled—preferably in the normal range—prior to surgery. Metabolic disturbances such as hypokalemia should be corrected. Patients should be evaluated for preexisting renal dysfunction (Chapter 31). Those above age 50 years should also be evaluated for the presence and severity of coexisting atherosclerotic disease, especially of the coronary arteries (Chapter 20).

What antihypertensive agents are most useful for controlling blood pressure perioperatively in these patients?

The most useful agents in renovascular hypertension are those that decrease renin-angiotensin system activity, namely ACE inhibitors, beta-blockers, and centrally acting agents that decrease sympathetic activity. Three oral ACE inhibitors are currently available (captopril, enalapril, and lisinopril), and one is available as an intravenous preparation (enalaprilat). Captopril has a half-life of approximately 2 hours, while the others have significantly longer half-lives (10–12 hours). Side effects include transient hypotension, hyperkalemia, neutropenia, angioedema, urticaria, and rashes. ACE inhibitors can cause acute renal failure in patients with bilateral renal artery stenosis. Their role in perioperative blood pressure management is restricted to the preoperative period.

In contrast, β-adrenergic blocking drugs can be readily used intra- and postoperatively for blood pressure control. They are especially effective because secretion of renin is partly mediated by β_1-adrenergic receptors. Although parenteral selective β_1-blocking agents such as metoprolol and esmolol would be expected to be most effective, nonselective agents such as propranolol appear equally effective. Esmolol may be the agent of choice because of its short half-life and titratability.

Direct vasodilators such as nitroprusside and nitroglycerin are also invaluable in controlling intraoperative hypertension. The role of saralasin, an angiotensin II receptor antagonist, is limited because of its partial agonist activity.

What are the important intraoperative considerations for the anesthesiologist?

Revascularization of a kidney is a major procedure, with the potential for major blood loss, fluid shifts, and hemodynamic changes. One of several procedures may be performed, including transaortic renal endarterectomy, aortorenal bypass (using a saphenous vein, synthetic graft, or segment of the hypogastric artery), a splenic to (left) renal artery bypass, a hepatic or gastroduodenal to (right) renal artery bypass, or excision of the stenotic segment with reanastomosis of the renal artery to the aorta. Rarely, nephrectomy may be performed. Regardless of the exact procedure, an extensive retroperitoneal dissection usually necessitates relatively large volumes of intravenous fluid replacement. Large-bore intravenous access is mandatory because of the potential for extensive blood loss. Heparinization contributes to increased blood loss. Depending on the surgical technique, aortic cross-clamping with its associated hemodynamic consequences often complicates anesthetic management (Chapter 21). Direct intra-arterial and central venous pressure monitoring are mandatory. Pulmonary artery pressure monitoring is indicated for patients with poor ventricular function (Chapter 6). The choice of anesthetic technique is generally determined by the patient's cardiovascular function.

Urinary output should be followed carefully. Mea-sures to protect the affected as well as the normal kidney against ischemic injury are necessary. Generous hydration together with solute diuresis with mannitol are generally advisable (Chapter 31). Topical cooling of the affected kidney during the anastomosis may also be employed.

What are the important postoperative considerations?

Although in most patients hypertension is ultimately cured or significantly improved, arterial blood pressure is often quite labile in the early postoperative period. Close hemodynamic monitoring should be continued well into the postoperative period. Reported operative mortality rates range from 1% to 6%, and most deaths are associated with myocardial infarction. The latter probably reflects the relatively high prevalence of coronary artery disease in older patients with renovascular hypertension.

SUGGESTED READINGS

Bastron RD, Deutsch S: *Anesthesia and the Kidney.* Grune & Stratton, 1976.

Burke GR, Guylyassy PF: Surgery in the patient with renal disease and related electrolyte disorders. Med Clin North Am 1979;63:1191. An excellent review of the preoperative evaluation.

Schrier RW (editor): *Renal and Electrolyte Disorders,* 3rd ed. Little, Brown, 1986.

Stanski DR, Watkins WD: *Drug Disposition in Anesthesia.* Grune and Stratton, 1982.

Stoelting RK, Dierdorf SE, McCammon RL: *Anesthesia and Co-existing Disease.* Churchill Livingstone, 1988.

Wood M, Wood AJJ: *Drugs and Anesthesia: Pharmacology for the Anesthesiologist,* 2nd ed. Williams & Wilkins, 1990.

33

Anesthesia for Genitourinary Surgery

Urologic procedures account for 10–20% of most anesthetic practices. Patients undergoing genitourinary procedures may be of any age, but most are elderly and many have coexisting medical illnesses, especially renal dysfunction. Anesthetic management of patients with renal impairment is discussed in Chapter 32, and the effects of anesthesia on renal function are discussed in Chapter 31. This chapter reviews the anesthetic management of common urologic procedures. Use of the lithotomy position, the transurethral approach, and extracorporeal shock waves (lithotripsy) complicates many of these procedures. Moreover, advances in surgical technique are allowing more patients to undergo radical procedures for urologic cancer, urinary diversion with bladder reconstruction, and renal transplantation.

CYSTOSCOPY

Preoperative Considerations

Cystoscopy is the most commonly performed urologic procedure. Indications for cystoscopy include hematuria, recurrent urinary infections, and urinary obstruction. Bladder biopsies, extraction of renal stones, and placement or manipulation of ureteral catheters can also be performed through the cystoscope.

Anesthetic management varies with the age and gender of the patient and the purpose of the procedure. General anesthesia is necessary for most children. Because of a short urethra, topical anesthesia in the form of viscous lidocaine with or without sedation is used for diagnostic studies in most women. Operative cystoscopies involving biopsies, cauterization, or manipulation of ureteral catheters require regional or general anesthesia. Most males require regional or general anesthesia even for diagnostic studies.

Intraoperative Considerations

A. Lithotomy Position: Next to the supine position, this is the most commonly used position for patients undergoing any type of surgery. It is most commonly used for urologic and gynecologic procedures. Failure to properly position patients can result in iatrogenic injuries. Two persons are required to safely

move the patient's legs simultaneously up or down. Straps around the ankles usually hold the legs in position (Figure 33–1). The strap supports should be padded, and the legs should hang freely. Injury to the common peroneal nerve, resulting in loss of dorsiflexion of the foot, may result if the lateral thigh rests on the strap support. If the legs are allowed to rest on medially placed strap supports, compression of the saphenous nerve can result in numbness along the medial calf. Excessive flexion of the thigh against the groin can injure the obturator and, less commonly, the femoral nerves.

The lithotomy position is associated with major physiologic alterations. Functional residual capacity decreases, predisposing to atelectasis and hypoxia. This effect is accentuated by the head-down (Trendelenburg) position. Elevation of the legs increases venous return acutely and may exacerbate congestive heart failure. Conversely, rapid lowering of the legs acutely decreases venous return and can result in hypotension. Vasodilatation from either general or regional anesthesia accentuates the hypotension. For this reason, blood pressure measurements should always be taken immediately after the legs are lowered.

B. Choice of Anesthesia:

1. General anesthesia—Because of the short duration (15–20 minutes) and the outpatient setting of most cystoscopies, general anesthesia is usually employed. Most patients are apprehensive about the procedure and prefer to be asleep. Any anesthetic technique suitable for outpatients may be used (Chapter 44). Oxygen saturation should be closely monitored when obese or elderly patients or those with marginal pulmonary reserve are placed in the lithotomy or Trendelenburg position.

2. Regional anesthesia—Both epidural and spinal blocks can provide satisfactory anesthesia. However, satisfactory sensory blockade may require 15–20 minutes for epidural anesthesia compared to 5 minutes for spinal anesthesia. Consequently, most clinicians prefer spinal anesthesia, especially for procedures lasting more than 30 minutes with elderly and high-risk patients. The sensory level following anesthetic injection should be well established ("fixed") before the patient is moved into the lithotomy position. Although the matter is controversial, some believe that prema-

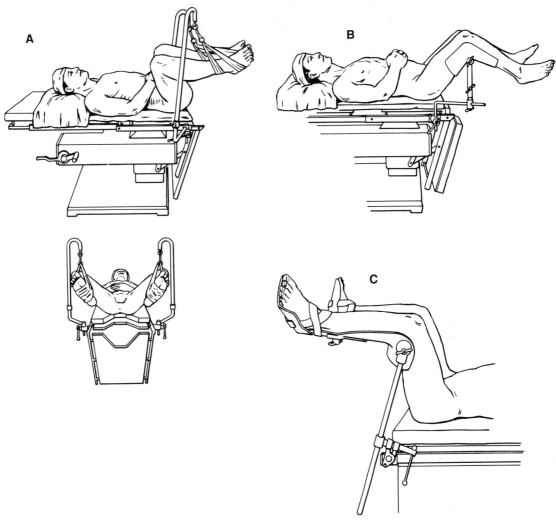

Figure 33–1. The lithotomy position. **A:** Strap stirrups. **B:** Bier-Hoff stirrups. **C:** Allen stirrups. (Modified and reproduced, with permission, from *Martin JT: Positioning in Anesthesia.* Saunders, 1988.)

ture elevation of the legs following intrathecal injection of a hyperbaric anesthetic solution may result in a high spinal level of anesthesia that may lead to severe hypotension and respiratory compromise. A sensory level to T10 provides excellent anesthesia for nearly all cystoscopic procedures. Regional anesthesia, however, does not abolish the obturator reflex (external rotation and adduction of the thigh secondary to stimulation of the obturator nerve by electrocautery current through the lateral bladder wall). The reflex (muscle contraction) is reliably blocked only by muscle paralysis during general anesthesia.

TRANSURETHRAL RESECTION OF THE PROSTATE

Preoperative Considerations

Benign prostatic hypertrophy frequently leads to symptomatic bladder outlet obstruction in men over the age of 60 years. Because conservative treatment is generally unsuccessful, most patients eventually ask for surgical relief. One of four operations may be selected to remove the hypertrophied and hyperplastic prostatic tissue: suprapubic (transvesical) prostatectomy, perineal prostatectomy, retropubic prostatectomy, or transurethral resection of the prostate (TURP). With the possible exception of the suprapubic approach, morbidity and mortality rates are generally comparable. Nonetheless, the transurethral approach is nearly always selected for patients with prostate glands weighing less than 40–50 g. An alternative approach is chosen if the prostate is over 80 g. Patients with advanced prostatic carcinoma may also present for transurethral resections to relieve symptomatic urinary obstruction. Regardless of its cause, long-standing obstruction can lead to impaired renal function.

Patients undergoing TURP should be carefully evaluated for coexistent cardiac and pulmonary disease as well as renal dysfunction (Chapters 20, 23, and 32). These patients have a relatively high (30–60%) prevalence of both cardiovascular and pulmonary disorders. The procedure is reported to carry a 0.5–6% mortality rate. Common causes of death include myocardial infarction, pulmonary edema, and renal failure.

Although a type and screen (Chapter 29) is adequate for most patients if the gland is not large, blood should be available and crossmatched for anemic patients as well as patients with large glands (> 30–40 g). Prostatic bleeding can be difficult to control through the cystoscope.

Intraoperative Considerations

The procedure is performed by passing a loop through a special cystoscope (resectoscope). Using continuous irrigation and direct visualization, prostatic tissue is resected by applying a cutting current to the loop. Because of the characteristics of the prostate and the large amounts of irrigation fluid often used, TURP can be associated with a number of serious complications (Table 33–1).

A. TURP Syndrome: Transurethral prostatic resection often opens the extensive network of venous sinuses in the prostate and potentially allows systemic absorption of the irrigating fluid. The absorption of large amounts of fluid results in a constellation of symptoms and signs commonly referred to as the TURP syndrome (Table 33–2). This syndrome presents intraoperatively or postoperatively as headache, restlessness, confusion, cyanosis, dyspnea, arrhythmias, hypotension, or seizures. Moreover, it can be rapidly fatal. The manifestations are primarily those of circulatory fluid overload, water intoxication, and occasionally toxicity from the solute in the irrigating fluid.

Electrolyte solutions cannot be used for irrigation during TURP because they disperse the electrocautery current. Water provides excellent visibility because its hypotonicity lyses red blood cells, but significant absorption can readily result in acute water intoxication. Water irrigation is generally restricted to transurethral resection of bladder tumors only. For TURP, near-isotonic nonelectrolyte irrigating solutions such as glycine 1.5% (230 mosm/L) or a mixture of sorbitol 2.7% and mannitol 0.54% (195 mosm/L) are most commonly used. Less commonly used solutions include mannitol 3%, sorbitol 3.3%, dextrose 2.5–4%, and urea 1%. Because all these fluids are still hypotonic, significant absorption of water can nevertheless occur. Solute absorption can also occur because the irrigation fluid is under pressure.

Table 33–1. Major complications associated with TURP.

Hemorrhage
TURP syndrome
Bladder perforation
Hypothermia
Septicemia
Disseminated intravascular coagulation

Table 33–2. Manifestations of the TURP syndrome.

Hyponatremia
Hypo-osmolality
Fluid overload
Congestive heart failure
Pulmonary edema
Hypotension
Hemolysis
Solute toxicity
Hyperglycinemia (glycine)
Hyperammonemia (glycine)
Hyperglycemia (sorbitol)
Intravascular volume expansion (mannitol)

Absorption of irrigation fluid appears to be dependent on the duration of the resection as well as the height (pressure) of the irrigation fluid. Most resections last 45–60 minutes, and on the average 20 mL/min of the irrigating fluid is absorbed. Pulmonary congestion or florid pulmonary edema can readily result from the absorption of large amounts of irrigation fluid, especially in patients with limited cardiac reserve. The hypotonicity of these fluids also results in acute hyponatremia and hypo-osmolality, which can lead to serious neurologic manifestations (Chapter 28). Symptoms of hyponatremia usually do not develop until the serum sodium concentration decreases below 120 meq/L. Marked hypotonicity in plasma ($[Na^+] <$ 100 meq/L) may also result in acute intravascular hemolysis (Chapter 29).

Toxicity may also arise from absorption of the solutes in these fluids. Marked hyperglycinemia has been reported with glycine solutions and is thought to contribute to circulatory depression and central nervous system toxicity. Plasma glycine concentrations in excess of 1000 mg/L have been recorded (normal is 13–17 mg/L). Glycine is known to be an inhibitory neurotransmitter in the central nervous system and has also been implicated in rare instances of transient blindness following TURP. Hyperammonemia, presumably from the degradation of glycine, has also been documented in a few patients with marked central nervous system toxicity following TURP. Blood ammonia levels in some patients exceeded 500 μmol/L (normal: 5–50 μmol/L). It has been suggested that arginine deficiency predisposes to central nervous system toxicity following absorption of glycine solution. Arginine is a critical intermediate in the conversion of ammonia to urea (Chapter 32). Laboratory studies suggest that addition of arginine to glycine irrigating solutions may protect against hyperammonemia and central nervous system toxicity. The use of large amounts of sorbitol or dextrose irrigating solutions can lead to hyperglycemia, which can be marked in diabetic patients. Absorption of mannitol solutions causes intravascular volume expansion and exacerbates fluid overload.

Treatment of TURP syndrome depends on early recognition and should be based on the severity of symptoms. The absorbed water must be eliminated, and hypoxemia and hypoperfusion must be avoided. Symptomatic hyponatremia resulting in seizures or coma should be treated with hypertonic saline (Chapter 28). Seizure activity can be terminated with small doses of midazolam (2–4 mg), diazepam (3–5 mg), or thiopental (50–100 mg). Phenytoin, 10–20 mg/kg intravenously (no faster than 50 mg/min), should also be considered to provide more sustained anticonvulsant activity. Endotracheal intubation is generally advisable to prevent aspiration until the patient's mental status normalizes. The amount and rate of hypertonic saline solution (3% or 5%) to correct the hyponatremia to a safe level should be based on the patient's serum sodium concentration (Chapter 28). Hypertonic saline solution should not be given at a rate faster than 100 mL/h so as not to exacerbate circulatory fluid overload.

B. Hypothermia: Large volumes of irrigating fluids at room temperature can be a major source of heat loss in patients. Irrigating solutions should be warmed to body temperature prior to use to prevent hypothermia. Postoperative shivering associated with hypothermia is especially undesirable, since it can dislodge clots and promote postoperative bleeding.

C. Bladder Perforation: The incidence of bladder perforation during TURP is estimated to be approximately 1%. Perforation may result from the resectoscope going through the bladder wall or from overdistention of the bladder with irrigation fluid. Most bladder perforations are extraperitoneal and are signaled by poor return of the irrigating fluid. Awake patients will typically complain of nausea, diaphoresis, and retropubic or lower abdominal pain. Large extraperitoneal and most intraperitoneal perforations are usually even more obvious, presenting as sudden unexplained hypotension with generalized abdominal pain (in awake patients). Regardless of the anesthetic technique employed, perforation should be suspected in settings of sudden hypotension or hypertension, especially with bradycardia (vagally mediated).

D. Coagulopathy: Disseminated intravascular coagulation (DIC) has on rare occasions been reported following TURP and is thought to result from the release of thromboplastins from the prostate into the circulation during surgery. A dilutional thrombocytopenia can also develop during surgery as part of the TURP syndrome from absorption of irrigation fluids. Rarely, patients with metastatic carcinoma of the prostate develop a coagulopathy from primary fibrinolysis; the tumor is thought to secrete a fibrinolytic enzyme in such instances. The diagnosis of coagulopathy may be suspected from diffuse uncontrollable bleeding but must be confirmed by laboratory tests (see Case Discussion, Chapter 34). The treatment of DIC in this setting may require heparin in addition to replacement of clotting factors and platelets. Consultation with a hematologist is advisable.

E. Septicemia: The prostate is often colonized with bacteria and may harbor chronic infection. Extensive surgical manipulation of the gland together with the opening of venous sinuses can allow entry of organisms into the bloodstream. Bacteremia following transurethral surgery is not uncommon and can lead to septicemia or septic shock (Chapter 48). Prophylactic antibiotic therapy (most commonly gentamicin) prior to TURP may decrease the likelihood of bacteremic and septic episodes.

F. Choice of Anesthesia: Either spinal or epidural anesthesia with a T10 sensory level provides excellent anesthesia and good operating conditions for TURP. When compared to general anesthesia, regional anesthesia appears to decrease surgical blood loss and reduce the incidence of postoperative venous thrombosis; it is also less likely to mask symptoms and signs of the TURP syndrome or bladder perforation. The possibility of vertebral metastasis must considered in patients with carcinoma, especially those with back pain. Metastatic disease to the lumbar spine is a contraindication to regional anesthesia. Acute hyponatremia from the TURP syndrome may delay or prevent emergence from general anesthesia.

G. Monitoring: Evaluation of mental status in the awake patient is the best monitor for detection of early signs of the TURP syndrome and bladder perforation. A decrease in arterial oxygen saturation may be an early sign of fluid overload. Temperature monitoring should be used during long resections to detect hypothermia. Blood loss is especially difficult to assess because of the use of irrigating solutions, so clinical signs of hypovolemia must be relied upon (Chapter 29). Blood loss averages 200–300 mL but rarely can be life-threatening. Decreases in hematocrit may simply reflect hemodilution from absorption of irrigation fluid.

EXTRACORPOREAL SHOCK WAVE LITHOTRIPSY

Extracorporeal shock wave lithotripsy (ESWL) is employed for disintegration of calculi in the kidneys or the upper two-thirds of the ureters (above the iliac crest). One of several techniques may be used to focus high-energy shock waves at the renal calculus. With Dornier HM3 units, the patient is placed in a hydraulic chair, immersed in a heated water bath, and positioned with the aid of two image intensifiers such that the stone is in the second focus of an elliptical reflector, while the source of the shock waves is in the first focus (Figure 33–2). Newer units such as the Siemens Lithostar require only a small amount of mineral oil on the skin to acoustically couple the patient to the energy source. The latter is enclosed in a water-filled casing and comes in contact with the patient via a plastic membrane.

Shock waves are most commonly generated by discharging an underwater capacitor beneath the patient in the first focus of the elliptical reflector. Newer units generate shock waves electromagnetically or from

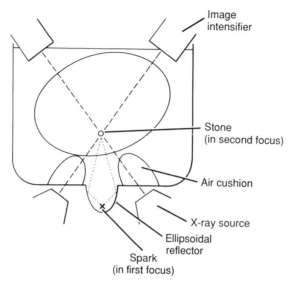

Figure 33–2. Schematic representation of a lithotripsy unit.

piezoelectric crystals. Because tissue has the same acoustic density as water, the waves travel through the body without damaging tissue. However, the change in acoustic impedance at the tissue-stone interface creates shear and tear forces on the stone. The stone is fragmented enough by the waves to allow its passage down the urinary tract. Ureteral stents are often placed cystoscopically prior to the procedure to facilitate the passage of large particles of stone. Tissue destruction can occur if the waves are focused at air-tissue interfaces such as in the lung and intestine. Inability to position the patient so that lung and intestine are away from the wave focus is a contraindication to the procedure. Other contraindications include urinary obstruction below the stone, untreated infection, a bleeding diathesis, and pregnancy. The presence of a nearby aortic aneurysm or spinal prosthetic device is considered a relative contraindication in some centers.

Preoperative Considerations

Patients with a history of cardiac arrhythmias and those with a pacemaker are at risk of developing arrhythmias induced by the shock waves. Shock waves can damage the internal components of some pacemakers. Synchronization of the shock waves to the R wave from the ECG decreases the incidence of arrhythmias. The shock waves are usually timed to be 20 ms after the R wave to correspond to the ventricular refractory period (Chapter 19).

Intraoperative Considerations

A. Effects of Immersion: Immersion into a heated water bath (36–37 °C) initially results in vasodilatation that can transiently lead to hypotension. Arterial blood pressure, however, subsequently rises as venous blood is redistributed centrally from the hydrostatic pressure of water on the legs and abdomen.

The sudden increase in venous return can precipitate congestive heart failure in patients with marginal cardiac reserve. Moreover, the increase in intrathoracic blood volume significantly reduces functional residual capacity (30–60%) and predisposes some patients to hypoxemia.

B. Choice of Anesthesia: Pain during lithotripsy is from dissipation of a small amount of energy as shock waves enter the body through the skin. The pain is therefore localized to the skin and proportionate to the intensity of the shock waves. Lithotripsy with units employing a water bath (Dornier HM3) requires 1000–2000 relatively high-intensity shock waves (18–22 kV) that most patients do not tolerate without either regional or general anesthesia. In contrast, lithotripsy with units that are coupled directly to the skin utilizes 2000–3000 lower-intensity shock waves (10–18 kV) that usually require only light sedation.

C. Regional Anesthesia: Continuous epidural anesthesia is commonly used for ESWL using a water bath. A T6 sensory level assures adequate anesthesia, as renal innervation is derived from T10 to L2. Supplementation of the block with fentanyl, 50–100 µg epidurally, is often useful. Light sedation is also generally desirable for most patients. Supplemental oxygen by face mask or nasal cannula is also useful in avoiding hypoxemia. Because of the potential for post-dural puncture headache in a seated patient and less control over the sensory level with the latter, epidural anesthesia is usually preferred over spinal anesthesia. Regional anesthesia greatly facilitates positioning and monitoring. Prior intravascular volume expansion with 1000–1500 mL of lactated Ringer's injection prevents severe postural hypotension following epidural activation, positioning in the hydraulic chair, and immersion in the warm bath.

A major disadvantage of regional anesthesia is the

inability to control diaphragmatic movement. Excessive diaphragmatic excursion during spontaneous ventilation can move the stone in and out of the wave focus and may prolong the procedure. This problem can be partially solved by asking the patient to breathe in a more rapid but shallow respiratory pattern. Bradycardia from high sympathetic blockade also prolongs the procedure when shock waves are coupled to the ECG.

D. General Anesthesia: General endotracheal anesthesia allows control of diaphragmatic excursion and is preferred by many patients. The procedure is complicated by the inherent risks associated with placing a supine anesthetized patient in a chair, elevating and then lowering the chair into a water bath to shoulder depth, and then reversing the sequence at the end. A light general anesthetic technique in conjunction with a muscle relaxant is preferable. The muscle relaxant assures patient immobility and control of diaphragmatic movement. High-frequency jet ventilation during ESWL may be used to reduce diaphragmatic excursions to a minimum, but studies have failed to substantiate a decrease in the number of shocks required or in radiation exposure from fluoroscopy. As with regional anesthesia, intravenous fluid loading with 1000 mL of lactated Ringer's injection is generally advisable prior to moving patients upright into the hydraulic chair to prevent postural hypotension.

E. Monitoring: Electrocardiograph pads should be attached securely with water-proof dressing prior to immersion. Even with R wave-triggered shocks, supraventricular arrhythmias can still occur and may require treatment. Changes in functional residual capacity with immersion mandate close monitoring of oxygen saturation, especially in patients at high risk for developing hypoxemia (Chapter 22).

F. Fluid Management: Intravenous fluid therapy is typically generous. Following the initial intravenous fluid bolus (above), an additional 1000–2000 mL of lactated Ringer's injection is usually given with a small dose of furosemide (10–20 mg) to maintain brisk urinary flow and flush the stone debris. Patients with poor cardiac reserve require more conservative fluid therapy.

RADICAL SURGERY FOR UROLOGIC MALIGNANCIES

Improved survival rates for patients with urologic cancer following radical resections have resulted in an increase in number of procedures performed for prostatic, bladder, testicular, and renal cancer.

Preoperative Considerations

The highest incidence of urologic cancer occurs in elderly males. The association of cigarette smoking with carcinoma of the bladder and possibly of the kidney contributes to coexistent coronary artery and chronic obstructive pulmonary disease in many of these patients. Impaired renal function may be age-related or secondary to urinary tract obstruction. Patients undergoing retroperitoneal lymph node dissection for testicular cancer, although typically 15–35 years old, are often at increased risk of morbidity from the residual effects of preoperative chemotherapy. In addition to bone marrow suppression, specific organ toxicity such as renal impairment following cisplatin, pulmonary fibrosis following bleomycin, and cardiomyopathy following doxorubicin may be present.

Intraoperative Considerations

Radical resection of these cancers typically last 3–4 hours or longer and frequently requires blood transfusion. General endotracheal anesthesia with a muscle relaxant provides optimal operating conditions. Controlled hypotensive anesthesia may reduce intraoperative blood loss and transfusion requirements (Chapter 13). Supplementation of general anesthesia with spinal or continuous epidural anesthesia facilitates the induced hypotension and decreases general anesthetic requirements. Moreover, an epidural catheter provides a highly effective route for postoperative analgesia (Chapter 18). Epidural narcotics often provide more effective, longer-lasting pain relief with greater preservation of respiratory function when compared with parenteral narcotics.

Close monitoring of intravascular volume and blood loss is essential during these procedures. Intra-arterial pressure monitoring is indicated if controlled hypotension is used, if the patient has significant cardiovascular disease, or if rapid blood loss is encountered during the procedure. Central venous pressure monitoring is advisable in the majority of patients, while pulmonary artery pressure monitoring is indicated for those with decreased cardiac reserve (Chapter 6). Urinary output should be monitored continuously and correlated with the progress of the operation, as the urinary path is interrupted at some point during most of these procedures.

Special Considerations

A. Retroperitoneal Lymph Node Dissections: This operation is usually performed for staging and treatment of some testicular cancers. A thoracoabdominal incision (extending from the posterior axillary line over the eighth to tenth ribs to a paramedian line halfway between the xiphoid and the umbilicus) is most commonly used to gain access to the retroperitoneum. Alternatively, the transabdominal approach is chosen using a midline incision (directly from the xiphoid to the pubis).

Patients receiving bleomycin preoperatively appear to be at increased risk of developing postoperative pulmonary insufficiency. Although still controversial, the use of high inspired oxygen concentrations and perhaps excessive intravenous fluid administration contributes to the development of the adult respiratory distress syndrome (ARDS) postoperatively in these cases. Anesthetic management requires use of the lowest inspired concentration of oxygen compatible with an acceptable hemoglobin oxygen saturation ($> 90\%$). Positive end-expiratory pressure (PEEP), 5–10 cm H_2O, may optimize oxygenation. Because nitrous oxide has been associated with bone marrow suppression, some clinicians prefer to use an air-oxygen mixture.

Evaporative and redistributive fluid losses ("third spacing") are considerable as a result of the large wound and the extensive surgical dissection. Fluid replacement should be sufficient to maintain an adequate urinary output (> 0.5 mL/kg/h); the combined use of both colloid and crystalloid solutions in a ratio of 1:2 or 1:3 may be more effective in preserving urinary output than crystalloid alone. Mannitol (0.25–0.5 g/kg) is usually given prior to dissection near the renal arteries. Mannitol is thought to prevent ischemic renal injury from surgically induced spasm of the renal arteries by preserving renal blood and tubular flow.

The postoperative pain associated with thoracoabdominal incisions is severe and typically associated with considerable splinting. Aggressive postoperative analgesia is necessary to avoid atelectasis. Continuous epidural analgesia (with intercostal nerve blocks, if necessary) is particularly efficacious in this setting. Because ligation of intercostal arteries during left-sided dissections has rarely resulted in paraplegia, it may be prudent to document normal motor function postoperatively prior to institution of epidural anesthesia. The arteria radicularis magna (artery of Adamkiewicz), which is supplied by these vessels and is responsible for most of the arterial blood to the lower half of the spinal cord (Chapter 21), arises on the left side in most individuals.

B. Radical Nephrectomy: During a radical nephrectomy, the renal artery and vein are ligated, and the kidney, adrenal, and perinephric fat are removed en bloc with the surrounding (Gerota's) fascia. Most patients undergoing this procedure have a tumor that is confined to the kidney. In some medical centers, complicated resections of tumors with vena caval invasion are also successfully performed.

The surgical approach may utilize a thoracoabdominal, transabdominal, or flank incision, depending on tumor size and the presence or absence of a tumor thrombus. A flank incision requires the patient to be in a modified lateral decubitus position (Chapter 24) with a kidney rest under the iliac crest. The table is then hyperextended to open the flank space. The thoracoabdominal approach is used for large tumors and when a thrombus is present. Tumor extension into the inferior vena cava, hepatic vein, or right atrium greatly complicates anesthetic management and predisposes to potentially catastrophic pulmonary embolization. Cardiopulmonary bypass may be necessary with a large atrial thrombus. A pneumothorax can develop following the flank approach if the pleura is entered, and that complication should be excluded by a postoperative chest x-ray. Chest tubes are routinely placed only with the thoracoabdominal approach.

C. Urinary Diversion: Urinary diversion is most commonly performed immediately following radical cystectomy. Several procedures are currently used, but all entail implanting the ureters into a segment of bowel. The bowel segment is either left in situ (ureterosigmoidostomy) or divided with its mesenteric blood supply intact and attached to a cutaneous stoma or, less commonly, the urethra. Moreover, the bowel may function merely as a conduit (ileal conduit) or be reconstructed to form a continent reservoir (such as a Kock ileal reservoir).

Good anesthetic management is dependent on keeping the patient well hydrated and maintaining a brisk urinary output. If the procedure follows a radical cystectomy, central venous pressure monitoring is invaluable. The point at which the ureters are divided should be noted to prevent overzealous fluid administration in response to an abrupt decrease in urine output. When regional anesthesia is being utilized, unopposed parasympathetic activity due to sympathetic blockade often results in a very contracted, hyperactive bowel that makes construction of a continent ileal reservoir technically difficult. The use of a large dose of anticholinergic (glycopyrrolate, 1 mg) or papaverine (50–100 mg as a slow intravenous infusion) often alleviates this problem.

RENAL TRANSPLANTATION

The success of renal transplantation, which is largely due to recent advances in immunosuppressive therapy, has greatly improved the quality of life for patients with end-stage renal disease. With present immunosuppressive regimens, cadaveric transplants have achieved almost the same 3-year graft survival rates (80–90%) as living related donor grafts. Additionally, restrictions on candidates for renal transplantation have gradually decreased. Infection and cancer are at present the only remaining absolute contraindications. Advanced age (> 60 years) and severe cardiovascular disease are relative contraindications.

Preoperative Considerations

Preoperative optimization of the patient's medical condition with dialysis is mandatory (Chapter 32). Current organ preservation techniques allow ample time (24–48 hours) for preoperative dialysis of cadaveric recipients. Living-related transplants are performed electively with the donor and recipient anesthetized simultaneously but in separate rooms. The recipient's serum potassium concentration should be below 5.5 meq/L, and existing coagulopathies should be corrected.

Intraoperative Considerations

The transplant is carried out by placing the donor kidney retroperitoneally in the iliac fossa and anastomosing the renal vessels to the iliac vessels and the ureter to the bladder. Nephrectomy is performed only in the presence of intractable hypertension or chronic infection. Immunosuppression is started on the day of surgery with combinations of corticosteroids, cyclosporine, and azathioprine. Some centers avoid cyclosporine in the first few days and use instead antithymocyte globulin or monoclonal antibodies directed against specific subsets of T lymphocytes.

A. Choice of Anesthesia: Although both spinal and epidural anesthesia have been successfully employed, most transplants are usually done under general anesthesia. All general anesthetic agents, including methoxyflurane and enflurane, have been employed without any apparent detrimental effect on graft function; nonetheless, these two agents are best avoided (Chapter 32). Atracurium may be the muscle relaxant of choice, since it is not dependent on renal excretion for elimination. Alternatively, vecuronium may be used with only modest prolongation of its effects.

B. Monitoring: Central venous pressure monitoring is very useful in ensuring adequate hydration but avoiding fluid overload. Normal saline or half-normal saline solutions are commonly used. A urinary catheter is placed preoperatively. A brisk urine flow following the arterial anastomosis generally indicates good graft function. The diuresis that follows may resemble nonoliguric renal failure (Chapter 32). If the graft ischemic time was prolonged, an oliguric phase may precede the diuretic phase, in which case fluid therapy must be adjusted appropriately. The judicious use of mannitol (0.25–0.5 g/kg) may be indicated in such cases. Hyperkalemia has been reported after release of the vascular clamp following completion of the arterial anastomosis. Release of potassium contained in the preservative solution has been implicated in those cases. Serum electrolyte concentrations should be monitored closely after completion of the anastomosis. Hyperkalemia may be suspected from peaking of the T wave on the ECG. Most patients can generally be extubated immediately after the procedure.

CASE DISCUSSION: HYPOTENSION IN THE RECOVERY ROOM

A 69-year-old man with a history of an inferior myocardial infarction was admitted to the recovery room following TURP under general anesthesia. The procedure took 90 minutes and was reported as uncomplicated. On admission, the patient is extubated but still unresponsive, and vital signs are stable. Twenty minutes later, he is noted to be awakening but restless. He begins to shiver intensely; his blood pressure decreases to 80/35 mm Hg; and his respirations increase to 40 breaths/min. The bedside monitor shows a sinus tachycardia of 140 beats/min and an oxygen saturation of 92%.

What is the differential diagnosis?
The differential diagnosis of hypotension following TURP should always include the following:

(1) Hemorrhage
(2) TURP syndrome
(3) Bladder perforation
(4) Myocardial infarction or ischemia
(5) Septicemia
(6) DIC

Other possibilities (Chapter 47) are less likely in this setting but should always considered, especially when the patient fails to respond to appropriate measures (see below).

Based on the history, what is the most likely diagnosis?
A diagnosis cannot be made with reasonable certainty at this point, and the patient requires further evaluation. Nonetheless, the hypotension and shivering must be treated rapidly because of the history of coronary artery disease. The hypotension seriously compromises coronary perfusion, and the shivering markedly increases myocardial oxygen demand (Chapter 20).

What diagnostic aids would be helpful?
A quick examination of the patient is extremely useful in narrowing down the possibilities. Hemorrhage from the prostate should be apparent from effluent of the continuous bladder irrigation system placed at the end of the procedure. Although relatively little blood in the urine makes it look red, brisk hemorrhage is often apparent as grossly bloody drainage. Occasionally, the drainage may be scant because of clots blocking the drainage catheter; irrigation of the catheter is indicated in such cases.

Clinical signs of peripheral perfusion are invaluable. Hypovolemic patients have decreased peripheral (radial) pulses, and their extremities are usually cool and may be cyanotic. Poor perfusion is consistent with hemorrhage, bladder perforation, DIC, and severe myocardial ischemia or infarction. A full bounding peripheral pulse with warm extremities is suggestive but not always present in septicemia (Chapter 48). Signs of fluid overload should be searched for, such as jugular venous distention, pulmonary crackles, and an S_3 gallop. Fluid overload is more consistent with TURP syndrome but may also be seen in with myocardial infarction or ischemia.

The abdomen should be examined for signs of perforation. A rigid and tender or distended abdomen is very suggestive of perforation and should prompt immediate evaluation for laparotomy. When the abdomen is soft and nontender, perforation can reasonably be excluded.

Further evaluation requires laboratory measurements, an ECG, and a chest x-ray. Blood should be immediately obtained for arterial blood gas analysis and measurements of hematocrit, hemoglobin, electrolytes, glucose, a platelet count, and prothrombin and partial thromboplastin tests. If DIC is suggested by diffuse oozing, fibrinogen and fibrin split product measurements will confirm the diagnosis. Ionized calcium and magnesium levels are indicated if the patient develops seizure activity. A 12-lead ECG should be evaluated for signs of ischemia, electrolyte abnormalities (Chapter 29), or an evolving myocardial infarction. A chest x-ray should be obtained to search for evidence of pulmonary congestion, aspiration, pneumothorax, or cardiomegaly.

While laboratory measurements are being performed, what therapeutic and diagnostic measures should be undertaken?

Immediate measures aimed at avoiding hypoxemia and hypoperfusion should be instituted. Oxygen supplementation protects against hypoxemia and may increase oxygen delivery to tissues. If hypoventilation or respiratory distress is apparent, endotracheal intubation is indicated. Frequent blood pressure measurements should be obtained. If signs of fluid overload are absent, a diagnostic fluid challenge with 500 mL of crystalloid or 250 mL of colloid is helpful. A favorable response, as indicated by an increase in blood pressure and decrease in heart rate, is suggestive of hypovolemia and an indication for additional fluid boluses. Obvious bleeding in the setting of hypotension necessitates blood transfusion. Absence of a quick response should prompt further evaluation with invasive monitors. Administration of an inotrope, such as dopamine or dobutamine, is appropriate while the evaluation is being completed. Dobutamine may be preferable because it causes less tachycardia. Direct intra-arterial pressure measurement is invaluable in this setting. Central venous access should be established to measure central venous pressure and for possible placement of a pulmonary artery catheter. The latter is useful in patients with a history of congestive heart failure and when clinical signs are ambiguous. Cardiac output can then be measured by thermodilution, and pulmonary capillary wedge pressure measurements can be used to guide fluid or vasodilator therapy (see below).

If signs of fluid overload are present, intravenous furosemide in addition to an inotrope is indicated. Further treatment with vasodilator therapy should only be initiated after full hemodynamic monitoring is established.

The patient's axillary temperature is 35.5°C. Does the absence of obvious fever exclude sepsis?

No. Anesthesia is commonly associated with altered temperature regulation. A rise in temperature may be delayed or even absent, particularly in patients who are hypothermic from heat losses during surgery (Chapter 42). Moreover, correlation between axillary and core temperatures is quite variable (Chapter 6). A high index of suspicion is therefore required to diagnose sepsis. Leukocytosis is common following surgery and is not a reliable indicator of sepsis in this setting.

The mechanism of shivering in patients recovering from anesthesia is poorly understood. Although shivering is common in patients who become hypothermic during surgery (and presumably functions to raise body temperature back to normal), its relation to body temperature is inconsistent. Anesthetics probably alter the normal behavior of hypothalamic thermoregulatory centers in the brain. In contrast, infectious agents, circulating toxins, or immune reactions cause the release of cytokines (interleukin-1 and tumor necrosis factor) that stimulate the hypothalamus to synthesize prostaglandin PGE_2. The latter in turn activates neurons responsible for heat production, resulting in intense shivering.

How can the shivering be stopped?

Regardless of its cause, shivering has the undesirable effects of markedly increasing oxygen consumption (100–200%) and CO_2 production. Both cardiac output and minute ventilation must therefore also increase. These effects are often poorly tolerated by patients with limited cardiac or pulmonary reserve. Although the ultimate therapeutic goal is to correct the underlying problem (such as hypothermia or sepsis), additional measures are indicated in this patient. Supplemental oxygen therapy (high FIO_2) helps prevent hypoxemia from the low mixed venous oxygen tension commonly associated with shivering; a low mixed venous oxygen tension tends to accentuate the effects of any intrapulmonary shunting (Chapter 22). Unlike other opioid agonists, meperidine in small doses (20–50 mg intravenously) frequently terminates shivering regardless of the cause. Chlorpromazine, 10–25 mg, and butorphanol, 1–2 mg, may also be effective. These agents may have specific actions on temperature regulation centers in the hypothalamus. Shivering associated with sepsis and immune reactions can also be blocked by inhibitors of prostaglandin synthetase (aspirin, acetaminophen, and nonsteroidal anti-inflammatory agents) as well as glucocorticoids. Acetaminophen, which can be given rectally, is generally preferred perioperatively because it does not affect platelet function. Rectal suppositories are, however, generally avoided following prostatic surgery to prevent bleeding from minor trauma to the gland during insertion.

Outcome

Examination of the patient reveals warm extremities with a good pulse considering the low blood pressure. The abdomen is soft and nontender. The irrigation fluid from the bladder was only slightly pink. A diagnosis of probable septicemia is made. Blood cultures are obtained and antibiotic therapy is initiated to cover gram-negative organisms and enterococci (the most common pathogens). The patient receives intravenous gentamicin, 80 mg, and ampicillin, 500 mg, and an intravenous dopamine infusion is started. The shivering ceases following administration of meperidine, 20 mg intravenously. The blood pressure increases to 110/60 mm Hg and the pulse slows to 110 beats/min following a 1000 mL intravenous fluid bolus and 5 μg/kg/min of dopamine. The serum sodium concentration was found to be 130 meq/L. Four hours later, the dopamine was no longer needed, and the patient recovered uneventfully.

SUGGESTED READINGS

Gissen D: Anesthesia for extracorporeal shock wave lithotripsy. Semin Anesth 1987;6:57.

Martin JT: *Positioning in Anesthesia,* 2nd ed. Saunders, 1988.

Marx GF, Orkin LR: Complications associated with transurethral surgery. Anesthesiology 1962;23:802. A classic review of the problems with this surgical approach.

Skinner DG, Lieskovsky G: *Genitourinary Cancer.* Saunders, 1988. Describes the various surgical procedures in detail and includes a chapter on anesthetic management.

34

Hepatic Physiology & Anesthesia

The liver, which weighs approximately 1500–1600 g in adults, is the largest organ in the body. It is responsible for a seemingly endless number of complex and interrelated functions. Fortunately, because of the liver's large functional reserves, clinically significant hepatic dysfunction following anesthesia and surgery is uncommon. Such dysfunction is limited chiefly to patients with preexisting hepatic impairment and to those with rare idiosyncratic reactions to halogenated volatile anesthetics. This chapter reviews normal hepatic physiology, laboratory evaluation of hepatic function, and the effects of anesthesia on hepatic function. The anesthetic management of patients with liver disease is discussed in the following chapter.

FUNCTIONAL ANATOMY

The liver is made up of 50,000–100,000 discrete functional units called lobules. Each lobule is composed of plates of hepatocytes arranged cylindrically around a central vein (Figure 34–1) and receives blood from branches of both the hepatic artery and the portal vein. Blood from both sources commingles in the sinusoidal channels, which lie between the cellular plates and serve as capillaries. Two types of cells line the hepatic sinusoids: endothelial cells and macrophages (also called Kupffer cells). The space of Disse lies between the sinusoidal capillaries and the hepatocytes. Venous drainage from the central veins of hepatic lobules coalesces to form the hepatic veins, which empty into the inferior vena cava (Figure 34–2).

Bile canaliculi originate between hepatocytes within each plate and join to form bile ducts. An extensive system of lymphatic channels also forms within the plates and is in direct communication with the space of Disse.

VASCULAR FUNCTIONS OF THE LIVER

Control of Hepatic Blood Flow

Normal hepatic blood flow is about 1500 mL/min, of which 25–30% is derived from the hepatic artery and 70–75% from the portal vein (Figure 34–2). The total blood flow from this dual supply represents 25–30% of total cardiac output. Hepatic arterial flow appears dependent on metabolic demand postprandially (autoregulation), while flow through the portal vein is dependent on blood flow to the gastrointestinal tract and the spleen. Although autoregulation of hepatic arterial flow may not be appreciable during fasting, a reciprocal though somewhat limited mechanism exists such that a decrease in either hepatic arterial or portal venous flow results in a compensatory increase in the other.

Splanchnic blood vessels receive sympathetic innervation from T3–T11 via the splanchnic nerves. Both α- and β-adrenergic receptors are present in the hepatic arterial circulation, but only α receptors are present in the portal circulation. Sympathetic activation results in vasoconstriction of the hepatic artery and mesenteric vessels, decreasing hepatic blood flow.

Reservoir Function

Portal vein pressure is normally only about 7–10 mm Hg, but the low resistance of the hepatic sinusoids allows relatively large blood flows through the portal vein. Small changes in hepatic venous tone (and pressure) thus can result in large changes in hepatic blood volume, allowing the liver to act as a blood reservoir.

Normal hepatic blood volume is about 450 mL (almost 10% of total blood volume). A decrease in hepatic venous pressure, as occurs during hemorrhage, shifts blood from hepatic veins and sinusoids into the central venous circulation and augments circulating blood volume as much as 300 mL. In patients with congestive heart failure, the increase in central venous pressure is transmitted to the hepatic veins and causes blood to accumulate within the liver. As much as 1 L of blood can effectively be removed from the circulation in this way at the expense of causing hepatic congestion.

Blood-Cleansing Function

The Kupffer cells lining the sinusoids are part of the monocyte-macrophage (reticuloendothelial) system. Their phagocytic activity is responsible for removing colonic bacteria entering the bloodstream from the portal circulation. Cellular debris and particulate matter in the blood are also phagocytosed.

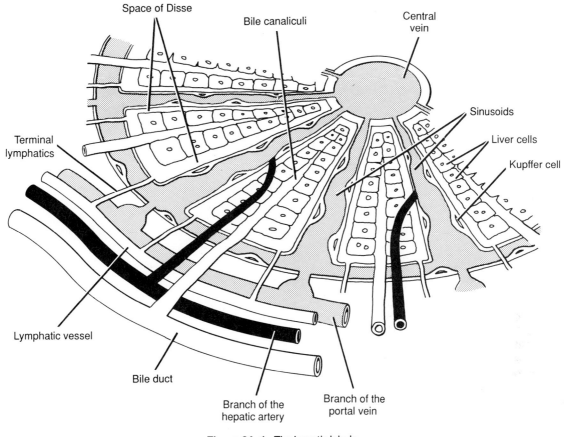

Figure 34–1. The hepatic lobule.

METABOLIC FUNCTIONS

The abundance of enzymatic pathways in the liver allow it to play a key role in the metabolism of carbohydrates, fats, proteins, and other substances (Figure 34–3).

Carbohydrate Metabolism

The final products of carbohydrate digestion are glucose, fructose, and galactose. Hepatic conversion of fructose and galactose into glucose makes glucose metabolism the final common pathway for all carbohydrates.

All cells utilize glucose to produce energy in the form of ATP via glycolysis (anaerobically) or the citric acid cycle (aerobically). The liver (and adipose tissue) can also utilize the phosphogluconate pathway, and the latter not only provides energy but also produces an important cofactor in the synthesis of fatty acids. Glucose absorbed following a meal is normally stored as glycogen. When glycogen storage capacity is exceeded, excess glucose is converted into fat. Glycogen is a readily available source of glucose that does not contribute to intracellular osmolality. Only the liver

and (to a lesser extent) muscle are able to store significant amounts of glycogen. Insulin enhances glycogen synthesis, while epinephrine and glucagon enhance glycogenolysis. Because hepatic glycogen stores are normally only about 70 g while glucose consumption averages 150 g/d, glycogen stores are depleted after 24 hours of fasting. After this period of fasting, de novo synthesis of glucose (gluconeogenesis) is necessary to provide an uninterrupted supply of glucose for other organs.

The liver is unique in its large capacity to form glucose from lactate, amino acids (mainly alanine), and glycerol (derived from fat metabolism). Hepatic gluconeogenesis is responsible for maintaining a normal blood glucose concentration. Glucocorticoids, catecholamines, glucagon, and thyroid hormone greatly enhance gluconeogenesis, while insulin inhibits it.

Fat Metabolism

When carbohydrate stores are saturated, the liver converts the excess ingested carbohydrates (and proteins) into fat. The fatty acids thus formed can be used immediately for fuel or stored in adipose tissue or the

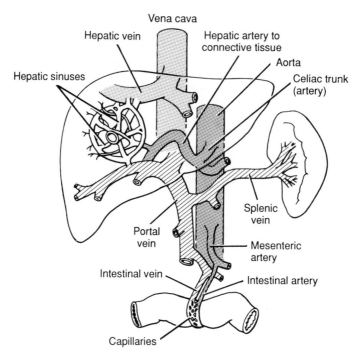

Figure 34–2. Hepatic blood flow. (Modified and reproduced, with permission, from Guyton AC: Textbook of Medical Physiology, 7th ed Saunders, 1986.)

liver for later consumption. Nearly all cells utilize directly, as an energy source, fatty acids derived from ingested fats or those synthesized from intermediary metabolites of carbohydrates and protein. Only red blood cells and the renal medulla can utilize only glucose. Neurons normally utilize only glucose, but after a few days of starvation neurons can switch to fatty acids as an energy source.

Fatty acids derived from fats are oxidized first into acetylcoenzyme A (acetyl-CoA), which is then oxidized via the citric acid cycle to produce ATP. The liver is capable of high rates of fatty acid oxidation and as a result forms acetoacetic acid from excess acetyl-CoA. The acetoacetate released by hepatocytes serves as alternative circulating and readily available fuel (by reconversion into acetyl-CoA) for other cell types. Glucagon increases fatty acid oxidation while insulin inhibits it.

Acetyl-CoA is also used by the liver for production of the cholesterol and phospholipids which are necessary in the synthesis of cellular membranes throughout the body. Hepatic synthesis of lipoproteins is also important in lipid transport by blood.

Protein Metabolism

The liver performs a critical role in protein metabolism. Without this function, death usually occurs within several days. The steps involved include (1) deamination of amino acids, (2) formation of urea (to eliminate the ammonia produced from deamination),

(3) interconversions between nonessential amino acids, and (4) formation of plasma proteins.

Deamination is necessary for conversion of excess amino acids into carbohydrates and fats. The enzymatic processes (most commonly transamination) convert amino acids into their respective keto acids and produce ammonia as a by-product. The deamination of alanine plays a major role in hepatic gluconeogenesis. Although deamination also occurs to a minor extent in the kidneys (primarily glutamine; see Chapter 30), the liver is the principal site of deamination. With the exception of branched-chain amino acids (leucine, isoleucine, and valine), the liver normally deaminates most of the amino acids derived from dietary proteins.

The ammonia formed from deamination (as well as that produced by colonic bacteria and absorbed through the gut) is highly toxic to tissues. Through a series of enzymatic steps, the liver combines two molecules of ammonia with CO_2 to form urea. The urea thus formed readily diffuses out of the liver and can then be excreted by the kidneys.

Hepatic transamination of the appropriate keto acid allows formation of nonessential amino acids and compensation for any dietary deficiency in these amino acids. Essential amino acids, by definition, cannot be readily synthesized through this mechanism and must be supplied exogenously.

Nearly all plasma proteins with the notable exception of immunoglobulins are formed by the liver. Quantitatively, the most important of these proteins are

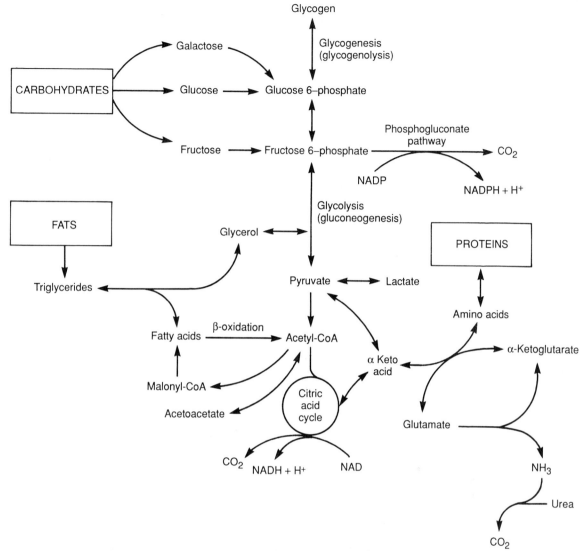

Figure 34–3. Important metabolic pathways in hepatocytes. Although small amounts of ATP are derived directly from some intermediary reactions, the overwhelming majority of ATP produced is the result of oxidative phosphorylation of the reduced forms of nicotinamide adenine dinucleotide (NADH) and nicotinamide adenine dinucleotide phosphate (NADPH).

albumin and coagulation factors. Albumin is responsible for maintaining a normal plasma oncotic pressure and is the principal binding and transport protein for a large number of hormones and drugs. Consequently, changes in albumin concentration can affect the concentration of the pharmacologically active, unbound fraction of many drugs.

Nearly all coagulation factors (I, II, and V–XIII) are produced by the liver. Vitamin K is a necessary cofactor in the synthesis of prothrombin (factor II) and factors VII, IX, and X. The liver also produces plasma cholinesterase (pseudocholinesterase), an enzyme that hydrolyses esters, including some local anesthetics and succinylcholine. Other important proteins formed

by the liver include antithrombin III, α_1-antitrypsin, transferrin, haptoglobin, and ceruloplasmin.

Drug Metabolism

Many exogenous substances, including most drugs, undergo hepatic biotransformation. The end products of these reactions are generally either inactivated or more water-soluble substances that can be readily excreted in bile or urine. Hepatic biotransformations are often categorized as one of two types of reactions: (1) Phase I reactions modify reactive chemical groups through mixed-function oxidases or the cytochrome P-450 enzyme systems, resulting in oxidation, reduction, deamination, sulfoxidation, dealkylation, or methylation. Barbiturates and benzodiazepines are inactivated by phase I reactions. (2) Phase II reactions, which may or may not follow a phase I reaction, involve conjugation of the substance with glucuronide, sulfate, taurine, or glycine. The conjugated compound can then be readily eliminated in urine or bile.

Some enzyme systems, like those of cytochrome P-450, can be induced by a few drugs. Ethanol, barbiturates, ketamine, and perhaps benzodiazepines (eg, diazepam) are capable of enzyme induction, increasing production of the enzymes that metabolize those drugs. This can result in increased tolerance to the drugs' effects. Moreover, enzyme induction often promotes tolerance to other drugs that are metabolized by the same enzymes (cross-tolerance). Conversely, some agents, such as cimetidine and chloramphenicol, can prolong the effects of other drugs by inhibiting these enzymes.

Products of phase I reactions may in a few instances be more active or even cytotoxic. Such reactions are thought to be important in the toxicity of acetaminophen, isoniazid, and perhaps halothane (see below).

The metabolism of a few drugs—including lidocaine, meperidine, morphine, and propranolol—is highly dependent on hepatic blood flow. These drugs have very high rates of hepatic extraction from the circulation. As a result, a decrease in their metabolic clearance usually reflects decreased hepatic blood flow rather than hepatocellular dysfunction.

Other Metabolic Functions

The liver plays a major role in hormone, vitamin, and mineral metabolism. Normal thyroid function is dependent on hepatic formation of the more active triiodothyronine (T_3) from thyroxine (T_4). Degradation of thyroid hormone is principally hepatic. The liver is also the major site of degradation for insulin, steroid hormones (estrogen, aldosterone, and cortisol), glucagon, and antidiuretic hormone. Hepatocytes are the principal storage sites for vitamins A, B_{12}, E, and D. Lastly, hepatic production of transferrin and haptoglobin is important in iron metabolism, while ceruloplasmin is important in copper metabolism.

BILE FORMATION & EXCRETION

Bile plays an important role in fat absorption and in the excretion of bilirubin and many drugs. Hepatocytes in each lobule continuously secrete fluid containing bile salts, cholesterol, phospholipids, conjugated bilirubin, and other substances into bile canaliculi. Bile ducts from all the lobules join to form the common bile duct (Figure 34–4). Biliary flow from the common bile duct into the duodenum is controlled by the sphincter of Oddi. The gallbladder communicates with the common bile duct via the cystic duct and serves as a reservoir for bile. Through active sodium transport and passive water reabsorption, the gall-bladder concentrates biliary fluid between meals. Cholecystokinin, a

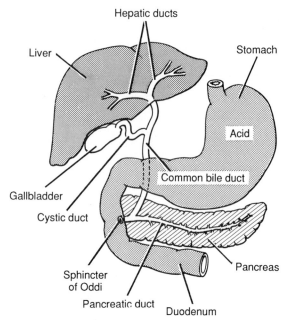

Figure 34–4. The biliary system. (Modified and reproduced, with permission, from Guyton AC: Textbook of Medical Physiology, 7th ed. Saunders, 1986.)

hormone released by the intestinal mucosa in response to fat and protein, causes contraction of the gallbladder, relaxation of the sphincter of Oddi, and propulsion of bile into the small intestine.

Fat Absorption

The bile salts formed by hepatocytes from cholesterol and secreted into bile are essential for emulsifying and facilitating the intestinal absorption of lipids. Defects in this mechanism interfere with the absorption of the fat-soluble vitamins: A, D, E, and K. Because of normally limited stores of vitamin K, a deficiency can develop in a few days. Vitamin K deficiency is manifested as a coagulopathy due to impaired formation of prothrombin and of factors VII, IX, and X.

Bilirubin Excretion

Bilirubin is the end product of hemoglobin metabolism. It is formed from degradation of the heme ring in reticuloendothelial cells (macrophages). The bilirubin is then released into blood, where it readily binds albumin. Hepatic uptake of bilirubin from the circulation is passive, but binding to intracellular proteins traps the bilirubin inside hepatocytes. Inside the hepatocyte, bilirubin is then conjugated (primarily with glucuronide) and actively excreted into bile canaliculi. A small fraction of the conjugated bilirubin is reabsorbed into the bloodstream. Half the bilirubin secreted into the intestine is converted by colonic bacteria into urobilinogen. A small amount of this substance is normally reabsorbed by the intestine, only to be excreted into bile again (enterohepatic recirculation). Urobilinogen is also renally excreted to a minor extent.

LIVER FUNCTION TESTS

Unfortunately, the most commonly performed liver function tests are neither very sensitive nor very specific. Many tests such as serum transaminase measurements reflect hepatocellular integrity more than hepatic function. Only two routine tests truly measure hepatic synthetic function: serum albumin concentration and prothrombin time (PT). Moreover, because of the liver's large functional reserves, cirrhosis may be present with few or no laboratory abnormalities.

No one test reflects overall hepatic function. Each test generally reflects one aspect of hepatic function and must be interpreted in conjunction with the other tests along with clinical assessment of the patient.

Liver abnormalities can often be divided into either parenchymal disorders or obstructive disorders based on laboratory tests (Table 34–1). Obstructive disorders primarily affect biliary excretion of substances, while parenchymal disorders result in generalized hepatocellular dysfunction.

Serum Bilirubin

The normal total bilirubin concentration (conjugated and unconjugated) is less than 1.5 mg/dL and reflects the balance between production and biliary excretion. Jaundice is usually clinically obvious when total bilirubin exceeds 3 mg/dL. A predominantly conjugated hyperbilirubinemia (> 50%) is associated with increased urinary urobilinogen and may reflect hepatocellular dysfunction, intrahepatic cholestasis, or extrahepatic biliary obstruction. Hyperbilirubin-

emia that is chiefly unconjugated may be seen with hemolysis or with congenital or acquired defects in bilirubin conjugation.

Serum Aminotransferases (Transaminases)

These enzymes are released into the circulation as a result of hepatocellular injury or death. Two aminotransferases are most commonly measured: serum aspartate aminotransferase (AST), also known as glutamic-oxaloacetic transaminase (SGOT); and serum alanine aminotransferase (ALT), also called glutamic pyruvic-transferase (SGPT). AST is present in many tissues, including the liver, heart, skeletal muscle, and kidneys. ALT is primarily located in the liver and is more specific for hepatic dysfunction. Normal AST and ALT levels are below 35–45 units/L. Mild elevations (< 300 units/L) can be seen with cholestasis or metastatic liver disease. Absolute levels generally correlate poorly with degree of hepatic injury.

Serum Alkaline Phosphatase

Alkaline phosphatase is produced by the liver, bone, small bowel, kidneys, and placenta and is excreted into bile. Normal serum alkaline phosphatase activity is generally 45–125 units/L in most laboratories. Most of the circulating enzyme is normally derived from bone, but with biliary obstruction more hepatic alkaline phosphatase is synthesized and released into the circulation. Although mild elevations (up to twice normal) may be seen with hepatocellular injury or hepatic metastatic disease, higher levels are indicative of intrahepatic cholestasis or biliary obstruction.

Increased serum alkaline phosphatase levels may also be encountered with pregnancy (Chapter 40) or bone disease (Paget's disease or bone metastases). Simultaneous measurements of serum 5'-nucleotidase or γ-glutamyl transpeptidase levels are helpful in excluding an extrahepatic source of alkaline phosphatase elevations. Although both enzymes can also be released from extrahepatic tissues, the combination of an elevated 5'-nucleotidase or γ-glutamyl transpeptidase level together with an elevated alkaline phosphatase level strongly suggests hepatobiliary disease. In fact, elevated serum γ-glutamyl transpeptidase activity is the most sensitive indicator of hepatobiliary disease.

Table 34–1. Abnormalities in liver tests.[1]

	Parenchymal (Hepatocellular) Dysfunction	Biliary Obstruction or Cholestasis
AST (SGOT)	↑ to ↑↑↑	↑
ALT (SGPT)	↑ to ↑↑↑	↑
Albumin	0 to ↓↓↓	0
Prothrombin time	0 to ↑↑↑	0 to ↑↑[2]
Bilirubin	0 to ↑↑↑	0 to ↑↑↑
Alkaline phosphatase	↑	↑ to ↑↑↑
5'-Nucleotidase	0 to ↑	↑ to ↑↑↑
γ-Glutamyl transpeptidase	0 to ↑↑↑	↑↑↑

[1]Adapted from Wilson JD et al (editors): *Harrison's Principles of Internal Medicine,* 12th ed. McGraw-Hill, 1991.
[2]Usually corrects with vitamin K.
Key:
  ↑ = Increases
  0 = No change
  ↓ = Decreases

Serum Albumin

The normal serum albumin concentration is 3.5–5.5 g/dL. Because its half-life is about 2–3 weeks, albumin concentration may initially be normal with acute liver disease. Albumin values less than 2.5 g/dL are generally indicative of chronic liver disease or malnutrition. Increased losses of albumin in the urine (nephrotic syndrome) or the gastrointestinal tract (protein-losing enteropathy) can also produce hypoalbuminemia.

Prothrombin Time

The PT, which is normally 11–14 seconds (depending on the control), measures the activity of fibrinogen, prothrombin, and factors V, VII, and X. The relatively short half-life of factor VII (4–6 hours) makes the PT useful in evaluating hepatic synthetic function of patients with acute or chronic liver disease. Prolongations of the PT greater than 3–4 seconds from the control are considered significant. Because only 20–30% of normal factor activity is required for normal coagulation, prolongation of the PT usually reflects severe liver disease unless vitamin K deficiency is present. Failure of the PT to correct following parenteral administration of vitamin K implies severe liver disease; correction normally requires 24 hours.

EFFECT OF ANESTHESIA ON HEPATIC FUNCTION

Hepatic Blood Flow

Hepatic blood flow usually decreases during regional and general anesthesia. Multiple factors are probably responsible, including both direct and indirect effects of anesthetic agents, the type of ventilation employed, and the type of surgery being performed.

All volatile anesthetic agents reduce portal hepatic blood flow. This decrease is greatest with halothane and least with isoflurane. Moreover, isoflurane appears to be the only volatile agent causing significant direct arterial vasodilatation that can increase hepatic arterial blood flow. Nonetheless, even with isoflurane, total hepatic blood flow decreases because the decrease in portal blood flow usually offsets any increase in hepatic artery flow. All anesthetic agents indirectly reduce hepatic blood flow in proportion to any decrease in mean arterial blood pressure or cardiac output. Decreases in cardiac output reduce hepatic blood flow via reflex sympathetic activation, which vasoconstricts both the arterial and the venous splanchnic vasculature. If an adequate intravascular volume is maintained, spinal and epidural anesthesia therefore decrease hepatic blood flow primarily by lowering arterial blood pressure, while general anesthesia usually decreases it through reductions in blood pressure and cardiac output and sympathetic stimulation.

The hemodynamic effects of ventilation can also have a significant impact on hepatic blood flow. Controlled positive pressure ventilation with high mean airway pressures reduces venous return to the heart and decreases cardiac output; both mechanisms can compromise hepatic blood flow. The former increases hepatic venous pressure, while the latter can reduce blood pressure and increase sympathetic tone. Positive end-expiratory pressure (PEEP) further accentuates these effects. Spontaneous ventilation therefore may be more advantageous in maintaining hepatic blood flow. Hypoxemia decreases hepatic blood flow via sympathetic activation. Hypocapnia, hypercapnia, acidosis, and alkalosis have variable effects owing to the complex interaction between direct effects (increased flow with hypercapnia and acidosis but decreased flow with hypocapnia and alkalosis), secondary effects on the sympathetic system (activation with hypercapnia and acidosis), the ventilatory mode (spontaneous versus controlled ventilation), and the anesthetic agent used.

Surgical procedures near the liver can reduce hepatic blood flow up to 60%. Although the mechanisms are not clear, they most likely involve sympathetic activation, local reflexes, and direct compression of vessels in the portal and hepatic circulations.

Metabolic Functions

The effects of the various anesthetic agents on hepatic intermediary metabolism (carbohydrate, fat, and protein) are poorly defined. An endocrine stress response secondary to fasting and surgical trauma is generally observed. This state is characterized by elevated circulating levels of catecholamines, glucagon, and cortisol. Mobilization of carbohydrate stores and proteins results in hyperglycemia and a negative nitrogen balance, respectively. The endocrine stress response may be at least partially blunted by regional anesthesia, deep general anesthesia, or pharmacologic blockade of the sympathetic system.

Drug Metabolism

Although halothane has been reported to directly inhibit the metabolism of several drugs (phenytoin, warfarin, and ketamine), it is probably the decreased hepatic blood flow associated with halothane and other anesthetics that is responsible for altered pharmacokinetics of other drugs (fentanyl, verapamil, and propranolol).

Biliary Function

Anesthetic interactions with bile formation and storage have not been reported. However, all narcotics can potentially cause spasm of the sphincter of Oddi and increase biliary pressure (fentanyl > morphine > meperidine > butorphanol > nalbuphine). The effects of alfentanil are similar to those of fentanyl but more short-lived. Intravenous opioid administration can therefore induce biliary colic or result in false-positive cholangiograms. Sphincter spasm may be less likely when the narcotic is given slowly in small increments. Halothane and to a lesser extent enflurane may further blunt the increase in biliary pressure following opioid administration.

Liver Function Tests

Mild postoperative liver dysfunction in healthy individuals is not uncommon if sensitive tests are employed. A combination of factors is probably responsible, including decreased blood flow due to anesthesia, sympathetic stimulation, and the surgical procedure itself. Procedures in close proximity to the liver frequently result in modest elevations in lactate dehydrogenase and transaminase concentrations regard-

Table 34–2. Causes of postoperative jaundice.

Prehepatic (increased bilirubin production)
Large hematomas
Transfusion
  Senescent red cell breakdown
  Delayed hemolytic reactions
Hepatic (hepatocellular dysfunction)
Underlying liver disease
Ischemic or hypoxemic injury
Drug-induced
Gilbert's syndrome
Intrahepatic cholestasis
Posthepatic (biliary obstruction)
Postoperative cholecystitis
Postoperative pancreatitis
Retained common bile duct stone

---

less of the anesthetic agent or technique employed.

Significant postoperative elevations in liver function tests are usually due to underlying liver disease or the surgical procedure itself. Persistent abnormalities in liver function tests may be indicative of viral hepatitis (usually transfusion-related), sepsis, idiosyncratic drug reactions, or surgical complications. Postoperative jaundice can be due to a variety of factors (Table 34–2), but the most common cause is overproduction of bilirubin due to resorption of a large hematoma or red cell breakdown following transfusion. Nonetheless, all other causes should be considered. Correct diagnosis requires a careful review of preoperative liver function as well as intraoperative and postoperative events such as transfusions, sustained hypotension or hypoxemia, and drug exposure.

HEPATIC DYSFUNCTION ASSOCIATED WITH HALOGENATED ANESTHETICS

Halothane, the first halogenated volatile anesthetic, was introduced in 1956, and shortly afterward the first cases of "halothane hepatitis" were reported. Since then, this entity has been widely recognized, and cases associated with methoxyflurane, enflurane, and isoflurane have been described.

Several mechanisms have been proposed for halothane-associated hepatitis, including the formation of hepatotoxic metabolic intermediates and immune hypersensitivity. Antibodies directed against hepatocyte components have been identified in some patients. A genetic susceptibility has been shown in rats and may also be operative in humans. Reductive metabolism under hypoxic conditions can produce hepatotoxic intermediates in some strains of laboratory animals. In contrast, oxidative metabolism, which produces trifluoroacetic acid, appears to be responsible in other models; trifluoroacetylation of tissue proteins can cause hepatotoxicity.

Halothane-associated hepatitis is a diagnosis of exclusion. Viral hepatitis—including that due to hepatitis viruses (types A, B, and C), cytomegalovirus,

Epstein-Barr virus, and herpes viruses—should be excluded. The severity of this syndrome can vary from an asymptomatic elevation in serum transaminases to fulminant hepatic necrosis. Although the incidence of the mild form of this syndrome may be as high as 20% in adults following a second exposure to halothane, the incidence of fatal hepatic necrosis is estimated to be approximately 1:35,000. Epidemiologic studies have identified several risk factors that are associated with this syndrome, including middle age, obesity, female sex, and a repeat exposure to halothane (especially within 28 days). Prepubertal children appear to be more resistant to this entity, with reported incidences of 1:200,000–1:80,000.

Hepatitis due to enflurane or isoflurane is very rare (estimated to be 1:500,000–1:300,000); indeed, the association between hepatitis and these two agents—especially isoflurane—is still questioned by many investigators.

CASE DISCUSSION: COAGULOPATHY IN A PATIENT WITH LIVER DISEASE

A 52-year-old man with a long history of alcohol abuse presents for a splenorenal shunt after three major episodes of upper gastrointestinal hemorrhage from esophageal varices. Coagulation studies reveal a prothrombin time of 17 seconds (control: 12 seconds) and a partial prothrombin time of 43 seconds (control: 29 seconds). The platelet count is 95,000/μL.

Describe the mechanisms involved in normal coagulation.

Coagulation, often referred to as secondary hemostasis, involves formation of a fibrin clot, which usually binds and strengthens a platelet plug (primary hemostasis; see Chapter 21). Fibrin can be formed via one of two mechanisms (pathways) that involve activation of soluble coagulation precursor proteins in blood (Table 34–3). Regardless of which pathway is activated, the coagulation cascade ends in the conversion of fibrinogen to fibrin. The intrinsic pathway (Figure 34–5) is usually triggered by the interaction between subendothelial collagen with circulating Hageman factor (XII), high-molecular-weight kininogen (HMWK), and prekallikrein (PK). The latter two substances are also involved in the formation of bradykinin. The extrinsic pathway of the coagulation cascade is triggered by the release of a tissue lipoprotein (thromboplastin) from the membranes of injured cells.

Thrombin plays a central role in coagulation because it not only activates platelets (Chapter 21) but also accelerates conversion of factors V, VII, and XIII

Table 34–3. Coagulation factors.

Factor		Approximate Half-Life (hours)
I	Fibrinogen	100
II	Prothrombin	80
III	Tissue thromboplastin	—
IV	Calcium	—
V	Proaccelerin	18
VII	Proconvertin	6
VIII	Antihemophilic factor	10
IX	Christmas factor	24
X	Stuart factor	50
XI	Plasma thromboplastin antecedent	25
XII	Hageman factor	60
XIII	Fibrin-stabilizing factor	90

to their active forms. Conversion of prothrombin to thrombin is markedly accelerated by activated platelets. Thrombin then converts fibrinogen to soluble fibrin monomers that polymerize on the platelet plug. Cross-linking of fibrin polymers by factor XIII is necessary to form a strong, insoluble fibrin clot. Finally, retraction of the clot (which requires platelets) expresses fluid with the clot and helps pull the walls of the damaged blood vessel together.

What prevents coagulation of blood in normal tissues?

The coagulation process is limited to injured areas by localization of platelets to the injured area and maintenance of normal blood flow in uninjured areas. The latter is important in clearing activated coagulation factors, which are taken up by the monocyte-macrophage scavenger system. That system includes hepatic Kupffer cells (see above). Additionally, multiple inhibitors of coagulation are normally present in plasma, including antithrombin III and proteins C and S. Antithrombin III complexes with and inactivates circulating coagulation factors (with the notable exception of factor VII), while protein C specifically inactivates factors V and VIII. Heparin exerts its anticoagulant activity by augmenting the activity of antithrombin III.

What is the role of the fibrinolytic system in normal hemostasis?

The fibrinolytic system is normally activated simultaneously with the coagulation cascade. It functions to help maintain the fluidity of blood during coagulation and is also responsible for clot lysis once tissue repair begins. When a clot is formed, a large amount of plasminogen is incorporated into the clot. Plasminogen is then activated either by tissue plasminogen activator (tPA), which is usually released by damaged endo-

thelial cells, or by Hageman factor and thrombin. Activation results in formation of plasmin, which then degrades fibrin and fibrinogen as well as other coagulation factors. Urokinase (found in urine) and streptokinase (a product of bacteria) are also potent activators of plasminogen. The action of plasmin is localized because (1) plasminogen is incorporated into the clot and (2) free plasmin is rapidly neutralized by a circulating α_2-plasmin inhibitor. Plasmin degrades fibrin and fibrinogen into small fragments. These fibrin degradation products possess anticoagulant activity because they compete with fibrinogen for thrombin; they are normally cleared by the monocyte-macrophage system. The drug aminocaproic acid inhibits the binding of plasmin to fibrin.

How are coagulation tests helpful in evaluating hemostasis?

The diagnosis of coagulation abnormalities can be facilitated by measurement of the partial prothrombin time (PTT), thromboplastin time (PT), thrombin time (TT), and fibrinogen level (Table 34–4). The PTT measures the intrinsic pathway (factors I, II, V, VIII, IX, X, XI, and XII). The whole blood clotting time and activated clotting time (ACT) also measure the intrinsic pathway. In contrast, the PT measures the extrinsic pathway (factors I, II, V, and VII). The TT specifically measures conversion of fibrinogen to fibrin (factors I and II). The normal plasma fibrinogen level is 200–400 mg/dL (5.9–11.7 μmol/L). Since heparin therapy affects chiefly the intrinsic pathway, in low doses it usually only prolongs the PTT. In high doses, heparin also prolongs the PT. In contrast, warfarin primarily affects vitamin K-dependent factors (II, VII, IX, and X), so the PT is prolonged at usual doses and the PTT is prolonged only at high doses.

What are the most common causes of abnormal coagulation?

Coagulation defects can be acquired or hereditary. Acquired defects are by far the most common. In addition to anticoagulant drug therapy (heparin or warfarin) and vitamin K deficiency (see above), acquired defects are frequently encountered in patients with

Table 34–4. Coagulation test abnormalities.

	PT	PTT	TT	Fibrinogen
Advanced liver disease	↑	↑	N or ↑	N or ↓
DIC	↑	↑	↑	↓
Vitamin K deficiency	↑ ↑	↑	N	N
Warfarin therapy	↑ ↑	↑	N	N
Heparin therapy	↑	↑ ↑	↑	N
Hemophilia				
Factor VIII deficiency	N	↑	N	N
Factor IX deficiency	N	↑	N	N
Factor VII deficiency	↑	N	N	N
Factor XIII deficiency	N	N	N	N

EXTRINSIC PATHWAY

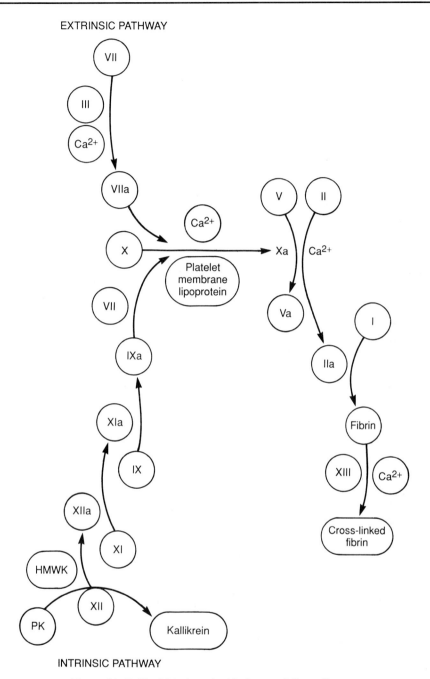

INTRINSIC PATHWAY

Figure 34–5. The intrinsic and extrinsic coagulation pathways.

liver disease, disseminated intravascular coagulation (DIC), or massive blood transfusion (Chapter 29).

What is the pathophysiology of coagulation defects in patients with liver disease?

Patients with advanced liver disease often develop a multifactorial coagulopathy. Three major causes are usually responsible: (1) vitamin K deficiency (impaired storage or absorption), (2) impaired synthesis of coagulation factors, and (3) splenic sequestration of platelets due to hypersplenism. To complicate matters further, patients with cirrhosis typically have multiple potential bleeding sites (esophageal varices, gastritis, peptic ulcers, and hemorrhoids) and frequently require multiple blood transfusions. With severe liver disease, patients may also have decreased synthesis of coagulation inhibitors and fail to clear activated coagulation factors and fibrin split products (impaired Kupffer cell function); the coagulation defect resembles and becomes indistinguishable from disseminated intravascular coagulation (DIC).

What is the pathophysiology of DIC?

In DIC, the coagulation cascade is activated by the release of endogenous tissue thromboplastin or thromboplastin-like substances or by direct activation of factor XII by endotoxin or foreign surfaces. Widespread deposition of fibrin in the microcirculation results in consumption of coagulation factors, secondary fibrinolysis, thrombocytopenia, and a microangiopathic hemolytic anemia. Diffuse bleeding and in some cases thromboembolic phenomena usually follow. Treatment is generally aimed at the underlying cause. Supportive measures include transfusion of coagulation factors and platelets. Heparin therapy is controversial but may benefit patients with thromboembolic phenomena.

What hereditary defects should be considered in the differential diagnosis of abnormal secondary hemostasis?

The most common inherited defect in secondary hemostasis is factor VIII deficiency (hemophilia A). This X-linked abnormality is estimated to affect 1:10,000 males. Disease severity is generally inversely related to factor VIII activity. Most symptomatic patients experience hemarthrosis, bleeding into deep tissues, and hematuria. Symptomatic patients generally have less than 5% of normal factor VIII activity. Classically,

patients present with a prolonged PTT but a normal PT and bleeding time. The diagnosis is confirmed by measuring factor VIII activity in blood. Afflicted patients generally do not experience increased bleeding during surgery when factor VIII levels are over 30%, but most authors recommend increasing factor VIII levels to more than 50% prior to surgery. Normal (fresh frozen) plasma, by definition, is considered to have 1 unit of factor VIII activity per milliliter. In contrast, cryoprecipitate has 5–10 units/mL, while factor VIII concentrates have approximately 40 units/mL. Each unit of factor VIII transfused is estimated to raise factor VIII levels 2% per kilogram of body weight. Twice-a-day transfusions are generally recommended following surgery because of the relatively short half-life of factor VIII (8–12 hours).

Hemophilia B (also known as Christmas disease) is due to an X-linked hereditary deficiency of factor IX. The disease is very similar to hemophilia A but much less common (1:100,000 males). Measurement of factor IX levels establishes the diagnosis. Perioperative factor IX concentrates are generally recommended to maintain factor IX activity at more than 30% of normal.

Factor XIII deficiency is extremely rare but notable in that the PTT, PT, TT, and bleeding times are normal. The diagnosis requires measurement of factor XIII levels. Since only 1% of normal factor XIII activity is generally required, patients are treated by a single transfusion of fresh frozen plasma.

SUGGESTED READINGS

Brown BR: *Anesthesia in Hepatic and Biliary Tract Disease.* Davis, 1988. The only text on anesthesia and liver disease.

Stock JGL, Strunin L: Unexplained hepatitis following halothane. Anesthesiology 1985;63:424. Summarizes studies on halothane hepatitis.

Stoelting RK, Dierdorf SE, McCammon RL: *Anesthesia and Co-Existing Disease,* 2nd ed. Churchill Livingstone, 1988.

Anesthesia for Patients With Liver Disease

35

The prevalence of liver disease appears to be increasing in the United States. Mortality rates from cirrhosis have been on the rise over the last few decades, perhaps related to high alcohol consumption as well as percutaneous (sexual and transfusion-associated) transmission of hepatitis viruses. Cirrhosis is a major cause of death of men in their fourth and fifth decades. The incidence of cirrhosis in some autopsy series is as high as 5%. Unfortunately, because of the liver's remarkable functional reserves, clinical manifestations are often absent until extensive hepatic damage has already occurred. In patients with compensated or occult liver disease, minor stress may precipitate overt hepatic dysfunction. The adverse effects of anesthesia and surgery on hepatic blood flow (Chapter 34) can precipitate hepatic dysfunction in these patients.

This chapter discusses the anesthetic management of patients with known liver disease. With some important exceptions, the anesthetic considerations tend to be similar in both acute and chronic liver disease. Although patients with cholelithiasis often have minimal hepatic impairment, the effects of anesthesia on the biliary system also require comment.

HEPATITIS

ACUTE HEPATITIS

Acute hepatitis is usually due to viral infection, a drug reaction, or exposure to a hepatotoxin. The illness represents acute hepatocellular injury with variable amounts of cell necrosis. Clinical manifestations generally depend both on the severity of the inflammatory reaction and, more importantly, on the amount of necrosis. Mild inflammatory reactions may present as asymptomatic elevations in the serum transaminases, while massive hepatic necrosis presents as acute hepatic failure.

Viral Hepatitis

Viral hepatitis is most commonly due to hepatitis A, hepatitis B, or hepatitis C viruses (previously called blood-borne non-A, non-B). At least two other hepatitis viruses have also been recently identified: hepatitis D (delta virus) and hepatitis E (enteric non-A, non-B) viruses. Hepatitis types A and E are transmitted by the oral-fecal route, while types B and C are transmitted percutaneously (Chapter 29) and by contact with body fluids. Hepatitis D is unique in that it may be transmitted by either route and requires the presence of hepatitis B virus in the host to be infective. Other viruses, including Epstein-Barr, herpes simplex, cytomegalovirus, and coxsackieviruses, can also cause hepatitis, but their effects on other organs are also prominent.

Patients with viral hepatitis often have a 1- to 2-week mild prodromal illness (fatigue, malaise, low-grade fever, or nausea and vomiting) that may or may not be followed by jaundice. The jaundice typically lasts 2–12 weeks, but complete recovery, as evidenced by serum transaminase measurements, usually takes 4 months. Because clinical manifestations overlap, serologic testing is necessary to determine the etiologic viral agent. The clinical course tends to be more complicated and prolonged with hepatitis B and C viruses. Less commonly, cholestasis (see below) is the major manifestation. Rarely, patients can develop fulminant hepatitis (massive hepatic necrosis). The incidence of chronic active hepatitis (see below) is 3–10% following hepatitis B and 10–50% following hepatitis C. A small percentage of patients (mainly immunosuppressed patients and those on chronic hemodialysis regimens) become asymptomatic infectious carriers following hepatitis B or C infection. Depending on the patient group studied, anywhere between 0.3% and 30% of patients remain infectious and have persistence of the B surface antigen (HBsAg) in their blood. Approximately 1% of patients with hepatitis C infection become asymptomatic infectious carriers. Infectious carriers pose a major health hazard to operating room personnel. In addition to precautions for avoiding direct contact with blood and secretions (gloves, mask, protective eyewear, and not recapping needles), vaccination is highly effective against hepatitis B infection.

Drug-Induced Hepatitis

Drug-induced hepatitis (Table 35–1) can result from direct dose-dependent toxicity of a drug (or a metabo-

Table 35–1. Drugs and substances associated with hepatitis.

Toxic
Alcohol
Acetaminophen
Salicylates
Tetracyclines
Trichloroethylene
Vinyl chloride
Carbon tetrachloride
Yellow phosphorus
Poisonous mushrooms
Amanita
Galerina
Idiosyncratic
Volatile anesthetics
Halothane
Phenytoin
Sulfonamides
Rifampin
Indomethacin
Toxic and idiosyncratic
Methyldopa
Isoniazid
Sodium valproate
Amiodarone
Primarily cholestatic
Chlorpromazine
Chlorpropamide
Oral contraceptives
Anabolic steroids
Erythromycin estolate
Methimazole

lite), from an idiosyncratic drug reaction, or from a combination of the two causes. The clinical course often resembles viral hepatitis, making diagnosis difficult. Alcoholic hepatitis is probably the most commonly encountered type of drug-induced hepatitis, but the cause may not be obvious from the history. Chronic alcohol ingestion can also result in hepatomegaly from fatty infiltration of the liver, which reflects (1) impaired fatty acid oxidation, (2) increased uptake and esterification of fatty acids, and (3) diminished lipoprotein synthesis and secretion. A few drugs such as chlorpromazine and oral contraceptives characteristically cause cholestatic-type reactions (see below). Ingestion of potent hepatotoxins, such as carbon tetrachloride and certain species of mushrooms *(Amanita, Galerina),* are often associated with acute hepatic failure.

Preoperative Considerations

All elective surgery should be postponed until the hepatitis has resolved, as indicated by normal liver function tests. Studies indicate increased perioperative mortality (up to 10% with laparotomy) and morbidity (12%) during acute viral hepatitis. Although the risk with alcoholic hepatitis may not be as great, acute alcohol toxicity greatly complicates anesthetic management. Moreover, alcohol withdrawal during surgery may be associated with a mortality rate as high as 50%. Only truly emergent surgery should be considered in such instances. Patients with hepatitis are at risk for deterioration of hepatic function and the devel-

opment of complications from hepatic failure, such as encephalopathy or the hepatorenal syndrome (see below).

If a surgical procedure is necessary during acute hepatitis, the preanesthetic evaluation should focus on determining the cause and the degree of hepatic impairment. Information should be obtained regarding recent drug exposures, including alcohol intake, intravenous drug abuse, recent transfusions, and prior anesthetics. The presence of nausea or vomiting should be noted. Mental status changes usually indicate severe hepatic impairment. With alcoholic patients, inappropriate behavior or obtundation may be signs of acute intoxication, while tremulousness and irritability usually reflect withdrawal. Hypertension and tachycardia are often also prominent with the latter.

Laboratory evaluation should include BUN, serum electrolytes, and serum creatinine, glucose, transaminases, bilirubin, alkaline phosphatase, and albumin as well as prothrombin time (PT) and platelet count. Serum should be checked also for HBsAg whenever possible. A blood alcohol level is useful if the history or mental status is compatible with intoxication. Hypokalemia and metabolic alkalosis are not uncommon and are usually due to vomiting. Concomitant hypomagnesemia may be present in chronic alcoholics and predisposes to arrhythmias. The elevation in serum transaminases does not necessarily correlate with the amount of necrosis. The serum alanine aminotransferase (ALT) is generally higher than the serum aspartate aminotransferase (AST) except in alcoholic hepatitis, where the reverse occurs. Bilirubin and alkaline phosphatase are usually only moderately elevated, except with the cholestatic variant of hepatitis. The PT is the best indicator of hepatic synthetic function (Chapter 34). Persistent prolongation greater than 3 seconds following vitamin K administration is indicative of severe hepatic dysfunction. Hypoglycemia may also be seen in such cases. Hypoalbuminemia is usually not present except in protracted cases, with malnutrition, or when chronic liver disease is present.

If a patient with acute hepatitis must undergo emergent operation, dehydration and electrolyte abnormalities should be corrected. Vitamin K or fresh frozen plasma (FFP) may be necessary to correct a coagulopathy. When immediate correction is necessary, FFP is indicated. Premedication is generally not given to minimize drug exposure and avoid precipitating hepatic encephalopathy in patients with advanced liver disease. In contrast, benzodiazepines and thiamine are indicated for alcoholic patients with acute withdrawal.

Intraoperative Considerations

The goal of intraoperative management is to preserve existing hepatic function and avoid factors that may be detrimental to the liver. Drug selection and dosage should be individualized. Some patients with viral hepatitis may exhibit increased central nervous system sensitivity to anesthetics, while alcoholic patients will often display cross-tolerance to both intravenous and volatile anesthetics. Alcoholic patients also require close cardiovascular monitoring, because the cardiac depressant effects of alcohol are additive to those of anesthetics; moreover, many alcoholics develop an alcoholic cardiomyopathy.

By definition, all anesthetics are central nervous system depressants, and for that reason the fewest number of agents should be used. Inhalational anesthetics are generally preferable to intravenous agents because most of the latter are dependent on the liver for metabolism or elimination. Standard induction doses of intravenous induction agents can generally be used, since their action is terminated by redistribution rather than metabolism or excretion. A prolonged duration of action, however, may be encountered with large or repeated doses of intravenous agents, especially opioids. Isoflurane is the volatile agent of choice because it has the least effect on hepatic blood flow (Chapter 34). Factors known to reduce hepatic blood flow, such as hypotension, excessive sympathetic activation, and high mean airway pressures during controlled ventilation, should be avoided. Regional anesthesia may be employed in the absence of coagulopathy provided hypotension is avoided.

CHRONIC HEPATITIS

Chronic hepatitis is defined as persistent hepatic inflammation for longer than 6 months, as evidenced by elevated aminotransferase. Patients can usually be classified as having one of three distinct syndromes based on a liver biopsy: chronic persistent hepatitis, chronic lobular hepatitis, or chronic active hepatitis. Those with **chronic persistent hepatitis** manifest chronic inflammation of portal tracts with preservation of normal cellular architecture on the biopsy; this type rarely if ever progresses to cirrhosis. Clinically, these patients present with acute hepatitis (usually hepatitis B or C) that has a protracted course but eventually resolves. A recently described variant called **chronic lobular hepatitis** is characterized by acute hepatitis that resolves but is followed by recurrent exacerbations; however, like chronic persistent hepatitis, chronic lobular hepatitis rarely progresses to cirrhosis.

Patients with **chronic active hepatitis** have chronic hepatic inflammation with destruction of normal cellular architecture (piecemeal necrosis) on the biopsy. Evidence of cirrhosis is often present initially (20–50% of patients) or eventually develops. Although chronic active hepatitis appears to have many causes, it occurs most commonly as a sequela of hepatitis B or hepatitis C. Other postulated causes include drugs (methyldopa, oxyphenisatin, isoniazid, and nitrofurantoin) and autoimmune disorders. Both immunologic factors and a genetic predisposition appear to be responsible in most cases. Patients usually present with a history of fatigue and recurrent jaundice; extrahepatic manifestations, such as arthritis and serositis, are not uncommon. Manifestations of cirrhosis eventually predominate in patients with progressive disease. Laboratory tests may show only a mild elevation in serum aminotransferase activity and often correlate poorly with disease severity. Patients with HBsAg-negative chronic active hepatitis usually have a favorable response to immunosuppressants and are usually managed with long-term corticosteroids therapy with or without azathioprine.

Anesthetic Management

Patients with chronic persistent or chronic lobular hepatitis should be treated similarly to those with acute hepatitis (see above). In contrast, those with chronic active hepatitis should be assumed to have cirrhosis already and treated accordingly (see below). Patients with HBsAg-negative chronic active hepatitis may also present problems related to other autoimmune manifestations (such as diabetes or thyroiditis) as well as long-term corticosteroid therapy (Chapter 36).

CIRRHOSIS

Cirrhosis is a serious and progressive disease that eventually results in hepatic failure. The most common cause of cirrhosis in the United States is alcohol (Laennec's cirrhosis). Other causes include chronic active hepatitis (postnecrotic cirrhosis), chronic biliary inflammation or obstruction (biliary cirrhosis), chronic right-sided congestive heart failure (cardiac cirrhosis), hemochromatosis, Wilson's disease, and α_1-antitrypsin deficiency. Regardless of the cause, hepatocyte necrosis is followed by fibrosis and nodular regeneration. Distortion of the liver's normal cellular and vascular architecture obstructs portal venous flow and leads to the development of portal hypertension, while impairment of the liver's normal synthetic and other diverse metabolic functions results in multisystem disease. Clinically, signs and symptoms often do not correlate with disease severity. Manifestations are typically absent initially, but jaundice and ascites eventually develop in most patients. Other signs include spider angiomas, palmar erythema, gynecomastia, and splenomegaly. Moreover, cirrhosis is generally associated with the development of three major complications: (1) variceal hemorrhage from portal hypertension, (2) intractable fluid retention in the form of ascites and the hepatorenal syndrome, and (3) hepatic encephalopathy or coma. Approximately 10% of patients also develop at least one episode of spontaneous bacterial peritonitis, and some may eventually develop hepatocellular carcinoma.

A few diseases can produce hepatic fibrosis without hepatocellular necrosis or nodular regeneration. They result mainly in portal hypertension and its associated complications (see below); hepatocellular function is often but not always preserved. These disorders include schistosomiasis, idiopathic portal fibrosis (Banti's syndrome), and congenital hepatic fibrosis. Obstruction of the hepatic veins or inferior vena cava (Budd-Chiari syndrome) can also cause portal hypertension. The latter may be the result of venous thrombosis (hypercoagulable state), a tumor thrombus (renal carcinoma), or occlusive disease of the sublobular hepatic veins.

Preoperative Considerations

The detrimental effects of anesthesia and surgery on hepatic blood flow are discussed in Chapter 34. Patients with cirrhosis are at increased risk for deterioration of liver function because of their limited functional reserves. Successful anesthetic management of these patients is dependent on recognizing the multisystem nature of cirrhosis and controlling or preventing its complications (Table 35–2).

A. Gastrointestinal Manifestations: Portal hypertension (> 10 mm Hg) leads to the development of extensive portosystemic venous collaterals. Four major collateral sites are generally recognized: gastroesophageal, hemorrhoidal, periumbilical, and retroperitoneal. Portal hypertension is often apparent

Table 35–2. Manifestations of cirrhosis.

Gastrointestinal
  Portal hypertension
    Ascites
    Esophageal varices
    Hemorrhoids
    Gastrointestinal bleeding
Circulatory
  Hyperdynamic state (high cardiac output)
  Systemic arteriovenous shunts
Pulmonary
  Increased intrapulmonary shunting
  Decreased functional residual capacity
  Pleural effusions
  Restrictive ventilatory defect
  Primary respiratory alkalosis
Renal
  Increased proximal reabsorption of sodium
  Increased distal reabsorption of sodium
  Impaired free water clearance
  Decreased renal perfusion
  Hepatorenal syndrome
Hematologic
  Anemia
  Coagulopathy
  Hypersplenism
    Thrombocytopenia
    Leukopenia
Infectious
  Spontaneous bacterial peritonitis
Metabolic
  Hyponatremia
  Hypokalemia
  Hypoalbuminemia
  Hypoglycemia
Neurologic
  Encephalopathy

Table 35–3. Child's classification for evaluating hepatic reserve.[1]

Risk Group	A	B	C
Bilirubin (mg/dL)	<2.0	2.0–3.0	>3.0
Serum albumin (g/dL)	>3.5	3.0–3.6	<3.0
Ascites	None	Controlled	Poorly controlled
Encephalopathy	Absent	Minimal	Coma
Nutrition	Excellent	Good	Poor
Mortality rate (%)	2–5	10	50

[1]Adapted from Child CG: *The Liver and Portal Hypertension.* Saunders, 1964.

preoperatively as evidenced by dilated abdominal wall veins (caput medusae). Massive bleeding from gastroesophageal varices is a major cause of morbidity and mortality in patients with cirrhosis. In addition to the effects of acute blood loss, the increased nitrogenous load (from the breakdown of blood in the intestinal tract) can precipitate hepatic encephalopathy. Endoscopy is important in identifying the site of bleeding because patients with varices often bleed from other sites such as a peptic ulcer or gastritis, which require different therapy.

The treatment of variceal bleeding is generally supportive (medical) once the cause of the bleeding is established by endoscopy. Blood loss should be replaced with intravenous fluids and blood products (Chapter 29). Vasopressin infusion (0.1–0.9 units/min intravenously), balloon tamponade (with a Sengstaken-Blakemore tube), or endoscopic sclerosis of the varices usually stops the bleeding. High doses of vasopressin can result in congestive heart failure or myocardial ischemia. When the bleeding fails to stop or recurs, emergency surgery may be indicated. Surgical risk has been shown to correlate with the degree of hepatic impairment, based on clinical and laboratory findings (Child's classification; see Table 35–3). Shunting procedures are generally performed on good-risk patients, while ablative surgery, esophageal transection, and gastric devascularization are reserved for high-risk patients. Nonselective shunts (portacaval and proximal splenorenal) have generally been abandoned in favor of selective shunts (distal splenorenal). The latter also decompress the varices but do not impair hepatic blood flow as much and are less likely to cause encephalopathy postoperatively (see below).

B. Hematologic Manifestations: Anemia, thrombocytopenia, and, less commonly, leukopenia may be present. The causes of the anemia are usually multifactorial and include blood loss, increased red cell destruction, bone marrow suppression, and nutritional deficiencies. Congestive splenomegaly (from portal hypertension) is largely responsible for the thrombocytopenia and leukopenia. Coagulation factor deficiencies arise as a result of decreased hepatic synthesis. Enhanced fibrinolysis secondary to decreased clearance of activators of the fibrinolytic system may also contribute to the coagulopathy.

The need for preoperative blood transfusions should be balanced against the obligatory increase in nitrogen load. Protein breakdown from excessive blood transfusions can precipitate encephalopathy. The hematocrit should generally be increased to 30% preoperatively by transfusions when blood loss is expected during surgery. Coagulopathy should be corrected before surgery. Clotting factors should be replaced with FFP and platelet transfusions given immediately before operation for counts less than $100,000/\mu L$. Cryoprecipitate may be necessary for severe coagulation defects.

C. Circulatory Manifestations: Cirrhosis is typically characterized by a hyperdynamic circulatory state. Cardiac output is often increased, and generalized peripheral vasodilatation is present. Arteriovenous shunting can occur in both the systemic and pulmonary circulations. The arteriovenous shunting together with the decrease in blood viscosity from anemia are at least partly responsible for the increased cardiac output. In contrast, patients with a superimposed alcoholic cardiomyopathy readily develop congestive heart failure.

D. Respiratory Manifestations: Disturbances in pulmonary gas exchange as well as ventilatory mechanics are often present. Hyperventilation is common and results in a primary respiratory alkalosis. Hypoxemia is frequently present and is due to right-to-left shunting (up to 40% of cardiac output). Shunting is due to an increase in both pulmonary arteriovenous communications (absolute) and ventilation/perfusion mismatching (relative). Elevation of the diaphragm from ascites decreases lung volumes, especially functional residual capacity, and predisposes to atelectasis. Moreover, large amounts of ascites produce a restrictive ventilatory defect that increases the work of breathing.

Review of the chest x-ray and arterial blood gas measurements is very useful preoperatively because atelectasis and hypoxemia are often not evident on clinical examination. Paracentesis should be considered for patients with massive ascites and pulmonary compromise.

E. Renal Manifestations and Fluid Balance: Derangements of fluid and electrolyte balance are manifested as ascites, edema, electrolyte disturbances, or the hepatorenal syndrome. Important mechanisms thought to be responsible for ascites include (1) portal hypertension, which increases the hydrostatic pressure and favors transudation of fluid across bowel; (2) hypoalbuminemia, which decreases plasma oncotic pressure and also favors fluid transudation; (3) seepage of protein-rich lymphatic fluid from the serosal surface of the liver secondary to distortion and obstruction of lymphatic channels in the liver; and (4) avid renal sodium (and often water) retention (see below). Both "underfilling" and "overflow" theories have been proposed to explain the sodium retention.

The "underfilling" theory proposes that although the measurable total extracellular fluid and plasma volumes are increased in cirrhotic patients with ascites, "effective plasma volume" is decreased: sodium retention is secondary to relative hypovolemia and secondary hyperaldosteronism. The apparent discrepancy between the measured and "effective" plasma volumes may be accounted for by an increase in splanchnic blood volume. In contrast to underfilling, the "overflow" theory holds that the primary abnormality is sodium retention by the kidneys and that the ascites represents transudation secondary to an expanded plasma volume.

Regardless of the mechanisms involved, patients with cirrhosis and ascites have decreased renal perfusion, altered intrarenal hemodynamics, enhanced proximal and distal sodium reabsorption, and often an impairment of free water clearance. Hyponatremia and hypokalemia are common. The former is dilutional, while the latter is due to excessive urinary potassium losses (from secondary hyperaldosteronism or diuretics). The most severe expression of these abnormalities is seen with development of the hepatorenal syndrome.

The hepatorenal syndrome is a functional renal defect in patients with cirrhosis that usually follows gastrointestinal bleeding, aggressive diuresis, sepsis, or major surgery. It is characterized by progressive oliguria, azotemia, intractable ascites, and a very high mortality rate. Treatment is supportive and often unsuccessful unless liver transplantation is undertaken.

Judicious perioperative fluid management in patients with advanced liver disease is therefore critical. The importance of preserving renal function perioperatively cannot be overemphasized. Overzealous preoperative diuresis should be avoided, and acute intravascular fluid deficits should be corrected with colloid infusions. Diuresis of ascites and edema fluid should be accomplished over several days. Loop diuretics are employed only when bed rest, sodium restriction (< 2 g NaCl/d), and spironolactone are ineffective. Daily body weight measurements are useful in preventing intravascular volume depletion during diuresis. For patients with both ascites and peripheral edema, no more than 1 kg/d should be lost during diuresis; while for those with ascites alone, no more than 0.5 kg/d should be lost. Hyponatremia (serum $[Na^+] < 130$ meq/L) also necessitates water restriction, while potassium deficits require replacement preoperatively. Prophylactic perioperative mannitol infusions may be effective in preventing renal failure, but this has not been conclusively demonstrated.

F. Central Nervous System Manifestations: Hepatic encephalopathy is characterized by alterations in mental status with fluctuating neurologic signs (asterixis, hyperreflexia, or an inverted plantar reflex) and characteristic electroencephalographic changes (symmetric high-voltage slow-wave activity). Some patients also have elevated intracranial pressure. The metabolic encephalopathy appears to be related to both the amount of hepatocellular damage present as well as the degree of shunting of portal blood away from the liver and directly into the systemic circulation. The accumulation of substances originating in the gastrointestinal tract but normally metabolized by the liver has been implicated. These proposed toxins include ammonia, methionine metabolites (mercaptans), short-chain fatty acids, and phenols. Other reported abnormalities include increased blood levels of aromatic amino acids, decreased blood levels of branched-chain amino acids, increased permeability of the blood-brain barrier, and abnormally high levels of γ-aminobutyric acid in the brain. Factors known to precipitate hepatic encephalopathy include gastrointestinal bleeding, increased dietary protein intake, hypokalemic alkalosis (from vomiting or diuresis), infections, and worsening liver function.

Encephalopathy should be aggressively treated preoperatively. Precipitating causes should be corrected. Oral lactulose or neomycin is useful in reducing intestinal ammonia absorption. Patients with a history of encephalopathy are very sensitive to all central nervous system depressants and should not receive premedication.

Intraoperative Considerations

Patients with cirrhosis may also pose a health hazard to operating room personnel. Patients with postnecrotic cirrhosis due to hepatitis B or C who are carriers of the virus may be infectious. Extra caution is indicated in preventing contact with blood and body fluids from these patients (see above).

A. Drug Responses: The response to anesthetic agents is unpredictable in patients with cirrhosis. Changes in central nervous system sensitivity, volumes of distribution, protein binding, drug metabolism, and drug elimination are common. Thiopental clearance is often unaltered because its decreased metabolism is balanced by a decrease in protein binding. Many patients display enhanced central nervous system sensitivity to thiopental, while those with an alcoholic history may show tolerance. An increase in the volume of distribution for highly ionized drugs, such as muscle relaxants, is due to the expanded extracellular fluid compartment; an apparent resistance may be observed, necessitating larger than normal loading doses. However, for relaxants dependent on hepatic elimination (pancuronium and vecuronium), reduced plasma clearance necessitates smaller than normal maintenance doses. There may be a prolonged duration of action for succinylcholine as a result of reduced levels of pseudocholinesterase, but it is rarely of clinical consequence.

B. Anesthetic Technique: Because portal venous blood flow is reduced in cirrhosis, the liver becomes very dependent on hepatic arterial perfusion. Preservation of hepatic arterial blood flow and avoidance of agents with potentially adverse effects on hepatic function are critical (Chapter 34). Regional anesthesia may be used in patients without thrombocytopenia or coagulopathy if hypotension is avoided. A barbiturate induction followed by isoflurane in oxygen or an oxygen-nitrous oxide mixture is most commonly employed for general anesthesia (see above). The use of halothane is best avoided so as not to confuse the diagnosis if liver function tests deteriorate postoperatively. Opioid supplementation reduces the dose of the volatile agent required, but the half-lives of opioids are often significantly prolonged, leading to prolonged respiratory depression. Atracurium is the relaxant of choice owing to its unique nonhepatic metabolism.

Preoperative nausea, vomiting, upper gastrointestinal bleeding, and abdominal distention due to massive ascites require preoxygenation and a rapid-sequence induction with cricoid pressure. For unstable patients and those with active bleeding, either an awake intubation or a rapid-sequence induction with cricoid pressure using ketamine and succinylcholine should be used.

C. Monitoring: Close respiratory and cardiovascular monitoring is necessary for patients undergoing abdominal procedures. Pulse oximetry should be supplemented with arterial blood gas measurements to evaluate acid-base status. Patients with large right-to-left intrapulmonary shunts may not tolerate the addition of nitrous oxide and often require positive endexpiratory pressure (PEEP) to prevent hypoxemia.

Intra-arterial pressure monitoring is generally indicated for most patients. Rapid changes in blood pressure occur as a result of excessive bleeding, rapid intercompartmental fluid shifts, and surgical manipulations. Five-lead electrocardiographic monitoring of patients receiving vasopressin infusions is necessary to detect ischemia from coronary vasoconstriction. Intravascular volume status is often difficult to assess without central venous or pulmonary artery pressure monitoring. Such monitoring is critical in preventing the hepatorenal syndrome. Urinary output must be followed closely; mannitol or low-dose dopamine should be considered for persistently low urine outputs in spite of adequate intravascular fluid replacement (Chapter 29).

D. Fluid Replacement: Although most patients are on sodium restriction preoperatively, preservation of intravascular volume and urine output take priority intraoperatively. The use of predominantly colloid intravenous fluids may be preferable in order to avoid sodium overload (Chapter 28). Intravenous fluid replacement should take into account the excessive bleeding and fluid shifts that often occur in these patients during abdominal procedures. Venous engorgement from portal hypertension, adhesions from previous surgery, and coagulopathy are responsible for excessive bleeding, while evacuation of ascites and prolonged surgical manipulations result in large fluid shifts. Intravenous colloid fluid replacement is often necessary to prevent profound hypotension and renal shutdown following the removal of large amounts of ascitic fluid.

Because most patients are anemic preoperatively, red cell transfusions should be given on the basis of 1 unit for each unit of blood loss. Whole blood, when available, may be preferable to packed red blood cells.

Coagulation factor and platelet deficiencies should be replaced with FFP and platelet transfusions, respectively. Citrate toxicity readily occurs in patients with cirrhosis due to impaired metabolism of the citrate anticoagulant in blood products. Intravenous calcium is often necessary to reverse the negative inotropic effects of a drop in the blood ionized calcium concentration.

HEPATOBILIARY DISEASE

Hepatobiliary disease is often characterized by cholestasis, the suppression or stoppage of bile flow. The most common cause of cholestasis is extrahepatic obstruction of the biliary tract (obstructive jaundice). The biliary obstruction is usually due to a gallstone, stricture, or tumor in the common hepatic duct. Patients with complete or near-complete obstruction present with progressive jaundice, a dark urine with pale stools, or pruritus. In contrast, gallstone disease (cholelithiasis) limited to the gallbladder typically presents as biliary colic secondary to obstruction of the cystic duct and cholecystitis. Passage of a gallstone through the common duct, however, may also produce transient jaundice. In either case, concomitant chills or high fever is usually indicative of an ascending bacterial infection of the biliary system (cholangitis). Less commonly, the gallstone can obstruct the pancreatic duct and cause acute pancreatitis.

Obstructive jaundice must be differentiated from intrahepatic cholestasis. The latter is due to suppression or obstruction of bile flow at the level of the hepatocyte or bile canaliculus. Intrahepatic cholestasis most commonly results from viral hepatitis or an idiosyncratic drug reaction (most commonly reactions to phenothiazines or oral contraceptives). The treatment for extrahepatic obstruction is usually surgical, whereas that for intrahepatic cholestasis is medical. Although pruritus (due to retained bile salts) is a prominent feature of intrahepatic cholestasis, correct diagnosis may not be possible based on clinical or laboratory grounds. Both entities produce a predominantly conjugated (> 50%) hyperbilirubinemia and moderate to marked elevations of serum alkaline phosphatase (Chapter 34). Imaging studies (ultrasound, cholangiograms, radioisotopic or CT scans) are necessary to confirm extrahepatic biliary obstruction preoperatively.

Preoperative Considerations

Patients most commonly present to the operating room for cholecystectomy or relief of extrahepatic biliary obstruction. Those scheduled for cholecystectomy after resolution of an attack of cholecystitis do not require special treatment. However, controversy has existed about performing a cholecystectomy during an acute attack of cholecystitis. Recent evidence suggests that although mortality and morbidity rates are similar for early versus delayed operation, a significant number of patients become worse or develop another attack prior to the scheduled surgery. Current practices favor early operation in patients who are a good surgical risk as well as those who fail to improve with medical management. Preoperative preparation should include adequate hydration with intravenous fluids, nasogastric suction, and antibiotics. Acalculous cholecystitis, which most frequently occurs in critically ill patients, is associated with a high risk of gangrene and perforation; emergency operation is indicated in all these patients.

Patients with extrahepatic biliary obstruction from whatever cause readily develop vitamin K deficiency. Vitamin K should be given parenterally but requires 24 hours for a full response. Failure of the PT to correct prior to surgery necessitates FFP. High bilirubin levels are associated with an increased risk of postoperative renal failure; generous preoperative hydration and possibly intravenous mannitol should be given. Long-standing extrahepatic obstruction (> 1 year) produces secondary biliary cirrhosis and portal hypertension (see above).

Intraoperative Considerations

Because all opioids can cause spasm of the sphincter of Oddi to varying degrees (Chapter 34), their use has been questioned when an intraoperative cholangiogram is contemplated. Opioid-induced sphincteric spasm may theoretically result in a falsely positive intraoperative cholangiogram and needless exploration of the common bile duct. Although this point may have been over-emphasized in the past, opioids are be best withheld in the anesthetic protocol until after the cholangiogram.

In patients with biliary tract obstruction, a prolonged duration of action of drugs primarily dependent on biliary excretion should be anticipated. Agents dependent on renal elimination are preferable. Urinary output should be monitored with an indwelling catheter. Maintenance of perioperative diuresis is desirable (see above).

Patients with acalculous cholecystitis and those with severe cholangitis are critically ill and have a high perioperative mortality rate. Invasive hemodynamic monitoring optimizes their anesthetic care (Chapter 6).

HEPATIC SURGERY

Common hepatic procedures include repair of lacerations, drainage of abscesses, and resections for tumors. Liver transplantation is now also performed in many centers. Anesthetic management for all these procedures can be potentially complicated by large amounts of blood loss. Multiple large-bore intravenous catheters with fluid (blood) warmers are necessary; rapid infusion devices facilitate management when massive blood transfusion is necessary. Hypotensive anesthesia is generally avoided because of its potentially deleterious effects on remaining liver tissue. Hypoglycemia may occur following large liver resections. Drainage of an abscess or cyst may be complicated by peritoneal contamination, with spillage of its contents. In the case of a hydatid cyst, spillage can cause anaphylaxis due to *Echinococcus* antigens.

CASE DISCUSSION: LIVER TRANSPLANTATION

A 23-year-old woman develops fulminant hepatic failure after ingesting wild mushrooms. She is not expected to survive without a liver transplant.

How are donor livers procured?

Donors are individuals 2 months to 45 years of age who fulfill the criteria for brain death (Chapter 48) and have no evidence of hepatic dysfunction; most are victims of motor vehicle accidents. Selection of a donor organ for a given patient is generally based only on ABO blood type and organ size. The number of liver transplantations is generally limited by the availability of suitable donor organs. The liver is removed from the donor in the operating room while the circulation is intact. Every effort is made to minimize the period of warm ischemia; prolonged hypotension or hypoxia precludes transplantation. As soon as the liver is removed, it is flushed with a cold preservative solution and packed in ice; donor life-support systems are then discontinued. Current preservation techniques allow a maximum total ischemic time of 20 hours.

What are the most common indications for liver transplantation?

Orthotopic liver transplantation is performed in patients with end-stage liver disease who begin to experience life-threatening complications. Transplantation may also occasionally be performed in patients with fulminant hepatic failure (from viral hepatitis or a hepatotoxin) when survival with medical management alone is judged unlikely. In order of decreasing frequency, the most common indications for liver transplantation in children are biliary atresia, inborn errors of metabolism (usually α_1-antitrypsin deficiency, Wilson's disease, tyrosinemia, and Crigler-Najjar type I syndrome), and postnecrotic cirrhosis. The most common indications in adults are postnecrotic (nonalcoholic) cirrhosis, primary liver malignancies, primary biliary cirrhosis, and sclerosing cholangitis. Some controversy exists over the justification for expenditure of scarce organs in transplanting patients with alcoholic cirrhosis, because they often revert to habitual drinking afterward.

Why are these operations so lengthy?

These procedures usually require 8–12 hours of surgery that can be divided into three phases: a dissection phase, an anhepatic phase, and a revascularization phase.

(1) Dissection (preanhepatic) phase: Through a wide subcostal incision, the liver is dissected so that it remains attached only by the inferior vena cava, the portal vein, the hepatic artery, and the common bile duct. Previous abdominal procedures greatly prolong the duration of and increase the blood loss associated with this phase.

(2) Anhepatic phase: Once the liver is freed, the inferior vena cava is clamped above and below the liver, as are the hepatic artery, portal vein, and common bile duct. The liver is then completely excised. Venovenous bypass (see below) may or may not be employed during this phase. The donor liver is then anastomosed to the supra- and infrahepatic inferior venae cavae and the portal vein.

(3) Revascularization and biliary reconstruction (neohepatic or postanhepatic) phase: Following completion of the venous anastomoses, venous clamps are removed and the circulation to the new liver is completed by anastomosing the hepatic artery. Lastly, the common bile duct of the donor liver is then usually connected to the recipient via a choledochocholedochostomy or Roux-en-Y choledochojejunostomy.

What major problems complicate anesthesia for liver transplantation?

These include the multisystem nature of cirrhosis (Chapter 34), major (often massive) blood loss throughout the procedure, the hemodynamic consequences of clamping and unclamping the inferior vena cava and portal vein, the metabolic consequences of the anhepatic phase, and the risks of air embolism and hyperkalemia when circulation to the new liver is fully established.

What factors contribute to and complicate the large blood loss?

Preoperative coagulation defects, thrombocytopenia, and previous abdominal surgery greatly increase blood loss. Extensive venous collaterals between the portal and systemic venous circulations (see above) also probably contribute to increased bleeding from the abdominal wall. Hypothermia, coagulopathies, citrate intoxication, and the potential transmission of infectious agents complicate massive blood transfusion. Typical transfusion requirements consist of 15–30 units of red blood cells, 15–30 units of FFP, 15–25 units of platelets, and 10–20 units of cryoprecipitate. Blood salvaging techniques can be extremely useful in reducing (by 25–30%) the number of donor red cell units required (Chapter 29).

How are the circulatory effects of venous clamping managed?

When the inferior vena cava and portal vein are clamped, marked decreases in cardiac output and hypotension are typically encountered. Moreover, the increase in distal venous pressure can markedly increase bleeding and impair renal perfusion and often promotes edema and ischemia of intestines. Some patients (usually children) tolerate caval clamping because of extensive transdiaphragmatic collateral venous channels. To avoid these problems, most surgeons now routinely utilize the technique of venovenous bypass in adults and in children weighing over 10 kg. This technique involves cannulating the inferior vena cava and the portal vein and diverting their blood flow (1–3 L/min) away from the liver and back to the heart, usually via an axillary vein. The pump and tubing are designed in such a way that heparinization of the patient is not necessary. Venovenous bypass can prevent severe hypotension, intestinal edema, ischemia, the build-up of acid metabolites, and postoperative renal dysfunction. Prophylactic measures such as mannitol or low-dose dopamine (2–3 μg/kg/min) prior to and during venous clamping may be beneficial in preserving renal function but are unproved. Temporary inotropic support (in addition to blood and fluid replacement) is often required transiently until effective venovenous bypass is established. Technical considerations have prevented the routine use of venovenous bypass for small children. The use of venovenous bypass is not without risk; it increases operative time; can be associated with air embolism, thromboembolic complications, and brachial plexus injuries; and may contribute to hypothermia.

What physiologic derangements are associated with the anhepatic phase?

When the liver is removed, the large citrate load from blood products is no longer metabolized and results in hypocalcemia and secondary myocardial depression (Chapter 29). Periodic calcium chloride administration (200–500 mg) is necessary but should be guided by ionized calcium concentration measurements to avoid hypercalcemia. Electrocardiographic signs of hypocalcemia are unreliable (Chapter 28). Progressive acidosis is also encountered because acid metabolites from the intestines (and lower body) are not cleared by the liver. Sodium bicarbonate therapy is therefore also necessary and should similarly be guided by arterial blood gas analysis. Excessive $NaHCO_3$ administration results in hypernatremia, hyperosmolality, and accentuation of the metabolic alkalosis that typically follows massive blood transfusions (Chapter 29). Although hypoglycemia can occur during the anhepatic phase, hyperglycemia is a more common occurrence. The large amounts of transfused blood products given usually provide a large glucose load. Glucose-containing intravenous solutions are therefore not used unless hypoglycemia is documented.

Pulmonary and systemic (paradoxic) air embolism can occur when the circulation is fully reestablished to the donor liver because air often enters hepatic sinusoids after harvesting. Systemic air embolism probably reflects the fact that many of these patients have extensive arteriovenous communications. Venous air embolism can be detected as a sudden increase in end-expired nitrogen concentration (Chapter 26). The incidence of air embolism is decreased by infusing cold lactated Ringer's injection through the portal vein while the venous anastomoses are being constructed. Additionally, after completion of the portal and suprahepatic caval anastomoses but prior to completion of the infrahepatic caval anastomosis, the portal vein clamp is released; blood from the portal vein then "flushes out" any air remaining in the liver, which can now escape through the incomplete infrahepatic caval anastomotic site. Marked hypotension is often encountered during this period and requires inotropic support as well as intravenous fluid replacement. After "flushing," venous clamps are reapplied until infrahepatic caval anastomosis is completed. The anhepatic phase ends when the three venous clamps are removed and the liver donor liver is perfused. Thromboembolic phenomena are also described following reperfusion.

What problems may be anticipated during the revascularization phase?

Perfusion of the donor liver by the recipient's blood uniformly results in a transient increase in serum potassium concentration of usually 1–2 meq/L and increased systemic acidosis. Acidosis accentuates the hyperkalemia (Chapter 28). Reperfusion releases potassium from any remaining preservative solution (100–110 meq/L of K^+) still within the liver as well as potassium released from tissues distal to venous clamps. Unclamping may also release a large acid load from ischemic tissue in the lower body (especially without venovenous bypass); prophylactic administration of $NaHCO_3$ is advocated by some.

When the circulation to the new liver is established, the sudden increase in blood volume, acidosis, and hyperkalemia can produce either tachyarrhythmias or, more commonly, bradyarrhythmias. In addition to $CaCl_2$ and $NaHCO_3$, inotropic support is also often required. Occasionally, the release of large amounts of tissue plasminogen activator can produce fibrinolysis, which may be detected by thromboelastography. Aminocaproic acid, 1 g intravenously, which inhibits the action of plasmin on fibrin, is indicated in those instances.

What factors have contributed to the recent success of liver transplantation?

One-year survival rates for liver transplantations exceed 80–90% in some centers. Currently, 5-year survival rates are 50–60%. The success of this procedure has been largely due to use of cyclosporine for immunosuppressant therapy. Cyclosporine suppresses both humoral and cell-mediated immunity by inhibiting interleukin-2 production. Cyclosporine is usually initially combined with corticosteroids and azathioprine. The use of OKT-3, a monoclonal antibody directed against lymphocytes, is also very promising. Additional factors may include greater understanding and experience with transplantation, the safe use of venovenous bypass, and the introduction of rapid infusion devices that allow transfusion of up to 2 L/min of warmed blood.

What is adequate venous access for these procedures?

Bleeding is a recurring problem during each phase of liver transplantation. Adequate venous access is paramount in anesthetic management. Three to five 14-gauge or larger intravenous catheters are necessary. Specialized 8.5F catheters can be placed in antecubital veins and used in conjunction with rapid infusion devices. Catheters should generally not be placed in the arm to be used for venovenous bypass. All transfusion lines should pass through a warming device that heats fluids to normal body temperature to prevent hypothermia. Blood replacement can range anywhere from one to 35 times the patient's entire blood volume.

What monitoring techniques are most useful during surgery?

All patients require direct intra-arterial pressure monitoring. A central venous or pulmonary artery catheter should be used to guide fluid replacement. The latter is preferred for most adult patients. Urine output should be monitored carefully throughout surgery via an indwelling urinary catheter.

Laboratory measurements constitute an important part of intraoperative monitoring. Serial hematocrit measurements are mandatory to guide red blood cell replacement. Similarly, frequent measurements of arterial blood gases, serum electrolytes, serum ionized calcium, and serum glucose are necessary to detect and appropriately treat severe metabolic derangements (see above). Coagulation can be monitored by measuring PT, PTT, and fibrinogen and by platelet counts, or by thromboelastography. The latter not only measures overall clotting and platelet function but can also detect fibrinolysis.

What anesthetic technique may be used for liver transplantation?

Premedication is usually administered unless the patient is in an advanced stage of hepatic encephalopa-

thy. Intramuscular injections are avoided in patients with coagulopathy. Oral diazepam, 5–15 mg, or lorazepam, 2–3 mg, can be used for adults, while diazepam, 0.1–0.2 mg/kg, can be used orally for children. Because many if not most patients can be considered as having a "full stomach" (recent oral intake, marked abdominal distention, or recent upper gastrointestinal bleeding), general anesthesia is usually induced via a rapid-sequence induction with cricoid pressure. The semi-upright position during induction prevents rapid oxygen desaturation and facilitates ventilation until the abdomen is open. Thiopental, 4–5 mg/kg, ketamine, 1–2 mg/kg, or etomidate, 0.3–0.4 mg/kg, may be used. Succinylcholine, 1.5 mg/kg, is usually employed to facilitate rapid intubation. Hyperventilation may be beneficial in patients with severe encephalopathy because they may have increased intracranial pressure (Chapter 25). Anesthesia is usually maintained with a volatile agent, usually isoflurane, and an intravenous opioid, usually fentanyl. The concentration of the volatile agent should be limited to less than 1 MAC in patients with severe encephalopathy (Chapter 25). Nitrous oxide is usually avoided or used only until just prior to perfusion of the donor graft to prevent expansion of intravascular air bubbles. Nitrous oxide can also cause marked distention of the bowel. The choice of muscle relaxant is generally not important because patients are routinely left intubated at the end of the procedure.

What problems are encountered postoperatively?

Patients often have a very complicated postoperative course. Problems that may be encountered include persistent hemorrhage, fluid overload, metabolic abnormalities (metabolic alkalosis and hypokalemia), respiratory failure, paralysis of the right hemidiaphragm (secondary to injury of the right phrenic nerve), renal failure, systemic infections, and surgical complications such as bile leaks or thrombosis of the hepatic or portal vessels. Renal dysfunction is often multifactorial in origin; contributory factors include periods of hypotension, impaired renal perfusion when the inferior vena cava is clamped (resulting in high pressures in the renal veins), and cyclosporine or antibiotic nephropathy. Prophylactic antibiotics and antifungal agents are routinely given in many centers. Rejection of the transplant is generally not a problem until 1–6 weeks after surgery.

SUGGESTED READINGS

Abdul-Rasool I, Khoury GF: Anesthesia for liver transplantation. Semin Anesth 1987;6:143.

Brown BR: *Anesthesia in Hepatic and Biliary Tract Disease.* Davis, 1988. The only recent text on the subject.

Gelman S: *Anesthesia and Organ Transplantation.* Saunders, 1987.

Katz J, Benumof JL, Kadis LB: *Anesthesia and Uncommon Diseases,* 3rd ed. Saunders, 1990. Contains a good chapter on liver disease.

Khoury GF, Abdul-Rasool I: The cardiovascular and metabolic changes during liver transplantation: Anesthetic considerations. Semin Anesth 1987;6:309.

Vickers MD: *Medicine for Anaesthetists,* 3d ed. Blackwell, 1989.

Wilson JD et al (editors): *Harrison's Principles of Internal Medicine,* 12th ed. McGraw-Hill, 1991. The sections on liver disease are outstanding.

Anesthesia for Patients With Endocrine Disease

36

The underproduction or overproduction of hormones can have dramatic physiologic and pharmacologic consequences. Therefore, it is not surprising that endocrinopathies affect anesthetic management. This chapter presents the dysfunction of four endocrine organs: the pancreas, the thyroid, the parathyroids, and the adrenal gland. A brief review of normal physiology is followed by an examination of the clinical manifestations and anesthetic implications of abnormal hormonal activity. Obesity and carcinoid syndrome are also considered.

THE PANCREAS

Physiology

Adults normally secrete approximately 50 units of insulin each day from the B (β) cells of the islets of Langerhans in the pancreas. The rate of insulin secretion is primarily determined by the plasma glucose level. Insulin has multiple metabolic effects, including (1) increased glucose and potassium entry into adipose and muscle cells; (2) increased glycogen, protein, and fatty acid synthesis; and (3) decreased glycogenolysis, gluconeogenesis, ketogenesis, lipolysis, and protein catabolism.

In general, insulin stimulates anabolism while its lack is associated with catabolism and a negative nitrogen balance (Table 36–1).

DIABETES MELLITUS

Clinical Manifestations

Diabetes mellitus is characterized by impairment of carbohydrate metabolism due to a deficiency of insulin activity, which leads to hyperglycemia and glycosuria. The diagnosis is based on an elevated fasting plasma glucose (> 140 mg/dL) or 2-hour postprandial plasma glucose (> 200 mg/dL). Diabetes is clinically classified as insulin-dependent (type I) or non-insulin-dependent (type II) (Table 36–2). Long-term com-

Table 36–1. Endocrine effects of insulin.[1]

Effects on liver
  Anabolic effects:
    Promotes glycogenesis
    Increases synthesis of triglycerides, cholesterol, and VLDL
    Increases protein synthesis
    Promotes glycolysis
  Anticatabolic effects:
    Inhibits glycogenolysis
    Inhibits ketogenesis
    Inhibits gluconeogenesis
Effects on muscle
  Promotes protein synthesis:
    Increases amino acid transport
    Stimulates ribosomal protein synthesis
  Promotes glycogen synthesis:
    Increases glucose transport
    Enhances activity of glycogen synthetase
    Inhibits activity of glycogen phosphorylase
Effects on fat
  Promotes triglyceride storage:
    Induces lipoprotein lipase, making fatty acids available for absorption into fat cells
    Increases glucose transport into fat cells, thus increasing availability of α-glycerol phosphate for triglyceride synthesis
    Inhibits intracellular lipolysis

[1]Reproduced, with permission, from Greenspan FS (editor): *Basic & Clinical Endocrinology*, 3rd ed. Appleton & Lange, 1991.

Table 36–2. Classification of diabetes mellitus.[1]

	Insulin-Dependent (Type I)	Non-Insulin-Dependent (Type II)
Usual age at onset	Juvenile	Adult
Insulin production	Very low	Normal or high
Body habitus	Lean	Obese
Treatment	Insulin	Diet, oral agents, insulin
Response to insulin	Sensitive	Resistant
Likelihood of ketosis	Prone	Resistant
Hereditary influence	Moderate	Great

[1]These characterizations are only generally valid. There is significant overlap between the two types. Note that non-insulin-dependent diabetes may be treated with insulin.

plications of diabetes include hypertension, myocardial infarction, peripheral and cerebral vascular disease, peripheral and autonomic neuropathies, and renal failure. There are three life-threatening acute complications: diabetic ketoacidosis, hyperosmolar nonketotic coma, and hypoglycemia.

Decreased insulin activity allows the catabolism of free fatty acids into ketone bodies (acetoacetate and β-hydroxybutyrate). Accumulation of these organic acids results in an anion gap metabolic acidosis **(diabetic ketoacidosis)**. Diabetic ketoacidosis can be easily distinguished from lactic acidosis, which is identified by the presence of elevated plasma lactate ($>$ 6 mmol/L) and the absence of urine and plasma acetone. Clinical manifestations of ketoacidosis include changes in sensorium, dyspnea (attempting to compensate for the metabolic acidosis), abdominal pain, nausea, and vomiting. The treatment of diabetic ketoacidosis depends upon correcting the hyperglycemia, total body potassium deficit, and dehydration with a continuous infusion of insulin, potassium, and isotonic fluids.

Ketoacidosis is not a feature of **hyperosmolar nonketotic coma** because enough insulin is available to prevent ketone body formation. Instead, a hypoglycemic diuresis results in dehydration and hyperosmolality. Severe dehydration eventually leads to renal failure, lactic acidosis, and a predisposition to form intravascular thromboses. Hyperosmolality, frequently exceeding 360 mosm/L, alters cerebral water balance, causing mental status changes and seizures. Treatment includes fluid resuscitation and relatively small doses of insulin.

Hypoglycemia in the diabetic patient is the result of an excess of insulin relative to carbohydrate intake. Furthermore, some diabetic patients are unable to counter hyperglycemia by secreting glucagon or epinephrine **(counterregulatory failure)**. The conspicuous dependence of the brain on glucose as an energy source makes it the organ most susceptible to episodes of hypoglycemia. If hypoglycemia is not treated, mental status changes can progress from faintness or confusion to convulsions and permanent coma. Systemic manifestations of hypoglycemia result from catecholamine discharge and include diaphoresis, tachycardia, and nervousness. Most of the signs and symptoms of hypoglycemia will be masked by general anesthesia. Although "normal" plasma glucose levels are ill-defined and depend on age and sex, hypoglycemia can generally be considered to be less than 50 mg/dL.

Anesthetic Considerations

A. Preoperative: The perioperative morbidity of diabetic patients is related to preoperative end-organ damage. In particular, the cardiovascular and renal systems demand close examination. Myocardial ischemia may be evident on an ECG despite a negative history ("silent" myocardial infarction). Painless myocardial ischemia, orthostatic hypotension, lack of

heart rate variability, resting tachycardia, early satiety, neurogenic bladder, and impotence may indicate **diabetic autonomic neuropathy.** This autonomic neuropathy may limit the heart's ability to compensate for intravascular volume changes and may predispose patients to cardiovascular instability and even sudden cardiac death. Furthermore, autonomic dysfunction contributes to delayed gastric emptying. Premedication with a histamine antagonist or metoclopramide would be especially prudent in an obese diabetic patient with autonomic dysfunction (Chapter 15).

Renal dysfunction is manifested first by proteinuria and later by elevated serum creatinine. In fact, most type I diabetics have evidence of renal failure by age 30. Because of a high incidence of infections referable to a compromised immune system, strict attention to aseptic technique must accompany the placement of all intravenous catheters and invasive monitors.

B. Intraoperative: The primary goal of intraoperative blood sugar management is to avoid hypoglycemia. While attempting to maintain euglycemia is imprudent, unacceptably loose blood sugar control ($>$ 300 mg/dL) also carries risk. Hyperglycemia may be associated with infection (phagocyte dysfunction) and poor wound healing. More importantly, hyperglycemia may worsen neurologic outcome following an episode of cerebral ischemia. Unless hyperglycemia is treated aggressively in type I diabetic patients, metabolic control may be lost, particularly in the face of major surgery and sepsis. Finally, tight control of the pregnant patient has been shown to improve fetal outcome. Nonetheless, because of the brain's dependence on glucose as an energy supply, there is no doubt that hypoglycemia must be avoided.

There are several perioperative management regimens for diabetic patients. In the most common, the patient receives a fraction—usually half—of the total morning insulin dose in the form of intermediate-acting insulin (Table 36–3). To lessen the risk of hypoglycemia, insulin is administered *after* intravenous access has been established and the morning blood glucose level is checked. For example, a patient who normally takes 20 units of NPH (intermediate-acting) and 10 units of regular (short-acting) insulin each morning and whose blood sugar is at least 150 mg/dL would receive 15 units of NPH subcutaneously or intramuscularly before surgery along with an infusion of 5% dextrose solution (1.5 mL/kg/h). Dedication of a small-gauge intravenous line for the dextrose infusion prevents interference with other intraoperative fluids and drugs. Supplemental dextrose can be administered if the patient becomes hypoglycemic ($<$ 100 mg/dL). Ten grams of dextrose (20 mL of 50% dextrose solution) usually raises an adult's plasma glucose by 30–40 mg/dL. On the other hand, intraoperative hyperglycemia ($>$ 200 mg/dL) is treated with intravenous regular insulin according to a sliding scale. One unit of regular insulin given to an adult usually lowers plasma glucose by 25–30 mg/dL. *It must be stressed that these dosages are approximations and do not apply to pa-*

Table 36–3. Two common techniques for perioperative insulin management in diabetes mellitus.

	Bolus Administration	Continuous Infusion
Preoperative	D_5W (1.5 mL/kg/h) NPH insulin (half usual AM dose)	D_5W (1 mL/kg/h) Regular insulin: $\text{Units/h} = \dfrac{\text{Plasma glucose}}{150}$
Intraoperative	Regular insulin (as per sliding scale)	Same as preoperative
Postoperative	Same as intraoperative	Same as preoperative

tients in catabolic states (eg, sepsis, hypothermia).

An alternative method is to administer short-acting insulin as a continuous infusion. The advantages of this technique include more precise and predictable control of insulin delivery than can be achieved with a subcutaneous or intramuscular injection of NPH insulin, particularly in conditions associated with poor skin and muscle perfusion. Ten units of regular insulin can be added to 1 L of 5% dextrose solution and infused at a rate of 1.5 mL/kg/h (1 unit/h/70 kg). Mixing the glucose and the insulin ensures that if the intravenous line malfunctions, the patient cannot receive insulin or glucose alone. However, infusing the 5% dextrose (1 mL/kg/h) and insulin (50 units of regular insulin in 250 mL of normal saline) through separate intravenous lines provides greater flexibility. As blood sugars fluctuate, the rate of insulin infusion can be adjusted according to the following formula:

Units regular insulin per hour =

$$\frac{\text{Plasma glucose (mg/dL)}}{150}$$

For example, if the plasma glucose rose to 300 mg/dL, the rate of regular insulin infusion should be 2 units/h (10 mL/h of the insulin solution described above) while the glucose infusion would remain unchanged. Adding 30 meq of KCl to each liter of dextrose might be prudent, since insulin shifts potassium intracellularly. The effect of insulin absorption to intravenous tubing can be minimized by flushing the line before beginning the infusion. Similarly, some anesthesiologists suggest placing the insulin infusion in a glass bottle. Because individual insulin needs can vary dramatically, any formula should only be used as a guideline.

If the patient is taking an oral hypoglycemic agent preoperatively instead of insulin, the drug can be continued until the day of surgery. Because of the long duration of action of some of these drugs (that of chlorpropamide is 1–3 days), a glucose infusion is begun and blood sugars are monitored as if intermediate-acting insulin has been given. Many of these patients will require some exogenous insulin during the intraoperative and postoperative periods. This is because anesthesia and surgery cause elevations in catecholamines, glucocorticoids, and growth hor-

mone. Each of these imbalances contributes to stress hyperglycemia, which increases insulin requirements. Nonetheless, some type II diabetics will tolerate minor, brief surgical procedures without any exogenous insulin.

The key to any management regimen is to monitor blood glucose levels frequently and appreciate the variation between patients. Diabetics vary in their ability to produce endogenous insulin. "Brittle" type I diabetics may need to have their glucose measured every hour, while every 2 or 3 hours is sufficient for many type II diabetics. Likewise, insulin requirements vary with the stress of the surgical procedure. Patients receiving insulin in the morning but not going to surgery until the afternoon are prone to hypoglycemia despite a dextrose infusion. Unless an arterial line is available, drawing multiple blood specimens and sending them to the laboratory is time-consuming, expensive, and traumatic to the patient's veins. Portable spectrophotometers are capable of determining the glucose concentration in a drop of blood obtained from a finger stick within 1 minute. These devices measure the color conversion of a glucose oxidase-impregnated strip that has been exposed to the patient's blood for a specified period. Their accuracy depends to a large extent upon the care with which the measurements are made. Monitoring urine sugar is not accurate enough for intraoperative management.

Diabetic patients who require NPH (neutral protamine Hagedorn) or protamine zinc insulin are at a much greater risk of allergic reactions to protamine sulfate, including anaphylactic shock and death. Unfortunately, surgeries that require heparinization and subsequent reversal with protamine (eg, coronary artery bypass grafting) are more common in diabetic patients. These patients should receive a small protamine test dose of 1–5 mg over 5–10 minutes prior to the full reversal dose.

C. Postoperative: Close monitoring of the diabetic's blood sugar must continue postoperatively. One reason for this is the individual variation in onset and duration of action of insulin preparations (Table 36–4). For example, the onset of action of regular insulin may be less than 1 hour, but its duration of action may exceed 6 hours. NPH insulin typically has an onset of action within 2 hours, but the action can last longer than 24 hours. Another reason for close monitoring is the progression of stress hyperglycemia in the recov-

Table 36–4. Summary of bioavailability characteristics of the insulins.[1,2]

	Insulin Type	Onset	Peak Action	Duration
Short-acting	Regular, Actrapid, Velosulin	15–30 min	1–3 hours	5–7 hours
	Semilente, Semitard	30–60 min	4–6 hours	12–16 hours
Intermediate-acting	Lente, Lentard, Monotard, NPH, Insulatard	2–4 hours	8–10 hours	18–24 hours
Long-acting	Ultralente, Ultratard, PZI	4–5 hours	8–14 hours	25–36 hours

[1]Reproduced, with permission, from Greenspan FS (editor): *Basic & Clinical Endocrinology*, 3rd ed. Appleton & Lange, 1991.
[2]There is considerable patient-to-patient variation.

ery period. If large volumes of lactate-containing intravenous fluids have been administered intraoperatively, blood sugar will tend to rise 24–48 hours postoperatively when the liver converts the lactate to glucose. Diabetic outpatients should be admitted to a hospital overnight if persistent nausea and vomiting prevent oral intake.

THE THYROID

Physiology

Dietary iodine is absorbed by the gastrointestinal tract, converted to iodide ion, and actively transported into the thyroid gland. Once inside, iodide is oxidized back to iodine, which is bound to the amino acid tyrosine. The end result is two hormones—triiodothyronine (T_3) and thyroxine (T_4)—which are bound to proteins and stored within the thyroid. Although the gland releases more T_4 than T_3, the latter is more potent and is less protein-bound. Most T_3 is formed peripherally from partial deiodination of T_4. An elaborate feedback mechanism controls thyroid hormone synthesis and involves the hypothalamus (thyrotropin-releasing hormone), the anterior pituitary (thyroid-stimulating hormone), and autoregulation (thyroid iodine concentration).

Thyroid hormone increases carbohydrate and fat metabolism by activating the adenylyl cyclase system. It is an important factor in determining growth and metabolic rate. An increase in metabolic rate is accompanied by a rise in oxygen consumption and CO_2 production, indirectly increasing minute ventilation. Heart rate and contractility are also increased, presumably from an alteration in adrenergic receptor physiology as opposed to an increase in catecholamine levels.

HYPERTHYROIDISM

Clinical Manifestations

Hyperthyroidism can be caused by Graves' disease, toxic multinodular goiter, thyroiditis, thyroid-stimulating hormone (TSH)-secreting pituitary tumors, functioning thyroid adenomas, or overdosage of thyroid replacement hormone. Clinical manifestations of hyperthyroidism include weight loss, heat intolerance, muscle weakness, diarrhea, hyperactive reflexes, and nervousness. A fine tremor, exophthalmos, or goiter may be noted. Cardiac signs range from sinus tachycardia to atrial fibrillation and congestive heart failure. The diagnosis of hyperthyroidism is confirmed by abnormal thyroid function tests, which may include an elevation in total (bound and unbound) serum thyroxine, serum triiodothyronine, and free (unbound) thyroxine.

Medical treatment of hyperthyroidism relies upon drugs that inhibit hormone synthesis (eg, propylthiouracil and methimazole), prevent hormone release (eg, potassium or sodium iodide), or mask the signs of adrenergic overactivity (eg, propranolol). While β-adrenergic antagonists do not affect thyroid gland function, they do decrease the peripheral conversion of thyroxine to triiodothyronine. Radioactive iodine destroys thyroid cell function but is not recommended for pregnant patients and may result in hypothyroidism. Subtotal thyroidectomy is a surgical alternative to medical therapy.

Anesthetic Considerations

A. Preoperative: All elective surgical procedures, including subtotal thyroidectomy, should be postponed until the patient is rendered euthyroid with medical treatment. The days of a "thyroid steal" induction with covertly administered medications are past. Preoperative assessment should include normal thyroid function tests, and a resting heart rate less than 85 beats/min has been recommended. Benzodiazepines are a good choice for preoperative sedation. Antithyroid medications and β-adrenergic antagonists are continued through the morning of surgery.

B. Intraoperative: Cardiovascular function and body temperature should be closely monitored in patients with a history of hyperthyroidism. Patients' eyes should be well protected, since the exophthalmos of Graves' disease increases the risk of corneal abrasion or ulceration. The head of the operating table may be raised 15–20 degrees to aid venous drainage and decrease blood loss, though doing so increases the risk of venous air embolism. An armored endotracheal tube passed beyond the goiter will lessen the risk of kinking and airway obstruction.

Ketamine, pancuronium, indirect-acting adrenergic agonists, and other drugs that stimulate the sympathetic nervous system are avoided because of the possibility of exaggerated elevations in blood pressure and heart rate. Thiopental may be the induction agent of choice, since it possesses some antithyroid activity at high dosages. Hyperthyroid patients can be chronically hypovolemic and vasodilated and are prone to an exaggerated hypotensive response during induction. However, adequate anesthetic depth must be obtained before laryngoscopy or surgical stimulation to avoid tachycardia, hypertension, and ventricular dysrhythmias.

Hyperthyroid patients display accelerated drug biotransformation and, theoretically, may be more susceptible to hepatic injury from halothane or kidney toxicity from enflurane. Muscle relaxants should be administered cautiously, because thyrotoxicosis is associated with an increased incidence of myopathies and myasthenia gravis. Hyperthyroidism does not increase anesthetic requirements—ie, there is no change in minimum alveolar concentration (MAC).

C. Postoperative: The most serious threat to hyperthyroid patients in the postoperative period is **thyroid storm,** which is characterized by hyperpyrexia, tachycardia, altered consciousness (agitation delirium, and coma), and hypotension. The onset is usually 6–24 hours after surgery but can occur intraoperatively, mimicking malignant hyperthermia. However, in contrast to malignant hyperthermia, thyroid storm is not associated with muscle rigidity, elevated creatine kinase, or a marked degree of lactic and respiratory acidosis. Treatment includes hydration and cooling; intravenous propranolol (0.5-mg increments until the heart rate is < 100/min); propylthiouracil (250 mg every 6 hours orally or by nasogastric tube) followed by sodium iodide (1 g intravenously over 12 hours); and correction of any precipitating cause (eg, infection). Cortisol (100–200 mg every 8 hours) is recommended to prevent complications due to coexisting adrenal gland suppression. Thyroid storm is a medical emergency that requires aggressive management and monitoring (see Case Discussion, Chapter 47).

Subtotal thyroidectomy is associated with several potential surgical complications. **Recurrent laryngeal nerve palsy** will result in hoarseness (unilateral) or aphonia and stridor (bilateral). Vocal cord function may be evaluated by laryngoscopy immediately following "deep" extubation. Failure of one or both cords to move may require intubation and exploration of the wound. **Hematoma formation** may cause airway compromise from collapse of the trachea in patients with tracheomalacia. Dissection into the compressible soft tissues of the neck may make intubation difficult. Immediate treatment includes opening the neck wound and evacuating the clot, then reassessing the need for reintubation. **Hypoparathyroidism** from unintentional removal of the parathyroid glands will cause acute hypocalcemia within 24–72 hours (see clinical man-

ifestations of hypoparathyroidism, below). Unintentional **pneumothorax** is a possible complication of neck exploration.

HYPOTHYROIDISM

Clinical Manifestations

Hypothyroidism can be caused by autoimmune disease (eg, Hashimoto's thyroiditis), thyroidectomy, radioactive iodine, antithyroid medications, iodine deficiency, or failure of the hypothalamic-pituitary axis (secondary hypothyroidism). Hypothyroidism during neonatal development results in cretinism, a condition marked by physical and mental retardation. Clinical manifestations in the adult are usually subtle and include weight gain, cold intolerance, muscle fatigue, constipation, hypoactive reflexes, dull facial expression, and depression. Heart rate, myocardial contractility, and cardiac output are decreased. Extremities are cool and mottled owing to peripheral vasoconstriction. Pleural, abdominal, and pericardial effusions are common. The diagnosis of hypothyroidism may be confirmed by a low free thyroxine level. Primary hypothyroidism is differentiated from secondary disease by an elevation in TSH. The treatment of hypothyroidism consists of oral replacement therapy with a thyroid hormone preparation.

Myxedema coma results from extreme hypothyroidism and is characterized by impaired mentation, hypoventilation, hypothermia, hyponatremia (due to inappropriate antidiuretic hormone secretion), and congestive heart failure. It is more common in elderly patients and may be precipitated by infection, surgery, or trauma. Myxedema coma is a life-threatening disease that has been successfully treated with intravenous thyroid hormones. A loading dose of T_3 or T_4 (eg, 300–500 μg of levothyroxine sodium in patients without heart disease) is followed by a maintenance infusion (eg, 50 μg of levothyroxine per day). The ECG must be monitored during therapy to detect myocardial ischemia or dysrhythmias. Steroid replacement (eg, hydrocortisone, 100 mg intravenously every 8 hours) is routinely given in case of coexisting adrenal gland suppression. Some patients may require ventilatory support.

Anesthetic Considerations

A. Preoperative: Patients with uncorrected severe hypothyroidism (T_4 < 1 μg/dL) or myxedema coma should not undergo elective surgery and should be treated with thyroid hormone prior to emergency surgery. While a euthyroid state is ideal, mild to moderate hypothyroidism does not appear to be an absolute contraindication to surgery. In fact, hypothyroid patients with symptomatic coronary artery disease may benefit from a delay in thyroid therapy until after coronary artery bypass surgery.

Hypothyroid patients usually do not require much preoperative sedation and may be prone to drug-induced respiratory depression. Consideration should be given to premedicating these patients with histamine H_2 antagonists and metoclopramide because of their slowed gastric emptying times. Patients who have been rendered euthyroid may receive their usual dosage of thyroid medication on the morning of surgery; however, most commonly used preparations have long half-lives.

B. Intraoperative: Hypothyroid patients are more susceptible to the hypotensive effect of anesthetic agents because of their diminished cardiac output, blunted baroreceptor reflexes, and decreased intravascular volume. For this reason, ketamine is often recommended for induction of anesthesia. Coexistent primary adrenal insufficiency or congestive heart failure should be considered in cases of refractory hypotension. Decreased cardiac output may speed the rate of induction with an inhalational anesthetic, but hypothyroidism does not significantly decrease minimum alveolar concentration. Other potential problems include difficulty during intubation due to a large tongue, hypothermia from decreased basal metabolic rate, hypoglycemia, and hyponatremia.

C. Postoperative: Recovery from general anesthesia may be delayed in hypothyroid patients by slowed drug biotransformation, hypothermia, and respiratory depression. These patients often require prolonged mechanical ventilation.

THE PARATHYROID GLANDS

Physiology

Parathyroid hormone is the principal regulator of calcium homeostasis. It increases serum calcium by promoting bone resorption, limiting renal excretion, and indirectly enhancing gastrointestinal absorption by its effect on vitamin D metabolism. Parathyroid hormone decreases serum phosphate by increasing renal excretion. The effects of parathyroid hormone on calcium serum levels are countered by calcitonin, a hormone excreted by the thyroid (Table 36–5). Ninety-

nine percent of total body calcium is in the skeleton. Of the calcium in the blood, 40% is bound to proteins and 60% is ionized or complexed to organic ions. Unbound, ionized calcium is physiologically more important.

HYPERPARATHYROIDISM

Clinical Manifestations

Causes of **primary hyperparathyroidism** include adenoma, carcinoma, and hyperplasia of the parathyroid gland. **Secondary hyperparathyroidism** is an adaptive response to hypocalcemia produced by diseases such as renal failure or intestinal malabsorption syndromes. **Ectopic hyperparathyroidism** is due to production of a parathyroid hormone-like substance by a carcinoma (eg, hepatoma or bronchogenic carcinoma). Most of the clinical manifestations of hyperparathyroidism are due to hypercalcemia (Table 36–6). Other causes of hypercalcemia include bone metastases, vitamin D intoxication, milk-alkali syndrome, sarcoidosis, and prolonged immobilization (Chapter 28). The treatment of hyperparathyroidism depends upon the cause, but surgical removal of the four glands is usually required.

Anesthetic Considerations

Preoperative evaluation should include an assessment of volume status to avoid hypotension during induction. Hydration with normal saline and diuresis with furosemide usually decreases serum calcium levels to acceptable levels (< 14 mg/dL, 7 meq/L, or 3.5 mmol/L). More aggressive therapy with plicamycin (mithramycin), glucocorticoids, calcitonin, or dialysis may rarely be necessary. Hypoventilation should be avoided, since acidosis increases ionized calcium. Elevated calcium levels can cause cardiac dysrhythmias. The response to muscle relaxants may be altered in patients with preexisting muscle weakness due to the effects of calcium at the neuromuscular junction. Osteoporosis predisposes patients to vertebral compression during laryngoscopy and bone fractures during transport. The postoperative complications of parathyroidectomy are similar to those described above for subtotal thyroidectomy.

Table 36–5. Actions of major calcium-regulating hormones.[1]

	Bone	Kidney	Intestine
Parathyroid hormone (PTH)	Increases resorption of calcium and phosphate	Increases reabsorption of calcium; decreases reabsorption of phosphate; increases conversion of $25OHD_3$ to $1,25(OH)_2D_3$; decreases reabsorption of bicarbonate	No direct effects
Calcitonin (CT)	Decreases resorption of calcium and phosphate	Decreases reabsorption of calcium and phosphate; questionable effect on vitamin D metabolism	No direct effects
Vitamin D	Maintains Ca^{2+} transport system	Decreases reabsorption of calcium	Increases absorption of calcium and phosphate

[1]Reproduced, with permission, from Greenspan FS (editor): *Basic & Clinical Endocrinology*, 3rd ed. Appleton & Lange, 1991.

Table 36–6. Effects of hyperparathyroidism.

Organ System	Clinical Manifestations
Cardiovascular	Hypertension, ventricular dysrhythmias, ECG changes (shortened QT interval)[1]
Renal	Impaired renal concentrating ability, hyperchloremic metabolic acidosis, polyuria, dehydration, polydipsia, renal stones, renal failure
Gastrointestinal	Ileus, nausea and vomiting, peptic ulcer disease, pancreatitis
Musculoskeletal	Muscle weakness, osteoporosis
Neurologic	Mental status changes (delirium, psychosis, coma)

[1]The QT interval may be prolonged at serum calcium levels > 16 mg/dL.

HYPOPARATHYROIDISM

Clinical Manifestations

Hypoparathyroidism is usually due to deficiency of parathyroid hormone following parathyroidectomy. Clinical manifestations of hypoparathyroidism are a result of hypocalcemia (Table 36–7). Other causes of hypocalcemia include renal failure, hypomagnesemia, vitamin D deficiency, and acute pancreatitis (Chapter 28). Hypoalbuminemia decreases total serum calcium (a 1 g/dL drop in serum albumin causes a 0.8 mg/dL fall in total serum calcium), but ionized calcium, the active entity, is unaltered. Neuromuscular irritability can be clinically confirmed by the presence of Chvostek's sign (painful twitching of the facial musculature following tapping over the facial nerve) or Trousseau's sign (carpopedal spasm following inflation of a tourniquet above systolic blood pressure for 3 minutes). These signs are occasionally present in normal individuals. Treatment of symptomatic hypocalcemia consists of intravenous administration of calcium chloride.

Anesthetic Considerations

Serum calcium should be normalized in any patient with cardiac manifestations of hypocalcemia. Anesthetics that depress the myocardium should be avoided in these patients. Alkalosis from hyperventilation or sodium bicarbonate therapy will further decrease ionized calcium. Although citrate-containing blood

Table 36–7. Effects of hypoparathyroidism.

Organ System	Clinical Manifestations
Cardiovascular	Hypotension, congestive heart failure, ECG changes (prolonged QT interval)
Neurologic	Neuromuscular irritability (laryngospasm, inspiratory stridor, tetany, seizures), perioral paresthesia, mental status changes (dementia, depression, psychosis)
Musculoskeletal	Muscle cramps, weakness

products do not usually lower serum calcium significantly, they should not be administered rapidly in patients with preexisting hypocalcemia. Other theoretic considerations include avoidance of 5% albumin solutions (which might bind and lower ionized calcium), the possibility of coagulopathy, and a sensitivity to nondepolarizing muscle relaxants.

THE ADRENAL GLAND

Physiology

The adrenal gland is divided into two parts. The **adrenal cortex** secretes androgens, mineralocorticoids (eg, aldosterone), and glucocorticoids (eg, cortisol). The **adrenal medulla** secretes catecholamines (epinephrine, norepinephrine, and dopamine). The adrenal androgens have insignificant relevance for anesthetic management and will not be considered further.

Aldosterone is chiefly involved with fluid and electrolyte balance. Aldosterone secretion causes sodium to be reabsorbed in the distal renal tubule in exchange for potassium and hydrogen ions. The net effect is an expansion in extracellular fluid volume due to fluid retention, a decrease in plasma potassium, and metabolic alkalosis. Aldosterone secretion is stimulated by the renin-angiotensin system (specifically, angiotensin II), pituitary ACTH, and hyperkalemia. Hypovolemia, hypotension, congestive heart failure, and surgery result in an elevation of aldosterone concentrations.

Glucocorticoids are essential for life and have multiple physiologic effects. Metabolic actions include enhanced gluconeogenesis and inhibition of peripheral glucose utilization. These anti-insulin effects tend to raise blood glucose and worsen diabetic control. Glucocorticoids are required for vascular and bronchial smooth muscle to be responsive to catecholamines. Because these hormones are structurally related to aldosterone, they tend to promote sodium retention and potassium excretion (a mineralocorticoid effect). ACTH from the anterior pituitary is the principal regulator of glucocorticoid secretion. Secretion of ACTH and glucocorticoids exhibits a diurnal rhythm, is stimulated by stress, and is inhibited by circulating glucocorticoids. Endogenous production of cortisol, the most important glucocorticoid, averages 20 mg/d.

The structure, biosynthesis, physiologic effects, and metabolism of **catecholamines** are discussed in Chapter 12. Eighty percent of adrenal catecholamine secretion in humans is in the form of epinephrine. Catecholamine release is regulated mainly by cholinergic preganglionic fibers of the sympathetic nervous system that innervate the adrenal medulla. Stimuli include hypotension, hypothermia, hypoglycemia, hypercapnia, hypoxemia, pain, and fear.

MINERALOCORTICOID EXCESS

Clinical Manifestations

Intrinsic hypersecretion of aldosterone by the adrenal cortex (**primary aldosteronism,** or Conn's syndrome) can be due to a unilateral adenoma (aldosteronoma), bilateral hyperplasia, or carcinoma of the adrenal gland. Some diseases stimulate aldosterone secretion by affecting the renin-angiotensin system. For example, congestive heart failure, hepatic cirrhosis with ascites, nephrotic syndrome, and some forms of hypertension (eg, renal artery stenosis) can cause **secondary aldosteronism.** Although both primary and secondary aldosteronism are characterized by increased levels of aldosterone, only the latter is associated with increased renin activity. Clinical manifestations of mineralocorticoid excess include an elevation in blood pressure, hypervolemia, hypokalemia, muscle weakness, and metabolic alkalosis. Prolonged hypokalemia may lead to a renal concentrating defect and polyuria. Alkalosis will lower ionized calcium levels and can cause tetany. Serum sodium is often normal.

Anesthetic Considerations

Fluid and electrolyte disturbances can be corrected preoperatively with supplemental potassium and spironolactone. This aldosterone antagonist is a potassium-sparing diuretic with antihypertensive properties. Intravascular volume can be assessed preoperatively by testing for orthostatic hypotension or measuring cardiac filling pressures. However, correction of plasma potassium does not guarantee normal total body potassium.

MINERALOCORTICOID DEFICIENCY

Clinical Manifestations
& Anesthetic Considerations

Atrophy or destruction of both adrenal glands results in a combined deficiency of mineralocorticoids and glucocorticoids (see Glucocorticoid Deficiency, below). Nonetheless, unilateral adrenalectomy, diabetes, or heparin therapy occasionally causes isolated hypoaldosteronism. These patients are hyperkalemic, acidotic, and usually hypotensive (the opposite of mineralocorticoid excess). Preoperative preparation includes treatment with an exogenously administered mineralocorticoid (eg, fludrocortisone).

GLUCOCORTICOID EXCESS

Clinical Manifestations

Glucocorticoid excess may be due to exogenous administration of steroid hormones, intrinsic hyperfunction of the adrenal cortex (eg, adrenocortical adenoma), ACTH production by a nonpituitary tumor (ectopic ACTH syndrome), or hypersecretion by a pituitary adenoma (Cushing's disease). Regardless of the cause, an excess of corticosteroids produces **Cushing's syndrome,** characterized by muscle wasting and weakness, osteoporosis, central obesity, abdominal striae, glucose intolerance, hypertension, and mental status changes.

Anesthetic Considerations

Patients with Cushing's syndrome tend to be volume-overloaded and have hypokalemic metabolic alkalosis resulting from the mineralocorticoid activity of glucocorticoids. These abnormalities should be corrected preoperatively with supplemental potassium and spironolactone. Patients with osteoporosis are at risk for fracture during positioning, while preoperative weakness may indicate an increased sensitivity to muscle relaxants. If the cause of Cushing's syndrome is exogenous glucocorticoids, the patient's adrenal glands may not be able to respond to perioperative stresses and supplemental steroids are indicated (see Glucocorticoid Deficiency, below). Likewise, patients undergoing adrenalectomy require intraoperative glucocorticoid replacement (intravenous hydrocortisone succinate, 100 mg every 8 hours). Other complications of adrenalectomy include significant blood loss during resection of a highly vascularized tumor and unintentional penetration of the pleura, causing pneumothorax.

GLUCOCORTICOID DEFICIENCY

Clinical Manifestations

Primary adrenal insufficiency (Addison's disease) is caused by destruction of the adrenal gland, which results in a combined mineralocorticoid and glucocorticoid deficiency. Clinical manifestations are due to aldosterone deficiency (hyponatremia, hypovolemia, hypotension, hyperkalemia, and metabolic acidosis) and cortisol deficiency (weakness, fatigue, hypoglycemia, hypotension, and weight loss). Etomidate suppresses adrenal function by inhibiting two enzymes that are essential for the production of corticosteroid hormones (Chapter 8).

Secondary adrenal insufficiency is a result of inadequate ACTH secretion by the pituitary. The most common cause of secondary adrenal insufficiency is iatrogenic administration of exogenous glucocorticoids. Mineralocorticoid secretion is usually adequate in this disease, so that fluid and electrolyte disturbances are usually not present. However, acute adrenal insufficiency (addisonian crisis) can be triggered in steroid-dependent patients who do not receive increased doses during periods of stress (eg, infection, trauma, or surgery). The clinical features of this medical emergency include circulatory collapse, fever, hypoglycemia, and depressed mentation.

Anesthetic Considerations

The key to the anesthetic management of patients with glucocorticoid deficiency is to ensure adequate steroid replacement therapy during the perioperative period. Because the risk of supplementation is probably quite low, all patients who have received potentially suppressing doses of steroids (ie, the daily equivalent of 5 mg of prednisone) by any route of administration (topical, inhalational, or oral) for a period of more than 1 week any time in the previous 12 months should be considered unable to respond appropriately to surgical stress.

What represents "adequate" steroid coverage is controversial. While adults normally secrete 20 mg of cortisol daily, this may increase to over 300 mg under conditions of maximal stress. Thus, one recommendation is to administer 100 mg of hydrocortisone phosphate every 8 hours beginning the evening before or on the morning of surgery. An alternative low-dose regimen (25 mg of hydrocortisone at the time of induction followed by an infusion of 100 mg during the subsequent 24 hours) achieves plasma cortisol levels equal to or higher than those reported in healthy patients undergoing similar elective surgery. This second regimen might be especially appropriate for diabetic patients, in whom glucocorticoid administration often interferes with control of blood sugar.

CATECHOLAMINE EXCESS

Clinical Manifestations

Pheochromocytoma is a catecholamine-secreting tumor consisting of cells originating from the embryonic neural crest (chromaffin tissue) that accounts for 0.1% of all cases of hypertension. While the tumor is usually benign and localized in a single adrenal gland, 20–30% are either malignant, bilateral, or extra-adrenal. The cardinal manifestations of pheochromocytoma are paroxysmal headache, hypertension, sweating, and palpitations. Unexpected intraoperative hypertension and tachycardia are occasionally the first indications of an undiagnosed pheochromocytoma. The pathophysiology, diagnosis, and treatment of these tumors require an understanding of catecholamine metabolism and of the pharmacology of adrenergic agonists and antagonists (see Chapter 12 Case Discussion).

Anesthetic Considerations

Preoperative assessment should focus on the adequacy of adrenergic blockade and volume replacement. Specifically, resting arterial blood pressure, orthostatic blood pressure and heart rate changes, ventricular ectopy, and electrocardiographic evidence of ischemia should be evaluated. The goal of preoperative sedation is to prevent anxiety-induced release of catecholamines. Potentially life-threatening variations in blood pressure—particularly during induction and manipulation of the tumor—indicate the need for direct arterial pressure monitoring.

Intubation should not be attempted until a deep level of anesthesia has been established. Intraoperative hypertension can be effectively treated with phentolamine or nitroprusside. The latter is favored by some anesthesiologists because of a more rapid onset of action, a shorter duration of action, and increased familiarity with the drug. Hypotension is often treated with phenylephrine. Inadequate intravascular volume, which can be assessed perioperatively with pulmonary artery pressure monitoring, is a common cause of hypotension after tumor removal. Anesthetic drugs or techniques that stimulate the sympathetic nervous system (eg, ephedrine, ketamine, hypercapnia), potentiate the dysrhythmic effects of catecholamines (eg, halothane), inhibit the parasympathetic nervous system (eg, pancuronium), or release histamine (eg, atracurium, morphine sulfate) may precipitate hypertension and are best avoided.

OBESITY

Obesity is arbitrarily defined as an excess of ideal body weight by 20% or more. Ideal body weight, which is determined from actuarial tables, depends upon height, sex, and body frame size. Morbidly obese patients weigh twice as much as their ideal body weight. The body mass index (BMI) is an alternative measure of obesity. For a patient 1.8 meters tall and weighing 70 kg, the BMI would be as shown in the following formula:

$$BMI = \frac{Weight\ (kg)}{Height\ (m)^2} = \frac{70\ kg}{1.8^2} = \frac{70}{3.24} = 21.6\ kg/m^2$$

A BMI greater than 27.5 kg/m^2 is by definition obesity; morbid obesity is by definition a BMI greater than 40 kg/m^2.

Clinical Manifestations

Obesity is associated with many diseases, including type II diabetes mellitus, coronary artery disease, and cholelithiasis. However, even in the absence of obvious coexisting disease, morbid obesity has profound physiologic consequences. Oxygen demand, CO_2 production, and alveolar ventilation are elevated because metabolic rate is proportionate to body weight. Excessive adipose tissue over the thorax decreases chest wall compliance even though lung compliance may remain normal. Increased abdominal mass forces the diaphragm cephalad, yielding lung volumes suggestive of restrictive lung disease. Reductions in lung volumes are accentuated by the supine and Trendelenburg positions. In particular, functional residual capacity may fall below closing capacity. If this occurs, some alveoli will close during normal tidal volumes, causing a ventilation-perfusion mismatch.

While obese patients are often found to be hypoxemic, only a few are hypercapnic. **Pickwickian syndrome** (obesity-hypoventilation syndrome) is a complication of extreme obesity characterized by hypercapnia, cyanosis-induced polycythemia, right-sided heart failure, and somnolence. These patients appear to have blunted respiratory drive and often suffer from obstructive sleep apnea.

The heart is also exposed to an increased work load, since cardiac output and blood volume rise in order to perfuse additional fat stores. The elevation in cardiac output (0.1 L/min/kg of adipose tissue) is achieved through an increase in stroke volume—as opposed to heart rate—and frequently results in arterial hypertension and left ventricular hypertrophy. Elevations in pulmonary blood flow and pulmonary artery vasoconstriction due to persistent hypoxemia can lead to pulmonary hypertension and cor pulmonale.

Obesity is also associated with gastrointestinal pathophysiology, including hiatal hernia, gastroesophageal reflux, poor gastric emptying, and hyperacidic gastric fluid. The extent of fatty infiltration of the liver is often not reflected by abnormalities in liver function tests.

Anesthetic Considerations

A. Preoperative: For the reasons outlined above, obese patients are at an increased risk of developing aspiration pneumonitis. Routine pretreatment with H_2 antagonists and metoclopramide should be considered. Premedication with respiratory depressant drugs must be avoided in patients with evidence of preoperative hypoxemia, hypercapnia, or obstructive sleep apnea. Intramuscular injections are often unreliable owing to the thickness of the overlying adipose tissue.

Preoperative evaluation of morbidly obese patients undergoing major surgery should attempt to assess cardiopulmonary reserve with a chest radiograph, an ECG, arterial blood gases, and pulmonary function tests. Classic physical signs of cardiac failure (eg, sacral edema) may be difficult to identify. Blood pressures must be taken with an appropriately sized cuff (Chapter 6). Intravenous and intra-arterial access sites should be checked in anticipation of technical difficulties. Obscured landmarks, difficult positioning, and extensive layers of adipose tissue may make regional anesthesia impossible using standard equipment and techniques. The airway should receive particular attention, since these patients are often difficult to intubate as a result of limited mobility of the temporomandibular and atlanto-occipital joints, a narrowed upper airway, and a shortened distance between the mandible and sternal fat pads.

B. Intraoperative: Owing to the risk of aspiration, obese patients are usually intubated for all but the shortest of general anesthetics. Furthermore, controlled ventilation with large tidal volumes often provides better oxygenation than shallow, spontaneous respirations. If intubation appears likely to be difficult, keeping the patient awake and intubating with a fiberoptic bronchoscope is strongly recommended. Because breath sounds may be difficult to appreciate, confirmation of tracheal intubation may require detection of end-tidal CO_2. Even controlled ventilation may require relatively high inspired oxygen concentrations to prevent hypoxemia, especially in the lithotomy, Trendelenburg, or prone positions. Subdiaphragmatic

abdominal laparotomy packs may cause further deterioration of pulmonary function and a reduction of arterial blood pressure by impairing venous return. The addition of positive end-expired pressure (PEEP) may worsen pulmonary hypertension in some morbidly obese patients.

Volatile anesthetics may be metabolized more extensively in obese patients. This is of particular concern with respect to the defluorination of methoxyflurane, halothane, and enflurane. Increased metabolism and a predisposition to hypoxia may explain the increased incidence of halothane hepatitis in obese patients. Theoretically, larger fat stores provide an increased volume of distribution for lipid-soluble drugs, which might prolong elimination. However, distribution to the fat tissue group is so slow for volatile anesthetics that increasing the fat "reservoir" has little clinical effect. Water-soluble drugs are not distributed to fat tissue, and if their dosage is based upon weight instead of body surface area, higher peak plasma levels should be expected.

The technical difficulties associated with regional anesthesia have been mentioned. Although dosage requirements for epidural and spinal anesthesia are difficult to predict, obese patients usually require 20–25% less local anesthetic due to epidural fat and distended epidural veins. A high level of blockade can easily result in respiratory compromise. Continuous epidural anesthesia has the advantage of providing pain relief and lessening respiratory complications in the postoperative period.

C. Postoperative: Respiratory failure is the major postoperative problem of morbidly obese patients. The risk of postoperative hypoxemia is increased by preoperative hypoxemia and by surgery involving the thorax or upper abdomen (especially vertical incisions). Extubation should be delayed until the effects of muscle relaxants are completely reversed and the patient is fully awake. An obese patient should remain intubated until there is no doubt that an adequate airway and tidal volume will be maintained. If the patient is extubated in the operating room, supplemental oxygen should be provided during transportation to the recovery room. A 45-degree modified sitting position will "unload" the diaphragm and improve ventilation and oxygenation. The risk of hypoxemia extends for several days into the postoperative period, and providing supplemental oxygen should be routinely considered. Other common postoperative complications in obese patients include wound infection and pulmonary embolism.

CARCINOID SYNDROME

Carcinoid syndrome is the complex of signs and symptoms caused by the secretion of vasoactive substances (eg, serotonin, kallikrein, and histamine) from enterochromaffin tumors (**carcinoid tumors**). Since most of these tumors are located in the gastrointestinal tract, their metabolic products are released into the portal circulation and destroyed by the liver before they can cause systemic effects. However, the products of nonintestinal tumors (eg, pulmonary, ovarian) or hepatic metastases bypass the portal circulation and can cause a variety of clinical manifestations.

Clinical Manifestations

The most common manifestations of carcinoid syndrome are cutaneous flushing, bronchospasm, profuse diarrhea, dramatic swings in arterial blood pressure, and supraventricular dysrhythmias (Table 36–8). Carcinoid syndrome is associated with right-sided heart disease due to valvular and myocardial plaque formation. Lung metabolism of serotonin evidently prevents involvement of the left side of the heart. The diagnosis of carcinoid syndrome is confirmed by detection of serotonin metabolites in the urine (5-hydroxyindole-acetic acid). Treatment varies depending upon tumor location but may include surgical resection, symptomatic relief, or specific serotonin and histamine antagonists.

Anesthetic Considerations

The key to anesthetic management of these patients is to avoid anesthetic techniques or agents that could cause tumor release of vasoactive substances. For example, hypotension, which may itself cause hormone release, should be treated with volume expansion. Catecholamine administration has been associated with kallikrein activation. Regional anesthesia may limit perioperative stress and the subsequent release of vasoactive agents. Clearly, histamine-releasing drugs (eg, morphine, atracurium, tubocurarine) should be avoided. Surgical manipulation of the tumor can cause a massive release of hormones. Monitoring should include an arterial line and central venous or pulmonary artery catheter because of the hemodynamic instability and intrinsic heart disease caused by carcinoid syndrome. Alterations in carbohydrate metabolism may lead to unsuspected hypoglycemia or hyperglycemia. Consultation with an endocrinologist may help clarify the role of antihistamine, antiserotonin drugs (eg, methysergide), or antikallikrein drugs (eg, corticosteroids) in a specific patient.

Table 36–8. Principal mediators of carcinoid syndrome and their clinical manifestations.

Mediator	Clinical Manifestations
Serotonin	Vasoconstriction (coronary artery spasm, hypertension), increased intestinal tone, water and electrolyte imbalance (diarrhea), tryptophan deficiency (hypoproteinemia, pellagra)
Kallikrein	Vasodilatation (hypotension, flushing), bronchoconstriction
Histamine	Vasodilatation (hypotension, flushing), dysrhythmias, bronchoconstriction

CASE DISCUSSION: MULTIPLE ENDOCRINE NEOPLASIA (MEN)

An isolated thyroid nodule is discovered during physical examination of a 36-year-old woman complaining of diarrhea and headaches. Workup of the tumor reveals an elevated calcitonin level, which leads to the diagnosis of medullary cancer, and hypercalcemia. During induction of general anesthesia for total thyroidectomy, the patient's blood pressure rises to 240/140 mm Hg and her heart rate approaches 140 beats/min, with frequent premature ventricular contractions. The surgery is canceled, an arterial line is placed, and the patient is treated with intravenous phentolamine, propranolol, lidocaine, and sodium nitroprusside.

What is the probable cause of this patient's hypertensive crisis during induction of general anesthesia?

Multiple endocrine neoplasia is a group of syndromes characterized by tumor formation in several endocrine organs. MEN type I consists of pancreatic (gastrinomas, insulinomas), pituitary (chromophobes), and parathyroid tumors. MEN type II consists of medullary thyroid carcinoma, pheochromocytoma, and hyperparathyroidism (type IIa) or multiple mucosal neuromas (type IIb or type III). The hypertensive episode in this case may be due to a previously undiagnosed pheochromocytoma. The pheochromocytoma in MEN is often bilateral.

What is calcitonin and why is it associated with medullary cancer?

Calcitonin is a polypeptide manufactured by the parafollicular cells (C cells) in the thyroid gland. It is secreted in response to increases in plasma ionic calcium and tends to lower calcium levels by affecting kidney and bone function. Therefore, it acts as an antagonist of parathyroid hormone.

Why is this patient hypercalcemic if calcitonin lowers serum calcium?

An excess or deficiency of calcitonin has minor effects in humans compared with parathyroid disorders. This patient's hypercalcemia may be due to coexisting primary hyperparathyroidism (MEN type IIa).

Are headache and diarrhea consistent with the diagnosis of multiple endocrine neoplasia?

The history of headaches suggests the possibility of pheochromocytoma, while diarrhea may be due to calcitonin or one of the other peptides often produced by medullary thyroid carcinoma (eg, ACTH, somato-statin, β-endorphin).

What follow-up is required for this patient?

Because of the life-threatening hemodynamic changes associated with pheochromocytoma, this en-tity must be medically controlled before surgery can be considered (see Chapter 12 Case Discussion). Because MEN syndromes are hereditary, family members should be screened for early signs of pheochromocy-toma, thyroid cancer, and hyperparathyroidism.

SUGGESTED READINGS

Brown BR (editor): *Anesthesia and the Patient With Endocrine Disease*. Davis, 1980. Medical, surgical, and anesthetic considerations in endocrine disease. Good chapters on diabetes mellitus and thyroid disease.

Brown BR (editor): *Anesthetics and the Obese Patient*. Davis, 1982. Excellent discussions of the pathophysiology of obesity.

Cooper JR, Brodsky JB: Anesthetic management of the morbidly obese patient. Semin Anesth 1987;6:260.

Greenspan FS (editor): *Basic & Clinical Endocrinology*, 3Rd ed. Appleton & Lange, 1991. Physiology, anatomy, and medical management of endocrine disease.

Hirsch IB et al: Perioperative management of surgical patients with diabetes mellitus. Anesthesiology 1991;74:346. Specific recommendations for perioperative blood glucose management. See editorial in the same issue.

Pullerits F, Balfe JW: Anaesthesia for pheochromocytoma. Can J Anaesth 1988;35:526.

Roizen MF (editor): Anesthesia for patients with endocrine disease. Anesthesiol Clin North Am 1987;5:245. Covers many endocrinopathies, including pheochromocytoma, carcinoid syndrome, and insulinoma. Two chapters review the effects of anesthesia on endocrine function.

Anesthesia for Patients With Neuromuscular Disease

37

Although neuromuscular disorders are relatively uncommon, patients present to the operating room with some regularity for diagnostic studies, for treatment of complications, or for surgical management of unrelated disorders. Diminished respiratory muscle strength and enhanced sensitivity to muscle relaxants predispose these patients to postoperative ventilatory failure. A basic understanding of the major disorders and their potential interaction with anesthetic agents is necessary to avoid postoperative morbidity of this nature.

MYASTHENIA GRAVIS

Myasthenia gravis is characterized by weakness and easy fatigability of skeletal muscle. The incidence of myasthenia is about 1:10,000 and is highest in women during their third decade; in men, it typically presents in the sixth and seventh decades. The weakness is thought to be due to autoimmune destruction or inactivation of postsynaptic acetylcholine receptors at the neuromuscular junction. Antibodies against the acetylcholine receptor in neuromuscular junctions are found in over 80% of patients with myasthenia gravis. Nearly 65% also have a "hyperplastic" thymic gland, while another 10% have thymomas. Other autoimmune disorders (hypothyroidism, hyperthyroidism, rheumatoid arthritis) are present also in 10% of patients.

The course of the disease is marked by exacerbations and remissions. Remissions may be partial or complete. The weakness can be asymmetric, confined to one group of muscles, or generalized. Ocular muscles are most commonly affected, resulting in ptosis and diplopia. With bulbar involvement, laryngeal and pharyngeal muscle weakness can result in dysarthria, difficulty in swallowing, problems clearing secretions, or pulmonary aspiration. Severe disease is usually also associated with proximal muscle weakness (primarily in the neck and shoulders) and involvement of respiratory muscles. Muscle strength characteristically improves with rest but deteriorates rapidly with repeated effort. Infection, stress, surgery, and pregnancy have unpredictable effects on the disease but often lead to exacerbations.

Treatment is with anticholinesterase drugs, immunosuppressants, glucocorticoids, plasmapheresis, and thymectomy. Anticholinesterase drugs are the most commonly used agents. By inhibiting the breakdown of acetylcholine by tissue cholinesterase, they increase the amount of acetylcholine at the neuromuscular junction. Pyridostigmine is the most commonly used agent; when given orally, it has an effective duration of 3–4 hours. Excessive administration of an anticholinesterase may precipitate cholinergic crisis, which is characterized by increased weakness and excessive muscarinic effects, including salivation, diarrhea, miosis, and bradycardia. An edrophonium test can be used to differentiate a cholinergic from a myasthenic crisis. Increased weakness after up to 10 mg of intravenous edrophonium is indicative of cholinergic crisis, whereas increasing strength implies myasthenic crisis. Therapy with immunosuppressants, corticosteroids, and plasmapheresis has had variable results. Thymectomy is usually reserved for patients with generalized weakness and those with a radiographically evident thymic tumor. Up to 80% of patients will show clinical improvement following thymectomy, but improvement may be delayed up to several years.

Anesthetic Considerations

Patients with myasthenia may present for thymectomy or for unrelated surgical or obstetric procedures. In all cases, patients should be under the best possible medical control prior to operation. Patients scheduled for thymectomy often have deteriorating muscle strength, while those undergoing other elective procedures may be well controlled or in remission. Adjustments in anticholinesterase medication, immunosuppressants, or steroid therapy may be necessary. An edrophonium test may be necessary to rule out cholinergic crisis (see above). Management of anticholinesterase therapy in the perioperative period is controversial but should probably be individualized. Potential problems in continuing such therapy include changing patient requirements following surgery, increased vagal reflexes, and the possibility of disrupting bowel anastomoses secondary to hyperperistalsis. Moreover, because these agents also inhibit plasma cholinesterase, they can prolong the duration of ester-type local anesthetics and succinylcholine. Conversely, patients with advanced generalized disease may deteriorate significantly when anticholinesterase agents are withheld.

Preoperative evaluation should focus on the recent course of the disease, the muscle groups affected, drug therapy, and coexisting illnesses. Patients with respiratory muscle or bulbar involvement are at increased risk for pulmonary aspiration. Premedication with metoclopramide or an H_2 blocker may decrease this risk, but supporting studies are lacking in this group of patients. Because some patients with myasthenia are often very sensitive to respiratory depressants, premedication with opioids, benzodiazepines, and similar drugs is usually omitted.

With the exception of muscle relaxants, standard anesthetic agents may be used in patients with myasthenia gravis. Marked respiratory depression, however, may be encountered following even moderate doses of barbiturates or narcotics. A volatile agent-based anesthetic is generally most satisfactory. Deep anesthesia with a volatile agent alone in myasthenics often provides sufficient relaxation for endotracheal intubation as well as most surgical procedures. Muscle relaxants should generally be avoided. The response to succinylcholine is unpredictable. Patients may manifest a relative resistance, a prolonged effect, or an unusual response (phase II block; see Chapter 9). Many patients are exquisitely sensitive to nondepolarizing muscle relaxants. Even a defasciculating dose in some patients can result in nearly complete paralysis. If a muscle relaxant is necessary, small doses of a short-acting nondepolarizing agent (atracurium, vecuronium, or mivacurium) may be preferable. Neuromuscular blockade should be monitored very closely with a nerve stimulator. Ventilatory function should be evaluated carefully prior to extubation. Patients with bulbar involvement may be at greatest risk for postoperative respiratory failure. Disease duration more than 6 years, concomitant pulmonary disease, a vital capacity less than 40 mL/kg, and a pyridostigmine dose greater than 750 mg/d have been suggested as predictive of the need for postoperative ventilation following transsternal thymectomy.

Women with myasthenia can experience increased weakness in the last trimester of pregnancy and the early postpartum period. Epidural anesthesia is generally preferable for these patients because it avoids potential problems with respiratory depression and muscle relaxants during general anesthesia. However, excessively high levels of motor blockade can also result in hypoventilation. Babies of myasthenic mothers may show transient myasthenia for 1–3 weeks, sometimes necessitating controlled mechanical ventilation.

MYASTHENIC SYNDROME

This unusual disorder, also called Eaton-Lambert syndrome, is a paraneoplastic syndrome characterized by proximal muscle weakness that typically affects the lower extremities. The myasthenic syndrome is usually associated with small-cell carcinoma of the lung or, less commonly, other metastatic cancers, sarcoidosis, or autoimmune disorders. In contrast to myasthenia gravis, the muscle weakness improves with repeated effort and is unaffected by anticholinesterase drugs. Guanidine hydrochloride often produces marked improvement. A prejunctional defect in the release of acetylcholine is postulated. Some patients also manifest signs of an autonomic defect, such as orthostatic hypotension, gastroparesis, or urinary retention.

Patients with the myasthenic syndrome are very sensitive to both depolarizing and nondepolarizing muscle relaxants. The response to other drugs used in anesthesia is usually normal. Volatile agents alone are usually sufficient to provide muscle relaxation for both intubation and most surgical procedures. Muscle relaxants should be given only in small increments and with careful neuromuscular monitoring. The management of autonomic defects is discussed in Chapter 27.

MUSCULAR DYSTROPHIES

The muscular dystrophies are a group of hereditary disorders characterized by progressive weakness and degeneration of muscle. Sporadic cases are presumably due to mutations. Duchenne's muscular dystrophy is the most common and most severe form. Other major variants include Becker's, facioscapulohumeral, and limb-girdle dystrophies.

Duchenne's Muscular Dystrophy

Duchenne's muscular dystrophy is an X-linked recessive disorder that affects males almost exclusively. It has an incidence of approximately 1–3 cases per 10,000 live male births and most commonly presents between 3 and 5 years of age. Patients characteristically develop proximal muscle weakness which is manifested as a gait disturbance. Fatty infiltration typically causes enlargement of calf muscles (pseudohypertrophy). Progressive weakness and contractures eventually result in kyphoscoliosis. By age 12, most patients are confined to wheelchairs. Intellectual impairment is common but generally nonprogressive. Plasma creatine kinase (CK) levels are 10–100 times normal even early in the disease and are thought to reflect an abnormal increase in the permeability of muscle cell membranes. Female carriers often also have high plasma CK levels. Plasma myoglobin concentration may also be elevated. The diagnosis is confirmed by muscle biopsy.

Degeneration of the respiratory muscles interferes with an effective coughing mechanism and leads to retention of secretions and frequent pulmonary infections. The combination of marked kyphoscoliosis and muscle wasting produces a severe restrictive ventilatory defect. Pulmonary hypertension is common with disease progression. Degeneration of cardiac muscle is common but results in congestive cardiomyopathy in only 10% of patients. Mitral regurgitation secondary to papillary muscle dysfunction can also be documented in 25% of patients. Electrocardiographic abnormalities include prolongation of the PR interval, QRS and ST segment abnormalities, and prominent R waves over the right precordium with deep Q waves over the left precordium. Atrial arrhythmias are common. Death is usually due to recurrent pulmonary infections and respiratory failure.

Becker's Muscular Dystrophy

This less common disorder (1:30,000 male births) is also an X-linked recessive muscular dystrophy. Its manifestations are virtually identical to those of Duchenne's muscular dystrophy except that they usually present later in life (adolescence) and progress more slowly. Patients often reach the fourth or fifth decade. Death is usually from respiratory complications.

Facioscapulohumeral Dystrophy

Facioscapulohumeral dystrophy is an autosomal dominant variant with an incidence of approximately 1:100,000. It affects males and females with equal frequency. Patients usually present in the second or third decade of life with weakness that is confined chiefly to the muscles of the face and shoulders. Muscles in the lower extremities are less commonly affected. The disease is slowly progressive and has a variable course. Plasma CK levels are usually normal or only slightly elevated. Cardiac involvement is rare, but atrial paralysis has been reported in a few patients. The latter resulted in loss of all atrial electrical activity and an inability to atrially pace the heart; ventricular pacing was still possible. Longevity is minimally affected in most of these patients.

Limb-Girdle Dystrophy

Several variants are classified under this heading. Inheritance is usually autosomal recessive. Most patients present in the second or third decade of life with muscle weakness that may involve the shoulder girdle (Erb's type), the hip girdle (Leyden-Möbius), or both. The disease tends to be very slowly progressive. Plasma CK levels are usually elevated. Cardiac involvement can present as frequent arrhythmias or congestive heart failure but is relatively uncommon. Respiratory complications occur only after long-standing disease (> 30 years).

Anesthetic Considerations

A. Duchenne's and Becker's Muscular Dystrophies: In addition to the muscle weakness, anesthetic management of these patients is complicated by both cardiac and pulmonary manifestations. An association with malignant hyperthermia has been suggested but is controversial. Preoperative premedication is best avoided, because patients may be at increased risk for aspiration from respiratory muscle weakness or gastric hypomotility. Succinylcholine has been used safely in some patients but is best avoided

because of unpredictable responses and the risks of inducing severe hyperkalemia or triggering malignant hyperthermia. Although some patients exhibit a normal response to nondepolarizing muscle relaxants, others may be very sensitive. Marked respiratory and circulatory depression may be seen with volatile anesthetics in patients with advanced disease. Regional or local anesthesia may therefore be preferable in these patients. Respiratory complications are largely responsible for perioperative morbidity. Patients with vital capacities less than 30% of predicted appear to be at greatest risk and often require temporary postoperative mechanical ventilation.

B. Other Forms of Muscular Dystrophy: Patients with facioscapulohumeral and limb-girdle muscular dystrophy generally have normal responses to anesthetic agents. Nonetheless, because of the great variability and overlap between the various forms of muscular dystrophy, nondepolarizing muscle relaxants should be used cautiously while succinylcholine should be avoided (see above).

MYOTONIAS

Myotonic disorders are characterized by sustained contractions of muscles after voluntary or mechanical stimulation. Myotonic contractions often fail to relax even following neural blockade and administration of a nondepolarizing muscle relaxant. These contractions are thought to be a result of increased sodium conductance in the muscle cell membrane or impaired calcium reuptake into the sarcoplasmic reticulum following contraction. Infiltration of the muscle with a local anesthetic often induces relaxation of a myotonic contraction.

Myotonic Muscular Dystrophy

Myotonic muscular dystrophy is the most common form of myotonia (1:10,000). The disease presents in the second or third decade of life and involves skeletal, cardiac, and smooth muscle. Myotonia is the principal manifestation early in the disease, but as the disease slowly progresses, muscle weakness and atrophy become most prominent. Plasma CK levels are usually normal or slightly elevated. Multi-organ dysfunction in some patients is evidenced by presenile cataracts, frontal baldness, hypersomnolence with sleep apnea, or endocrine dysfunction leading to pancreatic, adrenal, thyroid, or gonadal insufficiency. Involvement of respiratory muscles decreases vital capacity. Gastrointestinal hypomotility can predispose to pulmonary aspiration. Uterine atony can prolong labor and increases the incidence of a retained placenta. Cardiac manifestations, which are often present before other clinical symptoms appear, consist of atrial arrhythmias, varying degrees of heart block, and, later in the course of the disease, deteriorating ventricular function. Chronic hypoxemia in some patients may lead to cor pulmonale.

Although treatment of myotonic dystrophy is primarily supportive, phenytoin may be used in some patients to suppress myotonic contractions. Phenytoin does not appear to worsen cardiac conduction abnormalities.

Myotonia Congenita & Paramyotonia Congenita

Less common forms of myotonia include myotonia congenita and paramyotonia. Myotonia congenita is usually manifested early in life and is characterized by frequent generalized myotonic contractions. The disorder is confined to skeletal muscle and produces minimal or no weakness or atrophy. Most patients require antimyotonic therapy with phenytoin, procainamide, or quinine. Cardiac involvement is absent, and patients have a normal life span.

Paramyotonia congenita is a very rare disorder characterized by transient stiffness (myotonia) and weakness after exposure to cold temperatures. Serum potassium concentration may rise following an attack similar to hyperkalemic periodic paralysis (see below).

Anesthetic Considerations

Patients with myotonic muscular dystrophy are at risk for pulmonary aspiration as well as postoperative respiratory and cardiac failure. Patients are often very sensitive to even small doses of opioids and sedatives; premedication should therefore be avoided. Aspiration prophylaxis is also probably indicated (Chapter 15). Regional anesthesia can be employed but does not prevent myotonic contractions. Enhanced respiratory and circulatory depression should be expected during general anesthesia. Even patients without overt muscle weakness may develop cardiac conduction abnormalities perioperatively, perhaps necessitating temporary cardiac pacing. Succinylcholine is contraindicated because it can precipitate intense myotonic contractions; trismus can prevent opening the mouth for intubation, while myotonic contraction of respiratory, chest wall, or laryngeal muscles can make ventilation difficult or impossible. An association between myotonia and malignant hyperthermia has been suggested but is not well established. The response to nondepolarizing muscle relaxants is usually reported to be normal. Nondepolarizing muscle relaxants, however, do not consistently prevent or relieve myotonic contractions. Some reports suggest that reversal of nondepolarizing relaxants can induce myotonic contractions, while others have disputed this observation. The postoperative shivering commonly associated with volatile agents can induce myotonic contractions in the recovery room. Small doses of meperidine can often prevent such shivering and perhaps also the myotonic contractions.

Anesthetic management of patients with myotonia congenita and paramyotonia is complicated only by an abnormal response to depolarizing muscle relaxants (see above), troublesome intraoperative myotonic contractions, and the need to avoid hypothermia. Infiltration of muscles in the operative field with a dilute local anesthetic may alleviate refractory myotonic contractions.

FAMILIAL PERIODIC PARALYSIS

This group of rare disorders is characterized by sudden attacks of transient muscle weakness or paralysis. Symptoms usually begin in childhood. The attacks generally last a few hours and typically spare respiratory muscles. Secondary abnormalities in serum potassium concentration are common and are thought to reflect abnormal sodium and potassium transport across cell membranes. Hypokalemic, hyperkalemic, and normokalemic variants are generally recognized. Muscle strength and serum potassium concentration are usually normal between attacks, though frequent attacks can lead to progressive long-term weakness in some patients. The disorders are generally inherited as autosomal dominant traits.

Hypokalemic Periodic Paralysis

The hypokalemic variant is most common and may be inherited, occur sporadically, or be associated with hyperthyroidism. Up to 10% of hyperthyroid Latin and Oriental men have episodes of hypokalemic periodic paralysis. Attacks are usually characterized by weakness or paralysis of limb muscles and last 3–4 hours; the weakness is typically proximal and may be asymmetric. Rarely, respiratory muscles may be affected. Paralysis can be precipitated by high sodium or carbohydrate loads, exposure to cold temperatures, or rest following intense exercise. Hypokalemia characteristically occurs during the onset of the attack, is often manifested by electrocardiographic changes (Chapter 28), and may precipitate arrhythmias.

Acute attacks are treated with oral or intravenous potassium chloride. Severe attacks require intravenous potassium, 5 meq at a time, administered slowly every 10–15 minutes with electrocardiographic monitoring. Glucose solutions should be avoided, as uptake of glucose by cells can exacerbate the hypokalemia and weakness. Mannitol, 20–25% solutions, may also be given to acutely increase the serum potassium concentration. Chronic acetazolamide therapy is usually effective in preventing attacks. Its efficacy may be related to the metabolic acidosis it produces.

Hyperkalemic & Normokalemic Periodic Paralysis

Patients with these types of periodic paralysis are prone to shorter (1–2 hours) but more frequent attacks. Myotonia is often also a prominent feature. Attacks are most often precipitated by fasting or by rest following exercise. The muscle weakness usually involves limb muscles but can also affect cranial and respiratory muscles. Cardiac arrhythmias can occur during attacks. Some patients have modest hyperkalemia between or during attacks, while others have normal or even low serum potassium during episodes of weakness. Patients are said to have the hyperkalemic variant in the first case and the normokalemic variant in the second. Both groups probably represent the same disorder, because potassium administration precipitates attacks in both.

Glucose administration may hasten recovery following attacks of hyperkalemic and normokalemic periodic paralysis. Most attacks are not severe and do not require additional treatment. For unclear reasons, attacks can be prevented by thiazide diuretic therapy.

Anesthetic Considerations

Regardless of the type of periodic paralysis, anesthetic management of patients with the disorder is directed toward preventing attacks. Careful electrocardiographic monitoring is necessary to detect attacks and arrhythmias during anesthesia. Glucose-containing intravenous fluids should not be used in patients with hypokalemic paralysis, while such solutions may be beneficial for patients with hyperkalemic and normokalemic paralysis (see above). Neuromuscular function should be carefully monitored during general anesthesia. The response to muscle relaxants is unpredictable. Increased sensitivity to nondepolarizing relaxants is especially apt to be encountered in patients with hypokalemic periodic paralysis. Succinylcholine is contraindicated in hyperkalemic paralysis and perhaps other variants as well because of the risk of hyperkalemia. Shivering hypothermia may trigger attacks and should also be avoided.

CASE DISCUSSION: ANESTHESIA FOR MUSCLE BIOPSY

A 16-year-old boy with progressive proximal muscle weakness is suspected of having a primary myopathy and is scheduled for biopsy of the quadriceps muscle.

What other potential abnormalities should concern the anesthesiologist?

The diagnosis of myopathy can be difficult and may include any one of several hereditary, inflammatory, endocrine, metabolic, or toxic disorders. A muscle biopsy may be necessary to supplement clinical, laboratory, nerve conduction, and electromyographic findings and help establish the diagnosis. Although the cause of the myopathy in this case is not yet clear, the clinician must always consider potential problems that can be associated with primary myopathies.

Respiratory muscle involvement should always be suspected in patients with muscle weakness. Pulmonary reserve can be assessed clinically by questions regarding dyspnea and activity level. Pulmonary function tests (Chapter 22) are indicated if significant dyspnea on exertion is present. An increased risk of pulmonary aspiration is suggested by a history of dysphagia, regurgitation, recurrent pulmonary infections, or abdominal distention. Cardiac abnormalities may be manifested as arrhythmias, mitral valve prolapse, or cardiomyopathy. A 12-lead ECG is also helpful in excluding conduction abnormalities. A chest x-ray can evaluate inspiratory effort, the pulmonary parenchyma, and cardiac size; gastric distention secondary to smooth muscle or autonomic dysfunction may also be evident. Preoperative laboratory evaluation should have excluded a metabolic cause with measurement of serum sodium, potassium, magnesium, calcium, and phosphate concentrations. Similarly, thyroid, adrenal, and pituitary disorders should have been excluded. Plasma CK measurement may not be helpful, but very high levels (10 times normal) generally suggest a muscular dystrophy or polymyositis.

What anesthetic technique should be used?

The choice of anesthesia should be based on both patient and surgical requirements. Most muscle biopsies can be performed under local or regional anesthesia with supplemental intravenous sedation using small doses of midazolam. Since most procedures are performed on an outpatient basis, spinal and epidural anesthesia are usually avoided. A femoral nerve block (Chapter 17) can provide excellent anesthesia for biopsy of the quadriceps muscle; a separate injection may be necessary for the lateral femoral cutaneous nerve to anesthetize also the anterolateral thigh. General anesthesia should be reserved for uncooperative patients or for times when local anesthesia proves to be inadequate. The anesthesiologist must therefore always be prepared with a plan for general anesthesia.

What agents may be safely used for general anesthesia?

The same principles discussed in the preceding chapter should be applied. Major goals include preventing pulmonary aspiration, avoiding excessive respiratory or circulatory depression, avoiding muscle relaxants if possible, and perhaps avoiding agents known to trigger malignant hyperthermia. A normal response to a previous general anesthetic in the patient or a family member may be reassuring but does not guarantee the same response this time. General anesthesia may be induced and maintained with a combination of a barbiturate (thiopental or methohexital), benzodiazepine (midazolam), or opioid (alfentanil) and nitrous oxide. Patients at increased risk for aspiration should be intubated (see above). When a muscle relaxant is necessary, a short-acting nondepolarizing agent (atracurium, vecuronium, or mivacurium) should be used. Succinylcholine should generally be avoided because of the unknown risk of an unusual response (myotonic contractions, prolonged duration, or phase II block), inducing severe hyperkalemia, or triggering malignant hyperthermia.

SUGGESTED READINGS

Katz J, Benumof JL, Kadis LB: *Anesthesia and Uncommon Diseases,* 3rd ed. Saunders, 1990.

Pollard BJ, Harrison MJ: *Anaesthesia for Uncommon Disease.* Blackwell, 1989.

Stoelting RK, Dierdorf SF, McCammon RL: *Anesthesia and Co-Existing Disease.* Churchill Livingstone, 1988.

Anesthesia for Ophthalmic Surgery

38

Eye surgery provides several unique challenges for the anesthesiologist, including regulation of intraocular pressure, prevention of the oculocardiac reflex and management of its consequences, control of intraocular gas expansion, and an awareness of potential systemic effects of ophthalmic drugs. An understanding of the mechanisms and management of these potential problems can favorably influence surgical outcome. This chapter also considers specific techniques of general and regional anesthesia in ophthalmic surgery.

INTRAOCULAR PRESSURE DYNAMICS

Physiology of Intraocular Pressure

The eye can be considered as a hollow sphere with a rigid wall. If the contents of the sphere increase, the intraocular pressure (normal: 12–20 mm Hg) must rise. For example, glaucoma is caused by an obstruction to aqueous humor outflow. Similarly, intraocular pressure will rise if the volume of blood within the globe is increased. A rise in venous pressure will increase intraocular pressure by decreasing aqueous drainage and increasing choroidal blood volume. Ex-

treme changes in arterial blood pressure and ventilation can also affect intraocular pressure (Table 38–1). Any anesthetic event that alters these parameters can affect intraocular pressure (eg, laryngoscopy, intubation, airway obstruction, coughing, Trendelenburg position).

Alternatively, decreasing the size of the globe without a proportionate change in the volume of its contents will increase intraocular pressure. Pressure on the eye from a tightly fitted mask, improper prone positioning, or retrobulbar hemorrhage can lead to marked increases in pressure.

Intraocular pressure helps maintain the shape and therefore the optical properties of the eye. Temporary variations in pressure are usually well tolerated in normal eyes. In fact, blinking raises intraocular pressure by 5 mm Hg and squinting by 26 mm Hg. However, even transient episodes of increased intraocular pressure in patients with low ophthalmic artery pressure (eg, deliberate hypotension, arteriosclerotic involvement of the retinal artery) may jeopardize retinal perfusion and cause retinal ischemia.

When the globe is open during certain surgical procedures (Table 38–2) or after traumatic perforation, intraocular pressure approaches atmospheric pressure. Any factor that normally increases intraocular pressure will tend to decrease intraocular volume by causing drainage of aqueous or extrusion of vitreous through the wound. The latter is a serious complication that can permanently worsen vision.

Effect of Anesthetic Drugs on Intraocular Pressure

Most anesthetic drugs either lower or have no effect on intraocular pressure (Table 38–3). Inhalational an-

Table 38–1. The effect of cardiac and respiratory variables on intraocular pressure (IOP).

Variable	Effect on IOP
Central venous pressure Increase Decrease	↑↑↑ ↓↓↓
Arterial blood pressure Increase Decrease	↑ ↓↓
PaCO₂ Increase (hypoventilation) Decrease (hyperventilation)	↑↑ ↓↓
PaO₂ Increase Decrease	0 ↑

Key:
↓ = Decrease (mild, moderate, marked)
↑ = Increase (mild, moderate, marked)
0 = No effect

Table 38–2. "Open eye" surgical procedures.

Cataract extraction
Corneal laceration repair
Corneal transplant (penetrating keratoplasty)
Peripheral iridectomy
Removal of foreign body
Ruptured globe repair
Secondary intraocular lens implant
Trabeculectomy (and other filtering procedures)
Vitrectomy (anterior and posterior)
Wound leak repair

Table 38–3. The effect of anesthetic agents on intraocular pressure (IOP).

Drug	Effect on IOP
Inhalational anesthetics Halothane, enflurane, isoflurane Nitrous oxide	 ↓ ↓ ↓
Intravenous anesthetics Barbiturates Benzodiazepines Ketamine Narcotics	 ↓ ↓ ↓ ↓ ? ↓
Muscle relaxants Depolarizers (succinylcholine) Nondepolarizers	 ↑ ↑ 0 or ↓

Key:
↓ = Decline (mild, moderate)
↑ = Rise (mild, moderate)
0 = No change
? = Conflicting reports

esthetics decrease intraocular pressure in proportion to the depth of anesthesia. The decrease has multiple causes: a drop in blood pressure reduces choroidal volume, relaxation of the extraocular muscles lowers wall tension, and pupillary constriction facilitates aqueous outflow. Intravenous anesthetics also decrease intraocular pressure. A possible exception is ketamine, which raises arterial blood pressure and does not relax extraocular muscles.

Topically administered anticholinergic drugs result in pupillary dilatation (mydriasis), which may precipitate angle-closure glaucoma. However, premedication doses of systemically administered atropine are not associated with intraocular hypertension even in patients with glaucoma. The bulky, quaternary ammonium structure of glycopyrrolate may provide a greater margin of safety.

Succinylcholine increases intraocular pressure by 5–10 mm Hg for 5–10 minutes after administration. The principal mechanism of this rise is prolonged contracture of the extraocular muscles. Unlike other skeletal muscle, extraocular muscles contain cells with multiple neuromuscular junctions. Repeated depolarization of these cells by succinylcholine causes prolonged contracture. The resulting increase in intraocular pressure may have several effects. It will cause spurious measurements of intraocular pressure during examinations under anesthesia in glaucoma patients, potentially leading to unnecessary surgery. Furthermore, a rise in intraocular pressure may cause extrusion of ocular contents through an open surgical or traumatic wound. A final effect of prolonged contracture of the extraocular muscles is an abnormal **forced duction test** for 20 minutes. This maneuver evaluates the cause of extraocular muscle imbalance and may influence the type of strabismus surgery performed. Congestion of choroidal vessels may also contribute to the rise in intraocular pressure. Nondepolarizing muscle relaxants do not increase intraocular pressure.

THE OCULOCARDIAC REFLEX

Traction on extraocular muscles or pressure on the eyeball can elicit cardiac dysrhythmias ranging from bradycardia and ventricular ectopy to sinus arrest or ventricular fibrillation. This reflex consists of a trigeminal afferent (V_1) and a vagal efferent pathway. The oculocardiac reflex is most common in pediatric patients undergoing strabismus surgery. Nonetheless, it can be evoked in all age groups and during a variety of procedures, including cataract extraction, enucleation, and retinal detachment repair.

Anticholinergic medication is often helpful in the prevention of the oculocardiac reflex. Intravenous atropine or glycopyrrolate immediately prior to surgery is more effective than intramuscular premedication. Of course, anticholinergic medications can be hazardous in elderly patients, who often have some degree of coronary artery disease. Retrobulbar blockade or deep inhalational anesthesia may also be of value, but these procedures impose risks of their own. In fact, retrobulbar blockade can elicit the oculocardiac reflex. The need for any routine prophylaxis is controversial.

Management of the oculocardiac reflex when it occurs consists of the following procedures: (1) immediate notification of the surgeon and cessation of stimulation; (2) confirmation of adequate ventilation, oxygenation, and depth of anesthesia; (3) administration of intravenous atropine (10 μg/kg) if the conduction disturbance persists; and (4) in recalcitrant episodes, infiltration of the rectus muscles with local anesthetic. The reflex fatigues ("self-extinguishes") with repeated traction on the extraocular muscles.

INTRAOCULAR GAS EXPANSION

A gas bubble may be injected by the ophthalmologist into the posterior chamber during vitreous surgery. Intravitreal air injection will tend to flatten a detached retina and allow anatomically correct healing. The air bubble is absorbed within 5 days by gradual diffusion through adjacent tissue and into the bloodstream. If the patient is breathing nitrous oxide, the bubble will increase in size. This is because nitrous oxide is 35 times more soluble in blood than nitrogen (Chapter 7). Thus, nitrous oxide tends to diffuse into an air bubble more rapidly than nitrogen (the major component of air) is absorbed by the bloodstream. If the bubble expands after the eye is closed, intraocular pressure will rise.

Sulfur hexafluoride (SF_6) is an inert gas that is less soluble in blood than nitrogen and much less soluble than nitrous oxide. Its longer duration of action (up to 10 days) in comparison with an air bubble can provide an advantage to the ophthalmologist. Bubble size doubles within 24 hours after injection because nitrogen from inhaled air enters the bubble more rapidly than the sulfur hexafluoride diffuses into the bloodstream.

Even so, unless high volumes of pure sulfur hexafluoride are injected, the slow bubble expansion does not usually raise intraocular pressure. However, if the patient is breathing nitrous oxide, the bubble will rapidly increase in size and may lead to intraocular hypertension. A 70% inspired nitrous oxide concentration will almost triple the size of a 1-mL bubble and may double the pressure in a closed eye within 30 minutes. Subsequent discontinuation of nitrous oxide will lead to reabsorption of the bubble, which has become a mixture of nitrous oxide and sulfur hexafluoride. The consequent fall in intraocular pressure may precipitate another retinal detachment.

These complications involving the intraocular expansion of gas bubbles can be avoided *by discontinuing nitrous oxide at least 15 minutes prior to the injection of air or sulfur hexafluoride*. Depth of anesthesia should be maintained by substituting other anesthetic agents. Nitrous oxide should be avoided until the bubble is absorbed (5 days after air and 10 days after sulfur hexafluoride injection).

SYSTEMIC EFFECTS OF OPHTHALMIC DRUGS

Topically applied eye drops are absorbed by vessels in the conjunctival sac and the nasolacrimal duct mucosa. (See Case Discussion, Chapter 11.) One drop (typically 1/20 mL) of 10% **phenylephrine** contains 5 mg of drug. Compare this with the intravenous dose of phenylephrine (0.05–0.1 mg) used to treat an adult patient with hypotension. Topically applied drugs are absorbed at a rate intermediate between absorption following intravenous and subcutaneous injection (toxic subcutaneous dose of phenylephrine = 10 mg). Children and the elderly are at particular risk for the toxic effects of topically applied medications and should only receive 2.5% phenylephrine (Table 38–4). Coincidentally, these patients are the ones most apt to require eye surgery.

Echothiophate is an irreversible cholinesterase inhibitor used in the treatment of glaucoma. Topical application leads to systemic absorption and a reduction in plasma cholinesterase activity. Because succinylcholine is metabolized by this enzyme, echothiophate will prolong succinylcholine's duration of action. However, paralysis usually does not exceed 20 or 30 minutes, and postoperative apnea is unlikely (Chapter 9). The inhibition of cholinesterase activity lasts for 3–7 weeks after discontinuation of echothiophate drops. Muscarinic side effects—such as bradycardia during induction—can be prevented with intravenous anticholinergic drugs (atropine, glycopyrrolate).

Epinephrine eye drops can cause hypertension, tachycardia, and ventricular dysrhythmias. The dysrhythmogenic effects of epinephrine are potentiated by halothane. Direct instillation of epinephrine into the anterior chamber of the eye has not been associated with cardiovascular toxicity.

Timolol, a nonselective β-adrenergic antagonist, reduces intraocular pressure by decreasing aqueous humor production. Topically applied timolol eye drops, commonly used to treat glaucoma, have in rare cases been associated with atropine-resistant bradycardia, hypotension, and bronchospasm during general anesthesia.

Table 38–4. The systemic effects of ophthalmic medications.

Drug	Mechanism of Action	Systemic Effect
Acetylcholine	Cholinergic agonist (miosis)	Bronchospasm, bradycardia, hypotension
Azetazolamide	Carbonic anhydrase inhibitor (decreases IOP)	Diuresis, hypokalemic metabolic acidosis
Atropine	Anticholinergic (mydriasis)	Central anticholinergic syndrome (see Chapter 11 Case Discussion)
Cyclopentolate	Anticholinergic (mydriasis)	Disorientation, psychosis, convulsions
Echothiophate	Cholinesterase inhibitor (miosis, decreases IOP)	Prolongation of succinylcholine paralysis, bronchospasm
Epinephrine	Sympathetic agonist (mydriasis, decreases IOP)	Hypertension, bradycardia, tachycardia, headache
Phenylephrine	Alpha-adrenergic agonist (mydriasis, vasoconstriction)	Hypertension, tachycardia, dysrhythmias
Scopolamine	Anticholinergic (mydriasis, vasoconstriction)	Central anticholinergic syndrome (see Chapter 11 Case Discussion)
Timolol	Beta-adrenergic blocking agent (decreases IOP)	Bradycardia, asthma, congestive heart failure

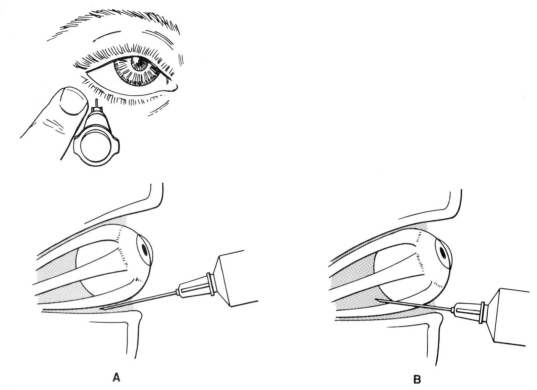

A   B

Figure 38–1. *A:* During administration of a retrobulbar block, the patient looks supranasally as a needle is advanced 1.5 cm along the inferotemporal wall of the orbit. ***B:*** The needle is then redirected upward and nasally toward the apex of the orbit and advanced until its tip penetrates the muscle cone.

TECHNIQUES OF GENERAL ANESTHESIA FOR OPHTHALMIC SURGERY

The choice between general and local anesthesia should be made jointly by the patient, anesthesiologist, and surgeon. Some patients refuse even to discuss local anesthesia. This apprehension is often due to the fear of being awake during a surgical procedure or the recollection of pain during prior regional techniques. Although there is no conclusive evidence that one form of anesthesia is safer than the other, local anesthesia seems to be less stressful. General anesthesia is indicated in uncooperative patients, since even small head movements can prove disastrous during microsurgery. In other patients, local anesthesia is contraindicated for surgical reasons. In any event, a definitive decision must be made. "Local-general anesthesia"—a technique of deep sedation without adequate airway control—should be avoided because it imposes the combined risks of both local and general anesthesia.

PREMEDICATION

Patients undergoing eye surgery may be apprehensive, especially if they have undergone multiple procedures and there is a possibility of permanent blindness. Pediatric patients often have associated congenital disorders (eg, rubella syndrome, Goldenhar's syndrome, Down's syndrome). Adult patients are usually elderly, with a myriad of systemic illnesses (eg, hypertension, diabetes mellitus, and coronary artery disease). All of these factors must be considered in the selection of premedication.

INDUCTION

The choice of induction technique for eye surgery usually depends more on the patient's other medical problems than on the patient's eye disease or the type of surgery contemplated. One exception is the patient with a ruptured globe. The key to inducing anesthesia in a patient with an open eye injury is controlling intraocular pressure with a "smooth induction." Specifically, coughing during intubation must be avoided by achieving a deep level of anesthesia and, most importantly, profound paralysis. The intraocular pressure response to laryngoscopy and endotracheal intubation can be somewhat blunted with intravenous lidocaine (1.5 mg/kg) or fentanyl (3–5 μg/kg). A nondepolarizing muscle relaxant is used instead of succinylcholine because of the latter's influence on intraocular pressure. Most patients with open globe injuries have "full stomachs" and require a modified rapid-sequence induction technique (see Case Discussion).

MONITORING & MAINTENANCE

Eye surgery necessitates positioning the anesthesiologist away from the patient's airway. For this reason, pulse oximetry is mandatory for all ophthalmologic procedures. Continuous monitoring for breathing circuit disconnections or unintentional extubation is also crucial. The possibility of dysrhythmias due to the oculocardiac reflex increases the importance of constantly scrutinizing the electrocardiograph. In contrast to most pediatric surgery, infant body temperature often rises during ophthalmic surgery because of head-to-toe draping and insignificant body surface exposure. End-tidal CO_2 analysis helps to differentiate this from malignant hyperthermia.

The pain and stress evoked by eye surgery are considerably less than during a major intra-abdominal procedure. A lighter level of anesthesia would be satisfactory if the consequences of patient movement were not so catastrophic. The lack of cardiovascular stimulation inherent in most eye procedures combined with the need for adequate anesthetic depth can result in hypotension in elderly individuals. This problem is usually avoided by ensuring adequate intravenous hydration, administering small doses of ephedrine (2–5 mg), or establishing intraoperative paralysis with nondepolarizing muscle relaxants. The latter allows maintenance of a lighter level of anesthesia.

Emesis due to vagal stimulation is a common postoperative problem, particularly following strabismus surgery. The Valsalva effect and the increase in central venous pressure that accompany vomiting can be detrimental to the surgical result and increase the risk of aspiration. Intraoperative administration of intravenous metoclopramide (10 mg in adults) or small doses of droperidol (20 μg/kg) may be beneficial.

EXTUBATION & EMERGENCE

Modern suture material and wound closure techniques lessen the risk of postoperative wound dehiscence. Nonetheless, most anesthesiologists and ophthalmologists prefer a smooth emergence from general anesthesia. Coughing on the endotracheal tube can be prevented by extubating the patient during a moderately deep level of anesthesia. As the end of the surgical procedure approaches, muscle relaxation is reversed and spontaneous respirations return. Anesthetic agents are left on during suction of the airway. Nitrous oxide is discontinued, and intravenous lidocaine (1.5 mg/kg) can be given to transiently blunt cough reflexes. Extubation proceeds 1–2 minutes after the lidocaine and during spontaneous respiration of 100% oxygen. Proper airway control is crucial until the patient's cough and swallowing reflexes return. Obviously, this technique is not suitable in patients at increased risk for aspiration (see Case Discussion).

Severe postoperative pain is unusual following eye surgery. Scleral buckling procedures, enucleation, and ruptured globe repair are the most painful operations. Small doses of intravenous narcotics (eg, 15–25 mg of meperidine for an adult) are usually sufficient. Severe pain may signal intraocular hypertension, corneal abrasion, or other surgical complications.

TECHNIQUES OF REGIONAL ANESTHESIA FOR OPHTHALMIC SURGERY

Regional anesthesia for eye surgery usually consists of a retrobulbar block, a facial nerve block, and intravenous sedation. While less invasive than general anesthesia with endotracheal intubation, local anesthesia is not without possible complications. Additionally, the block may not provide adequate akinesia or analgesia of the eye, or the patient may be unable to lie perfectly still for the duration of the surgery. For these reasons, equipment and personnel required to treat the complications of local anesthesia and to induce general anesthesia must be readily available. Formerly, the term "local-standby" described the anesthesiologist's role in these cases. However, this term has been replaced by **"monitored anesthesia care,"** since the anesthesiologist should be continually monitoring the patient during surgery and not just "standing by."

RETROBULBAR BLOCKADE

In this technique, local anesthetic is injected behind the eye into the cone formed by the extraocular muscles (Figure 38–1). A blunt-tipped 25-gauge needle penetrates the lower lid at the junction of the middle and lateral one-third of the orbit (usually 0.5 cm medial to the lateral canthus). The patient is instructed to stare supranasally as the needle is advanced 3.5 cm toward the apex of the muscle cone. After aspiration to preclude intravascular injection, 2–5 mL of local anesthetic are injected and the needle is removed. Choice of local anesthetic varies, but lidocaine and bupivacaine are most common. Hyaluronidase, a hydrolyzer of connective tissue polysaccharides, is frequently added to enhance the retrobulbar spread of the local anesthetic.

Complications of retrobulbar injection of local anesthetics include retrobulbar hemorrhage, globe perforation, optic nerve atrophy, frank convulsions, oculocardiac reflex, and respiratory arrest. Forceful injection of local anesthetic into the ophthalmic artery causes retrograde flow toward the brain and may instantaneously result in a seizure. The **post-retrobulbar apnea syndrome** is probably due to injection of local anesthetic into the optic nerve sheath with spread into the cerebrospinal fluid. The central nervous system is exposed to high concentrations of local anesthetic, leading to apprehension and unconsciousness. Apnea occurs within 20 minutes and resolves within an hour. In the meantime, treatment is supportive, with positive-pressure ventilation to prevent hypoxemia, bradycardia, and cardiac arrest. *Adequacy of ventilation must be constantly monitored in patients who have received retrobulbar anesthesia.* Retrobulbar injection is usually not performed in patients with bleeding disorders (due to the risk of retrobulbar hemorrhage), extreme myopia (the longer globe increases the risk of perforation), or an open eye injury (the pressure from injecting fluid behind the eye may cause extrusion of intraocular contents through the wound).

FACIAL NERVE BLOCK

A facial nerve block prevents squinting of the eyelids during surgery and allows placement of a lid speculum. There are several techniques of facial nerve block: van Lint, Nadbath, O'Brien, and Atkinson (Figure 38–2). The major complication of these blocks is subcutaneous hemorrhage.

INTRAVENOUS SEDATION

Several techniques of intravenous sedation have been described for eye surgery. The particular drug employed is less important than the dosage. Deep sedation increases the risk of apnea and unintentional patient movement during surgery. Nonetheless, the retrobulbar and facial nerve blocks can be quite uncomfortable. Some anesthesiologists administer a small dose of a short-acting barbiturate (eg, 10–20 mg of methohexital or 25–75 mg of thiopental) to produce a brief state of unconsciousness during the regional block. Others, feeling that the risks of respiratory arrest and aspiration are unacceptable, limit their doses to provide some relaxation and amnesia. Midazolam (1–3 mg) with or without fentanyl (12.5–25 μg) is a common regimen. Doses vary considerably between patients and should be administered in small increments. Regardless of the technique employed, ventilation and oxygenation must be continuously monitored

(preferably by pulse oximetry), and equipment to provide positive-pressure ventilation must be immediately available.

CASE DISCUSSION: AN APPROACH TO A PATIENT WITH AN OPEN EYE & A FULL STOMACH

A 12-year-old boy presents to the emergency room after being shot in the eye with a pellet gun. A brief examination by the ophthalmologist reveals intraocular contents presenting at the wound. The boy is scheduled for emergency repair of the ruptured globe.

What should be stressed in the preoperative evaluation of this patient?

Aside from taking a routine history and performing a physical examination, one should establish as accurately as possible the time of last oral intake in relation to the injury. The patient must be considered to have a full stomach if the injury occurred within 8 hours after the last meal even if the patient has not eaten for several hours since the injury. This is because gastric emptying is delayed by the pain and anxiety that follows trauma.

What is the significance of a full stomach in a patient with an open globe injury?

Managing patients who have sustained penetrating eye injuries provides a challenge to anesthesiologists because of the need to develop an anesthetic plan that is consistent with at least two conflicting objectives. One obvious objective is to prevent further damage to the eye by avoiding increases in intraocular pressure. A second important objective is to prevent pulmonary aspiration in a patient with a full stomach.

However, many of the common strategies utilized to achieve these objectives are in direct conflict with one another (Tables 38–5 and 38–6). For example, while regional anesthesia (eg, retrobulbar block) minimizes the risk of aspiration pneumonitis, it is contraindicated in patients with penetrating eye injuries because injecting local anesthetic behind the globe increases intraocular pressure and may lead to expulsion of intraocular contents. Therefore, these patients require general anesthesia despite the increased risk of aspiration pneumonitis.

What preoperative preparation should be considered in this patient?

The goal of preoperative preparation is to minimize the risk of aspiration pneumonitis by decreasing gas-

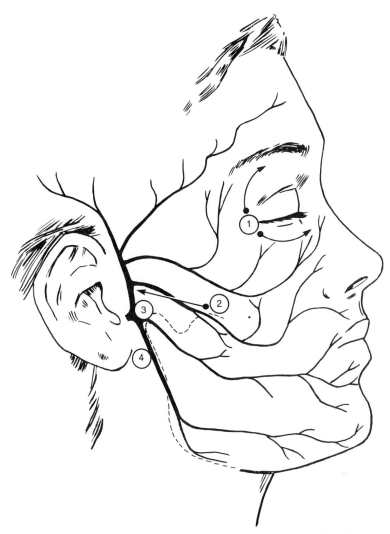

Figure 38–2. There are many techniques of facial nerve block, including (1) van Lint, (2) Atkinson, (3) O'Brien, and (4) Nadbath.

Table 38–5. Strategies to prevent increases in intraocular pressure.

(1) Avoid direct pressure on the globe
    a. Patch eye with Fox shield
    b. No retrobulbar or peribulbar injections
    c. Careful face mask technique
(2) Avoid increases in central venous pressure
    a. Prevent coughing during induction and intubation
    b. Ensure a deep level of anesthesia and relaxation prior to laryngoscopy[1]
    c. Avoid head-down positions
    d. Extubate deep[1]
(3) Avoid pharmacologic agents that increase IOP
    a. Succinylcholine
    b. Ketamine (?)

[1]These strategies are not recommended in patients with full stomachs.

Table 38–6. Strategies to prevent aspiration pneumonitis.

(1) Regional anesthesia with minimal sedation[1]
(2) Premedication
    a. Metoclopramide
    b. Histamine H_2 antagonists
    c. Antacids
(3) Evacuation of gastric contents
    a. Nasogastric tube[1]
(4) Rapid-sequence intubation
    a. Cricoid pressure
    b. A rapid-acting induction agent
    c. Succinylcholine[1]
    d. Avoidance of positive-pressure ventilation
    e. Intubation as soon as possible
(5) Extubation awake

[1]These strategies are not recommended in patients with penetrating eye injuries.

tric volume and acidity. Aspiration in patients with eye injuries is prevented by proper selection of pharmacologic agents and anesthetic techniques. Evacuation of gastric contents with a nasogastric tube may lead to coughing, retching, and other responses that can dramatically increase intraocular pressure.

Metoclopramide increases lower esophageal sphincter tone, speeds gastric emptying, lowers gastric fluid volume, and exerts an antiemetic effect. It should be given intravenously (10–20 mg) as soon as possible and repeated every 2–4 hours until surgery.

Ranitidine (50 mg intravenously) and cimetidine (300 mg intravenously) are H_2 histamine receptor antagonists that inhibit gastric acid secretion. Because they have no effect on the pH of gastric secretions in the stomach prior to their administration, they have limited value in patients presenting for emergency surgery.

Unlike H_2 receptor antagonists, antacids have an immediate effect. Unfortunately, they increase intragastric volume. Nonparticulate antacids (preparations of sodium citrate, potassium citrate, and citric acid) lose effectiveness within 30–60 minutes and should be given immediately prior to induction (15–30 mL orally).

Which induction agents are recommended in patients with penetrating eye injuries?

The ideal induction agent for patients with full stomachs would provide a rapid onset of action in order to minimize the risk of regurgitation. Ketamine, thiopental, propofol, and etomidate have equally rapid onsets of action (ie, one arm-to-brain circulation time).

Furthermore, the ideal induction agent would not increase the risk of ocular expulsion by raising intraocular pressure. In fact, most intravenous induction agents lower intraocular pressure. While investigations of the effects of ketamine on intraocular pressure have provided conflicting results, ketamine is not recommended in penetrating eye injuries owing to the high rate of blepharospasm and nystagmus.

Although etomidate may prove valuable in some patients with cardiac disease, it is associated with an incidence of myoclonus ranging from 10% to 60%. An episode of severe myoclonus perhaps contributed to complete retinal detachment and vitreous prolapse in one patient with an open globe injury and limited cardiovascular reserve.

Propofol and thiopental have a rapid onset of action and decrease intraocular pressure. However, neither prevents the hypertensive response to laryngoscopy and intubation. Similarly, neither prevents the increase in intraocular pressure that accompanies laryngoscopy and intubation. Prior administration of fentanyl (3–5 μg/kg), alfentanil (20 μg/kg), esmolol (0.5–1 mg/kg), or lidocaine (1.5 mg/kg) attenuate this response with varying degrees of success.

How does the choice of muscle relaxant differ in these patients from other patients at risk for aspiration?

The choice of muscle relaxant in patients with penetrating eye injuries has provided controversy for over 3 decades. Succinylcholine definitely increases intraocular pressure. Although there is conflicting research, it is probably most prudent to conclude that this rise in pressure is *not* consistently and reliably prevented by pretreatment with a nondepolarizing agent, "self-taming" doses of succinylcholine, lidocaine, or diazepam. Contradictory findings by various investigators utilizing different regimens are probably due to differences in dosages and timing of the pretreatment drugs.

Some anesthesiologists argue that the relatively small and transient rise in intraocular pressure caused by succinylcholine is insignificant when compared to changes caused by laryngoscopy and intubation. They claim that a slight rise in intraocular pressure is a small price to pay for two distinct advantages that succinylcholine offers: (1) a rapid onset of action that decreases the risk of aspiration, and (2) profound muscle relaxation that decreases the chance of a Valsalva response during intubation. Furthermore, these advocates of succinylcholine usually point to the lack of case reports documenting further eye injury when succinylcholine has been used.

Nondepolarizing muscle relaxants do not increase intraocular pressure. However, currently available nondepolarizing agents do not provide an onset of action as rapid as that achieved with succinylcholine. A slow onset of action increases the time until an endotracheal tube can be placed into the trachea, thus increasing the risk of aspiration. This disadvantage may be partially overcome by administering a large dose, but at the cost of a long duration of action and an increased incidence of side effects. Vecuronium (0.2–0.28 mg/kg) is a good choice of muscle relaxant in this situation owing to its intermediate duration of action and lack of cardiovascular side effects. Regardless of the muscle relaxant chosen, intubation should not be attempted until a level of paralysis is achieved that will definitely prevent coughing on the endotracheal tube.

How do induction strategies vary in pediatric patients?

A hysterical child with a penetrating eye injury and a full stomach provides an anesthetic challenge for which there is no perfect solution. Once again, the dilemma is due to the need to avoid increases in intraocular pressure yet minimize the risk of aspiration. For example, screaming and crying can lead to tremendous increases in intraocular pressure. However, attempting to sedate children with rectal suppositories or intramuscular injections often heightens their state of agitation and may worsen their eye injury. Likewise, although preoperative sedation may increase the risk of aspiration by obtunding airway reflexes, it is often necessary for establishing an intravenous line for a rapid-sequence induction. An ideal strategy would be to painlessly administer enough sedation to allow placement of an intravenous line yet maintain a level of consciousness adequate to protect airway reflexes. While this solution is currently hard to achieve, the introduction of new drugs and innovative delivery systems, such as opioid-containing lollipops, may provide some acceptable alternatives in the near future. In the meantime, the prudent strategy is to do everything possible to avoid aspiration even at the cost of further eye damage.

Are there special considerations during extubation and emergence?

Patients at risk for aspiration during induction are also at risk during extubation and emergence. Therefore, extubation must be delayed until the patient is awake and has intact airway reflexes (eg, spontaneous swallowing and coughing on the endotracheal tube). Deep extubation risks unrecognized vomiting and aspiration. Intraoperative administration of antiemetic medication and nasogastric tube suctioning may decrease the incidence of emesis during emergence, but they do not guarantee an empty stomach.

SUGGESTED READINGS

Bruce RA, McGoldrick KE, Oppenheimer P: *Anesthesia for Ophthalmology.* Aesculapius, 1982. A detailed discussion of all aspects of ophthalmic anesthesia.

Morrison JD, Mirakhur RK, Craig HJL: *Anaesthesia for Eye, Ear, Nose, and Throat Surgery.* Churchill Livingstone, 1985. Chapters 10–15 are a summary of the literature concerning eye anesthesia.

Murphy DF: Anesthesia and intraocular pressure. Anesth Analg 1985;64:520. A comprehensive review article on the determinants of intraocular pressure.

Wolf GL: Anesthesia for ophthalmologic surgery. Lecture 136 in: *37th Annual Refresher Course Lectures.* American Society of Anesthesiologists, 1986. A concise presentation of the major points of interest to the clinical anesthesiologist.

Zahl K, Meltzer MA (editors): Regional anesthesia for intraocular surgery. Ophthalmol Clin North Am 1990;3:No. 1. Contains useful illustrations of technique of retrobulbar blocks.

Anesthesia for the Trauma Patient

Trauma is the leading cause of death in Americans 1–35 years of age. One-third of all hospital admissions in the United States are directly related to trauma. Because many trauma victims require immediate surgery, anesthesiologists can directly affect the survival of these patients. In fact, the role of the anesthesiologist is often that of primary resuscitator, while providing anesthesia becomes a secondary activity. This chapter presents a framework for the initial assessment of the trauma victim and anesthetic considerations in the treatment of patients with injuries of the head and spine, chest, abdomen, and extremities. Burn trauma is the subject of the Case Discussion at the end of the chapter.

INITIAL ASSESSMENT

The initial assessment of the trauma patient can be divided into primary and secondary surveys. The primary survey resembles the sequence suggested for cardiopulmonary resuscitation: *A*irway, *B*reathing, and *C*irculation. If the function of any of these three systems is impaired, resuscitation must be initiated immediately. In critically ill patients, resuscitation and assessment proceed simultaneously by a team of trauma practitioners. The principles of cardiopulmonary resuscitation are presented in detail in Chapter 46. Trauma resuscitation includes two additional phases: control of hemorrhage and definitive repair of the injury. The primary survey is followed by a more comprehensive secondary survey of the patient.

PRIMARY SURVEY

Airway

A cervical spine fracture must be assumed in trauma patients, particularly if there is known injury above the level of the clavicle. To avoid neck hyperextension, the jaw thrust maneuver is the preferred means of establishing an airway. Oral and nasal airways may help maintain airway patency. Cervical spine injury is ruled out by examining a cross-table lateral radiograph and a swimmer's view.

While a simple jaw thrust may alleviate airway obstruction due to unconsciousness (Figure 46–1), a major trauma patient is *always* considered to be at increased risk for aspiration, and the airway must be secured as soon as possible with an endotracheal tube. Neck hyperextension must be avoided during endotracheal intubation if there is any possibility of cervical fracture. For this reason, nasal intubation is usually preferred in the spontaneously breathing patient in whom cervical spine injury is suspected. Oral intubation, with cricoid pressure, is reserved for patients who are apneic, do not have a cervical fracture, or are suspected of having a basilar skull fracture. The cervical spine can also be protected by applying axial traction during laryngoscopy. Patients with evidence of laryngeal fracture (neck crepitations, hematoma, poor phonation) require placement of a tracheostomy instead of endotracheal intubation. If an esophageal obturator has been placed in the field, it should not be removed until the trachea has been intubated because of the likelihood of regurgitation (Chapter 46).

Obstruction due to upper airway trauma often requires an aggressive approach. Facial or neck injuries that preclude endotracheal intubation are indications for emergency cricothyrotomy (see Chapter 5 Case Discussion).

Breathing

Most critically ill trauma patients require assisted— if not controlled—ventilation. Bag-valve devices (self-inflating bag with a nonrebreathing valve) usually provide adequate ventilation immediately after intubation and during periods of patient transport. A 100% oxygen concentration is delivered until oxygenation is assessed by arterial blood gases. If the patient arrives in the operating room already intubated, correct positioning of the endotracheal tube must be reconfirmed. Patients suspected of sustaining head trauma are hyperventilated to decrease intracranial pressure. Ventilation may be compromised by pneumothorax, flail chest, obstruction of the endotracheal tube, or direct pulmonary injury.

Circulation & Fluid Resuscitation

The term **"shock"** denotes circulatory failure leading to inadequate vital organ perfusion and oxygen

Table 39–1. Classification of shock by mechanism and common causes.[1]

Hypovolemic shock
Loss of blood (hemorrhagic shock)
  External hemorrhage
    Trauma
    Gastrointestinal tract bleeding
  Internal hemorrhage
    Hematoma
    Hemothorax or hemoperitoneum
Loss of plasma
  Burns
  Exfoliative dermatitis
Loss of fluid and electrolytes
  External
    Vomiting
    Diarrhea
    Excessive sweating
    Hyperosmolar states (diabetic ketoacidosis, hyperosmolar nonketotic coma)
  Internal ("third-spacing")
    Pancreatitis
    Ascites
    Bowel obstruction
Cardiogenic shock
Dysrhythmia
  Tachyarrhythmia
  Bradyarrhythmia
"Pump failure" (secondary to myocardial infarction or other cardiomyopathy)
Acute valvular dysfunction (especially regurgitant lesions)
Rupture of ventricular septum or free ventricular wall
Obstructive shock
Tension pneumothorax
Pericaridal disease (tamponade, constriction)
Disease of pulmonary vasculature (massive pulmonary emboli, pulmonary hypertension)
Cardiac tumor (atrial myxoma)
Left atrial mural thrombus
Obstructive valvular disease (aortic or mitral stenosis)
Distributive shock
Septic shock
Anaphylactic shock
Neurogenic shock
Vasodilator drugs
Acute adrenal insufficiency

[1]Reproduced, with permission, from Ho MT, Saunders CE: *Current Emergency Diagnosis & Treatment*, 3rd ed. Appleton & Lange, 1990.

delivery. While there are many causes of shock (Table 39–1), in the trauma patient it is usually due to hypovolemia. Physiologic responses to hemorrhage range from tachycardia, poor capillary perfusion, and a decrease in pulse pressure to hypotension, tachypnea, and delirium (Table 39–2). Serum hematocrit and hemoglobin concentrations are not accurate indicators of acute blood loss. The hemodynamic volatility of these patients demands invasive arterial blood pressure monitoring. The degree of hypotension on presentation to the emergency room and operating room correlates strongly with the mortality rate.

Obvious sites of hemorrhage should be identified and controlled with direct pressure on the wound. Occult bleeding in the thorax, abdomen, or extremities is more difficult to assess and manage. Pneumatic anti-shock garments can decrease bleeding in the abdomen and lower extremities, increase peripheral vascular resistance, and augment perfusion of the heart and brain.

The mainstay of therapy of hemorrhagic shock is intravenous fluid resuscitation. Multiple short (1.5–2 inches), large-bore (14–16 gauge, or 7F) catheters are placed in whichever veins are easily accessible. Although central lines may provide useful information regarding volume status, they are time-consuming and introduce the possibility of life-threatening complications (eg, pneumothorax). Peripheral lines are sufficient for initial resuscitation.

Massive hemorrhage depletes the intravascular fluid compartment. Fluid shifts intravascularly from the interstitial compartment to maintain cardiovascular integrity, and interstitial fluid also moves into cells. This intracellular translocation is best explained by a depletion of ATP due to cellular hypoxia (anaerobic metabolism only supplies two ATP moieties per glucose molecule, compared with 36 ATPs from aerobic metabolism). ATP depletion leads to dysfunction of the ATP-dependent Na^+-K^+ pump. The end result is cellular edema.

The choice of initial fluid therapy is determined chiefly by availability. While fully crossmatched whole blood is ideal, typing and crossmatching take time. Type-specific blood may cause minor antibody reactions but is appropriate therapy as soon as it is available. Uncrossed type O-negative packed red blood cells should be reserved for life-threatening blood loss that cannot be adequately replaced by other fluids (ie, exsanguination). Complications associated with massive blood transfusions are discussed in Chapter 29.

Crystalloid solutions are readily available and inexpensive. However, resuscitation requires large quantities because most crystalloid solution does not remain in the intravascular compartment. Lactated Ringer's injection is less likely to cause hyperchloremic acidosis than normal saline, though calcium in the former makes it incompatible with blood transfusions. Dextrose-containing solutions may exacerbate ischemic brain damage and should be avoided in the absence of documented hypoglycemia. Hypertonic solutions such as 7.5% saline may eventually be shown to have a place during emergency resuscitation.

Colloid solutions are much more expensive than crystalloids, but they more effectively restore intravascular volume. Nonetheless, the interstitial fluid deficit associated with hypovolemic shock may be better treated with a crystalloid solution. Albumin is usually selected over dextran or starch solutions because of the fear of inducing a coagulopathy—a problem that has been well documented with dextran solutions.

Whichever fluid is chosen, it must be warmed prior to administration. Rapid infusion systems that use large-bore tubing and rapidly warm fluids can be invaluable during massive transfusions. A warming blanket and heated humidifier will also help maintain body temperature. Hypothermia worsens acid-base disorders, coagulopathies (platelet sequestration and red

Table 39–2. Clinical classification of shock.[1,2]

	Pathophysiology	Clinical Manifestations
Mild (<20% of blood volume lost)	Decreased peripheral perfusion only of organs able to withstand prolonged ischemia (skin, fat, muscle, and bone). Arterial pH normal.	Patient complains of feeling cold. Postural hypotension and tachycardia. Cool, pale, moist skin; collapsed neck veins; concentrated urine.
Moderate (20–40% of blood volume lost)	Decrease central perfusion of organs able to tolerate only brief ischemia (liver, gut, kidneys). Metabolic acidosis present.	Thirst. Supine hypotension and tachycardia (variable). Oliguria or anuria.
Severe (>40% of blood volume lost)	Decreased perfusion of heart and brain. Metabolic acidosis is severe. Respiratory acidosis may also be present.	Agitation, confusion, or obtundation. Supine hypotension and tachycardia are invariably present. Rapid, deep respiration.

[1]Reproduced, with permission, from Ho MT, Saunders CE: *Current Emergency Diagnosis & Treatment,* 3rd ed. Appleton & Lange, 1990.
[2]These clinical findings are most consistently observed in hemorrhagic shock but apply to other types of shock as well.

blood cell deformities), and myocardial function. It also shifts the oxygen-hemoglobin curve to the left and decreases the metabolism of lactate, citrate, and some anesthetic drugs. The amount of fluid administered is based upon improvement of clinical signs, particularly blood pressure, pulse pressure, and heart rate. Central venous pressure and urinary output also provide indications of restoration of vital organ perfusion.

Inadequate organ perfusion interferes with aerobic metabolism and results in lactic acid production and metabolic acidosis. Sodium bicarbonate, which dissociates into bicarbonate ion and CO_2, may temporarily worsen intracellular acidosis because cell membranes are relatively insoluble to bicarbonate compared with CO_2. Acid-base imbalances will eventually resolve with hydration and improved organ perfusion. Lactate will be metabolized in the liver to bicarbonate, and H^+ will be excreted by the kidneys.

Hypotension in patients with hypovolemic shock should be aggressively treated with intravenous fluids, *not* vasopressors. Exceptions to this dictum include coexisting cardiogenic shock (eg, pump damage due to direct myocardial injury), severe hypotension unresponsive to fluid therapy, or cardiac arrest. Some clinicians advocate a low-dose infusion of dopamine (2 μg/kg/min) in an attempt to increase renal blood flow.

Regional anesthesia is usually impractical in hemodynamically unstable patients with life-threatening injuries. If possible, hypovolemia should be corrected prior to induction of general anesthesia. In unstable patients, "anesthesia" may consist primarily of muscle relaxants, with general anesthetic agents titrated as tolerated (mean arterial pressure > 50–60 mm Hg) in an effort to at least provide amnesia. Drugs such as ketamine and nitrous oxide that indirectly stimulate cardiac function in normal patients often display cardiodepressant properties in shock patients who already have maximal sympathetic stimulation. Obviously,

drugs that tend to lower blood pressure (eg, tubocurarine) should be avoided in patients in hypovolemic shock. The rate of rise of alveolar concentration of inhalational anesthetics is greater in shock because of lower cardiac output and increased ventilation (Chapter 7). Higher alveolar anesthetic partial pressures lead to higher arterial partial pressures and greater myocardial depression. Likewise, the effects of intravenous anesthetics are exaggerated since they are injected into a smaller intravascular volume. The key to the safe management of shock patients is to administer small incremental doses of whichever agents are selected.

Shock that is refractory to aggressive fluid therapy may be due to uncontrolled hemorrhage that exceeds the rate of transfusion, cardiogenic shock (eg, pericardial tamponade, myocardial contusion, myocardial infarction), neurogenic shock (eg, brain stem dysfunction, spinal cord transection), septic shock (a late complication), pulmonary failure (eg, pneumothorax, hemothorax), or severe acidosis or hypothermia.

SECONDARY SURVEY

In the secondary survey, the patient is evaluated from head to toe and indicated studies (radiographs, laboratory tests, invasive diagnostic procedures) are obtained. The neurologic examination includes evaluation of consciousness, pupillary signs, motor function, and sensory loss. Fixed dilated pupils do not necessarily imply irreversible brain damage. The patient should be undressed and examined for any hidden injuries. The chest is inspected for fractures and functional integrity (flail chest). Diminished breath sounds may reveal a pneumothorax, which is an indication for chest tube placement. Similarly, distant heart sounds, a narrow pulse pressure, and distended neck veins may signal pericardial tamponade, calling for pericardiocentesis. However, a normal examination does not definitely eliminate the possibility of these problems. Examination of the abdomen should consist of inspection, auscultation, and palpation. Peritoneal lavage may confirm intra-abdominal hemorrhage. The extremities are examined for fractures, dislocations, and peripheral pulses.

ANESTHETIC CONSIDERATIONS PERTAINING TO SPECIFIC ANATOMIC REGIONS

HEAD & SPINAL CORD TRAUMA

Any trauma victim with altered consciousness must be considered to have a brain injury. The level of consciousness is assessed by serial Glasgow Coma Scale evaluations (Table 26–1). Other signs of brain damage include restlessness, convulsions, and cranial nerve dysfunction (eg, nonreactive pupil). The classic Cushing triad (hypertension, bradycardia, and respiratory disturbances) is a late and unreliable sign that usually just precedes brain herniation. Hypotension is rarely due to head injury alone. Patients suspected of sustaining head trauma should not receive any premedication that will alter their mental status (eg, sedatives, analgesics) or neurologic examination (eg, anticholinergic-induced pupillary dilatation).

Brain injuries are often accompanied by increased intracranial pressure due to cerebral hemorrhage or edema. Intracranial hypertension is controlled by a combination of fluid restriction (except in the presence of hypovolemic shock), diuretics (eg, mannitol, 0.5 g/kg), steroids (eg, dexamethasone, 1 mg/kg), barbiturates, and deliberate hypocapnia ($PaCO_2$ of 26–30 mm Hg). The latter requires endotracheal intubation, which also protects against aspiration due to altered airway reflexes. Hypertension or tachycardia during intubation can be attenuated with intravenous lidocaine or fentanyl. Awake intubations cause a precipitous rise in intracranial pressure. Nasal passage of an endotracheal tube or nasogastric tube in patients with basal skull fractures risks cribriform plate perforation and cerebrospinal fluid infection. Slight elevation of the head will improve venous drainage and decrease intracranial pressure. Anesthetic agents that increase intracranial pressure should be avoided (eg, ketamine).

Autoregulation of cerebral blood flow is usually impaired in areas of brain injury. Therefore, arterial hypertension can worsen cerebral edema and increase intracranial pressure. Likewise, episodes of arterial hypotension will cause regional cerebral ischemia. In general, cerebral perfusion pressure (the difference between mean arterial pressure at the level of the brain and the larger of central venous pressure or intracranial

pressure) should be maintained above 50 mm Hg. Deliberate hypocapnia can improve autoregulation.

Severely head-injured patients are more prone to arterial hypoxemia due to pulmonary shunting and ventilation/perfusion mismatching. These changes may be due to aspiration, atelectasis, or direct neural effects on the pulmonary vasculature. Intracranial hypertension may predispose to pulmonary edema due to an increase in sympathetic outflow.

The degree of physiologic derangement following spinal cord injury is proportionate to the height of the lesion. Great care must be taken to prevent further injury during transportation and intubation. Lesions of the cervical spine may involve the phrenic nerves (C3–5), resulting in apnea. Loss of intercostal function limits pulmonary reserve and the ability to cough. High thoracic injuries will eliminate sympathetic innervation of the heart (T1–4), leading to bradycardia. Acute high spinal cord injury can cause **spinal shock,** a condition characterized by loss of sympathetic tone in the capacitance and resistance vessels below the level of the lesion. In fact, venous distention in the legs is a sign of spinal cord injury. Hypotension in these patients requires aggressive fluid therapy tempered by the possibility of pulmonary edema after the acute phase has resolved. Succinylcholine is safe during the first 48 hours following the injury but is associated with life-threatening hyperkalemia afterward. **Autonomic hyperreflexia** is associated with lesions above T5 but is not a problem during acute management.

CHEST TRAUMA

Trauma to the chest may severely compromise the function of the heart or lungs, leading to cardiogenic shock or hypoxia. A **simple pneumothorax** is an accumulation of air between the parietal and visceral pleura. The ipsilateral collapse of lung tissue results in a severe ventilation/perfusion abnormality and hypoxia. The overlying chest wall is hyperresonant to percussion; breath sounds are decreased or absent; and a chest x-ray confirms lung collapse. Nitrous oxide will expand a pneumothorax and is contraindicated in these patients. Treatment includes placement of a chest tube in the fourth or fifth intercostal space, anterior to the midaxillary line. A persistent air leak following chest tube placement may indicate injury to a major bronchus.

A **tension pneumothorax** develops from air entering the pleural space through a one-way valve in the lung or chest wall. In either case, air is forced into the thorax with inspiration but cannot escape during expiration. As a result, the ipsilateral lung completely collapses and the mediastinum and trachea are shifted to the contralateral side. A simple pneumothorax may develop into a tension pneumothorax when positive-pressure ventilation is instituted. Venous return and expansion of the contralateral lung are impaired. Clinical signs include ipsilateral absence of breath sounds and hyperresonance to percussion, contralateral tracheal shift, and distended neck veins. Insertion of a 14-gauge over-the-needle catheter (3–6 cm long) into the second intercostal space at the midclavicular line will convert a tension pneumothorax to an open pneumothorax. Definitive treatment includes chest tube placement as described above.

Multiple rib fractures may compromise the functional integrity of the thorax, resulting in **flail chest.** Hypoxia is often worsened in these patients by underlying pulmonary contusion or hemothorax. **Pulmonary contusion** results in worsening respiratory failure over time. **Hemothorax** is differentiated from pneumothorax by dullness to percussion over silent lung fields.

Cardiac tamponade is a life-threatening chest injury that must be recognized early. The presence of Beck's triad (neck vein distention, hypotension, and muffled heart tones), pulsus paradoxus (a > 10 mm Hg decline in blood pressure during spontaneous inspiration), and a high index of suspicion will help make the diagnosis. Pericardiocentesis provides temporary relief. This is performed by directing a 16-gauge over-the-needle catheter (at least 15 cm long) from the xiphochondral junction toward the tip of the left scapula at a 45-degree angle. Electrocardiographic changes during pericardiocentesis indicate overadvancement of the needle into the myocardium. Definitive treatment of pericardial tamponade requires thoracotomy. Anesthetic management of these patients should maximize cardiac inotropy, chronotropy, and preload. For these reasons, ketamine is a favored induction agent.

Myocardial contusion is usually diagnosed by electrocardiographic changes consistent with ischemia (ST segment elevation) and cardiac enzyme elevations (creatine kinase MB [muscle band] determinations). Patients are at increased risk for dysrhythmias such as heart block and ventricular fibrillation. Elective surgery should be postponed until all signs of heart injury resolve. Other possible chest injuries following trauma include traumatic aortic rupture, valvular disruption, septal rupture, traumatic diaphragmatic herniation, and esophageal rupture.

Adult respiratory distress syndrome (ARDS) is a later pulmonary complication of trauma that has multiple causes: sepsis, direct thoracic injury, aspiration, head injury, fat embolism, massive transfusion, and oxygen toxicity. Clearly, the trauma patient is often at risk for several of these factors. Even with advances in technology, the mortality rate of ARDS approaches 50%.

ABDOMINAL TRAUMA

Intra-abdominal injury is often indicated by the presence of a penetrating wound to the abdomen or lower thorax, paralytic ileus, or peritoneal irritation (eg, muscle guarding or percussion tenderness). The diagnosis may be confirmed by free air on an abdominal x-ray or a bloody aspirate from peritoneal lavage. Management of abdominal trauma usually includes an exploratory laparotomy. Nitrous oxide is avoided to prevent intraoperative bowel distention. A nasogastric tube will help prevent gastric dilatation but should be placed orally if a cribriform plate fracture is suspected. Significant blood replacement should be anticipated, particularly when abdominal trauma is associated with pelvic fractures or retroperitoneal hemorrhage.

EXTREMITY TRAUMA

Extremity injuries can be life-threatening because of associated vascular injuries and secondary infectious complications. Vascular injuries can lead to massive hemorrhage and threaten extremity viability. For example, a femoral fracture can be associated with three units of occult blood loss, and closed pelvic fractures can cause hypovolemic shock. Delay of treatment or indiscriminate positioning can worsen dislocations and further compromise neurovascular bundles. **Fat emboli** are associated with pelvic and long bone fractures and may cause pulmonary insufficiency, dysrhythmias, skin petechiae, and mental deterioration within 1–3 days after the traumatic event. The laboratory diagnosis of fat embolism depends upon elevation of serum lipase, fat in the urine, and thrombocytopenia.

Modern surgical techniques frequently allow the reimplantation of severed extremities and digits. If these are isolated injuries, a regional technique (eg, brachial plexus block) is often recommended to increase peripheral blood flow by interrupting sympathetic innervation. If general anesthesia is chosen, the patient should be kept warm, and emergence shivering must be avoided in order to maximize perfusion.

CASE DISCUSSION: ANESTHETIC MANAGEMENT OF THE BURN PATIENT

A 43-year-old man who suffered a major thermal burn 7 days previously is scheduled for excision and grafting under general anesthesia.

How are burn injuries classified?

Burn injuries are described according to the percentage of body surface area involved and the depth of the skin destroyed. Survival is influenced by the percentage surface area involved and the age of the patient (Figure 39–1). The "rule of nines" divides the body's surface area into areas of 9% or multiples of 9%. For example, in adults the upper extremities and the head

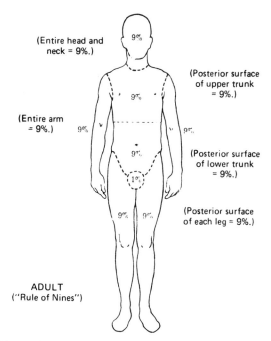

Figure 39–2. Estimation of body surface area in burns. (Reproduced, with permission, from Schroeder SA et al: *Current Medical Diagnosis & Treatment 1991.* Appleton & Lange, 1991.)

are 9% each, while the lower extremities, the front of the chest and abdomen, and the back of the trunk are

each 18% (Figure 39–2). The surface area of one side of the patient's hand represents 1% of total body surface area.

First-degree burns are limited to the epithelium, while second-degree burns extend into the dermis and third-degree burns destroy the entire skin thickness. Since third-degree burns devastate nerve endings, they are not as painful as second-degree burns. A "major" thermal burn is considered to be a second-degree burn involving at least 25% of body surface area or a third-degree burn of at least 10% body surface area. Electrical burns are typically more serious than superficial inspection would indicate because of underlying tissue damage.

How should one describe the pulmonary pathophysiology associated with major burn injuries?

Pulmonary function can be directly or indirectly affected. Direct inhalational injury is usually limited to upper airway edema that can lead to life-threatening airway obstruction. Nonetheless, lower airways can also be subjected to direct thermal insult (eg, steam) or can be injured by exposure to smoke and toxic products of combustion. Indications of inhalational injury include stridor, hoarseness, facial burns, singed nasal hair or eyebrows, soot in sputum or in the oropharynx, respiratory distress, or a history of combustion in a closed space.

Major burns can alter pulmonary function even in the absence of direct lung injury. For example, per-

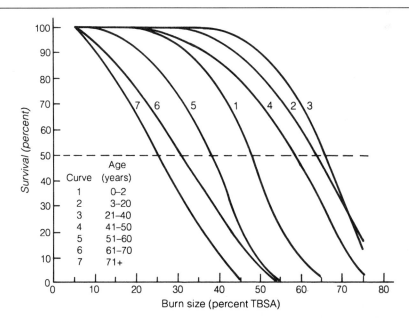

Figure 39–1. Sigmoid curves showing survival of humans as a function of total percentage of body surface burned and age. Survival curves estimated by probit analysis for five different age categories. (Reproduced, with permission, from Merrell SW et al: Increased survival after major thermal injury. Am J Surg 1987;154:623.)

meability can be increased throughout the entire microvascular system and may contribute to the development of pulmonary edema and adult respiratory distress syndrome. Circumferential burns of the thorax may decrease chest wall compliance and further increase peak inspiratory pressures.

Carbon monoxide inhalation shifts the oxygen-hemoglobin curve to the left (interfering with the unloading of oxygen at tissues) and decreases oxyhemoglobin saturation. PaO_2 and skin color may remain normal, but carboxyhemoglobin concentration will be increased. Carbon monoxide has an affinity for hemoglobin 200 times greater than that of oxygen. Administration of 100% oxygen will shorten the half-life of carboxyhemoglobin from 4 hours in room air to less than 1 hour.

Metabolism is markedly increased during the healing phase of a burn injury. This hypermetabolic state is reflected by increased oxygen consumption and CO_2 production. Therefore, alveolar ventilation must be proportionately increased and supplemental oxygen supplied.

What cardiovascular effects are associated with major burn injuries?

Increases in permeability at the site of injury and throughout the microvasculature cause a tremendous shift of fluid from the plasma volume to the interstitial space. Despite red blood cell destruction, hematocrit may rise owing to the contraction of intravascular volume. This decrease in intravascular volume is most pronounced during the first 24 hours and is typically replaced with crystalloid solutions (eg, lactated Ringer's injection, 2–4 mL/kg per percent of body surface burned). Cardiac output declines as a result of the contraction of plasma volume and a circulating myocardial depressant factor. Perfusion of vital organs is monitored by measurement of urinary output through a Foley catheter. If volume replacement does not provide an adequate diuresis (1 mL/kg/h), inotropic support with dopamine may be beneficial.

After 24–48 hours, capillary integrity returns to normal, and colloid solutions will remain intravascular. Interstitial fluid reabsorption, increased metabolic demands, and high levels of circulating catecholamines may lead to high-output failure. Blood pressure and heart rate are typically elevated.

What electrolyte derangements can be found in burn patients?

Hyperkalemia due to tissue destruction may complicate management during the acute resuscitation phase. Later, renal wasting and gastric losses may result in hypokalemia. Topical antibiotic therapy may also cause electrolyte imbalances. Mafenide acetate inhibits carbonic anhydrase, causing hyperchloremic acidosis. Another topical medication, silver nitrate, decreases serum sodium, chloride, and potassium levels. Significant methemoglobinemia is a rare complication

of topical silver nitrate therapy. Electrical burns are associated with such severe muscle cell damage that myoglobinuria can lead to renal failure.

Which monitors would be useful during this excision and grafting procedure?

Excision of dead tissue after a major burn injury is usually associated with significant blood loss. This is especially true if surgery is delayed more than a few days after the burn or if the burn is not limited to areas that can be isolated with tourniquets. In these situations, at least two large-bore intravenous lines, an arterial line, and often a central venous catheter or pulmonary artery catheter are indicated. A central triple-lumen catheter can be helpful in patients with difficult intravenous access. If possible, a noninvasive blood pressure unit should be used as a backup to the arterial line, which may malfunction if the patient is frequently repositioned.

Electrocardiograph skin electrodes will not stick to burned areas, and they interfere with chest wall excision. As an alternative, needle electrodes are often sutured in place. Patients with respiratory insufficiency should be monitored with pulse oximetry if a suitable probe location is available.

Heat loss through denuded skin is a serious problem in the burn patient and should be closely monitored. Hypothermia can be minimized by using warming blankets and heat lamps, increasing operating room temperature, humidification of inspired gases, and warming intravenous fluids.

Are there any special intubation considerations in these patients?

Burn victims with inhalational injury will often be intubated prior to surgery. Indications for early intubation include hypoxemia not correctable with a face mask, upper airway edema that may progress to obstruction, or the presence of copious secretions. Impending airway obstruction or severe facial contractures call for an awake fiberoptic intubation. Precautions to prevent emesis and aspiration should be considered in the acute resuscitation phase, during episodes of sepsis, or if the patient is receiving large doses of narcotics. Tracheostomies have been associated with increased morbidity in burn patients.

How does a burn injury affect the pharmacology of anesthetic drugs?

Succinylcholine is contraindicated in burn patients. Its administration has caused cardiac arrest owing to dramatic increases in serum potassium levels. Prolonged muscle depolarization following succinylcholine appears to be related to an increase in postjunctional acetylcholine receptors. This response has even been documented in patients with less than a 10% body surface area burn. In contrast, burn patients require higher than normal doses of nondepolarizing muscle relaxants. This resistance is due to altered protein binding and an increased number of extrajunctional acetylcholine receptors, which bind nondepolarzing drug without causing a neuromuscular effect.

Volatile anesthetics will exacerbate myocardial depression but are useful after the acute phase. Because of the potential for serious dysrhythmias, halothane is best avoided if epinephrine-soaked bandages are being used to decrease blood loss.

SUGGESTED READINGS

Advanced Trauma Life Support Course for Physicians. American College of Surgeons, 1984. An integral portion of the ATLS course provided by the American College of Surgeons.

Fitch W, Barker J: *Head Injury and the Anaesthetist.* Elsevier, 1985. Reviews all aspects of the head-injured patient, including anesthetic considerations.

Kirby RR, Brown DL: *Anesthesia for Trauma.* Little, Brown, 1987. Includes two chapters on battlefield anesthesia.

Lamb JD: Anesthetic considerations for major thermal injury. Can Anaesth Soc J 1985;32:84.

Martyn JA (editor): *Acute Management of the Burned Patient.* Saunders, 1990.

Shires GT: *Principles of Trauma Care.* McGraw-Hill, 1985. Includes a concise chapter on anesthetic considerations.

Stene JK, Grande CM (editors): *Trauma Anesthesia.* Williams & Wilkins, 1991. Covers all the expected areas and includes an interesting chapter on information management systems.

Walt AJ: *Early Care of the Injured Patient.* Saunders, 1982. Emphasizes surgical considerations.

40

Maternal & Fetal Physiology & Anesthesia

Pregnancy produces profound physiologic changes that alter the usual responses to anesthesia. Moreover, anesthetic care of the pregnant patient is unique in that two patients are cared for simultaneously: the parturient and the fetus. Failure to take these facts into consideration can have disastrous consequences.

This chapter reviews the normal physiologic changes associated with pregnancy, labor, and delivery. Uteroplacental physiology and its response to common anesthetic agents are also discussed. Much of this knowledge forms the basis for current anesthetic practices for labor and delivery (Chapter 41). Lastly, care of the neonate in the obstetric suite or the intensive care unit requires an understanding of the physiologic transition from fetal to neonatal life.

PHYSIOLOGIC CHANGES DURING PREGNANCY

Pregnancy affects virtually every organ system (Table 41–1). Many of these physiologic changes appear to be adaptive and useful to the mother in tolerating the stresses of pregnancy, labor, and delivery. Other changes lack obvious benefits but nonetheless require special consideration in caring for the parturient.

Central Nervous System

The minimal alveolar concentration (MAC) progressively decreases during pregnancy—at term, by as much as 40% for all general anesthetic agents. Changes in maternal hormonal and endogenous opiate levels have been implicated. Progesterone, which is sedating when given in pharmacologic doses, increases up to 20 times normal at term and is probably at least partly responsible for this observation. A surge in β-endorphin levels during labor and delivery is also probably contributory.

At term, pregnant patients also often display enhanced sensitivity to local anesthetics during regional anesthesia. This phenomenon may be partly hormonally mediated but may also be related to engorgement of the epidural venous plexus. Distention of the epidural venous plexus is secondary to partial obstruction of the inferior vena cava by the enlarging uterus. The resulting increase in epidural blood volume has

three major effects: (1) a decrease in spinal cerebrospinal fluid volume, (2) a decrease in the potential volume of the epidural space, and (3) an increase in epidural (space) pressure. The first two effects enhance sensitivity (greater cephalad spread with the same dose) to local anesthetic solutions during spinal and epidural anesthesia, respectively, while the last may predispose to a higher incidence of dural puncture with epidural anesthesia (Chapter 16). Bearing down during labor further accentuates all these effects. Positive epidural pressures have been recorded in parturients and complicate identification of the epidural space without dural puncture. Engorgement of the epidural veins also increases the likelihood of placing an epidural catheter in a vein, resulting in an unintentional intravascular injection (Chapter 16).

Respiratory System

Oxygen consumption and minute ventilation progressively increase during pregnancy. Tidal volume and, to a lesser extent, respiratory rate increase. By

Table 40–1. Physiologic changes associated with pregnancy.

Parameter	Change
Neurologic	
MAC	−40%
Respiratory	
Oxygen consumption	+20%
Minute ventilation	+50%
Tidal volume	+40%
Respiratory rate	+15%
PaO_2	+10%
$PaCO_2$	−15%
HCO_3^-	−15%
FRC	−20%
Cardiovascular	
Blood volume	+35%
Plasma volume	+45%
Cardiac output	+40%
Stroke volume	+30%
Heart rate	+15%
Peripheral resistance	−15%
Hematologic	
Hemoglobin	−20%
Clotting factors	+50–250%
Renal	
GFR	+50%

term, oxygen consumption has increased about 20%, while minute ventilation has increased 50%. $PaCO_2$ decreases to about 32 mm Hg, but respiratory alkalosis is prevented by a compensatory decrease in plasma bicarbonate concentration. Hyperventilation usually also increases PaO_2 slightly. The P-50 (Chapter 22) for hemoglobin increases from 27 to 30 mm Hg. The increase in cardiac output (see below), together with the latter observation, enhances oxygen delivery to tissues.

The maternal respiratory pattern changes as the uterus enlarges. In the third trimester, elevation of the diaphragm is compensated by an increase in the anteroposterior diameter of the chest. Thoracic breathing is favored over abdominal breathing. Both vital capacity and closing capacity are minimally affected, but functional residual capacity decreases up to 20% at term. This decrease is principally due to a reduction in expiratory reserve volume as a result of larger than normal tidal volumes (Chapter 22).

The combination of a decreased functional residual capacity and an increased oxygen consumption leads to rapid oxygen desaturation during periods of apnea (Chapter 22). Preoxygenation prior to induction of general anesthesia is mandatory to avoid hypoxemia in pregnant patients. Closing volume exceeds functional residual capacity in up to half of all pregnant women when they are supine at term. Under these conditions, atelectasis and hypoxemia readily occur. Parturients should not lie flat without supplemental oxygen. Lastly, the decrease in functional residual capacity coupled with the increase in minute ventilation accelerates the uptake of all inhalation anesthetics.

Capillary engorgement of the respiratory mucosa during pregnancy predisposes the upper airways to trauma, bleeding, and obstruction. Gentle laryngoscopy and the use of small endotracheal tubes (6–7 mm) should be employed during general anesthesia.

Cardiovascular System

Cardiac output and blood volume increase to meet accelerated maternal and fetal metabolic demands. An increase in plasma volume in excess of the increase in red cell mass causes a dilutional anemia. Hemoglobin concentration, however, usually remains greater than 11 g/dL. Moreover, in terms of tissue oxygen delivery, the reduction in hemoglobin concentration is offset by the increase in cardiac output and the rightward shift of the hemoglobin dissociation curve (above). A decrease in systemic vascular resistance by the second trimester decreases both diastolic and, to a lesser degree, systolic blood pressure.

At term, maternal blood volume has increased by 1000–1500 mL in most women (about 90 mL/kg blood volume at term), allowing them to easily tolerate the blood loss associated with delivery. The average blood loss during vaginal delivery is 400–500 mL, compared to 800–1000 mL for a cesarean section. Blood volume does not return to normal until 1–2 weeks after delivery.

The increase in cardiac output (40% at term) is due to increases in both heart rate (15%) as well as stroke volume (30%). Most of these effects are observed in the first and, to a lesser extent, the second trimester. In the third trimester, cardiac output does not appreciably rise, except during labor. The greatest increases in cardiac output are seen during labor and immediately after delivery (see below). Cardiac output often does not return to normal until 2 weeks after delivery.

Decreases in cardiac output can occur in the supine position after the 28th week of pregnancy (some authors suggest even earlier). Such decreases have been shown to result from impeded venous return to the heart as the enlarging uterus compresses the inferior vena cava. Up to 15% of women at term develop the **supine hypotension syndrome,** characterized by hypotension associated with pallor, sweating, or nausea and vomiting. The cause of this syndrome appears to be complete or near-complete occlusion of the inferior vena cava by the gravid uterus. Turning the patient on her side typically restores venous return from the lower body and corrects the hypotension in such instances. The gravid uterus also compresses the aorta in most parturients when they are supine. This latter effect decreases blood flow to the lower extremities and, more importantly, the uteroplacental circulation.

Aortocaval compression is an important but preventable cause of fetal distress. The combination of systemic hypotension (due to decreased venous return), increased uterine venous pressure, and uterine arterial hypoperfusion can severely compromise uterine and placental blood flows. When combined with the hypotensive effects of regional or general anesthesia, aortocaval compression can readily produce fetal asphyxia. Parturients with a 28-week or longer gestation should not be placed supine without left uterine displacement. This maneuver is most readily accomplished by placing a wedge (>15 degrees) under the right hip.

Chronic partial caval obstruction in the third trimester predisposes to venous stasis, phlebitis, and edema in the lower extremities. Moreover, compression of the inferior vena cava below the diaphragm distends and increases blood flow through collateral venous drainage, ie, the paravertebral venous plexus (including the epidural veins) and to a minor degree the abdominal wall.

Lastly, elevation of the diaphragm shifts the heart's position in the chest, resulting in the appearance of an enlarged heart on chest x-ray, and a left axis deviation on the ECG. Reversible electrocardiographic changes and a systolic flow murmur (grade I or II) are also common.

The Kidney

Renal plasma flow and the glomerular filtration rate increase as much as 50% during the first trimester and remain elevated thereafter. Serum creatinine and BUN decrease to 0.5–0.6 mg/dL and 8–9 mg/dL, respectively. A decreased renal tubular threshold for glucose and amino acids is common and often results in mild glycosuria (1–10 g/d) or proteinuria (< 300 mg/d).

Gastrointestinal System

Gastroesophageal reflux and esophagitis are common during pregnancy. Upward displacement of the stomach by the uterus promotes incompetence of the gastroesophageal sphincter and retards pyloric emptying. Elevated progesterone levels reduce gastric motility and possibly the tone of the gastroesophageal sphincter, while placental gastrin secretion causes hypersecretion of gastric acid. These factors, together with an increase in intragastric pressure during the last trimester, place the parturient at high risk for regurgitation and pulmonary aspiration. Even worse, nearly all parturients have a gastric pH under 2.5, and over 60% have gastric volumes greater than 25 mL; both factors have been associated with an increased risk for severe aspiration pneumonitis. Narcotics and anticholinergics reduce lower esophageal sphincter pressure and may facilitate gastroesophageal reflux. These physiologic effects together with recent food ingestion just prior to labor and the delayed gastric emptying associated with labor pains predispose parturients to nausea and vomiting.

The Liver

Overall hepatic function and blood flow are unchanged. Elevations in serum alkaline phosphatase are due to its secretion by the placenta. A mild decrease in serum albumin is due to an expanded plasma volume. A 25–30% decrease in serum pseudocholinesterase activity is also present at term but rarely produces significant prolongation of succinylcholine's action. The breakdown of ester-type local anesthetics is not appreciably altered. Pseudocholinesterase activity may not return to normal until up to 6 weeks postpartum.

Hematologic

Pregnancy is associated with a hypercoagulable state that may be beneficial in limiting blood loss at delivery. Fibrinogen and factor VII, VIII, and X concentrations all increase. In addition to the dilutional anemia (above), leukocytosis (up to 21,000/μL) and a 20% decrease in platelet count may be encountered during the third trimester.

Metabolic

Complex metabolic and hormonal changes occur during pregnancy. Altered carbohydrate, fat, and protein metabolism favors fetal growth and development. Elevated levels of human placental lactogen and cortisol are probably responsible for the relative insulin resistance associated with pregnancy. Pancreatic B cell hyperplasia occurs in response to an increased demand for insulin secretion.

THE UTEROPLACENTAL CIRCULATION

A normal uteroplacental circulation (Figure 40–1) is critical in the development and maintenance of a healthy fetus. Uteroplacental insufficiency is an important cause of intrauterine fetal growth retardation and when severe can result in fetal demise. The integrity of this circulation is, in turn, dependent on both adequate uterine blood flow and normal placental function.

Uterine Blood Flow

At term, uterine blood flow represents about 10% of the cardiac output, or 700 mL/min (compared to 50 mL/min in the nonpregnant uterus). Eighty percent of uterine blood flow normally supplies the placenta, while the remainder goes to the myometrium. Pregnancy maximally dilates the uterine vasculature, so that autoregulation is absent. Uterine blood flow is not usually significantly affected by respiratory gas tensions.

Blood flow is directly proportionate to the difference between uterine arterial and venous pressures but inversely proportionate to uterine vascular resistance. Although not under appreciable neural control, the uterine vasculature has an abundant supply of α-adrenergic and some β-adrenergic receptors.

Three major factors decrease uterine blood flow during pregnancy: (1) hypotension, (2) vasoconstriction, and (3) uterine contractions. Hypotension during pregnancy is most commonly caused by aortocaval compression, hypovolemia, or sympathetic blockade as a result of regional anesthesia. Stress-induced release of endogenous catecholamines (sympathoadrenal activation) during labor causes uterine arterial vasoconstriction. Any drug with α-adrenergic activity (phenylephrine) is also capable of decreasing uterine blood flow by vasoconstriction. Ephedrine, which has predominantly β-adrenergic activity, is therefore the vasopressor of choice for hypotension during pregnancy. Paradoxically, hypertensive disorders are often associated with decreased uterine blood flow due to generalized vasoconstriction. Uterine contractions decrease blood flow by elevating uterine venous pressure and, when intense, by compressing arterial vessels as they traverse the myometrium. Hypertonic contractions during labor or during oxytocin infusions can critically compromise uterine blood flow.

Placental Function

The fetus is dependent on the placenta for respiratory gas exchange, nutrition, and waste elimination. The placenta is formed by both maternal and fetal tissues and derives a blood supply from each. The resulting exchange membrane has a functional area of about 1.8 m².

A. Physiologic Anatomy: The placenta (Figure 40–2) is composed of projections of fetal tissue (villi)

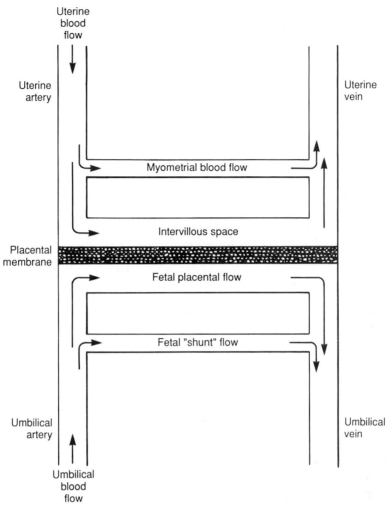

Figure 40–1. The uteroplacental circulation. (Modified and reproduced, with permission, from Schnider S, Levinson G: *Anesthesia for Obstetrics,* 2nd ed. Williams & Wilkins, 1987.)

that lie in maternal vascular spaces (intervillous spaces). As a result of this arrangement, the fetal capillaries within villi are able to exchange substances with the maternal blood that bathes them. Maternal blood in the intervillous spaces is derived from spiral branches of the uterine artery and drains into the uterine veins. Fetal blood within villi is derived from umbilical cord via two umbilical arteries and is returned to the fetus via a single umbilical vein.

B. Placental Exchange: Placental exchange can occur by one of five mechanisms:

1. Diffusion–Respiratory gases and small ions are transported by diffusion. Most drugs used in anesthesia have molecular weights well under 1000 and consequently can diffuse across the placenta. Lipid-soluble agents, such as thiopental, diffuse most rapidly, while highly ionized drugs, such as all the muscle relaxants, diffuse poorly owing to their electri-

cal charge. Drugs that are highly protein-bound, such as bupivacaine, also diffuse poorly across the placenta.

2. Bulk flow–Water moves across by bulk flow.

3. Active transport–Amino acids, vitamins, and some ions (calcium and iron) utilize this mechanism.

4. Pinocytosis–Large molecules such as immunoglobulins are transported by pinocytosis.

5. Breaks–Breaks in the placental membrane and mixing of maternal and fetal blood are probably responsible for Rh sensitization (Chapter 29).

Fetal Oxygen Balance

Of all the substances exchanged across the placenta, oxygen has the lowest storage to utilization ratio. At term, fetal oxygen consumption averages about 21 mL/min, yet fetal oxygen stores are normally estimated to be only 42 mL. Fortunately, because of multiple adaptive mechanisms, the normal fetus at term can

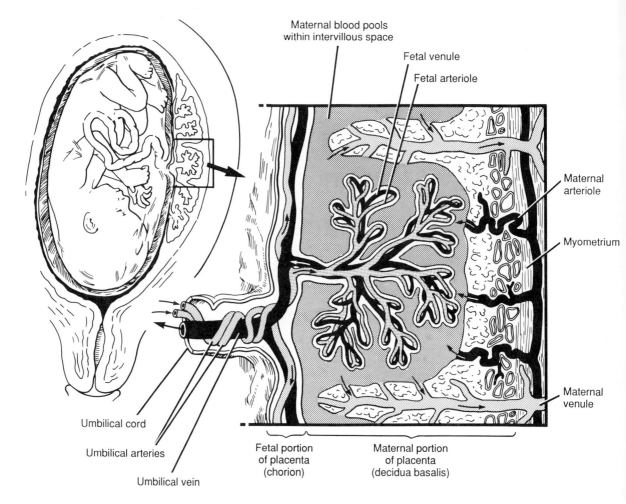

Maternal blood pools
within intervillous space

Fetal venule

Fetal arteriole

Maternal
arteriole

Myometrium

Maternal
venule

Umbilical cord

Umbilical arteries

Umbilical vein

Fetal portion
of placenta
(chorion)

Maternal portion
of placenta
(decidua basalis)

Figure 40–2. The placenta.

survive 10 minutes instead of the expected 2 minutes of total oxygen deprivation. Partial or complete oxygen deprivation can result from umbilical cord compression, umbilical cord prolapse, placental abruption, severe maternal hypoxemia, or hypotension. Compensatory mechanisms include (1) redistribution of blood flow primarily to the brain, heart, and placenta; (2) decreased oxygen consumption; and (3) anaerobic metabolism.

Transfer of oxygen across the placenta is dependent on the ratio of maternal uterine to fetal umbilical blood flows. Animal studies suggest that the reserve for oxygen transfer is small even during normal pregnancy. Well-oxygenated fetal blood from the placenta has a PaO_2 of only 40 mm Hg. To aid oxygen transfer, the fetal hemoglobin oxygen dissociation curve is shifted to the left such that fetal hemoglobin has greater affinity for oxygen compared to maternal hemoglobin (whose curve is already shifted to the right; see above). Additionally, fetal hemoglobin concentration is usually 15 g/dL (compared to approximately 12 g/dL in the mother).

Effect of Anesthetic Agents on Uteroplacental Blood Flow

Intravenous anesthetic agents have variable effects on uteroplacental blood flow. Barbiturates are typically associated with small reductions in uterine blood flow due to mild to moderate, dose-dependent decreases in maternal blood pressure. A small induction dose of a barbiturate, however, can produce greater reductions in blood flow as a result of sympathoadrenal activation (due to light anesthesia). Ketamine does not appreciably alter uteroplacental blood flow; its hypertensive effect typically counteracts any vasoconstriction. The effects of midazolam, propofol, and etomidate on uteroplacental circulation are not well described.

Volatile inhalation anesthetics decrease blood pressure and, consequently, uteroplacental blood flow. In concentrations of less than 1 MAC, however, their effects are generally minor. Halothane and isoflurane may dilate the uterine arteries. Nitrous oxide has minimal effects.

High blood levels of local anesthetics—particularly

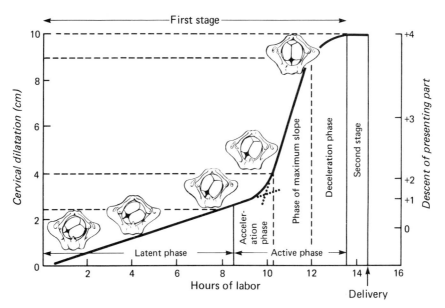

Figure 40–3. The course of normal labor. (Reproduced, with permission, from Pernoll ML, Benson RC [editors]: *Current Obstetric & Gynecologic Diagnosis & Treatment,* 6th ed. Appleton & Lange, 1987.)

lidocaine—cause uterine arterial vasoconstriction. Such levels are seen only with unintentional intravascular injections and occasionally following paracervical blocks (where the injection site is in close proximity to the uterine arteries). Spinal and epidural anesthesia typically do not decrease uterine blood flow provided hypotension is avoided. Moreover, uterine blood flow during labor may actually improve in preeclamptic patients following epidural anesthesia; a reduction in circulating endogenous catecholamines is probably responsible in such instances. The addition of epinephrine to local anesthetic solutions does not appreciably alter uterine blood flow. Intravascular uptake of the epinephrine from the epidural space may result in only minor systemic β-adrenergic effects.

THE PHYSIOLOGY OF NORMAL LABOR

True labor begins when sporadic, haphazard (Braxton Hicks) uterine contractions increase in strength (25–60 mm Hg), coordination, and frequency (15–20 minutes apart). Following progressive cervical dilatation, the contractions propel first the fetus and then the placenta. By convention, labor is divided into three stages: The first stage is defined by the onset of true labor and ends with complete cervical dilatation; the second stage begins with full cervical dilatation, is characterized by fetal descent, and ends with complete delivery of the fetus; the third stage extends from the birth of the baby to the delivery of the placenta.

The first stage is further divided, based on the rate of cervical dilatation, into a slow **latent phase** followed

by a faster **active phase** (Figure 40–3). The latent phase is characterized by progressive cervical effacement and minor dilatation (2–3 cm). The subsequent active phase is characterized by more frequent contractions (3–5 minutes apart) and progressive cervical dilatation up to 10 cm. The first stage usually lasts 10–12 hours in nulliparous patients and about 6–8 hours in multiparous patients.

Contractions during the second stage occur 1.5–2 minutes apart and last 1–1.5 minutes. Although contraction intensity does not appreciably change, the parturient, by bearing down, can greatly augment intrauterine pressure and facilitate expulsion of the fetus. The second stage usually lasts less than 2 hours, while the third stage typically takes 15–30 minutes.

The course of labor is monitored by uterine activity, cervical dilatation, and fetal descent. "Uterine activity" is the frequency of uterine contractions and the pressure they generate within. The latter may be measured directly, with a catheter inserted through the cervix, or indirectly, with a tocodynamometer applied externally around the abdomen. Cervical dilatation and fetal descent are assessed by pelvic examination. Prolongation of the latent phase is most commonly caused by excessive sedation or analgesia, while prolongation of the active phase and the second stage of labor are most often due to cephalopelvic disproportion, fetal malpresentation, or malposition.

Effect of Labor on Maternal Physiology

During intense painful contractions, maternal minute ventilation increases up to 300%. Oxygen consumption also increases another 60% above third-trimester values. With excessive hyperventilation, $PaCO_2$ may fall below 20 mm Hg. Marked hypocapnia can cause hypoventilation and transient maternal and fetal hypoxemia in between contractions.

Each contraction places an additional burden on the heart by displacing 300–500 mL of blood from the uterus into the central circulation (analogous to an autotransfusion). Cardiac output rises 45% over third-trimester values. However, the greatest strain on the heart occurs immediately after delivery, when intense uterine contraction and involution suddenly relieve inferior vena caval obstruction and increase cardiac output as much as 80% above prelabor values.

Effect of Anesthetic Agents on Uterine Activity and Labor

A. Inhalation Agents: Halothane, enflurane, and isoflurane depress uterine activity equally at equipotent doses. All three cause dose-dependent uterine relaxation. Low doses (< 0.5 MAC) of these agents, however, do not interfere with oxytocin's effect on the uterus. Higher doses can result in uterine atony and increase blood loss at delivery. Nitrous oxide has minimal if any effects.

B. Parenteral Agents: Narcotics minimally decrease the progression of labor, while ketamine appears to have little effect.

C. Regional Anesthesia: The effects of regional anesthesia are complex, predominantly indirect, and somewhat controversial. Direct effects are only observed with toxic systemic levels of local anesthetics, which can result in tetanic contractions. Indirect effects relate to the duration of labor and the efficiency of maternal expulsive efforts. The traditional view is that regional anesthesia administered early in the course of labor significantly prolongs it, whereas a regional block given once labor is well established has little effect. Studies suggest that epidural (or spinal) anesthesia up to a T10 sensory level has little effect on labor provided that (1) the parturient is already in the active phase, (2) epinephrine-containing solutions are not used (controversial), and (3) hypotension and aortocaval compression are avoided. Moreover, decreases in uterine activity are said to be readily reversible with an oxytocin infusion.

Controversy exists regarding whether regional anesthesia increases the incidence of low forceps deliveries. Regional anesthesia removes the urge to bear down during the second stage and appears to blunt a reflex increase in endogenous oxytocin levels from distention of the lower birth canal (Ferguson reflex). With proper coaching, the patient who is unable to feel contractions during the second stage can usually expel the fetus without the use of forceps, particularly if more time is allowed for the second stage.

D. Vasopressors: Uterine muscle has both α and β receptors. Alpha$_1$-receptor stimulation causes uterine contraction, while β_2-receptor stimulation produces relaxation. Alpha-adrenergic agents such as methoxamine and phenylephrine, in addition to caus-

ing uterine arterial constriction, can produce tetanic uterine contractions. In contrast, ephedrine appears to have little effect on uterine contractions. The use of epinephrine-containing local anesthetic solutions for epidural anesthesia can theoretically prolong the first stage of labor if absorption of epinephrine from the epidural space results in significant systemic β-adrenergic effects. Although somewhat controversial, prolongation of labor is generally not clinically observed with dilute epinephrine-containing local anesthetics.

FETAL PHYSIOLOGY

Because the placenta is responsible for respiratory gas exchange, the lungs receive little blood flow in the fetus, and the pulmonary and systemic circulations are parallel instead of in series, as in the adult (Figures 40–4 and 40–5). This arrangement is made possible by two cardiac shunts—the foramen ovale and the ductus arteriosus:

(1) Well-oxygenated blood from the placenta mixes with venous blood returning from the lower body and flows via the inferior vena cava into the right atrium.
(2) Right atrial anatomy preferentially directs flow from the inferior vena cava through the foramen ovale into the left atrium.
(3) Left atrial blood is then pumped by the left ventricle to the upper body (mainly the brain and the heart).
(4) Poorly oxygenated blood from the upper body returns via the superior vena cava to the right atrium.
(5) Right atrial anatomy preferentially directs flow from the superior vena cava into the right ventricle
(6) Right ventricular blood is pumped into the pulmonary artery.
(7) Because of high pulmonary vascular resistance, 95% of the flow ejected from the right ventricle is shunted across the ductus arteriosus, into the descending aorta, and back to the placenta and lower body.

The parallel circulation results in unequal ventricular flows; the right ventricle ejects two-thirds of the combined ventricular outputs, while the left ventricle ejects only one-third.

Blood from the placenta is diluted with blood from the lower body and can pass through the liver (via the ductus venosus) before reaching the heart. The latter may be important in allowing relatively rapid hepatic degradation of drugs (or toxins) absorbed from the maternal circulation.

In contrast to the fetal circulation, which is established very early during intrauterine life, maturation of the lungs lags behind. Extrauterine life is not possible until after 24–26 weeks of gestation, when pulmonary capillaries are formed and come to lie in close approximation to an immature alveolar epithelium. At 30

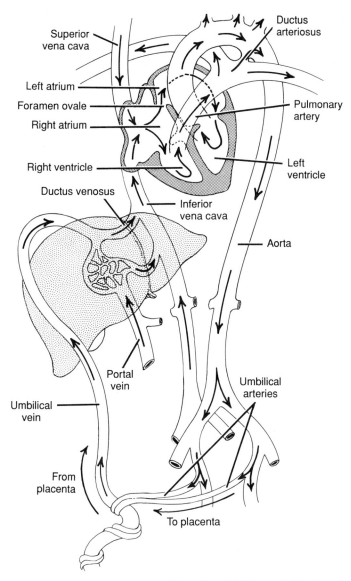

Figure 40–4. The fetal circulation before and after birth. (Reproduced, with permission, from Ganong WF: *Review of Medical Physiology,* 14th ed. Appleton & Lange, 1991.)

weeks, the cuboidal alveolar epithelium flattens out and begins to produce pulmonary surfactant. This substance provides alveolar stability and is necessary to maintain normal lung expansion after birth (Chapter 22). Sufficient pulmonary surfactant is usually present after 34–38 weeks of gestation. Administration of corticosteroids to the mother can accelerate fetal surfactant production.

PHYSIOLOGIC TRANSITION OF THE FETUS AT BIRTH

The most profound adaptive changes at birth involve the circulatory and respiratory systems. Failure to

make this transition successfully results in fetal death or permanent neurologic damage.

At term, the fetal lungs are developed but contain about 90 mL of a plasma ultrafiltrate. During expulsion of the fetus at delivery, this fluid is normally squeezed from the lungs by the forces of the pelvic muscles and the vagina acting on the baby (the vaginal squeeze). Any remaining fluid is reabsorbed by the pulmonary capillaries and lymphatics. Small (preterm) neonates and neonates delivered via cesarean section do not benefit from the "vaginal squeeze" and thus typically have greater difficulty in maintaining respirations (transient tachypnea of the newborn). Respiratory efforts are normally initiated within 30 seconds after birth and become sustained within 90 sec-

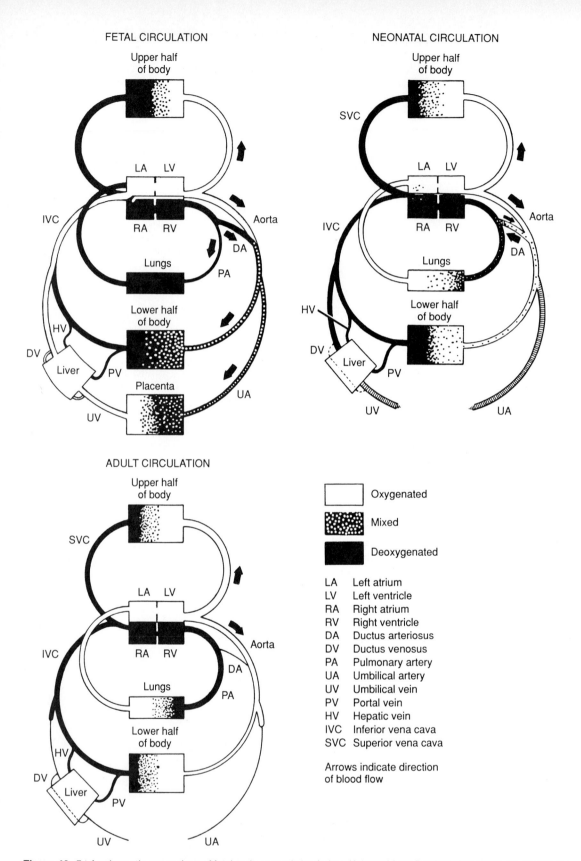

Figure 40–5. A schematic comparison of fetal and neonatal circulation. (Adapted from Danforth DN, Scott JR: *Obstetrics and Gynecology,* 5th ed. Lippincott, 1986.)

onds. Mild hypoxia and acidosis as well as stimulation—cord clamping, pain, touch, and noise—help initiate and sustain respirations, while the outward recoil of the chest at delivery aids in filling the lungs with air.

Lung expansion increases both alveolar and arterial oxygen tensions and decreases pulmonary vascular resistance. The increase in oxygen tension is a potent stimulus for pulmonary arterial vasodilatation. The resultant increase in pulmonary blood flow and augmented flow to the left heart elevates left atrial pressure and functionally closes the foramen ovale. The increase in arterial oxygen tension also causes the ductus arteriosus to contract and functionally close. Other chemical mediators that may play a role in ductal closure include catecholamines, acetylcholine, bradykinin, prostaglandins, and perhaps leukotrienes. The overall result is elimination of right-to-left shunting and establishment of the adult circulation (Figure 40–5). Anatomic closure of the ductus arteriosus does not usually occur until about 2 weeks, while closure of the foramen ovale takes months if it occurs at all.

Hypoxia or acidosis during the first few days of life can prevent or reverse these physiologic changes, resulting in persistence of (or return to) the fetal circulation. A vicious circle is established where the right-to-left shunting promotes hypoxemia and acidosis, which in turn promote more shunting (Figure 40–6). Right-to-left shunting may occur across the foramen ovale, the ductus arteriosus, or both. Unless this circle is broken, neonatal demise can occur rapidly.

CASE DISCUSSION: POSTPARTUM TUBAL LIGATION

A 36-year-old woman is scheduled for bilateral tubal ligation 12 hours after delivery of a healthy baby.

Is this patient still at increased risk for pulmonary aspiration?

Controversy exists over when the increased risk for pulmonary aspiration diminishes following pregnancy. Certainly, many factors contributing to delayed gastric emptying are alleviated shortly after delivery: mechanical distortion of the stomach is relieved, labor pains cease, and the circulating progesterone level rapidly declines. Additionally, a period of 8–12 hours of elective fasting is possible. Some studies suggest that the risk of pulmonary aspiration as judged by gastric volume and gastric fluid pH (see above) normalizes within 24 hours. Unfortunately, even these studies report up to a 30–60% incidence of either a gastric volume greater than 25 mL or a gastric fluid pH less than 2.5. Most clinicians therefore still consider the postpartum patient at increased risk for pulmonary aspiration and take appropriate precautions (Chapters 15 and 41). It is not known when the risk returns to that associated with elective surgical patients. Although some physiologic changes associated with pregnancy may require up to 6 weeks for resolution, the increased risk for pulmonary aspiration probably returns to "normal" well before that time.

Other than aspiration risk, what factors determine the "optimal" time for postpartum sterilization?

The decision when to perform postpartum tubal ligation (or laparoscopic fulguration) is complex and varies according to patient and obstetrician preferences as well as local practices. Additionally, the decision may be based on whether the patient had a vaginal delivery or caesarean section and whether an anesthetic was administered for labor (epidural anesthesia) or delivery (epidural or general anesthesia).

Postpartum tubal ligation (or fulguration) may be performed immediately following delivery of the baby and repair of the uterus during a cesarean section, delayed 8–48 hours following delivery to allow an elective fasting period, or deferred until after the postpartum period (generally 6 weeks). Many obstetricians

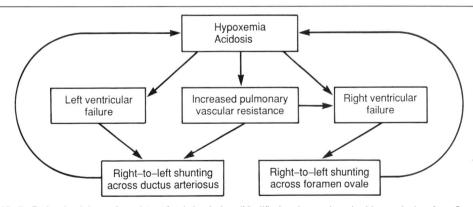

Figure 40–6. Pathophysiology of persistent fetal circulation. (Modified and reproduced, with permission, from Gregory GA: *Pediatric Anesthesia,* 2nd ed. Churchill Livingstone 1989.)

are reluctant to do immediate postpartum sterilizations because the patient may change her mind later, especially if something happens to the baby. Furthermore, they want to ensure that the patient is stable, especially after a complicated delivery. On the other hand, sterilization is technically much easier to perform in the immediate postpartum period because of the enlargement of the uterus and tubes. Moreover, postpartum sterilization saves the patient an additional hospitalization. Postpartum sterilizations following natural vaginal delivery are generally performed within 48 hours of delivery, because bacterial colonization of the reproductive tract thereafter is thought to increase the risk of postoperative infection.

What factors determine selection of an anesthetic technique for postpartum sterilization?

When general or continuous epidural anesthesia is administered for a cesarean section, the same technique can easily be continued for immediate sterilization (provided that the patient is stable). When continuous epidural anesthesia was administered for labor and vaginal delivery, the epidural catheter may be left in place up to 48 hours for subsequent tubal ligation. The delay allows a period of elective fasting (see above). A T4–5 sensory level with regional anesthesia is usually necessary to ensure a pain-free anesthetic experience. Lower sensory levels (as low as T10) may be adequate but sometimes fail to prevent pain during surgical traction on viscera.

When the patient has not had anesthesia for delivery, postpartum sterilization may be performed under either regional or general anesthesia. Because of the increased risk for pulmonary aspiration, regional anesthesia usually is preferred for bilateral tubal ligation via a minilaparotomy. Many clinicians prefer spinal over epidural anesthesia in this setting because of the risk of unintentional intravascular or intrathecal injections with the latter (Chapter 16). Moreover, the risk of a precipitous decrease in blood pressure following spinal anesthesia may be significantly diminished following delivery (especially when preceded by an intravenous fluid bolus). Additionally, the incidence of post-dural puncture headache is as low as 1% when a 25-gauge or smaller needle is used. Dosage requirements for regional anesthesia generally return to normal within 24–36 hours after delivery. Tetracaine, 7–10 mg, bupivacaine, 8–12 mg, or lidocaine, 60–90 mg, may be used for spinal anesthesia. For epidural anesthesia, 15–20 mL of lidocaine 1.5–2%, chloroprocaine 3%, or bupivacaine 0.5% are most commonly used.

In contrast, when laparoscopic tubal fulguration is planned, general endotracheal anesthesia is usually preferred. Insufflation of gas during laparoscopy impairs pulmonary gas exchange and predisposes to nausea, vomiting, and possibly pulmonary aspiration. Endotracheal intubation generally ensures adequate ventilation and protects the airway.

What are important considerations for postpartum patients undergoing general anesthesia?

Preoperative concerns include a decreased blood hemoglobin concentration and the persistent increased risk of pulmonary aspiration (see above). Anemia is nearly always present as a result of the physiologic effects of pregnancy combined with blood loss during and following delivery. Hemoglobin concentrations are usually greater than 9 g/dL, but levels as low as 7 g/dL are generally considered safe. Fortunately, sterilization procedures are rarely associated with significant blood loss.

The risk of pulmonary aspiration is diminished by a minimum of 8 hours of fasting, premedication with an H_2 histamine blocker (ranitidine), a clear antacid (sodium citrate), or metoclopramide (Chapters 15 and 41). Additionally, induction of anesthesia should employ a rapid-sequence technique with cricoid pressure prior to endotracheal intubation, and the patient should be extubated only when she is awake. Decreased plasma cholinesterase levels persist after delivery (see above) and generally prolong the effect of succinylcholine by only 3–5 minutes. High concentrations of volatile agents should be avoided because of the at least theoretic risk of increasing uterine blood loss or inducing postpartum hemorrhage secondary to uterine relaxation. Intravenous narcotics may be used to supplement inhalation agents. Intravenous drugs administered intraoperatively to mothers who are breast feeding appear to have minimal if any effects on their neonates. Nonetheless, it may be prudent to avoid breast feeding 12–24 hours following general anesthesia.

SUGGESTED READINGS

Albright GA: *Anesthesia in Obstetrics,* 2nd ed. Butterworths, 1986.

Creasy RK, Resnik R: *Maternal-Metal Medicine: Principles and Practice.* Saunders, 1984. This text and the next one include good chapters on maternal and fetal physiology.

Danforth DN, Scott JR: *Obstetrics and Gynecology,* 5th ed. Lippincott, 1986.

Ramanathan S: *Obstetric Anesthesia.* Lea & Febiger, 1988.

Shnider S, Levinson G: *Anesthesia for Obstetrics,* 2nd ed. Williams & Wilkins, 1987. The most widely read textbook on obstetric anesthesia.

Obstetric Anesthesia

41

Obstetric anesthesia is a demanding but gratifying subspecialty of anesthesiology. Although most parturients are young and healthy, they nonetheless represent a high-risk group of patients for the reasons discussed in the preceding chapter. This chapter concerns itself with the practice of obstetric anesthesia; techniques for anesthesia during labor, vaginal delivery, and cesarean section are presented, as well as procedures for neonatal resuscitation. The suggested procedures are intended to serve as guidelines consistent with our current understanding of maternal and fetal physiology.

GENERAL APPROACH TO THE OBSTETRIC PATIENT

All patients entering the obstetric suite potentially require anesthesia, whether planned or as an emergency. The anesthesiologist should therefore be aware of the presence and relevant history of all patients in the suite. Pertinent historical items include age, parity, duration of the pregnancy, and any complicating factors. Patients definitely requiring anesthetic care (for labor or cesarean section) should undergo a detailed preanesthetic evaluation (Chapter 1).

All women in true labor should be kept NPO and managed with intravenous fluids (usually lactated Ringer's injection with dextrose) to prevent dehydration. An 18-gauge or larger intravenous catheter should be employed in case rapid transfusion should become necessary. Blood should be sent for typing and screening (Chapter 29). Regardless of the time of last oral intake, all patients are considered to have a full stomach and to be at risk for pulmonary aspiration. Prophylactic administration of a clear antacid (15–30 mL of 0.3-M sodium citrate) every 3 hours should be considered to maintain gastric pH greater than 2.5 and to decrease the likelihood of severe aspiration pneumonitis. An H_2-blocking drug (ranitidine, 100–150 mg) or metoclopramide, 10 mg, should also be considered in patients expected to receive general or regional anesthesia. H_2-blockers reduce both gastric volume and pH but have no effect on the gastric con-

tents already present. Metoclopramide accelerates gastric emptying, decreases gastric volume, and increases lower esophageal sphincter tone. All patients should ideally have a tocodynamometer and fetal heart rate monitor. The supine position should be avoided unless a left uterine displacement device ($>$ 15-degree wedge) is placed under the right hip.

ANESTHESIA FOR LABOR & VAGINAL DELIVERY

PAIN PATHWAYS DURING LABOR

Pain during the first stage of labor is due to uterine contractions and cervical dilatation. Visceral afferent fibers carry these impulses along sympathetic nerves to the spinal cord, where they enter at T10–L1. The onset of perineal pain at the end of the first stage signals the beginning of fetal descent and the second stage of labor. Sensory innervation of the perineum is provided by the pudendal nerve (S2–4). Afferent impulses from all levels ascend in the spinal cord to the brain, where sensations of pain and suffering are perceived (Chapter 18).

PSYCHOLOGIC & NONPHARMACOLOGIC TECHNIQUES

Psychologic and nonpharmacologic techniques are based on the premise that the pain of labor can be suppressed by reorganizing one's thoughts. Patient education and positive conditioning about the birthing process are central to most such techniques. Pain during labor tends to be accentuated by fear of the unknown or previous unpleasant experiences. With the most popular (Lamaze) technique, a deep breath at the beginning of each contraction is followed by rapid shallow breathing for the duration of each contraction. The parturient also concentrates on an object in the room and attempts to focus her thoughts away from the pain. Nonpharmacologic techniques include hypnosis, transcutaneous electrical nerve stimulation, and acupuncture (Chapter 18). The success of all these techniques varies considerably from patient to patient, but most patients require additional forms of pain relief.

PARENTERAL AGENTS

Nearly all narcotic analgesics and sedatives cross the placenta and can have an effect on the fetus. Concern over fetal depression limits the use of these agents to the early stages of labor or to situations in which regional anesthetic techniques are not available. Central nervous system depression in the neonate may be manifested by a prolonged time to sustain respirations, respiratory acidosis, or an abnormal neurobehavioral examination. Moreover, loss of beat-to-beat variability in the fetal heart rate (seen with most central nervous system depressants) complicates the evaluation of fetal well-being during labor (see below). The degree and significance of these effects depend on the specific agent, the dose, the time elapsed between its administration and delivery, and fetal maturity. Premature neonates exhibit the greatest sensitivity.

Meperidine is the most commonly used narcotic and can be given in doses of 10–25 mg intravenously or 25–50 mg intramuscularly, usually up to a total of 100 mg. Maximal maternal and fetal respiratory depression are seen in 10–20 minutes following intravenous administration and in 1–3 hours following administration by the intramuscular route. Consequently, meperidine is usually administered early in labor when delivery is not expected for at least 4 hours. The use of agents with mixed agonist-antagonist activity (butorphanol and nalbuphine) does not appear to be advantageous in avoiding respiratory depression or excessive sedation.

Promethazine (25–50 mg intramuscularly) and **hydroxyzine** (50–100 mg intramuscularly) can be useful alone or in combination with meperidine. Both drugs reduce anxiety, narcotic requirements, and the incidence of nausea and do not add appreciably to neonatal depression. A significant disadvantage of hydroxyzine is pain at the injection site following intramuscular administration.

Diazepam is no longer used during labor because of its potential to cause prolonged neonatal depression, especially in doses higher than 10 mg. Experience with midazolam during labor is limited. The amnestic properties of benzodiazepines makes them undesirable agents for parturients, who usually want to remember the experience of delivery.

Low-dose intravenous **ketamine** is a powerful analgesic. In doses of 10–15 mg intravenously, good analgesia can be obtained in 2–5 minutes without loss of consciousness. Unfortunately, fetal depression may be associated with doses greater than 1 mg/kg. Consequently, low-dose ketamine is most useful just prior to delivery or as an adjuvant to regional anesthesia. Ketamine's reputation for producing hallucinations has recently decreased its popularity.

INHALATION ANALGESIA

This once popular technique involves giving subanesthetic doses of a volatile agent (isoflurane, enflurane, methoxyflurane, or halothane), nitrous oxide, or both, during the late first stage and second stage of labor. The gas may be self-administered (via special apparatus) but is safest when given by an experienced anesthetist (via mask and anesthesia machine). Ideally, the patient remains awake, free of pain, and cooperative, with intact laryngeal reflexes; the anesthetist must remain in constant communication with the parturient. Overdosage with loss of protective airway reflexes and vomiting can lead to pulmonary aspiration and is a major hazard of this technique. Confusion, excitement, or drowsiness is indicative of overdosage and the need to reduce the concentration. When given alone in oxygen, these agents are carefully titrated, with concentration limits of 50% for nitrous oxide, 1% for enflurane, and 0.7% for isoflurane. Supplementation with a pudendal nerve block or perineal infiltration of a local anesthetic is helpful during the second stage.

PUDENDAL NERVE BLOCK

Pudendal nerve blocks are most often given by obstetricians to provide perineal anesthesia during the second stage of labor when other forms of anesthesia are not employed or prove to be inadequate. A guide (Iowa trumpet) is used to place the needle transvaginally underneath the ischial spine on each side; the needle is advanced 1.5 cm into the sacrospinous ligament, and 10 mL of 1% lidocaine or 2% chloroprocaine is injected following aspiration.

REGIONAL ANESTHETIC & ANALGESIC TECHNIQUES

Regional techniques employing either the epidural or intrathecal route (Chapter 16) are currently the most popular methods of pain relief during labor and delivery. These techniques can provide excellent pain relief yet allow the mother to be awake and cooperative during labor. Although intraspinal opioids or local anesthetics alone can provide satisfactory analgesia, techniques utilizing combinations of the two have proved to be the most satisfactory in the majority of parturients. Moreover, the apparent synergy between the two types of agents decreases dose requirements and provides excellent analgesia with few maternal side effects and little or no neonatal depression (see below).

Table 41–1. Intraspinal narcotic dosages for labor and delivery.

Agent	Intrathecal	Epidural
Morphine	0.5–1 mg	7.5–10 mg
Meperidine	10 mg	100 mg
Fentanyl	5–25 μg	50–200 μg
Sufentanil	3–10 μg	10–50 μg

1. INTRASPINAL NARCOTICS ALONE

Preservative-free narcotics may be given intraspinally as a single injection or intermittently via an epidural or intrathecal catheter (Table 41–1). These techniques are most useful for high-risk patients who may not tolerate the functional sympathectomy associated with spinal or epidural anesthesia (Chapter 16). This group includes patients with significant cardiovascular disease such as hypovolemia, aortic stenosis, tetralogy of Fallot, Eisenmenger's syndrome, or pulmonary hypertension. Intraspinal narcotics, when used alone, do not produce motor blockade (and thus do not impair the ability of the parturient to push the baby out) and do not cause maternal hypotension (sympathectomy). Disadvantages include less complete analgesia, lack of perineal relaxation, and side effects that can include pruritus, nausea, vomiting, sedation, and respiratory depression (Chapter 18). Side effects often improve with low doses of naloxone (0.2 mg/h intravenously).

Epidural Narcotics Alone

Relatively high doses (≥7.5 mg) of morphine are required for satisfactory analgesia during labor. The resulting analgesia is slow in onset (30–60 minutes) but of long duration (up to 24 hours). Unfortunately, such doses are associated with a high incidence of significant side effects (see above). Epidural meperidine, 100 mg, provides consistently good but relatively brief analgesia (1–4 hours). Epidural fentanyl, 50–200 μg, or sufentanil, 10–50 μg, usually produces relatively rapid analgesia (5–10 minutes) with few side effects, but it has a short duration (1–2 hours). Although "single-shot" epidural narcotics do not appear to cause significant neonatal depression, caution should be exercised following repeated administrations. Combinations of a lower dose of morphine, 2.5 mg, with fentanyl, 25–50 μg, or sufentanil, 10–20 μg, may result in a more rapid onset and prolongation of analgesia (4–5 hours) with fewer side effects.

Intrathecal Narcotics Alone

Intrathecal morphine in doses of 0.5–1 mg can produce satisfactory and prolonged (6–8 hours) analgesia during the first stage of labor. Unfortunately, as with the epidural route, the onset of analgesia is slow (45–60 minutes), and these doses are associated with a relatively high incidence of side effects (see above). Furthermore, some patients may experience a postdural puncture headache. The combination of morphine, 0.25 mg, and fentanyl, 25 μg, or sufentanil, 5–10 μg, may result in a more rapid onset of analgesia (5 minutes) but a shorter duration (4–5 hours). Intermittent boluses of meperidine, 10 mg, fentanyl, 5–10 μg, or sufentanil, 3–10 μg, via a 28- or 32-gauge intrathecal catheter can also provide satisfactory analgesia for labor. Intraspinal meperidine appears to have some weak local anesthetic properties.

2. LOCAL ANESTHETICS WITH & WITHOUT NARCOTICS

Lumbar epidural, caudal, and spinal (intrathecal) anesthesia (Chapter 16) can be used safely during labor and delivery. Pain relief during the first stage requires a T10–L1 sensory level, while that during the second stage requires blockade of both T10–L1 and S2–4. Continuous lumbar epidural anesthesia is the most versatile technique, because it can be used for pain relief for the first stage of labor as well as anesthesia for subsequent vaginal delivery or cesarean section, if necessary. "Single-shot" epidural, spinal, and caudal anesthesia may be appropriate when pain relief is initiated just prior to vaginal delivery (the second stage).

Absolute contraindications to regional anesthesia include infection over the injection site, coagulopathy, hypovolemia, true allergies to local anesthetics, and the patient's refusal of or inability to cooperate with regional anesthesia (Chapter 16). Preexisting neurologic disease, back disorders, and some forms of heart disease (Chapter 20) are relative contraindications. A previous cesarean section through a low transverse incision is no longer considered a contraindication to regional anesthesia during labor. Concern over the anesthesia masking the pain associated with uterine rupture (see below) may not be justified, because dehiscence of a lower segment scar frequently does not cause pain even without epidural anesthesia; moreover, changes in uterine tone and contraction pattern may be more reliable signs.

Prior to the performance of any regional block, appropriate equipment and supplies for resuscitation should be checked and made immediately available. Minimum supplies include an oxygen supply, suction, a mask with a positive-pressure device for ventilation, a functioning laryngoscope, endotracheal tubes (6 or 7 mm), oral or nasal airways, intravenous fluids, ephedrine, thiopental, and succinylcholine. The capability for frequent monitoring of at least blood pressure and heart rate is mandatory. A pulse oximeter should also be readily available.

Lumbar Epidural Anesthesia

Epidural anesthesia is generally administered only when labor is well established (see below). It may be advantageous to place an epidural catheter early when the patient is comfortable and can be positioned easily, but one should wait to inject local anesthetics until labor is progressing well and the patient becomes uncomfortable. Although criteria for initiation of epidural anesthesia tend to vary somewhat, commonly used criteria include the following: (1) no fetal distress; (2) good regular contractions 3–4 minutes apart; (3) adequate cervical dilatation, ie, 5–6 cm for nulliparous patients and 4–5 cm for multiparous patients; and (4) engagement of the fetal head.

Epidural anesthesia can generally be administered earlier to parturients who are receiving an oxytocin infusion once a good contraction pattern is achieved.

A. Technique: The technique of epidural anesthesia is described in Chapter 16. Parturients are most commonly positioned on their sides for the block. In obese patients, the sitting position is often more useful for identifying the midline. When epidural anesthesia is being given for vaginal delivery (second stage), the sitting position is useful in ensuring good sacral spread.

Because the epidural space pressure may be positive in some parturients (Chapter 40), correct identification of the epidural space may be difficult, and unintentional dural puncture may readily occur. Some clinicians advocate the midline approach, while others favor the paramedian approach. Placement of the epidural catheter at the L3–4 or L4–5 interspace is generally optimal for achieving a T10–S5 neural blockade.

B. Choice of Local Anesthetic: Anesthetic solutions in common usage include lidocaine 1–2%, chloroprocaine 2–3%, and bupivacaine 0.25–0.5%. The effect of epinephrine-containing solutions on the course of labor is controversial. Some clinicians only use epinephrine-containing solutions for intravascular test doses because of their theoretic potential for slowing the progression of labor (Chapter 40) and adversely affecting the fetus; others use only very dilute concentrations of epinephrine such as 1:800,000 or 1:400,000. Studies comparing these various agents have failed to find any differences in neonatal Apgar scores (see below), acid-base status, or neurobehavioral evaluations. In spite of the potential cardiotoxicity of bupivacaine (Chapter 14), its long duration of action makes it a particularly valuable agent for labor. Chloroprocaine is valuable for its almost immediate onset of action, but controversy over its potential for neurotoxicity has caused some clinicians to abandon it. Studies suggest that cases of chloroprocaine neurotoxicity were related to a relatively high concentration of sodium bisulfite used as an antioxidant in its solutions and a very low pH. New formulations of chloroprocaine do not contain bisulfite. Some practitioners add sodium bicarbonate to local anesthetic solutions (1 meq/10 mL of lidocaine or chloroprocaine and 0.1 meq/10 mL of bupivacaine) to increase the concentration of the nonionized free base and produce a faster onset and more rapid spread of epidural anes-

thesia. The clinical utility of this practice remains controversial. The use of local anesthetic-opioid mixtures is discussed below.

C. Epidural Activation for the First Stage of Labor: Epidural injection of local anesthetic may be done either before or after the catheter is placed. Activation through the needle may facilitate catheter placement. The following sequence is suggested for epidural activation:

1. Administer a 500- to 1000-mL intravenous bolus of lactated Ringer's injection. Glucose-free intravenous fluid boluses are used to avoid maternal hyperglycemia and hypersecretion of insulin by the fetus. When placental transfer of glucose ceases abruptly following delivery, persistent high circulating levels of insulin in the neonate can result in transient hypoglycemia.

2. Test for unintentional subarachnoid or intravascular placement of the needle or catheter with a 3- to 4-mL test dose of a local anesthetic with 1:200,000 epinephrine (controversial; see below).

3. If after 5 minutes signs of intravascular or intrathecal injection are absent (see below), give an additional 4–8 mL of local anesthetic to achieve a T10–L1 sensory level.

4. Monitor with frequent blood pressure measurements for 20–30 minutes or until the patient is stable.

5. Repeat steps 2–4 when pain recurs until the first stage of labor is completed; alternatively, a continuous epidural infusion technique may be employed using 0.125% bupivacaine or 0.5% lidocaine at an initial rate of 10 mL/h, subsequently adjusted according to the patient's needs.

D. Epidural Activation During the Second Stage of Labor: Activation for the second stage of labor extends the block to include the S2–4 dermatomes. Whether a catheter is already in place or epidural anesthesia is just being initiated, the following steps should be undertaken:

1. Give a 1000- to 1500-mL intravenous bolus of lactated Ringer's injection.

2. The epidural space is identified in the sitting position; if the patient already has an epidural catheter in place, she is placed a semiupright or sitting position.

3. Give a 3- or 4-mL test dose of local anesthetic with 1:200,000 epinephrine (see below).

4. If after 5 minutes signs of an intravascular or intrathecal injection are absent, give 10–15 mL of additional local anesthetic at a rate not faster than 5 mL every 30 seconds.

5. Lay the patient supine with left uterine displacement and monitor blood pressure every 1–2 minutes for the first 15 minutes, then every 5 minutes thereafter.

E. Prevention of Unintentional Intravascular and Intrathecal Injections: The safe administration of epidural anesthesia is critically dependent on avoiding unintentional intrathecal or intravascular injections. Unintentional intravascular or intrathecal placement of an epidural needle or catheter is possible even when aspiration fails to yield blood or cerebrospinal fluid, respectively. The incidence of unintentional intravascular or intrathecal placement of an epidural catheter is 5–15% and 0.5–2.5%, respectively. Even a properly placed catheter can subsequently erode into an epidural vein or an intrathecal position. Each time local anesthetic is injected through an epidural catheter, this possibility should be excluded.

Test doses of lidocaine, 45–60 mg, bupivacaine, 12.5 mg, or chloroprocaine, 100 mg, can be given to exclude unintentional intrathecal placement. Signs of sensory and motor blockade usually become apparent within 2–3 minutes and 3–5 minutes, respectively, if the injection is intrathecal.

Test dose techniques for unintentional intravascular injections may not be reliable in parturients. The best method for detecting intravascular injections is controversial in obstetric anesthesia. In nonpregnant patients, the intravascular injection of a local anesthetic solution with epinephrine, 15–20 μg, consistently increases the heart rate by 20–30 beats/min within 60–90 seconds if the catheter (or epidural needle) is intravascular. This technique is not always reliable in parturients because they often have marked spontaneous baseline variations in heart rate with contractions. In fact, bradycardia has been reported in a parturient following intravenous injection of epinephrine, 15 μg. Moreover, 15-μg doses of epinephrine intravenously reduce uterine blood flow in animal studies and have been associated with fetal distress in humans. Alternative methods of detecting unintentional intravascular catheter placement include eliciting tinnitus or perioral numbness following a 100-mg test dose of lidocaine, eliciting a chronotropic effect following injection of isoproterenol, 5 μg, or injecting 1 mL of air while monitoring with a precordial Doppler (Chapter 26). With the possible exception of the precordial Doppler, false-negative responses may be encountered with all methods; false-positives can also be observed. The use of dilute local anesthetic solutions and slow injection rates may also enhance detection of unintentional intravascular injections before catastrophic complications develop.

F. Management of Complications Associated With Epidural Anesthesia:

1. Hypotension–Hypotension is generally defined as a 20–30% decrease in blood pressure or a systolic pressure less than 100 mm Hg. Hypotension is the most common side effect of regional anesthesia. It is primarily due to decreased sympathetic tone and is greatly accentuated by aortocaval compression (Chapter 40) and an upright or semiupright position. Treatment should be aggressive and consists of left uterine displacement, an intravenous fluid bolus, intravenous boluses of ephedrine, 5–15 mg, and supplemental oxygen. Use of the head-down (Trendelenburg) position is controversial because of its potentially detrimental effects on pulmonary gas exchange (Chapter 22).

2. Unintentional intravascular injections–Early recognition of intravascular injections (see above), detected by the use of small incremental doses of local anesthetic, may prevent more serious local anesthetic toxicity such as seizures or cardiovascular collapse. Intravascular injections of toxic doses of lidocaine or chloroprocaine usually present as seizures. Thiopental in small doses (50–100 mg) may prevent seizures and will terminate frank seizure activity. Maintenance of a patent airway and adequate oxygenation are of paramount importance. Intubation with succinylcholine and cricoid pressure may be necessary. Intravascular injections of bupivacaine can cause rapid and profound cardiovascular collapse as well as seizure activity. Pregnant patients appear to be more susceptible to the cardiotoxic effects of bupivacaine than nonpregnant patients. Cardiac resuscitation may be exceedingly difficult and is especially aggravated by acidosis and hypoxia. Bretylium appears to be useful in reversing bupivacaine-induced decreases in the threshold for ventricular tachycardia.

3. Unintentional intrathecal injection–If dural puncture is recognized immediately after injection of local anesthetic, an attempt to aspirate the local anesthetic may be tried but is usually unsuccessful. The patient should be gently placed supine with left uterine displacement. Head elevation accentuates hypotension and should be avoided. The hypotension should be treated aggressively with intravenous fluids and ephedrine. A high spinal level can also result in diaphragmatic paralysis, which necessitates intubation and ventilation with 100% oxygen.

4. Post-dural puncture headache–Headache frequently follows unintentional dural puncture in parturients. Oral analgesics, epidural saline injection (50–100 mL), and caffeine and sodium benzoate, 500 mg intravenously, may be effective in patients with mild headaches. Patients with moderate to severe headaches usually require an epidural blood patch (10 mL) (Chapter 16). Prophylactic epidural blood patches are advocated by some clinicians.

G. Lumbar Epidural Anesthesia With Mixtures of Local Anesthetics and Narcotics:
The addition of narcotics to local anesthetic solutions for epidural anesthesia has dramatically changed the practice of obstetric anesthesia. The synergy between epidural narcotics and local anesthetic solutions appears to be due to separate sites of action, namely, opiate receptors and neuronal axons, respectively. When the two are combined, very low concentrations of both local anesthetics and narcotics can be used. Following a 10-mL initial bolus, these mixtures are then most commonly given as continuous epidural infusions at a rate of 10–15 mL/h. The initial bolus is usually bupivacaine, 0.0625–0.125%, with fentanyl, 50 μg, or sufentanil, 5–20 μg. The most widely used infusion mixtures are bupivacaine, 0.0625–0.125%, plus fentanyl, 1–2 μg/mL, or sufentanil, 1 μg/mL. These dilute mixtures generally do not produce motor blockade. More-

over, they do not appear to have any adverse effects on the fetus. Patient-controlled epidural analgesia using these mixtures has been advocated by some clinicians but appears to offer few clear advantages over continuous infusions for parturients.

Caudal Anesthesia

Lumbar epidural anesthesia is generally superior to caudal anesthesia because the former is technically easier to perform and requires less local anesthetic. Moreover, early paralysis of the pelvic muscles during caudal anesthesia may interfere with normal rotation of the fetal head. The principal advantage of caudal anesthesia is the rapidity of onset of perineal anesthesia when it is administered just prior to delivery. The technique for caudal anesthesia in pregnant patients differs only in that once the needle is positioned in the sacral canal—and prior to injection—rectal examination may be necessary to exclude accidental puncture of the fetus. Fifteen to 20 mL of local anesthetic is required for a T10–S5 nerve block, and a catheter may be left in place.

Some authors have advocated the combined used of both a lumbar epidural and a caudal catheter. The lumbar catheter is used for labor, while the caudal catheter is used for delivery. The purported advantage is improved anesthesia with less total drug requirement.

Spinal Anesthesia

Spinal anesthesia given just prior to delivery—also known as saddle block—provides profound anesthesia for vaginal delivery. A 500- to 1000-mL fluid bolus is given prior to the procedure, which is performed with the patient in the sitting position. Use of either a 25- or 26-gauge regular or a 22-gauge Whitacre spinal needle decreases the likelihood of post-dural puncture headache. Hyperbaric tetracaine, 3–4 mg, or lidocaine, 20–40 mg, usually provides excellent perineal anesthesia. A T10 sensory level can be obtained with slightly larger amounts of local anesthetic. The intrathecal injection should be given slowly over 30 seconds and in between contractions to minimize excessive cephalad spread. Three minutes after injection, the patient is placed in the lithotomy position with left uterine displacement.

PARACERVICAL BLOCK

Paracervical blocks are seldom performed nowadays, usually by obstetricians only when regional anesthetic techniques are not available. They are associated with an unacceptably high rate (up to 33%) of fetal bradycardia. The technique involves injecting local anesthetic (5 mL) submucosally in the vagina on either side of the cervix at the 3 o'clock and 9 o'clock positions. Visceral sensory fibers from the uterus, cervix, and upper vagina are blocked at these positions as they pass through the inferior hypogastric (pelvic) ganglia and plexus. The close proximity of the injection site to the uterine artery is thought to result in uterine arterial vasoconstriction and high fetal blood levels of the local anesthetic.

GENERAL ANESTHESIA

Because of the inherent risk of aspiration, general anesthesia for vaginal delivery is indicated only when emergency operation is necessary. Most indications for general anesthesia generally share the need for uterine relaxation. Intravenous nitroglycerin, 50–100 μg intravenously, has recently been shown to be effective in inducing uterine relaxation and may obviate the need for general anesthesia. Indications for general anesthesia include fetal distress during the second stage, tetanic uterine contractions, breech extraction, version and extraction, manual removal of a retained placenta, replacement of an inverted uterus, and psychiatric patients who become uncontrollable.

Suggested Technique for Vaginal Delivery:

(1) Place a wedge under the right hip for left uterine displacement.

(2) Preoxygenate the patient for 3–5 minutes as monitors are applied. Defasciculation with curare or another nondepolarizer is usually not necessary, because most pregnant patients do not fasciculate following succinylcholine. Moreover, fasciculations do not appear to favor regurgitation, because any increase in intragastric pressure is matched by a similar increase in the lower esophageal sphincter.

(3) Once all monitors are applied and the obstetrician is ready, proceed with a rapid-sequence induction while cricoid pressure is applied and intubate with a 6- to 7-mm endotracheal tube. Thiopental, 4 mg/kg, and succinylcholine, 1.5 mg/kg, are most commonly used unless the patient is hypovolemic or hypotensive, in which case ketamine, 1 mg/kg, is substituted for thiopental.

(4) After successful intubation, use 1–2 MAC of any potent volatile inhalational agent (Chapter 7) in 100% oxygen while carefully monitoring blood pressure.

(5) If skeletal muscle relaxation is necessary, atracurium, vecuronium, or a succinylcholine infusion may be used.

(6) Once the fetus and placenta are delivered, the volatile agent is decreased to less than 0.5 MAC or discontinued; an oxytocin infusion is started (20–40 units/L of intravenous fluid); and a nitrous oxide-opioid technique can be used.

(7) An attempt to aspirate gastric contents may be made via an orogastric tube to decrease the likelihood of pulmonary aspiration on emergence.

(8) At the end of the procedure, skeletal muscle relaxants (if given) are reversed, the gastric tube (if placed) is removed, and the patient is extubated awake.

Table 41–2. Major indications for cesarean section.

Labor unsafe for mother and fetus
  Increased risk of uterine rupture
    Previous classic cesarean section
    Previous extensive myomectomy or uterine
      reconstruction
  Increased risk of maternal hemorrhage
    Central or partial placenta previa
    Abruptio placentae
    Previous vaginal reconstruction
Dystocia
  Abnormal fetopelic relations
    Fetopelvic disproportion
    Abnormal fetal presentation
      Transverse or oblique lie
      Breech presentation
  Dysfunctional uterine activity
Immediate or emergent delivery necessary
  Fetal distress
  Umbilical cord prolapse
  Maternal hemorrhage
  Amnionitis
  Genital herpes with ruptured membranes
  Impending maternal death

ANESTHESIA FOR CESAREAN SECTION

Common indications for cesarean section are listed in Table 41–2. The choice of anesthesia for cesarean section is determined by multiple factors, including the indication for operating, its urgency, patient and obstetrician preferences, and the skills of the anesthetist. Cesarean section rates have been steadily increasing in recent years (up to 25% of all deliveries), and regional anesthesia has become the preferred technique.

Advantages of regional anesthesia include (1) less neonatal exposure to potentially depressant drugs; (2) a decreased risk of maternal pulmonary aspiration; (3) an awake mother at the birth of her child, with the father also present if desired; and (4) the option of using intraspinal opioids for postoperative pain relief. The choice between spinal and epidural anesthesia is often based on physician preferences. Epidural anesthesia is preferred over spinal anesthesia in most hospitals because of the more gradual decrease in blood pressure associated with epidural anesthesia. Continuous epidural anesthesia also allows better control over the sensory level. Conversely, spinal anesthesia is easier to perform, has a more rapid, predictable onset, and may produce a more intense (complete) block. The recent introduction of continuous intrathecal catheters now also allows better control over the sensory level with spinal anesthesia. Regardless of the regional technique chosen, the ability to administer a general anesthetic at any time during the procedure is mandatory.

General anesthesia offers (1) a very rapid and reliable onset, (2) control over the airway and ventilation, and (3) potentially less hypotension than regional anesthesia. Its principal disadvantages are the risk of pulmonary aspiration, an inability to intubate the patient, and the potential for fetal depression. With present anesthetic techniques, fetal depression is usually not clinically significant with general anesthesia. However, the administration of large doses of intravenous agents prior to delivery can result in neonatal depression. Long uterine incision-to-delivery times (> 90 seconds) are associated with fetal hypoxia and acidosis regardless of the type of anesthesia.

REGIONAL ANESTHESIA

Cesarean section requires a T4 sensory level. Because of the associated high sympathetic blockade, all patients should receive a 1500- to 2000-mL bolus of lactated Ringer's injection prior to neural blockade. After injection of the anesthetic, the patient is placed supine with left uterine displacement; supplemental oxygen (40–50%) is given; and blood pressure is measured every 1–2 minutes until it stabilizes. Prophylactic administration of intramuscular ephedrine (25 mg) may be indicated only for spinal anesthesia, as precipitous hypotension is often seen. Hypotension following epidural anesthesia typically has a slower onset and can be treated with increments of ephedrine (5–15 mg intravenously), additional intravenous fluid, and more uterine tilt. Slight Trendelenburg positioning facilitates achieving a T4 sensory level and may also help prevent severe hypotension. Extreme degrees of Trendelenburg may interfere with pulmonary gas exchange.

1. SPINAL ANESTHESIA

The patient is usually placed in the lateral decubitus position, and a hyperbaric solution of tetracaine, 7–10 mg, lidocaine 60–90 mg, or bupivacaine, 8–12 mg, is injected. Addition of fentanyl, 10–20 μg, or sufentanil, 5–10 μg, to the local anesthetic solution enhances the intensity of the block and prolongs its duration without adversely affecting neonatal outcome. Addition of preservative-free morphine, 0.1–0.25 mg, can prolong postoperative analgesia up to 24 hours but requires special monitoring for delayed postoperative respiratory depression (Chapter 18).

2. EPIDURAL ANESTHESIA

Epidural anesthesia for cesarean section is generally most satisfactory when an epidural catheter is employed. The catheter facilitates achieving an initial T4 sensory level, allows supplementation if necessary, and provides an excellent route for postoperative narcotic administration. After a negative test dose, a total of 15–20 mL of local anesthetic is injected slowly in 5-mL increments (see above). Lidocaine 1.5–2% (with or without 1:200,000 epinephrine), chloroprocaine 3%, or bupivacaine 0.5% is most commonly used. Addition of fentanyl, 50–100 µg, or sufentanil, 20–30 µg, greatly enhances the intensity of the block and prolongs its duration without adversely affecting neonatal outcome. Sodium bicarbonate may be added to the local anesthetic solution to accelerate onset of anesthesia (see above). If pain develops as the sensory level recedes, additional local anesthetic is given in 5-mL increments to maintain a T4 sensory level. "Patchy" anesthesia prior to delivery of the baby can be treated with ketamine, 10–20 mg intravenously, or 30% nitrous oxide; after delivery, intravenous narcotic supplementation may also be used provided excessive sedation and loss of consciousness are avoided. Intolerable pain in spite of a seemingly adequate sensory level and unresponsive to these measures necessitates general anesthesia with endotracheal intubation (see below). Nausea can be treated with droperidol, 0.625 mg intravenously.

Epidural morphine, 5 mg, at the end of surgery provides good to excellent pain relief postoperatively for up to 24 hours. An increased incidence (3.5–30%) of recurrent herpes simplex labialis infection has been reported 2–5 days following epidural morphine in some studies. Postoperative analgesia can also be provided by continuous epidural infusions of fentanyl, 50–75 µg/h, or sufentanil, 10–20 µg/h, at a rate of approximately 10 mL/h. Epidural butorphanol, 2 mg, can also provide effective postoperative pain relief, but marked somnolence is often a troublesome side effect.

GENERAL ANESTHESIA

Pulmonary aspiration of gastric contents (incidence: 1:500–400) and failed endotracheal intubation (incidence: 1:300) during general anesthesia are the major causes of maternal morbidity and mortality. Every effort should be made to ensure optimal conditions prior to the start of anesthesia and to follow measures aimed at preventing these complications.

All patients should receive prophylaxis against severe nonparticulate aspiration pneumonia with 30 mL of 0.3-M sodium citrate 15 minutes prior to induction. Patients with additional risk factors predisposing to aspiration should also receive ranitidine, 100–150 mg, or metoclopromide, 10 mg, 1–2 hours prior to induction; such factors include morbid obesity, symptoms of gastroesophageal reflux, a potentially difficult airway, or emergent surgical delivery without an elective fasting period.

Anticipation of a difficult endotracheal intubation may help reduce the incidence of failed intubations. Examination of the neck, mandible, dentition, and oropharynx often helps predict which patients may be

difficult (Chapter 5). The higher incidence of failed intubations in pregnant patients compared to nonpregnant surgical patients may be due to airway edema (Chapter 40), a full dentition, or large breasts that can obstruct the laryngoscope handle in patients with short necks. A variety of laryngoscope blades, a short laryngoscope handle, at least one extra styled endotracheal tube (6 mm), and Magill forceps (for nasal intubation) should be readily available. When a difficult airway is suspected, alternatives to the standard rapid-sequence induction should be considered such as regional anesthesia or awake fiberoptic techniques (Chapter 5). Moreover, a clear plan should be formulated for a failed endotracheal intubation following induction of anesthesia (Figure 41–1). Note that the health of the mother takes priority over delivery of the fetus. In the absence of fetal distress, the patient should be awakened, and an awake intubation regional or local (infiltration) anesthesia may be tried. In the presence of fetal distress, if spontaneous or positive ventilation with cricoid pressure is possible, delivery of the fetus may be attempted. In such instances, a potent volatile agent in oxygen is employed for anesthesia, but once the fetus is delivered, nitrous oxide can be added to reduce the concentration of the volatile agent. Inability to ventilate the patient at any time mandates immediate cricothyrotomy or tracheostomy.

Suggested Technique for Cesarean Section

(1) The patient is placed supine with a wedge under the right hip for left uterine displacement.

(2) Preoxygenation is accomplished with 100% oxygen for 3–5 minutes while monitors are applied. Defasciculation is generally not necessary (see above).

(3) The patient is prepared and draped for surgery.

(4) When the surgeons are ready, a rapid-sequence induction with cricoid pressure is performed using 4 mg/kg of thiopental and 1.5 mg/kg of succinylcholine. Ketamine, 1 mg/kg, is used instead of thiopental in hypovolemic patients.

(5) Surgery is begun only after proper placement of the endotracheal tube is confirmed by capnography.

(6) Fifty percent nitrous oxide in oxygen with a low concentration of a volatile agent (up to 0.5% halothane, 1% enflurane, or 0.75% isoflurane) is used for maintenance. The low dose of volatile agent helps ensure amnesia but is generally not enough to cause excessive uterine relaxation or prevent uterine contraction following oxytocin. A muscle relaxant of intermediate duration (vecuronium, 0.05 mg/kg, or atracurium, 0.5 mg/kg) is used for relaxation.

(7) After the neonate and placenta are delivered, 10–

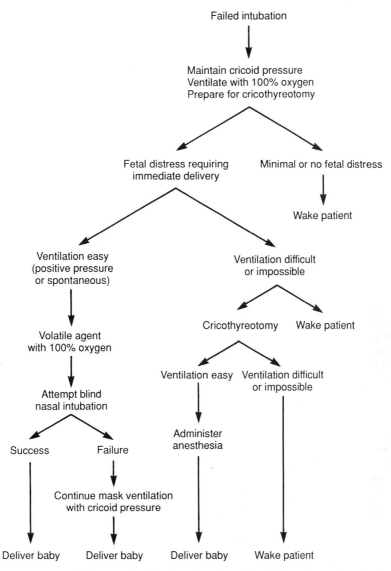

Figure 41–1. An algorithm for a difficult intubation in obstetric patients. (Modified and reproduced, with permission, from Shnider SM, Levinson G, in: *Anesthesia,* 3rd ed. Miller RD (editor). Churchill Livingstone, 1990.)

20 units of oxytocin is added to each liter of intravenous fluid.

(8) If the uterus does not contract readily, a narcotic should be given, and the halogenated agent is discontinued. Methergine, 0.2 mg intramuscularly, may also be given but can increase arterial blood pressure.

(9) An attempt to aspirate gastric contents may be made via an oral gastric tube to decrease the likelihood of pulmonary aspiration on emergence.

(10) At the end of surgery, muscle relaxants are completely reversed, the gastric tube (if placed) is removed, and the patient is extubated awake.

ANESTHESIA FOR EMERGENCY CESAREAN SECTION

Indications for emergency cesarean section include massive bleeding (placenta previa or abruptio placentae), severe fetal distress, umbilical cord prolapse, or uterine rupture. The patient must be rushed to the operating room for a "crash" cesarean section under general anesthesia. Even if the patient has an epidural catheter in place, the delay in establishing adequate epidural anesthesia generally prohibits its use. Moreover, regional anesthesia is contraindicated in hypovolemic or hypotensive patients. Adequate preoxygenation may be achieved rapidly by four maximal breaths with 100% oxygen while monitors are being applied. Ketamine, 1 mg/kg, should be substituted for thiopental in hypotensive or hypovolemic patients.

ANESTHESIA FOR THE COMPLICATED PREGNANCY

ANTEPARTUM HEMORRHAGE

Placenta Previa

Placenta previa complicates 0.5% of pregnancies and often occurs in patients who have had previous cesarean section or uterine myomectomy. The placenta may completely cover the internal cervical os (central or complete placenta previa), may partially cover the os (partial placenta previa), or may be close to the internal cervical os without extending beyond its edge (low-lying or marginal placenta). Placenta previa usually presents as painless vaginal bleeding. Although the bleeding often stops spontaneously, severe hemorrhage can occur at any time. When the gestation is less than 37 weeks in duration and the bleeding is mild to moderate, the patient is usually treated with bed rest and observation. After 37 weeks of gestation, delivery is usually accomplished via cesarean section. Patients with low-lying placenta may occasionally be allowed to deliver vaginally if the bleeding is mild.

All parturients with vaginal bleeding are assumed to have placenta previa until proved otherwise. An abdominal ultrasound examination greatly facilitates localization of the placenta, but direct examination with a vaginal speculum may be necessary to confirm the diagnosis. However, the examination itself can precipitate exsanguinating hemorrhage. A "double setup" is therefore employed in such instances: The patient is placed in the lithotomy position for the examination (and possible vaginal delivery) and is simultaneously prepared for a "crash" cesarean section if profuse bleeding occurs. An anesthesiologist must therefore be present. The patient should have two large-bore intravenous catheters in place; intravascular volume deficits must be replaced; and blood must be available for transfusion. A central venous line is often useful. Preoxygenation is established as preparation for a "crash" cesarean section under general anesthesia is made (see above).

A history of a previous placenta previa or cesarean section increases the risk of placenta accreta in subsequent pregnancies. In this condition, the placenta becomes adherent to the uterus and becomes difficult or impossible to separate from it. Hysterectomy may be required to control profuse bleeding following separation of the placenta.

Abruptio Placentae

Premature separation of the placenta complicates approximately 1–2% of pregnancies. Patients usually experience painful vaginal bleeding. The diagnosis is made by excluding placenta previa. Most abruptions result in mild to moderate bleeding and are managed with vaginal delivery if the fetus is over 37 weeks of gestational age. The bleeding may remain concealed inside the uterus and cause underestimation of blood loss. Severe abruptio placentae can cause coagulopathy, especially following fetal demise. The coagulopathy is thought to be due to activation of circulating plasminogen (fibrinolysis) and the release of tissue thromboplastins that precipitate disseminated intravascular coagulation. Severe abruption is a life-threatening emergency that necessitates a "crash" emergency cesarean section under general anesthesia (see above). Massive blood transfusion, including replacement of coagulation factors and platelets, are often necessary.

Uterine Rupture

Uterine rupture is relatively uncommon (1:3000–1000 deliveries) but can occur during labor as a result of (1) dehiscence of a scar from a previous (usually classic) cesarean section, extensive myomectomy, or uterine reconstruction; (2) intrauterine manipulations or use of forceps (iatrogenic); or (3) spontaneous rupture following prolonged labor in patients with hypertonic contractions (especially with oxytocin infusions), fetopelvic disproportion, or a very large, thin, and weakened uterus. Uterine rupture can present either as frank hemorrhage or as hypotension with occult bleeding into the abdomen. Even when epidural anesthesia is employed for labor, uterine rupture is often heralded by the abrupt onset of continuous abdominal pain and hypotension. The use of dilute concentrations of local anesthetics for epidural anesthesia during labor may facilitate early recognition. Treatment requires volume resuscitation and immediate laparotomy under general anesthesia.

PRETERM LABOR

Preterm labor by definition occurs between the 20th and 37th weeks of gestation and is the most common complication of the third trimester. Approximately 7% of liveborn infants in the United States are delivered before term. Important contributory maternal factors include extremes of age, inadequate prenatal care, unusual body habitus, increased physical activity, and medical illnesses or complications during pregnancy.

Because of their small size and incomplete development, preterm infants, especially those under 30 weeks of gestational age or weighing less than 1500 g, experience a greater number of complications than term infants. They are more vulnerable to asphyxia. Their soft, poorly calcified cranium predisposes to intracranial hemorrhage during vaginal delivery. Preterm infants with a breech presentation are especially prone to prolapse of the umbilical cord during labor. Moreover, inadequate pulmonary surfactant production frequently leads to the idiopathic respiratory distress syndrome (hyaline membrane disease) after delivery. Surfactant levels are generally adequate only after the 35th week of gestation (Chapter 40).

When preterm labor occurs before 35 weeks of gestation, tocolytic therapy is usually initiated. Labor is inhibited until the lungs mature and sufficient pulmonary surfactant is produced as judged by amniocentesis. The most commonly used tocolytics are β_2-adrenergic agonists (usually ritodrine or terbutaline). Most agents also have some β_1-adrenergic receptor activity. Maternal side effects include tachycardia, arrhythmias, myocardial ischemia, mild hypotension, hyperglycemia, hypokalemia, and, rarely, pulmonary edema. Other tocolytic agents include magnesium sulfate, ethanol, and calcium channel blockers.

When tocolytic therapy fails to stop labor, anesthesia often becomes necessary. The goal during vaginal delivery of a preterm fetus is a slow controlled delivery with minimal pushing by the mother. A large episiotomy and low forceps are often employed. Spinal or epidural anesthesia allows complete pelvic relaxation. Cesarean section is currently performed for fetal distress, breech presentation, intrauterine growth retardation, or failure of labor to progress. Regional or general anesthesia may be employed. Because preterm infants may be more sensitive to all central nervous system depressants, regional anesthesia may be preferable. Residual effects from β-adrenergic agonists may complicate general anesthesia. Halothane, pancuronium, ketamine, and ephedrine should be used cautiously (if at all). Hypokalemia is usually due to an intracellular uptake of potassium and rarely requires treatment; however, it may increase sensitivity to muscle relaxants. Lastly, preterm newborns are often depressed at delivery and frequently need resuscitation. Preparations for resuscitation should be completed prior to delivery.

ABNORMAL FETAL POSITIONS & PRESENTATIONS

Abnormal fetal positions and presentations increase maternal and fetal morbidity and mortality as well as the likelihood that anesthesia will be required.

Occiput Posterior

When the fetal occiput fails to spontaneously rotate anteriorly, the persistent occiput posterior results in a more prolonged and painful labor. Manual or forceps rotation is usually necessary but increases the likelihood of maternal and fetal injuries. Regional anesthesia can be used to provide perineal analgesia and pelvic relaxation, allowing manual or forceps rotation followed by forceps delivery.

Transverse Lie

A transverse lie occurs when the fetus fails to present with either the head or as a breech. It typically leads to dysfunctional labor and predisposes to cord prolapse when the membranes rupture. Cesarean section is indicated when membranes rupture in a parturient with a persistent transverse lie.

Breech Presentation

Breech presentations complicate 3–4% of deliveries and significantly increase both maternal and fetal morbidity and mortality rates. The incidence of cord prolapse is up to 10% in complete and incomplete breech delivery. Because the shoulders or head can become trapped after vaginal delivery of the body, some obstetricians employ cesarean section for all breech presentations. Manual or forceps-assisted partial breech extraction is usually necessary with vaginal delivery. The need for breech extraction does not appear to be increased when epidural anesthesia is used for labor—if labor is well established prior to epidural activation. Epidural anesthesia may lessen the likelihood of a trapped head because the former relaxes perineum. The fetal head can also become trapped in the uterus during cesarean section; general endotracheal anesthesia with a volatile agent may be necessary to relax the uterus even if epidural anesthesia is already established.

MULTIPLE GESTATIONS

Multiple gestations account for one birth in 90 and are commonly associated with two complications: breech presentation and prematurity. Anesthesia may be necessary for version, extraction, or cesarean section. The second baby (and any subsequent ones) is often more depressed and asphyxiated than the first baby. Regional anesthesia provides effective pain relief during labor, minimizes the need for central nervous system depressants, and may shorten the interval between the first and second baby. Some studies suggest that the acid-base status of the second twin is better when epidural anesthesia is used. However, patients with multiple gestations are more prone to develop hypotension from aortocaval compression, especially after regional anesthesia. Left lateral uterine displacement and intravenous fluid loading are mandatory prior to regional anesthesia. Either regional or general anesthesia may used for cesarean section; regional anesthesia may be associated with less neonatal depression.

PREGNANCY-INDUCED HYPERTENSION

The syndrome of pregnancy-induced hypertension, also called preeclampsia, consists of hypertension, proteinuria ($>$ 500 mg/d), and edema occurring after the 20th week of gestation and resolving within 48 hours after delivery. Hypertension induced by pregnancy is usually defined as a systolic blood pressure greater than 140 mm Hg or diastolic pressure greater than 90 mm Hg; or, alternatively, as a consistent increase in systolic or diastolic pressure by 30 mm and 15 Hg, respectively, above the patient's normal baseline. When seizures occur, the syndrome is termed eclampsia. In the United States, preeclampsia and eclampsia complicate approximately one in 10–15 and one in 10,000–15,000 pregnancies, respectively. Moreover, they cause or contribute to 20–40% of cases maternal deaths and 20% of perinatal deaths.

Pathophysiology & Manifestations

Pregnancy-induced hypertension affects chiefly primigravidas, but it can occur in multiparous women, especially those with vascular disorders. The pathophysiology of this multisystem disease remains obscure but appears to be related to decreased placental perfusion. Placental ischemia is thought to result in (1) altered prostaglandin metabolism (increased thromboxane and decreased prostacyclin production), (2) secretion of a renin-like substance that results in hypersecretion of angiotensin and aldosterone, and (3) release of tissue thromboplastins.

Major manifestations of pregnancy-induced hypertension include (1) generalized vasospasm, (2) reduced intravascular volume, (3) hypertension, (4) decreased glomerular filtration, and (5) generalized edema (Table 42–3). Severe pregnancy-induced hypertension substantially increases both maternal and fetal morbidity and mortality and is defined by a blood pressure greater than 160/110 mm Hg, proteinuria in excess of 5 g/d, oliguria ($<$ 500 mL/d), pulmonary edema, central nervous system manifestations (headache, visual disturbances, or seizures), hepatic tenderness, or the HELLP syndrome (*h*emolysis, *e*levated *l*iver enzymes, and a *l*ow *p*latelet count). The most common causes of death are pulmonary edema and cerebral hemorrhage.

Treatment

Treatment consists of bed rest, sedation, antihypertensive drugs (usually hydralazine or methyldopa), and magnesium sulfate to treat hyperreflexia and prevent convulsions. Therapeutic magnesium levels are 4–6 meq/L. Definitive treatment is delivery of the fetus and placenta.

Anesthetic Management

Patients with mild pregnancy-induced hypertension generally only require extra caution during anesthesia; standard anesthetic practices may be used (see above).

Table 41–3. Complications of pregnancy-induced hypertension.

Neurologic
  Headache
  Visual disturbances
  Hyperexcitability
  Seizures
  Intracranial hemorrhage
  Cerebral edema
Pulmonary
  Upper airway edema
  Pulmonary edema
Cardiovascular
  Decreased intravascular volume
  Increased arteriolar resistance
  Hypertension
  Heart failure
Hepatic
  Impaired function
  Elevated enzymes
Renal
  Proteinuria
  Sodium retention
  Decreased glomerular filtration
  Renal failure
Hematologic
  Coagulopathy
    Thrombocytopenia
    Platelet dysfunction
    Prolonged partial thromboplastin time
  Microangiopathi hemolysis

However, patients with severe disease are critically ill and require stabilization prior to any anesthetic. Hypertension should be controlled and hypovolemia corrected before anesthesia. In the absence of coagulopathy, continuous epidural anesthesia is the anesthetic of choice for most patients with pregnancy-induced hypertension during labor, vaginal delivery, and cesarean section. A bleeding time, platelet count, and coagulation profile should be checked prior to the institution of regional anesthesia in patients with severe pregnancy-induced hypertension. Continuous epidural anesthesia has been shown to decrease catecholamine secretion and improve uteroplacental perfusion in these patients provided hypotension is avoided. Colloid fluid boluses prior to epidural activation may be more effective than crystalloids in correcting the hypovolemia. A central venous line or, in severe cases, a pulmonary artery catheter should ideally be used to guide volume replacement. Use of an epinephrine-containing test dose for epidural anesthesia is controversial because of its questionable reliability (see above) and the risk of exacerbating hypertension. Hypotension should be treated with small doses of vasopressors (ephedrine, 5 mg) because patients tend to be very sensitive to these agents. Intra-arterial blood pressure monitoring is indicated in patients with severe hypertension during both general and regional anesthesia. Intravenous nitroprusside, trimethaphan, or nitroglycerin is usually necessary to control blood pressure during general anesthesia. Labetalol (up to 1 mg/kg) can also be effective in controlling the hypertensive response to intubation and does not appear to alter placental blood flow. Because magnesium potentiates muscle relaxants, doses of nondepolarizing muscle relaxants should be reduced in patients receiving magnesium therapy and guided by a peripheral nerve stimulator.

HEART DISEASE

The marked cardiovascular changes associated with pregnancy, labor, and delivery often cause pregnant patients with heart disease (2% of parturients) to decompensate during this period. Although most patients have rheumatic heart disease, an increasing number of parturients are presenting with congenital heart lesions. Anesthetic management is directed toward employing techniques that minimize the added stresses of labor and delivery (Chapter 40). Specific management of the various lesions is discussed elsewhere (Chapter 20). Most patients can be divided into one of two groups. Patients in the first group include those with mitral valve disease, aortic insufficiency, or congenital lesions with left-to-right shunting. These patients benefit from regional techniques, particularly continuous epidural anesthesia. The induced sympathectomy reduces both preload and afterload, relieves pulmonary congestion, and in some cases increases forward flow (cardiac output).

Patients in the second group include those with aortic stenosis, congenital lesions with right-to-left or bidirectional shunting, or primary pulmonary hypertension. Regional anesthesia is generally detrimental in this group. Reductions in venous return (preload) or afterload are usually poorly tolerated. These patients are better managed with intraspinal narcotics alone (see above), systemic medications, pudendal nerve blocks, and, if necessary, general anesthesia.

AMNIOTIC FLUID EMBOLISM

Amniotic fluid embolism is a rare (1:20,000 deliveries) but potentially lethal complication (86% mortality rate in some series) that can occur during labor and delivery. Entry of amniotic fluid into the maternal circulation can occur through any break in the uteroplacental membranes. Such breaks may occur during normal delivery or cesarean section or following placental abruption, placenta previa, or uterine rupture. Three major manifestations are observed: (1) pulmonary embolism, (2) DIC, and (3) uterine atony. Although the diagnosis can be firmly established only by demonstrating fetal elements in the maternal circulation (usually at autopsy), it is clinically suggested by sudden respiratory distress and circulatory collapse. Treatment is directed at aggressive cardiopulmonary resuscitation and delivery of the fetus.

FETAL & NEONATAL RESUSCITATION

FETAL RESUSCITATION

Resuscitation of the neonate starts during labor. Any compromise of the uteroplacental circulation readily produces fetal asphyxia (Chapter 40). Intrauterine asphyxia during labor is the most common cause of neonatal depression. Fetal monitoring throughout labor is helpful in identifying which babies may be at risk, detecting fetal distress, and evaluating the effect of acute interventions.

1. FETAL HEART RATE MONITORING

Fetal heart rate monitoring, supplemented by fetal scalp blood sampling, is presently the most useful technique. Correct interpretation of heart rate patterns is crucial. Three parameters are evaluated: baseline heart rate, baseline variability, and the relationship to uterine contractions (deceleration patterns). Heart rate monitoring is most accurate when fetal scalp electrodes are used, but the latter requires rupture of the membranes and is not without complications (amnionitis or fetal injury).

Baseline Heart Rate

The mature fetus normally has a baseline heart rate of 120–160 beats/min. An increased baseline heart rate may be due to prematurity, mild fetal hypoxia, chorioamnionitis, maternal fever, maternally administered drugs (anticholinergics or β agonists), or, rarely, hyperthyroidism. A decreased baseline heart rate may be due to a postterm pregnancy, fetal heart block, or fetal asphyxia.

Baseline Variability

The healthy mature fetus normally displays a baseline beat-to-beat (R wave to R wave) variability of 3–6 beats/min. Baseline variability, which can only be properly assessed with scalp electrodes, has become an important sign of fetal well-being and represents a normally functioning autonomic system. Sustained decreased baseline variability is a prominent sign of fetal asphyxia. Central nervous system depressants (narcotics, barbiturates, benzodiazepines, or magnesium sulfate), parasympatholytics (atropine), prematurity, fetal dysrhythmias, and anencephaly also decrease baseline variability.

Deceleration Patterns

A. Early (Type I) Decelerations: (Figure 41–2A.) This type of deceleration (usually 10–40 beats/min) is thought to be a vagal response to compression of the fetal head or stretching of the neck during uterine contractions. The heart rate forms a

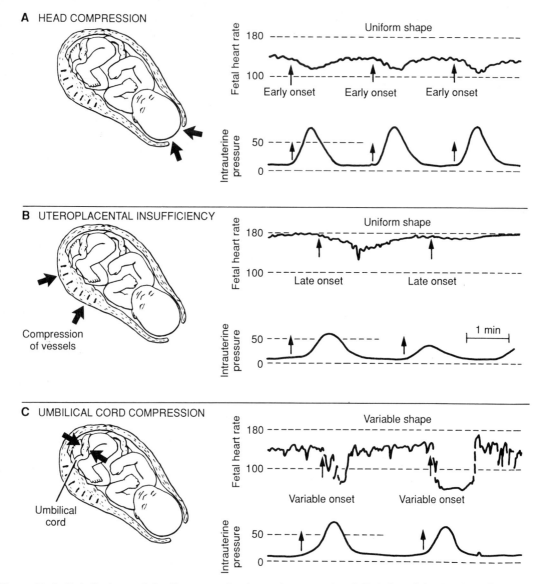

A HEAD COMPRESSION

Fetal heart rate

180 — — — — — — — — — — — — — — — — — Uniform shape — — — — — — — — —

100 —

Early onset   Early onset   Early onset

Intrauterine pressure

50 — — —

0 —

B UTEROPLACENTAL INSUFFICIENCY

Fetal heart rate

180 — — — — — — — — — — — — — — — — Uniform shape — — — — — — — — — —

100 —

Late onset   Late onset

Compression of vessels

Intrauterine pressure

50 — — —   1 min

0 —

C UMBILICAL CORD COMPRESSION

Fetal heart rate

180 — — — — — — — — — — — — — — — — Variable shape — — — — — — — — —

100 —

Variable onset   Variable onset

Umbilical cord

Intrauterine pressure

50 — — —

0 —

Figure 41–2. Periodic changes in fetal heart rate related to uterine contraction. **A:** Early (type I) decelerations. **B:** Late (type II) decelerations. **C:** Variable (type III) decelerations. (Modified and reproduced, with permission, from Danforth DN, Scott JR: *Obstetrics and Gynecology,* 5th ed. Lippincott, 1986.)

smooth mirror image of the contraction. Early decelerations are generally not associated with fetal distress.

B. Late (Type II) Decelerations: (Figure 42–2B.) Late decelerations are associated with fetal compromise and are characterized by a decrease in heart rate that coincides with or follows the peak of uterine contractions. Late decelerations may be as few as 5 beats/min and are thought to be due to the effect of a decrease in arterial oxygen tension on chemoreceptors or the sinoatrial node. Late decelerations with normal variability may be observed following acute insults (maternal hypotension or hypoxemia) and are usually reversible with treatment. Late decelerations with decreased variability are associated with prolonged asphyxia and are an indication for fetal scalp sampling (see below). Complete abolition of variability in this setting is an ominous sign signifying severe decompensation and the need for immediate delivery.

C. Variable (Type III) Decelerations: (Figure 42–2C.) These decelerations are variable in onset, duration, and magnitude (often > 30 beats/min). They are typically abrupt in onset and are thought to be related to umbilical cord compression and acute intermittent decreases in umbilical blood flow. Variable decelerations are typically associated with fetal asphyxia when they are greater than 70 beats/min or last more than 60 seconds or when the pattern persists for more than 30 minutes.

2. FETAL BLOOD SAMPLING

Fetal blood can be obtained and analyzed via a small scalp puncture once the membranes are ruptured. A pH higher than 7.20 is usually associated with a vigorous neonate, whereas a pH less than 7.20 is often but not always associated with a depressed neonate. Because of wide overlap, fetal blood sampling can be interpreted correctly only in conjunction with heart rate monitoring.

3. TREATMENT OF THE FETUS

Aggressive treatment of intrauterine fetal asphyxia is necessary to prevent fetal demise or permanent neurologic damage. All interventions are directed at restoring an adequate uteroplacental circulation. Aortocaval compression, maternal hypoxemia or hypotension, or excessive uterine activity (during oxytocin infusions) must be corrected. Changes in maternal position, supplemental oxygen, intravenous ephedrine or fluid, or adjustments in an oxytocin infusion often correct the problem. Persistent evidence of asphyxia necessitates immediate delivery.

NEONATAL RESUSCITATION

1. GENERAL CARE OF THE NEONATE

In the first 30 seconds, the neonate should be placed in a radiant warmer, in slight Trendelenburg position; the nose, mouth, and pharynx are suctioned with a bulb syringe, and the skin is dried with a sterile towel. Breathing should begin within 30 seconds and should be sustained within 90 seconds. Respirations should be 30–60/min and the heart rate 120–160 beats/min. Respirations are assessed by auscultation of the chest, while heart rate is determined by either auscultation of the precordium or palpation of the pulse at the base of the umbilical cord.

In addition to respirations and heart rate, color, tone, and reflex irritability should be evaluated. The Apgar score (Table 41–4), recorded at 1 minute and again at 5 minutes after delivery, remains the most valuable assessment of the neonate. The 1-minute score correlates with survival, while the 5-minute score is related to neurologic outcome.

Neonates with Apgar scores of 8–10 are vigorous and may only require gentle stimulation (flicking the foot, rubbing the back, and drying). A catheter should also be gently passed through each nostril to rule-out choanal atresia.

2. MECONIUM-STAINED NEONATES

The presence or absence of meconium in the amniotic fluid dictates the immediate management of the neonate at birth. Fetal distress, especially after 42 weeks of gestation, is often associated with release of thick meconium into the fluid. Fetal gasping during stress results in entry of a large amount of meconium-tainted amniotic fluid into the lungs. When the neonate initiates respiration at birth, the meconium moves from the trachea and large airways down toward the periphery of the lung. Thick or particulate meconium obstructs small airways and causes severe respiratory distress.

When thick (pea soup) meconium is present in the amniotic fluid, the obstetrician should suction the nose and mouth with a suction bulb when the head is out but prior to delivery of the shoulders. Once the delivery is completed, the neonate is placed in a radiant warmer and, ideally, intubated and suctioned before the first breath is taken. Tracheal suctioning of the thick meconium is accomplished by a special suctioning device attached to the endotracheal tube as the tube is withdrawn. If meconium is aspirated, the procedure should be repeated until no meconium is obtained—but no more than three times, after which it is usually of no further benefit. The infant should then be given supplemental oxygen by face mask and observed closely. The stomach should also be suctioned to prevent passive regurgitation of any meconium. Newborns with meconium aspiration have an increased incidence of pneumothorax (10% compared with 1% for all vaginal deliveries).

Table 41–4. Apgar score.

Sign	Points		
	0	1	2
Heart rate (beats/min)	Absent	< 100	> 100
Respiratory effort	Absent	Slow, irregular	Good, crying
Muscle tone	Flaccid	Some flexion	Active motion
Reflex irritability	No response	Grimace	Crying
Color	Blue or pale	Body pink, extremities blue	All pink

3. CARE OF THE DEPRESSED NEONATE

Resuscitation of the depressed neonate requires two or more persons—one to manage the airway and ventilation and another to perform chest compressions if necessary. A third person greatly facilitates the placement of intravascular catheters and the administration of fluids or drugs.

Because the most common cause of neonatal depression is intrauterine asphyxia, the emphasis in resuscitation is on respiration. Hypovolemia is also a contributing factor in a significant number of neonates. Factors associated with hypovolemia include early clamping of the umbilical cord, prematurity, maternal hemorrhage, placental transection during cesarean section, sepsis, and a twin-to-twin transfusion.

Failure of the neonate to quickly respond to respiratory resuscitative efforts mandates vascular access and blood gas analysis; pneumothorax and congenital anomalies of the airway, including tracheoesophageal fistula (1:5000–3000 live births), and congenital diaphragmatic hernia (1:4000–2000) should also be considered.

Grouping by **Apgar score** greatly facilitates resuscitation: (1) mildly asphyxiated neonates (Apgar score of 5–7) usually need only stimulation while oxygen is blown across the face; (2) moderately asphyxiated neonates (Apgar score of 3–4) require temporary assisted positive-pressure ventilation with mask and bag; and (3) severely depressed neonates (Apgar score of 0–2) should be immediately intubated, and chest compressions may be required.

Guidelines for Ventilation

Indications for positive-pressure ventilation include (1) apnea, (2) heart rate less than 100 beats/min, and (3) persistent central cyanosis on 100% oxygen by mask. Assisted ventilation by bag and mask should be at a rate of 40 breaths/min with 100% oxygen. Initial breaths may require peak pressures of up to 40 cm H_2O, but pressures should not exceed 30 cm H_2O subsequently. Adequacy of ventilation should be checked by auscultation and chest excursions. Gastric decompression may facilitate ventilation. If after 30 seconds the heart rate is over 100 beats/min and spontaneous ventilations become adequate, assisted ventilation is no longer necessary. If the heart rate is less than 60 beats/min, the neonate is intubated and chest compressions are started. If the heart rate is 60–100 beats/min, the neonate can be observed provided ventilation is adequate; failure of the heart rate to rise above 80 beats/min is an indication for chest compressions.

Intubation (Figure 42–3) is performed with a Miller 00 or 0 laryngoscope blade, using a 2.5- to 3.5-mm endotracheal tube. Correct endotracheal tube size is indicated by a small leak with 20 cm H_2O pressure. Right endobronchial intubation should be excluded by chest auscultation.

Guidelines for Chest Compressions

Indications for chest compressions are (1) a heart rate less than 60 beats/min and (2) a heart rate less than 80 beats/min that does not increase with adequate ventilation.

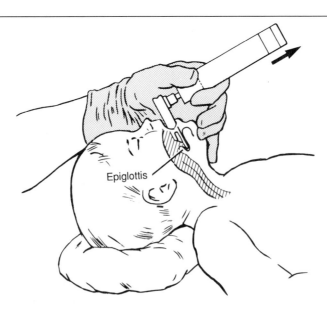

Figure 41–3. Intubation of the neonate. The head is placed in neutral position, and the laryngoscope handle is held with the thumb and index finger as the chin is supported with the remaining fingers. Pressure applied over the hyoid bone with the little finger will bring the larynx into view. A straight blade such as a Miller 0 usually provides the best view. Laryngoscope blades with a built-in channel that allows oxygen to be delivered at the tip may decrease the risk of hypoxia during laryngoscopy.

therefore be measured. Normal blood pressure depends on birth weight and varies from 50/25 mm Hg for neonates weighing 1–2 kg to 70/40 mm Hg for those weighing over 3 kg. A low blood pressure suggests hypovolemia. Volume expansion may be accomplished with type O-negative blood crossmatched with maternal blood or with 10 mL/kg of either 5% albumin or lactated Ringer's injection.

Drug Therapy

Drugs should be administered in the smallest possible volume. Sodium bicarbonate should generally only be given for a metabolic acidosis documented by blood gas measurements. During prolonged resuscitation (> 5 minutes)—particularly if blood gas measurements are not readily available—2 meq/kg of sodium bicarbonate may be given empirically; the infusion rate should not exceed 1 meq/kg/min to avoid hypertonicity and intracranial hemorrhage. Vasopressors (see below) are most effective when arterial pH is higher than 7.20.

A. Epinephrine, 0.01–0.03 mg/kg (0.1–0.3 mL/kg of a 1:10,000 solution), should be given for asystole or a spontaneous heart rate of less than 80 beats/min in spite of adequate ventilation and chest compressions. The epinephrine may be given down the endotracheal tube if venous access is not available. Atropine, 0.03 mg/kg, can be used for reflex bradycardia (as during instrumentation of the airway). Epinephrine or isoproterenol in doses of 0.1–1 μg/kg/min is indicated for persistent bradycardia, hypotension, and signs of a low cardiac output.

B. Calcium, 30 mg/kg of $CaCl_2$ or 100 mg/kg of calcium gluconate, should probably be given only to neonates suspected of magnesium intoxication from maternal magnesium sulfate therapy. These neonates are usually hypotensive and hypotonic and appear vasodilated.

C. Naloxone, 0.01 mg/kg intravenously or 0.02 mg/kg intramuscularly, is given to reverse the respiratory depressant effect of narcotics given to the mother in the last 4 hours of labor. Withdrawal may be precipitated in babies of narcotic addicts.

D. Glucose, 4 mL/kg of a 10% solution, is given for documented hypoglycemia. Blood glucose can be readily measured at the bedside with chemical reagent strips. Hyperglycemia should be avoided as it appears to worsen hypoxic neurologic deficits.

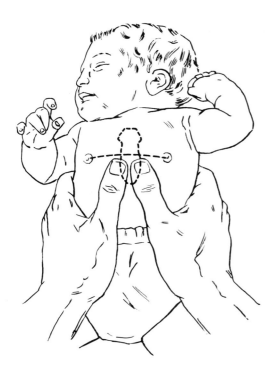

Figure 41–4. Chest compressions in the neonate. The neonate is held with both hands as each thumb is placed between the lower and middle third of the sternal body and the remaining fingers encircle the chest. The sternum is compressed 1/2 to 3/4 inches (1–cm) at a rate of 120 /min. (Modified and reproduced, with permission, from: Neonatal life support, Part VI. JAMA 1986;255:2969.)

Cardiac compressions at a rate of 120/min should be started (Figure 42–4). The technique described for infants (Chapter 46) may be used for large neonates. The heart rate should be checked periodically. Chest compressions should be stopped when the spontaneous heart rate exceeds 80 beats/min.

Vascular Access

Cannulation of the umbilical vein with a 3.5F or 5F umbilical catheter is easiest and the preferred technique. The tip of the catheter should be just below skin level yet should allow free backflow of blood; further advancement may result in infusion of hypertonic solutions directly into the liver. Umbilical artery cannulation allows measurement of blood pressure and facilitates blood gas measurements but is more difficult and time-consuming.

Volume Resuscitation

Recommended indications include (1) pallor that persists after oxygenation, (2) a faint pulse with an adequate heart rate, and (3) a poor response to resuscitation. Neonatal blood pressure generally correlates with intravascular volume. Blood pressure should

CASE DISCUSSION: APPENDICITIS IN A PREGNANT WOMAN

A 31-year-old woman with a 24-week gestation presents for an appendectomy.

How does pregnancy complicate the management of this patient?

Nearly 1–2% of all pregnant patients require surgery during their pregnancy. Appendectomy (1:1500 pregnancies) and cholecystectomy (1: 2000–10,000 pregnancies) are the most commonly performed abdominal procedures. The physiologic effects of pregnancy can alter the manifestations of the disease process and make diagnosis difficult. Patients may therefore present with advanced or complicated disease. The physiologic changes associated with pregnancy (Chapter 40) further predispose the patient to increased morbidity and mortality. Moreover, both the surgery and the anesthesia can adversely affect the fetus.

What are the potentially detrimental effects of surgery and anesthesia on the fetus?

The procedure can have both immediate and long-term undesirable effects on the fetus. Hypotension, hypovolemia, severe anemia, hypoxemia, and marked increases in sympathetic tone can seriously compromise the transfer of oxygen and other nutrients across the uteroplacental circulation and promote intrauterine fetal asphyxia. The stress of the procedure may also precipitate preterm labor. Preterm labor often follows intra-abdominal surgery near the uterus. Long-term detrimental effects relate to possible teratogenic effects on the developing fetus.

When is the fetus most sensitive to teratogenic influences?

Three stages of susceptibility are generally recognized. In the first 2 weeks of intrauterine life, teratogens have either a lethal or no effect on the embryo. The third to eighth weeks are the most critical period, when organogenesis takes place; drug exposure during this period can produce major developmental abnormalities. From the eighth week onward, organogenesis is complete, and organ growth takes place. Teratogen exposure during this last period usually results in only minor morphologic abnormalities but can produce significant physiologic abnormalities and growth retardation. Although the teratogenic influences of anesthetic agents have been extensively studied in animals, retrospective human studies have not been conclusive. A notable exception is the benzodiazepine group, which has been linked to congenital anomalies. Nonetheless, as with all drugs, exposure to anesthetic agents should be kept to a minimum in terms of the number of agents, dosage, and duration of exposure.

What would be the most ideal anesthetic technique in this patient?

By the end of the second trimester, most of the physiologic changes associated with pregnancy have taken place. Regional anesthesia may therefore be preferable to general anesthesia to decrease the risks of pulmonary aspiration and failed intubation and minimize drug exposure to the fetus. Drug exposure is least (probably negligible) with spinal anesthesia. Moreover, spinal anesthesia may be preferable to epidural anesthesia because it is not associated with unintentional intravascular injections or potentially large intrathecal doses of local anesthetic. On the other hand, general anesthesia guarantees patient comfort and, when a volatile agent is used, may even suppress preterm labor (Chapter 40).

Although regional anesthesia is preferable in most instances, the choice between regional and general anesthesia must be individualized according to the patient, the anesthesiologist, and the type of surgery. Spinal anesthesia is usually satisfactory for appendectomies, while general anesthesia is more satisfactory for cholecystectomies. The same techniques and doses used for the parturient (see above) should be followed.

Are any special monitors indicated perioperatively?

In addition to standard monitors (Chapter 6), fetal heart rate and uterine activity should be monitored with a Doppler and tocodynamometer during induction of anesthesia, emergence, and recovery, and, whenever possible, during surgery. When regular organized uterine activity is detected, early treatment with a β-adrenergic agonist such as ritodrine usually aborts the preterm labor.

When should elective operations be performed during pregnancy?

All elective operations should be postponed until 6 weeks after delivery. Only emergency procedures that pose an immediate threat to the mother or fetus should be routinely performed. The timing of semielective procedures, such as those for cancer, valvular heart disease, or intracranial aneurysms, must be individualized and must balance the threat to maternal health versus fetal well-being.

SUGGESTED READINGS

Albright GA: *Anesthesia in Obstetrics: Maternal, Fetal, and Neonatal Aspects,* 2nd ed. Butterworths, 1986.

Crawford JS: *Principles and Practice of Obstetric Anaesthesia,* 5th ed. Blackwell, 1984.

Datta S: *Anesthetic and Obstetric Management of High-Risk Pregnancy.* Mosby Year Book, 1990.

Datta S, Ostheimer GW: *Common Problems in Obstetric Anesthesia.* Mosby Year Book, 1987.

Gibbs C et al: Obstetric anesthesia: A national survey. Anesthesiology 1986;65:298. A summary of obstetric anesthesia practices in the 1980s.

James FM: *Obstetric Anesthesia: The Complicated Patient,* 2nd ed. Davis, 1988.

Ostheimer GW: *Manual of Obstetric Anesthesia.* Churchill Livingstone, 1984.

Ramanathan S: *Obstetric Anesthesia.* Lea & Febiger, 1988.

Shnider SM, Levinson G: *Anesthesia for Obstetrics,* 2nd ed. Williams & Wilkins, 1987.

Standards and guidelines for cardiopulmonary resuscitation and emergency cardiac care. Part VI: Neonatal advanced life support. JAMA 1986;255:2969. American Heart Association guidelines for neonatal resuscitation based on the recommendations of experts.

42

Pediatric Anesthesia

Neonates ($<$ 30 days of age), infants (1–12 months of age), and children (1–12 years of age) are not merely "small adults." Their successful anesthetic management depends upon an appreciation of the physiologic, anatomic, and pharmacologic differences between each group (Table 42–1). These differences necessitate modification of anesthetic equipment and techniques. In addition, pediatric patients are prone to illnesses that require unique surgical and anesthetic strategies.

PHYSIOLOGIC DIFFERENCES

Cardiovascular System

The cardiac output of neonates and infants is dependent on heart rate, since stroke volume is relatively fixed by a noncompliant and poorly developed left ventricle. Although basal heart rate is higher than in adults (Table 42–2), activation of the parasympathetic

Table 42–1. Characteristics of neonates and infants that differentiate them from adult patients.

Physiologic
  Cardiac output is heart rate-dependent
  Lower blood pressure
  Faster heart rate
  Faster respiratory rate
  Lower lung compliance
  Greater chest wall compliance
  Lower functional residual capacity
  Higher ratio of body surface area to body weight
  Higher total body water content
Anatomic
  Noncompliant left ventricle
  Residual fetal circulation
  Difficult venous and arterial cannulation
  Large head and tongue
  Narrow nasal passages
  Anterior ad cephalad larynx
  Long epiglottis
  Short trachea and neck
  Prominent adenoids and tonsils
  Weak intercostal and diaphragmatic muscles
  High resistance to airflow
Pharmacologic
  Immature hepatic biotransformation
  Decreased protein binding
  Rapid rise in F_A/F_I
  Rapid induction and recovery
  Increased minimum alveolar concentration
  Larger volume of distribution for water-soluble drugs
  Immature neuromuscular junction

Table 42–2. Age-related changes in vital signs.[1]

Age	Respiratory Rate	Heart Rate	Arterial Blood Pressure	
			Systolic	Diastolic
Neonate	40	140	65	40
12 months	30	120	95	65
3 years	25	100	100	70
12 years	20	80	110	60

[1]Values are mean averages derived from numerous sources. Normal ranges vary by as much as 25–50%.

nervous system, anesthetic overdose, or hypoxia can cause profound bradycardia and reductions in cardiac output. The slowing of heart rate with age contrasts with rising systolic and diastolic blood pressures. The sympathetic nervous system and baroreceptor reflexes are not fully mature. The infant cardiovascular system maintains less catecholamine stores and displays a blunted response to exogenous catecholamines. The vascular tree is less able to respond to hypovolemia with vasoconstriction. Thus, the hallmark of intravascular fluid depletion in neonates and infants is hypotension without tachycardia.

The high heart rates of neonates are beyond the monitoring capability of some adult electrocardiograph units. Smaller electrode pads interfere less with sterile surgical areas. Accurate measurement of blood pressure is a problem in unstable neonates. Blood pressure cuffs must be properly fitted (see Figure 6–9), and Korotkoff sounds may be difficult to auscultate at lower pressures. Newer oscillometric and Doppler technologies provide reliable noninvasive solutions. A precordial stethoscope provides an inexpensive means of monitoring heart rate, quality of heart sounds, and airway patency.

Respiratory System

The respiratory rate is elevated in neonates but gradually falls to adult levels by adolescence. Tidal volume and dead space per kilogram remain constant. Small alveoli are associated with low lung compliance. In contrast, the cartilaginous chest wall of the neonate is very compliant. The combination of these two factors leads to chest wall collapse during inspiration and relatively low residual lung volumes during expiration.

This decrease in functional residual capacity is important because it limits oxygen reserves during periods of apnea (eg, intubation) and increases the likelihood of atelectasis. Alveolar maturation is not complete until late childhood. Hypoxic and hypercapnic ventilatory drives are not well developed in neonates and infants. In fact, in contrast to adults, hypoxia and hypercapnia depress respiration.

Many anesthesia ventilators designed for adult patients cannot reliably provide the low tidal volumes and rapid rates required by neonates and infants. Unintentional delivery of large tidal volumes to a small child can generate enormous peak airway pressures and cause extensive barotrauma. Small tidal volumes can be manually delivered with greater sensitivity with a 1-L breathing bag compared to a 3-L adult bag. Spirometers are less accurate at lower tidal volumes. Additionally, the gas lost in long breathing tubes with high compliance becomes quite significant compared to a child's small tidal volume. For this reason, pediatric tubing is usually shorter and stiffer. Equipment dead space, a critical determinant of rebreathing in children, is minimized by a septum that divides the inspiratory and expiratory gas in the Y-piece.

During spontaneous ventilation, even the low resistance of a circle system can become a significant obstacle for a sick neonate to overcome. Some anesthesiologists prefer the Mapleson D circuit or the Bain system (Chapter 3). In general, respiration is controlled during anesthesia of neonates and infants. Airway pressure monitoring may provide early evidence of obstruction due to a kinked endotracheal tube or advancement of the tube into a main stem bronchus.

End-tidal CO_2 analysis allows assessment of the adequacy of ventilation, confirmation of endotracheal tube placement, and early warning of malignant hyperthermia. However, the small tidal volumes and rapid respiratory rates of small infants can present difficulties with some capnograph models. Furthermore, the size of some flow-through sensors may lead to kinking of the endotracheal tube or hypercapnia due to increased equipment dead space.

Metabolism & Temperature Regulation

Pediatric patients have a larger surface area per kilogram than adults (increased surface area/weight ratio). Metabolism and its associated parameters (oxygen consumption, CO_2 production, cardiac output, and alveolar ventilation) correlate better with surface area than with weight. The higher surface area is also responsible for increased heat loss to the environment. This problem is compounded by cold operating rooms, wound exposure, intravenous fluid administration, dry anesthetic gases, and the direct effect of anesthetic agents on temperature regulation. Hypothermia is a serious problem that has been associated with delayed awakening from anesthesia, cardiac irritability, respiratory depression, increased pulmonary vascular resistance, and altered drug responses. The major mech-

anism for heat production in neonates is **nonshivering thermogenesis** by metabolism of brown fat. Even this is severely limited in premature infants and in sick neonates who possess deficit fat stores.

Temperature must be closely monitored in pediatric patients. Monitoring site selection is considered in Chapter 6. There are several ways to prevent hypothermia, including maintaining a warm operating room environment (26 °C or higher), warming and humidifying inspired gases, utilizing a warming blanket and warming lights, and warming all intravenous fluids. The room temperature required for a neutral thermal environment varies with age, being highest in premature newborns.

Care must be taken to prevent unintentional skin burns from overzealous warming efforts.

Gastrointestinal Tract

To avoid excessive dehydration, preoperative fluid restriction is more lenient in pediatric patients. Regular formula feedings are continued in neonates and infants until 6–8 hours before surgery. Clear fluids are offered until 4 hours before induction. However, several studies have documented low gastric pH (< 2.5) and relatively high residual volumes in pediatric patients scheduled for elective outpatient surgery, suggesting that children may be at a higher risk of aspiration than previously thought. Overnight fasting is usually recommended in patients over 1 year of age.

Renal Function, Glucose Homeostasis, & Fluid Requirements

By 6 months of age, healthy infants possess almost normal kidney function. On the other hand, premature neonates may possess multiple renal defects, including decreased creatinine clearance; impaired sodium retention, glucose excretion, and bicarbonate reabsorption; and poor diluting and concentrating ability. These abnormalities increase the importance of meticulous attention to fluid administration in the early days of life. Impaired glucose excretion is offset by a tendency toward hypoglycemia in neonates who are premature, those who are small for gestational age, those who have received hyperalimentation, or those who have diabetic mothers. All of the foregoing should have frequent serum glucose determinations.

Neonates and infants have a proportionately higher total water content (70–75%) than adults (50–60%). In particular, the extracellular fluid compartment is enlarged. These differences affect fluid therapy and clinical pharmacology. Fluid therapy can be divided into maintenance, deficit, and replacement requirements. A formula for determining **maintenance fluid requirements** in adult and pediatric patients was presented in Chapter 29: 4 mL/kg/h for the first 10 kg;. 2 mL/kg/h for the second 10 kg; and 1 mL/kg/h for each remaining kg. The choice of maintenance fluid remains controversial. A solution such as $D_5 1/2NS$ with 20 meq/L of KCl provides adequate dextrose and electrolytes at these maintenance infusion rates. $D_5 1/4NS$ may be a better maintenance fluid choice in neonates because of their limited ability to handle sodium loads. Some neonates may require $D_{10}W$ maintenance solutions to prevent hypoglycemia.

In addition to a maintenance infusion, any **preoperative fluid deficits** must be replaced. For example, if a 5-kg infant has not received oral or intravenous fluids for 4 hours prior to surgery, a deficit of 80 mL has accrued (5 kg × 4 mL/kg/h × 4 h). In contrast to adults, infants respond to dehydration with decreased blood pressure but without increased heart rate. Preoperative fluid deficits are typically administered with hourly maintenance requirements in aliquots of 50% in the first hour and 25% in the second and third hours. In the example above, a total of 60 mL would be given the first hour (80/2 + 20), and 40 mL in the second and third hours (80/4 + 20). Large quantities of dextrose-containing solutions are avoided to prevent hyperglycemia. Preoperative fluid deficits are usually replaced with a balanced salt solution (eg, lactated Ringer's injection) or 1/2NS. Normal saline has the disadvantage of being a more acidic solution than lactated Ringer's injection. Fluid overload is diagnosed by prominent veins, flushed skin, increased blood pressure, decreased serum sodium, and a loss of the folds in the upper eyelids.

Replacement requirements are subdivided into blood loss and third space loss. The blood volume of premature neonates (100 mL/kg), full-term neonates (85–90 mL/kg), and infants (80 mL/kg) is proportionately higher than that of adults (65–70 mL/kg). An initial hematocrit of 55% in the healthy full-term neonate gradually falls to as low as 30% in the 3-month-old infant before rising to 35% by 6 months. Hemoglobin type is also changing during this period: from a 75% concentration of HbF (high oxygen affinity, low PaO_2, poor tissue unloading) at birth to almost 100% HbA (low oxygen affinity, high PaO_2, good tissue unloading) by 6 months. **Blood loss** is typically replaced with non-glucose-containing crystalloid (eg, 3 mL of lactated Ringer's injection for each milliliter of blood lost) or colloid solutions (eg, 1 mL of 5% albumin per milliliter of blood lost) until the patient's hematocrit reaches a predetermined lower limit. In premature and sick neonates, this may be as high as 40% or 50%, while in older children a hematocrit of 25–30% is generally well tolerated. Because of their small intravascular volume, neonates and infants are at an increased risk of some of the electrolyte disturbances that can accompany rapid blood transfusion such as hyperglycemia, hyperkalemia, and hypocalcemia.

Third space loss is impossible to measure and must be estimated by the extent of the surgical procedure. One popular guideline is 2 mL/kg/h for relatively atraumatic surgery (strabismus correction) and up to 6–10 mL/kg/h for traumatic procedures (abdominal abscess). Third space loss is usually replaced with lactated Ringer's injection. Thus, intraoperative fluid management considers maintenance requirements (4:2:1 rule), preoperative deficit (duration of NPO), blood loss, and third-space loss. Other fluid losses, such as copious nasogastric suctioning, may become significant in some diseases.

Precise delivery of small volumes of fluid is facilitated by programmable infusion pumps and intravenous sets with burets and microdrips. Drugs are flushed through low dead-space tubing to minimize unnecessary fluid administration.

ANATOMIC DIFFERENCES

Cardiovascular System

The anatomy of the fetal circulation and the transition to an extrauterine vascular system are discussed in Chapter 40. Cannulation of tiny pediatric veins can be a trying ordeal. This is particularly true for infants who have spent weeks in a neonatal intensive care unit and have few veins left unscarred. Even healthy 1-year-old children can prove a challenge because of extensive subcutaneous fat. The saphenous vein has a consistent location at the ankle and, with experience, can usually be cannulated even if it is not visible or palpable. Twenty-four-gauge over-the-needle catheters are adequate in neonates and infants when blood transfusions are not anticipated. All air bubbles should be removed from the intravenous line, since a high incidence of patent foramen ovale increases the risk of paradoxic air embolism. In emergency situations where intravenous access is impossible, fluids can be effectively infused through an 18-gauge needle inserted into the medullary sinusoids within the tibial bone. This **intraosseous infusion** can be used for all medications normally given intravenously with equally rapid results (Chapter 46).

Invasive monitoring (eg, arterial cannulation, central venous catheterization) requires considerable expertise. Some anesthesiologists avoid pulmonary artery catheterization in infants because of the presence of a patent foramen ovale and the predictable relationship between right- and left-sided filling pressures in most of these patients. The right radial artery is often chosen for cannulation in the neonate since its preductal location mirrors the oxygen content of the carotid and retinal arteries.

Respiratory System

There are many differences between adult and pediatric anatomy that affect mask ventilation and intubation. In the neonate and infant, these include a proportionately larger head and tongue, narrow nasal passages, an anterior and cephalad larynx (opposite a vertebral level of C4 versus C6 in adults), a long epiglottis, and a short trachea and neck (Figure 42–1). These factors contribute to making infants obligate nasal breathers. The cricoid cartilage is the narrowest point of the airway in children younger than 5 years of age, as opposed to the glottis in the adult. One millimeter of edema will have a proportionately greater effect

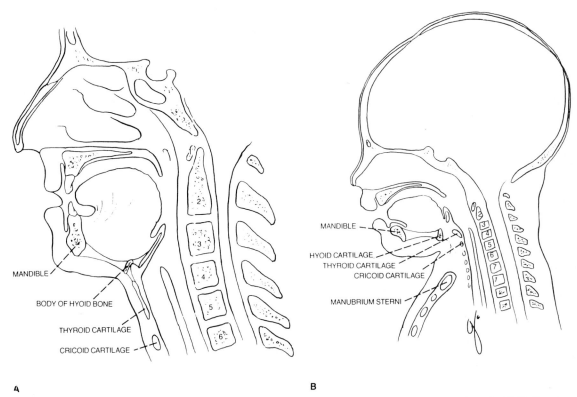

Figure 42–1. Sagittal section of the infant *(A)* and adult *(B)* airway. (Reproduced, with permission, from Snell RS, Katz J: *Clinical Anatomy for Anesthesiologists.* Appleton & Lange, 1988.)

in children because of their smaller tracheal diameters. In older children, prominent adenoid and tonsillar tissue can obstruct visualization of the larynx.

These anatomic differences influence anesthetic technique. A prominent occiput tends to place the head in a flexed position prior to intubation. This is easily corrected by slightly elevating the shoulders with towels and placing the head on a doughnut-shaped pillow. Oral airways often help displace an oversized tongue, while nasal airways can traumatize small nares or prominent adenoids. Specially contoured masks minimize dead space (Figure 5–7). Compression of submandibular soft tissues should be avoided during mask ventilation to prevent upper airway obstruction. Straight laryngoscope blades aid intubation of the anterior larynx in infants and young children. Endotracheal tubes that pass through the glottis may still impinge upon the cricoid cartilage, causing postoperative edema, stridor, croup, and airway obstruction. Uncuffed endotracheal tubes are usually selected for children under the age of 10 in order to decrease the risk of postintubation croup and to provide a leak to minimize the risk of accidental barotrauma. Endotracheal tube inside diameter is initially estimated by a formula based on age:

$$4 + \frac{Age}{4} = \text{Tube diameter in mm}$$

For example, a 4-year-old child would be predicted to require a 5-mm tube (4 + 4 ÷ 4 = 5). This formula provides only a rough guideline, however. Exceptions include premature (2.5–3 mm) and full-term neonates (3–3.5 mm). Endotracheal tubes 0.5 mm larger or smaller than predicted should be readily available. Correct tube size is confirmed by easy passage into the larynx and the development of a gas leak at 10–25 cm H_2O pressure. No leak indicates an oversized tube that should be replaced to prevent postoperative edema, while an excessive leak may preclude adequate ventilation and contaminate the operating room with anesthetic gases. There is also a formula to estimate endotracheal length:

$$12 + \frac{Age}{2} = \text{Length of cut tube in cm}$$

Again, this formula provides only a guideline, and the result must be confirmed by auscultation and clinical judgment. To avoid endobronchial intubation, the tip of the endotracheal tube should pass only 1–2 cm beyond an infant's glottis. An alternative technique is to intentionally place the tip of the endotracheal tube into the right main stem bronchus and then withdraw it until breath sounds are equal.

Several anatomic characteristics decrease the efficiency of respiration in neonates and infants, including weak intercostal and diaphragmatic musculature due to a paucity of type I fibers, horizontal and pliable ribs, and a protuberant abdomen. The paucity of small airways and alveoli is responsible for a high total resistance to air flow.

PHARMACOLOGIC DIFFERENCES

Pediatric drug dosing is typically based upon a per kilogram recommendation (see Inside Back Cover for a table of pediatric drug doses). A child's weight can be roughly estimated based upon age:

50th percentile weight (kg) = (Age × 2) + 9

However, weight does not take into account the disproportionate size of the pediatric intravascular and extracellular fluid compartments, the immaturity of hepatic biotransformation pathways, increased organ blood flow, decreased protein binding, or higher metabolic rate. These variables must be considered on an individual basis.

Inhalational Anesthetics

High alveolar ventilation, relatively low functional residual capacity (ie, a high ratio of minute ventilation to functional residual capacity), and a large vessel-rich group contribute to a rapid rise in alveolar anesthetic concentration. Furthermore, the blood/gas coefficients of isoflurane and halothane are lower in neonates than in adults. These factors result in rapid induction and recovery from general anesthesia. The minimum alveolar concentration is higher in infants than in neonates or adults. The blood pressure of neonates and infants tends to be more sensitive to volatile anesthetics, probably due to undeveloped compensatory mechanisms (eg, vasoconstriction and tachycardia) and exaggerated myocardial depression. Prepubertal children are at much less risk for halothane-induced hepatic dysfunction than adults.

Nonvolatile Anesthetics

Some barbiturates and opioid agonists appear to be more toxic in neonates than in adults. Possible explanations include easier entry across the blood-brain barrier, decreased metabolic capability, or increased sensitivity of the respiratory centers. For example, morphine sulfate should be used with caution in neonates, since conjugation is reduced and impaired renal function decreases the rate of clearance of morphine metabolites. In contrast, neonates and infants appear to be more resistant to the effects of ketamine. The cytochrome P-450 pathway is mature at 1 month. Pediatric patients have relatively high rates of biotransformation and elimination as a result of high hepatic blood flow.

Muscle Relaxants

Infants require higher doses of succinylcholine per kilogram than adults because of their larger volume of distribution (expanded extracellular space). This discrepancy disappears if dosage is based upon body surface area. Children are more prone to cardiac dysrhythmias, myoglobinemia, and malignant hyperthermia after succinylcholine than are adults. Bradycardia is prevented by preceding the succinylcholine with intravenous atropine.

The response of neonates to nondepolarizing muscle relaxants is quite variable. Immaturity of the neuromuscular junction (particularly in premature neonates) tends to increase sensitivity, while an expanded extracellular compartment dilutes drug concentration. Duration of action will be prolonged in neonates if the drug depends on hepatic metabolism (eg, vecuronium). In contrast, atracurium does not depend on hepatic biotransformation and has a shorter duration of effect in infants. As with adults, the effect of incremental doses of muscle relaxant should be monitored with a peripheral nerve stimulator. Nondepolarizing blockade can be reversed with neostigmine (up to 70 μg/kg) or edrophonium (1 mg/kg) along with an anticholinergic agent.

PEDIATRIC ANESTHETIC TECHNIQUES

Preoperative Interview

The art of pediatric anesthesia begins during the preoperative interview. Depending upon their age, past surgical experiences, and maturity, children suffer from varying degrees of terror when faced with the prospect of surgery. In contrast to adults, who are usually most concerned with the possibility of death, children are principally worried about pain and separation from their parents. An established physician-patient relationship can go a long way toward reassuring the frightened child. One successful strategy is to demystify the process of anesthesia and surgery by explaining in age-appropriate terms what lies ahead. For example, one might bring an anesthesia mask for the child to play with during the interview and describe it as something the astronauts use. Unfortunately, in this day of outpatient and morning-of-admission surgery, it is often difficult for an anesthesiologist to break through the barriers erected by pediatric patients. For this reason, it is often helpful if someone the child trusts (eg, a parent, nurse, or surgeon) remains in attendance during preanesthetic preparations and induction of anesthesia.

Premedication

There is great variation in the recommendations for premedication of pediatric patients. Premedication is often omitted for neonates, infants, outpatients, and older children. One possible exception is the neonate or infant with congenital heart disease. Morphine sulfate (0.1 mg/kg) may prevent perioperative crying and its associated increased oxygen consumption, pulmonary vasoconstriction, and hypercyanotic episodes. Many anesthesiologists routinely premedicate young children with anticholinergic drugs (eg, atropine 0.01–0.02 mg/kg) to lessen the likelihood of bradycardia during induction and accumulation of secretions that can be life-threatening in small airways and endotracheal tubes. This is often administered intramuscularly but can also be given orally or rectally. Other anesthesiologists prefer to give atropine intravenously at induction.

Children who appear likely to exhibit uncontrollable separation anxiety can be given a sedative such as pentobarbital (4–6 mg/kg intramuscularly) or chloral hydrate (50–100 mg/kg orally). Pentobarbital is discussed in Chapter 8.

Chloral hydrate is a relatively safe and effective hypnotic drug. Its therapeutic action is due to an active metabolite (trichloroethanol) with a half-life that can exceed 9 hours. Chloral hydrate has little effect on respiration or blood pressure in the recommended dosage range. However, overdosage can result in severe respiratory depression. Undesirable central nervous system effects may include paradoxic excitement, disorientation, and paranoid behavior. If there is no response after 30 minutes, half the initial dose may be repeated. Maximum effect is usually achieved within 1 hour, but sedation may last from 2 hours to several hours. Ingestion is characterized by an unpleasant taste and gastric irritation. Possible side effects include vomiting (15% of patients), delirium, bradypnea, and airway obstruction. Vomiting may result in insufficient sedation. Rectal suppositories are also available.

Rectal methohexital (25–30 mg/kg of 10% solution) can be administered to children weighing less than 20 kg by the anesthesiologist in the presence of the parents. Within 10 minutes, the child will be asleep and can be taken to the operating room for a "steal induction." One investigator has reported better systemic absorption by using a 1% solution of methohexital, as evidenced by more rapid onset and longer recovery time. As with adults, the best preoperative preparation is a personal interview with the anesthesiologist. Other premedication considerations are discussed in the case study presented in Chapter 8.

Induction

General anesthesia is usually induced by an intravenous or inhalational technique. Induction with intramuscular ketamine (5–10 mg/kg) is reserved for specific situations such as combative children. Intravenous induction is preferred if the patient comes to the operating room with an intravenous line or appears to be cooperative enough to allow an awake venous cannulation. The same induction sequence can be used as in adults: a rapid-acting barbiturate (eg, thiopental, 3–6 mg/kg) followed by a muscle relaxant (eg, succinylcholine, vecuronium, atracurium). If succinylcholine is chosen to aid intubation, atropine should be administered to prevent bradycardia. The advantages of an intravenous technique include familiarity with the agents, availability of intravenous access if emergency drugs need to be administered, and rapidity of induction in the child at risk for aspiration.

Most children do not arrive in the operating room with an intravenous line in place, and most dread the prospect of being stuck with a needle. Modern potent volatile anesthetics can render small children unconscious within minutes. This is usually easier in children who have been sedated prior to entering the operating room and who are sleepy enough to be induced without ever knowing what has happened ("steal induction"). Alternatives to frightening a child with a black mask include insufflation of the anesthetic gases over the face, substituting a clear face mask, placing a drop of food flavoring on the inside of the mask (eg, oil of orange), and allowing the child to sit during the early stages of induction.

Typically, the child is coaxed into breathing an odorless mixture of nitrous oxide (70%) and oxygen (30%). Halothane or another volatile anesthetic is added to the anesthetic gas mixture in 0.5% increments every 3–5 breaths. After unconsciousness has been achieved, an intravenous line can be started by an assistant and a muscle relaxant administered.

Alternatively, the anesthesiologist can deepen the level of anesthesia by increasing the concentration of volatile anesthetic and intubate the patient without supplemental relaxation. The possibility of severe cardiac depression or laryngospasm without intravenous access detracts from this technique. Intramuscular succinylcholine (4–6 mg/kg, not to exceed 150 mg) and atropine (0.02 mg/kg, not to exceed 0.4 mg) should be available if laryngospasm or bradycardia occurs before an intravenous line is established.

With either inhalational approach, nitrous oxide should be discontinued prior to intubation so that the patient's lungs will contain a high inspired oxygen concentration and adequate arterial oxygen saturations will be maintained during this period of apnea. Positive-pressure ventilation prior to intubation sometimes causes gastric distention, resulting in impairment of lung expansion. Placement of a nasogastric tube will decompress the stomach but must be done without traumatizing fragile mucous membranes.

Maintenance

Anesthesia is maintained in pediatric patients with the same agents as in adults. Although the minimum alveolar concentration is higher in children than in adults, neonates may be particularly susceptible to the cardiodepressant effects of general anesthetics. Nondepolarizing muscle relaxants are usually required for optimal surgical conditions. Nonetheless, almost all patients can tolerate and are entitled to anesthesia during operative procedures. Intraoperative fluid therapy, body temperature management, ventilation, and monitoring have been discussed.

Emergence & Recovery

Pediatric patients are particularly vulnerable to two postanesthetic complications: laryngospasm and postintubation croup. **Laryngospasm** is a forceful, involuntary spasm of laryngeal musculature caused by stimulation of the superior laryngeal nerve (Chapter 5).

Laryngospasm can usually be avoided by extubating the patient either awake (ie, eye opening) or while deeply anesthetized (spontaneously breathing but not coughing). Extubation during the interval between these extremes is hazardous. Treatment of laryngospasm includes gentle positive pressure ventilation, intravenous lidocaine (1–1.5 mg/kg), or paralysis with a small dose of succinylcholine (eg, 0.25 mg/kg) and controlled ventilation. Laryngospasm is usually an immediate postoperative event but may occur in the recovery room as the patient wakes up and chokes on pharyngeal secretions. For this reason, recovering pediatric patients should be positioned in the lateral position so that oral secretions pool and drain away from the cords. As soon as the child begins to regain consciousness, it is comforting to have the parents come to the bedside.

Postintubation croup is due to glottic or tracheal edema. Because the narrowest part of the pediatric airway is the cricoid cartilage, this is the most susceptible area. Croup is less common with endotracheal tubes that are uncuffed and small enough to allow a slight gas leak at 10–25 cm H_2O pressure. Postintubation croup is associated with early childhood (age 1–4), repeated intubation attempts, size of endotracheal tube, duration of surgery, head and neck procedures, and excessive movement of the tube (eg, coughing with the tube in place or moving the patient's head). Intravenous dexamethasone (0.1–0.5 mg/kg) may prevent edema formation, while inhalation of nebulized racemic epinephrine (0.5 mL of a 2.25% solution in 2.5 mL normal saline) is effective treatment. Although postintubation croup is a later complication than laryngospasm, it almost always appears within 3 hours after extubation.

PATHOPHYSIOLOGY & ANESTHETIC CONSIDERATIONS IN SPECIFIC PEDIATRIC DISORDERS

PREMATURITY

Pathophysiology

Prematurity is defined as birth before 38 weeks of gestation or at a weight of less than 2500 g. The multiple medical problems of this subset of neonates are usually due to immaturity of major organ systems or intrauterine asphyxia. Pulmonary complications include hyaline membrane disease, apneic spells, and bronchopulmonary dysplasia. Patent ductus arteriosus leads to shunting, pulmonary edema, and congestive heart failure. Persistent hypoxemia or shock may result in an ischemic gut and necrotizing enterocolitis. Prematurity increases susceptibility to infection, hypothermia, intracranial hemorrhage, and kernicterus

compared to full-term neonates. Premature neonates also have an increased incidence of congenital anomalies.

Anesthetic Considerations

The small size (often less than 1000 g) and tenuous medical condition of premature neonates demand meticulous anesthetic technique. Obviously, special attention must be paid to airway control, fluid management, and temperature regulation. The problem of **retinopathy of prematurity** deserves special consideration. While hyperoxia is associated with this blinding disease, the presence of fetal hemoglobin and treatment with vitamin E may be protective. Oxygenation should be continuously monitored with pulse oximetry or transcutaneous oxygen analysis. Normal PaO_2 is 60–80 mm Hg in neonates. Excessive inspired oxygen concentrations are avoided by blending with air or nitrous oxide. Other risk factors associated with retinopathy of prematurity include multiple blood transfusions, apnea requiring artificial ventilation, parenteral nutrition, hypoxemia, hypercapnia and hypocapnia.

Anesthetic requirements of premature neonates are reduced. Opioid agonists such as fentanyl are often favored over volatile anesthetics due to the latter's tendency to cause myocardial depression. Even nitrous oxide can cause significant cardiovascular depression. Muscle relaxants provide good surgical conditions, and ventilation is controlled.

Premature infants less than 60 weeks postconception are prone to episodes of apnea up to 24 hours postoperatively. In fact, even term infants can (rarely) experience apneic spells following general anesthesia. **Postanesthetic apnea** may be prevented in infants at high risk by intravenous administration of caffeine or aminophylline. Nonetheless, elective or outpatient procedures should be deferred until the preterm infant reaches the age of at least 60 weeks postconception. If surgery must be performed in these infants, monitoring with pulse oximetry for 12–24 hours postoperatively is mandatory.

Sick premature neonates often receive multiple aliquots of blood during their stay in the pediatric intensive care unit. Their immunocompromised status predisposes them to clinically significant cytomegalovirus infection following transfusion. Signs of infection include generalized lymphadenopathy, fever, pneumonia, hepatitis, hemolytic anemia, and thrombocytopenia. Preventive measures include using cytomegalovirus-seronegative donor blood or frozen blood cells.

CONGENITAL DIAPHRAGMATIC HERNIA

Pathophysiology

During fetal development, the gut can herniate into the thorax through one of three possible diaphragmatic defects: the left or right posterolateral foramen of

Bochdalek or the anterior foramen of Morgagni. Left-sided herniation is the most common type. While the ipsilateral lung is especially impaired, the herniated gut can compress and retard the maturation of both lungs. A reduction in alveoli and bronchioli (**pulmonary hypoplasia**) is accompanied by marked elevation in pulmonary vascular resistance. Hallmarks of diaphragmatic herniation include hypoxemia, a scaphoid abdomen, and evidence of bowel in the thorax by auscultation or radiography.

Anesthetic Considerations

Gastric distention must be minimized by placement of a nasogastric tube and avoidance of high levels of positive-pressure ventilation. The neonate is preoxygenated and intubated awake, often without the aid of muscle relaxants. Anesthesia is maintained with low concentrations of volatile agents or opioids, muscle relaxants, and air as tolerated. Hypoxemia and expansion of air in the bowel contraindicate the use of nitrous oxide. If possible, peak inspiratory airway pressures should be less than 30 cm H_2O. A sudden fall in lung compliance, blood pressure, or oxygenation may signal a *contralateral* (usually right-sided) pneumothorax and indicate chest tube placement. Arterial blood gases are monitored by sampling a preductal artery. Aggressive attempts at expansion of the ipsilateral lung following surgical decompression are detrimental. Postoperative prognosis parallels the extent of pulmonary hypoplasia and the presence of other congenital defects.

TRACHEOESOPHAGEAL FISTULA

Pathophysiology

There are several types of tracheoesophageal fistula. The most common is the combination of an upper esophagus that ends in a blind pouch and a lower esophagus that connects to the trachea. Breathing results in gastric distention, while feeding leads to choking and coughing. Aspiration pneumonia and the coexistence of other congenital anomalies (eg, cardiac) are common.

Anesthetic Considerations

These neonates tend to have copious pharyngeal secretions that require frequent suctioning before and during surgery. Positive-pressure ventilation is avoided prior to intubation, since the resulting gastric distention may interfere with lung expansion. Intubation is often performed awake and without muscle relaxants. These infants are often dehydrated and malnourished due to poor oral intake. The key to successful management is correct endotracheal tube position. Ideally, the tip of the tube lies between the fistula and the carina, so that anesthetic gases preferentially pass into the lungs instead of the stomach. This is impossible if the fistula connects to the carina or a main stem bronchus. In these situations, intermittent

venting of a gastrostomy tube that has been placed preoperatively may permit positive-pressure ventilation without excessive gastric distention. Suctioning of the gastrostomy tube and upper esophageal pouch tube helps to prevent aspiration pneumonitis. Surgical division of the fistula and esophageal anastomosis is performed with the patient in the left lateral position. A precordial stethoscope should be placed in the dependent axilla, since main stem bronchus obstruction during surgical retraction is not uncommon. A drop in oxygen saturation indicates that the retracted lung needs to be reexpanded. Surgical traction can also compress the great vessels, trachea, heart, and vagus nerve. Blood should be immediately available for transfusion. Postoperative complications include gastroesophageal reflux, aspiration pneumonitis, tracheal compression, and anastomotic leakage.

HYPERTROPHIC PYLORIC STENOSIS

Pathophysiology

Hypertrophic pyloric stenosis interferes with emptying of gastric contents. Persistent vomiting depletes sodium, potassium, chloride, and hydrogen ions, causing **hypochloremic metabolic alkalosis.** Initially, the kidney tries to compensate for the alkalosis by excreting sodium bicarbonate in the urine. Later, as hyponatremia and dehydration worsen, the kidneys must conserve sodium even at the expense of hydrogen ion excretion (**paradoxic aciduria).** Correction of the volume deficit and metabolic alkalosis requires hydration with a sodium chloride solution supplemented with potassium. Because lactate is metabolized to bicarbonate, lactated Ringer's injection should not be used.

Anesthetic Considerations

Surgery should be postponed until fluid and electrolyte abnormalities have been corrected. The stomach should be emptied with a large nasogastric or orogastric tube. Techniques of intubation and induction may vary, but in all cases one must consider the patient's high risk for aspiration. Pyloromyotomy is a short procedure that requires muscle relaxation. These neonates may be at increased risk for respiratory depression and hypoventilation in the recovery room due to persistent metabolic or cerebrospinal fluid alkalosis.

INFECTIOUS CROUP & ACUTE EPIGLOTTITIS

Pathophysiology

Croup is obstruction of the airway characterized by a barking cough. One type of croup, postintubation croup, has already been discussed. Another type is due to viral infection. **Infectious croup** usually follows an upper respiratory infection in children aged 3 months to 3 years. The airway *below* the epiglottis (laryngo-tracheobronchitis) is involved. Infectious croup progresses slowly and rarely requires intubation. In contrast, **acute epiglottitis** is a bacterial infection (*Haemophilus influenzae* type B) most commonly affecting 2- to 6-year-old children—but rarely adults—that rapidly progresses from a sore throat to dysphagia and complete airway obstruction. Endotracheal intubation and antibiotic therapy can be lifesaving.

Anesthetic Considerations

Children with impending airway obstruction due to epiglottitis or severe infectious croup (ie, cyanosis and intercostal retractions) present in the operating room for definitive diagnosis by laryngoscopy and intubation. A preoperative lateral neck radiograph may show a characteristic "thumblike" epiglottic shadow but is time-consuming and unnecessary. Total obstruction can occur at any moment, and adequate preparations for tracheostomy must be made prior to induction of general anesthesia. Laryngoscopy should not be performed before induction of anesthesia because of the possibility of laryngospasm. In most cases, inhalational induction is performed with the patient in the sitting position with a volatile anesthetic and a high concentration of oxygen. Oral intubation with an endotracheal tube one-half to one size smaller than usual is attempted as soon as an adequate depth of anesthesia is established. The oral tube may be replaced with a well-secured nasal endotracheal tube at the end of the procedure, since the latter is better tolerated in the postoperative period. If intubation is impossible, rigid bronchoscopy or emergency tracheostomy must be performed.

GASTROSCHISIS & OMPHALOCELE

Pathophysiology

Gastroschisis and omphalocele are congenital disorders characterized by defects in the abdominal wall that allow external herniation of viscera. They differ in location, the presence of a hernial sac, and associated congenital anomalies (Table 42–3). Perioperative management centers around prevention of hypothermia, infection, and dehydration. These problems are usually more serious in gastroschisis, since the protective hernial sac is absent.

Anesthetic Considerations

The stomach is decompressed with a nasogastric tube before induction. Intubation can be accomplished with the patient awake or asleep and with or without muscle relaxation. Nitrous oxide should be avoided to prevent further bowel distention. Muscle relaxation is required for replacement of bowel into the abdominal cavity. A one-stage closure is not always possible, since it can decrease pulmonary compliance and reduce lower extremity blood flow. Third space fluid losses are aggressively replaced with a balanced salt solution and 5% albumin. The neonate remains intubated after the procedure and is weaned from the ventilator over the next 1–2 days in the intensive care unit.

TONSILLECTOMY & ADENOIDECTOMY

Pathophysiology

Lymphoid hyperplasia can lead to upper airway obstruction, obligate mouth breathing, and even pulmonary hypertension with cor pulmonale. Although these extremes of pathology are unusual, all children undergoing tonsillectomy or adenoidectomy should be considered to be at increased risk for perioperative airway problems.

Anesthetic Considerations

Surgery should be postponed if there is evidence of acute infection or suspicion of a bleeding dysfunction (eg, recent aspirin ingestion). Preoperative administration of an anticholinergic will decrease pharyngeal secretions. A history of airway obstruction or apnea suggests an inhalation induction without paralysis until the ability to ventilate with positive pressure is established. A reinforced or preformed endotracheal tube (eg, RAE tube) lessens the risk of kinking by the surgeon's self-retaining mouth gag. Blood transfusion is usually not necessary, but the anesthesiologist must be wary of occult blood loss. Meticulous but gentle inspection and suctioning of the pharynx precedes extubation. Although deep extubation lessens the chance of laryngospasm and may prevent blood clot dislodgment from coughing, most anesthesiologists prefer an awake extubation because of the risks of aspiration. Postoperative vomiting is common. The

Table 42–3. Characteristics of gastroschisis and omphalocele.

Characteristic	Gastroschisis	Omphalocele
Location	Lateral to umbilicus	Base of umbilicus
Hernial sac	Absent	Present
Associated congenital anomalies	None	Trisomy 21, cardiac anomalies, diaphragmatic hernia, bladder anomalies

anesthesiologist must be alert in the recovery room for postoperative bleeding, which may be evidenced by restlessness, pallor, tachycardia, or hypotension. If reoperation is necessary to control bleeding, intravascular volume must first be restored. Evacuation of stomach contents with a nasogastric tube is followed by a rapid-sequence induction with cricoid pressure.

TRISOMY 21 SYNDROME
(Down's Syndrome)

Pathophysiology

An additional part or whole chromosome 21 results in the most common congenital pattern of human malformation: Down's syndrome. Characteristic abnormalities of interest to the anesthesiologist include a short neck, irregular dentition, mental retardation, hypotonia, and a large tongue. Associated abnormalities include congenital heart disease in 40% of patients (most commonly endocardial cushion defects), subglottic stenosis, tracheoesophageal fistula, chronic pulmonary infections, and seizures. These neonates are often premature and small for gestational age.

Anesthetic Considerations

Because of anatomic differences, these infants have consistently difficult airways. The size of endotracheal tube required is typically smaller than predicted by age. Respiratory complications such as postoperative stridor and apnea are common. Neck flexion during laryngoscopy and intubation may result in atlanto-occipital dislocation due to the congenital laxity of these ligaments. The possibility of associated congenital diseases must always be considered. As in all pediatric patients, care must be taken to avoid air bubbles in the intravenous line because of possible right-to-left shunts (paradoxic air embolus). Whether there is an exaggerated heart rate response to atropine in trisomy 21 syndrome is controversial, but that effect appears to be unlikely.

PRUNE BELLY SYNDROME

Pathophysiology

Prune belly syndrome is caused by agenesis of the abdominal musculature, which results in a thin-walled, protuberant abdomen. Associated anomalies include club feet, cryptorchidism, and other genitourinary tract abnormalities.

Anesthetic Considerations

Patients with prune belly syndrome have multiple pulmonary complications associated with their inability to cough effectively. They are at risk for aspiration and are often intubated awake. Muscle relaxants

are not necessary. If renal anomalies are present, overhydration must be avoided.

CYSTIC FIBROSIS

Pathophysiology

Cystic fibrosis is a hereditary disease of exocrine glands primarily affecting the pulmonary and gastrointestinal systems. Abnormally thick and viscous secretions coupled with decreased ciliary activity lead to pneumonia, wheezing, and bronchiectasis. Pulmonary function studies reveal increased residual volume and airway resistance with decreased vital capacity and expiratory flow rate. Malabsorption syndrome may lead to dehydration and electrolyte abnormalities.

Anesthetic Considerations

Premedication should not include respiratory depressants. Anticholinergic drugs are controversial, but they have been used in large series without ill effects. Induction with inhalational anesthetics may be prolonged in patients with severe pulmonary disease. Intubation should not be performed until the patient is deeply anesthetized in order to avoid coughing and stimulation of mucous secretions. Aggressive suctioning throughout the anesthesia and before extubation minimizes the accumulation of pulmonary secretions. Intraoperative hyperventilation will cause shallow respirations postoperatively and should be avoided. Outcome is favorably influenced by aggressive preoperative and postoperative respiratory therapy that includes bronchodilators, incentive spirometry, postural drainage, and pathogen-specific antibiotic therapy.

CONGENITAL LOBAR EMPHYSEMA

Pathophysiology

Congenital lobar emphysema is characterized by hyperinflation of one or several lobes of the lung. Bronchial cartilage dysplasia, the most common cause, allows large airways to collapse during expiration. The air that remains trapped in the lung acts like a pneumothorax, causing compression of neighboring lobes, mediastinal shift, and impairment of venous return to the heart. Hypoxemia and hypotension can deteriorate to cardiorespiratory arrest. Management often requires lobectomy.

Anesthetic Considerations

The key to successful anesthetic management of these patients is to avoid anything that will worsen lung hyperinflation or hypotension. For example, nitrous oxide is contraindicated. Gentle assistance of ventilation is probably preferable to controlled positive-pressure ventilation. Intravenous ketamine offers myocardial contractility advantages over volatile anesthetics. If induction of anesthesia is accompanied by severe hypotension or hypoxemia, immediate thoracotomy will allow herniation of the lobe outside the thorax and relieve intrathoracic pressure.

SCOLIOSIS

Pathophysiology

Scoliosis is lateral rotation and curvature of the vertebrae and a deformity of the rib cage. It is classified by etiology: idiopathic, congenital, neuromuscular, traumatic, etc. Scoliosis can affect cardiac and respiratory function. Elevated pulmonary vascular resistance from chronic hypoxia causes pulmonary hypertension and right ventricular hypertrophy. Respiratory abnormalities include reduced lung volumes and chest wall compliance. PaO_2 is reduced as a result of ventilation/perfusion mismatching, while an increased $PaCO_2$ signals severe disease.

Anesthetic Considerations

Preoperative evaluation should include pulmonary function tests, arterial blood gases, and electrocardiography. Corrective surgery is complicated by the prone position, significant blood loss, and the possibility of paraplegia. Spinal cord function can be monitored with somatosensory evoked potentials (Chapter 6) or by waking the patient intraoperatively to test lower limb muscle strength. Patients with severe respiratory disease are often left intubated postoperatively. Patients with scoliosis due to muscular dystrophy are predisposed to malignant hyperthermia, cardiac dysrhythmias, and untoward effects of succinylcholine (hyperkalemia, myoglobinuria, and sustained muscular contractures).

CASE DISCUSSION: MASSETER SPASM & MALIGNANT HYPERTHERMIA

A 4-year-old boy is scheduled for strabismus correction. Inhalational induction with nitrous oxide and halothane is followed by the intravenous administration of atropine and succinylcholine. Rigidity of the masseter muscle prevents mouth opening and intubation.

What is malignant hyperthermia?

Malignant hyperthermia is a rare, often inherited syndrome characterized by an acute hypermetabolic state. Although most cases occur in pediatric patients, all ages can be affected. Signs and symptoms of a crisis include tachycardia, dysrhythmias, hypercapnia, tachypnea, cyanosis, mottling of the skin, skeletal muscle rigidity, and high body temperature. Laboratory findings include myoglobinuria, decreased mixed venous oxygen tension, and elevated serum calcium, potassium, creatine kinase (drawn at 6, 12, and 24 hours after the episode), and myoglobin concentrations. Arterial blood gas analysis reveals a mixed metabolic and respiratory acidosis. Part of the problem in diagnosing malignant hyperthermia is its variable presentation during or after an anesthetic. For instance, although the disorder was originally termed malignant hyperthermia, fever is an inconsistent and often late sign.

While the precise cellular origin of malignant hyperthermia is poorly understood, recent investigations have identified an increase in phospholipase A_2 activity in muscle cells of susceptible patients. This enzyme alteration may be responsible for an increase in intracellular glycolysis and calcium ion concentrations. In any event, abnormal excitation-contraction coupling results in prolonged actin and myosin interaction and irreversible muscle contracture. This leads to increased oxygen consumption and CO_2 production. Attempts by muscle cells to reduce intracellular calcium concentration deplete ATP stores, leading to cellular edema (eg, cerebral edema) and lactate production (lactic acidosis).

How should an episode of malignant hyperthermia be treated?

Since succinylcholine and volatile anesthetics are considered to be the principal "triggering agents," they should be immediately discontinued. Even trace amounts of anesthetics absorbed by soda lime, breathing tubes, and breathing bags may be detrimental. The patient should be aggressively ventilated with 100% oxygen to minimize the effects of hypercapnia, metabolic acidosis, and increased oxygen consumption. If fever is present, cooling measures such as high gas flows, decreasing room temperature, ice water packs over major arteries, and administration of chilled normal saline are beneficial. An arterial line will provide precise blood pressure monitoring and access to serial arterial blood gas measurements. Inducing a brisk diuresis with furosemide may lessen the risk of renal damage due to myoglobinuria. Nonetheless, the mainstay of therapy of a malignant hyperthermia crisis is *immediate* administration of intravenous dantrolene.

Describe the mechanism of action of dantrolene, its recommended dosage, and its possible side effects.

Dantrolene directly interferes with muscle contraction by inhibiting calcium ion release from the sarcoplasmic reticulum. This *intracellular* dissociation of excitation-contraction coupling contrasts with the depolarizing and nondepolarizing muscle relaxants that antagonize the *extracellular* neuromuscular junction.

The dose of dantrolene is 2.5 mg/kg given intravenously every 5 minutes until symptoms subside—to a maximum of 10 mg/kg. Dantrolene is packaged as 20 mg of lyophilized powder to be dissolved in 60 mL of sterile water. Depending on the total dose required, reconstitution can be time-consuming. The dose is repeated every 8 hours for 24–72 hours.

Dantrolene is a relatively safe drug. Although chronic therapy for spastic disorders has been associated with hepatic dysfunction, the most serious complication following acute administration is generalized muscle weakness that may result in respiratory insufficiency or aspiration pneumonitis. Dantrolene can cause phlebitis in small peripheral veins and should be given through a central venous line if one is available. The safety and efficacy of dantrolene call for its immediate use in this potentially life-threatening disease.

What is the differential diagnosis of masseter spasm during intubation?

Both myotonia and malignant hyperthermia can cause trismus that typically lasts for 2–3 minutes following administration of succinylcholine. The two disorders can be differentiated by the medical history, neurologic examination, and electromyography. The incidence of masseter spasm following succinylcholine administration in pediatric patients at some medical centers may be higher than 1%. Although many of these patients will not develop classic signs of malignant hyperthermia, about 50% may prove to be "MH-susceptible" by muscle biopsy. The safest course is to assume that masseter spasm is due to malignant hyperthermia and to postpone elective surgery. However, if there are no other signs of malignant hyperthermia and if monitoring and treatment capabilities are readily available, some anesthesiologists will allow surgery to continue and utilize a "safe" anesthetic.

Which patients should be suspected of being susceptible to malignant hyperthermia?

Several musculoskeletal diseases are associated with a relatively high incidence of malignant hyperthermia. These include Duchenne's muscular dystrophy, neuroleptic malignant syndrome, and central core disease. King-Denborough syndrome (short stature, mental retardation, and musculoskeletal abnormalities) is consistently associated with malignant hyperthermia. Other possible clues to susceptibility include a family history of anesthetic complications, intolerance to caffeine-containing foods, or a history of unexplained fevers or muscular cramps. As previously mentioned, any patient who develops trismus during induction of anesthesia should be suspected of being susceptible to malignant hyperthermia.

How is susceptibility to malignant hyperthermia confirmed?

Patients who have survived an unequivocal episode of malignant hyperthermia are considered susceptible. If the diagnosis remains in doubt postoperatively, a fresh section of living skeletal muscle is biopsied and exposed to a caffeine, halothane, or combination caffeine-halothane bath. A positive muscle contracture response confirms with 95% reliability that the patient is susceptible. An elevated serum creatine kinase level implies susceptibility only in patients with relatives known to be susceptible.

What other diseases can present like malignant hyperthermia?

Surgery and anesthesia can precipitate **thyroid storm** in hyperthyroid patients. Its signs include tachycardia, hyperthermia, and labile blood pressure. Thyroid storm usually develops postoperatively, as opposed to the typical intraoperative presentation of malignant hyperthermia (Chapter 36). **Pheochromocytoma** is associated with dramatic increases in heart rate and blood pressure but not end-tidal CO_2. **Sepsis** shares several characteristics with malignant hyperthermia, including fever, tachypnea, tachycardia, and metabolic acidosis. This can be a difficult differential diagnosis if there is no obvious primary site of infection. However, malignant hyperthermia is associated with more dramatic degrees of metabolic acidosis and venous desaturation than any of the other diseases.

What constitutes a "safe" anesthetic in patients who are susceptible to malignant hyperthermia?

Thiopental and pancuronium appear to be protective, since they raise the triggering threshold for malignant hyperthermia. Other safe drugs include opiate agonists, droperidol, benzodiazepines, and ester-type local anesthetics. Nitrous oxide, ketamine hydrochloride, and amide-type anesthetics may be weak triggering agents but are considered by most experts to be safe. Finally, an adequate supply of dantrolene should always be available wherever general anesthesia is provided. Prophylactic use of intravenous dantrolene prior to induction of general anesthesia in susceptible patients is probably not necessary if a "safe" anesthetic is administered. Further information about malignant hyperthermia can be obtained from the Malignant Hyperthermia Association of the United States (Box 3231, Darien, CT 06820).

MALIGNANT HYPERTHERMIA
PROTOCOL

1. Discontinue inhalational anesthetic and succinylcholine. *Call for help!*
2. Hyperventilate with 100% O_2 at high flows.
3. Administer sodium bicarbonate, 1–2 meq/ kg IV.
4. Mix dantrolene sodium with sterile distilled water and administer 2.5 mg/kg IV *as soon as possible.*
5. Institute cooling measures (lavage, blanket, cold IV solutions).
6. Treat persistent ventricular arrhythmias wtih procainamide, 200 mg IV.
7. Administer additional doses of dantrolene if needed.
8. Change anesthetic tubing and soda lime.
9. Monitor urine output, K^+, Ca^{2+}, blood gases, $ETCO_2$, clotting studies.
10. Treat severe hyperkalemia with dextrose, 25–50 g IV, and regular insulin, 10–20 units IV.
11. Consider invasive monitoring of arterial blood pressure and central venous pressure.
12. If necessary, consult on-call physicians at-

MEDIC ALERT HOTLINE:
(209) 634–4917

SUGGESTED READINGS

Berry FA (editor): *Anesthetic Management of Difficult and Routine Pediatric Patients.* Churchill Livingstone, 1986. Good chapters on airway management and malignant hyperthermia.

Cook DR, Marcy JH (editors): *Neonatal Anesthesia.* Appleton Davies, 1988.

Gregory GA (editor): *Pediatric Anesthesia,* 2nd ed. Churchill Livingstone, 1989. Good chapters on intensive care, neuroanesthesia, and pain management.

Motoyama EK (editor): *Smith's Anesthesia For Infants And Children,* 5th ed. Mosby-Year Book, 1990. A classic work with new chapters on organ transplantation, regional anesthesia, blood conservation, and other subspecialty areas.

Roy WL, Lerman J: Laryngospasm in paediatric anaesthesia. Can J Anesth 1988;35:93.

Ryan JF et al (editors): *A Practice of Anesthesia for Infants and Children.* Grune & Stratton, 1986. Heavily illustrated and referenced.

Saint-Maurice C, Schulte-Steinberg O (editors): *Regional Anaesthesia in Children.* Appleton & Lange, 1990. Regional anesthesia in children is gaining acceptance.

Steward DJ: Manual of Pediatric Anesthesia, 3rd ed. Churchill Livingstone, 1989.

Tiret L et al: Complications related to anaesthesia in infants and children: A prospective survey of 40,240 anaesthetics. Br J Anaesth 1988;61:263.

Yaster M, Maxwell LG: Pediatric regional anesthesia. Anesthesiology 1989;70:324.

Geriatric Anesthesia

43

In the 1980 census, people aged 65 or older made up 11.3% of the population in the United States and consumed 29% of total health-care expenditures. By 2040, the elderly population may increase to 24% of the population and account for 50% of such expenditures. Half of these individuals will require surgery before they die, despite being at a threefold risk of perioperative death. As with pediatric patients, optimal anesthetic management of geriatric patients depends upon an understanding of normal changes in physiology, anatomy, and response to pharmacologic agents that accompany aging. In fact, there are many similarities between elderly and pediatric patients (Table 43–1). However, compared with pediatric patients, older people show a wider range of variation in these parameters. The relatively high frequency of serious physiologic abnormalities in elderly patients demands an especially careful preoperative evaluation.

ANATOMIC & PHYSIOLOGIC CHANGES ASSOCIATED WITH AGING

CARDIOVASCULAR SYSTEM

It is important to distinguish between changes in physiology that normally accompany aging and the pathophysiology of age-related diseases (Table 43–2). For example, atherosclerosis is pathologic—it is not present in healthy elderly patients. On the other hand, a reduction in arterial elasticity due to fibrosis of the media is part of the normal aging process. Reduced arterial compliance results in increased afterload, elevated systolic blood pressure, and left ventricular hy-

Table 43–1. Similarities between elderly and pediatric patients.

Decreased ability to increase heart rate in response to hypovolemia, hypotension, or hypoxia
Decreased lung compliance
Decreased arterial oxygen tension
Impaired ability to cough
Decreased renal tubular function
Increased susceptibility to hypothermia

pertrophy. The left ventricular wall thickens at the expense of the left ventricular cavity. In the absence of coexisting disease, diastolic blood pressure remains unchanged or decreases. Similarly, while cardiac output typically declines with age, it appears to be maintained in well-conditioned, healthy individuals. Increased vagal tone and decreased sensitivity of adrenergic receptors lead to a decline in heart rate. Maximal heart rate declines by approximately one beat per minute per year of age over 50. Fibrosis of the conduction system and loss of sinoatrial node cells increase the incidence of dysrhythmias.

Elderly patients undergoing evaluation for surgery have been shown to have an increased incidence of abnormal mean pulmonary wedge pressures, pulmonary hypertension, and left ventricular dysfunction (Figure 43–1). Diminished cardiac reserve in many elderly patients may be manifested as exaggerated drops in blood pressure during induction of general anesthesia. A prolonged circulation time delays the onset of intravenous drugs but speeds induction with inhalational agents. Similar to infants, elderly patients have an impaired ability to respond to hypovolemia, hypotension, or hypoxemia with an increase in heart rate.

RESPIRATORY SYSTEM

Elasticity is also decreased in lung tissue, allowing overdistention of alveoli and collapse of small airways. The former reduces the alveolar surface area, which decreases the efficiency of gas exchange. Airway collapse increases **residual volume** (the volume of air remaining in the lungs at the end of a forced expiration) and **closing capacity** (the volume of air in the lungs at which small airways begin to close). Even in normal individuals, closing capacity exceeds **functional residual capacity** (the volume of air remaining in the lungs at the end of a normal expiration) at age 45 in the supine position and age 65 in the sitting position. When this happens, some airways are closed during part of normal tidal breathing. The additive effect of these emphysema-like changes is said to decrease arterial oxygen tension by an average rate of 0.35 mm Hg per year. However, there is a wide range of arterial oxygen tensions in elderly preoperative patients (Figure 43–2). Other pulmonary effects of aging are summarized in Table 43–2.

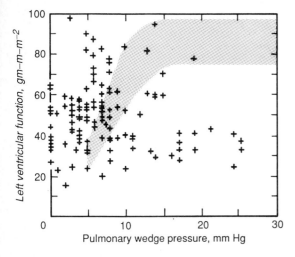

Figure 43–1. Abnormal mean pulmonary wedge pressures, pulmonary hypertension, and left ventricular dysfunction is common in elderly patients presenting for surgery. (Redrawn and reproduced, with permission, from Del Guercio LRM, Cohn JD: Monitoring operative risk in elderly. JAMA 1980;243:1350.)

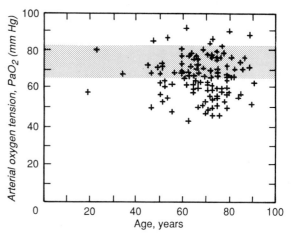

Figure 43–2. There is a wide range of arterial oxygen tensions in elderly preoperative patients. (Redrawn and reproduced, with permission, from Del Guercio LRM, Cohn JD: Monitoring operative risk in elderly. JAMA 1980;243:1350.)

Mask ventilation may be more difficult in edentulous patients, while arthritis of the temporomandibular joint or cervical spine may make intubation challenging. On the other hand, absence of upper teeth often improves visualization of the vocal cords during laryngoscopy.

Prevention of perioperative hypoxemia includes higher inspired oxygen concentrations, small increments of positive end-expiratory pressure, and aggressive pulmonary toilet. Aspiration pneumonia is a common and potentially life-threatening complication in elderly patients. One reason for this predisposition is a progressive decrease in protective laryngeal reflexes with age. Ventilatory impairment in the recovery room is more common in elderly patients. Thus, those with severe preexisting respiratory disease and those who have just had major abdominal surgery should usually be left intubated postoperatively. In addition, pain control techniques that facilitate postoperative pulmonary function should be seriously considered (eg, epidural opioids, intercostal nerve blocks).

RENAL FUNCTION

Renal blood flow and kidney mass (eg, glomerular number and tubular length) decrease with age. These changes are particularly prominent in the renal cortex. Renal function as determined by glomerular filtration rate and creatinine clearance is reduced (Table 43–2). Serum creatinine is unchanged because of a decrease in muscle mass and creatinine production, while BUN gradually increases (0.2 mg/dL per year). Impairment of sodium handling, concentrating ability, and diluting capacity predisposes elderly patients to dehydration or fluid overload.

As renal function declines, so does the kidney's ability to excrete drugs. The decreased capacity to handle water and electrolyte loads makes proper fluid management more critical. This is further complicated by the common use of diuretics in the elderly population. To this end, serum electrolytes, cardiac filling pressures, and urine output are more frequently monitored.

GASTROINTESTINAL SYSTEM

Hepatic blood flow and liver mass decline with age. The rate of biotransformation, albumin production, and plasma cholinesterase synthesis is slowed. Gastric pH tends to rise, while gastric emptying is prolonged. These factors may affect drug pharmacokinetics.

NERVOUS SYSTEM

Cerebral blood flow and brain mass decrease with age. Neuronal loss is prominent in the cerebral cortex. The synthesis of some neurotransmitters is reduced. Degeneration of peripheral nerve cells results in prolonged conduction velocity and skeletal muscle atrophy.

Dose requirements for local (Cm: minimum anesthetic concentration) and general (MAC: minimum alveolar concentration) anesthetics are reduced. Spinal anesthesia tends to have a longer duration, while the dosage requirement for epidural anesthesia may be reduced. Elderly patients often take more time to recover completely from the central nervous system effects of general anesthesia, especially if they were confused or disoriented preoperatively. This is particularly important in geriatric outpatient surgery, where socio-

Table 43–2. Physiologic changes with age as opposed to age-related diseases.

Normal Physiologic Changes	Common Pathophysiology
CARDIOVASCULAR	

Decreased arterial elasticity
   Elevated afterload
   Elevated systolic blood pressure
   Left ventricular hypertrophy
Decreased adrenergic activity
   Decreased resting heart rate
   Decreased maximal heart rate
   Decreased baroreceptor reflex
	Atherosclerosis
	Coronary artery disease
	Essential hypertension
	Congestive heart failure
	Cardiac dysrhythmias
	Aortic stenosis

RESPIRATORY	

Decreased pulmonary elasticity
   Decreased alveolar surface area
   Increased residual volume
   Increased closing capacity
   Ventilation/perfusion mismatching
   Decreased arterial oxygen tension
Increased chest wall rigidity
Decreased muscle strength
   Decreased cough
   Decreased maximal breathing capacity
Blunted response to hypercapnia and hypoxia
	Emphysema
	Chronic bronchitis
	Pneumonia
	Lung cancer
	Tuberculosis

RENAL	

Decreased renal blood flow
   Decreased renal plasma flow
   Decreased glomerular filtration rate
Decreased renal mass
Decreased tubular function
   Impaired sodium handling
   Decreased concentration ability
   Decreased diluting capacity
   Impaired fluid handling
   Decreased drug excretion
Decreased renin-aldosterone responsiveness
   Impaired potassium excretion
	Diabetic nephropathy
	Hypertensive nephropathy
	Prostatic obstruction
	Congestive heart failure

economic factors such as lack of a caretaker at home necessitate a higher level of self-care.

MUSCULOSKELETAL

Skin atrophies with age and is prone to trauma from adhesive tape, electrocautery pads, and electrocardiographic electrodes. Veins are often frail and easily ruptured by intravenous infusions. Arthritic joints may interfere with positioning (eg, lithotomy) or regional anesthesia (eg, subarachnoid block).

CHANGES IN RESPONSES TO DRUGS ASSOCIATED WITH AGING

Aging produces both pharmacokinetic (the relationship between drug dose and plasma concentration) and pharmacodynamic (the relationship between plasma concentration and clinical effect) changes. Distribution is affected by a decrease in total body water and a doubling of body fat in older patients. As a result, the volume of distribution is diminished for water-soluble drugs, leading to a higher plasma concentration, and enlarged for lipid-soluble drugs, causing a lower plasma concentration. These changes in volume of distribution may affect elimination half-life. For example, as the volume of distribution expands, elimination half-life is prolonged unless the rate of clearance is also increased.

Distribution and elimination are also affected by altered plasma protein binding. Albumin, which tends to bind acidic drugs (eg, barbiturates, benzodiazepines, and opioid agonists), typically decreases with age. Alpha$_1$ acid glycoprotein, which binds basic drugs (eg, local anesthetics), is increased. Protein-bound drug cannot interact with end-organ receptors and is unavailable for metabolism or excretion. Thus, drugs that are dependent upon renal or hepatic clearance may display prolonged elimination half-lives.

The principal pharmacodynamic change associated with aging is a reduced anesthetic requirement. This is represented by lower minimum alveolar concentrations.

INHALATIONAL ANESTHETICS

The MAC for inhalational agents is reduced by 4% per decade of age over 40 years. For example, the MAC of halothane in an 80-year-old person would be expected to be $0.65 \, (0.77 - [0.77 \times 4\% \times 4])$. Onset of action will be more rapid if cardiac output is depressed, while it will be delayed if there is a significant ventilation/perfusion abnormality (Chapter 7). The myocardial depressant effects of volatile anesthetics are exaggerated in elderly patients, while the tachycardiac tendencies of isoflurane and enflurane are attenuated.

NONVOLATILE ANESTHETIC AGENTS

In general, the elderly patient display a lower dose requirement for barbiturates, opioid agonists, and benzodiazepines. For example, peak sodium thiopental plasma levels do not appear to decrease as rapidly in geriatric patients. This may be explained by a slower distribution from the central compartment to the rapidly equilibrating compartment. In any event, pharmacokinetic and not pharmacodynamic differences are responsible. This is in contrast to opioid agonists, which display pharmacokinetic (prolonged elimination half-life) and pharmacodynamic (increased brain sensitivity) alterations. Because diazepam tends to accumulate in fat stores, its volume of distribution is larger in older patients and its elimination from the body is therefore slowed. A half-life of over 36 hours can cause confusion for days following diazepam administration. Although midazolam is water-soluble at acidic pH, it is lipid-soluble at physiologic pH and undergoes similar pharmacokinetic changes. Lorazepam is less lipid-soluble than diazepam, and its elimination half-life remains relatively unchanged.

MUSCLE RELAXANTS

The effect of nondepolarizing muscle relaxants that depend upon renal excretion (eg, pancuronium and tubocurarine) may be slightly prolonged in the elderly owing to decreased drug clearance. The dosage requirement and recovery time of atracurium are not affected by age. Elderly men—but not elderly women—may display a slightly prolonged effect from succinylcholine owing to their lower plasma cholinesterase levels.

CASE DISCUSSION: THE ELDERLY PATIENT WITH A FRACTURED HIP

An 86-year-old nursing home patient is scheduled for open reduction and internal fixation of a subtrochanteric fracture of the femur.

How should this patient be evaluated for the risk of perioperative morbidity?

Anesthetic risk correlates much better with the presence of coexisting disease than chronologic age. Therefore, preanesthetic evaluation should concentrate on the identification of age-related diseases (Table 43–2) and an estimation of physiologic reserve. There is a tremendous physiologic difference between a patient who walks three blocks to a grocery store on a regular basis and one who is bedridden, even though both may be the same age. Obviously, any condition that may be amenable to preoperative therapy (eg, bronchodilator administration) must be identified and addressed. At the same time, lengthy delays may compromise surgical repair and increase overall morbidity.

What are some of the considerations in selection of premedication for this patient?

In general, elderly patients require lower doses of premedication. The pharmacodynamic and pharmacokinetic reasons for this have been explained. Nonetheless, hip fractures are painful, particularly during movement to the operating room. Unless contraindicated by severe concomitant disease, a narcotic premedication may be valuable. Anticholinergic medication is rarely needed, since aging is accompanied by atrophy of the salivary glands. These patients should always be considered to be at risk for aspiration, since narcotic premedication and the pain from their injury will decrease gastric emptying. Therefore, pretreatment with an H_2 antagonist or an oral nonparticulate antacid is indicated (Chapter 15).

What factors might influence the choice between regional and general anesthesia?

Advancing age is not a contraindication for either regional or general anesthesia. However, each technique has its advantages and disadvantages in the elderly population. For hip surgery, regional anesthesia can be achieved with a subarachnoid or epidural block extending to the T8 sensory level. Both of these require patient cooperation and the ability to lie still for the duration of the surgery. Unless regional anesthesia is accompanied by heavy sedation, postoperative confusion and disorientation are less troublesome than after general anesthesia. Cardiovascular changes are usually limited to a fall in arterial blood pressure as sympathetic block is established. While this fall can be minimized by prophylactic fluid loading, a patient with borderline heart function may decompensate when the block dissipates and sympathetic tone returns. Reduced afterload can result in profound hypotension in patients with aortic stenosis, a common valvular lesion in the elderly population. Patients with coronary artery disease may experience an increase in myocardial oxygen demand as a result of reflex tachycardia or a decrease in supply caused by lower coronary artery perfusion.

Are there any specific advantages or disadvantages to a regional technique in elderly patients having hip surgery?

A major advantage in regional anesthesia—particularly for hip surgery—is a lower incidence of postoperative thromboembolism. Presumably this is due to peripheral vasodilation and maintenance of venous blood flow in the lower extremities. Additionally, local anesthetics inhibit platelet aggregation and stabilize endothelial cells. Regional anesthesia is considered by many anesthesiologists to maintain respiratory function better than general anesthesia. Unless the anesthetic level involves the intercostal musculature, ventilation and the cough reflex are well maintained.

Technical problems associated with regional anesthesia in the elderly include altered landmarks due to degeneration of the vertebral column and the difficulty of obtaining adequate patient positioning. To avoid having the patient lie on the fracture, a hypobaric solution can be injected subdurally. Postpuncture headache is less of a problem in the elderly population.

If the patient refuses regional anesthesia, is general anesthesia acceptable?

General anesthesia is an acceptable alternative to regional block. One advantage is that the patient can be induced in bed and moved over to the operating room table after intubation, avoiding the pain of positioning. A disadvantage is that the patient is unable to provide feedback regarding pressure points on the unpadded orthopedic table.

What specific factors should be considered during induction and maintenance of general anesthesia with this patient?

Intravenous induction agents should be administered slowly, since a slow blood circulation time will delay the onset of action. It is important to remember that because a hip fracture can be associated with over 1 L of occult blood loss, induction with sodium thiopental may lead to an exaggerated drop in arterial blood pressure. Thus, although the patient may be at risk for aspiration, the usual rapid-sequence induction should be modified to minimize cardiovascular changes. An acceptable compromise allows slower drug administration and gentle mask ventilation while maintaining firm cricoid pressure until satisfactory endotracheal tube position is confirmed. Initial hypotension may be replaced by hypertension and tachycardia during laryngoscopy and intubation. This roller coaster volatility in blood pressure increases the risk of stroke and myocardial ischemia and can be avoided by preceding airway instrumentation with lidocaine (1.5 mg/kg), esmolol (0.3 mg/kg), or alfentanil (5–15 μg/kg).

Intraoperative paralysis with a nondepolarizing muscle relaxant provides improved surgical conditions and allows maintenance of a lighter plane of anesthesia. Deliberate hypotension may lessen intraoperative blood loss and is not contraindicated solely on the basis of age (see Chapter 13 Case Discussion).

SUGGESTED READINGS

Davenport HT (editor): *Anaesthesia and the Aged Patient.* Blackwell, 1988. The British prospective.

Felts JA (editor): *Anesthesia and the Geriatric Patient.* Saunders, 1986. Specific issues of clinical importance such as thermoregulation in the elderly, diabetic management, and considerations during cranial vascularization procedures.

Krechel SW (editor): *Anesthesia and the Geriatric Patient.* Grune & Stratton, 1984. Physiologic changes and basic anesthetic management.

Stephen CR, Assaf RAE (editors): *Geriatric Anesthesia: Principles and Practice.* Butterworths, 1986.

44

Outpatient Anesthesia

Vincent Valdez, MD & G. Edward Morgan, MD*

One of the most dramatic transformations in health care delivery during the past decade has been a shift from inpatient to outpatient surgery (also called ambulatory surgery). The economic savings afforded by not admitting patients the night before or keeping them in hospital the night after surgery have provided the primary impetus for this change. Other advantages of outpatient surgery include less risk of nosocomial infection, earlier ambulation, and patient convenience. As would be expected, the trend toward outpatient surgery has affected the practice of anesthesia. This chapter highlights anesthetic considerations in outpatient surgical care during the preoperative, intraoperative, and postoperative periods.

PREOPERATIVE CONSIDERATIONS

SURGICAL CASE SELECTION

The appropriateness of performing a particular surgical procedure on an outpatient ambulatory basis depends upon the resources of the facility, the estimated duration of the procedure, and the level of postoperative care the patient will probably require. For example, a free-standing surgical facility might not allow as difficult an operation as an outpatient surgery department within a hospital, because of the possibility that the patient may require admission postoperatively. Since the duration of surgery and anesthesia does not correlate well with recovery room time, many centers now feel comfortable in accepting patients for outpatient surgery that extends beyond the traditional recommendation of a 2-hour maximum. Clearly, outpatient surgery is inappropriate if a patient will require extensive postoperative care related to a preexisting

medical condition or the nature of the surgery. Some outpatient surgical centers do not accept cases complicated by infection because of the lack of isolation facilities. Finally, outpatient surgery is often mandated by third-party payers (eg, Medicare) to avoid the expense of "unnecessary" inpatient care.

The controversy surrounding outpatient case selection is typified by tonsillectomies and adenoidectomies. Approximately 3% of patients requiring these procedures experience postoperative bleeding, with many requiring transfusion and reoperation. Posttonsillectomy hemorrhage is often delayed for more than 12 hours after surgery. For these reasons, many centers schedule these operations in the morning to allow maximal in-hospital observation, while others do not allow tonsillectomies to be performed in the outpatient setting.

PATIENT SELECTION

As with surgical procedures, the guidelines for patient selection have become much more liberal. While only ASA class 1 or class 2 patients were formerly considered candidates for outpatient surgery, many centers currently allow medically stable ASA 3 patients. Even an ASA 4 patient may be eligible if the procedure is quite limited in nature or if hospital admission would place the patient at increased risk. An example of this situation would be an immunosuppressed cancer patient requiring insertion of a Hickman catheter for chemotherapy.

The ability of a patient to cooperate with written preoperative and postoperative instructions and the availability of a responsible adult to accompany the patient home are often as important as the patient's medical condition in determining the suitability of outpatient surgery. The possibility of overnight hospital admission must be understood and accepted by the patient.

Age is not a contraindication to outpatient surgery with the following exceptions: (1) premature infants less than 60 weeks postconception (some centers use 44 weeks as the cutoff time); (2) infants with a history

*Associate Professor of Anesthesiology, University of Southern California, Los Angeles.

of bronchopulmonary dysplasia or apneic episodes who are still symptomatic; and (3) siblings of infants who have died of sudden infant death syndrome. All three of these groups are at increased risk of postoperative apnea and should be monitored for at least 24 hours after surgery. Elderly patients may require more time than young adults to fully recover psychomotor skills. Nonetheless, children and elderly patients benefit most from outpatient surgery because they are most susceptible to the adverse psychologic effects associated with hospital admission.

LABORATORY TESTING & PREOPERATIVE EVALUATION

The need for laboratory testing does not depend on whether surgery is performed as an outpatient or inpatient. Outpatients should receive the same level of perioperative care, including laboratory testing, as would be required for an inpatient. One of the frustrations of outpatient anesthesia is having to cancel a scheduled procedure because of an inadequate preoperative workup, unexpected laboratory abnormalities, or failure of the patient to follow preoperative instructions (eg, NPO orders). Because of the logistical problems in evaluating an outpatient prior to the day of surgery to ascertain what is really required, excessive laboratory testing is often ordered. Much of this confusion and expense could be eliminated if patients were evaluated by an anesthesiologist before the day of surgery. This could take the form of the usual preoperative history and physical examination, a telephone interview, or a screening questionnaire. Even a cursory history and physical examination is a more effective screening procedure for disease than a battery of laboratory tests.

PREMEDICATION

The considerations for outpatient premedication are similar to those for inpatients except for the added goal of rapid emergence (see Chapter 8 Case Discussion). Intramuscular injection of long-acting agents such as morphine sulfate or lorazepam can easily be switched to intravenous administration of shorter-acting drugs such as fentanyl or midazolam. In general, judicious use of short-acting agents does not significantly prolong recovery time. Of course, withholding all sedative premedication is an alternative in most patients. As with inpatients, the most effective premedication is an informative preoperative interview.

Outpatients have been shown to be at increased risk for aspiration pneumonitis because of increased acidity and volume of gastric secretions. However, the administration of H_2 histamine antagonists or other protective drugs is not routinely recommended by most authorities.

INTRAOPERATIVE CONSIDERATIONS

ANESTHETIC TECHNIQUES & PHARMACOLOGIC CONSIDERATIONS

1. GENERAL ANESTHESIA

Most common induction techniques do not interfere with wakeup times except following the shortest of cases. Specifically, thiopental, etomidate, methohexital, and inhalation inductions are acceptable. Ketamine has been associated with prolonged emergence in some patients. Outpatient surgery is not a contraindication to intubation, but many cases are brief enough to allow mask ventilation. Anesthesia may be maintained with volatile agents, small boluses of short-acting opioids, or continuous infusions of intravenous anesthetics. Enflurane appears to be an exception to the lack of correlation between anesthesia time and recovery time and should probably be avoided during cases exceeding 1 or 2 hours. Anesthesia may be supplemented with nitrous oxide.

A continuous drip of succinylcholine or careful titration of an intermediate-duration nondepolarizing muscle relaxant (eg, vecuronium, atracurium) provides intraoperative relaxation and reduces the requirements for anesthesia. Outpatients appear to be at increased risk for postoperative myalgias following succinylcholine.

Newer agents that may further reduce recovery time include propofol, alfentanil, desflurane, mivacurium, and flumazenil (a benzodiazepine antagonist).

2. REGIONAL ANESTHESIA

The advantages of regional anesthesia in outpatient surgery include less alteration in central nervous system function and a degree of postoperative pain relief. Depending upon the type of regional block, postoperative complications such as emesis or urinary retention appear to be reduced compared with general anesthesia. A potential disadvantage of regional anesthesia is the amount of time required to perform some blocks. Possible techniques range from spinal or epidural anesthesia to peripheral nerve block or local infiltration. Post-dural puncture headache appears to be more common in outpatients than in inpatients. Techniques that may be associated with occult complications (eg, pneumothorax following supraclavicular block) should be avoided. Local anesthetic agents should be chosen carefully to prevent prolonged muscle relaxation in the postoperative period. Even with regional anesthesia, psychomotor function may be impaired for several hours after surgery if sedative drugs are administered.

POSTOPERATIVE CONSIDERATIONS

POSTOPERATIVE COMPLICATIONS

Postoperative complications that are relatively insignificant for an inpatient can prevent an outpatient from becoming "home ready" and jeopardize discharge from an ambulatory surgical unit. Factors that have been associated with postoperative complications include female gender, no previous exposure to general anesthesia, endotracheal intubation, and surgical time in excess of 20 minutes.

Emesis is a common problem which, if protracted, can require hospital admission. The incidence is increased with anesthetic techniques that require high doses of opioids, certain types of surgery (eg, strabismus surgery, laparoscopy), postoperative pain, and a predisposition to motion sickness. Patients at increased risk benefit from routine prophylaxis with an antiemetic agent. Droperidol (0.01–0.05 mg/kg intravenously) is an effective agent, but its adult dose should be limited to less than 1.25 mg to prevent postoperative drowsiness. Metoclopramide (10 mg intravenously) has the advantage of not prolonging the recovery from general anesthesia.

Postoperative **pain** can be controlled with intravenous analgesics or local nerve block. Although intraoperative administration of short-acting opioid agonists may increase the incidence of postoperative nausea and vomiting, recovery from anesthesia is not prolonged by low doses (eg, fentanyl, 2 μg/kg). Even lower doses are often effective at controlling pain in the recovery room (fentanyl, 0.5 μg/kg). Infiltration with local anesthetic during surgery may effectively decrease postoperative discomfort following inguinal hernia repair, circumcision, and tubal ligation. Postoperative **myalgia** due to succinylcholine may be lessened by pretreatment with a nondepolarizing muscle relaxant.

Prolonged somnolence is unusual unless long-acting anesthetic agents have been administered (see Chapter 9 Case Discussion). **Headache** is a common postoperative problem and appears to be increased following administration of volatile anesthetic agents. **Urinary retention** can follow general anesthesia as well as spinal or epidural blockade. This is especially a problem in elderly men with prostatic hypertrophy. Simple bladder catheterization may prove to be traumatic and require consultation with a urologist. **Sore throat** and **hoarseness** are not unusual following endotracheal intubation. **Postintubation croup** is usu-

Table 44–1. Criteria defining "home readiness."[1]

Orientation to person, place, and time
Stable vital signs for 30–60 minutes
Ability to ambulate unassisted
Ability to tolerate oral fluids[2]
Ability to void[2]
Absence of significant pain or bleeding

[1]These criteria assume normal preoperative function.
[2]These may not be mandatory in all patients.

ally limited to pediatric patients and is discussed in Chapter 42.

DISCHARGE CRITERIA

Recovery from anesthesia can be divided into at least three stages: (1) emergence and awakening, (2) "home readiness," and (3) complete psychomotor recovery.

Discharge from an outpatient surgical center is conditioned upon achieving a minimum level of "home readiness" (Table 44–1). Currently available cognitive and psychomotor tests (Trieger test, digit symbol substitution test) are not routinely recommended for this purpose. Recovery of proprioception, sympathetic tone, and motor function are additional criteria following regional anesthesia. For example, intact proprioception of the big toe, minimal orthostatic changes, and normal plantar flexion of the foot are important signals of recovery following spinal anesthesia.

All outpatients must be discharged home in the company of a responsible adult who will stay with them overnight. Patients must be provided with written postoperative instructions that include how to obtain emergency help and routine follow-up care. The assessment of "home readiness" is the responsibility of the physician, preferably an anesthesiologist, who is familiar with the patient. The authority to discharge a patient home can be delegated to a nurse if preapproved discharge criteria are rigorously applied.

"Home readiness" does not imply the ability to make important decisions, to drive, or to return to work. These "street fitness" activities require complete psychomotor recovery which are often not achieved until 24–72 hours postoperatively.

Some outpatient centers use a system of postoperative follow-up procedures involving the use of patient questionnaires or phone contacts the day after discharge.

CASE DISCUSSION: OUTPATIENT LAPAROSCOPY

A 35-year-old woman is scheduled for elective laparoscopic sterilization in an outpatient facility. Her only known medical problem is obesity.

What are the most frequent complications following general anesthesia for pelvic laparoscopy?

The most common complications are similar to those following other outpatient procedures: myalgia, sore throat, dizziness, nausea, incisional pain, and headache.

What surgical complications are associated with pelvic or abdominal laparoscopy?

To prepare for laparoscopy, the surgeon inserts a trocar into the abdomen and distends the cavity with a gas (eg, carbon dioxide or nitrous oxide). Introduction of the trocar may cause **hemorrhage** if a major abdominal vessel is lacerated or **peritonitis** if a viscus is perforated. Electrofulguration during laparoscopy has been associated with **bowel burns** and bowel gas **explosions.** Significant intraoperative hemorrhage may go unrecognized because of the limitations of laparoscopic visualization. The occurrence of some of these complications may force conversion to open laparotomy.

How does the abdominal insufflation of gas affect the anesthetic management of these patients?

Gas insufflation raises abdominal pressure and interferes with normal ventilation and oxygenation. Atelectasis and a decreased functional residual capacity may lead to **hypoxemia.** This can be exacerbated by placing the patient in the Trendelenburg position, which is often requested by the surgeon during pelvic laparoscopy. Furthermore, if CO_2 is used as the filling gas, **hypercapnia** may be worsened by its absorption into the bloodstream. Impaired venous return to the heart may lead to **hypotension.** Reverse Trendelenburg position, required for laparoscopic cholecystectomy, will exaggerate circulatory impairment. An elevation in abdominal pressure may increase the risk of **aspiration** by raising gastric pressure and altering the function of the gastroesophageal junction. Pneumoperitoneum has been associated with **pneumothorax, pneumomediastinum,** and **air embolism.**

Should all patients be intubated for pelvic laparoscopy?

This is a controversial question. Many experienced anesthesiologists feel comfortable in ventilating healthy laparoscopy patients with a mask despite the potential problems of hypoventilation and aspiration. Risk factors that would favor intubation include a Trendelenburg position of greater than 10 degrees, abdominal pressures exceeding 20 mm Hg, pelvic adhesions, or preexisting cardiopulmonary dysfunction. An additional advantage of intubation is the ability to suction gastric contents, which decreases the risk of gastric perforation, aspiration, and postoperative nausea. The obese patient presented here would benefit from intubation to lessen the likelihood of hypoxemia, hypercapnia, and aspiration. End-tidal CO_2 should be monitored to ensure adequate ventilation and detect CO_2 embolism.

What are some alternatives to general anesthesia for pelvic laparotomy?

Epidural and spinal anesthesia have been associated with a lower incidence of postoperative emesis and shorter discharge times. One disadvantage is the occasional occurrence of shoulder pain due to referred diaphragmatic irritation. Some patients will experience a sense of respiratory distress while trying to maintain spontaneous ventilation in the face of abdominal distention and the Trendelenburg position. Laparoscopic clip sterilizations can also be performed with local anesthesia infiltrated in the subumbilical and suprapubic regions.

SUGGESTED READINGS

Weintraub HD, Levy M (editors): Outpatient anesthesia. Anesthesiol Clin North Am 1987;5:1. Covers many areas, including preoperative testing, regional anesthesia, dental surgery, pain management, and legal considerations.

Wetchler BV (editor): *Anesthesia for Ambulatory Surgery,* 2nd ed. Lippincott, 1991. Even includes a chapter on planning and marketing an outpatient facility.

White PF (editor): *Outpatient Anesthesia.* Churchill Livingstone, 1990. Includes excellent chapters on pediatric outpatient anesthesia and postoperative pain management.

Section V
Special Problems

Anesthetic Complications

45

Perioperative morbidity and mortality are usually related to the interaction of three factors: (1) the patient's preoperative condition, (2) the surgical procedure, and (3) anesthetic management. The risk classification system of the American Society of Anesthesiologists (ASA) attempts to quantify the first factor (Chapter 1). In other attempts, investigators have identified specific preoperative risk factors (eg, a prior myocardial infarction). However, any scheme that ignores the specific surgical procedure anticipated or anesthetic considerations cannot fully assess perioperative risk. For example, the potential for morbidity in an ASA class 3 patient who has suffered a prior myocardial infarction is greater during a lung resection than during a hernia repair. Furthermore, the likelihood of postoperative morbidity is increased if the patient has recently eaten and this is not considered in planning anesthetic management.

Earlier chapters have discussed the risks and alternative anesthetic techniques associated with specific preoperative medical problems and types of surgical procedures. However, complications due to errors in anesthetic management can occur despite an adequate knowledge of didactic material. This chapter reviews the incidence, causes, and prevention of anesthetic accidents. Complications associated with patient positioning and anaphylactic drug reactions are also discussed. The chapter concludes with an examination of occupational hazards of anesthesiology such as chronic exposure to trace concentrations of anesthetic gases, infectious complications, and substance abuse.

ANESTHETIC ACCIDENTS

Incidence

There are several reasons why it is difficult to accurately measure the incidence of anesthetic accidents. First, it is often impossible to distribute the responsibility for a poor outcome between the patient's inherent disease, the surgical procedure, and the anesthetic

management. In fact, all three can contribute to poor outcomes. Second, it is difficult to find a measurable event. Death is the clearest end point, but perioperative death is so rare that a very large series of patients must be studied in order to assemble conclusions that have statistical significance. Finally, medicolegal fears hinder accurate reporting.

Nonetheless, many studies have attempted to determine the incidence of anesthetic deaths. It is clear that most perioperative fatalities are due to the patient's preoperative disease or the surgical procedure. The mortality rate referable primarily to anesthesia *appears* to have dropped during the last 30 years from 1 or 2 deaths per 3000 anesthetic experiences to a current rate of 1 or 2 per 20,000 experiences. These statistics should be viewed with considerable skepticism, however, since they are derived from different countries using different methodologies. Recent studies indicate that the anesthetic mortality rate in some institutions may be even less than 1:20,000. This decline may be due to the availability and utilization of new monitoring equipment, greater knowledge of anesthetic physiology and pharmacology, or improved surgical and medical care.

Causes

Anesthetic mishaps can be categorized as preventable or unpreventable. Examples of the latter include sudden death syndrome, fatal idiosyncratic drug reactions, or any poor outcome that occurs despite proper management. However, studies of anesthetic-related deaths or "near misses" demonstrate that most such accidents are preventable. Of these preventable incidents, most involve human error (Table 45–1) as opposed to equipment malfunctions (Table 45–2). Of course, some rate of human error is inevitable, and the occurrence of preventable accidents is not synonymous with incompetence.

Most serious anesthetic complications are associated with adverse respiratory events. Problems of airway management include inadequate ventilation, pre-

Table 45–1. Common human errors leading to preventable anesthetic accidents.

Unrecognized breathing circuit disconnection
Mistaken drug administration
Airway mismanagement
Anesthesia machine misuse
Fluid mismanagement
Intravenous line disconnection

Table 45–3. Factors associated with human and equipment errors.

Factor	Example
Inadequate preparation	No machine checkout or pre-operative evaluation; haste and carelessness
Inadequate experience and training	Unfamiliarity with the anesthetic technique or equipment
Environmental limitations	Inability to visualize surgical field; poor communication with surgeons
Physical and emotional factors	Fatigue; personal problems

mature extubation, and unrecognized esophageal intubation. Breathing circuit disconnection is a problem especially with mechanical ventilation and usually occurs at the endotracheal tube connector. New anesthesia machines with built-in low circuit pressure alarms and end-tidal CO_2 analysis should reduce the likelihood of this problem. Hypoxemia from failing to ventilate a paralyzed patient has probably been the most common cause of intraoperative cardiac arrest. Aspiration pneumonitis is discussed in the "Case Discussion" following Chapter 15.

Most accidents related to the anesthesia machine also involve an element of human error: gas flow control changes, vaporizer errors, gas supply problems, and unnoticed fail-safe activation. Unintentional administration of the wrong drug (**"syringe swap"**) often involves muscle relaxants or their reversal agents. Similar-appearing prefilled syringes containing resuscitation drugs are also easily confused. The administration of inappropriate doses of the correct drug may be as important a problem as syringe swap. Drug syringes and ampules in the work area should be restricted to only those needed for the specific case under way and should be consistently diluted to the same concentration for each use and clearly labeled.

Another generalization about serious anesthetic accidents is that there are usually other factors associated with their occurrence (Table 45–3). For instance, the impact of most equipment failures is lessened—if not totally avoided—by routine preoperative checkouts and personnel training. An error such as esophageal intubation results in a serious complication such as brain damage when it goes unrecognized due to inadequate monitoring or a lack of vigilance. Another type of human error occurs when the most critical problem is ignored because attention is inappropriately focused on a less important problem or an incorrect solution (**fixation error**). Many anesthetic fatalities occur only after a series of coincidental circumstances, misjudgments, and technical errors (the **mishap chain**).

Prevention

Strategies to reduce the incidence of serious anesthetic complications include (1) better monitoring and anesthetic technique, (2) improved education, (3) more comprehensive protocols and standards of practice, and (4) active risk management programs. Better monitoring and anesthetic techniques imply closer patient contact, more comprehensive monitoring equipment, and better-designed anesthesia machines and work spaces. The fact that most accidents occur during the maintenance phase of anesthesia—rather than during induction or emergence—implies a failure of vigilance. Inspection, auscultation, and palpation of the patient is a never-ending responsibility. Instruments should supplement but never replace the anesthesiologist's own senses.

A major goal of the Society for Education in Anesthesia is to improve resident training. Of course, education must continue beyond residency as new drugs, techniques, and equipment are developed. Part of this continuing education requirement includes awareness of recommended monitoring standards (Chapter 6), equipment checkouts (Chapter 4), preoperative evaluation (Tables 1–3 and 1–4), postoperative follow-up (Figure 1–3), and relief exchanges (Table 45–4). The medicolegal obligations that accompany the establishment of specific standards are part of the cost of patient safety.

Risk management and continuous quality improvement programs at the departmental level should reduce

Table 45–2. Common equipment malfunctions leading to preventable anesthetic accidents.

Breathing circuit
Monitoring device
Ventilator
Anesthesia machine
Laryngoscope

Table 45–4. A relief exchange protocol should review all the types of information another anesthesiologist would need to assume full responsibility for the patient's care.

1. Preoperative patient summary (eg, pertinent findings in history, physical examination, laboratory)
2. Surgical and anesthetic plan (eg, estimated duration of case, anesthetic technique)
3. Progress report (eg, estimated blood loss, volume replacement, response to anesthetics, problems encountered)
4. Suggested approach to potential problems (eg, drug choice for deepening anesthesia, raising blood pressure, or increasing muscle relaxation)
5. Vital signs confirmation and monitoring check by each individual (eg, blood pressure, heart rate and rhythm, breath sounds, anesthetic gas concentrations)

Table 45–5. Physiologic effects of common patient positions.

Position	Organ System	Effects
Supine Horizontal[1]	Cardiac	Equalization of pressures throughout the arterial system. Increased right-sided filling and cardiac output. Decreased heart rate and peripheral vascular resistance.
	Respiratory	Gravity increases perfusion of dependent (posterior) lung segments. Abdominal viscera displace diaphragm cephalad. Spontaneous ventilation favors dependent lung segments, while controlled ventilation favors independent (anterior) segments. Functional residual capacity decreases and may fall below closing volume in older patients.
Trendelenburg	Cardiac	Activation of baroreceptors, generally causing decreased cardiac output, peripheral vascular resistance, heart rate, and blood pressure.
	Respiratory	Marked decreases in lung capacities due to shift of abdominal viscera. Increased ventilation-perfusion mismatching and atelectasis. Increased likelihood of regurgitation.
	Other	Increase in intracranial pressure and decrease in cerebral blood flow due to cerebral venous congestion. Increase in intraocular pressure in patients with glaucoma.
Reverse Trendelenburg	Cardiac	Preload, cardiac output, and arterial pressure decrease. Baroreflexes increase sympathetic tone, heart rate, and peripheral vascular resistance.
	Respiratory	Spontaneous respiration requires less work. Functional residual capacity increases.
	Other	Cerebral perfusion pressure and blood flow may decrease.
Lithotomy	Cardiac	Autotransfusion from leg vessels increases circulating blood volume and preload. Lowering legs has opposite effect. Effect on blood pressure and cardiac output depends on volume status.
	Respiratory	Decreases vital capacity. Increases likelihood of aspiration.
Prone	Cardiac	Pooling of blood in extremities and compression of abdominal muscles may decrease preload, cardiac output, and blood pressure
	Respiratory	Compression of abdomen and thorax decreases total lung compliance and increases work of breathing.
	Other	Extreme head rotation may decrease cerebral venous drainage and cerebral blood flow.
Lateral decubitus	Cardiac	Cardiac output unchanged unless venous return obstructed (eg, kidney rest). Arterial blood pressure may fall as a result of decreased vascular resistance (right > left side).
	Respiratory	Decreased volume of dependent lung. Increased perfusion of dependent lung. Increased ventilation of dependent lung in awake patients (no $\dot{V}/\dot{Q}$ mismatch). Decreased ventilation of dependent lung in anesthetized patients ($\dot{V}/\dot{Q}$ mismatch). Further decreases in dependent lung ventilation with paralysis and an open chest (Chapter 24).
Sitting	Cardiac	Pooling of blood in lower body decreases central blood volume. Cardiac output and arterial blood pressure fall despite a rise in heart rate and systemic vascular resistance.
	Respiratory	Lung volumes and functional residual capacity increase. Work of breathing increases.
	Other	Cerebral blood flow decreases.

[1]The effects described for the horizontal position are in comparison with a patient standing erect. All other positions are compared with the horizontal position.

Table 45–6. Complications associated with patient positioning.

Complication	Position	Prevention
Air embolism	Sitting, prone, reverse Trendelenburg	Maintain venous pressure at the wound > 0 (Chapter 27).
Alopecia	Supine, lithotomy, Trendelenburg	Normotension, padding, and occasional head turning.
Backache	Any	Lumbar support, padding, and slight hip flexion.
Corneal abrasion	Especially prone	Taping and lubricating eye.
Digit amputation	Any	Check for protruding digits before changing table configuration.
Nerve palsies		
Brachial plexus	Any	Avoid stretching or direct compression at neck or axilla.
Common peroneal	Lithotomy, lateral decubitus	Pad lateral aspect of upper fibula.
Radial	Any	Avoid compression of lateral humerus.
Ulnar	Any	Padding at elbow.
Retinal ischemia	Prone, sitting	Avoid pressure on globe.
Skin necrosis	Any	Padding over bony prominences.

anesthetic morbidity and mortality by addressing equipment, in-training, and staffing issues. Specific responsibilities of peer review committees include identification and prevention of potential problems, formulating departmental policies, ensuring the availability of properly functioning anesthetic equipment, enforcing standards required for clinical privileges, and evaluating the appropriateness of patient care. The latter is judged by a quality improvement system that should impartially review complications and ensure physician competence.

PATIENT POSITIONING

Changes of body position have physiologic consequences that can be exaggerated in disease states. For example, whereas getting out of bed in the morning is usually well tolerated, it may cause dizziness or even syncope in patients with marginal cardiac reserve. Similarly, general and regional anesthesia may limit the cardiovascular response to such a change. Even positions that are safe for short periods may eventually lead to complications in individuals who are not able to move in response to pain. For example, the alcoholic patient who passes out on a hard floor may waken with a brachial plexus injury. Similarly, regional and general anesthesia abolish protective reflexes and predispose patients to injury.

Postural hypotension, the most common physiologic consequence of positioning, can be minimized by (1) avoiding abrupt or extreme position changes (eg, the sitting position), (2) reversing the position if vital signs deteriorate, (3) keeping the patient as well hydrated as possible, and (4) having drugs available to counter any anticipated reaction. While maintaining a

minimal level of anesthesia will lessen the likelihood of hypotension, coincidental movement of the endotracheal tube during positioning may cause the patient to cough and become hypertensive. Table 45–5 summarizes the major physiologic effects of common patient positions. These effects are generalizations that may vary depending upon the patient's volume status and cardiac reserve.

Many complications have been associated with improper patient positioning (Table 45–6). Most result from the physiologic changes described above (eg, air embolism), ischemic injury (eg, nerve injury), or crush injury (eg, finger amputation). These are best prevented by (1) evaluating the patient's postural limitations during the preanesthetic visit; (2) padding of pressure points, susceptible nerves, and any area of the body that is *potentially* in contact with the operating room table or its attachments; (3) avoiding flexion or extension of a joint to its limit; (4) having an awake individual mimic the position to ensure comfort; and (5) understanding the potential complications of each position. Periods during which the patient is being transported pose a particular threat if monitoring is interrupted for any reason. Similarly, monitors are often disconnected during patient repositioning.

Postoperative peripheral nerve injury is presumed to be due to improper patient positioning. Specifically, nerve injuries are usually assumed to be caused by a pressure or traction mechanism. Nonetheless, large reviews of perioperative nerve injuries reveal that their precise cause is often obscure. The most common injuries involve the ulnar nerve, the brachial plexus, or the femoral and sciatic nerves. Certain positions predispose to specific nerve injuries. For example, improper lithotomy positioning is associated with damage to the peroneal nerve.

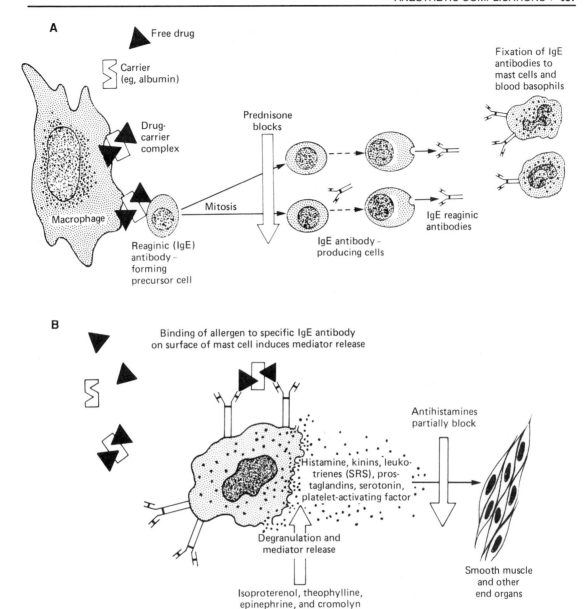

Figure 45–1. A: Induction of IgE-mediated allergic sensitivity to drugs and other allergens. **B:** Response of IgE-sensitized cells to subsequent exposure to allergens. (Reproduced, with permission, from Katzung BG (editor): *Basic & Clinical Pharmacology*, 4th ed. Appleton & Lange, 1989.)

ALLERGIC DRUG REACTIONS

Anaphylaxis is an exaggerated response to a foreign substance (eg, anesthetic drugs or volume expanders) that is mediated by an antigen-antibody reaction (type I hypersensitivity reaction). Even low-molecular-weight drugs can trigger an anaphylactic reaction by binding to a carrier protein (eg, albumin). The drug-carrier complex stimulates the production of IgE antibodies that fix to mast cells and basophils (Figure 45–

1). Reexposure to the antigen results in antibody binding and release of a variety of chemical mediators, including (1) leukotrienes (slow-reacting substance of anaphylaxis), (2) histamine, (3) prostaglandins, (4) kinins, and (5) platelet-activating factor. These mediators have many physiologic effects (Table 45–7) that result in the clinical manifestations of anaphylaxis (Table 45–8).

Anaphylactoid reactions resemble anaphylaxis but do not depend upon IgE antibody interaction with anti-

Table 45–7. Physiologic effects of anaphylactic mediators.

	Leukotrienes	Histamine	Prostaglandins	Kinins	Platelet-Activating Factor
Increased capillary permeability	•	•	•	•	•
Vasodilatation	•	•	•	•	•
Bronchospasm	•	•	•	•	
Coronary spasm	•	•	•		
Myocardial depression	•				

gen. For example, a drug can activate the complement system or directly release histamine from mast cells (eg, urticaria following high-dose morphine sulfate). Although the mechanisms differ, anaphylactic and anaphylactoid reactions can be clinically indistinguishable and equally life-threatening. Treatment must be immediate and tailored to the severity of the reaction (Table 45–9).

Factors that may predispose patients to these reactions include (1) youth, (2) pregnancy, (3) a history of atopy, and (4) previous drug exposure. Laboratory identification of patients who have experienced an adverse allergic reaction or who may be particularly susceptible is often aided by (1) intradermal skin testing, (2) leukocyte or basophil degranulation testing (histamine release test), or (3) radioallergosorbent testing (RAST). The latter is capable of measuring drug-specific IgE antibody in the serum. Prophylactic pretreatment with histamine antagonists (Chapter 15), cromolyn sodium, and corticosteroids decreases the severity of the reaction.

OCCUPATIONAL HAZARDS IN ANESTHESIOLOGY

1. CHRONIC EXPOSURE TO ANESTHETIC GASES

Chapter 2 began with the statement, "Anesthesiologists spend more time in operating rooms than any other group of physicians." One result of this fact is greater exposure to the risks of the operating room environment. For instance, the long-term effects of trace anesthetic gases have been addressed in several epidemiologic studies. These studies have varied in validity of experimental design and have produced conflicting and somewhat sketchy results. While well-established conclusions are lacking, some generalizations have been offered:

(1) Female anesthesia personnel who work in the operating room *may* be at a slightly increased risk of spontaneous abortion and of having offspring with congenital abnormalities.
(2) Female anesthesia personnel *may* be at a slightly increased risk of cancer.
(3) Male and female anesthesia personnel *may* be at a higher risk of hepatic disease not totally explained as serum hepatitis.
(4) Female operating room personnel *may* be at an increased risk of renal disease.
(5) Dentists and dental assistants *may* be at an increased risk of neurologic disease due to exposure to nitrous oxide.

It is important to emphasize that *none* of these conclusions have been definitively proved. Laboratory studies have failed to convincingly link trace concentrations of modern anesthetic agents to mutagenic, carcinogenic, or teratogenic consequences in animal models. However, the potential for adverse effects due to occupational exposure to anesthetic agents has led to proposals by the National Institute for Occupational Safety and Health of less than 25 ppm nitrous oxide and 0.5 ppm halogenated anesthetics (2 ppm if the halogenated agent is used alone). Achieving these low levels depends upon efficient scavenging equipment, adequate operating room ventilation, and conscientious anesthetic technique. Monitoring trace gas levels requires special equipment (eg, infrared analyzer or gas chromatography), since most people cannot detect the odor of volatile agents at a concentration of less than 30 ppm (of course, nitrous oxide is essentially odorless).

Table 45–8. Clinical manifestations of anaphylaxis.

Organ System	Signs and Symptoms
Cardiovascular	Hypotension,* tachycardia, dysrhyrhmias
Pulmonary	Bronchospasm,* cough, dyspnea, pulmonary edema, laryngeal edema, hypoxemia
Dermatologic	Urticaria,* facial edema, pruritus

*Key signs during general anesthesia.

Table 45–9. Treatment of anaphylactic and anaphylactoid reactions.

Discontinue drug administration
Administer 100% oxygen
Epinephrine (0.01–0.5 mg IV or IM)[1]
Intravenous fluids (1–2 L lactated Ringer's injection)
Aminophylline (5–6 mg/kg IV)
Diphenhydramine (50–75 mg IV)

[1]The dose and route of epinephrine depends upon the severity of the reaction.

2. INFECTIOUS COMPLICATIONS

Hospital workers are exposed to many infectious diseases prevalent in the community (eg, respiratory viral infections, rubella, tuberculosis). Anesthesia personnel are at particular risk for acquiring herpetic whitlow and hepatitis B. **Herpetic whitlow** is infection of the finger with herpes simplex virus type 1 or 2. Infection usually involves direct contact of previously traumatized skin with contaminated oral secretions. Painful vesicles appear at the site of infection. The diagnosis is confirmed by the appearance of giant epithelial cells or nuclear inclusion bodies in a smear taken from the base of a vesicle, the presence of a rise in herpes simplex virus titer, or identification of the virus with antiserum. Treatment is conservative and includes topical application of 5% acyclovir ointment. Prevention rests upon wearing gloves when contacting oral secretions. Patients at risk for harboring the virus include those suffering from immunosuppression, cancer, malnutrition, and other infections.

The prevalence of **hepatitis B** serologic markers is several times higher in anesthesia personnel (15–50%) than in the general population (3–5%). The risk of infection is proportionate to the number of years in practice. Fulminant hepatitis (1% of acute infections) carries a 60% mortality rate. Chronic active hepatitis ($<$ 5% of all cases) is associated with an increased incidence of cirrhosis of the liver and hepatocellular carcinoma. Transmission of the virus is chiefly through contact with blood products or body fluids. The diagnosis is confirmed by detection of hepatitis B surface antigen (HBsAg). Uncomplicated recovery is signaled by the disappearance of HBsAg and the appearance of antibody to the surface antigen (anti-HBs). A hepatitis vaccine is available and is recommended for prophylaxis of anesthesia personnel. The appearance of anti-HBs after a three-dose regimen indicates successful immunization.

Hepatitis non-A, non-B is another important occupational hazard in anesthesiology. Four to 8 percent of non-A, non-B infections occur in health care workers. One-half of these infections lead to chronic hepatitis. In fact, non-A, non-B hepatitis is the most common cause of nonalcoholic cirrhosis in the United States. While there is no vaccine to protect against non-A, non-B hepatitis, one causative agent (hepatitis C virus) has been recently identified. Screening of donor blood for antibodies to hepatitis C should decrease the incidence of non-A, non-B hepatitis following blood transfusion.

Anesthesia personnel appear to be at a low risk of occupationally contracting **AIDS.** Nonetheless, because there are a few documented reports of transmission of human immunodeficiency virus (HIV) from infected patients to health care workers, the Centers for Disease Control has proposed guidelines that apply to all categories of patient contact. These **universal precautions,** which are equally valid for protection from hepatitis B infection, are as follows:

(1) Needle precautions.
(2) Use of gloves and other barriers during contact with open wounds and body fluids.
(3) Frequent hand-washing.
(4) Proper techniques for disinfection or disposal of contaminated materials.
(5) Particular caution by pregnant health-care workers, and no contact with patients by workers who have exudative or weeping dermatitis.

3. SUBSTANCE ABUSE

Anesthesiology may be the highest-risk medical specialty for drug addition. Reasons for this include (1) the stress of anesthetic practice, (2) the easy availability of drugs with addiction potential, and (3) curiosity aroused by the frequent example of patients' "euphoria" after receiving opioids and sedatives. The likelihood of developing a substance abuse problem is increased by coexisting personal problems (eg, marital or financial difficulties) and a family history of alcoholism or drug addition.

The voluntary use of mood-altering drugs is a disease. If left untreated, substance abuse often leads to death due to intentional or unintentional drug overdose. One of the greatest challenges in treating this illness is identifying the afflicted individual, since **denial** is a consistent feature. Unfortunately, changes evident to an outside observer are often vague and late signs: reduced involvement in social activities, subtle changes in appearance, extremes of mood swings, and altered work habits. Treatment begins with an intervention plan with the goal of enrolling the individual in a formal rehabilitation program. The potential for retaining medical licensure and reentering the mainstream of practice provides powerful motivation. Experienced diversion programs report a success rate of approximately 70%. Long-term compliance often involves continued participation in support groups (eg, Alcoholics Anonymous), random urine testing, and oral naltrexone therapy (a long-acting narcotic antagonist). Effective prevention strategies are difficult to formulate but may include better control of drug availability and education about the severe consequences of substance abuse.

CASE DISCUSSION: UNEXPLAINED INTRAOPERATIVE TACHYCARDIA & HYPERTENSION

A 73-year-old man is scheduled at midnight for emergency relief of an intestinal obstruction with strangulation due to a volvulus. The patient has a history of a myocardial infarction 1 month ago which was complicated by intermittent congestive heart failure. The blood pressure is 160/90 mm Hg; pulse 110 beats/min, respiratory rate 22/min, temperature 38.8 °C.

Why is this case an emergency?

Strangulation of the bowel begins with venous obstruction but can quickly progress to arterial occlusion, ischemia, infarction, and perforation. Acute peritonitis could lead to sepsis, shock, and multi-organ failure—obviously a poor prognosis in this elderly patient. However, a few hours could be well spent optimizing the patient's fluid status (eg, dehydration) and cardiovascular parameters (eg, tachycardia) before rushing to the operating room. Furthermore, a complex and high-risk case such as this requires extra operating room setup time in preparation of medications, monitors, and other anesthetic equipment.

The patient is immediately rushed to an available operating room which has been set up for a possible open heart case.

What special monitoring would be appropriate for this patient?

Because of the history of recent myocardial infarction and congestive heart failure, an arterial line and a pulmonary artery catheter would be useful. Large fluid shifts should be anticipated, and a beat-to-beat monitor of blood pressure is needed. Furthermore, information regarding myocardial supply (diastolic blood pressure) and demand (systolic blood pressure, left ventricular wall stress, and heart rate) should be continuously available. A central venous pressure may give misleading information owing to the potential discrepancy between right- and left-sided pressures in a patient with significant left ventricular dysfunction. Further monitoring could include transesophageal echocardiography for early detection of myocardial ischemia and assessment of ventricular wall motion.

An arterial line is easily placed, but the pulmonary artery catheter gives only an intermittent pulmonary artery tracing.

What cardiovascular medications could be useful during induction and maintenance of general anesthesia?

A continuous intravenous infusion of nitroglycerin could beneficially alter the myocardial supply/demand balance. Esmolol might be useful in decreasing the heart rate, but caution is suggested by the history of congestive heart failure. Drugs causing tachycardia or extremes in arterial blood pressure should obviously be avoided.

A nitroglycerin drip is begun, and the patient's vital signs remain stable throughout a "standard thiopental induction." During the laparotomy, gradual increases in heart rate and blood pressure are noted. The rate of administration of nitroglycerin is increased, and ST segment elevations appear on the ECG. The heart rate

is now 130/min and the blood pressure 220/140 mm Hg. The pulmonary artery catheter tracing is consistent with a right ventricular location. The concentration of volatile anesthetic is increased, and propranolol is administered intravenously in 1-mg increments. This results in a decline in heart rate to 115 beats/min but a rise in blood pressure to 250/160 mm Hg. Suddenly, the rhythm converts to ventricular tachycardia, with a profound drop in blood pressure. As lidocaine is being administered and the defibrillation unit prepared, the rhythm degenerates into ventricular fibrillation.

What could explain this series of events?

A differential diagnosis of pronounced tachycardia and hypertension might include pheochromocytoma, malignant hyperthermia, or thyroid storm. In this case, further inspection of the "nitroglycerin" infusion revealed that the intravenous tubing had been mislabeled. In fact, while the tubing was labeled nitroglycerin, the infusion bag was labeled epinephrine.

How does this explain the paradoxic response to propranolol?

Propranolol is a nonselective β-adrenergic antagonist. Thus, it blocks the tachycardia due to epinephrine's β_1 stimulation and the dilatation of blood vessels due to β_2 stimulation but does not affect alpha-induced vasoconstriction. The net result is a decrease in heart rate but an increase in blood pressure.

Why wasn't the patient hypertensive during induction?

It was surprising that a "standard thiopental induction" would not result in profound hypotension in this dehydrated elderly patient with a history of heart disease. The epinephrine infusion may have masked the hypotensive effects of induction, resulting in relatively stable vital signs.

What is the cause of the ventricular tachycardia?

An overdose of epinephrine could result in life-threatening ventricular dysrhythmias. A high concentration of volatile anesthetic could have further sensitized the myocardium to the dysrhythmogenic effects of epinephrine. Additionally, the malpositioned tip of the pulmonary artery catheter could have irritated the endothelium and conduction pathways in the right ventricle.

What other factors may have contributed to this anesthetic mishap?

Many factors may have indirectly contributed to this end result, including the timing of the case at night (ie, physician fatigue), the lack of preparation (ie, patient fine-tuning), the use of drugs prepared by another anesthesiologist, and the decision to proceed with induction and surgery despite unsatisfactory positioning of the pulmonary artery catheter. The end result of this chain of coincidence, misjudgment, and an unhealthy patient resulted in a poor outcome.

SUGGESTED READINGS

Anderton JM, Keen RI, Neave R (editors): *Positioning the Surgical Patient*. Butterworths, 1988. Many line drawings.

Brown DL (editor): *Risk and Outcome in Anesthesia*. Lippincott, 1988.

Cheney FW et al: Standard of care and anesthesia liability. JAMA 1989;261:1599. Review of over 1000 malpractice actions for anesthesia-related injuries.

Eichhorn JH: Prevention of intraoperative anesthesia accidents and related severe injury through safety monitoring. Anesthesiology 1989;70:572. Examines several aspects of anesthetic risk, including the effects of new monitors and monitoring standards.

Fisher M McD (editor): Adverse reactions. Clin Anesthesiol 1984;2:451. Untoward effects of the major anesthetic drug groups are discussed, along with malignant hyperthermia and anaphylactoid reactions.

Gravenstein N (editor): *Manual of Complications during Anesthesia*. Lippincott, 1991. Noteworthy chapters on quality assurance and occupational hazards.

Gravenstein JS, Holzer JF (editors): *Safety and Cost Containment in Anesthesia*. Butterworths, 1988. The economic implications of anesthesia safety and mishaps.

Lunn JN (editor): *Epidemiology in Anaesthesia: The Techniques of Epidemiology Applied to Anaesthetic Practice*. Edward Arnold, 1986. Studies of anesthetic risk, operating room pollution, and halothane hepatitis.

Martin JT (editor): *Positioning in Anesthesia and Surgery*. Saunders, 1987. Physiologic effects and complications.

Orkin FK, Cooperman LH (editors): *Complications in Anesthesiology*. Lippincott, 1983. See next comment.

Taylor TH, Major E (editors): *Hazards and Complications of Anaesthesia*. Churchill Livingstone, 1987. Two definitive works describing anesthetic hazards, risks, and complications.

Peters JD et al: *Anesthesiology and the Law*. Health Administration Press, 1983. A sobering discussion of medical liability, anesthetic mishaps, and the standard of care concept, utilizing practical case illustrations.

Pierce E, Cooper J: Equipment-related anesthetic incidents. Int Anesthesiol Clin 1984;22:133.

Weinger MB, Englund CE: Ergonomic and human factors affecting anesthetic vigilance and monitoring performance in the operating room environment. Anesthesiology 1990;73:995.

46

Cardiopulmonary Resuscitation

One goal of anesthesiology is to maintain the function of vital organ systems during surgery. It is not surprising that anesthesiologists have also played a major role in the development of cardiopulmonary resuscitation techniques outside the operating room. Cardiopulmonary resuscitation should be considered any time an individual cannot adequately oxygenate or perfuse vital organs—not only following cardiac or respiratory arrest.

This chapter presents an overview of the American Heart Association recommendations for establishing and maintaining the **ABCs** of cardiopulmonary resuscitation: *a*irway, *b*reathing, and *c*irculation. However, it is not intended as a substitute for a formal course in either life support without the use of special equipment (Basic Life Support) or with the use of special equipment and drugs (Advanced Cardiac Life Support).

Resuscitation of neonates is discussed in Chapter 41.

A: AIRWAY

Basic Techniques

Although the "a" of *ABC* represents "airway" for mnemonic purposes, the approach to the patient must always include an initial *a*ssessment. Before cardiopulmonary resuscitation is initiated, unresponsiveness is established and the airway assessed. The patient is positioned supine on a firm surface. The airway is most commonly obstructed by posterior displacement of the tongue or epiglottis and is opened by one of two maneuvers. The **head-tilt, chin-lift** is easily performed, while a **jaw-thrust** without head-tilt is preferred whenever a cervical spine injury is suspected (Figure 46–1). Basic airway management is discussed in detail in Chapter 5.

If vomitus or a foreign body is visible in the mouth of an unconscious patient, it should be swept out with the index finger.* If the patient is conscious or if the foreign body cannot be removed by a finger sweep, the **Heimlich maneuver** is recommended. This subdiaphragmatic abdominal thrust elevates the diaphragm, expelling a blast of air from the lungs that displaces the foreign body (Figure 46–2). Complica-

tions of the Heimlich maneuver include rib fracture, trauma to the internal viscera, and regurgitation.

Advanced Techniques

A. Esophageal Obturator Airways: More sophisticated airway management requires specialized equipment. Oral and nasopharyngeal airways, face masks, laryngoscopes, and endotracheal tubes are described in Chapter 5. The **esophageal obturator airway** and the **esophageal gastric tube airway** are simple but less effective alternatives to endotracheal intubation. A blocked distal end and the face mask connection of these tubes differ from endotracheal tube design (Figure 46–3). Esophageal airways are purposely introduced into the esophagus, not the trachea. Because of the distal cuffs and blind ends of these airways, fresh gas is not permitted to enter the stomach. A good mask seal will force air flow through the trachea and into the lungs.

Because esophageal airways are easier to place by less experienced personnel, their use "in the field" by paramedical personnel continues. However, these devices have generally fallen out of favor because they are associated with numerous complications, including inadequate ventilation. Insertion into the trachea would be as disastrous as esophageal intubation with an endotracheal tube. The risk of esophageal perforation contraindicates their use in patients suspected of having esophageal trauma or disease.

In the hospital setting, an esophageal airway is usually replaced with an endotracheal tube. If possible, suction should be immediately available, since esophageal airway removal often induces regurgitation. For the same reason, it is recommended that the esophageal airway be left in place until proper endotracheal tube placement is confirmed. Unfortunately, the presence of the esophageal obturator airway in the oropharynx often makes endotracheal intubation difficult or impossible.

B. Cricothyrotomy (Cricothyroidotomy): Some causes of airway obstruction may not be relieved by conventional methods. Furthermore, intubation may be technically impossible to perform (eg, severe facial trauma), or repeated attempts may be unwise (cervical spine trauma). In these circumstances, cricothyrotomy or tracheostomy may be necessary. **Cricothyrotomy** involves placing a large intravenous catheter or a commercially available cannula (eg, Nu-Trake) into the

---

*However, placing a finger in the mouth of a conscious patient is not recommended!

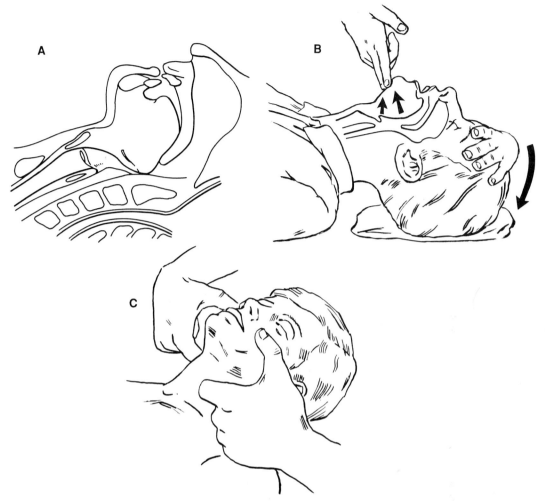

Figure 46–1. Loss of consciousness is often accompanied by loss of submandibular muscle tone **(A).** Occlusion of the airway by the tongue can be relieved by a head-tilt/chin-lift **(B),** or a jaw thrust **(C).** In patients with possible cervical spine injury, the angles of the jaw should be lifted anteriorly without hyperextending the neck. (Courtesy of American Heart Association.)

trachea through the midline of the cricothyroid membrane (Figures 46–4 and 46–5). Proper location is confirmed by aspiration of air. While a cannula such as the Nu-Trake is large enough to allow adequate ventilation with a self-inflating resuscitation bag, a 12- or 14-gauge catheter requires a driving pressure of 50 psi to generate sufficient gas flow **(transtracheal jet ventilation).**

Various systems are available that connect a high-pressure source of oxygen (eg, central wall oxygen, tank oxygen, or the anesthesia machine fresh gas outlet) to the catheter (Figure 46–6). A hand-operated jet injector or the oxygen flush valve of an anesthesia machine controls ventilation. The addition of a pressure regulator minimizes the risk of barotrauma.

Regardless of which transtracheal jet ventilation system is chosen, it must be readily available, must utilize noncompliant tubing, and must have secure connections. Direct connection of a 12- or 14-gauge intravenous catheter to the anesthesia circle system does not allow adequate ventilation owing to the high compliance of the corrugated breathing tubing and breathing bag. Likewise, it is impossible to reliably deliver acceptable ventilation through a 12- or 14-gauge catheter with a self-inflating resuscitation bag.

Adequacy of ventilation—particularly expiration—is judged by observation of chest wall movement and auscultation of breath sounds. Acute complications include pneumothorax, subcutaneous emphysema, mediastinal emphysema, bleeding, esophageal puncture, aspiration, and respiratory acidosis. Long-term complications include tracheomalacia, subglottic stenosis, and vocal cord changes. Cricothyrotomy is not generally recommended in children under 10 years of age.

Tracheostomy can be performed in a more controlled environment after oxygenation has been se-

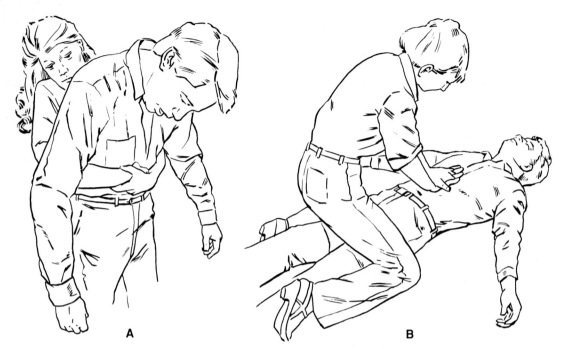

Figure 46–2. The Heimlich maneuver can be performed with the victim standing **(A)** or lying down **(B)**. The hands are positioned slightly above the navel and well below the xiphoid process. The fist is then pressed into the abdomen with a quick upward thrust. The maneuver may need to be repeated. (Courtesy of American Heart Association.)

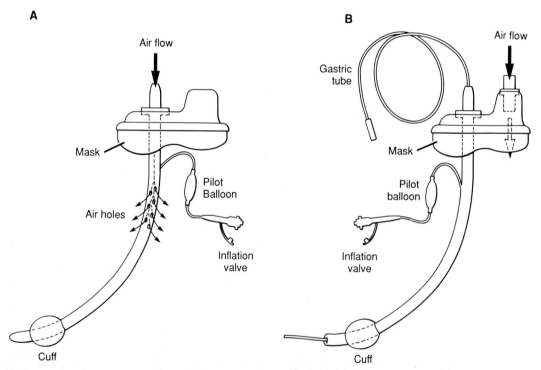

Figure 46–3. Esophageal obturator airway **(A)** and the esophageal gastric tube airway **(B)**. Note the blocked distal ends and the face mask connections of these tubes, which differ from endotracheal tube design.

A. Locate the cricothyroid membrane.

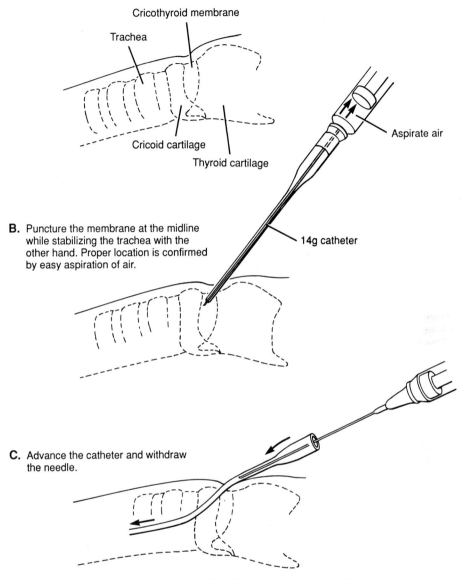

B. Puncture the membrane at the midline while stabilizing the trachea with the other hand. Proper location is confirmed by easy aspiration of air.

C. Advance the catheter and withdraw the needle.

Figure 46–4. Percutaneous cricothyrotomy with a 14-gauge over-the-needle intravenous catheter.

cured by cricothyrotomy. A detailed description of tracheostomy is beyond the scope of this text.

B: BREATHING

Assessment of spontaneous breathing should immediately follow establishment of the airway. Ventilation should not be delayed for intubation if a patent airway is established by a jaw-thrust maneuver. Apnea is confirmed by observing chest movement, listening for breath sounds, and feeling air flow. Regardless of the

airway and breathing methods employed, a specific regimen of ventilation has been proposed for the apneic patient. Initially, two breaths are slowly administered (1–1½ seconds each). If these breaths cannot be delivered, the airway is still obstructed and the head and neck need repositioning or a foreign body is present that must be removed.

Mouth-to-mouth or **mouth-to-mask** rescue breathing must be immediately instituted in the breathless patient, even in the hospital setting when the crash cart is "on its way." Pinching the nose allows formation of an airtight seal between the rescuer's lips and the out-

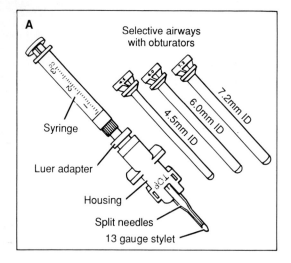

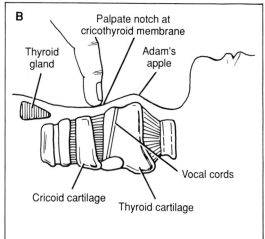

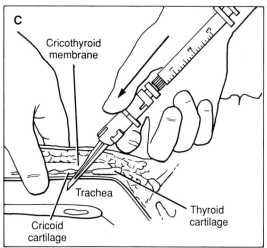

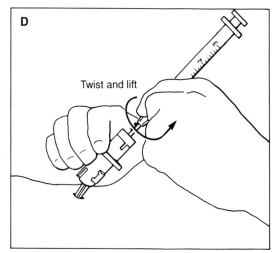

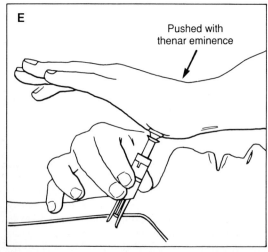

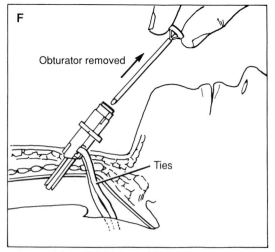

Figure 46–5. The Nu-Trake is a commercially available kit for cricothyrotomy **(A).** The neck is hyperextended and the cricothyroid membrane is identified and exposed **(B).** The needle punctures the membrane, and easy aspiration of air confirms entry into the trachea **(C).** The stylet and syringe are removed, leaving the housing on the overlying skin **(D).** An airway and obturator are inserted by pushing with the thenar eminence against the cap of the obturator **(E).** The obturator is removed **(F)** and a resuscitation bag or anesthesia breathing system is attached.

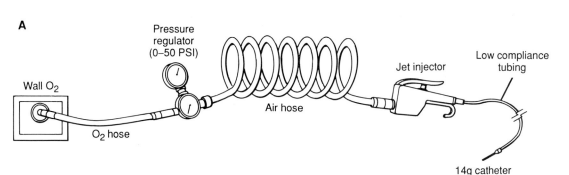

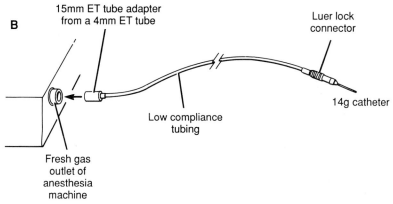

Figure 46–6. Two systems for transtracheal jet ventilation after cricothyrotomy (Figure 46–4). A jet ventilator and pressure regulator *(A)* provide better control of the inspiratory cycle. Both systems use noncompliant tubing and a high-pressure source of oxygen.

side of the victim's mouth. Successful rescue breathing (800–1200 mL tidal volume in an adult) is confirmed by observing the chest rising and falling with respiration and hearing and feeling the escape of air during expiration. The most common cause of inadequate mouth-to-mouth ventilation is inadequate airway control. **Mouth-to-mouth-and-nose** breathing is more effective in infants and small children.

A rescuer's exhaled air has an oxygen concentration of only 16–17%, but that much oxygen is far better than no oxygen at all. This low inspired oxygen concentration, combined with low cardiac output and intrapulmonary shunting during resuscitation, invariably results in hypoxemia. **Supplemental oxygen,** preferably 100%, should always be used if available.

Mouth-to-mask breathing has a hygienic advantage over mouth-to-mouth since the rescuer's lips form a seal with an intervening mask. Devices that avoid mouth-to-mouth breathing should be immediately available everywhere in the hospital. Ventilation with a mask may be performed more easily in some patients because the rescuer may be able to adjust the airway or make an airtight seal more effectively. Furthermore, some mouth-to-mask devices allow the delivery of supplemental oxygen.

A self-inflating **bag-valve-mask** device is described in Chapter 3. These devices are often less effective than mouth-to-mask or **bag-valve-endotracheal tube** ventilation because of the difficulty inexperienced personnel may have in maintaining an airway and seal with one hand while simultaneously delivering an adequate tidal volume with the other.

Endotracheal intubation should be attempted as soon as practical. Attempts at intubation should not interrupt ventilation longer than 30 seconds. Cricoid pressure is indicated to lessen the possibility of regurgitation and aspiration during intubation. After intubation, the patient can be ventilated with a self-inflating bag capable of delivering high oxygen concentrations. Since two hands are now available to squeeze the bag, ventilation should be satisfactory.

Pressure-cycled ventilators may be prematurely terminated by the thoracic pressure associated with chest compressions, while volume-cycled ventilators may be unable to develop necessary airway pressures. Manually triggered constant-pressure (time-cycled) devices are capable of delivering high flows of 100% oxygen and high inspiratory pressures. The chest must be constantly observed for signs of unintentional overexpansion. Special care must be taken not to overinflate the lungs of an infant or child.

The ratio of physiologic dead space to tidal volume (V_D/V_T) reflects the efficiency of CO_2 elimination. V_D/V_T increases during cardiopulmonary resuscitation as a result of low pulmonary blood flow and high alveolar pressures. Thus, minute ventilation must be increased by 50–100% to prevent arterial hypercapnia.

CIRCULATION

After successful delivery of two initial breaths (each 1–1½ seconds in duration), the circulation must be assessed. If the patient has an adequate pulse (carotid artery in an adult or child, brachial artery in an infant) or blood pressure, then breathing is continued at 12 breaths/min for an adult (older than 8 years), 16 breaths/min for a child (1–8 years old), or 20 breaths/min for an infant (< 1 year of age). If the patient is pulseless or severely hypotensive, the circulatory system must be supported by a combination of external chest compressions, intravenous drug administration, and defibrillation. Initiation of chest compressions is triggered by the inadequacy of peripheral perfusion, while drug choices and defibrillation energy levels often depend upon electrocardiographic diagnosis of dysrhythmias.

External Chest Compression

Chest compressions should be *immediately* initiated in the pulseless patient. The xiphoid process is located and the heel of the rescuer's hand is placed over the lower half of the sternum. The other hand is placed over the hand on the sternum with the fingers interlaced or extended. The rescuer's shoulders should be positioned directly over the hands with the elbows locked into position and arms extended, so that the weight of the upper body is used for compressions. With a downward thrust, the adult sternum is depressed 4–5 cm (2–3 cm in a child) and then allowed to return to its normal position. For an infant, compressions (1–2 cm) are made with the index and middle

fingers on the sternum one fingerbreadth below the nipple line. Compression time and release time should be equal. If the resuscitation is performed by one rescuer, two breaths are administered every 15 compressions (15:2). With two rescuers, one breath is administered every 5 compressions (5:1), pausing 1–1½ seconds for the ventilation. Every minute, 80–100 cardiac compressions should be performed regardless of the number of rescuers. A slightly higher compression rate of 100–120/min is suggested for infants. The adequacy of cardiac output can be estimated by monitoring end-tidal CO_2 or arterial pulsations.

External cardiac compressions probably support circulation primarily by a **thoracic pump** mechanism. The rise in intrathoracic pressure is transmitted to extrathoracic arteries but not to thinner-walled extrathoracic veins, which tend to collapse. The resulting extrathoracic arteriovenous pressure gradient causes forward blood flow. Compression of the heart between the sternum and the spine (the **cardiac pump** theory) may also contribute to flow. Although properly performed chest compressions can maintain a systolic blood pressure of 100 mm Hg, cardiac output is reduced to 25–33% of normal.

Intravenous Access

While some resuscitation drugs are well absorbed following administration down an endotracheal tube (eg, lidocaine, epinephrine, atropine, but *not* sodium bicarbonate), establishing reliable intravenous access for drugs and fluids is a high priority. A preexisting internal jugular or subclavian line is ideal for venous access during resuscitation. Peripheral intravenous sites are associated with a significant delay between drug administration and delivery to the heart, since peripheral blood flow is drastically reduced during resuscitation. Antecubital or femoral lines are preferred

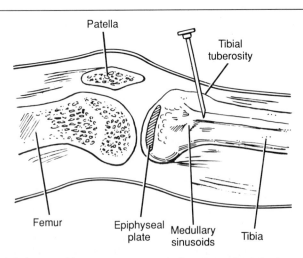

Figure 46–7. Intraosseous infusions provide emergency access to the venous circulation in pediatric patients by way of the large medullary venous channels. The needle is directed away from the epiphyseal plate to minimize the risk of injury.

to dorsal hand or saphenous sites. Cardiac chest compressions may have to be briefly interrupted to establish an internal jugular line if the response to peripherally administered drugs is inadequate.

If intravenous cannulation is difficult, an intraosseous infusion can provide emergency vascular access in children under 3 years of age. A rigid 18-gauge spinal needle with a stylet or a small bone marrow trephine needle can be inserted into the distal femur or proximal tibia. If the tibia is chosen, a needle is inserted 2–3 cm below the tibial tuberosity at a 45-degree angle away from the epiphyseal plate (Figure 46–7). Once the needle is advanced through the cortex, it should stand upright without support. Proper placement is confirmed by the ability to aspirate marrow through the needle and a smooth infusion of fluid. This route is as effective as intravenous access for fluid therapy and medications. However, because of the risks of osteomyelitis and compartment syndrome, intraosseous infusions should be replaced by a conventional intravenous route as soon as possible.

Dysrhythmia Recognition

Successful pharmacologic and electrical treatment of cardiac arrest depends on definitive identification of the underlying dysrhythmia. Representative rhythm strips for several important dysrhythmias are presented on pp 672 and 678, along with key identification and management criteria. Interpretation in resuscitation situations is complicated by artifact and variations in monitoring techniques (eg, lead systems and equipment).

Drug Administration

Many of the drugs administered during cardiopulmonary resuscitation have been described elsewhere in this text. Table 46–1 summarizes the cardiovascular actions, indications, and dosages of drugs commonly used during resuscitation.

Calcium chloride and sodium bicarbonate are conspicuously absent from this table. Calcium (2–4 mg/kg of the chloride salt) is recommended only in the treatment of documented hypocalcemia, hyperkalemia, hypermagnesemia, or calcium channel blocker overdosing. Sodium bicarbonate (0.5–1 meq/kg) is no longer considered a first-line drug and should be considered only in specific situations such as preexisting metabolic acidosis or hyperkalemia. Sodium bicarbonate elevates $PaCO_2$ and may exacerbate respiratory acidosis. Because CO_2 readily crosses cell membranes, arterial hypercapnia will result in intracellular tissue acidosis. Furthermore, bicarbonate administration can lead to detrimental alterations in osmolality and the oxygen-hemoglobin dissociation curve. Therefore, effective ventilation and circulatory support are the treatments of choice for the respiratory and metabolic acidosis that accompany resuscitation.

Intravenous fluid therapy with either colloid or balanced salt solutions (eg, normal saline) is indicated in patients with intravascular volume depletion (eg, acute blood loss, diabetic ketoacidosis, thermal burns). Dextrose-containing solutions may lead to a hyperosmotic diuresis or may worsen neurologic outcome. They should be avoided unless hypoglycemia is suspected. Likewise, free water administration (eg, D_5W) may lead to cerebral edema.

Defibrillation & Cardioversion

Normal sinus rhythm depends upon spontaneous depolarization of the sinoatrial node (automaticity) and subsequent spread of electrical activity throughout the heart in an organized and coordinated fashion (conduction). Cardiac dysrhythmias are usually due to disturbances in automaticity or conduction. Applying an external electrical current to the heart can be beneficial in converting some dysrhythmias to normal sinus rhythm.

Successful defibrillation and cardioversion depend upon proper electrode placement, energy level, and timing in relation to the cardiac cycle. One paddle (4.5 cm in diameter in infants; 8 cm in children; 10–13 cm in adults) is placed to the right of the upper sternum just below the clavicle and the other in the midaxillary line just to the left of the nipple (the standard or anterolateral electrode placement). Conductive pads or gel must be placed between the paddles and the patient to prevent skin burns. The paddles should not be placed within 12 cm of a permanent pacemaker. Energy requirements depend upon the dysrhythmia (Table 46–2). Initially, low energy levels are attempted for cardioversion (25–75 J), with rapid advancement to defibrillation levels if unsuccessful (200–360 J). Note that body weight is an insignificant factor in determining energy requirements except in children. Defibrillation is indicated for ventricular fibrillation and pulseless ventricular tachycardia. Synchronized cardioversion is useful for patients who are hemodynamically stable but unresponsive to intravenous drug therapy for supraventricular dysrhythmia or ventricular tachycardia associated with a pulse.

A single precordial thump with the hypothenar aspect of a fist dropped from a height of 10 cm should be delivered to the center of the sternum in witnessed cardiac arrests if a defibrillator is unavailable. Nonetheless, some authorities doubt the efficacy of the precordial thump.

RECOMMENDED RESUSCITATION PROTOCOLS

A resuscitation team leader integrates the assessment of the patient, including electrocardiographic diagnosis, with the electrical and pharmacologic therapy (Table 46–3). This individual must have a firm grasp of the guidelines for cardiac arrest presented in the Advanced Cardiac Life Support algorithms (Figures 46–8 to 46–14).

Table 46–1. The cardiovascular effects, indications, and dosages of resuscitation drugs.

Drug	Cardiovascular Effects	Indications	Initial Dose		Comments
			Adult	Pediatric	
Epinephrine	Alpha- and β-adrenergic agonist Peripheral vasoconstriction Increases cerebral blood flow Increases coronary blood flow Coarsens ventricular fibrillation Increases blood pressure Increases heart rate Increases automaticity Positive inotropy	Ventricular fibrillation, pulseless ventricular tachycardia, electro-mechanical dissociation, ventricular asystole Severe hypotension	0.5–1 mg 1 μg/kg	0.01 mg/kg 1 μg/kg	Epinephrine doses are repeated every 5 minutes as necessary. An infusion of epinephrine (eg, 1 mg in 250 mL of D_5W, 4 μg/mL) can be titrated to effect in adults (1–10 μg/min) or children (0.1–1 μg/kg/min).
Atropine	Anticholinergic (parasympatholytic) Increases sinoatrial node rate Increases sinoatrial node automaticity Increases atrioventricular node conduction	Symptomatic bradycardia, artrioventricular block Ventricular asystole	0.5 mg 1 mg	0.02 mg/kg 0.02 mg/kg	Atropine doses are repeated every 5 minutes to a total dose of 2 mg in adults or 1 mg in children. The minimum pediatric dose is 0.1 mg.
Lidocaine	Decreases rate of phase 4 depolarization (decreases automaticity) Depresses conduction in reentry pathways Elevates ventricular fibrillation threshold Reduces disparity in action potential durations between normal and ischemic tissue Reduces action potential and effective refractory period duration	Ventricular tachycardia, ventricular fibrillation, premature ventricular contractions Postinfarction prophylaxis	1 mg/kg 1.5 mg/kg	1 mg/kg Not applicable	Lidocaine doses can be repeated every 8 minutes to a total dose of 3 mg/kg. After infarction or successful resuscitation, a continuous infusion (eg, 1 g in 500 ml D_5W, 2 mg/mL) should be run at a rate of 20–50 μg/kg/min (2–4 mg/min in most adults). Therapeutic blood levels are usually 1.5–6 μg/mL
Bretylium	Possesses a triphasic adrenergic effect: (1) Initially, releases norepinephrine (tachycardia, hypertension) (2) Then, postganglionic adrenergic blockade (bradycardia, postural hypotension) (3) Finally, inhibition of catecholamine reuptake (potentiates exogenous catecholamines) Elevates ventricular fibrillation threshold Depresses ventricular defibrillation threshold Reduces disparity in action potential duration between normal and ischemic tissue Prolongs action potential and effective refractory period duration	Ventricular tachycardia Ventricular fibrillation	5–10 mg/kg over 10 minutes 5 mg/kg by rapid bolus injection		For refractory or recurrent ventricular tachycardia, a second dose of 5–10 mg/kg can be administered slowly after 1–2 hours. Drug levels can be maintained by a continuous infusion (eg, 500 mg in 250 mL D_5W, 2 mg/mL) at a rate of 2 mg/min in adults. For persistent ventricular fibrillation, the second dose is increased to 10 mg/kg and repeated at 15- to 30-minute intervals to a maximum dose of 30 mg/kg.
Procainamide	Decreases rate of phase 4 depolarization (decreases automaticity) Depresses intraventricular conduction	Ventricular tachycardia, premature ventricular contractions	100 mg	Not applicable	Procainamide should not be administered at a rate greater than 20 mg/min due to vasodilating and negative inotropic side

(continued)

Table 46–1. (Continued)

Drug	Cardiovascular Effects	Indications	Initial Dose Adult	Initial Dose Pediatric	Comments
Procainamide (cont'd)	Depresses conduction in reentry pathways Depresses rate of phase 0 depolarization (decreases excitability) Prolongs action potential and effective refractory period duration Elevates ventricular fibrillation threshold				effects. The initial 100-mg dose can be repeated every 5 minutes until the dysrhythmia is suppressed, hypotension occurs, the QRS widens by 50%, or a total dose of 1 g has been administered. A maintenance infusion (eg, 1 g in 500 mL D_5W, 2 mg/mL) at 1–4 mg/min should be titrated to effect (usual therapeutic blood levels are 4–10 μg/mL). Procainamide is not recommended for children.
Verapamil	Inhibition of slow calcium channel activity Decreases rate of phase 4 depolarization Slows atrioventricular node conduction Blocks atrioventricular node reentry pathways Reduces action potential and effective refractory period duration Negative inotropy Peripheral and coronary vasodilatation	Paroxysmal supraventricular tachycardia (narrow QRS), slowing of ventricular response to atrial flutter/fibrillation	5–10 mg	0.1–0.3 mg/kg	The initial dose of verapamil can be repeated after 30 minutes if response is not adequate.
Isoproterenol	Beta-adrenergic agonist Increases contractility Increases heart rate and cardiac output (increases myocardial oxygen consumption) Decreases systemic vascular resistance Decreases diastolic arterial pressure (decreases myocardial oxygen supply)	Symptomatic refractory bradycardia, status asthmaticus, complete heart block	2–10 μg/min	0.1–1 μg/kg/min	Isoproterenol is delivered as an infusion (eg 1 mg in 500 mL D_5W, 2 μg/mL) and titrated to achieve a heart rate of 60 beats/min.

Table 46–2. Energy requirements for cardioversion and defibrillation.

Indications	Shocks (joules) First	Second	Third	Subsequent
Unstable atrial fibrillation (adult)	75–100	200	360	360
Unstable paroxysmal atrial tachycardia				
Adult	75–100	200	360	360
Child	0.5–1/kg	2/kg	4/kg	4/kg
Unstable atrial flutter (adult)	25	75–100	200	360
Ventricular tachycardia				
Pulse present				
Adult	50	100	200	360
Pulseless				
Adult	200	200–300	360	360
Child	0.5–1/kg	2/kg	4/kg	4/kg
Ventricular fibrillation				
Adult	200	200–300	360	360
Child	2/kg	4/kg	4/kg	4/kg

KEYS TO DYSRHYTHMIA
RECOGNITION AND MANAGEMENT[1]

I. BRADYCARDIAS

SINUS BRADYCARDIA

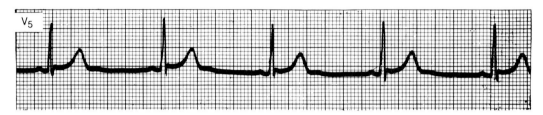

Recognition
1. Rate < 60/min (atrial = ventricular rate).
2. Regular rhythm.
3. Normal P waves and QRS complexes.
4. Each P wave is followed by one QRS complex (1:1).

Clinical Considerations
1. Heart rates less than 40/min usually indicate significant disease (eg, sick sinus syndrome, hypoxemia).
2. The need for treatment depends upon the adequacy of blood pressure and peripheral perfusion.

Management
1. If blood pressure is stable, observe or consider glycopyrrolate (0.1–0.2 mg IV).
2. If unstable, or signs of poor perfusion, give atropine (0.4–1 mg IV), ephedrine (5–20 mg IV), isoproterenol (2–10 µg/min), or consider pacemaker.

JUNCTIONAL BRADYCARDIA

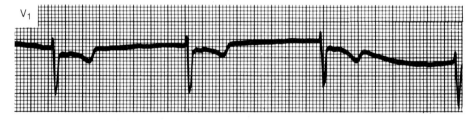

Recognition
1. Ventricular rate 40–60/min.
2. Regular or irregular rhythm.
3. P waves absent or abnormal morphology (eg, retrograde, inverted).
4. PR interval, if present, is short (<0.12 s).
5. QRS usually normal morphology.

Clinical Considerations
1. Junctional rhythms with normal heart rate are common during general anesthesia with volatile agents.
2. Blood pressure and cardiac output often fall as a result of loss of "atrial kick," particularly in patients with heart disease.

Management
1. Same as for sinus bradycardia.

[1]CPR should be initiated in any situation where inadequate perfusion of vital organs is suspected.

SECOND-DEGREE AV BLOCK
(Type I: Wenckebach)

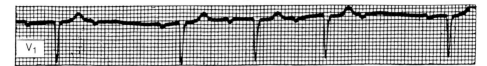

Recognition
1. Ventricular rate < atrial rate.
2. Atrial rhythm regular, ventricular rhythm irregular.
3. Progressive increase in PR interval and shortening of RR interval until nonconductive P wave.
4. QRS usually normal morphology.

Clinical Considerations
1. May be due to digitalis toxicity or myocardial ischemia.
2. Indicates AV node pathology.
3. Often reversible.

Management
1. Same as for sinus bradycardia.

SECOND-DEGREE AV BLOCK
(Type II)

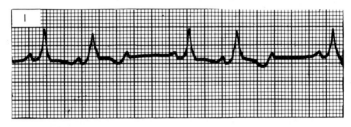

Recognition
1. Ventricular rate < atrial rate.
2. Atrial rhythm regular, ventricular rhythm regular or irregular.
3. Occasional nonconductive P wave without progressive lengthening of fixed PR interval.
4. QRS often widened.

Clinical Considerations
1. Indicates bundle of His disease.
2. More serious than type I block.

Management
1. Similar to that of sinus bradycardia, but transvenous pacemaker should be considered when stable because of the increased risk of progression of complete heart block.

THIRD-DEGREE AV BLOCK

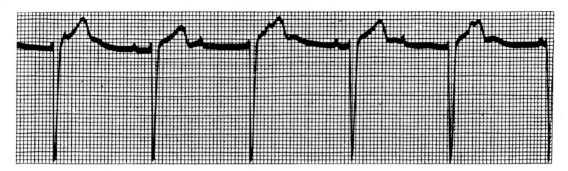

Recognition
1. Ventricular rate < atrial rate.
2. Ventricular rhythm usually regular.
3. Normal P waves that bear no temporal relationship to QRS waves.
4. QRS often widened.

Clinical Considerations
1. Complete heart block preventing any atrial impulses from reaching ventricle.
2. Usually associated with signs of inadequate cardiac output (eg, syncope).

Management
1. Similar to that of sinus bradycardia, but transvenous pacemaker should be considered when stable to increase heart rate and cardiac output.

II. TACHYCARDIAS

SINUS TACHYCARDIA

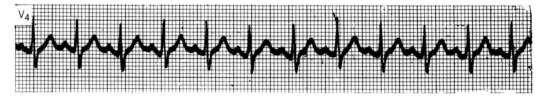

Recognition
1. Rate > 100/min (atrial = ventricular).
2. Rhythm regular.
3. Normal P wave and QRS.
4. Each P wave is followed by one QRS complex (1:1).

Clinical Considerations
1. May be associated with myocardial ischemia or congestive heart failure.
2. Common sign of inadequate anesthesia, hypovolemia, or hypercapnia.

Management
1. Determine if blood pressure is stable; *if so*, consider beta-blockade (eg, esmolol, 0.2–0.5 mg/kg IV) if signs of myocardial ischemia are present.
2. If blood pressure is unstable, give phenylephrine (1 µg/kg IV).

ATRIAL FLUTTER

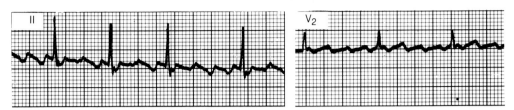

Recognition
1. Atrial rate usually 250–350 per min (ventricular < atrial).
2. Atrial rhythm regular, ventricular rhythm regular or irregular.
3. P waves appear "sawtoothed" (F waves).
4. AV block may be constant (eg, 2:1) or variable.
5. QRS usually normal.

Clinical Considerations
1. Usually a sign of significant heart disease.

Management
1. If stable, give verapamil (2.5–10 mg IV) or rapid atrial pacing (override pacing).
2. If unstable, begin cardioversion (Table 46–2).

ATRIAL FIBRILLATION

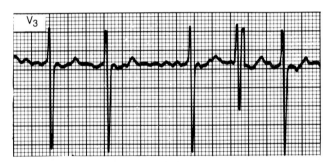

Recognition
1. Atrial rate too rapid to count (>350); ventricular rate variable.
2. Rhythm is irregularly irregular.
3. Irregular baseline undulations (f waves); no true P waves.
4. QRS may be normal or widened.

Clinical Considerations
1. Usually a sign of significant heart disease.
2. Digitalis often used to control ventricular response.
3. Patients are often anticoagulated to lessen risk of cerebral emboli.

Management
1. If stable, give esmolol (0.2–1 mg/kg IV), verapamil (2.5–10 mg IV), or digoxin (0.25–1 mg IV).
2. If unstable, cardioversion (see Table 46–2).

PAROXYSMAL SUPRAVENTRICULAR TACHYCARDIA

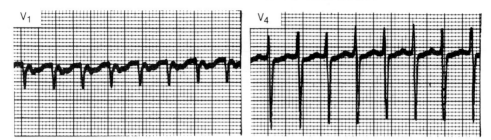

Recognition
1. Atrial rate 150–250; ventricular rate either equal or one-half atrial rate.
2. Atrial and ventricular rhythm are usually regular.
3. Isoelectric intervals between normal P waves.
4. Sudden onset and termination.
5. 1:1 or 2:1 block common.
6. QRS may be normal or widened.

Clinical Considerations
1. Often triggered during general anesthesia by stimulation of the sympathetic nervous system.
2. PAT with 2:1 block may indicate digitalis toxicity.

Management
1. If stable, give verapamil (2.5–10 mg IV except in patients with Wolff-Parkinson-White), esmolol (0.2–1 mg/kg IV), or adenosine (6 mg IV).
2. If unstable, give phenylephrine (1 μg/kg IV) and cardioversion (Table 46–2).

III. VENTRICULAR ECTOPY

PREMATURE VENTRICULAR CONTRACTIONS

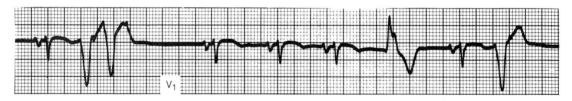

Recognition
1. Irregular rhythm.
2. Usually no P wave.
3. Compensatory pause follows (does not reset sinus node).
4. Bizarre QRS, often with right bundle branch block form.

Clinical Considerations
1. More likely to cause ventricular fibrillation if PVCs are multiple, multifocal, or occur during ventricular repolarization (vulnerable R-on-T period).

Management
1. Lidocaine (1.5 mg/kg IV repeated once, followed by lidocaine infusion of 1–4 mg/min).
2. Procainamide (20 mg/min to a maximum of 1000 mg).
3. Bretylium (5–10 mg/kg IV).

VENTRICULAR TACHYCARDIA

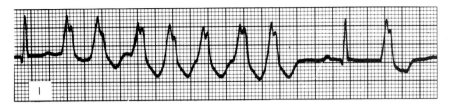

Recognition
1. Rate 100–220/min.
2. Rhythm regular or irregular.
3. P waves usually not present (if present, not temporally associated with QRS complexes).
4. QRS complexes appear like premature ventricular contractions (ventricular tachycardia is three or more premature ventricular contractions in succession).

Clinical Considerations
1. Usually associated with dramatic decline in blood pressure and cardiac output.

Management
1. If blood pressure is stable, deliver a precordial thump or give lidocaine (1.5 mg/kg IV repeated once).
2. If pulse is present but blood pressure is unstable, begin immediate cardioversion (Table 46–2).
3. If pulseless, treat as ventricular fibrillation.

VENTRICULAR FIBRILLATION

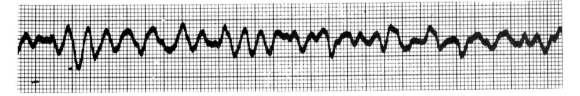

Recognition
1. Disorganized ventricular electrical activity.
2. Rate too rapid and disorganized to count.
3. Rhythm irregular.
4. No discernible P waves or QRS complexes.
5. Irregular undulations in electrocardiograph baseline.

Clinical Considerations
1. *Always* results in no effective cardiac output, and resuscitation must be started immediately.

Management
1. Defibrillation as soon as possible and repeated as necessary.
2. Epinephrine (0.5–1 mg IV) every 5 minutes.
3. Lidocaine (1 mg/kg IV).
4. Bretylium (10 mg/kg IV).

VENTRICULAR ASYSTOLE

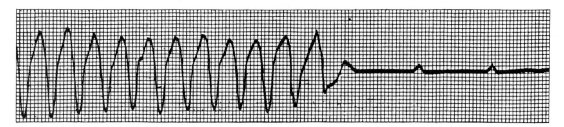

Recognition
1. Total absence of ventricular activity.
2. Absolutely flat baseline (except possible P waves).

Clinical Considerations
1. Consider possibility of fine ventricular fibrillation and need for defibrillation.
2. Poor prognosis.

Management
1. Epinephrine (0.5–1 mg IV) every 5 minutes.
2. Atropine (1 mg IV) every 5 minutes.
3. Pacemaker (external or transvenous).

CASE DISCUSSION: INTRAOPERATIVE HYPOTENSION & CARDIAC ARREST

A 16-year-old boy is rushed to the operating room for emergency laparotomy and thoracotomy after suffering multiple abdominal and thoracic stab wounds. In the field, paramedics intubated the patient, started two large-bore intravenous lines, began fluid resuscitation, and inflated a pneumatic antishock garment. Upon arrival in the operating room, the patient's blood pressure is unobtainable, heart rate is 128/min (sinus tachycardia), and respirations are being controlled by a bag-valve device.

What should be done immediately?

Cardiopulmonary resuscitation must be initiated immediately: External chest compressions should be started as soon as the arterial blood pressure is found to be inadequate for vital organ perfusion. Because the patient is already intubated, the location of the endotracheal tube should be confirmed with chest auscultation, and 100% oxygen should be delivered.

Which cardiopulmonary resuscitation sequence best fits this situation?

Pulselessness in the presence of sinus rhythm suggests severe hypovolemia, cardiac tamponade, ven-

tricular rupture, dissecting aortic aneurysm, tension pneumothorax, profound hypoxemia and acidosis, or pulmonary embolism. Epinephrine, 0.5–1 mg, should be administered intravenously.

What is the most likely cause of this patient's profound hypotension?

The history of multiple stab wounds strongly suggests hypovolemia. Fluids, preferably warmed, should be rapidly administered. Additional venous access can be sought as other members of the operating room team administer fluid through blood pumps or other rapid infusion devices. Five percent albumin or lactated Ringer's injection is acceptable until blood products are available.

What are the signs of tension pneumothorax and pericardial tamponade?

The signs of **tension pneumothorax**—the presence of air under pressure in the pleural space—include increasing peak inspiratory pressures, tachycardia and hypotension (decreased venous return), hypoxemia (atelectasis), distended neck veins, unequal breath sounds, tracheal deviation, and mediastinal shift away from the pneumothorax.

Pericardial tamponade (cardiac compression due to pericardial contents) should be suspected in any patient with narrow pulse pressure; pulsus paradoxus (a > 10 mm Hg drop in systolic blood pressure with inspiration); elevated central venous pressure with neck vein distention; equalization of central venous pressure, ventricular end-diastolic pressures, and

Table 46–3. Principles of management of cardiac arrest. **Note:** Many of the procedures will go forward simultaneously. The order shown below does not mandate that sequence in the code setting.[1]

Priorities	Equipment From Cart	Intervention
1. Recognition of arrest		1. Initiate CPR and call for help
2. Arrival of resuscitation team, emergency cart, monitor-defibrillator	2a. Cardiac board b. Mouth-to-mask or bag-valve-mask unit with O_2 tubing c. Oral airway d. Oxygen and regulator (if not already at bedside)	2a. Place patient on cardiac board. b. Ventilate with 100% O2 with oral airway and mouth-to-mask or bag-valve-mask device. c. Continue chest compressions.
3. Identification of team leader		3a. Assess patient. b. Direct and supervise team members. c. Solve problems. d. Obtain patient history and information about events leading up to the code.
4. Rhythm diagnosis	4. Cardiac monitor with quick-look paddles–defibrillator (limb leads, ECG machine–12 leads)	4a. Apply quick-look paddles first. b. Limb leads, but do not interrupt CPR.
5. Prompt defibrillation if indicated		5. Use correct algorithm.
6. Venous access	6a. Peripheral or central IV materials b. IV tubing, infusion fluid	6a. Peripheral: antecubital b. Central: internal jugular or subclavian
7. Drug administration	7. Drugs as ordered (and in anticipation, based on algorithms) for bolus and continuous infusion	7a. Use correct algorithm. b. Bolus or infusion.
8. Intubation	8a. Suction equipment b. Laryngoscope c. Endotracheal tube and other intubation equipment d. Stethoscope	8a. Connect suction equipment. b. Intubate patient (interrupt CPR no more than 30 seconds). c. Check tube position (listen for bilateral breath sounds). d. Hyperventilate and oxygenate.
9. Ongoing assessment of the patient's response to therapy during resuscitation		9. Assess frequently: a. Pulse generated with CPR. *(Is there a pulse?)* b. Adequacy of artificial ventilation. c. Spontaneous pulse after any intervention or rhythm change. *(Is there a pulse?)* d. Spontaneous breathing with return of pulse. *(Is there breathing?)* e. Blood pressure, if pulse is present. f. Decision to stop, if no response to therapy.
10. Documentation	10. Resuscitation record	10. Accurately record events while resuscitation is in progress.
11. Drawing arterial and venous blood specimens	11. Arterial puncture and venipuncture equipment	11a. Draw specimens. b. Treat as needed, based on results.
12. Controlling or limiting crowd		12. Dismiss those not required for bedside tasks.

[1]Courtesy of American Heart Association

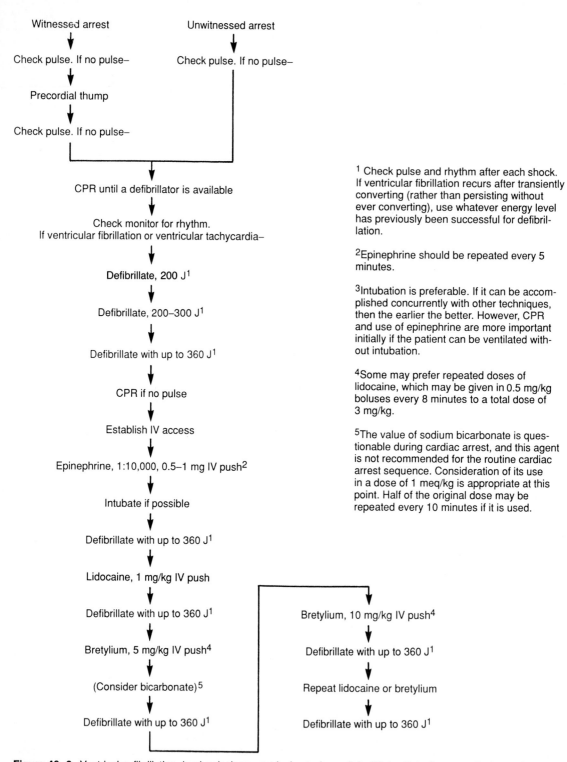

Figure 46–8. Ventricular fibrillation (and pulseless ventricular tachycardia). (**Note:** Pulseless ventricular tachycardia should be treated in the same way as ventricular fibrillation.) This sequence was developed to assist in teaching how to treat a broad range of patients with ventricular fibrillation or pulseless ventricular tachycardia. Some patients may require care not specified in this algorithm, which for that reason should not be construed rigidly. The flow of the algorithm assumes that ventricular fibrillation is continuing. (Courtesy of American Heart Association.)

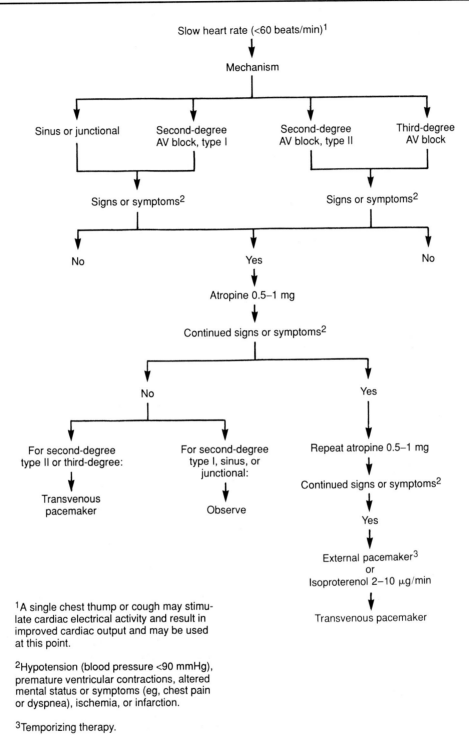

[1]A single chest thump or cough may stimulate cardiac electrical activity and result in improved cardiac output and may be used at this point.

[2]Hypotension (blood pressure <90 mmHg), premature ventricular contractions, altered mental status or symptoms (eg, chest pain or dyspnea), ischemia, or infarction.

[3]Temporizing therapy.

Figure 46–9. Bradycardia. This sequence was developed to assist in teaching how to treat a broad range of patients with bradycardia. Some patients may require care not specified in this algorithm, which for that reason should not be construed rigidly. (Courtesy of American Heart Association.)

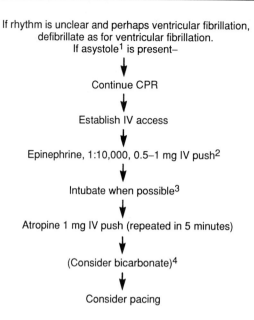

If rhythm is unclear and perhaps ventricular fibrillation,
defibrillate as for ventricular fibrillation.
If asystole[1] is present–

↓

Continue CPR

↓

Establish IV access

↓

Epinephrine, 1:10,000, 0.5–1 mg IV push[2]

↓

Intubate when possible[3]

↓

Atropine 1 mg IV push (repeated in 5 minutes)

↓

(Consider bicarbonate)[4]

↓

Consider pacing

[1]Asystole should be confirmed in two leads.

[2]Epinephrine should be repeated every 5 minutes.

[3]Intubation is preferable. If it can be accomplished concurrently with other techniques, then the earlier the better. However, CPR and use of epinephrine are more important initially if the patient can be ventilated without intubation. (Endotracheal epinephrine may be used).

[4]The value of sodium bicarbonate is questionable during cardiac arrest, and this agent is not recommended for the routine cardiac arrest sequence. Consideration of its use in a dose of 1 meq/kg is appropriate at this point. Half of the original dose may be repeated every 10 minutes if it is used.

Figure 46–10. Asystole (cardiac standstill). This sequence was developed to assist in teaching how to treat a broad range of patients with asystole. Some patients may require care not specified in this algorithm, which for that reason should not be construed rigidly. The flow of the algorithm assumes that asystole is continuing. (Courtesy of American Heart Association.)

atrial pressures; distant heart sounds; tachycardia; and hypotension. Many of these signs may be masked by concurrent hypovolemic shock.

Aggressive fluid administration and properly performed external cardiac compressions do not result in satisfactory carotid or femoral pulsations. What else should be done?

Because external chest compressions are often ineffective in trauma patients, an emergency thoracotomy should be performed as soon as possible in order to clamp the thoracic aorta, relieve a tension pneumothorax or pericardial tamponade, identify possible intrathoracic hemorrhage, and perform open-chest cardiopulmonary resuscitation. Cross-clamping of the thoracic aorta increases brain and heart perfusion while decreasing subdiaphragmatic hemorrhage. Lack of response to cross-clamping is a good predictor of demise. Direct cardiac massage is more effective than external chest compressions, particularly in the presence of pericardial tamponade.

What is the function of the pneumatic antishock garment, and how should it be removed?

Inflation of the bladders within a pneumatic antishock garment increases arterial blood pressure by elevating peripheral vascular resistance. Functionally, the suit resembles thoracic aorta cross-clamping by decreasing blood flow and hemorrhage in the lower half of the body. Complications of inflation of the abdominal section of the pneumatic antishock garment include visceral injury during external chest compressions, re-

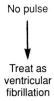

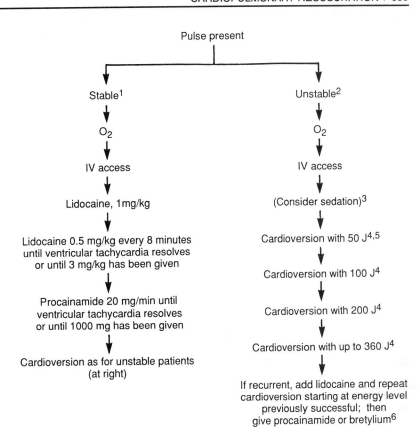

No pulse

Treat as
ventricular
fibrillation

Pulse present

Stable[1]

O_2

IV access

Lidocaine, 1mg/kg

Lidocaine 0.5 mg/kg every 8 minutes
until ventricular tachycardia resolves
or until 3 mg/kg has been given

Procainamide 20 mg/min until
ventricular tachycardia resolves
or until 1000 mg has been given

Cardioversion as for unstable patients
(at right)

Unstable[2]

O_2

IV access

(Consider sedation)[3]

Cardioversion with 50 J[4,5]

Cardioversion with 100 J[4]

Cardioversion with 200 J[4]

Cardioversion with up to 360 J[4]

If recurrent, add lidocaine and repeat
cardioversion starting at energy level
previously successful; then
give procainamide or bretylium[6]

[1]If patient becomes unstable at any time (see definition in next note),
move to "unstable" arm of algorithm.

[2]"Unstable" indicates symptoms (eg, chest pain or dyspnea), hypotension
(systolic blood pressure <90 mmHg), congestive heart failure, ischemia, or
infarction.

[3]Sedation should be considered in all patients, including those defined in
the previous note as unstable, except those who are hemodynamically
unstable (eg, hypotensive, in pulmonary edema, or unconscious).

[4]If hypotension, pulmonary edema, or unconsciousness is present,
unsynchronized cardioversion should be done to avoid delay associated
with synchronization.

[5]In the absence of hypotension, pulmonary edema, or unconsciousness,
a precordial thump may be employed prior to cardioversion.

[6]Once ventricular tachycardia has resolved, begin IV infusion of the
antiarrhythmic agent that has aided resolution of ventricular tachycardia.
If hypotension, pulmonary edema, or unconsciousness is present, use
lidocaine if cardioversion alone is unsuccessful, followed by bretylium.
In all other patients, the recommended order of therapy is lidocaine,
procainamide, and then bretylium.

Figure 46–11. Sustained ventricular tachycardia. This sequence was developed to assist in teaching how to treat a broad
range of patients with sustained ventricular tachycardia. Some patients may require care not specified in this algorithm,
which for that reason should not be construed rigidly. The flow of the algorithm assumes that ventricular tachycardia is
continuing. (Courtesy of American Heart Association.)

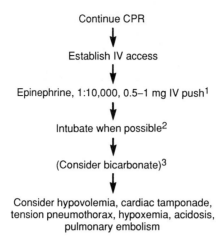

Continue CPR

↓

Establish IV access

↓

Epinephrine, 1:10,000, 0.5–1 mg IV push[1]

↓

Intubate when possible[2]

↓

(Consider bicarbonate)[3]

↓

Consider hypovolemia, cardiac tamponade,
tension pneumothorax, hypoxemia, acidosis,
pulmonary embolism

[1]Epinephrine should be repeated every 5 minutes.

[2]Intubation is preferable. If it can be accomplished concurrently with other
techniques, then the earlier the better. However, CPR and use of epinephrine
are more important initially if the patient can be ventilated without intubation.

[3]The value of sodium bicarbonate is questionable during cardiac arrest,
and this agent is not recommended for the routine cardiac arrest sequence.
Consideration of its use in a dose of 1 meq/kg is appropriate at this point.
Half of the original dose may be repeatedd every 10 minutes if it is used.

Figure 46–12. Electromechanical dissociation. This sequence was developed to assist in teaching how to treat a broad range of patients with electromechanical dissociation. Some patients may require care not specified in this algorithm, which for that reason should not be construed rigidly. The flow of the algorithm assumes that electromechanical dissociation is continuing. (Courtesy of American Heart Association.)

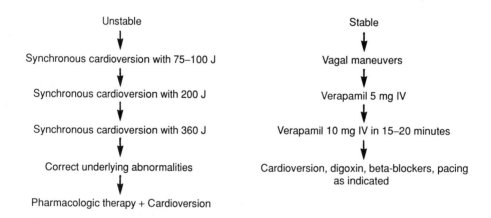

Unstable	Stable
↓	↓
Synchronous cardioversion with 75–100 J	Vagal maneuvers
↓	↓
Synchronous cardioversion with 200 J	Verapamil 5 mg IV
↓	↓
Synchronous cardioversion with 360 J	Verapamil 10 mg IV in 15–20 minutes
↓	↓
Correct underlying abnormalities	Cardioversion, digoxin, beta-blockers, pacing as indicated
↓	
Pharmacologic therapy + Cardioversion	

If conversion occurs but PSVT recurs, repeated electrical cardioversion is
not indicated. Sedation should be used as time permits.

Figure 46–13. Paroxysmal supraventricular tachycardia (PSVT). This sequence was developed to assist in teaching how to treat a broad range of patients with sustained PSVT. Some patients may require care not specified in this algorithm, which for that reason should not be construed rigidly. The flow of the algorithm assumes that PSVT is continuing. (Courtesy of American Heart Association.)

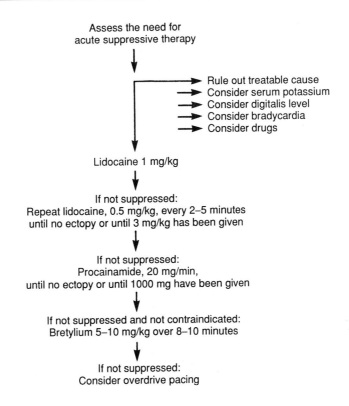

Assess the need for
acute suppressive therapy

Rule out treatable cause
Consider serum potassium
Consider digitalis level
Consider bradycardia
Consider drugs

Lidocaine 1 mg/kg

If not suppressed:
Repeat lidocaine, 0.5 mg/kg, every 2–5 minutes
until no ectopy or until 3 mg/kg has been given

If not suppressed:
Procainamide, 20 mg/min,
until no ectopy or until 1000 mg have been given

If not suppressed and not contraindicated:
Bretylium 5–10 mg/kg over 8–10 minutes

If not suppressed:
Consider overdrive pacing

Once ectopy is resolved, maintain as follows:

After lidocaine 1 mg/kg:	Lidocaine drip 2 mg/min
After lidocaine 1–2 mg/kg:	Lidocaine drip 3 mg/min
After lidocaine 2–3 mg/kg:	Lidocaine drip 4 mg/min
After procainamide:	Procainamide drip, 1–4 mg/min (check blood level)
After bretylium:	Bretylium drip 1 mg/min

Figure 46–14. Ventricular ectopy: acute suppressive therapy. This sequence was developed to assist in teaching how to treat a broad range of patients with ventricular ectopy. Some patients may require therapy not specified in this algorithm, which for that reason should not be construed rigidly. (Courtesy of American Heart Association.)

nal dysfunction, and altered lung volumes. The suit should be deflated only after restoration of hemodynamic parameters. Even then, deflation should be gradual, since it may be accompanied by marked hypotension and metabolic acidosis due to reperfusion of ischemic tissues.

SUGGESTED READINGS

Otto CW: Current concepts in cardiopulmonary resuscitation. Semin Anesth 1990;9:169.

Safar P, Bircher NG: *Cardiopulmonary Cerebral Resuscitation,* 3rd ed. Saunders, 1988. This manual on cardiopulmonary resuscitation prepared for the World Federation of Societies of Anaesthesiologists is in general agreement with American Heart Association recommendations.

Schleien CL et al: Controversial issues in cardiopulmonary resuscitation. Anesthesiology 1989;71:133. Rationale for the recommended techniques and pharmacology of CPR.

Standards and guidelines for cardiopulmonary resuscitation (CPR) and emergency cardiac care (ECC). JAMA 1986;255:2905. The consensus of the 1985 National Conference on Cardiopulmonary Resuscitation and Emergency Cardiac Care. Highlights changes from previous conferences.

Textbook of Advanced Cardiac Life Support. American Heart Association, 1987. The core text in American Heart Association courses in advanced cardiac life support.

47

Postanesthesia Care

Recovery rooms have been in existence for only 30–40 years in most medical centers. Prior to that time, many postoperative deaths occurred shortly after operation as patients were recovering from the effects of anesthesia and surgery. The realization that many of these deaths were preventable emphasized the need for specialized nursing care immediately following surgery. A nursing shortage in the United States following World War II may have also contributed to centralization of this care in the form of recovery rooms where one or more nurses could pay close attention to several patients at one time. As surgical procedures became increasingly complex and were performed on sicker patients, recovery room care was often extended beyond the first few hours after surgery, and some critically ill patients were kept in the recovery room overnight. The success of these early recovery rooms was a major factor in the evolution of modern surgical intensive care units (Chapter 48). Ironically, the recovery room has only recently received intensive care status in most hospitals, where they are now referred to as postanesthesia care units (PACUs).

At the conclusion of most operations, anesthetic agents are discontinued, monitors are disconnected, and the patient (often still anesthetized) is taken to the PACU. If the patient was intubated and ventilation is judged adequate, the endotracheal tube is also usually removed prior to transport. Following a report to the PACU nurse, the patient is left in the PACU until the major effects of anesthesia are judged to have worn off. This period is unfortunately characterized by a relatively high incidence of potentially life-threatening respiratory and circulatory complications. This chapter discusses the essential components of a modern PACU, the general care of patients recovering from anesthesia, and the most commonly encountered respiratory and circulatory complications.

THE POSTANESTHESIA CARE UNIT

Design

The PACU should be located near the operating rooms. A central location in the operating room area itself is desirable, since it ensures that the patient can be rushed back to surgery if needed or that members of the operating room staff can quickly attend to patients. Proximity to radiographic, laboratory, and other intensive care facilities on the same floor is also highly desirable. The transfer of critically ill patients in elevators or through long corridors can jeopardize their care, because emergencies may arise along the way.

An open ward design facilitates observation of all patients simultaneously. At least one enclosed patient space is desirable for patients needing isolation for infection control. A ratio of $1\frac{1}{2}$ PACU beds per operating room is customary. Each patient space should be well lighted and large enough to allow easy access to patients in spite of poles for intravenous infusions, a ventilator, or x-ray equipment; construction guidelines dictate a minimum of 7 ft between beds and 120 sq ft per patient. Multiple electrical outlets and at least one outlet for oxygen, air, and suction should be present at each space.

Equipment

Pulse oximetry (SpO_2) and electrocardiographic and automated blood pressure monitors for each space are desirable but not mandatory. Guidelines requiring a minimum of one set of monitors for every two beds are probably no longer acceptable, particularly since most PACU incidents leading to serious morbidity are related to inadequate monitoring. Mercury or aneroid back-up sphygmomanometers should also be readily available. Monitors with the capability for transducing at least two pressures simultaneously should be available for direct arterial, central venous, pulmonary artery, or intracranial pressure monitoring. Capnography is useful for intubated patients. Temperature-sensitive strips may be used to measure temperature in the PACU but are generally not sufficiently accurate to follow hypo- or hyperthermia; mercury or electronic thermometers should be used if an abnormality in temperature is suspected. A warming/cooling blanket and heating lamps should be available.

The PACU should have its own supplies of basic and emergency equipment, separate from that of the operating room. This includes oxygen cannulae, a selection of masks, oral and nasal airways, laryngoscopes, endotracheal tubes, and self-inflating bags for ventilation. An ample supply of catheters for vascular cannulation (venous, arterial, central venous, or pulmonary artery) is mandatory. Transvenous pacing catheters and a generator should also be available. A transthoracic pacing capability is also desirable. A defibrillation device and an emergency cart with drugs and supplies for advanced life support (Chapter 46) should be present and periodically inspected. Tracheostomy, chest tube, and vascular cutdown trays are also mandatory.

Respiratory therapy equipment for aerosol bronchodilator treatments, continuous positive airway pressure, and ventilators should be in close proximity to the recovery room. A bronchoscope for the PACU is desirable but not mandatory.

Staffing

The PACU should be staffed only by nurses specifically trained in the care of patients emerging from anesthesia. They should have expertise in airway management and advanced cardiac life support as well as problems commonly encountered in surgical patients relating to wound care, drainage catheters, and postoperative bleeding.

The PACU should be under the medical direction of an anesthesiologist. A physician assigned full-time to the PACU is desirable in busy centers but is not mandatory. The management of the patient in the PACU should not differ from management in the operating room and should be a coordinated effort between the surgeon and the anesthesiologist. Analgesia, the airway, and cardiac, pulmonary, and metabolic problems are still managed by the anesthesiologist, whereas those directly related to the surgical procedure itself are managed by the surgeon.

Based on the assumptions that the average PACU stay is 1 hour and the average procedure lasts 2 hours, a ratio of one recovery nurse for two patients is generally satisfactory. A minimum of two nurses ensures that if one patient requires continuous 1:1 nursing care, other patients will still be cared for adequately. The latter is also important medicolegally, because inadequate staffing is often cited as a major contributing factor to mishaps in the PACU. When the operating room schedule regularly includes pediatric patients or frequent short procedures, a ratio of one nurse to one patient is often needed. A charge nurse should be assigned to ensure optimal staffing at all times.

EMERGENCE FROM ANESTHESIA

Recovery from general or regional anesthesia is a time of great physiologic stress for many patients. Emergence from general anesthesia should ideally be a smooth and gradual awakening in a controlled environment. Unfortunately, it often begins in the operating room or during transport to the recovery room and is frequently characterized by airway obstruction, shivering, agitation, delirium, pain, nausea and vomiting, and autonomic lability. Even patients receiving spinal or epidural anesthesia can experience marked

decreases in blood pressure during transport or recovery; the sympatholytic effects of regional blocks prevent compensatory reflex vasoconstriction when patients are moved or when they sit up.

Following an inhalation-based anesthetic, the speed of emergence is directly proportionate to alveolar ventilation but inversely proportionate to the agent's blood solubility (Chapter 7). As the duration of anesthesia increases, emergence also becomes increasingly dependent on total tissue uptake, which is a function of agent solubility, the average concentration used, and the duration of exposure to the anesthetic. Recovery is therefore fastest from nitrous oxide. Of the currently available volatile agents, emergence is fastest following isoflurane anesthesia and slowest from prolonged deep anesthesia with halothane. Nonetheless, the commonest cause of delayed emergence from inhalation anesthesia is hypoventilation.

Emergence from an intravenous anesthetic is a function of its pharmacokinetics (Chapter 8). Recovery from most intravenous anesthetic agents is dependent chiefly on redistribution rather than on elimination half-life. However, as the total administered dose increases, cumulative effects become apparent in the form of prolonged emergence; the termination of action becomes increasingly dependent on the elimination or metabolic half-life. Under these conditions, advanced age or renal or hepatic disease can prolong emergence (Chapter 8).

The speed of emergence can also be influenced by preoperative medications. Premedication with agents that outlast the procedure may be expected to prolong emergence. The short duration of action of midazolam makes it a suitable premedication agent for short procedures. The effects of preoperative sleep deprivation or drug ingestion (alcohol, sedatives) can also be additive to those of anesthetic agents and can prolong emergence.

Transport From the Operating Room to the PACU

This period is usually complicated by a lack of adequate monitors, access to drugs, or resuscitative equipment. Patients should not leave the operating room unless they have a patent airway and adequate ventilation and are hemodynamically stable. Those at risk for hypoxemia (Chapter 22) should be transported with oxygen. As many as 30–50% of otherwise "normal" patients develop transient hypoxemia ($SpO_2 < 90\%$) during transport when supplemental oxygen is not given. Unstable patients should be left intubated and transported with a portable monitor and a supply of emergency drugs.

All patients should be taken to the PACU on a bed or gurney that can be placed in either the head-down (Trendelenburg) or head-up position. The head-down position is useful for hypovolemic patients, while the head-up position is useful for patients with underlying pulmonary dysfunction. Those at high risk for vomiting or upper airway bleeding, such as following tonsillectomy, should be transported in the lateral position. This position also helps to prevent airway obstruction.

General Care of the Patient in the PACU

Vital signs should be checked immediately on arrival. Subsequent blood pressure, pulse rate, and respiratory rate measurements are routinely made at least every 5 minutes for 15 minutes or until stable and every 15 minutes thereafter. At least one temperature measurement should also be obtained. After initial vital signs have been recorded, the anesthesiologist should give a brief report to the PACU nurse that includes the preoperative history (including mental status and any communication problems such language barriers, deafness, blindness, or mental retardation), pertinent intraoperative events (type of anesthesia, the surgical procedure, blood loss, fluid replacement, and any complications), expected postoperative problems, and postanesthesia orders (epidural catheter care, transfusion, postoperative ventilation, etc).

All patients recovering from general anesthesia should receive 30–40% oxygen during emergence because even "healthy" patients can develop transient hypoxemia (see above). Although one study suggests that the occurrence of the hypoxemia does not necessarily correlate with the level of consciousness, a pulse oximeter is becoming a standard monitor for *all* patients recovering from general anesthesia at least until they regain consciousness. Patients at increased risk for hypoxemia, such as those with underlying pulmonary dysfunction or those undergoing upper abdominal or thoracic procedures, should continue to be monitored with a pulse oximeter even after emergence (Chapter 22). A rational decision regarding continuing supplemental oxygen therapy at the time of discharge from the PACU can be made based on SpO_2 readings on room air. Arterial blood gas measurements should be obtained to confirm abnormal oximetry readings. Oxygen therapy should be carefully controlled in patients with chronic obstructive lung disease and a history of CO_2 retention (Chapter 23). Patients should generally be nursed in the head-up position whenever possible to optimize oxygenation (Chapter 22). Elevating the head of the bed, however, before the patient is responsive can lead to airway obstruction. In such cases, the oral or nasal airway should be left in place until the patient is awake. Deep breathing and coughing should be encouraged periodically.

Patients who are heavily sedated during regional anesthesia should also receive supplemental oxygen in the PACU. Sensory and motor levels should be periodically recorded following regional anesthesia to document dissipation of the block. Precautions in the form of padding or repeated warning may be necessary to prevent self-injury from uncoordinated arm movements following brachial plexus blocks. Blood pressure should be closely monitored following spinal and epidural anesthesia. Bladder catheterization may be necessary in patients who have had spinal or epidural anesthesia over 4 hours in duration.

A. Pain Control: Moderate to severe postoperative pain in the PACU can be managed with parenteral or intraspinal opioids, regional anesthesia, or specific nerve blocks (Chapter 18). When opioids are used, titration of small intravenous doses is generally safest. Although considerable variability may be encountered, most patients are quite sensitive to opioids within the first hour after general anesthesia. Adequate analgesia must be balanced against excessive sedation. Opioids of intermediate to long duration, such as meperidine, 10–20 mg (0.25–0.5 mg/kg in children), or morphine, 2–4 mg (0.025–0.05 mg/kg in children), are most commonly used. Analgesic effects usually peak within 4–5 minutes. Maximal respiratory depression, especially with morphine, may not be seen until 20–30 minutes later. When the patient is fully awake, patient-controlled analgesia (PCA) can be instituted (Chapter 18). Intramuscular administration of opioids has the disadvantage of delayed and variable onset (10–20 minutes) and delayed respiratory depression (up to 1 hour). When an epidural catheter has been placed, epidural administration of fentanyl, 50–100 μg, sufentanil, 20–30 μg, or morphine, 3–5 mg, can provide excellent pain relief in adults; however, the risk of delayed respiratory depression with morphine mandates special monitoring precautions for 12–24 hours afterward (Chapter 18). Wound infiltration with local anesthetic or intercostal, interscalene, epidural, or caudal anesthesia is often helpful when opioid analgesia alone is unsatisfactory (Chapter 18).

Mild to moderate pain can be treated intravenously with an opioid agonist-antagonist (butorphanol, 1–2 mg, or nalbuphine, 5–10 mg) or intramuscularly with ketorolac tromethamine, 30–60 mg (a parenteral nonsteroidal anti-inflammatory agent).

B. Agitation: Before the patient is fully responsive, pain is often manifested as postoperative restlessness. Serious systemic disturbances (such as hypoxemia, acidosis, or hypotension) or bladder distention should always be considered as well. Marked agitation necessitating restraints to avoid self-injury may also be seen, particularly in children. When serious physiologic disturbances have been excluded in children, cuddling and kind words from a sympathetic attendant or the parents (if they are allowed in the PACU) often calms the pediatric patient. Other contributory factors include marked preoperative anxiety and fear or drug effects (large doses of central anticholinergic agents, phenothiazines, or ketamine). Physostigmine, 1–2 mg intravenously (0.05 mg/kg in children), is most effective in treating delirium due to atropine and scopolamine but may also be useful in other cases. If serious systemic disturbances and pain can be excluded, persistent agitation may require sedation with intermittent intravenous doses of midazolam, 1–2 mg (0.05 mg/kg in children).

C. Nausea and Vomiting: Postoperative nausea and vomiting is common following general anesthesia. Nausea may also be seen with hypotension from spinal or epidural anesthesia. An increased incidence of nausea is reported following either opioid-based (balanced) anesthesia or intraperitoneal surgery. The highest incidence appears to be in young women. Increased vagal tone manifested as sudden bradycardia commonly precedes or coincides with emesis. Droperidol, 0.01 mg/kg intravenously, given intraoperatively significantly decreases the likelihood of postoperative nausea without significantly prolonging emergence; a second dose may be necessary if nausea occurs in the PACU. Metoclopromide, 0.15 mg/kg intravenously, is at least equally effective and may cause less drowsiness, especially in children. Ondansetron, 0.05–0.1 mg/kg intravenously, a selective 5-hydroxytryptamine (serotonin) antagonist, appears to be a promising antiemetic in postoperative patients and may be less likely to cause the acute extrapyramidal (dystonic) reactions occasionally encountered with the other two agents.

D. Shivering: Shivering can occur in the PACU as a result of intraoperative hypothermia or the effects of anesthetic agents. A cold ambient temperature in the operating room, prolonged exposure of a large wound, and the use of large amounts of unwarmed intravenous fluids or high flows of unhumidified gases result in significant heat loss. Shivering in such instances represents the body's effort to increase heat production and raise body temperature. Emergence from general anesthesia even following brief superficial procedures is also commonly associated with shivering. Although the shivering may be part of nonspecific neurologic signs (posturing, clonus, or Babinski's sign) sometimes observed during emergence, it is most often associated with the use of volatile anesthetics. Regardless of the mechanism, the incidence appears related to duration of surgery and the use of high concentrations of a volatile agent. The shivering occasionally can be intense enough to cause hyperthermia (38–39 °C) and a significant metabolic acidosis, both of which promptly resolve when the shivering stops. Shivering may also follow epidural injection of local anesthetics (Chapter 16). Other causes of shivering should be excluded, such as sepsis, drug allergy, or a transfusion reaction.

Shivering should be treated with warming lights or heating blankets to raise body temperature to normal. Intense shivering causes precipitous rises in oxygen consumption, CO_2 production, and cardiac output. These physiologic stresses are often poorly tolerated by patients with preexisting cardiac or pulmonary impairment. Small intravenous doses of meperidine, 10–20 mg, can dramatically abolish or reduce shivering. Intubated and mechanically ventilated patients can also be sedated and given a muscle relaxant until normothermia is reestablished and the effects of anesthesia have dissipated.

Discharge Criteria

All patients must be evaluated by an anesthesiologist prior to discharge from the PACU unless strict discharge criteria are adopted. Criteria for discharging patients from the PACU are established by the department of anesthesiology and the hospital's medical staff. They allow PACU nurses to determine when patients may be transferred without the presence of a physician provided all criteria have been met. Nonetheless, an anesthesiologist must take responsibility for the discharge and is noted in the patient's record as having done so. Criteria can vary according to whether the patient is going to be discharged to an intensive care unit, a regular ward, the outpatient department, or home.

Before discharge, patients should have been observed for respiratory depression for at least 30 minutes after the last dose of parenteral narcotic. Other minimum discharge criteria for patients recovering from general anesthesia include the following: (1) easy arousability, (2) full orientation, (3) the ability to maintain and protect the airway, (4) stable vital signs for at least 1 hour, (5) the ability to call for help if necessary, and (6) no obvious surgical complications (such as active bleeding). Controlling postoperative pain and reestablishing normothermia prior to discharge are also highly desirable. Scoring systems are widely used. Most assess color, consciousness, circulation, respiration, and motor activity (Table 47–1). The majority of patients meet discharge criteria after 60 minutes in the PACU. Patients to be transferred to other intensive care facilities need not meet all requirements.

Table 47–1. Postanesthetic recovery score.[1]
(Ideally, the patient should be discharged when the total score is 10.)

	Point Value
Color	
Pink	2
Pale or dusky	1
Cyanotic	0
Respiration	
Can breathe deeply and cough	2
Shallow but adequate exchange	1
Apnea or obstruction	0
Circulation	
Blood pressure within 20% of normal	2
Blood pressure within 20–50% of normal	1
Blood pressure deviating > 50% from normal	0
Consciousness	
Awake, alert, and oriented	2
Arousable but readily drifts back to sleep	1
No response	0
Activity	
Moves all extremities	2
Moves two extremities	1
No movement	0

[1]Based on Aldrete JA, Kronlik D: A postanesthetic recovery score. Anesth Analg 1970;49:924.

In addition to the above criteria, patients receiving regional anesthesia should also show signs of resolution of both sensory and motor blockade. Complete resolution of the block is desirable to avoid inadvertent injuries due to motor weakness or sensory deficits. Documenting resolution of the block is also important medicolegally.

Criteria for discharging ambulatory surgery patients to home care are discussed in Chapter 44.

RESPIRATORY COMPLICATIONS

Respiratory problems are the most frequently encountered complications in the PACU. The overwhelming majority are related to airway obstruction, hypoventilation, or hypoxemia. Because hypoxemia is the final common pathway to serious morbidity and mortality, it is anticipated that the increasing use of pulse oximetry in the PACU will lead to earlier recognition of these complications and fewer adverse outcomes.

Airway Obstruction

Airway obstruction in unconscious patients most commonly occurs when the tongue falls back against the posterior pharynx (Chapter 5). Other causes include laryngospasm; glottic edema; secretions, vomitus, or blood in the airway; or external pressure on the trachea (most commonly from a neck hematoma). Partial airway obstruction usually presents as sonorous respiration. Total obstruction causes cessation of airflow, an absence of breath sounds, and marked paradoxic movement of the chest. The abdomen and chest should normally rise together during inspiration; however, with airway obstruction, the chest descends as the abdomen rises during each inspiration (paradoxic chest movement). Patients with airway obstruction should receive supplemental oxygen while corrective measures are undertaken. A combined jaw-thrust and head-tilt maneuver pulls the tongue forward and opens the airway (Chapter 5). Insertion of an oral or nasal airway also often alleviates the problem. Nasal airways may be better tolerated than oral airways by patients during emergence and lessen the likelihood of trauma to the teeth when the patient bites down.

If the above maneuvers fail, laryngospasm should be considered. Laryngospasm is usually characterized by high-pitched crowing noises but may be silent, with complete glottic closure. Spasm of the vocal cords is more apt to occur following airway trauma, or repeated instrumentation, or stimulation from secretions or blood in the airway. The jaw-thrust maneuver, especially when combined with gentle positive airway pressure via a face mask, nearly always breaks laryngospasm. Insertion of an oral or nasal airway is also helpful in ensuring a patent airway down to the level of the vocal cords. Any secretions or blood in the hypopharynx should be suctioned to prevent recurrence. Refractory laryngospasm should be treated ag-

gressively with a small dose of succinylcholine (10–20 mg) and temporary positive-pressure ventilation with 100% oxygen to prevent severe hypoxemia. Endotracheal intubation may occasionally be necessary to reestablish ventilation; cricothyrotomy is indicated if intubation is unsuccessful in such instances.

Glottic edema following airway instrumentation is an important cause of airway obstruction in infants and young children. Intravenous glucocorticoids (dexamethasone, 0.5 mg/kg) or aerosolized racemic epinephrine (0.5 mL of a 2.25% solution with 3 mL of normal saline) may be useful in such cases. Postoperative wound hematomas following head and neck, thyroid, and carotid procedures can quickly compromise the airway; opening the wound immediately relieves tracheal compression. Rarely, gauze packing may be unintentionally left in the hypopharynx following oral surgery and can cause complete airway obstruction.

Hypoventilation

Hypoventilation, which is generally defined as a $PaCO_2$ greater than 45 mm Hg, is a common occurrence following general anesthesia. In most instances, the hypoventilation is mild, and many cases are overlooked. Significant hypoventilation is usually only clinically apparent when the $PaCO_2$ is greater than 60 mm Hg or arterial blood pH is less than 7.25. Signs include excessive or prolonged somnolence, airway obstruction, slow respiratory rate, tachypnea with shallow breathing, or labored breathing. Mild to moderate respiratory acidosis causes tachycardia and hypertension or cardiac irritability (via sympathetic stimulation), but a more severe acidosis produces circulatory depression (Chapter 30). If significant hypoventilation is suspected, arterial blood gas measurements should be obtained to assess its severity and guide further management.

Hypoventilation in the PACU is most commonly due to the residual depressant effects of anesthetic agents on respiratory drive (Chapters 7 and 8). Opioid-induced respiratory depression characteristically produces a slow respiratory rate, often with large tidal volumes. Excessive sedation is also often present, but the patient may be responsive and able to increase breathing on command. Biphasic or recurring patterns of respiratory depression have been reported with all opioids. Proposed mechanisms include variations in the intensity of stimulation during recovery and delayed release of the opioid from peripheral compartments such as skeletal muscle (or possibly the lungs with fentanyl) as the patient rewarms or begins to move. Secretion of intravenously administered opioids into gastric fluid followed by reabsorption has also been described but appears to be an unlikely explanation because of high hepatic extraction for most opioids.

Inadequate reversal, overdosage, pharmacologic interactions (such as with "mycin" antibiotics or magnesium therapy), altered pharmacokinetics (due to hypothermia, altered volumes of distribution, renal or hepatic dysfunction), or metabolic factors (such as hypokalemia or respiratory acidosis) can be responsible for residual muscle paralysis in the PACU (Chapter 10). Regardless of the cause, discoordinated breathing movements with shallow tidal volumes and tachypnea are usually apparent. The diagnosis can be made with a nerve stimulator (Chapter 6) in unconscious patients; awake patients can be asked to lift their head. The ability to sustain a head-lift for 5 seconds may be the most sensitive test for assessing the adequacy of reversal.

Splinting due to incisional pain and diaphragmatic dysfunction following upper abdominal or thoracic surgery, abdominal distention, or tight abdominal dressings are other factors that can contribute to hypoventilation. Increased CO_2 production from shivering, hyperthermia, or sepsis can also increase $PaCO_2$ even in normal patients recovering from general anesthesia. Marked hypoventilation and respiratory acidosis can result when these factors are superimposed on an impaired ventilatory reserve due to underlying pulmonary, neuromuscular, or neurologic disease.

Treatment should generally be directed at the underlying cause, but marked hypoventilation always requires controlled ventilation until contributory factors are identified and corrected. Obtundation, circulatory depression, or severe acidosis (arterial blood pH < 7.15) are immediate indications for endotracheal intubation. Antagonism of opioid-induced depression with naloxone is a two-edged sword; the abrupt increase in alveolar ventilation is usually also associated with sudden pain and sympathetic discharge. The latter can precipitate a hypertensive crisis, pulmonary edema, and myocardial ischemia or infarction. If naloxone is used, titration with small increments (0.04 mg in adults) may avoid complications by allowing partial reversal of the respiratory depression without significant reversal of the analgesia. Following naloxone, patients should be watched carefully for recurrence of the opioid-induced respiratory depression (renarcotization), since naloxone has a shorter duration than most opioids (Chapter 15). Alternatively, doxapram, 60–100 mg, followed by 1–2 mg/min intravenously, may be used (Chapter 15); doxapram does not reverse the analgesia, but it can also cause hypertension. If residual muscle paralysis is present, additional cholinesterase inhibitor may be given (Chapter 10). Residual paralysis in spite of a full dose of a cholinesterase inhibitor necessitates controlled ventilation until spontaneous recovery occurs. Judicious opioid analgesia (intravenous or intraspinal), epidural anesthesia, or intercostal nerve blocks are often beneficial in alleviating splinting following upper abdominal or thoracic procedures.

Hypoxemia

Mild hypoxemia is common in patients recovering from anesthesia unless supplemental oxygen is given during emergence (see above). Mild to moderate hypoxemia (PaO_2 50–60 mm Hg) in young healthy pa-

tients may be well tolerated initially, but with increasing duration or severity the initial sympathetic stimulation often seen is replaced with progressive acidosis and circulatory depression. Obvious cyanosis may be absent if the hemoglobin concentration is reduced. Clinically, hypoxemia may also be suspected from restlessness, tachycardia, or cardiac irritability (ventricular or atrial). Obtundation, bradycardia, hypotension, and cardiac arrest are late signs. The routine use of a pulse oximeter in the PACU facilitates early detection. Arterial blood gas measurements should be performed to confirm the diagnosis and guide therapy.

Hypoxemia in the PACU is usually caused by hypoventilation, increased right-to-left intrapulmonary shunting, or a combination of both. A decrease in cardiac output or an increase in oxygen consumption (as with shivering) will accentuate the hypoxemia. Diffusion hypoxia is an uncommon cause of hypoxemia when recovering patients are given supplemental oxygen (Chapter 7). Hypoxemia due to pure hypoventilation is also unusual in patients receiving supplemental oxygen unless marked hypercapnia or a concomitant increase in intrapulmonary shunting is present (Chapter 22). Increased intrapulmonary shunting (from a decreased functional residual capacity relative to closing capacity) is the most common cause of hypoxemia following general anesthesia (Chapter 22). The greatest reductions in FRC occur following upper abdominal or thoracic surgery. The loss of lung volume is often attributed to microatelectasis, since visible atelectasis is often not evident on a chest x-ray. A semi-upright position helps maintain FRC (Chapter 22).

Marked right-to-left intrapulmonary shunting ($Q_s/Q_t > 15\%$; see Chapter 22) is usually associated with radiographically discernible findings such as pulmonary atelectasis, parenchymal infiltrates, or a large pneumothorax. Causes include prolonged intraoperative hypoventilation with low tidal volumes, unintentional endobronchial intubation, lobar collapse from bronchial obstruction by secretions or blood, pulmonary aspiration, or pulmonary edema. Postoperative pulmonary edema most often presents as wheezing within the first 60 minutes after surgery; it may be due to left ventricular failure (cardiogenic), the adult respiratory distress syndrome (ARDS), or the sudden relief of prolonged airway obstruction (Chapter 48). In contrast to that associated with pulmonary edema, wheezing due to primary obstructive lung disease, which also often results in large increases in intrapulmonary shunting, is not associated with auscultatory crackles, edema fluid in the airway, or infiltrates on the chest x-ray. The possibility of a postoperative pneumothorax should always be considered following central line placement, intercostal blocks, rib fractures, neck dissections, tracheostomy, nephrectomies, or other retroperitoneal or intra-abdominal procedures where the diaphragm might be penetrated. Patients with subpleural blebs or large bullae can also develop pneumothorax during positive-pressure ventilation.

Oxygen therapy with or without positive-airway

pressure is the cornerstone of treatment (Chapter 48). In the PACU, most patients require only 30–40% oxygen until the effects of anesthesia have dissipated. This amount of oxygen is usually enough to prevent hypoxemia with even moderate hypoventilation and hypercapnia. Patients with underlying pulmonary or cardiac disease may require higher concentrations of oxygen; oxygen therapy should be guided by SpO_2 or arterial blood gas measurements. Oxygen concentration must be closely controlled in patients with chronic CO_2 retention to avoid suppressing their hypoxic drive to breathe (Chapter 23). Patients with severe or persistent hypoxemia should be given 100% oxygen via a nonrebreathing mask or an endotracheal tube until the cause is established and other therapies are instituted; controlled or assisted mechanical ventilation may also be necessary (Chapter 48). The chest x-ray (preferably an upright film) is invaluable in assessing lung volume and heart size and demonstrating a pneumothorax or pulmonary infiltrates. Infiltrates may initially be absent immediately following aspiration.

Additional treatment should be directed at the underlying cause. A chest tube should be inserted for any symptomatic pneumothorax or one that is greater than 15%. Bronchospasm should be treated with aerosolized bronchodilators and perhaps intravenous aminophylline (Chapter 23). Diuretics should be given for circulatory fluid overload. Cardiac function should be optimized (see below). Persistent hypoxemia in spite of 50% oxygen generally is an indication for positive end-expiratory pressure (PEEP) or continuous positive airway pressure (CPAP) (Chapter 48). Bronchoscopy is often useful in reexpanding lobar atelectasis caused by bronchial plugs or particulate aspiration.

Circulatory Complications

The most common circulatory disturbances in the PACU are hypotension and hypertension. The possibility that the circulatory abnormality is secondary to an underlying respiratory disturbance should always be considered (see above).

A. Hypotension: Hypotension is usually the result of decreased venous return to the heart or ventricular dysfunction. Hypovolemia is the most common cause of hypotension in the PACU. Absolute hypovolemia can result from inadequate intraoperative fluid replacement, continuing fluid sequestration by tissues ("third-spacing") or wound drainage, or postoperative bleeding. Venoconstriction during hypothermia may mask hypovolemia until the patient's temperature begins to rise again; subsequent venodilatation results in delayed hypotension. Relative hypovolemia is responsible for the hypotension associated with spinal or epidural anesthesia, venodilators, and α-adrenergic blockade; the increase in venous capacitance reduces venous return in spite of a previously normal intravascular volume in such instances. Hypotension due to sepsis and allergic reactions is usually due to both hypovolemia and vasodilatation.

Hypotension following a tension pneumothorax or cardiac tamponade is the result of impaired cardiac filling.

Ventricular dysfunction in previously healthy individuals is unusual unless it is associated with severe metabolic disturbances (hypoxemia, acidosis, or sepsis). Hypotension due to ventricular dysfunction is primarily encountered in patients with underlying heart disease and usually precipitated by fluid overload, myocardial ischemia, acute increases in afterload, or dysrhythmias.

Mild hypotension during recovery from anesthesia is common and usually reflects the decrease in sympathetic tone normally associated with sleep or residual effects of anesthetic agents. Significant hypotension is usually defined as a 20–30% reduction of blood pressure below the patient's baseline level and is indicative of a serious derangement requiring treatment. Treatment depends on the ability to assess intravascular volume (Chapter 29). An increase in blood pressure following a fluid bolus (250–500 mL crystalloid or 100–250 mL colloid) is generally confirmatory evidence for hypovolemia. With severe hypotension, a vasopressor or inotrope may be necessary to increase arterial blood pressure until the intravascular volume deficit is at least partially corrected. Signs of cardiac dysfunction should be sought in elderly patients and patients with known heart disease (Chapter 20). Failure of a patient to promptly respond to treatment mandates invasive hemodynamic monitoring (Chapter 6); manipulations of cardiac preload, contractility, and afterload are often necessary (Chapter 21). The presence of a tension pneumothorax, as suggested by hypotension with unilaterally decreased breath sounds, hyperresonance, and tracheal deviation, is an indication for immediate pleural aspiration even before x-ray confirmation. Similarly, hypotension due to cardiac tamponade (Chapter 21), usually following chest trauma or thoracic surgery, often necessitates immediate pericardiocentesis or thoracotomy.

B. Hypertension: Postoperative hypertension is common in the PACU and typically occurs within the first 30 minutes after admission. Noxious stimulation from incisional pain, endotracheal intubation, or bladder distention is usually responsible. Postoperative hypertension may also reflect sympathetic activation secondary to hypoxemia, hypercapnia, or metabolic acidosis. Patients with a history of systemic hypertension are likely to develop hypertension in the PACU even in the absence of an identifiable cause. The degree of preoperative control over blood pressure bears an inverse relationship to the incidence of postoperative hypertension in such patients. Fluid overload or intracranial hypertension can also occasionally present as postoperative hypertension.

Mild hypertension generally does not require treatment, but a reversible cause should be sought. Marked hypertension can precipitate postoperative bleeding, myocardial ischemia, heart failure, or intracranial hemorrhage. The decision about what degree of hypertension should be treated must be individualized. In general, blood pressure elevations greater than 20–30% of the patient's normal baseline or associated with adverse effects (such as ischemia, heart failure, or bleeding) should be treated. Mild to moderate elevations can be treated with intravenous hydralazine, labetalol, esmolol, or propranolol; sublingual nifedipine is also often useful (Chapter 20). Marked hypertension in patients with limited cardiac reserve requires direct intra-arterial pressure monitoring and should be treated with intravenous nitroprusside or nitroglycerin. The end point for treatment should be consistent with the patient's own normal blood pressure (Chapter 20).

CASE DISCUSSION: FEVER & TACHYCARDIA IN A YOUNG PATIENT

A 19-year-old man sustains a closed fracture of the femur in a motor vehicle accident. He is placed in traction for 3 days prior to surgery. During that time, a persistent low-grade fever (37.5–38.7 °C orally), mild hypertension (150–170/70–90 mm Hg), and tachycardia (100–126 beats/min) are noted. His hematocrit remains between 30% and 32.5%. Broad-spectrum antibiotic coverage is initiated. He is scheduled for open reduction and internal fixation of the fracture. When the patient is brought into the operating room, vital signs are as follows: blood pressure 162/95 mm Hg, pulse 150 beats/min, respirations 20 breaths/min, and oral temperature 38.1 °C. He is sweating and appears anxious in spite of intramuscular premedication with meperidine, 75 mg, and promethazine, 25 mg. On close examination, he is noted to have a slightly enlarged thyroid gland.

Should the surgical team proceed with the operation?

The proposed operation is elective; therefore, significant abnormalities should be diagnosed and properly treated preoperatively if possible in order to make the patient optimally ready for surgery. If the patient had an *open* fracture, the risk of infection would clearly mandate immediate operation. Even with a closed femoral fracture, needless cancellations or delays should be avoided because nonoperative treatment entails the risks of prolonged bed rest (with traction), including atelectasis, pneumonia, deep venous thrombosis, and potentially lethal pulmonary thromboembolism. In deciding whether or not to proceed with the surgery, the anesthesiologist must ponder the following questions:

(1) What are the most likely causes of the abnormalities based on the clinical presentation?
(2) What, if any, additional investigations or consultations might be helpful?

(3) How would these or other commonly associated abnormalities affect anesthetic management?
(4) Are the potential anesthetic interactions serious enough to delay surgery until a suspected cause is conclusively excluded?

The tachycardia of 150 beats/min and the low-grade fever therefore require further evaluation prior to surgery.

What are the likely causes of the tachycardia and fever in this patient?

These two abnormalities may reflect one process or separate processes (Tables 47–2 and 47–3). Moreover, although multiple factors can often be identified, their relative contribution is usually not readily apparent. Fever commonly follows major trauma; contributory factors can include the inflammatory reaction to the tissue trauma, superimposed infection (most commonly wound, pulmonary, or urinary), antibiotic therapy (drug reaction), or thrombophlebitis. Infection must be seriously considered because of the risk of bacterial seeding and infection of the metal fixation device placed during surgery. Although tachycardia is commonly associated with a low-grade fever, it is usually not of this magnitude in a 19-year-old patient. Moderate to severe pain, anxiety, hypovolemia, or anemia may be other contributory factors. Pulmonary fat embolism should also be considered in any patient with long bone fracture, especially when hypoxemia, tachypnea, or mental status changes are present (Chapter 48). Lastly, the possibly enlarged thyroid gland, sweating, and anx-

Table 47–2. Perioperative causes of tachycardia.

Anxiety
Pain
Fever
    See Table 47–3.
Respiratory
    Hypoxemia
    Hypercapnia
Circulatory
    Hypotension
    Anemia
    Hypovolemia
    Congestive heart failure
    Cardiac tamponade
    Tension pneumothorax
    Thromboembolism
Drug-induced
    Antimuscarinic agents
    Beta-adrenergic agonists
    Vasodilators
    Allergy
    Drug withdrawal
Metabolic disorders
    Hypoglycemia
    Thyrotoxicosis
    Pheochromocytoma
    Adrenal (addisonian) crisis
    Carcinoid syndrome
    Acute porphyria

Table 47–3. Perioperative causes of fever.

Infections
Immunologically mediated processes
  Drug reactions
  Blood reactions
  Tissue destruction (rejection)
  Connective tissue disorders
  Granulomatous disorders
Tissue damage
  Trauma
  Infarction
  Thrombosis
Neoplastic disorders
Metabolic disorders
  Thyroid storm (thyroid crisis)
  Adrenal (addisonian) crisis
  Pheochromocytoma
  Malignant hyperthermia
  Neuroleptic malignant syndrome
  Acute gout
  Acute porphyria

ious appearance together with both fever and tachycardia suggest thyrotoxicosis (Chapter 36).

What (if any) additional measures may be helpful in evaluating the fever and tachycardia?

Arterial blood gas measurements and a chest x-ray would be helpful in excluding fat embolism. A repeat hematocrit or hemoglobin concentration measurement would exclude worsening anemia; significant tachycardia may be expected when the hematocrit is below 25–27% (Hb < 8 g/dL) in most patients. The response to an intravenous fluid challenge with 250–500 mL of a colloid solution may be helpful; a decrease in heart rate after the fluid bolus is strongly suggestive of hypovolemia (Chapter 29). Similarly, response of the heart rate to sedation and additional opioid analgesia can be helpful in excluding anxiety and pain, respectively, as causes. Although a tentative diagnosis of hyperthyroidism can be made based on clinical grounds, confirmation requires measurement of serum thyroid hormones; the latter usually requires 24–48 hours in most hospitals. Signs of infection such as increased inflammation or purulence in a wound, purulent sputum, an infiltrate on the chest x-ray, pyuria, or leukocytosis with premature white cells on a blood smear (shift to the left) should prompt cultures and a delay of surgery until the results are obtained and correct antibiotic coverage is confirmed.

The patient is transferred to the PACU for further evaluation. A 12-lead ECG confirms sinus tachycardia of 150 beats/min. A chest x-ray is normal. Arterial blood gas measurements on room air are normal (pH 7.44, $PaCO_2$ 41 mm Hg, PaO_2 87 mm Hg, HCO_3^- 27 meq/L). The hemoglobin concentration is found to be 11 g/dL. Blood for thyroid function tests is sent to the laboratory. The patient is sedated intravenously with midazolam, 2 mg, and fentanyl, 50 μg, and is given 500 mL of 5% albumin. He appears relaxed and pain-free, but the heart rate decreases only to 144 beats/min. The decision is made to proceed with surgery using continuous lumbar epidural anesthesia with 2% lidocaine. Esmolol, 100 mg, is administered slowly until his pulse decreases to 120 beats/min, and a continuous esmolol infusion is administered at a rate of 300 μg/kg/h.

The procedure is completed in $3^{1}/_{2}$ hours. Although the patient did not complain of any pain during the procedure and was given only minimal additional sedation (midazolam, 2 mg), he is delirious upon admission to the PACU. The esmolol infusion is proceeding at a rate of 500 μg/kg/min. He has also received propranolol, 24 mg intravenously. Estimated blood loss was 500 mL, and fluid replacement consisted of 2 units of packed red blood cells, 1000 mL of hetastarch, and 9000 mL of lactated Ringer's injection. Vital signs are as follows: blood pressure 105/40 mm Hg, pulse 124 beats/min, respirations 30 breaths/min, and rectal temperature 38.8 °C. Arterial blood gas measurements are reported as follows: pH 7.37, $PaCO_2$ 37 mm Hg, PaO_2 91 mm Hg, HCO_3^- 22 meq/L.

What is the most likely diagnosis?

The patient is now obviously in a hypermetabolic state manifested by excessive adrenergic activity, fever, markedly increased fluid requirements, and a worsening mental status. The absence of major metabolic acidosis and lack of exposure to a known triggering agent exclude malignant hyperthermia (Chapter 42). Other possibilities include a transfusion reaction, sepsis, or an undiagnosed pheochromocytoma. The sequence of events makes the first two unlikely, while the decreasing prominence of hypertension (now replaced with relative hypotension) and increasing fever make the latter unlikely as well. The clinical presentation now strongly suggests thyroid storm.

Emergency endocrinologic consultation is obtained and the endocrinologist concurs with the diagnosis of thyroid storm. How is thyroid storm managed?

Thyroid storm (crisis) is a medical emergency that carries a 10–50% mortality rate. It is usually encountered in patients with poorly controlled or undiagnosed Graves' disease. Precipitating factors include (1) the stress of surgery and anesthesia, (2) labor and delivery, (3) severe infection, and, rarely, (4) thyroiditis 1–2 weeks following radioactive iodine administration. Manifestations usually include mental status changes (irritability, delirium, or coma), fever, tachycardia, and hypotension. Both atrial and ventricular arrhythmias are common, especially atrial fibrillation. Congestive heart failure develops in 25% of patients. Hypertension that often precedes hypotension, heat intolerance with profuse sweating, nausea and vomiting, and diarrhea may be prominent initially. Hypokalemia is present in up to 50% of patients. Levels of thyroid hormones are high in plasma but correlate poorly with the severity of the crisis. The sudden exacerbation of thyrotoxicosis may represent a rapid shift of the hormone from the protein-bound to the free state or increased responsiveness to thyroid hormones at the cellular level.

Treatment is directed toward reversing the crisis as well as its complications. Large doses of corticosteroids (dexamethasone intravenously, 10 mg stat followed by 2 mg every 6 hours), inhibit the synthesis, release, and peripheral conversion of thyroxine (T_4) to triiodothyronine (T_3) (Chapter 36). Corticosteroids also prevent relative adrenal insufficiency secondary to the hypermetabolic state. Propylthiouracil, 200–400 mg, followed by 100 mg every 2 hours, is used to inhibit thyroid hormone synthesis. Although methimazole inhibits thyroid hormone production and has a longer half-life, propylthiouracil is preferred because it also inhibits peripheral conversion of T_4 (see above). Intravenous preparations are not available for either agent, so they must be administered orally or via nasogastric tube. Iodide is given to inhibit release of thyroid hormones from the gland. The iodide may be given intravenously as sodium iodide, 1 g over 24 hours, or enterally as potassium iodide, 100–200 mg every 8 hours. Propranolol not only antagonizes the peripheral effects of the thyrotoxicosis but may also inhibit peripheral conversion of T_4. Combined β_1 and β_2 blockade is preferable to selective β_1 antagonism

(esmolol) because excessive β_2 receptor activity is responsible for the metabolic effects. Beta$_2$ receptor blockade also reduces muscle blood flow and may decrease heat production. Supportive measures include surface cooling (cooling blanket), acetaminophen (aspirin is not recommended because it may displace thyroid hormone from plasma carrier proteins), and generous intravenous fluid replacement. Vasopressors are often necessary to support arterial blood pressure. Digoxin is indicated in patients with atrial fibrillation to control the ventricular rate (Chapter 19) and those with congestive heart failure. A pulmonary artery catheter greatly facilitates management in patients with signs of congestive heart failure or persistent hypotension by allowing measurements of cardiac output and indices of ventricular filling pressures (Chapter 6). Beta-adrenergic blockade is contraindicated in patients with low cardiac output.

Propranolol, dexamethasone, propylthiouracil, and sodium iodide are given and the patient is admitted to the ICU, where treatment is continued. Over the next 3 days, his mental status markedly improves. The triiodothyronine and total thyroxine levels on the day of surgery were both elevated to 250 ng/dL and 18.5 μg/dL, respectively. He was discharged home 6 days later on a regimen of propranolol and propylthiouracil with a blood pressure of 124/80 mm Hg, a pulse of 92 beats/min, and an oral temperature of 37.3 °C.

SUGGESTED READINGS

Beal JM: *Intensive and Recovery Room Care.* Macmillan, 1982.

Eltringham R, Durkin M, Andrews S: *Postanesthetic Recovery.* Springer, 1983.

Frost EAM, Goldiner PL: *Postanesthetic Care.* Appleton & Lange, 1990. Contains detailed discussions of specific types of patients (cardiac, neurosurgical, obstetric, pediatric, burn, transplant, etc).

Israel JS, Dekornfeld TJ: *Recovery Room Care.* Year Book, 1987.

48

Critical Care

Critical care medicine—also referred to as intensive care—deals with potentially life-threatening illnesses. Anesthesiologists have played a major role in the development of this multidisciplinary subspecialty. Expertise in airway management, mechanical ventilation, administering potent fast-acting drugs, fluid resuscitation, and monitoring techniques gives the anesthesiologist the technical skills required. Moreover, the emphasis in anesthesia on physiology, pathophysiology, and pharmacology as well as the ability to make a rapid diagnosis and treat abrupt physiologic derangements provides an excellent foundation for dealing with critically ill patients. The critical care practitioner (intensivist) also requires a broad base of knowledge that crosses subspecialties in internal medicine, surgery, and pediatrics. Unlike traditional training in these subspecialties, which tends to emphasize one organ system, intensive care training also provides experience in treating patients with multi-organ dysfunction. The American Boards of Anesthesiology, Internal Medicine, Pediatrics, and Surgery recognize these requirements and now require specialized training for certification in critical care medicine.

The purpose of this chapter is only to provide a survey of critical care medicine. Many items have already been covered in other chapters. Only important topics not previously discussed will be presented.

ECONOMIC, ETHICAL, & LEGAL ISSUES IN CRITICAL CARE

COST

Critical care is very expensive. Intensive care beds constitute only 8–10% of all beds in most hospitals yet account for over 20% of hospital expenditures. In the United States, the average cost of a day in an intensive care unit is presently about $4000–5000. To justify this cost, clear benefits in terms of reductions in morbidity or mortality should be readily demonstrable. Unfortunately, supporting studies are few and often flawed by the use of historical controls. Disease severity, reversibility, preexisting health, and age are major determinants of outcome. A method of reliably predicting which patients benefit most from intensive care is needed. Several scoring systems based on the severity of physiologic derangements and preexisting health have been proposed, but none are entirely satisfactory. Survival is generally inversely related to the severity of illness and number of organ systems affected (see below).

ETHICAL & LEGAL ISSUES

The high cost and economic constraints increasingly applied by governments and third party payers, together with an increased awareness of ethical issues and legal precedents, have changed the practice of critical care medicine. Until recently, nearly all patients in the United States—even those who were clearly terminal—received maximal treatment (often contrary to the patient's or family's wishes) for fear of the possible legal repercussions of withholding treatment. "Heroic" measures such as cardiopulmonary resuscitation, mechanical ventilation, and vasopressor infusions were continued until the patient died.

Decisions about when to initiate or terminate treatment can be difficult. Ethically, any treatment that can reasonably be expected to reverse illness or restore health is justified, and withholding that treatment is unjustified. Conversely, if treatment will definitely not reverse a disease process or restore health, then the decision to initiate such treatment may not be justified and may be unethical. These complex decisions must involve the patient (or guardian) and the family and must be consistent with hospital policies and state law.

Fortunately, legal guidelines the practitioner can use in arriving at these decisions are available in nearly all states; although laws vary from state to state, they tend to be similar. The greatest problems are related to withholding treatment and discontinuing artificial life-support systems. Competent terminally ill patients have the right to refuse treatment and to ask that life-support machines be turned off. In most states, competent individuals can also make a "living will" to prevent needless prolongation of life if they become incompetent (eg, irreversible coma). Withholding treatment or discontinuing life supports from incompetent adults and minors requires permission of the spouse, guardian, or next of kin; in some cases, clarification from the courts may be necessary. "Do not resuscitate" (DNR) orders have been upheld by the courts in cases where resuscitation clearly offers no hope of curing or reversing the disease process responsible for imminent death.

Artificial support of respiration and the circulation complicates legal definitions of death. Until recently, most states required only a determination by a physician that irreversible cessation of respiratory and circulatory function had occurred. Nearly all states have added the concept of brain death to that definition.

Brain Death

Brain death is defined as irreversible cessation of all brain function; in some instances, specific reference is made to brainstem death. When there is no reasonable hope for recovery of brain function, establishing brain death gives relief from unjustifiable hope, prolonged anxiety, and financial burdens on families and society. It also allows more efficient utilization of medical resources and potentially allows the harvesting of organs for transplantation.

Brain death criteria can only be applied in the absence of hypothermia, metabolic or endocrine abnormalities, neuromuscular blockade, or drugs known to depress brain function. A toxicology screen is necessary if sufficient time (at least 3 days) has not elapsed to exclude a drug effect. Moreover, the patient should be observed long enough to establish with reasonable certainty the irreversible nature of the injury. Generally accepted clinical criteria for brain death include the following: (1) coma; (2) absent motor activity, including decerebrate and decorticate posturing (spinal cord reflexes may be preserved in some patients); (3) absent brainstem reflexes, including the pupillary, corneal, vestibulo-ocular (caloric), and gag reflexes; and (4) absence of spontaneous respirations for 3 minutes with the arterial CO_2 tension rising at least to 60 mm Hg (mild hypoxemia may also be necessary in patients with chronic CO_2 retention).

The examination should be performed at least twice (not less than 2 hours apart) by more than one physician (one of them preferably a neurologist or neurosurgeon). The apnea test should be reserved for last because of its detrimental effects on intracranial pressure (Chapter 25). Confirmatory tests may also be required in some centers; these may include an isoelectric EEG, absent brainstem auditory evoked potentials, or absence of cerebral perfusion as documented by angiographic or radioisotopic studies.

RESPIRATORY THERAPY

Respiratory therapy is an integral part of critical care medicine. This area encompasses oxygen therapy, me-

chanical ventilation, positive airway pressure therapy, and the application of various techniques to preserve or improve pulmonary function. The latter, which is not discussed in this section, includes administering aerosolized bronchodilators, clearing pulmonary secretions, reexpansion of atelectasis, and preserving normal lung volume.

OXYGEN THERAPY

Oxygen is medically indicated for both pulmonary and nonpulmonary disorders. The primary goal of oxygen therapy is to prevent tissue hypoxia (Table 48–1). Oxygen given alone or in a gas mixture (usually with air) can be used either as a supplement to inspired gases or as the sole source of oxygenation. When oxygen is administered to correct arterial hypoxemia, a tension of 60 mm Hg is generally considered minimally acceptable (Chapter 22). Lower tensions may be acceptable for patients with chronic hypoxemia and CO_2 retention. In contrast, much higher oxygen tensions are desirable for patients with hypotension, low hemoglobin, low cardiac output, carbon monoxide intoxication, or cyanide poisoning. In the latter case, oxygen administration not only protects against arterial hypoxemia but, more importantly, increases the amount of dissolved oxygen, which in such instances significantly contributes to tissue oxygen availability.

1. METHODS OF ADMINISTERING OXYGEN

Precise control over the inspired oxygen concentration is especially desirable in patients with respiratory disease. Delivering a constant enriched inspired oxy-

Table 48–1. Causes of tissue hypoxia.

Hypoxemia
Low inspired oxygen tension
Pulmonary
Hypoventilation
Low ventilation to perfusion ratios
Intrapulmonary shunting
Cardiac
Right-to-left intracardiac shunts
Low cardiac output
Impaired blood flow
Low cardiac output
Hypotension
Arterial occlusion
Impaired arterial oxygen carrying capacity
Low hemoglobin concentration
Abnormal hemoglobin
Carbon monoxide poisoning
Sickle cell anemia
Methemoglobinemia
Increased oxygen demand
Thyrotoxicosis
Malignant hyperthermia
Neuroleptic malignant syndrome
Impaired oxygen utilization
Cyanide poisoning

gen concentration requires a system that meets or exceeds the patient's peak tidal airflow rate (30–50 L/min). When patients have an artificial airway (endotracheal or tracheostomy tube), high-flow ventilator circuits allow precise control of inspired oxygen concentration between 21% and 100%. For patients without an artificial airway, less accurate techniques must be used. Humidification of inspired gases is discussed in Chapter 4.

Nasal Cannulas

When nasal cannulas are used, the inspired oxygen concentration is determined by oxygen flow rate, nasopharyngeal volume, and the patient's inspiratory flow rate (which depends both on tidal volume and on respiratory rate). Oxygen from the cannula fills the nasopharynx in between breaths; during each inspiration, oxygen is entrained from the nasopharynx into the trachea. Mouth breathing does not appreciably affect the inspired concentration as long as the passage between the nasopharynx and oropharynx is patent. The inspired oxygen concentration increases by approximately 3–4% per liter of oxygen given through nasal cannula in most adults. Inspired oxygen concentrations greater than 40–50% cannot be reliably achieved. Flow rates greater than 4–6 L/min for prolonged periods are poorly tolerated because of drying and crusting of the nasal mucosa.

Masks

A. Venturi Masks: These masks rely on the Bernoulli principle: Oxygen is passed through a narrowed orifice within the mask, and the subatmospheric pressure created by the accelerating oxygen stream entrains room air through openings (side ports) at right angles to the jet stream. By changing both the oxygen flow through the orifice and the size of the side openings, one can control the inspired oxygen concentration to within 1–2%. Because of the large volumes of air entrained, the performance of these masks is not appreciably affected by the patient's ventilatory pattern. Masks are available for delivering 24%, 28%, 35%, 40%, or 50% oxygen.

B. Open Masks: Simple open face masks can deliver up to 50–60% oxygen. A 6 L/min flow is necessary to prevent rebreathing of exhaled CO_2. Their major drawback is variability and lack of control over the inspired oxygen concentration.

C. Nonrebreathing Masks: When tightly fitting, these masks can provide close to 100% oxygen for nonintubated patients. An attached reservoir bag provides enough volume to meet the patient's inspiratory flow rate. One-way valves on the sides of the mask and between the mask and the reservoir prevent entrainment of room air into the mask and entry of exhaled gas into the reservoir, respectively. The oxygen flow into the reservoir should be enough to prevent it from completely collapsing during inspiration.

D. Partial Rebreathing Masks: These masks differ from the rebreathing mask only in that the one-way valve between the mask and the reservoir is miss-

ing. Oxygen concentrations up to 80% can be achieved.

Hyperbaric Oxygen

Hyperbaric oxygen therapy utilizes a pressurized chamber to expose the patient to oxygen tensions exceeding ambient barometric pressure (usually > 760 mm Hg). With a one-man hyperbaric chamber, 100% oxygen is used to pressurize the chamber. With a multi-place chamber that allows medical personnel to stay with the patient, air is used to pressurize the chamber while the patient receives 100% oxygen by mask or endotracheal tube. The most common established indications for hyperbaric oxygen are decompression sickness, gas embolism, gas gangrene, and carbon monoxide poisoning.

2. HAZARDS OF OXYGEN THERAPY

Oxygen therapy can result in both respiratory and nonrespiratory toxicity. Important factors include patient susceptibility, the inspired oxygen concentration, and duration of treatment.

Hypoventilation

This complication is primarily seen in patients with chronic obstructive pulmonary disease who have chronic CO_2 retention. These patients may have an altered respiratory drive that becomes at least partly dependent on the maintenance of relative hypoxemia (Chapter 23). Elevation of arterial oxygen tension to "normal" can cause severe hypoventilation in these patents.

Absorption Atelectasis

High concentrations of oxygen can cause pulmonary atelectasis in areas of low ventilation/perfusion ratios. When the more insoluble nitrogen is replaced by oxygen in these areas, alveolar volume decreases because of greater uptake of oxygen. Absorption atelectasis can produce a progressive increase in intrapulmonary shunting in patients receiving high concentrations of oxygen (80–100%).

Pulmonary Toxicity

Prolonged high concentrations of oxygen are known to damage the lungs. Toxicity is dependent both on the partial pressure of oxygen in the inspired gases and the duration of exposure. Alveolar rather than arterial oxygen tension is most important in the development of oxygen toxicity. Although 100% oxygen for up to 10–20 hours is generally considered safe (at sea level), concentrations greater than 50–60% for longer periods may lead to toxicity and are undesirable. Oxygen toxicity is thought to be due to intracellular generation of highly reactive oxygen metabolites (free radicals) such as superoxide and activated hydroxyl ions, singlet oxygen, and hydrogen peroxide. These molecules are cytotoxic because of their reaction with cellular DNA, sulfhydryl proteins, and lipids. Two cellular enzymes, superoxide dismutase and catalase, provide some protection by sequentially converting superoxide first to hydrogen peroxide and then to water. Additional protection may be provided by antioxidants and free radical scavengers such as glutathione peroxidase, ascorbic acid (vitamin C), and α-tocopherol (vitamin E); however, clinical evidence supporting the use of these vitamins in preventing pulmonary toxicity is lacking. Oxygen-mediated injury of the alveolar-capillary membrane produces a syndrome that is pathologically and clinically indistinguishable from adult respiratory syndrome (see below). Tracheobronchitis may also be present initially in some patients. Pulmonary oxygen toxicity in newborn infants is manifested as bronchopulmonary dysplasia.

Retrolental Fibroplasia

Oxygen therapy in neonates with immature retinas can lead to disorganized vascular proliferation, fibrosis, retinal detachment, and eventual blindness. Neonates of less than 36 weeks' gestational age are at greatest risk, but even those up to 44 weeks' gestational age may be at risk. In contrast to pulmonary toxicity, retrolental fibroplasia correlates better with arterial than with alveolar oxygen tension. Arterial oxygen tensions below 140 mm Hg are generally considered safe.

Hyperbaric Oxygen Toxicity

The high inspired tensions associated with hyperbaric oxygen therapy greatly accelerate oxygen toxicity. Latency of the toxicity is inversely related to the pressures employed as well as duration. At 2 atm of 100% oxygen, pulmonary manifestations (mainly dyspnea) are often apparent within 8 hours. Above 2 atm of 100% oxygen, neurologic signs predominate. Behavioral changes, nausea, vertigo, and muscular twitching may precede frank convulsions.

MECHANICAL VENTILATION

Mechanical ventilation replaces or supplements normal respiratory gas exchange in the lungs (Chapter 22). In most instances, the problem is primarily that of impaired CO_2 elimination (ventilatory failure). In other instances, mechanical ventilation may be used as an adjunct (usually to positive-pressure therapy; see below) in the treatment of hypoxemia (hypoxemic respiratory failure). The decision to initiate mechanical ventilation is a clinical one, but certain parameters have been suggested as guidelines (Table 48–2). Of the two available techniques, positive-pressure ventilation and negative-pressure ventilation, the former has much wider applications and is almost universally used.

Although negative-pressure ventilation does not require endotracheal intubation, it cannot overcome substantial increases in airway resistance or decreases in pulmonary compliance, and it also limits access to the patient.

Table 48–2. Guidelines suggesting the need for mechanical ventilation.

Respiratory gas tensions	Direct indices
	  Arterial oxygen tension < 50 mm Hg on room air
	  Arterial CO_2 tension > 50 mm Hg in the absence of metabolic alkalosis
	Derived indices
	  P_A-aO_2 gradient > 350 mm Hg
	  V_d/V_t > 0.6

Clinical indices	Respiratory rate > 35 breaths/min
Mechanical indices	Tidal volume < 5 mL/kg Vital capacity < 15 mL/kg Maximum inspiratory force < 25 cm H_2O

Lung inflation during positive-pressure ventilation is achieved by periodically applying positive pressure to the upper airway (Chapter 22) through an endotracheal or tracheostomy tube. Increased airway resistance and decreased lung compliance can be overcome by manipulating inspiratory gas flow and pressure. The major disadvantages of positive-pressure ventilation are its adverse circulatory effects and the risk of pulmonary barotrauma (see below). Reductions in cardiac output are primarily due to decreased venous return to the heart, while barotrauma is closely related to repetitive high peak inflation pressures. Nasal or oral (translargyneal) endotracheal intubation (Chapter 5) for mechanical ventilation appears to be relatively safe for at least 2–3 weeks. When compared with oral intubation, nasal intubation may be more comfortable for the patient, more secure (fewer instances of accidental extubation), and less likely to cause laryngeal damage. Nasal intubation, however, can result in significant nasal bleeding, transient bacteremia, submucosal dissection of the nasopharynx or oropharynx, and sinusitis or otitis media (from obstruction of the auditory tubes). If left in place for more than 3 weeks, both oral and nasal translaryngeal endotracheal tubes predispose to subglottic stenosis and therefore should generally be replaced by a cuffed tracheostomy tube.

1. POSITIVE-PRESSURE VENTILATORS

Positive-pressure ventilators periodically create a pressure gradient between the machine circuit and alveoli that results in inspiratory gas flow. Exhalation occurs passively. Ventilators and their control mechanisms can be powered pneumatically (by a pressurized gas source), electrically, or by both mechanisms. Gas flow is either derived directly from the pressurized gas source or produced by the action of a rotary or linear piston. This gas flow then either goes directly to the patient (single-circuit system) or, more commonly, compresses a reservoir bag or bellows that is part of the patient circuit (double-circuit system).

All ventilators have four phases: inspiration, the

changeover from inspiration to expiration, expiration, and the changeover from expiration to inspiration. Manipulation of these phases determines tidal volume, ventilatory rate, inspiratory time, and expiratory time.

Classification

The complexity of modern ventilators defies simple classification (Table 48–3). They are most commonly classified according to their inspiratory phase characteristics and their method of cycling from inspiration to expiration. Although most ventilators overlap, even with this simplified classification scheme, the concepts involved are clinically useful.

A. Inspiratory Characteristics:

1. Flow generators–Constant flow generators deliver a constant inspiratory gas flow regardless of airway circuit pressure (Figure 48–1). Constant flow is produced by the use of either a solenoid (on-off) valve with a high-pressure gas source (5–50 psi) or via a gas injector (Venturi) with a lower-pressure source. Ma-

Table 48–3. Criteria for classification of ventilators.

Power source
   Pneumatic
   Electric
   Pneumatic and electric
Control mechanism
   Pneumatic
   Electronic
   Fluidic
   Combination
Drive mechanism
   Single circuit
     Pneumatic
     Piston
   Double circuit
     Pneumatic
     Piston
Inspiratory characteristics
   Flow generator
     Constant
     Nonconstant
   Pressure generator
     Constant
     Nonconstant
Changeover from inspiration to expiration
   Time-cycled
   Pressure-cycled
   Volume-cycled
   Flow-cycled
   Combination
     Volume limiting
     Pressure limiting
Expiratory characteristics
   Positive end-expiratory pressure
   Zero end-expiratory pressure
   Negative end-expiratory pressure
   Expiratory retard
Changeover from expiration to inspiration
   Machine-triggered
     Controlled ventilation
     Intermittent mandatory ventilation
     Airway pressure release ventilation
   Patient-triggered
     Assist-control ventilation
     Synchronized intermittent mandatory ventilation
     Pressure support ventilation

chines with high-pressure gas sources allow inspiratory gas flow to remain constant in spite of large changes in airway resistance or pulmonary compliance. The performance of ventilators with gas injectors varies more with airway pressure. Nonconstant flow generators consistently vary inspiratory flow with each inspiratory cycle (such as by a rotary piston); a sine wave pattern is most common. Most modern ventilators behave like flow generators.

2. Pressure generators–Constant-pressure generators maintain airway pressure constant throughout inspiration and irrespective of inspiratory gas flow. Gas flow ceases when airway pressure equals the set inspiratory pressure (Figure 48–1). Pressure generators typically operate at low gas pressures (just above peak inspiratory pressure).

B. Changeover From Inspiration to Expiration:

1. Volume-cycled ventilators–This type of ventilator terminates inspiration when a preselected volume is delivered. Most adult ventilators are volume-cycled but also have secondary limits on inspiratory pressure to guard against pulmonary barotrauma. If inspiratory pressure exceeds the pressure limit, the machine cycles into expiration even if the selected volume has not been delivered. In reality, properly functioning cycled-volume ventilators still do not deliver the set volume to the patient. A percentage of the set tidal volume is always lost owing to expansion of the breathing circuit during inspiration. Circuit compliance is usually about 4–5 mL/cm H_2O; thus, if a pressure of 30 cm H_2O is generated during inspiration, 120–150 mL of the set tidal volume is lost to the circuit. Loss of tidal volume to the breathing circuit is therefore inversely related to lung compliance. For accurate measurement of the exhaled tidal volume, the spirometer must be placed at the endotracheal tube rather than the exhalation valve of the ventilator.

2. Pressure-cycled ventilators–This type of ventilator cycles into the expiratory phase when airway pressure reaches a predetermined level. Tidal volume and inspiratory time vary, being related to airway resistance and pulmonary and circuit compliance. A significant leak in the patient circuit can prevent the necessary rise in circuit pressure and machine cycling. Conversely, an acute increase in airway resistance, pulmonary compliance, or circuit compliance (kink) causes premature cycling and decreases the delivered tidal volume. Pressure-cycled ventilators are generally most useful for short-term use only (transport).

3. Time-cycled ventilators–Once a predetermined interval elapses from the start of inspiration, these ventilators cycle to the expiratory phase. Tidal volume is the product of the set inspiratory time and inspiratory flow rate. Time-cycled ventilators are commonly used for neonates and in the operating room.

4. Flow-cycled ventilators–The recent incorporation of microprocessors along with pressure and flow sensors into some ventilators allows multiple

FLOW GENERATOR PRESSURE GENERATOR

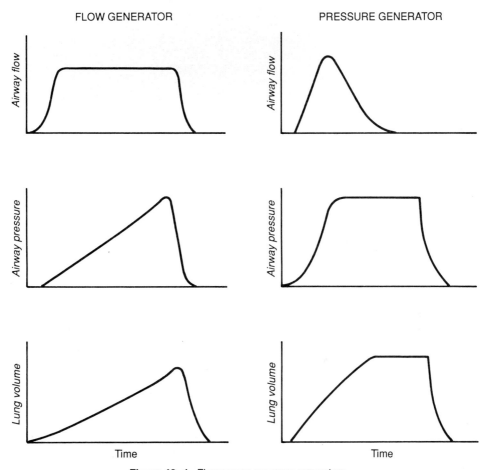

Figure 48–1. Flow versus pressure generators.

modes of operation. One such mode employs a closed-loop function that monitors inspiratory flow rate; when flow reaches a predetermined level, the ventilator cycles from inspiration into expiration (see Pressure Support Ventilation, below).

Ventilatory Modes

Ventilatory mode is defined by the method with which the ventilator cycles from expiration to inspiration as well as whether or not the patient is able to breathe spontaneously (see Table 48–4 and Figure 48–2). Most modern ventilators are capable of more than one ventilatory mode, and some can combine modes simultaneously (see below).

A. Controlled Ventilation: In this mode, the ventilator cycles from expiration to inspiration after a fixed time interval (time-cycled). The interval determines the ventilatory rate. This mode provides a fixed tidal volume and fixed rate (minute ventilation) regardless of patient effort. The patient cannot breathe spontaneously. Controlled ventilation is best reserved for patients capable of little or no ventilatory effort. Awake patients with active respiratory effort require sedation or muscle paralysis.

B. Assist-Control Ventilation: By incorporating a pressure sensor in the breathing circuit, the patient's inspiratory effort can be used to trigger inspiration. A sensitivity control allows selection of the inspiratory effort required. The ventilator is set for a minimum fixed ventilatory rate, but each patient effort of sufficient magnitude will trigger the set tidal volume (patient-time cycled). If spontaneous inspiratory efforts are not detected, the machine functions as if in the control mode.

C. Intermittent Mandatory Ventilation (IMV): IMV allows spontaneous respirations while the patient is on the ventilator. The principal physiologic advantage of IMV is a reduction in mean airway pressure (Table 48–5). A selected number of mechanical breaths (fixed tidal volume) is given to supplement spontaneous breathing. At high mandatory rates (10–12 breaths/min), IMV essentially provides all of the patient's ventilation, while at low rates (1–2 breaths/min) it provides minimal mechanical ventilation and allows patients to mostly breathe independently. The IMV rate is adjusted to maintain a normal arterial CO_2 tension. IMV has found greatest use as a weaning technique. Synchronized intermittent mandatory ventila-

Table 48–4. Ventilatory modes.

Ventilatory Mode	Trigger for Inspiratory Phase		Spontaneous Respirations	Fixed Minute Ventilation	Weaning Mode
	Time	Patient Effort			
Controlled	+			+	
Assist-controlled	+	+			
Intermittent mandatory ventilation (IMV)	+		+		+
Synchronized IMV	+	+	+		+
Pressure support		+	+		+
Mandatory minute ventilation	+		+	+	?
Inverse ratio ventilation	+			+	
Airway pressure release ventilation	+		+		
High-frequency jet ventilation	+				

tion (SIMV) times the mechanical breath, whenever possible, to coincide with the beginning of a spontaneous effort. Proper synchronization prevents superimposing (stacking) a mechanical breath in the middle of a spontaneous breath, resulting in a very large tide volume.

IMV circuits provide a continuous supply of gas flow for spontaneous ventilation in between mechanical breaths. Modern ventilators incorporate SIMV into their design, but older models must be modified by a parallel circuit, a continuous flow system, or a demand flow valve. Regardless of the system employed, proper functioning of one-way valves and sufficient gas flow are necessary to prevent an increase in the patient's work of breathing, especially when positive end-expiratory pressure is also used.

D. Mandatory Minute Ventilation (MMV): The patient is able to breathe spontaneously and receives mechanical breaths also, while the machine monitors the exhaled minute ventilation. In this mode, the machine then continuously adjusts the number of mechanical breaths so that the sum of spontaneous plus mechanical breaths equals the desired set minute ventilation. The role of this mode for weaning remains to be defined.

E. Pressure Support Ventilation (PSV): Pressure support ventilation was designed to augment the tidal volumes of spontaneously breathing patients and overcome any increased inspiratory resistance from the endotracheal tube and ventilator circuit (demand valves). Newer ventilators have this mode, which delivers sufficient gas flow with every inspiratory effort

Table 48–5. Possible advantages of IMV.

1. Lower mean airway pressure
   Less cardiovascular effects
   Less pulmonary barotrauma
   Allows the use of higher levels of PEEP
2. Facilitates weaning
3. Reduced sedation and muscle relaxant requirement
4. Greater patient comfort

to maintain a predetermined positive pressure throughout inspiration. The machine has a feedback (servo) loop that monitors inspiratory gas flow; when inspiratory flow decreases to 25% of initial peak flow, the machine cycles into the expiratory phase and airway pressure returns to baseline. The only setting on this mode is inspiratory pressure. The patient determines the respiratory rate, while tidal volume is determined by inspiratory gas flows and the patient's own inspiratory effort. The principal advantage of PSV is the ability to augment spontaneous tidal volume and decrease the work of breathing. Although the exact role of PSV has yet to be fully defined, it may be a most useful adjunct to SIMV and can be used to wean intubated patients with reliable respiratory drives.

F. Inverse I:E Ratio Ventilation (IRV): This mode reverses the normal inspiratory to expiratory time ratio to more than 1:1. This may be achieved (1) by an end-inspiratory pause, (2) by decreasing peak inspiratory flow, or (3) by limiting inspiratory pressure. This mode generally does not allow spontaneous breathing and in fact usually requires heavy sedation or muscle paralysis. Although questioned by many clinicians, its purported benefits include improved oxygenation, lower peak inspiratory pressures, and decreased dead space. Proponents suggest that IRV is more effective than PEEP or CPAP in alveolar recruitment (see below) and that it results in better distribution of ventilation. The increase in mean airway pressure associated with IRV is probably responsible for any improvement in oxygenation.

G. Airway Pressure Release Ventilation (APRV): Airway pressure release ventilation is a new ventilatory mode whose exact role has yet to elucidated. The technique was developed to overcome problems with high peak inspiratory pressures in patients with reduced lung compliance. With this mode of ventilation, continuous positive airway pressure (see below) is applied to the airway; periodic release of the CPAP to a lower level of positive pressure allows exhalations that augment spontaneous ventilation.

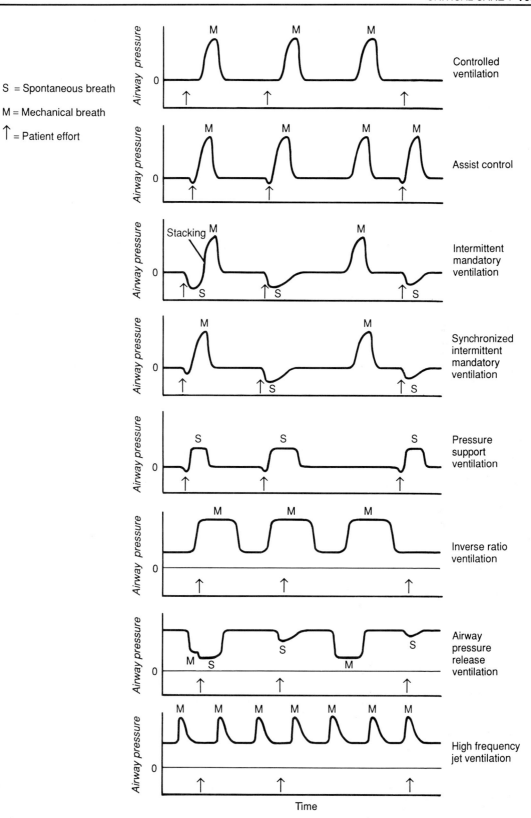

S = Spontaneous breath

M = Mechanical breath

↑ = Patient effort

Figure 48–2. Airway pressure waveforms of ventilatory modes.

Thus, with APRV, airway pressure decreases with spontaneous and mechanical exhalations. The rate and duration of CPAP release together with spontaneous respiratory activity determine minute ventilation. The principal advantage of APRV appears to be less circulatory depression and barotrauma.

H. High-Frequency Ventilation (HFV): Three forms of HFV are available. High-frequency positive-pressure ventilation (HFPPV) involves delivering small "conventional" tidal volumes at a rate of 60–120 breaths/min. High-frequency jet ventilation (HFJV) utilizes a small cannula at or in the airway through which gas is injected 80–300 times/min; gas entrainment (Bernoulli effect) may augment tidal volume. High-frequency oscillation (HFO) employs a driver (usually a piston) that creates to-and-fro gas movement in the airway at rates of 600–3000 times/min. The mechanism of gas exchange with these techniques, which employ tidal volumes below anatomic dead space, is not clear, but it is often described as augmented diffusion. HFJV has found widest use in the operating room and the intensive care unit. HFJV may be used for laryngeal, tracheal, and bronchial surgery as well as bronchoscopies. The technique can offer a nearly motionless field during thoracotomies and for lithotripsy. HFJV via cricothyrotomy (Chapter 46) is also extremely useful in emergency management of the airway when endotracheal intubation and positive-pressure ventilation are unsuccessful. In the intensive care unit, HFJV is can be useful in managing patients with bronchopleural and tracheoesophageal fistulas when conventional ventilation has failed. Adequate heating and humidification of inspired gases during prolonged HFV can be a problem.

2. DISCONTINUING MECHANICAL VENTILATION

The ease of weaning a patient from a ventilator is generally inversely related to the duration of the mechanical ventilation. The process that necessitated mechanical ventilation must be reversed or under control before weaning is attempted. Complicating factors should also be adequately dealt with, including bronchospasm, heart failure, infection, malnutrition, metabolic alkalosis, anemia, increased CO_2 production due to high carbohydrate loads (see below), altered mental status, and sleep deprivation. Underlying lung disease and respiratory muscle wasting from prolonged disuse are often major factors that complicate weaning.

Weaning from mechanical ventilation may be considered when patients no longer meet general criteria instituting for mechanical ventilation (Table 48–2). Clinical signs of improvement should be supported by laboratory and radiographic findings. The most useful weaning parameters are arterial blood gas tensions and the respiratory rate. Intact airway reflexes and a cooperative patient are also mandatory prior to completion of the weaning process unless the patient has a cuffed tracheostomy tube. Similarly, adequate oxygenation (arterial hemoglobin saturation > 90%) on 40–50% oxygen with less than 5 cm H_2O of positive end-expiratory pressure is imperative prior to extubation.

The most common weaning techniques utilize IMV, pressure support, or periods of spontaneous breathing alone on a T-piece or low levels of continuous positive airway pressure (CPAP). Mandatory minute ventilation has also been suggested as a weaning technique, but experience with it is more limited.

Weaning With IMV

With IMV the number of mechanical breaths is progressively decreased (by 1–2 breaths/min) as long as the arterial CO_2 tension and respiratory rate remain acceptable (generally < 45 mm Hg and < 30 breaths/min, respectively). In patients with acid-base disturbances or chronic CO_2 retention, arterial blood pH (> 7.35) is more useful than CO_2 tension. Blood gas measurements should be checked after a minimum of 15–20 minutes at each setting. When an IMV of 1–2 breaths is reached, mechanical ventilation is discontinued if arterial oxygenation remains acceptable.

Weaning With PSV

Weaning during PSV is accomplished by gradually decreasing the pressure support level by 2–3 cm H_2O while arterial blood gas tensions and respiratory rate are monitored (using the same criteria as for IMV). When a pressure support level less than 5 cm H_2O is reached, the patient can generally be extubated.

Weaning With a T-Piece or CPAP

T-piece trials allow observation while the patient breathes spontaneously without any mechanical breaths. The T-piece attaches directly to the endotracheal or tracheostomy tube and has corrugated tubing on the other two limbs. A humidified oxygen-air mixture flows into the proximal limb and exits from the distal limb. Sufficient gas flow must be given in the proximal limb to prevent the mist from being completely drawn back at the distal limb during inspiration; this ensures that the patient is receiving the desired oxygen concentration. The patient is then observed closely during this period; obvious signs of fatigue, chest retractions, tachypnea, marked tachycardia, dysrhythmias, or hypertension should terminate the trial. If the patient appears to tolerate the trial period, arterial blood gas tensions are checked after 15–20 minutes; if they are satisfactory, mechanical ventilation is discontinued permanently. If the patient has been intubated for a prolonged period or has severe underlying lung disease, sequential T-piece trials may be necessary: periodic trials of 10–20 minutes are initiated and progressively increased by 5–10 minutes per hour until the patient appears comfortable and maintains acceptable arterial blood gases.

Many patients develop progressive atelectasis during prolonged T-piece trials. The latter may reflect the absence of a normal "physiologic" positive end-expiratory pressure when the larynx is bypassed by an endotracheal tube. Many clinicians therefore have abandoned T-piece trials in favor of periods of spontaneous breathing alone on low levels (5 cm H_2O) of CPAP. The CPAP helps prevent atelectasis and maintain functional residual capacity (see below).

POSITIVE AIRWAY PRESSURE THERAPY

Positive airway pressure therapy generally consists of application of positive expiratory pressure to the airways; it may be used in patients breathing spontaneously as well as those receiving mechanical ventilation. The principal indication for positive airway pressure therapy is a symptomatic decrease in functional residual capacity (FRC), resulting in absolute or relative hypoxemia (Chapter 22). By increasing transpulmonary distending pressure (Chapter 22) during expiration, positive airway pressure therapy can increase lung volume, improve (increase) lung compliance, and reverse ventilation/perfusion mismatching. The latter is reflected in a decrease in venous admixture and an improvement in arterial oxygen tension.

Positive End-Expiratory Pressure

When the positive pressure is applied only during expiration, this form of therapy is referred to as positive end-expiratory pressure (PEEP). A pressurized expiratory valve is used during PEEP, such that exhalation occurs only above the selected pressure. Resistance to expiration is usually provided by a water column, spring tension, weighted ball, or pressurized balloon or diaphragm.

Continuous Positive Airway Pressure (CPAP)

When positive pressure is maintained during inspiration as well as expiration, this form of therapy is referred to as CPAP. Continuous positive airway pressure implies that the patient is able to breathe spontaneously. When the patient does not have an artificial airway, a tightly fitting face mask or a specially designed nasal mask can be used. The risks of gastric distention and regurgitation mandate that CPAP masks be used only on alert patients with intact airway reflexes and with pressures less than 14–15 cm H_2O (lower esophageal sphincter pressure in normal individuals). Expiratory pressures above 15 cm H_2O require an artificial airway.

CPAP Versus PEEP

The distinction between PEEP and CPAP is often confusing. While the latter usually implies spontaneous ventilation, CPAP can also be used during mechanical ventilatory modes that simultaneously allow mechanical and spontaneous ventilations (see

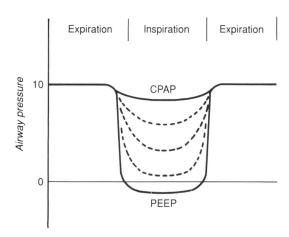

Figure 48–3. Airway pressure during PEEP and CPAP. Note that by increasing inspiratory gas flows, PEEP progressively becomes CPAP.

above). With "pure" PEEP, inspiratory gas flow can only take place when the patient decreases airway pressure below ambient (atmospheric) pressure. The inspiratory work of breathing is increased in direct proportion to the level of PEEP. In contrast, "pure" CPAP systems provide sufficient continuous or "on-demand" gas flows (60–90 L/min) to prevent inspiratory airway pressure from falling perceptibly below the expiratory level (Figure 48–3). Thus, when compared to PEEP, CPAP decreases the work of breathing but at the expense of a higher mean airway pressure. The characteristics of some CPAP demand valves still can significantly increase the inspiratory work of breathing.

Pulmonary Effects of PEEP & CPAP

The major effect of positive expiratory pressure on the lungs is to increase FRC. In patients with decreased lung volume, both PEEP and CPAP raise tidal ventilation above closing capacity (Chapter 22), improve lung compliance, and correct ventilation/perfusion abnormalities. The resulting decrease in intrapulmonary shunting improves arterial oxygenation. Their principal mechanism of action appears to be stabilization and recruitment of partially collapsed alveoli. Although neither PEEP nor CPAP decreases total extravascular lung water (Chapter 22), some authors suggest that they redistribute extravascular lung water from the interstitial space between alveoli and endothelial cells (Chapter 22) toward peribronchial and perihilar areas.

Excessive PEEP or CPAP, however, can overdistend alveoli (and bronchi), increasing dead space ventilation and reducing lung compliance; both effects increase the work of breathing. By compressing alveolar capillaries, overdistention of normal alveoli can also increase pulmonary vascular resistance. A higher incidence of pulmonary barotrauma is observed when PEEP or CPAP is added during mechanical ventilation, especially at PEEP levels greater than 20 cm H_2O. Disruption of alveoli allows air to track interstitially along bronchi into the mediastinum (pneumomediastinum). From the mediastinum, air can then rupture into the pleural space (pneumothorax) or the pericardium (pneumopericardium) or dissect along tissue planes subcutaneously (subcutaneous emphysema) or into the abdomen (pneumoperitoneum or pneumoretroperitoneum). Failure of an air leak to seal can result in a bronchopleural fistula (Chapter 24). Barotrauma may be most closely associated the higher peak inspiratory pressures that result as the level of PEEP or CPAP increases. Other factors that may increase the risk of barotrauma include underlying lung disease, a high rate of mechanical breaths, large tidal volumes, and young age.

Adverse Nonpulmonary Effects of PEEP & CPAP

Adverse nonpulmonary effects of PEEP and CPAP are primarily circulatory and are related to transmission of the elevated airway pressure to the contents of the chest. Fortunately, transmission is directly related to lung compliance; thus, patients with decreased lung compliance (most patients requiring PEEP) are least affected. Moreover, the use of IMV during mechanical ventilation minimizes the combined effect of mechanical breaths and PEEP on mean airway pressure.

Progressive reductions in cardiac output are often seen as mean airway pressure and, secondarily, mean intrathoracic pressure rise. The principal mechanism appears to be a progressive decrease in venous return to the heart. Other mechanisms may include leftward displacement of the interventricular septum (interfering with left ventricular filling) and an increase in pulmonary vascular resistance (increased right ventricular afterload) from overdistention of alveoli. Intravenous fluid administration usually at least partially offsets the effects of CPAP and PEEP on cardiac output. Circulatory depression is most often associated with end-expiratory pressures greater than 15 cm H_2O.

PEEP-induced elevations in central venous pressure and reductions in cardiac output decrease both renal and hepatic blood flow (Chapter 34). The increases in central venous pressure also aggravate intracranial hypertension (Chapter 25).

Optimum Use of PEEP & CPAP

The goal of positive-pressure therapy is to increase oxygen delivery to tissues. The latter is optimally accomplished only if adequate cardiac output and a hemoglobin concentration greater than 8–10 g/dL are maintained as well. Ideally, mixed venous oxygen tensions should be followed (Chapter 22). The salutary effect of PEEP (or CPAP) on arterial oxygen tension must be balanced against any detrimental effect on cardiac output (see above). PEEP or CPAP levels exceeding 15 cm H_2O usually require pulmonary artery pressure monitoring to properly assess circulatory

function and allow calculation of venous admixture (Chapter 22). Volume infusion or inotropic support may be necessary and should be guided by hemodynamic measurements.

Optimal PEEP is that amount above which the detrimental effects of PEEP overshadow any beneficial effect. Practically, PEEP is usually added in increments of 3–5 cm H_2O until the desired therapeutic end point is reached. The most commonly suggested end point is an arterial oxygen saturation of hemoglobin of greater than 90% on a nontoxic inspired oxygen concentration ($\leq 50\%$). Many clinicians favor reducing the inspired oxygen concentration to 40% and some even lower (to 30%) because of a potentially adverse effect of higher oxygen concentrations on venous admixture (see above). Alternatively, PEEP may be titrated to the calculated venous admixture. A shunt below 15% usually results in an acceptable oxygen tension on nontoxic oxygen concentration ($< 50\%$; see Chapter 22).

RESPIRATORY FAILURE

Respiratory failure may be defined as impairment of normal gas exchange severe enough to require acute therapeutic intervention. Definitions based on arterial blood gases (Table 48–2) may not apply to patients with chronic pulmonary diseases; dyspnea and progressive respiratory acidosis must also be present in patients with chronic CO_2 retention. Arterial blood gases typically follow one of several patterns in patients with respiratory failure (Figure 48–4). At one extreme, the derangement primarily affects oxygen transfer from the alveoli into blood (usually due to ventilation/perfusion mismatching), giving rise to hypoxemia (hypoxic respiratory failure); CO_2 elimination in these instances is typically normal or even enhanced. At the other extreme, the disorder primarily affects carbon elimination (pure ventilatory failure), resulting in hypercapnia; mismatching of ventilation to perfusion is typically absent or minimal. However, hypoxemia can also occur with pure ventilatory failure when arterial CO_2 tension reaches 75–80 mm Hg in patients breathing room air (see the alveolar gas equation in Chapter 22). Most patients with respiratory failure display a pattern in between these extremes.

Treatment

Regardless of the disorder, the treatment of respiratory failure is primarily supportive while the reversible components of underlying disease are being dealt with. Hypoxemia is treated with oxygen therapy and positive airway pressure (if FRC is decreased). Ventilatory failure is treated with mechanical ventilation. Other general measures include the following.

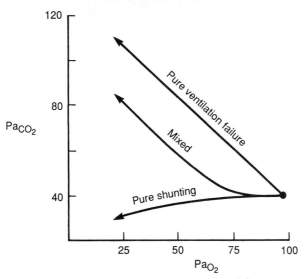

Figure 48–4. Arterial gas tension patterns during acute respiratory failure.

A. Chest Physiotherapy: This includes postural drainage and percussion to promote drainage and suctioning of secretions. Maximal inspiratory maneuvers are also helpful in postoperative patients in preventing atelectasis and improving oxygenation. Bronchoscopy is often useful in suctioning mucous plugs that may be responsible for persistent lobar collapse.

B. Bronchodilators in Patients With Reversible Airway Obstruction: Selective β_2-adrenergic agonists are most commonly used with or without aminophylline (Chapter 23). Aminophylline may also improve diaphragmatic contractility in patients with respiratory muscle weakness.

C. Eradicating Pulmonary and Systemic Infections With Antibiotics: Antibiotic selection is usually initially empiric but should subsequently be guided by culture results.

D. Adequate nutritional support (see below).

E. Correcting fluid overload and treating congestive heart failure (Chapters 20 and 21).

PULMONARY EDEMA

Pathophysiology

Pulmonary edema results from transudation of fluid, first from pulmonary capillaries into interstitial spaces and then from the interstitial spaces into alveoli. Fluid within the interstitial space and alveoli is collectively referred to as extravascular lung water. The movement of water across the pulmonary capillaries is similar to what occurs in other capillary beds (Chapter 28) and can be expressed by the Starling equation:

$$Q = K \times [(Pc - Pi) - \sigma(\pi c - \pi i)]$$

where Q is net flow across the capillary; Pc and Pi are capillary and interstitial hydrostatic pressures, respectively; and πc and πi are capillary and interstitial oncotic pressures, respectively; K is a filtration coefficient related to effective capillary surface area per mass of tissue; and σ is a reflection coefficient that expresses the permeability of the capillary endothelium to albumin. A σ with a value of 1 implies that the endothelium is completely impermeable to albumin, while a value of 0 indicates free passage. The pulmonary endothelium normally is partially permeable to albumin (Chapter 22), such that interstitial albumin concentration is approximately half that of plasma; therefore, πi must be about 14 mm Hg (half that of plasma). Pulmonary capillary hydrostatic pressure is dependent on vertical height in the lung (gravity) and normally varies from 0 to 15 mm Hg (average: 7 mm Hg). Since Pi is thought to be normally about −8 mm Hg, the forces favoring transudation of fluid (Pc, Pi, and πi) are normally almost balanced by the forces favoring reabsorption (πc). The net amount of fluid that normally moves out of pulmonary capillaries is small (about 10–20 mL/h in adults) and is rapidly removed by pulmonary lymphatics, which return it into the central venous system.

The alveolar epithelial membrane is normally permeable to water as well as gases but impermeable to albumin (proteins). A net movement of water from the interstitium into alveoli occurs only when the normally negative Pi becomes positive (relative to atmospheric pressure). Fortunately, because of the lung's unique ultrastructure (Chapter 22) and its capacity to increase lymph flow, its interstitium normally accommodates large increases in capillary transudation before Pi becomes positive. When this reserve capacity is exceeded, pulmonary edema develops.

Pulmonary edema is often divided into four stages:

Stage I: Only interstitial pulmonary edema is present, and it is often visible on a chest x-ray. Pulmonary compliance begins to decrease (Chapter 22).

Stage II: Fluid fills the interstitium and begins to fill the alveoli, being initially confined to the angles between adjacent septa (crescentic filling). Gas exchange may still remain relatively preserved.

Stage III: Alveolar flooding occurs such that many alveoli are completely flooded and no longer contain air. Flooding is most prominent in dependent areas of the lungs. Blood flow through the capillaries of flooded alveoli results in intrapulmonary shunting (Chapter 22). Hypoxemia and hypocapnia (due to dyspnea and hyperventilation) are characteristic.

Stage IV: Marked alveolar flooding spills over into the airways as froth. Gas exchange is severely compromised owing to both shunting and airway obstruction. Progressive hypercapnia and severe hypoxemia follow.

Causes of Pulmonary Edema

Pulmonary edema usually results from either an increase in the net hydrostatic pressure across the capillaries (hemodynamic edema) or an increase in the permeability of the alveolar-capillary membrane (permeability edema). The distinction can often be based on the protein content of the edema fluid. Edema fluid from the former has a low protein content, while fluid from the latter has a high protein content.

1. HEMODYNAMIC PULMONARY EDEMA

Significant elevations in Pc can increase extravascular lung water and result in pulmonary edema. As can be seen from the Starling equation, a decrease in πc can accentuate the effects of any increase in Pc. Two major mechanisms increase Pc, namely, pulmonary venous hypertension or a markedly increased pulmonary blood flow. Any elevation of pulmonary venous pressure is transmitted passively backward to the pulmonary capillaries and secondarily increases Pc. Pulmonary venous hypertension usually results from left ventricular failure, mitral stenosis, or left atrial obstruction. Increases in pulmonary blood flow that exceed the capacity of the pulmonary vasculature will also raise Pc. Marked increases in pulmonary blood flow can be the result of large left-to-right cardiac or peripheral shunts, hypervolemia (fluid overload), severe anemia, or exercise.

Treatment

The treatment of hemodynamic pulmonary edema is aimed at decreasing the pressure in the pulmonary capillaries. Generally, this includes measures to improve left ventricular function, correcting fluid overload, or reducing pulmonary blood flow. Pharmacologic treatments include diuretics, vasodilators, and inotropes (Chapter 21). Vasodilators, particularly nitrates, have proved extremely useful. By reducing preload, pulmonary congestion is relieved; and by reducing afterload (a lesser effect), cardiac output may be improved. Positive airway pressure therapy is also a useful adjunct (see above).

2. PERMEABILITY PULMONARY EDEMA & ADULT RESPIRATORY DISTRESS SYNDROME

Extravascular lung water increases in permeability pulmonary edema owing to enhanced permeability or disruption of the capillary-alveolar membrane. The protective effect of plasma oncotic pressure is lost as increased amounts of albumin "leak" into the pulmonary interstitium; normal—or even low—capillary hydrostatic pressures are unopposed and result in transudation of fluid into the lungs. Permeability edema may be seen with the acute lung injury often associated with various conditions (Table 48–6) and is commonly referred to as noncardiogenic pulmonary edema (NCPE) or adult respiratory distress syndrome (ARDS). Clinically, NCPE is the term usually reserved for the less severe form of the disorder in which the increased lung water is primarily confined to the interstitium.

Clinical Features of ARDS

Also known as shock lung, adult hyaline membrane disease, pump lung, or ventilator lung, ARDS is the clinical expression of severe permeability pulmonary edema. The diagnosis is based on both clinical and laboratory criteria (Table 48–7) and requires the exclusion of significant underlying left ventricular dysfunction or chronic pulmonary disease.

Central to the pathophysiology of ARDS is severe

Table 48–6. Causes of permeability pulmonary edema (ARDS).

Sepsis
Circulatory shock
Multiple trauma
DIC
Drug overdoses (heroin)
Pancreatitis
Thrombotic thrombocytopenic purpura
Head injury
Burns
Fat embolism
Amniotic fluid embolism
Multiple pulmonary emboli
Multiple blood transfusions
Cardiopulmonary bypass
Aspiration pneumonia
    Gastric
    Near-drowning
    Hydrocarbons
Diffuse infectious pneumonias
Oxygen toxicity
Smoke inhalation
Lung radiation
Pulmonary contusion

Table 48–7. Diagnosis of adult respiratory distress syndrome.

1. Clinical setting (see Table 48–6)
2. Exclusion of underlying cardiac and chronic pulmonary disease
3. Respiratory distress:
   Dyspnea
   ↑ Respiratory rate (> 35/min)
4. Laboratory findings:
   Arterial oxygen tension < 50 mm Hg on 60% oxygen
   Ventilation-perfusion mismatching:
   ↑ Venous admixture ($\dot{Q}_s/\dot{Q}_t$)
   ↑ Dead space ventilation (V_D/V_T)
   ↓ Lung compliance to < 50 mL/cm H_2O
5. Radiographic findings: early interstitial edema followed by alveolar edema

injury of the capillary-alveolar membrane. The heterogeneous causes of ARDS (Table 48–6) suggest that regardless of the type of injury, the lung responds in a similar fashion. While exact mechanisms remain elusive, research has focused on the release of membrane-bound phospholipids from the capillary endothelium and the activation of leukocytes and macrophages within the lungs. Activation of compliment and the coagulation cascade are also characteristic. The released phospholipids are converted by the endothelial cyclo-oxygenase and lipo-oxygenase enzyme systems into prostaglandins and leukotrienes, respectively. It is likely that prostaglandin metabolites mediate pulmonary vasoconstriction, altered vascular reactivity (loss of hypoxic pulmonary vasoconstriction), and airway constriction, while the lipo-oxygenase products are responsible for the capillary leak and activation of leukocytes. Release of various substances (oxygen free radicals and lysosomal proteases) by the activated leukocytes and pulmonary macrophages perpetuates lung injury. Destruction of alveolar epithelial cell (types I and II) is prominent. Alveolar flooding together with abnormalities in surfactant production result in diffuse collapse. The exudative phase of ARDS may rapidly resolve or persist for a varying period; it is often followed by a fibrotic phase (fibrosing alveolitis), which in some cases leads to permanent scarring.

ARDS is most commonly seen in the setting of sepsis and trauma. Patients present with severe dyspnea and labored respirations. Hypoxemia due to intrapulmonary shunting is a universal finding. Although dead space ventilation is increased, arterial CO_2 tension is typically decreased because of a marked increase in minute ventilation. Ventilatory failure may be seen initially in severe cases or may eventually develop owing to respiratory muscle fatigue or marked destruction of the capillary-alveolar membrane. Pulmonary hypertension and low or normal left ventricular filling pressures are characteristic hemodynamic findings. Multiple small filling defects on pulmonary angiography representing thromboemboli may occur and are associated with an increased mortality rate.

Treatment of ARDS

In addition to respiratory intensive therapy, treatment should also be directed at reversible processes such as sepsis or hypotension. Hypoxemia is treated with oxygen therapy and PEEP or CPAP. Milder cases may be treated with a CPAP mask, but most patients require intubation and at least some degree of mechanical ventilatory support. Early aggressive use of PEEP (or CPAP) allows reduction of the inspired oxygen concentration to nontoxic levels. Use of IMV may provide greater hemodynamic stability when high levels of positive expiratory pressure are required. Steroids are not beneficial in ARDS, and antibiotics should only be used to treat documented infections. For the occasional patient with refractory hypoxemia with or without hypercapnia, IRV, HFJV, or extracorporeal membrane oxygenation (ECMO) may be considered. Extensive pulmonary fibrosis complicates respiratory management and leads to residual pulmonary disability.

Morbidity and mortality from ARDS are usually due to the precipitating cause or complications rather than the respiratory failure itself. The most common serious complications are sepsis, renal failure, and gastrointestinal hemorrhage. Nosocomial pneumonia is especially common in patients with a protracted course. Colonization by gram-negative organisms, breach of mucocutaneous barriers by various catheters, malnutrition, and altered host immunity contribute to a high incidence of infection. Renal failure is usually due to volume depletion, sepsis, or nephrotoxins and substantially increases the mortality rate (to > 60%). Prophylaxis for gastrointestinal hemorrhage with sucralfate, antacids, or H_2 blockers may be indicated.

3. LESS COMMON FORMS OF PULMONARY EDEMA

Pulmonary edema can also be associated with severe neurologic injuries, high altitudes, sudden reexpansion of a collapsed lung, prolonged severe airway obstruction, or pulmonary lymphatic obstruction. Although poorly understood, neurogenic pulmonary edema appears to be related to a marked increase in sympathetic tone. Pulmonary edema following the relief of airway obstruction may be due to markedly negative interstitial hydrostatic pressures.

RENAL FAILURE

Acute renal failure is a rapid deterioration in renal function that is not immediately reversible by altering extrarenal factors, such as blood pressure, intravascular volume, cardiac output, or urinary flow. The hallmark of renal failure is azotemia (Chapter 32). Not all patients with acute azotemia have acute renal failure. Azotemia may be classified as prerenal, renal, and postrenal. Moreover, the diagnosis of acute renal failure (renal azotemia) is one of exclusion; thus, prerenal and postrenal causes must always be excluded.

PRERENAL AZOTEMIA

Prerenal azotemia occurs as a result of hypoperfusion of the kidneys; if untreated, it progresses to acute renal failure. Renal hypoperfusion is most commonly the result of a decrease in perfusion pressure, renal vasoconstriction, or both (Table 48–8). The diagnosis of prerenal azotemia is usually suspected from the clinical setting and confirmed by urinary laboratory indices (Table 48–9 and below). Treatment of prerenal azotemia is directed at correcting intravascular volume deficits, improving cardiac function, restoring a normal blood pressure, and reversing increases in renal vascular resistance. The hepatorenal syndrome is discussed in Chapter 35.

POSTRENAL AZOTEMIA

Azotemia due to urinary tract obstruction is referred to as postrenal azotemia. Obstruction of urinary flow from both kidneys is usually necessary for azotemia in these conditions (Table 48–8). Complete obstruction eventually develops into acute renal failure, while prolonged partial obstruction leads to chronic renal impairment. Rapid diagnosis and relief of acute ob-

Table 48–8. Reversible causes of azotemia.

Prerenal
  Decreased renal perfusion pressure
    Hypovolemia
    Decreased cardiac output
    Hypotension
  Increased renal vascular resistance
    Neural
    Humoral
    Pharmacologic
    Thromboembolic
Postrenal
  Urethral obstruction
  Bladder outlet obstruction
    Prostatic
    Bladder tumor
    Cystitis
    Neurogenic bladder
  Bilateral ureteral obstruction
    Intrinsic
      Calculi
      Tumor
      Blood clots
      Papillary necrosis
    Extrinsic compression
      Abdominal or pelvic tumor
      Retroperitoneal fibrosis
      Inadvertent ureteral ligations

Table 48–9. Urinary indices in azotemia.

Test	Prerenal	Renal	Postrenal
Urinary sodium (meq/L)	<20	>40	Variable
Urine/serum creatinine ratio	>40	<20	Variable
Fractional excretion of sodium	<1%	>3%	Variable

struction usually restores normal renal function. Obstruction may be suggested by a physical examination (distended bladder) or a plain x-ray film of the abdomen (revealing bilateral renal calculi) but is confirmed by demonstrating dilatation of the urinary tract proximal to the site of obstruction. Renal ultrasonography or cystoscopy with retrograde urograms is most commonly used.

REVERSIBLE AZOTEMIA VERSUS ACUTE RENAL FAILURE

The ability to differentiate prerenal and postrenal azotemia from acute renal failure is critical. Exclusion of postrenal azotemia requires visualization of the urinary tract, while exclusion of prerenal azotemia depends on the response to treatments aimed at improving renal perfusion. The latter may be facilitated by analysis of urinary composition (Table 48–9); urinary composition in postrenal azotemia is variable and depends on the duration and severity of obstruction. In prerenal azotemia, tubular concentrating ability is preserved and reflected by a low urinary sodium concentration and high urine/creatinine ratio. Calculation of the fractional excretion of filtered sodium (FENa) may also be extremely useful in the setting of oliguria:

$$FENa^+ = \frac{Urine\ sodium/Serum\ sodium}{Urine\ creatinine/Serum\ creatinine} \times 100\%$$

FENa is less than 1% in oliguric patients with prerenal azotemia but typically exceeds 3% in patients with oliguric acute renal failure. Values of 1–3% may be present in patients with nonoliguric acute renal failure. The use of diuretics increases urinary sodium excretion and invalidates the utility of FENa as a measure of tubular function. Once the diagnosis of acute renal failure is established, creatinine clearance (Chapter 32) may be used as an estimate of residual glomerular filtration.

Etiology of Acute Renal Failure

Causes of acute renal failure are listed in Table 48–10. Up to 50% of cases follow major trauma or surgery; in the majority of instances, ischemia and nephrotoxins are responsible. Acute renal failure associated with ischemia and nephrotoxins is generally referred to as acute tubular necrosis. Aminoglycosides

Table 48–10. Causes of acute renal failure.

Renal ischemia
 Hypotension
 Hypovolemia
 Impaired cardiac output
Nephrotoxins
 Endogenous pigments
  Hemoglobin (hemolysis)
  Myoglobin (rhabdomyolysis, crush injury, burns)
  ?Bilirubin
 Radiographic contrast agents
 Drugs
  Antibiotics (aminoglycosides, amphotericin)
  Nonsteroidal anti-inflammatory drugs
  Chemotherapeutic agents (cisplatin, methotrexate)
 Heavy metal poisoning
 Organic solvents
Intrinsic renal disease
 Vascular
  Glomerular disease
  Vasculitis
  Hypertension
  Thromboembolic disease
   Arterial
   Venous
 Interstitial nephritis

and x-ray contrast dyes are the most commonly implicated toxins in acute tubular necrosis, but nonsteroidal anti-inflammatory drugs may play an important role at least in some patients. Inhibition of prostaglandin synthesis by the latter group of agents decreases prostaglandin-mediated renal vasodilation; this effect allows unopposed renal vasoconstriction in patients with high circulating angiotensin II levels (Chapter 31). Other factors predisposing to acute renal failure include pre-existing renal impairment, advanced age, atherosclerotic vascular disease, diabetes, and dehydration.

Pathogenesis of Acute Renal Failure

The sensitivity of the kidneys to injury may be explained by their very high metabolic rate and ability to concentrate potentially toxic substances. The pathogenesis of acute renal failure is complex and probably has both a vascular and a tubular basis. Afferent arteriolar constriction, decreased glomerular permeability, or tubular obstruction from intraluminal debris or edema can all decrease glomerular filtration (Chapter 31). Renal ischemia or hypoxia is the likely triggering event in many instances. Activation of the renin-angiotensin system may also play an important role.

Oliguric Versus Nonoliguric Acute Renal Failure

Traditionally, acute renal failure is thought of as either oliguric (urinary volume < 400 mL/d) or anuric (< 100 mL/d). However, nonoliguric acute renal failure has been increasingly recognized and may account for up to 50% of all cases. Patients with nonoliguric acute renal failure typically have lower urinary sodium concentrations than oliguric patients (see above).

Moreover, they also appear to have a lower complication rate and to require shorter hospitalizations. Nonoliguric acute renal failure may therefore represent less severe renal injury. In some instances, it may be possible to convert oliguric acute renal failure into nonoliguric acute renal failure by administering mannitol, furosemide, or "renal" doses of dopamine ($1-3$ μg/kg/min). The resulting increase in urine output may be therapeutic or, what is more likely, may reflect lesser degrees of renal impairment.

Treatment of Acute Renal Failure

The course of acute renal failure is described in Chapter 32. Management is primarily supportive. Standard treatment includes restriction of fluid, sodium, potassium, and protein intake. Dialysis may be employed to treat or prevent uremic complications (Table 32–2). The high morbidity and mortality rates associated with acute renal failure favor the latter approach, but supporting studies are lacking. Sepsis remains the most common cause of death. Although peritoneal dialysis and hemodialysis can be equally effective, the latter provides more rapid correction of abnormalities and is indicated for markedly catabolic patients and those with severe derangements. Additionally, the immobilization and elevation of the diaphragm associated with continuous peritoneal dialysis may predispose to respiratory complications. Acute hemodialysis may be accomplished via a special high-flow central venous catheter or through separate arterial and venous catheters.

The recent introduction of techniques for continuous ultrafiltration of blood offers another alternative to standard periodic hemodialysis. Continuous arteriovenous hemofiltration (CAVH) is most effective in controlling fluid overload and may be better tolerated than hemodialysis in some critically ill patients. Using this technique, water and small solutes are continuously removed as blood flows (100–300 mL/min) under pressure (arterial blood pressure) past a semipermeable membrane. Continuous arteriovenous hemodialysis (CAVHD) also employs a countercurrent gravity flow of a dialysis solution to increase the clearance of urea and other uremic toxins and can be nearly as effective as standard hemodialysis.

SEPSIS

The reported incidence of hospital-acquired (nosocomial) infections in ICU patients ranges between 10% and 50%. Nosocomial infections are the leading cause of death in many ICUs. Moreover, strains of bacteria resistant to commonly used antibiotics are often responsible. Critically ill patients frequently have

Table 48–11. Common sources of infection in critically ill patients.

Urinary tract
Respiratory tract
    Lungs
    Sinuses
Gastrointestinal tract
Wounds
Intravascular catheters

demonstrable abnormal host defenses, including defective chemotaxis and phagocytosis, altered helper:suppressor T lymphocyte ratios, and impaired humoral immunity. Impaired immunity also predisposes to infections with unusual pathogens, including many endogenous and exogenous bacteria, fungi, viruses, and protozoans. Other host factors include age, drug therapy, integrity of mucosal and skin barriers, and underlying disease. Thus, advanced age (> 70 years), corticosteroid therapy, chemotherapy, prolonged use of invasive devices, respiratory failure, renal failure, and head trauma are established risk factors for nosocomial infections.

Most infections arise from the endogenous flora. Furthermore, many critical care patients eventually become colonized with resistant bacterial strains. The most common sources of infection are listed in Table 48–11. The urinary tract accounts for up to 40% of nosocomial infections. Urinary infections are usually due to gram-negative organisms and are associated with the use of indwelling catheters or urinary obstruction. Pneumonia is the leading cause of death in many ICUs. Nosocomial pneumonias are also most often due to gram-negative organisms. Retrograde colonization of the upper airway from the gastrointestinal tract followed by aspiration is the usual mechanism of entry for these bacteria; hematogenous origin is less common. The use of sucralfate instead of an H_2 antagonist (to prevent gastric mucosal ulceration) decreases gram-negative bacterial colonization of the upper airway. Preservation of gastric acidity appears to inhibit overgrowth of gram-negative organisms in the stomach and their migration up into the oropharynx. Prophylactic administration of aerosolized nonabsorbable antibiotic mixtures may also be effective in reducing colonization and nosocomial pneumonias.

Wounds are common sources of sepsis in postoperative and trauma patients; limited antibiotic prophylaxis appears to decrease the incidence of postoperative infections in some groups of patients. Although more commonly seen in postoperative patients, intra-abdominal infections (such as a perforated ulcer, diverticulitis, appendicitis, and acalculous cholecystitis) can also develop in critically ill nonsurgical patients. Intravascular catheter-related infections are most commonly due to *Staphylococcus aureus, Staphylococcus epidermidis,* and gram-negative rods. Bacterial sinusitis may be an unrecognized source of sepsis in nasally intubated patients. The diagnosis is suspected from purulent drainage and confirmed by x-ray films and cultures.

SEPTIC SHOCK

The pathophysiology of shock is characterized by inadequate tissue perfusion and widespread cellular dysfunction. Arterial hypotension is usually but not always (at least initially) present. In contrast to other forms of shock (hypovolemic, cardiogenic, neurogenic, or anaphylactic), cellular dysfunction in septic shock is not necessarily related to the hypoperfusion. Instead, both derangements are the result of uncontrolled and overwhelming infection.

Etiology & Pathogenesis

Septic shock is most commonly due to gram-negative infections arising from the genitourinary or gastrointestinal tracts but can also be seen with other pathogens. Other common sites of bacterial entry include the respiratory tract and skin. Bacteremia is usually present but may be absent, especially with gram-negative bacterial infections. In the latter instances, the release of a lipopolysaccharide component of the bacterial cell wall (endotoxin) is responsible for the shock syndrome. Endotoxemia triggers the formation of prostaglandins and leukotrienes and results in activation of leukocytes, platelets, complement, and the coagulation cascade. Generalized vasodilatation, increased capillary permeability, formation of fibrin-platelet aggregates, and tissue injury follow. Hypoperfusion from hypotension further aggravates injury through tissue hypoxia. At the cellular level, a defect in oxygen and normal fuel substrate utilization is also present.

The same processes in the pulmonary circulation favor the development of ARDS (see above). Even in the absence of ARDS, production of microthrombi and vasoactive substances are probably responsible for increases in pulmonary vascular resistance during sepsis.

Hemodynamic Subsets

The circulation in patients with septic shock is often described as either hyperdynamic or hypodynamic. In reality, both represent the same process, but their expression depends on preexisting cardiac function and intravascular volume. Systemic venodilatation results in a relative hypovolemia in all patients.

Hyperdynamic septic shock is characterized by normal or elevated cardiac output and profound vasodilatation (low systemic vascular resistance). Mixed venous oxygen saturation is characteristically high in the absence of hypoxemia. The latter is probably due to the high cardiac output as well as a metabolic defect in oxygen utilization (see above).

Hypodynamic septic shock is characterized by decreased cardiac output with low or normal systemic vascular resistance. It is more likely to be seen in severely hypovolemic patients and those with underlying cardiac disease. Myocardial depression is a prominent feature. Mixed venous oxygen saturation may be low in these patients. Pulmonary hypertension is also often prominent in septic shock. Elevation of pulmonary vascular resistance widens the normal pulmonary artery diastolic to wedge pressure gradient; large gradients have been associated with a higher mortality rate. The increase in pulmonary vascular resistance may contribute to right ventricular dysfunction (Chapter 19). Decreased myocardial contractility is often demonstrable even in hyperdynamic patients and is thought to be due to a circulating myocardial depressant factor.

Clinical Features

Manifestations of septic shock appear to be primarily related to host response rather than the infective agent. Septic shock classically presents with an abrupt onset of chills, fever, nausea (and often vomiting), decreased mental status, tachypnea, hypotension, and tachycardia. The patient may appear flushed and feel warm (hyperdynamic) or pale with cool and often cyanotic extremities (hypodynamic); in the latter case, a high index of suspicion is required. In old, debilitated patients and infants, the diagnosis often is less obvious and hypothermia may be seen. Leukocytosis with a leftward shift to premature cell forms is typical, but leukopenia can be seen with overwhelming sepsis and is an ominous sign. Progressive metabolic acidosis (usually lactic acidosis) is typically partially compensated by a concomitant respiratory alkalosis. Elevated lactate levels reflect both increased production resulting from poor tissue perfusion and decreased uptake by the liver and kidneys. Hypoxemia may herald the onset of ARDS. Oliguria is most commonly due to the combination of hypovolemia and hypotension but often progresses to acute renal failure (see above). Elevations in serum aminotransferases and bilirubin are due to hepatic dysfunction. Insulin resistance is uniformly present and produces hyperglycemia. Thrombocytopenia is common and often an early sign of sepsis. Laboratory evidence of disseminated intravascular coagulation is often present but is rarely associated with a bleeding diathesis. The latter only responds to control of the sepsis. Gastric mucosal stress ulceration is com-

Table 48–12. Selected empiric antibiotic regimens for septic shock based on probable origin.

Gentamicin + cefotaxine	Vancomycin + piperacillin + gentamicin
Immunocompromised or neutropenic patients	Cefazolin + vancomycin
Urosepsis	Ampicillin + gentamicin
Intra-abdominal sepsis	Clindamycin + gentamicin *or* Imipenem
Community-acquired pneumonia	Penicillin or erythromycin or cefotaxime
Nosocomial pneumonia Standard	Ceftazidime + gentamicin *or* Piperacillin + gentamicin
Probable aspiration AIDS patient	Clindamycin + gentamicin Add trimethoprim-sulfamethoxazole or pentamidine
Central venous catheter-related sepsis	Vancomycin + gentamicin
Splenectomy or functional asplenia	Penicillin + ceftriaxone
Cellulitis	Cefazolin or oxacillin
Meningitis	Penicillin or oxacillin or cefotaxime

INTRAVENOUS DOSAGES FOR SELECTED ANTIBIOTICS

Ampicillin	1–2 g every 4–6 hours
Cefazolin	1–2 g every 8 hours
Cefotaxime	1–2 g every 4–6 hours
Ceftriaxone	1–2 g every 6–8 hours
Ceftazidime	1–2 g every 8 hours
Clindamycin	600–900 mg every 8 hours
Gentamicin	1.5–2 mg/kg as loading dose, then 1–1.5 mg every 8 hours
Imipenem	0.5–1 g every 6–8 hours
Oxacillin	1–2 g every 4–6 hours
Penicillin G	1–2 million units every 4–6 hours
Pentamidine	4 mg/kg daily as single dose
Piperacillin	3 g every 4 hours
Trimethoprim-sulfamethoxazole	5 mg TMP and 25 mg SMZ per kg every 6–8 hours
Vancomycin	500 mg every 6 hours

mon. Respiratory and renal failure are the leading usual causes of death.

Treatment

Septic shock is a medical emergency and requires immediate intervention. Treatment is threefold: (1) control and eradication of the infection by intravenous antibiotics, drainage of abscesses, debridement of necrotic tissues, and removal of infected foreign bodies; (2) maintenance of adequate perfusion with intravenous fluids or inotropic agents; and (3) treatment of complications such as ARDS, renal failure, gastrointestinal bleeding, and DIC.

Antibiotic treatment must be initiated before pathogens are identified but after adequate cultures are obtained (usually of blood, urine, wounds, and sputum). Combination therapy with two or more antibiotics is generally indicated until pathogens are known. In most instances, the combination of a penicillin or cephalosporin with an aminoglycoside is adequate (Table 48–12). Additional diagnostic studies may be indicated, eg, thoracentesis, paracentesis, lumbar puncture, or CT scans. Debridement and drainage of surgical infections and abscesses should be undertaken expeditiously.

Tissue oxygenation and perfusion are maintained with oxygen therapy and intravenous fluids, respectively. Marked "third spacing" (Chapter 29) is characteristic of septic shock and is probably the result of increased systemic capillary permeability. A vasopressor should be used if intravenous fluids fail to rapidly restore adequate perfusion. Pulmonary artery catheterization greatly facilitates management in such instances. Dopamine is generally selected as an inotrope. Even in the absence of arterial hypotension, "renal" doses of dopamine may be helpful in maintaining urinary output and preventing renal failure in oliguric patients (see above). Hypotension refractory to intravenous fluids and dopamine usually responds to intravenous epinephrine or norepinephrine infusions. The use of corticosteroids, naloxone, and opsonins (fibronectin) in septic shock has been disappointing. In contrast, the use of monoclonal antibodies directed against the lipopolysaccharide component of endotoxin appears to improve survival in patients with gram-negative septic shock.

NUTRITIONAL SUPPORT

The importance of maintaining adequate nutrition in critically ill patients cannot be overemphasized. Malnutrition causes widespread organ dysfunction (Table 48–13) and increases perioperative morbidity and mortality rates. Moreover, nutritional repletion has been shown to be effective in improving wound heal-

Table 48–13. Physiologic effects of malnutrition.

Organ System	Effect
Pulmonary	Decreased diaphragmatic contractility Depressed hypoxic drive Decreased ventilatory response to CO_2
Cardiac	Decreased contractility Decreased response to inotropes Ventricular dilatation
Renal	Decreased GFR Impaired sodium excretion
Hepatic	Altered carbohydrate, protein, and fat metabolism Decreased protein synthesis Decreased drug metabolism Impaired bilirubin excretion
Hematologic	Anemia Coagulopathy
Immune	Depressed T cell function Impaired chemotaxis and phagocytosis

ing, restoring immune competence, and reducing morbidity and mortality rates in critically ill patients.

OVERVIEW OF NUTRITION

Maintenance of normal body mass, composition, structure, and function requires the periodic intake of water, specific nutrients, and energy substrates. Nutrients that cannot be synthesized from other nutrients are characterized as "essential." Remarkably, relatively few essential nutrients are required to form the thousands of compounds that form the body. Known essential nutrients include 8–10 amino acids, two fatty acids, 13 vitamins, and approximately 16 minerals (Table 48–14).

Energy is normally derived from dietary or endogenous carbohydrates, fats, and protein. Metabolic breakdown of these substrates yields the ATP required for normal cellular function. Dietary fats and carbohydrates normally supply most of the body's energy requirements. Dietary proteins provide amino acids for protein synthesis; however, when their supply exceeds both essential and nonessential amino acid requirements, they also function as energy substrates. The metabolic pathways of carbohydrate, fat, and amino acid substrates overlap such that some interconversions can occur through metabolic intermediates (Figure 34–3). Excess amino acids can therefore be converted to carbohydrate or fatty acid precursors. Excess carbohydrates are stored as glycogen in the liver and skeletal muscle. When glycogen stores are saturated (200–400 g in adults), excess carbohydrate is converted to fatty acids stored as triglycerides primarily in fat cells.

Normal Energy Requirements

Total energy requirements vary widely and depend on the basal metabolic rate (BMR), specific dynamic

Table 48–14. Parenteral nutritional requirements.[1]

	Approximate Daily Requirements (Adults)
Water	30 mL/kg
Calories	25–45 kcal/kg
Protein[2]	0.5–1.5 g/kg
Fat[3]	1–2 g/kg
Glucose	2–3 g/kg
Electrolytes	
Sodium	1–2 g
Potassium	2–4 g
Calcium	400 mg
Magnesium	300 mg
Chloride	2 g
Phosphate	400 mg
Vitamins	
A	1300 μg
B_1 (thiamine)	3 mg
B_2 (riboflavin)	3.6 mg
B_3 (niacin)	40 mg
B_5 (pantothenic acid)	15 mg
B_6 (pyridoxine)	4 mg
B_7 (biotin)	60 μg
B_9 (folic acid)	400 μg
B_{12} (cobalamin)	5 μg
C	100 mg
D	5 μg
E	10–15 mg
K	200 μg
Trace elements	
Copper	0.3–0.5 mg
Zinc	3–12 mg
Selenium	0.05–0.1 mg
Chromium	0.015 mg
Iron	1–2 mg
Manganese	2–5 mg
Iodine	0.15 mg
Molybdenum	0.01–0.5 mg

[1] Adapted from recommendations of the National Academy of Sciences (1989) and the Nutrition Advisory Group of the American Medical Association (1979).
[2] Essential amino acids: isoleucine, leucine, lysine, methionine, phenylalanine, threonine, tryptophan, valine, and perhaps arginine and histidine.
[3] Essential fatty acids: linoleic acid and linolenic acid.

action (energy required for digestion of meals), and a person's activity level. BMR is a specific measurement of energy expenditure in the morning immediately after awakening, 12 hours after the last meal, and in a state of thermal neutrality. Clinically, basal energy expenditure (BEE) in kilocalories can be estimated by the Harris-Benedict equation, using weight in kilograms, height in centimeters, and age in years:

Males: $\text{BEE} = 66 + (13.7 \times \text{Weight}) + (5 \times \text{Height}) - (6.8 \times \text{Age})$

Females: $\text{BEE} = 655 + (9.6 \times \text{Weight}) + (1.8 \times \text{Height}) - (4.7 \times \text{Age}).$

BEE is increased by temperature (13% per °C), and degree of stress (see below).

Organ-Specific Substrate Utilization

Variations in the ability to store glycogen and triglycerides, enzyme pathways, and membrane transport mechanisms result in differing substrate utilizations between organs. Neurons, red cells, and cells of the renal medulla normally utilize only glucose. The liver, heart, skeletal muscle, and renal cortex preferentially rely on fatty acid metabolism for energy.

Starvation

The physiology of starvation is such that the protein content of essential tissues is spared. As blood glucose concentration begins to fall during fasting, insulin secretion decreases while glucagon increases. Hepatic and, to a lesser extent, renal glycogenolysis and gluconeogenesis are enhanced (Chapter 34). Unfortunately, glycogen supplies are depleted within 24 hours, so that gluconeogenesis becomes increasingly important. The liver uses chiefly deaminated amino acids (alanine and glutamine) as precursors for glucose synthesis. Only neural tissue, renal medullary cells, and erythrocytes continue to utilize glucose, in effect sparing tissue proteins. Lipolysis in adipose tissue is enhanced, so that fats become the principal energy source. Glycerol from the triglycerides enters the glycolytic pathway, while fatty acids too are broken down to acetyl-CoA. Excess acetyl-CoA results in the formation of ketone bodies (ketosis). Some fatty acids can contribute to gluconeogenesis. Lactate is converted in the liver to glucose and metabolized to hydroxyl ion to neutralize the acid. If starvation is prolonged, the brain, kidneys, and muscle also begin to utilize ketone bodies efficiently. Glucose administration during starvation characteristically prevents or decreases protein breakdown as well as ketosis.

NUTRITION IN CRITICAL ILLNESS

Perioperative critical illnesses are usually characterized by starvation, tissue injury, and a neuroendocrine stress response. The response to injury involves increases in the secretion of catecholamines, cortisol, glucagon, thyroxine, angiotensin, aldosterone, growth hormone, ACTH, ADH, and TSH. Insulin secretion is at least initially decreased but may subsequently rise due to increasing levels of growth hormone.

Catecholamines, glucagon, and perhaps growth hormone promote glycogenolysis, while glucagon and possibly cortisol induce gluconeogenesis. Hyperglycemia is characteristic and reflects increased hepatic production as well as decreased utilization by peripheral tissues. Moreover, decreased tolerance to glucose loads occurs, apparently as a result of both decreased insulin secretion and peripheral resistance to its actions. Both effects are probably due to increased catecholamine secretion. Gluconeogenesis, glycolysis, and lipolysis are all increased. Both protein synthesis and breakdown are increased, but the latter ex-

Table 48–15. Acceptable weights (in pounds) for men and women.[1,2]

Height	Age	
	19–34 Years	35 Years and Older
5'0"	97–128	108–138
5'1"	101–132	111–143
5'2"	104–137	115–148
5'3"	107–141	119–152
5'4"	111–146	122–157
5'5"	114–150	126–162
5'6"	118–156	130–167
5'7"	121–160	134–172
5'8"	125–164	138–178
5'9"	129–169	142–183
5'10"	132–174	146–188
5'11"	136–179	151–194
6'0"	140–184	155–199
6'1"	144–189	159–205
6'2"	148–195	164–210

[1]Weights based on weighing in without shoes or clothes.
[2]Source: United States Department of Agriculture and United States Department of Health and Human Resources.

ceeds the former, so that there is a net loss of tissue protein. During sepsis, inability of muscle to utilize fat and carbohydrate results in increased protein breakdown. Moreover, the cells appear to rely more on branched-chain amino acids. Circulating levels of branched-chain amino acids decrease while levels of aromatic amino acids increase.

As is not the case with simple starvation, glucose administration during acute illnesses fails to suppress protein breakdown. Only an adequate intake of calories and proteins decreases protein catabolism.

Nutritional Assessment of Patients

Proper evaluation of nutritional status is central to nutritional support of critically ill patients. Tests include anthropometric measurements, cutaneous hypersensitivity, and laboratory determinations. Patients requiring close assessment include those with less than 80% acceptable body weight (Table 48–15) or weight loss exceeding 10% in the preceding 6 months; those with serum albumin less than 3 g/dL or serum transferrin less than 150 mg/dL; those with skin anergy; and those with low total lymphocyte counts (< 1200 cells/μL).

Comparison of body weight to acceptable body weight criteria and measurement of skinfolds are generally indicative of body fat stores. Midarm muscle circumference measurements and the urinary creatinine excretion to height index reflect skeletal protein muscle mass. Serum albumin and transferrin measurements are generally indicative of protein synthetic ability.

Calculating Energy Requirements

Caloric requirements are usually derived by means of the Harris-Benedict equation (see above). The result is multiplied by a stress factor according to the degree of tissue injury and severity of illness:

Stress factor = 1–1.25 for mild starvation
= 1.25–1.5 for moderate to severe illness
= 1.5–1.75 for severe illness

Most critically ill patients require 30–40 kcal/kg/d.

Calculating Protein Requirements

In contrast to nonstressed patients, who require about 0.5 g/kg/d of protein, critically ill patients generally require 0.75–1.5 g/kg/d. A kilocalorie:nitrogen ratio between 180:1 and 150:1 is generally suggested; a 180:1 ratio is most commonly used (1 g nitrogen = 6.25 g protein).

ENTERAL NUTRITION

The gastrointestinal tract is the route of choice for nutritional support when its functional integrity is intact. Enteral feedings can be used to provide complete or supplemental nutrition. Enteral nutrition is simpler, cheaper, less complicated, and associated with fewer complications than parenteral nutrition (see below). Moreover, enteral nutrition appears to better preserve gastrointestinal structure and function than the parenteral route, especially when glutamine-rich preparations are used.

Enteral feedings are most often given as a continuous infusion through a nasogastric tube, gastrostomy, or jejunostomy. Therapy is usually initiated at a rate of 25 mL/h and is increased slowly over the course of a few days until the desired caloric and protein goals are reached. Most enteral formulas contain polymeric mixtures of proteins, fats, and carbohydrates. Numerous preparations are available. Selection is based on lactose content, osmolality, and fat content. Some formulas are composed of elemental low-residue formulas. Elemental formulas are indicated in patients with short bowel syndrome, gastrointestinal fistula, and inflammatory bowel disease; they are readily absorbed and have low residues. Medium-chain triglycerides (MCT) are composed of 8- to 10-carbon fatty acids that do not require bile salts or pancreatic enzymes for absorption; MCT oils are indicated for patients with pancreatic insufficiency and cholestasis.

Diarrhea is the most common problem with enteral feedings and is usually related either to hyperosmolarity of the solution or lactose intolerance. The risk of regurgitation and pulmonary aspiration is decreased by the use of duodenal or jejunostomy tubes. Progressive abdominal distention or large gastric residual volumes are indicative of ileus and should prompt discontinuation of enteral feedings.

PARENTERAL NUTRITION

Total parenteral nutrition (TPN) is indicated if the gastrointestinal tract cannot be used or provides inade-

Table 48–16. Complications of TPN.

Catheter-related
  Pneumothorax
  Hemothorax
  Chylothorax
  Hydrothorax
  Air embolism
  Cardiac tamponade
  Thrombosis
    Subclavian vein
    Vena cava
  Pulmonary thromboembolism
  Catheter sepsis
Metabolic
  Cholestasis
  Hepatic dysfunction
  Hyperglycemia
    Hyperosmolar coma
    Diabetic ketoacidosis
  Excessive CO_2 production
  Hypoglycemia (due to interruption of infusion)
  Metabolic acidosis
  Hypernatremia
  Hyperkalemia
  Hypokalemia
  Hypocalcemia
  Hypophosphatemia
  Hyperlipidemia
  Pancreatitis
  Fat embolism syndrome
  Anemia
    Iron
    Folate
    B_{12}
    ?Copper
  Vitamin D deficiency
  Vitamin K deficiency
  Essential fatty acid deficiency
  Hypervitaminosis A
  Hypervitaminosis D

quate nutrition. TPN formulas utilize hyperosmolar solutions of amino acids and glucose mixed together. The hypertonic nature of these solutions requires central venous access. Electrolytes, trace elements, and a multivitamin preparation are added (Table 48–14). Parenteral glucose solutions provide only 3.4 kcal/g (compared to 4 kcal/g for the dry carbohydrate) because their glucose concentration is expressed as the monohydrate. Fats are given in the form a fat emulsion that can be infused separately or mixed with the glucose-amino acid solution. Available fat emulsions are derived from either soybean (Intralipid and Soyacal) or safflower seed oil (Liposyn II). Fat emulsions are available as either 10% (1.1 kcal/mL) or 20% (2 kcal/mL). Failure to give fat at least once a week may result in essential fatty acid deficiency, which is manifested as dermatitis, alopecia, hepatomegaly (fatty liver), and defective immunity.

The amount of amino acids given is determined by estimated protein requirements (see above), while glucose and fat are given to the desired caloric requirements (see above). Fat calories generally should account for 30–60% of desired caloric requirements. Excessive reliance on glucose exacerbates problems with hyperglycemia and

increases CO_2 production. The latter is often a problem in weaning patients with a compromised pulmonary reserve from mechanical ventilation.

Complications of TPN are either metabolic or related to central venous access (Table 48–16).

TPN must be modified for patients with significant hepatic or renal impairment. The amino acid load must be reduced to prevent encephalopathy in patients with hepatic insufficiency (Chapter 34). Plasma amino acid concentrations tend to be altered in these patients: Phenylalanine and methionine are usually elevated, while branched-chain amino acids (leucine, isoleucine and valine) are reduced. Amino acid formulations for patients with liver disease are therefore rich in branched-chain amino acids but low in aromatic amino acids.

Protein content must also be reduced in patients with renal failure. Increases in nitrogen load aggravate uremic symptoms (Chapter 32). Amino acid preparations for patients with renal failure therefore have increased essential to nonessential amino acid ratios. Additionally, total TPN volume and potassium content must be controlled. Effective TPN in patients with renal failure usually requires dialysis.

Monitoring patients on TPN

Initiation of TPN requires close metabolic monitoring. The most common problem is hyperglycemia. A gradual increase in glucose infusions lessens the severity of hyperglycemia and allows sufficient time for enhanced endogenous insulin secretion. Diabetic patients require the addition of insulin to the TPN solution. Conversely, abrupt withdrawal of TPN can precipitate hypoglycemia due to high circulating insulin levels; in these instances, 10% glucose should be temporarily used and gradually decreased. Serum glucose measurements should generally be measured every 4 hours until they stabilize. Other measurements (serum electrolytes, BUN, creatinine) are obtained daily. Calcium, phosphate, and magnesium concentrations and liver function tests (including albumin) should be checked weekly. The complete blood count (including a differential count) should also be followed. Lipid clearance should be checked by measuring a serum triglyceride level 6 hours after completion of a daily infusion (it should normalize). Twenty-four-hour nitrogen balance studies are useful in checking the efficacy of nutritional support:

Nitrogen balance = Input − Output
Nitrogen output = ([UUN] × 1.2 × Urinary volume)
+ 2 g

where [UUN] = urinary urea nitrogen concentration (g/L).

The 2 g in the above equation represents fecal and integumentary nitrogen losses. UUN is multiplied by 1.2, since twenty percent of the UUN is added, since urea nitrogen represents only 80% of urinary nitrogen losses. Ideally, TPN should result in a positive nitrogen balance.

PERIPHERAL PARENTERAL NUTRITION

When a 3–4% amino acid solution is added to a 5–10% dextrose solution, the resulting solution is still hypertonic but can generally be infused through a peripheral vein without irritation. Simultaneous infusion of a 1% fat emulsion through the same intravenous catheter further reduces the concentration and provides additional calories. Unfortunately, volume constraints usually limit caloric intake with peripheral parenteral nutrition to a maximum of 1500–1800 kcal/d.

CASE DISCUSSION: RESPIRATORY DISTRESS IN A YOUNG TRAUMA VICTIM

A 24 year-old man fractures his right femur in motorcycle vehicle accident. The day after admission, he is noted to be tachypneic (40 breaths/min). His blood pressure is 110/50 mm Hg, and his pulse is 140 beats/min. On examination, he is noted to be confused.

What is the differential diagnosis?

Dyspnea in a previous healthy trauma patient can be due to pneumothorax, hemothorax, pulmonary contusion, fat embolism, or other causes of ARDS (Table 48–6). A previously unrecognized head injury should also be considered, especially if neurologic findings predominate. Pulmonary thromboembolism is unlikely this early in the hospitalization. The most likely diagnosis in this setting is fat embolism syndrome, which classically presents with the triad of dyspnea, confusion, and petechiae. Its pulmonary manifestations are indistinguishable from other causes of ARDS. The syndrome usually occurs within 72 hours following long bone or pelvic fractures.

What is the pathophysiology of fat embolism?

Fat embolization is reported to occur in 30–90% of all patients with fractures. Most patients are asymptomatic, but others can develop life-threatening manifestations. Why only some patients develop the full fat embolism syndrome is not known. Two theories have been proposed for its pathogenesis. The most popular theory holds that fat globules are released by disruption of fat cells in the fractured bone and enter the circulation through tears in medullary vessels. Fat globules can be demonstrated throughout the circulation in both arterial and venous vessels. The fat globules may enter the arterial system by crossing open arteriovenous communications in the lungs or via a probe-patent foramen ovale (Chapter 26). Fat globules are most often found in the pulmonary, cerebral, and renal circulations and in the skin (petechiae).

An alternative theory proposes that the fat globules are chylomicrons resulting from the aggregation of circulating free fatty acids. Marked elevations in circulating levels of free fatty acids are often observed following major trauma. The source of the neutral fats may be either bone marrow or peripheral fat stores.

Regardless of their source, the increased free fatty acid levels can have a toxic effect on the capillary-alveolar membrane. The acute lung injury that follows is indistinguishable from that due to other causes of ARDS, resulting in the activation and aggregation of leukocytes in the pulmonary circulation and permeability pulmonary edema. Neurologic manifestations probably represent capillary damage in the cerebral circulation; cerebral edema may be present.

How can the diagnosis be established?

The fat embolism syndrome is for the most part a diagnosis of exclusion. The physical examination, arterial blood gas measurements, a complete blood count, and a chest x-ray are most useful. The diagnosis of fat embolism is suggested by petechiae on the chest, upper extremities, axillae, and conjunctiva. Unlike the confusion associated with other disorders, the confusion in patients with symptomatic fat embolism is characteristically disproportionate to the degree of hypoxemia. Neurologic findings may be insidious in onset and can consist of agitation, confusion, stupor, or coma. Hypoxemia may initially be absent, but patients can rapidly develop a severe hypocapnic, hypoxemic respiratory failure. Fat globules may be found in the retina, urine, or sputum, but these findings may also occur in asymptomatic patients. Thrombocytopenia is often present. Serum lipase activity may be elevated but bears no relationship to disease severity. The chest x-ray may be normal initially but eventually shows diffuse patchy pulmonary infiltrates.

In what other settings does fat embolism syndrome occur?

Although fat embolism syndrome is most frequently associated with fractures of the long bones and pelvis, it has been reported with other types of fractures as well as in other diverse settings. These include transfusions from cell saver devices, bone marrow transplantation, infusions of fat emulsions during TPN, lymphangiography, pancreatitis, and in burns.

What treatment is effective for fat embolism syndrome?

Treatment is twofold: prophylactic and supportive. Although somewhat controversial, fluid resuscitation and early stabilization of a fracture are reported to decrease the incidence of fat embolism syndrome. The cornerstone of treatment is supportive care with oxygen therapy and positive-pressure therapy (CPAP).

The latter can be administered via a special CPAP mask or endotracheal intubation (see above). Treatment with heparin or alcohol has generally been disappointing. The use of alcohol was based on the clinical impression that alcoholics rarely developed the fat embolism syndrome. High-dose corticosteroid therapy may be beneficial, especially in the presence of cerebral edema.

SUGGESTED READINGS

Chernow B: *The Pharmacologic Approach to Critically Ill Patients,* 2nd ed. Williams & Wilkins, 1988.

Civetta JM, Taylor RW, Kirby RR: *Critical Care.* Lippincott, 1988.

Hoyt JW, Tonnesen AS, Allen SJ: *Critical Care Practice.* Saunders, 1991.

Kirby RR, Banner MJ, Downs JB: *Clinical Application of Ventilatory Support.* Churchill Livingstone, 1990. An excellent foundation for understanding mechanical ventilators and their use.

Oh TE: *Intensive Care Manual,* 3rd ed. Butterworths, 1990. Concise but relatively complete.

Parrillo JE: *Current Therapy in Critical Care Medicine,* 2nd ed. BC Decker, 1990.

Schlichtig R, Ayres SM: *Nutitional Support of the Critically Ill.* Mosby-Year Book, 1988.

Shoemaker W et al: *Textbook of Critical Care,* 2nd ed. Saunders, 1989.

Silberman H: *Parenteral and Enteral Nutrition,* 2nd ed. Appleton & Lange, 1989.

Zapol WM, Lemaire F: *Adult Respiratory Distress Syndrome.* Marcel Dekker, 1990.

Index